D1746569

Ronald E. Goldstein's
Esthetics in Dentistry

THIRD EDITION

VOLUME 1

Principles of Esthetics
Esthetic Treatments
Esthetic Challenges of Missing Teeth

Ronald E. Goldstein's
Esthetics in Dentistry

THIRD EDITION

VOLUME 1

Principles of Esthetics
Esthetic Treatments
Esthetic Challenges of Missing Teeth

Edited by

Ronald E. Goldstein, DDS
Clinical Professor of Restorative Sciences at The Dental College of Georgia at Augusta University, Augusta, GA; Adjunct Clinical Professor of Prosthodontics, Boston University School of Dental Medicine, Boston; Adjunct Professor of Restorative Dentistry, University of Texas Health Science Center, San Antonio, TX; Former Visiting Professor of Oral and Maxillofacial Imaging and Continuing Education, University of Southern California, School of Dentistry, Los Angeles, CA; Private Practice, Atlanta, GA, USA

Stephen J. Chu, DMD, MSD, CDT
Adjunct Clinical Professor, Ashman Department of Periodontology and Implant Dentistry, Department of Prosthodontics, New York University College of Dentistry, New York, NY; Private Practice, New York, NY, USA

Ernesto A. Lee, DMD
Clinical Professor, University of Pennsylvania School of Dental Medicine, Philadelphia, PA; Former Director, Postdoctoral Periodontal Prosthesis Program, Penn Dental Medicine, University of Pennsylvania School of Medicine, Philadelphia, PA; Private Practice, Bryn Mawr, PA, USA

Christian F.J. Stappert, DDS, MS, PhD
Professor and Former Director of Postgraduate Prosthodontics, Department of Prosthodontics, University of Freiburg, Germany; Professor and Former Director of Periodontal Prosthodontics and Implant Dentistry, Department of Periodontics, University of Maryland School of Dentistry, Baltimore, MD, USA; Past Director of Aesthetics and Periodontal Prosthodontics, Department of Periodontology and Implant Dentistry, New York University College of Dentistry, New York, NY, USA; Private Practice, Zurich, Switzerland

WILEY Blackwell

This third edition first published 2018 © 2018 by John Wiley & Sons, Inc.

Edition History
1e 1976 Lippincott Williams & Wilkins; 2e 1998 B.C. Decker

All rights reserved. No part of this publication may be reproduced, stored in a retrieval system, or transmitted, in any form or by any means, electronic, mechanical, photocopying, recording or otherwise, except as permitted by law. Advice on how to obtain permission to reuse material from this title is available at http://www.wiley.com/go/permissions.

The right of Ronald E. Goldstein, Stephen J. Chu, Ernesto A. Lee and Christian F.J. Stappert to be identified as the authors of the editorial material in this work has been asserted in accordance with law.

Registered Office
John Wiley & Sons, Inc., 111 River Street, Hoboken, NJ 07030, USA

Editorial Office
111 River Street, Hoboken, NJ 07030, USA

For details of our global editorial offices, customer services, and more information about Wiley products visit us at www.wiley.com.

Wiley also publishes its books in a variety of electronic formats and by print-on-demand. Some content that appears in standard print versions of this book may not be available in other formats.

Limit of Liability/Disclaimer of Warranty

The contents of this work are intended to further general scientific research, understanding, and discussion only and are not intended and should not be relied upon as recommending or promoting scientific method, diagnosis, or treatment by physicians for any particular patient. In view of ongoing research, equipment modifications, changes in governmental regulations, and the constant flow of information relating to the use of medicines, equipment, and devices, the reader is urged to review and evaluate the information provided in the package insert or instructions for each medicine, equipment, or device for, among other things, any changes in the instructions or indication of usage and for added warnings and precautions. While the publisher and authors have used their best efforts in preparing this work, they make no representations or warranties with respect to the accuracy or completeness of the contents of this work and specifically disclaim all warranties, including without limitation any implied warranties of merchantability or fitness for a particular purpose. No warranty may be created or extended by sales representatives, written sales materials or promotional statements for this work. The fact that an organization, website, or product is referred to in this work as a citation and/or potential source of further information does not mean that the publisher and authors endorse the information or services the organization, website, or product may provide or recommendations it may make. This work is sold with the understanding that the publisher is not engaged in rendering professional services. The advice and strategies contained herein may not be suitable for your situation. You should consult with a specialist where appropriate. Further, readers should be aware that websites listed in this work may have changed or disappeared between when this work was written and when it is read. Neither the publisher nor authors shall be liable for any loss of profit or any other commercial damages, including but not limited to special, incidental, consequential, or other damages.

A catalogue record for this book is available from the Library of Congress and the British Library

ISBN 9781119272830

Cover images: (background) © Natapong Supalertsophon/Getty Images; (first inset image) courtesy of Christian Coachman, DDS, CDT; (other inset images) courtesy of Dr. Ronald E. Goldstein
Cover design by Wiley

Set in 10/12 pt MinionPro by SPi Global, Pondicherry, India
Printed and bound in Singapore by Markono Print Media Pte Ltd

10 9 8 7 6 5 4 3 2 1

Contents

List of Contributors ix
Contributors at Large xvii
Preface to Third Edition xix
Acknowledgments xxi

VOLUME 1

PART 1 PRINCIPLES OF ESTHETICS 1

1. Concepts of Dental Esthetics 3
   Ronald E. Goldstein and Gordon Patzer

2. Successful Management of Common Psychological Challenges 25
   Shirley Brown

3. Esthetic Treatment Planning: Patient and Practice Management Skills in Esthetic Treatment Planning 47
   Ronald E. Goldstein and Maurice A. Salama

4. Digital Smile Design: A Digital Tool for Esthetic Evaluation, Team Communication, and Patient Management 85
   Christian Coachman, Marcelo Calamita, and Andrea Ricci

5. Esthetics in Dentistry Marketing 113
   Roger P. Levin and Ronald E. Goldstein

6. Legal Considerations 131
   Edwin J. Zinman

7. Practical Clinical Photography 155
   Glenn D. Krieger

8. Creating Esthetic Restorations Through Special Effects 185
   Ronald E. Goldstein, Jason J. Kim, Pinhas Adar, and Adam Mieleszko

9. Proportional Smile Design 243
   Daniel H. Ward, Stephen J. Chu, and Christian F.J. Stappert

10. Understanding Color 271
    Rade D. Paravina

PART 2 ESTHETIC TREATMENTS 295

11. Cosmetic Contouring 297
    Ronald E. Goldstein

12. Bleaching Discolored Teeth 325
    So Ran Kwon and Ronald E. Goldstein

13. Adhesion to Hard Tissue on Teeth 355
    Roland Frankenberger, Uwe Blunck, and Lorenzo Breschi

14. Composite Resin Bonding 375
    Ronald E. Goldstein and Marcos Vargas

15. Ceramic Veneers and
Partial-Coverage Restorations 433
*Christian F.J. Stappert, Ronald E. Goldstein,
Fransiskus A. Tjiptowidjojo,
and Stephen J. Chu*

16. Crown Restorations 499
*Kenneth A. Malament, Ronald E. Goldstein,
Christian F.J. Stappert, Mo Taheri,
and Thomas Sing*

PART 3 ESTHETIC CHALLENGES OF MISSING TEETH 541

17. Replacing Missing Teeth with Fixed
Partial Dentures 543
*Jacinthe M. Paquette, Jean C. Wu,
Cherilyn G. Sheets, and Devin L. Stewart*

18. Esthetic Removable Partial Dentures 581
*Carol A. Lefebvre, Roman M. Cibirka,
and Ronald E. Goldstein*

19. The Complete Denture 611
Walter F. Turbyfill Jr

20. Implant Esthetics: Concepts,
Surgical Procedures, and Materials 637
Sonia Leziy and Brahm Miller

Appendices

Appendix A: Esthetic Evaluation Form A1
Appendix B: The Functional-Esthetic Analysis B1
Appendix C: Laboratory Checklist C1
Appendix D: Pincus Principles D1

Index i1

VOLUME 2

PART 4 ESTHETIC PROBLEMS OF INDIVIDUAL TEETH 667

21. Management of Stained and Discolored Teeth 669
*Ronald E. Goldstein, Samantha Siranli,
Van B. Haywood, and W. Frank Caughman*

22. Abfraction, Abrasion, Attrition, and Erosion 693
*Ronald E. Goldstein, James W. Curtis Jr,
Beverly A. Farley, Samantha Siranli,
and Wendy A. Clark*

23. Chipped, Fractured, or Endodontically
Treated Teeth 721
*Ronald E. Goldstein, Daniel C.N. Chan,
Michael L. Myers, and Gerald M. Barrack*

24. Endodontics and Esthetic Dentistry 749
*John West, Noah Chivian, Donald E. Arens, and
Asgeir Sigurdsson*

PART 5 ESTHETIC CHALLENGES OF MALOCCLUSION 809

25. Oral Habits 811
*Ronald E. Goldstein, James W. Curtis Jr,
Beverly A. Farley, and Daria Molodtsova*

26. Restorative Treatment of Diastema 841
*Barry D. Hammond, Kevin B. Frazier,
Anabella Oquendo, and Ronald E. Goldstein*

27. Restorative Treatment of Crowded Teeth 877
*Ronald E. Goldstein, Geoffrey W. Sheen,
and Steven T. Hackman*

28. Esthetics in Adult Orthodontics 897
Eladio DeLeon Jr

29. Surgical Orthodontic Correction
of Dentofacial Deformity 929
*John N. Kent, John P. Neary, John Oubre,
and David A. Bulot*

PART 6 ESTHETIC PROBLEMS OF SPECIAL POPULATIONS, FACIAL CONSIDERATIONS, AND SUPPORTING STRUCTURES 967

30. Pediatric Dentistry 969
    Claudia Caprioglio, Alberto Caprioglio, and Damaso Caprioglio

31. Geresthetics: Esthetic Dentistry for Older Adults 1015
    Linda C. Niessen, Ronald E. Goldstein, and Maha El-Sayed

32. Facial Considerations: An Orthodontic Perspective 1051
    David Sarver

33. Facial Considerations in Esthetic Restorations 1085
    Ronald E. Goldstein and Bruno P. Silva

34. Plastic Surgery Related to Esthetic Dentistry 1131
    Foad Nahai and Kristin A. Boehm

35. Cosmetic Adjuncts 1143
    Ronald E. Goldstein, Richard Davis, and Marvin Westmore

36. Esthetic Considerations in the Performing Arts 1153
    Ronald E. Goldstein and Daniel Materdomini

37. Periodontal Plastic Surgery 1181
    W. Peter Nordland and Laura M. Souza

PART 7 PROBLEMS OF THE EMERGENCY AND FAILURE 1213

38. Esthetic and Traumatic Emergencies 1215
    Ronald E. Goldstein and Shane N. White

39. Esthetic Failures 1235
    Ronald E. Goldstein, Azadeh Esfandiari, and Anna K. Schultz

PART 8 CHAIRSIDE PROCEDURES 1261

40. Tooth Preparation in Esthetic Dentistry 1263
    Ronald E. Goldstein, Ernesto A. Lee, and Wendy A. Clark

41. Impressions 1287
    Ronald E. Goldstein, John M. Powers, and Ernesto A. Lee

42. Esthetic Temporization 1311
    Ronald E. Goldstein and Pinhas Adar

43. The Esthetic Try-In 1331
    Ronald E. Goldstein and Carolina Arana

44. Cementation of Restorations 1355
    Stephen F. Rosenstiel and Ronald E. Goldstein

PART 9 TECHNICAL ADVANCES AND PROPER MAINTENANCE OF ESTHETIC RESTORATIONS 1367

45. Esthetic Principles in Constructing Ceramic Restorations 1369
    Robert D. Walter

46. Digital Impression Devices and CAD/CAM Systems 1387
    Nathan S. Birnbaum and Heidi B. Aaronson

47. Maintenance of Esthetic Restorations 1409
    Ronald E. Goldstein, Kimberly J. Nimmons, Anita H. Daniels, and Caren Barnes

Index i1

List of Contributors

Heidi B. Aaronson, DMD
Former Clinical Instructor
Tufts University School of Dental Medicine
Boston, MA;
Private Practice
Wellesley, MA
USA

Pinhas Adar, MDT, CDT
Adjunct Clinical Professor
Tufts University School of Dentistry
Adar International, Inc.
Atlanta, GA
USA

Carolina Arana, DMD, MPH
Private Practice
Decatur, GA
USA

Donald E. Arens, DDS, MSD (Deceased)
Former Professor Emeritus in Endodontics Indiana;
Indiana University School of Dentistry
Indianapolis, IN;
Former Visiting Professor of Endodontics
College of Dental Medicine
Nova SE University
Davie, FL
USA

Caren Barnes, RDH, BS, MS
Professor, Coordinator of Clinical Research
University of Nebraska Medical Center College
of Dentistry
Department of Dental Hygiene
Lincoln, NE
USA

Gerald M. Barrack, DDS
Private Practice
Ho-Ho-Kus, NJ
USA

Nathan S. Birnbaum, DDS
Associate Clinical Professor
Tufts University School of Dental Medicine
Boston, MA;
Private Practice
Medford, MA
USA

Uwe Blunck, DDS
Associate Professor
Department for Operative, Endodontic and
Preventive Dentistry
School of Dentistry
Charité-Universitaetsmedizin
Berlin
Germany

Kristin A. Boehm, MD, FACS
Assistant Clinical Professor Plastic & Reconstructive Surgery
Emory University School of Medicine
Atlanta, GA;
Private Practice
Atlanta, GA
USA

Lorenzo Breschi, DDS, PhD
Associate Professor
Department of Biomedical and Neuromotor Sciences
University of Bologna - Alma Mater Studiorum
Bologna
Italy

Shirley Brown, DMD, PhD
Rittenhouse Collaborative
Vector Group Consulting
Philadelphia, PA
USA

David A. Bulot, DDS, MD
Assistant Clinical Professor
LSU Oral and Maxillofacial Surgery
New Orleans, LA;
Private Practice
Baton Rouge, LA
USA

Marcelo Calamita, DDS, MS, PhD
Former Associate Professor of Prosthodontics at University
Braz Cubas;
University of Guarulhos
São Paulo
Brazil

Alberto Caprioglio, DDS, MS
Associate Professor and Chairman
Department of Orthodontics
School of Dentistry
University of Insubria
Varese
Italy

Claudia Caprioglio, DDS, MS
Visiting Professor Department of Orthodontics
Pediatric Dentistry University of Pisa
Pisa
Italy

Damaso Caprioglio, MD, MS
Former Full Professor of Orthodontics
University of Parma School of Dentistry
Parma;
Lecturer in Ethics
University of Parma
Parma
Italy

W. Frank Caughman, DMD, MEd
Professor Emeritus
The Dental College of Georgia at Augusta University
Augusta, GA
USA

Daniel C.N. Chan, DMD, MS, DDS
Chair Department of Restorative Dentistry
School of Dentistry
University of Washington
Seattle, WA
USA

Noah Chivian, DDS
Clinical Professor
Department of Endodontics
Rutgers School of Dental Medicine
Newark, NJ;
Adjunct Professor of Endodontics
University of Pennsylvania
School of Dental Medicine
Philadelphia, PA
USA

Stephen J. Chu, DMD, MSD, CDT
Adjunct Clinical Professor
Ashman Department of Periodontology & Implant Dentistry
Department of Prosthodontics
New York University College of Dentistry, New York;
Private Practice
New York, NY
USA

Roman M. Cibirka, DDS, MS
Former Assistant Professor
Department of Rehabilitation
The Dental College of Georgia at Augusta University
Augusta, GA
USA

Wendy A. Clark, DDS, MS
Clinical Assistant Professor
Department of Prosthodontics
University of North Carolina School of Dentistry
Chapel Hill, NC
USA

Christian Coachman, DDS, CDT
Private Practice
São Paulo
Brazil

James W. Curtis Jr, DMD
Director
Dental Education
Palmetto Health Dental Center
Columbia, SC
USA

Anita H. Daniels, RDH
Adjunct Clinical Instructor
University of Miami
Department of Dental Implants
School of Medicine
Miami, FL
USA

Richard Davis
Professional Hair Stylist
Atlanta, GA
USA

List of Contributors

Eladio DeLeon Jr, DMD, MS
Goldstein Chair of Orthodontics
The Dental College of Georgia at Augusta University
Augusta, GA
USA

Maha El-Sayed, BDS, DMD, MS
Private Practice
Atlanta, GA
USA

Azadeh Esfandiari, DMD
Private Practice
Atlanta, GA
USA

Beverly A. Farley, DMD (Deceased)
Formerly in Private Practice
Irmo, SC
USA

Roland Frankenberger, DMD, PhD
Professor and Chair
Department of Operative Dentistry and Endodontics
Medical Center for Dentistry
University of Marburg
Marburg
Germany

Kevin B. Frazier, DMD, EDS
Professor
Oral Rehabilitation
The Dental College of Georgia at Augusta University
Augusta, GA
USA

Ronald E. Goldstein, DDS
Clinical Professor
Department of Restorative Sciences
The Dental College of Georgia at Augusta University
Augusta, GA;
Adjunct Clinical Professor of Prosthodontics
Boston University School of Dental Medicine
Boston;
Adjunct Professor of Restorative Dentistry
University of Texas Health Science Center
San Antonio, TX;
Former Visiting Professor of Oral and Maxillofacial Imaging and Continuing Education
University of Southern California
School of Dentistry
Los Angeles, CA;
Private Practice
Atlanta, GA
USA

Steven T. Hackman, DDS
Formerly, Department of Oral Rehabilitation
The Dental College of Georgia at Augusta University
Augusta, GA
USA

Barry D. Hammond, DMD
Associate Professor and Director of Dental Continuing Education
The Dental College of Georgia at Augusta University
Augusta, GA
USA

Van B. Haywood, DMD
Professor
Department of Oral Rehabilitation
The Dental College of Georgia at Augusta University
Augusta, GA
USA

John N. Kent, DDS
Former Boyd Professor and Head
Department of Oral and Maxillofacial Surgery
LSU School of Dentistry and LSU School of Medicine at Shreveport;
Professor Emeritus, LSUSD and LSUHSC
New Orleans, LA
USA

Jason J. Kim, CDT
Clinical Assistant Professor
New York University College of Dentistry
Oral Design Center
New York, NY
USA

Glenn D. Krieger, DDS, MS
Private Practice
Lewisville, TX
USA

So Ran Kwon, DDS, MS, PhD, MS
Associate Professor
Center for Dental Research
Loma Linda University School of Dentistry
Loma Linda, CA
USA

Ernesto A. Lee, DMD
Clinical Professor
University of Pennsylvania School of Dental Medicine;
Director
Postdoctoral Periodontal Prosthesis Program
Penn Dental Medicine;
Private Practice
Bryn Mawr, PA
USA

Carol A. Lefebvre, DDS, MS
Dean and Professor
Oral Rehabilitation and Oral Biology
The Dental College of Georgia at Augusta University
Augusta University
Augusta, GA
USA

Roger P. Levin, DDS
CEO/President
Levin Group Inc.
Owings Mills, MD
USA

Sonia Leziy, DDS
Associate Clinical Associate Professor
University of British Columbia
Vancouver
British Columbia;
Private Practice
Vancouver
Canada

Kenneth A. Malament, DDS, MScD
Clinical Professor
Tufts University
Medford, MA
USA

Daniel Materdomini, CDT
DaVinci Dental Studios
Beverly Hills, CA
USA

Adam Mieleszko, CDT
Technical instructor
New York University College of Dentistry
New York, NY
USA

Brahm Miller, DDS, MSc
Associate Clinical Professor and Sessional Lecturer
University of British Columbia
Vancouver, British Columbia;
Private Practice
Vancouver
Canada

Daria Molodtsova, MS
Moscow
Russia

Michael L. Myers, DMD
Professor
Department of Oral Rehabilitation
The Dental College of Georgia at Augusta University
Augusta, GA
USA

Foad Nahai, MD, FACS
Clinical Professor of Plastic Surgery
Emory University
Atlanta GA;
Private Practice
Atlanta, GA
USA

John P. Neary, MD, DDS
Assistant Professor and Chairman
Department of Oral and Maxillofacial Surgery
LSU Health Sciences Center-New Orleans
New Orleans, LA;
Assistant Professor
LSU Department of General Surgery
LSU Health Sciences Center-New Orleans,
New Orleans, LA;
Former Adjunct Professor
University of Leon
Department of Maxillofacial and Plastic Surgery
Leon, Nicaragua;
Former Clinical Assistant Professor
Case-Western University
Department of Oral and Maxillofacial Surgery
Cleveland, OH
USA

Linda C. Niessen, DMD, MPH, MPP
Dean
Nova Southeastern University
Fort Lauderdale, FL
USA

Kimberly J. Nimmons, RDH, BS
Clinical Specialist
Atlanta, GA
USA

W. Peter Nordland, DMD, MS
Associate Professor of Periodontics
Loma Linda University
Loma Linda, CA;
Private Practice
Newport Beach, CA
USA

Annabella Oquendo, DDS
Clinical Assistant Professor
Cariology and Comprehensive Care
New York University College of Dentistry
New York, NY
USA

John Oubre, DDS
Private Practice
Lafayette, LA
USA

Jacinthe M. Paquette, DDS
Private Practice
Newport Beach, CA
USA

Rade D. Paravina, DDS, MS, PhD
Professor
Department of Restorative Dentistry and Prosthodontics;
Director
Houston Center for Biomaterials and Biomimetics;
Ralph C. Cooley Distinguished Professor
The University of Texas School of Dentistry at Houston
Houston, TX
USA

Gordon Patzer, PhD
Professor
Roosevelt University
Chicago, IL
USA

John M. Powers, PhD
Professor of Oral Biomaterials
Department of Restorative Dentistry and Biomaterials
UT Health Dental Branch
Houston, TX
USA

Andrea Ricci, DDS
Private Practice
Florence
Italy

Stephen F. Rosenstiel, BDS, MSD
Professor Emeritus
Ohio State University College of Dentistry
Columbus, OH
USA

Maurice A. Salama, DMD
Faculty
University of Pennsylvania
Philadelphia, PA;
Clinical Assistant Professor
Department of Periodontics
The Dental College of Georgia at Augusta University
Augusta, GA;
Visiting Professor of Periodontics at Nova Southeastern University
Fort Lauderdale, FL;
Private Practice
Atlanta, GA
USA

David Sarver, DMD, MS
Adjunct Professor
University of North Carolina
Department of Orthodontics
Chapel Hill, NC;
Clinical Professor
University of Alabama Department of Orthodontics
Birmingham, AL;
Private Practice
Birmingham, AL
USA

Anna K. Schultz, DMD
Private Practice
Atlanta, GA
USA

Geoffrey W. Sheen, DDS, MS
Department of Oral Rehabilitation
Dental College of Georgia
Augusta University
Augusta, GA
USA

Cherilyn G. Sheets, DDS
Clinical Professor
Department of Restorative Dentistry
University of Southern California
Ostrow School of Dentistry
Los Angeles, CA;
Private Practice
Newport Beach, CA
USA

Asgeir Sigurdsson, DDS, MS
Associate Professor and Chairman
Department of Endodontics
NYU College of Dentistry
New York, NY
USA

Bruno P. Silva, DMD, PhD
Clinical Assistant Professor
Department of Prosthodontics
University of Seville
School of Dentistry
Spain;
Private Practice
Seville
Spain

Thomas Sing, MDT
Visiting Lecturer
Postdoctoral Program for Prosthodontics
Tufts University
School of Dental Medicine
Boston, MA;
Visiting Lecturer
Harvard School of Dental Medicine
Boston, MA;
Private Practice
Boston, MA
USA

Samantha Siranli, DMD, PhD
Former Adjunct Faculty
Department of Oral Rehabilitation
The Dental College of Georgia
Augusta University
Augusta, GA;
Former Associate Professor of Prosthodontics
University of Pittsburgh
Pittsburgh, PA;
Private Practice
Washington, DC
USA

Laura M. Souza, DDS
Private Practice
San Diego, CA
USA

Christian F.J. Stappert, DDS, MS, PhD
Professor and Former Director of Postgraduate Prosthodontics
Department of Prosthodontics
University of Freiburg
Germany;
Professor and Former Director of Periodontal Prosthodontics
and Implant Dentistry
Department of Periodontics
University of Maryland School of Dentistry
Baltimore, MD;
Past Director of Aesthetics and Periodontal Prosthodontics
Department of Periodontology and Implant Dentistry
New York University College of Dentistry
New York, NY
USA;
Private Practice
Zurich
Switzerland

Devin L. Stewart, DDS
Private Practice
San Luis Obispo
Los Angeles, CA;
Former Clinical Instructor
Removable Department
UCLA
Los Angeles, CA
USA

Mo Taheri, DMD
Clinical Instructor
Tufts University
Medford, MA
USA

Fransiskus A. Tjiptowidjojo, DDS, MS
Adjunct Instructor
University of Detroit Mercy School of Dentistry
Department of Restorative Dentistry
Detroit, MI
USA

Walter F. Turbyfill Jr, DMD
Private Practice
Columbia, SC
USA

Marcos Vargas, DDS, MS
Professor
Department of Family Dentistry
The University of Iowa
Iowa City, IA
USA

Robert D. Walter, DDS, MSD
Associate Professor
School of Dentistry
Loma Linda University
Loma Linda, CA
USA

Daniel H. Ward, DDS
Former Assistant Clinical Professor
Department of Restorative and Prosthetic Dentistry
College of Dentistry
The Ohio State University
Columbus OH;
Private Practice
Columbus, OH
USA

John West, DDS, MSD
Affiliate Associate Professor
Department of Endodontics
School of Dentistry
University of Washington
Seattle, WA
USA

Marvin Westmore
Professional Makeup Artist and Licensed Aesthetician
Hollywood, CA
USA

Shane N. White, BDentSc, MS, MA, PhD
Professor
UCLA School of Dentistry
Los Angeles, CA
USA

Jean C. Wu, DDS
Former Lecturer
Restorative Dentistry Department
University of Tennessee
Memphis, TN;
Private Practice
Newport Beach, CA
USA

Edwin J. Zinman, DDS, JD
Former Lecturer
Department of Periodontology
UCSF School of Dentistry
San Francisco CA;
Private Law Practice
San Francisco, CA
USA

Contributors at Large

Wendy A. Clark, DDS, MS
Clinical Assistant Professor
Department of Prosthodontics
University of North Carolina School of Dentistry
Chapel Hill, NC
USA

Nadia Esfandiari, DMD
Private Practice
Atlanta, GA
USA

David A. Garber, DMD
Clinical Professor
Department of Periodontics
The Dental College of Georgia at Augusta University
Augusta, GA;
Clinical Professor
Department of Prosthodontics
Louisiana State University Department of Restorative Dentistry
Baton Rouge, LA;
University of Texas in San Antonio
San Antonio, TX;
Private Practice
Atlanta, GA
USA

Cary E. Goldstein, DMD
Clinical Professor
Department of Restorative Sciences
The Dental College of Georgia at Augusta University
Augusta, GA;
Private Practice
Atlanta, GA
USA

Henry Salama, DMD
Former Director and Clinical Assistant Professor
Department of Periodontics
Implant Research Center
University of Pennsylvania
Philadelphia, PA;
Private Practice
Atlanta, GA
USA

Maurice A. Salama, DMD
Faculty
University of Pennsylvania
Philadelphia, PA;
Clinical Assistant Professor
Department of Periodontics
The Dental College of Georgia at Augusta University
Augusta, GA;
Visiting Professor of Periodontics at Nova Southeastern University
Fort Lauderdale, FL;
Private Practice
Atlanta, GA
USA

Preface to Third Edition

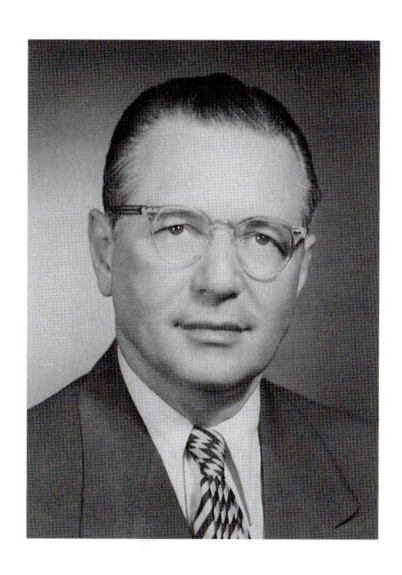

I owe so much of my career in esthetic dentistry to my first and most important mentor… my father, Dr Irving H. Goldstein, a great dentist, civic leader, and philanthropist. I learned so much watching him create the most beautiful smiles and only wish Dad had kept a photo library as I have done in my career. He taught me that being an average dentist was never an option… rather to always work to be the best, and at 84 years, I am still striving every day I practice.

I was first drawn to the study of esthetics a number of years before my 1969 article "The study of the need for esthetic dentistry" was published in the *Journal of Prosthetic Dentistry*. That article identified dentistry's lack of appreciation for the patients' appearances and their self-perception.

During the first half of the 1970s, I avidly pursued my study of esthetics, investigating every known aspect of dentofacial appearance. I became convinced of the huge untapped potential the field offered for improving patient outcomes and enhancing dental practice. Eventually, I was inspired to dedicate my professional career to promoting a comprehensive interdisciplinary approach to dentistry that united function and esthetics in total dentofacial harmony.

When the first edition of this text was published in 1976, the United States was in the midst of a celebration marking the 200th anniversary of our birth as a nation. It was an unprecedented national observance of the highly successful American Revolution. At the time, I considered the two events—both of considerable importance to me—distinct from one another. Since that time, however, I have come to recognize that, although the publishing of any textbook could never be considered in the same breath with the emergence of a nation, both events were indeed revolutionary.

Six decades ago, esthetics was considered, at best, a fortuitous by-product of a dental procedure—a bridesmaid, but certainly not a bride. In the years that have ensued, esthetics has taken its rightful place, along with functionality, as a bona fide objective of dental treatment. The revolution that has transpired has not only enhanced our knowledge of the field but also in methodology and technology. Today's patients are highly informed about the possibilities of esthetic dental restorations and fully expect that esthetics will be considered, from the inception of treatment to the final result.

Consumers know that dental esthetics play a key role in their sense of well-being, their acceptance by others, their success at work, in relationships, and their emotional stability. Informed by magazines, books, internet, and ongoing social media coverage, plus driven by the desire to live better lives, patients seek out dentists who can deliver superior esthetic services.

The ongoing effort to meet these demands with state-of-the-art and science treatment represents the continuation of that revolution. At the time this text book first appeared, I hoped that esthetics would eventually hold a preeminent position in our profession. That goal has been accomplished. Esthetics is recognized worldwide today as a basic principle of virtually all dental treatment.

We have been so fortunate in having over 75 world authorities helping to update the 47 chapters in two volumes. Virtually every phase of esthetic dentistry has now been included. It is my hope that, in some small way, this updated edition will serve to advance all aspects of the esthetic dental revolution and, in so doing, help patients and practitioners achieve even greater, more satisfying outcomes.

I feel so fortunate that three of the world's best known, talented, and respected academicians, clinicians, and teachers agreed to co-edit this third edition with me—Drs Steven Chu, Ernesto Lee, and Christian Stappert have continuingly contributed greatly in making the third edition more far-reaching into the high-tech worldwide revolution in esthetic dentistry.

Ronald E. Goldstein

Acknowledgments

So many people have worked on various aspects of this third edition that it would take far too much space to mention all of them. However, there were those who gave significant time to the project, and it is those people who I will attempt to thank at this time.

Most helpful in every way was the extraordinary 7-year effort of my personal editorial assistant, Annette Mathews. Annette's attention to detail and meticulous follow-through helped us greatly to complete this third edition. Despite the frustration of dealing with three different publishers, Annette helped coordinate with over 75 contributors, in addition to continuously proofreading the 47 chapters. I have had the pleasure of working with many individuals in my 60 years of practice, but none better than Annette. She wins the prize!

Others who assisted me on various aspects of the book were Daria Molodtsova, Candace Paetzhold, and Yhaira Grigsby.

My clinical office staff has always been generous with their help over the years. Those assistants who have been most helpful with this edition were Sondra Williams and Charlene Bennett.

It also takes a talented group of professionals for the day-to-day support necessary to sustain a lengthy project such as this text. I am most appreciative of the support from my long-time partners, David Garber and Maurice Salama. No one could ask for a more understanding and gifted friend than David. Maurice and Henry Salama have always been ready to lend a hand or help solve a dilemma as only they can. Wendy Clark, Nadia Esfandiari, and Maha El Sayed were particularly helpful during the writing and editing stages. Thanks also to Pinhas Adar, who has always been willing and available to help with technical or illustrative assistance. Thanks also to Zach Turner for his excellent illustrations throughout the text.

Last but not least, I must thank my busy but devoted family; my dentist sons Cary and Ken plus my dental daughter Cathy Goldstein Schwartz were particularly helpful in the second edition, and my physician son, Rick, managed to keep me healthy enough to complete the task.

I must pay the final tribute to my wife, Judy, who has continued to support and advise me throughout my career. She has put up with the tremendous hours over 60 years of writing articles and books and helped me through the good and bad times… fortunately more good than bad. My only promise to her was that this third edition of *Esthetics in Dentistry* will definitely be my last textbook as author or co-author.

Ronald E. Goldstein

PART I
PRINCIPLES OF ESTHETICS

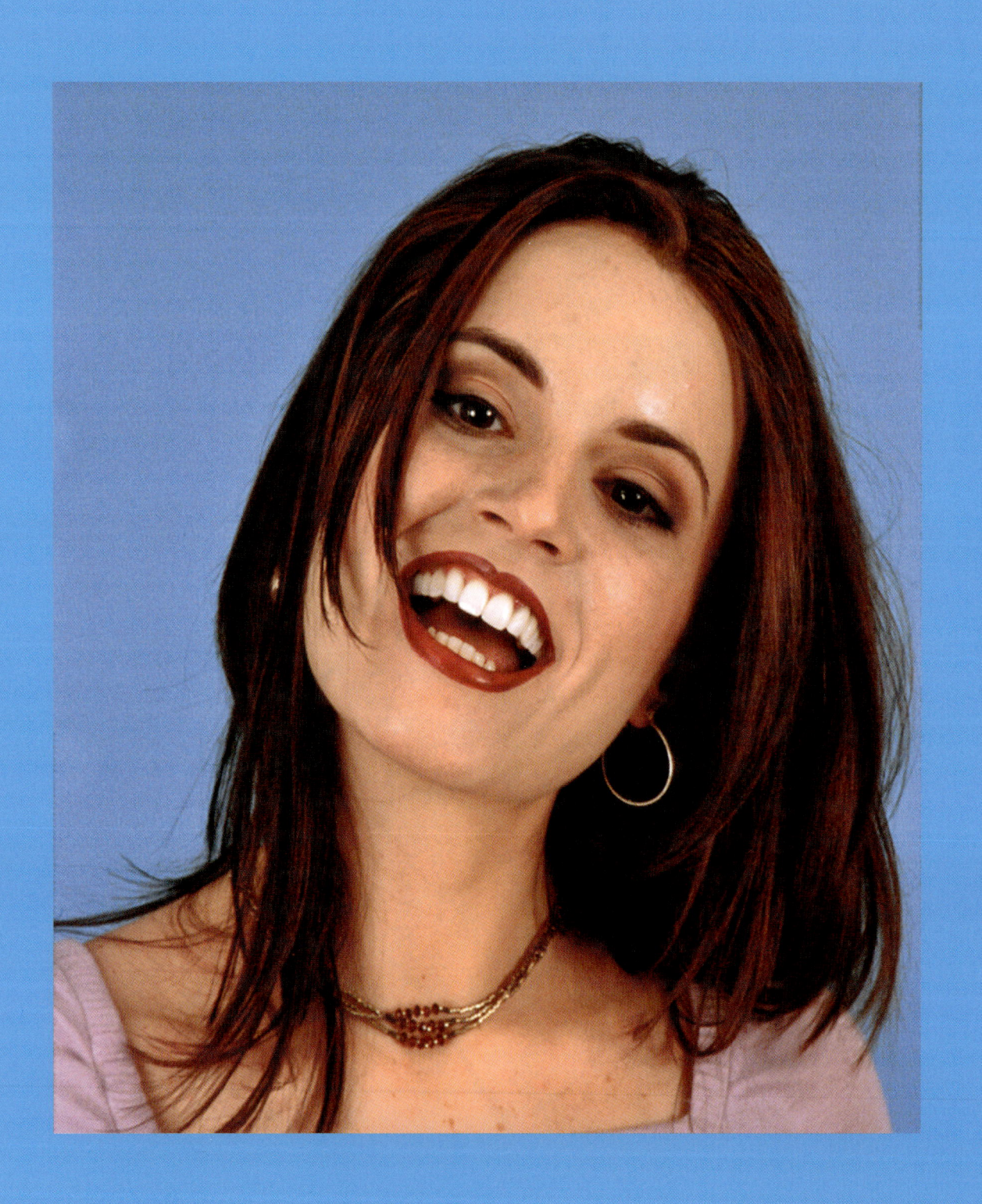

Chapter 1 Concepts of Dental Esthetics

Ronald E. Goldstein, DDS and Gordon Patzer, PhD

Chapter Outline

What is esthetics?	3	Personal values	11
Historical perspective of dental esthetics	4	Employment: a closer look	12
The social context of dental esthetics	5	The business of looking good	12
Esthetics: a health science and service	6	Patient response to abnormality	16
Understanding the patient's esthetic needs	8	Psychology and technology	16
Physical attractiveness phenomenon	8	Patient types and dentist alerts	16
Research methodology	9	Psychology and treatment planning	19
The importance of facial appearance	10	Predicting patient response	19
Functions of teeth	11	"Crossroads"	20

Beauty is in the eye of the beholder.

Margaret Hungerford

What is esthetics?

Mosby's Dental Dictionary defines esthetic dentistry as, "the skills and techniques used to improve the art and symmetry of the teeth and face to enhance the appearance as well as the function of the teeth, oral cavity, and face."[1] This definition positions appearance as a focal point of esthetic dentistry. Dental esthetics (also spelled aesthetics) connects with the principal aspect of appearance—physical attractiveness. Accordingly, esthetic dentistry provides benefits that extend far beyond total dental health toward total well-being throughout life.

Each of us has a general sense of beauty. Our own individual expression, interpretation, and experiences make it unique. In addition, we are also influenced by culture and self-image. What one culture perceives as disfigured may be beautiful to another. Chinese women once bound their feet, and Ubangis distend their lips. Individuals' sense of what is beautiful influences how they present themselves to others. Esthetics is not absolute, but extremely subjective.

Many factors and dimensions determine a person's appearance, among which physical attractiveness predominates and which esthetic dentistry can affect favorably. The entirety of the physical attractiveness aspect of appearance calls for the label, physical attractiveness phenomenon.

Gordon Patzer

Physical attractiveness phenomenon is a bias based on physical attractiveness. As discomforting as it may be for people to acknowledge, the reality lives. Individuals with an appearance of higher physical attractiveness *do* experience benefits throughout life that their counterparts of lower physical attractiveness *do not*. This takes place uniformly regardless of age, gender, race, ethnicity, socioeconomic level, geographical location, political structure, time in history, and so on. Indeed, esthetic dentistry naturally plays a critical role in a person's appearance, particularly in the link between dental esthetics and physical attractiveness. Therefore, it is reasonable to recognize esthetic dentistry as one dimension of physical attractiveness phenomenon. It is also reasonable to view the reality caused by, or at the least correlated with, physical attractiveness phenomenon to be significantly interrelated. In other words, esthetic dentistry possesses considerable capability, opportunity, and responsibility concerning the benefits and detriments that individuals experience throughout their lives.

Notions that esthetic dentistry is only about vanity and caters exclusively to the rich and famous fail tests of reality. Dental professionals who provide esthetic dentistry and recipients of these services readily offer evidence contrary to this. Yes, function matters tremendously. It is essential throughout dentistry, but coupling function with form that improves appearances matters even more. No, dental esthetics is not about vanity, the rich, or the famous. It is about realization that esthetic dentistry done well can contribute to the lives of all people in all walks of life far beyond the in-office, oral cavity, dental treatment received. As dental esthetics exert a key role in a person's looks, those looks carry influences internally concerning self-image, confidence, and happiness, and externally concerning what others see. In other words, at the same time that esthetic dentistry contributes to total dental health (making it a health science,) a person's ability to retain or to enhance appearances of his or her teeth contribute accordingly to the world's interactions with that person and vice versa.

Historical perspective of dental esthetics

Cosmetic dental treatment dates back more than four millennia. Throughout history, civilizations recognized that their accomplishments in the field of restorative and cosmetic dentistry were a measure of their level of competence in science, art, commerce, and trade. There are repeated references in history to the value of replacing missing teeth. In the El Gigel cemetery located in the vicinity of the great Egyptian pyramids, two molars encircled with gold wire were found. Gold was also used to splint anterior teeth and may be thought of as a luxurious way of saving teeth. This was one of the first pieces of evidence showing the Etruscan culture valued the smile as an important part of physical attractiveness. It was apparently a prosthetic device.[2] In the Talmudic Law of the Hebrews, tooth replacement is permitted for women. The Etruscans were well versed in the use of human teeth or teeth carved from animal's teeth to restore missing dentition[3] (Figure 1.1).

Other historical evidence that ancient cultures were concerned with cosmetic alteration of the teeth includes reference to the Japanese custom of decorative tooth-staining called *ohaguro* in 4000-year-old documents. Described as a purely cosmetic treatment, the procedure had its own set of implements, kept as a cosmetic kit. The chief result of the process was a dark brown or black stain on the teeth. Studies suggest that it might also have had a caries-preventive effect[4] (Figure 1.2).

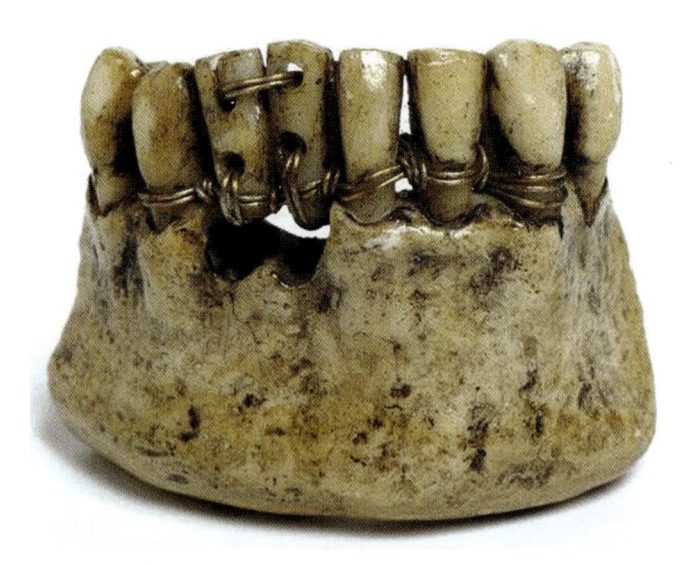

Figure 1.1 Over 4000 years ago, the Etruscans demonstrated the earliest treatment related to esthetic dentistry by using gold wire to save diseased teeth to maintain the beauty of the smile. This reproduction shows copper wire. Figure courtesy of the Royal College of Surgeons of Edinburgh.

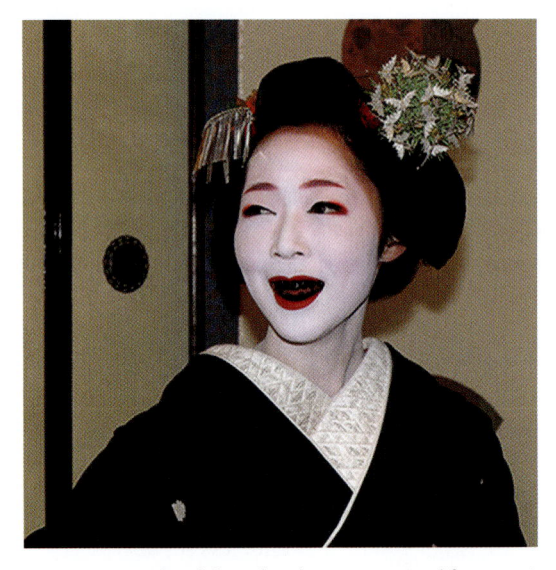

Figure 1.2 An example of dental esthetics practiced from ancient times in Japan, likely around 500 AD, called ohaguro, in which people stained their teeth to be black in color. This practice continued into the Meiji era, which ended in the early 20th century. Figure courtesy of Dr Peter Brown.

Smiles are evidenced as early as 3000 BCE.[1] A smile on the face of a statue of an early king of Abab is noted in the art of Sumer. Aboucaya noted in his thesis that the smile was absent or not very marked in early works of art and, when present, was almost always labial. The dentolabial smile, where the teeth are seen behind the lips, starts to emerge in the first decades of the 20th century. This is attributed to an increased emphasis of awareness of the body and art of cosmetics due to the evolution of social life and the change in habits and manners. Teeth began to play an increasingly important role as more attention was paid to the

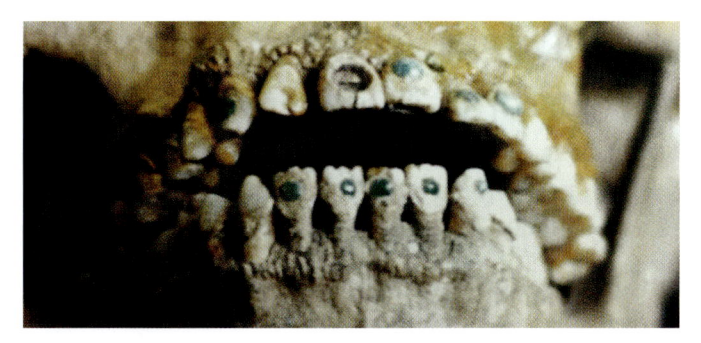

Figure 1.3 **(A)** This 2000-year-old Mayan skull provides some of the best evidence that jadeite inlays were used for cosmetic, rather than functional, purposes.

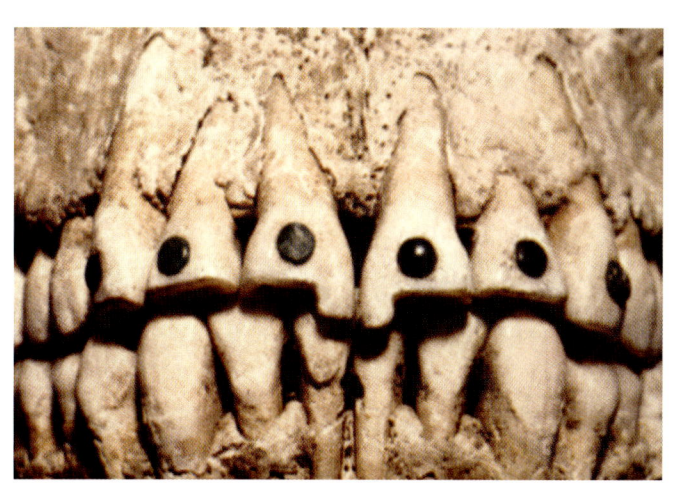

Figure 1.3 **(B)** Aside from jadeite inlays, the Mayans also valued using special tooth carvings to enhance physical appearance. However, there are still cultures that practice filing teeth for cosmetic enhancement (https://anthropology.net/2007/06/01/damien-hirsts-diamond-encrusted-skull-jeweled-skulls-in-archaeology/).

face, which exhibited more open and unrestricted expressions. The resulting emphasis on dental treatment and care also created an interest in the improvement of the esthetics of the smile.

At the height of the Mayan civilization, a system of dental decoration evolved in which some teeth were filed into complicated shapes and others were decorated with jadeite inlays (Figure 1.3A and B). These dental procedures were purely cosmetic and not restorative. Although the intent of these ancient attempts at cosmetic dentistry was strictly ornamental, there were sometimes beneficial side effects, such as the possible caries-preventive consequence of *ohaguro*. More often, however, the side effects were harmful. Some Mayans, seeking to brighten their smiles with jadeite, developed periapical abscesses because of careless or overenergetic "filers of the teeth," as their dentists were called. Today, dental esthetics is founded on a more ethically sound basis: the general improvement of dental health. But the same desires of those ancient men and women to submit to dental decoration as an outward portrayal of the inner self motivate today's adults to seek esthetic treatment. Distant history shows, without exception, labial smiles with lips closed and thus teeth not seen, rather than smiles with lips open and teeth visible. History made today and in the future likely will be substantially different, with quite dramatic changes over time with smiles more commonly showing teeth. Nevertheless, smiles with lips articulated to reveal teeth do not appear in history until the early 1900s, and then only very gradually and nearly only in images representing American history and, less so, history representing other Western cultures.

This change during history with smiles increasingly revealing teeth, albeit initially, parallels numerous other pertinent changes. First is the change regarding broader developments throughout populations particularly related to an individual's appearance in step with physical attractiveness phenomenon. Second, it is certainly reasonable to speculate that the change in smile appearances has been due in large part to esthetic capabilities within the dental profession, as well as changes in societal attitudes. It is certainly correct to attribute the interest in greater visibility of teeth, akin to the "American smile," wanted and displayed today and no doubt increasingly in the future, to these developments. Although esthetic dentistry can help achieve self-assurance, it must always be predicated on sound dental practice and keyed to total dental health. The limitations of esthetic treatment must also be communicated to the patient.

The social context of dental esthetics

A desire to look attractive is no longer taken as a sign of vanity. In an economically, socially, and sexually competitive world, a pleasing appearance is a necessity. In today's technology-driven society, social media contributes to a person's image being viewed more than ever. In addition, high definition has driven many television personalities to improve their physical appearance. As a result, more and more people are considering esthetic dentistry as a necessity to maintain an appealing look. The reason? Dr Johnnetta Cole, past president of Spellman College, tells the author, "Because people have to look at me."

Since the face is the most exposed part of the body, and the mouth a prominent feature, teeth are getting a greater share of attention. "Teeth are sexy" announced a leading fashion magazine, and it then went on to elaborate in nearly 500 words (Figure 1.4A and B). The headline was just the capstone of a string of magazine articles that drew new attention to teeth. Gradually, the public has been made more aware of the "aids to nature" that Hollywood stars have been using since movies began. They discovered that their favorite actors, models, and singers used techniques of dental esthetics to make themselves more presentable and attractive. Some followed the Hollywood lead and asked their dentists to give them teeth like those of some celebrities and thus learned of methods and materials that could improve their appearance.

In the United States today, we place a premium on health and vitality. In fact, these two words are now intertwined with images of beauty. Goleman and Goleman[5] reported that researchers found that attractive people win more prestigious and higher-paying jobs. At West Point, cadets with Clint Eastwood-style good looks—strong jaws and chiseled features—rise to higher military ranks before graduation than their classmates. They also found that good-looking criminals were less likely to be caught; if they did go to court, they were treated more leniently. Teachers were found to go easier when disciplining attractive children; both teachers and pupils consider attractive children as

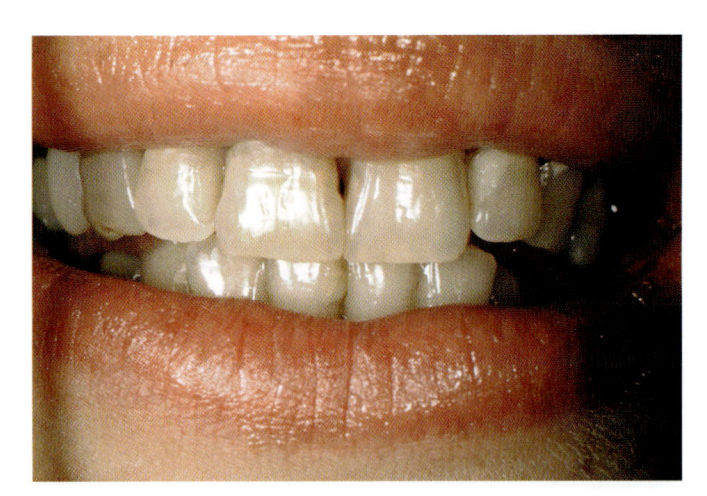

Figure 1.4 **(A)** Discolored teeth and leaking and discolored fillings marred the smile of this 24-year-old internationally known ice skating performer. (Note also the slight crowding of the front teeth, with the right lateral incisor overlapping the cuspid.)

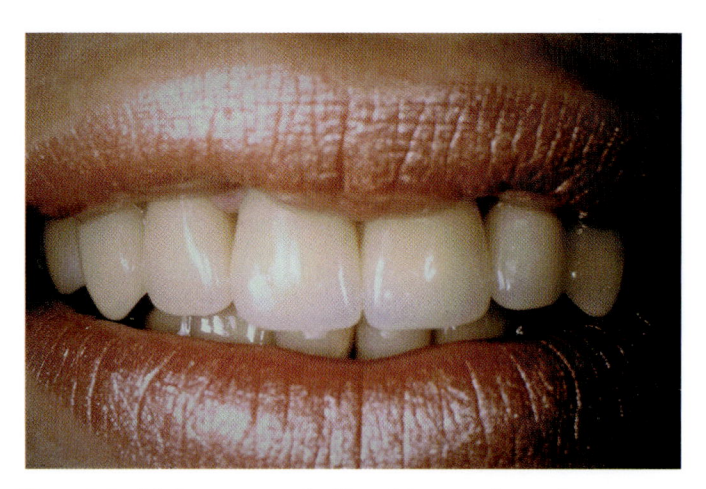

Figure 1.4 **(B)** A new sense of self-confidence and a much more appealing smile was the result of six full porcelain crowns. The teeth appear much straighter, and the lighter color brightens the smile and enhances the beauty of her face and lips.

smarter, nicer, and more apt to succeed at all things. Many studies on self-esteem have illustrated that body image was one of the primary elements in self-rejection.[3,6] Television reinforces in us an extraordinarily high standard of physical attractiveness, and Hollywood has long rewarded beauty and given us standards that are probably higher than most of us will ever achieve.

Society chooses leaders to set unspecified but pervasive standards of acceptable dress, behavior, and recreation. The swings of fashion filter down from the posh salons of couturiers patronized by the wealthy, or up from department store racks from which the majority buy their clothing. A catchphrase repeated on radio or television instantly becomes part of the national language, and songs that began as commercials wind up topping the popular music charts.

Uninfluenced by the esthetic standards set by society, many individuals want to change their appearance to emulate their chosen leaders. General social attitudes profoundly influence an individual's idea of what is attractive: "natural," "beautiful," and "good looking" hold different meanings within the population (Figure 1.5A and B). The female shown in Figure 1.5C was happy with her diastema, thinking it was "cute" and part of her personality. Occasionally, patients take extreme measures to call attention to the mouth in an attempt to achieve an attractive image (Figure 1.6). Therefore, it is the responsibility of the dentist to understand what the patient means when using a particular term, and to decide to what degree the patient's ideal may be realized. The patient's own feeling of esthetics and concept of self-image is most important.

Esthetic dentistry demands attention to the patient's desires and treatment of the patient's individual problems. Esthetic dentistry is the art of dentistry in its purest form. The purpose is not to sacrifice function but to use it as the foundation of esthetics.

The excellence of every art is its intensity, capable of making all disagreeables evaporate, from their being in close relationship with beauty and truth.

John Keats

Esthetics: a health science and service

Is esthetic dentistry a health science and a health service?[7] Or is it the epitome of vanity working its way into a superficial society?

The answer to these questions lie in the scientific facts gleaned from over a thousand studies proving the direct and indirect relationship of how looking one's best is a key ingredient to a positive self-image, which in turn relates to good mental health. The authors of a survey of nearly 30,000 people point to a relationship between psychosocial well-being and body image.[8] They found that feeling attractive, fit, and healthy results in fewer feelings of depression, loneliness, and worthlessness. This study also found that the earlier in life appearance is improved, the more likely it is that the person will go through life with a positive self-image. Sheets states that, "An impaired self-image may be more disabling developmentally than the pertinent physical defect."[9] For instance, adults who reported having been teased as children were more likely to have a negative self-evaluation than those who were not teased (Figure 1.7A and B).

According to Patzer, the face is the most important part of the body when determining physical attractiveness.[10] Specifically, "the hierarchy of importance for facial components appears to be mouth, eyes, facial structure, hair, and nose" (Table 1.1). Therefore, it becomes apparent that not only should esthetic dentistry be performed but it should also be performed as early as possible. It is not necessary for every dentist to master all of the treatments available. However, the advantages, disadvantages, possible results of treatment, maintenance required, and life expectancy of each treatment modality should be thoroughly understood by all dentists. A willingness to refer to another dentist when he or she is more capable of satisfying the patient's desires is both ethical and necessary for good patient relations. Your patient will likely return to you with trust and loyalty for your good judgment in referring for the specific esthetic treatment. The alternative is that your previously satisfied patient may leave you for another dentist if you

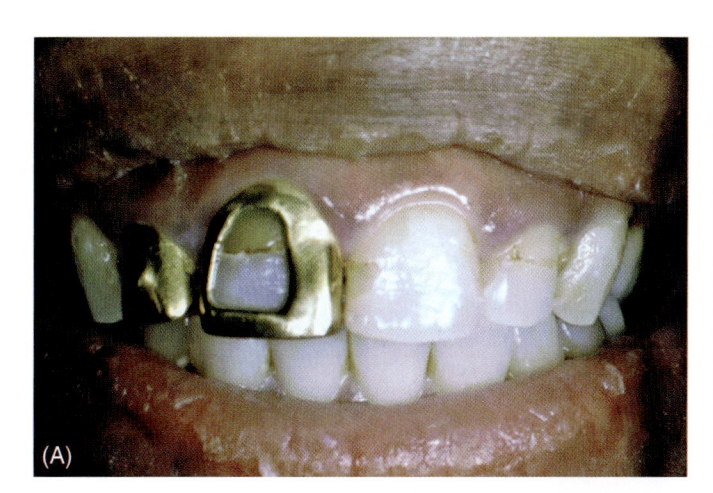

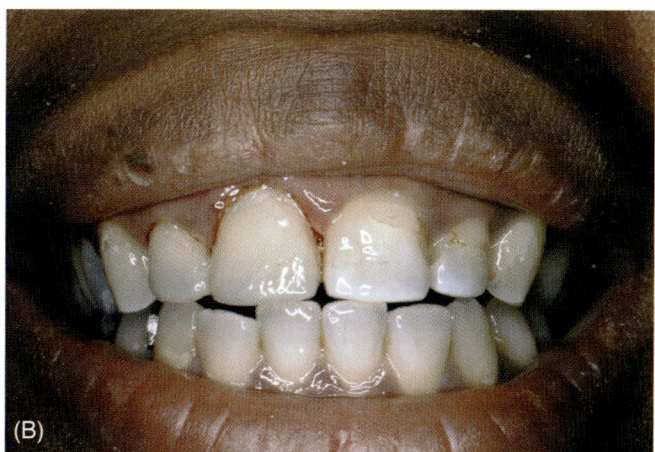

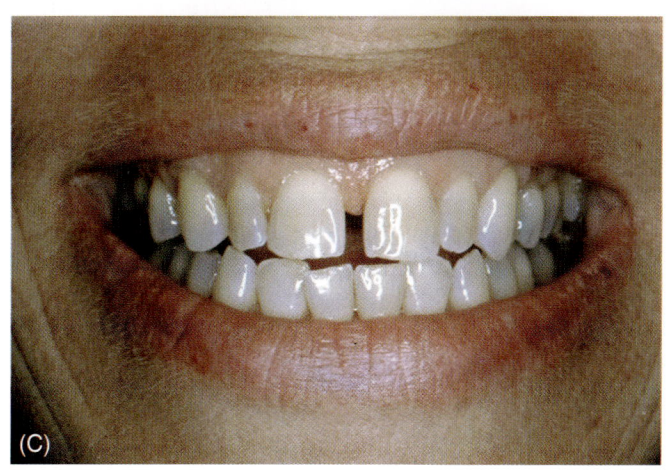

Figure 1.5 **(A–C)** Esthetic values change with social attitudes. (A) This patient once thought that showing gold was desirable, and it was accepted in her socioeconomic peer group. (B) When her status changed 10 years later, so did her attitude, and the gold crowns were removed. It is important to "wear" these temporary acrylic crowns for 1–3 months to make certain the patient will continue to like his or her new look. (C) This lady was happy with her diastema, thinking it was "cute" and part of her personality.

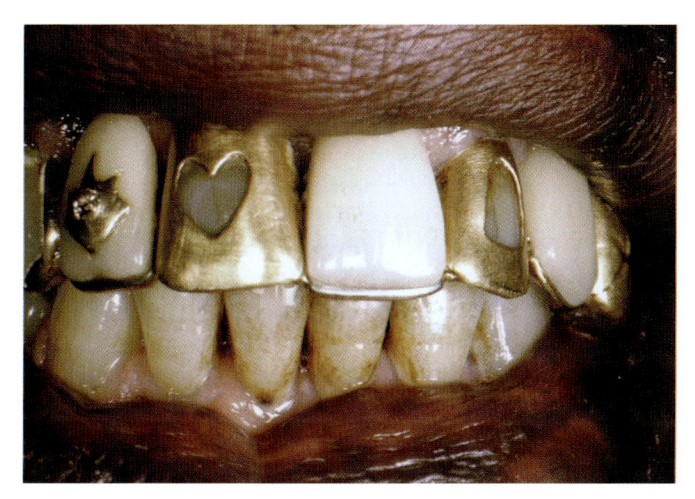

Figure 1.6 Example of an individual during contemporary times who defines good-looking teeth best when adorned with an inlaid diamond and multiple open-faced gold crowns depicting various shapes.

do not offer the requested treatments or belittle their effectiveness without offering an alternative. The fact is, all esthetic treatment modalities work on indicated patients. A good example would be a patient with teeth yellowed due to aging. If you do not provide vital tooth bleaching as one of your routine esthetic dentistry treatments, refer to a colleague who does provide this service. Most likely, the patient will return to your office for routine treatment. Patients may actually appreciate you more, realizing that you are more concerned with their well-being than your own.

Two questions seem in order. On the basis of the previous premise linking a great smile to overall success in life, are we as dentists doing all we should to motivate our patients to improve their smiles? Are we as a profession doing all we should to motivate the 50% of the population who do not normally visit the dentist to have their smiles esthetically improved? Based on the enormous amount of research showing the advantages of an attractive smile, the answer to both questions would seem to be "No." We can and should do much more to inform the public about why a great smile is an important asset and that we as a

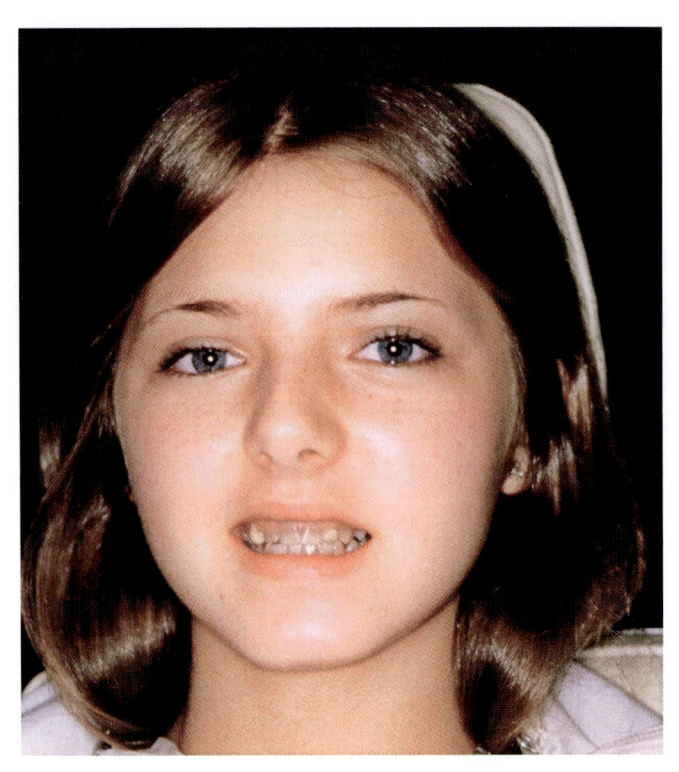

Figure 1.7 **(A)** This 13-year-old girl reported that boys "called her names," referring to her tetracycline-stained teeth.

Table 1.1 Numerical Ranking of Relative Importance of Face Components Using Three Different Research Methodologies

	Rank Order	Ratings by Self-Method	Ratings by Others Method	
			Dissected Photos	Intact Photos
Mouth	1	r = 0.54	r = 0.53	r = 0.72
Eyes	2	r = 0.51	r = 0.44	r = 0.68
Hair	3	r = 0.49	r = 0.34	Not assessed
Nose	4	r = 0.47	r = 0.31	r = 0.61

profession are the logical group to help accomplish this goal. Furthermore, we need to show how easy and painless it can be to achieve. One survey of dentists revealed 83% want greater effort by organized dentistry to promote the value of dentistry to the public.[11] Fitting promotional information can be delivered effectively online through popular social media alternatives as well as through radio, television, and print.

Understanding the patient's esthetic needs

A practicing dentist needs to be acquainted with certain generalities concerning the psychological significance of the patient's mouth. He or she should be familiar with basic considerations

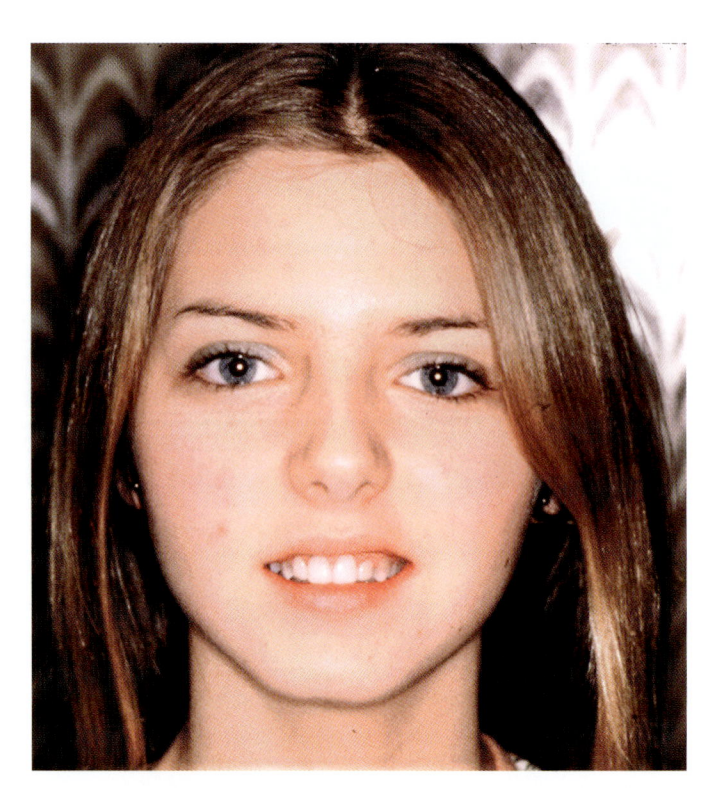

Figure 1.7 **(B)** Although bleaching was attempted, bonding the four maxillary incisors was required to properly mask the tetracycline stains. Unless attention is paid to esthetics in young people, severe personality problems may develop. Improving one's self-confidence through esthetic dentistry can make all the difference in having a positive outlook on life.

that apply to esthetic treatment as well as be aware of various problems that such treatments may incur. To be better equipped to anticipate any such problems, a better understanding of physical attractiveness phenomenon is essential.

Physical attractiveness phenomenon

Physical attractiveness is how pleasing someone or something looks. It is a reality perceived. And, as in nearly all of life, perception is more important than reality. However, given its esthetic essence, its variable/invariable nature constituted by tangibles and intangibles, perception of physical attractiveness is physical attractiveness. Modifiers qualify where and on which continuum the perceived physical attractiveness rates. Levels and descriptors range from low or extremely low to high or extremely high physical attractiveness, from very physically unattractive to very physically attractive, and so on.

Its basic definition applies equally to words used interchangeably—beauty, handsomeness, good looks, ugliness, cuteness, and so forth—as well as words used tangentially that express level and polarity such as gorgeous, stunning, head-turner, hunk, hottie, hot, voluptuous, pretty, homely, dog, pretty ugly. Sexiness does not define physical attractiveness. They are two different traits among many that can differentiate or describe a person. The terms are accordingly neither synonymous nor accurately interchanged. Sexiness expresses a level of sexual or erotic arousal.

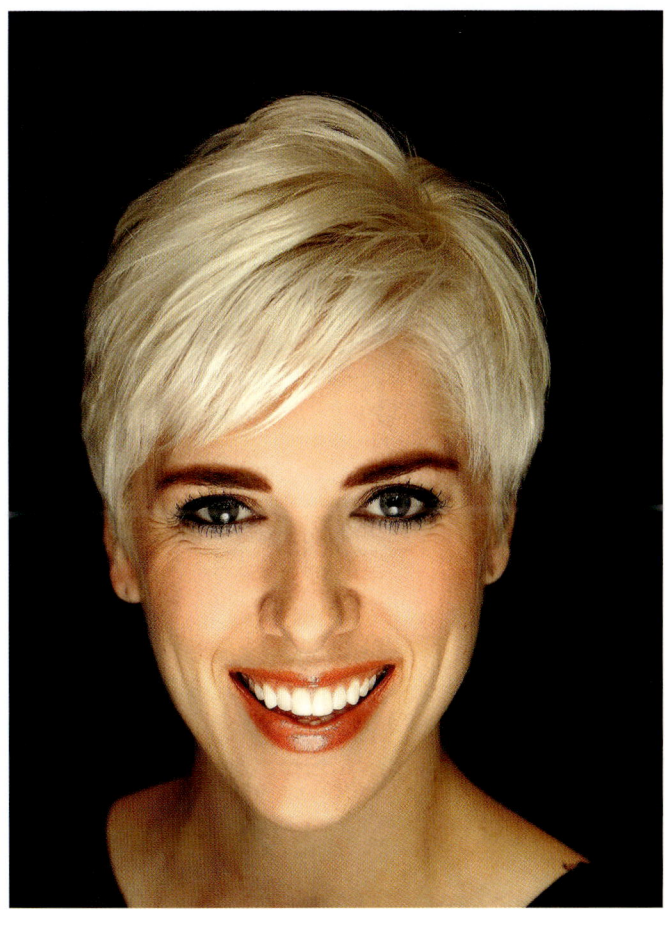

Figure 1.8 Although physical attractiveness and sexiness are two separate traits, this model represents a combination of both.

Table 1.2 Impressions About Persons of Higher and Lower Physical Attractiveness

Persons of Higher Physical Attractiveness		Persons of Lower Physical Attractiveness
Curious	rather than	Indifferent
Complex	rather than	Simple
Perceptive	rather than	Insensitive
Happy	rather than	Sad
Active	rather than	Passive
Amiable	rather than	Aloof
Humorous	rather than	Serious
Pleasure-seeking	rather than	Self-controlled
Outspoken	rather than	Reserved
Flexible	rather than	Rigid
More happy	rather than	Less happy
Better sex lives	rather than	Less good sex lives
Receive more respect	rather than	Receive less respect

A person whose appearance represents high or low physical attractiveness may or may not represent high or low sexiness. To be good-looking is not necessarily to be sexy nor vice versa. These two characteristics can certainly at times overlap and closely interrelate, but they are separate traits not unlike other distinguishing characteristics in these regards; whereby people viewed as more physically attractive are viewed concurrently more favorably on many other visual and nonvisual criteria (Figure 1.8). Although both men and women can be judged physically attractive with or without a great smile, so can they be judged as sexually appealing. However, there are definite attributes to the smile that can enhance one's attractiveness as well as one's sexiness.

Whether speaking about physical attractiveness or sexiness, teeth represent a key feature. Teeth add to or subtract from these desired appearances due to their prominent and inescapable presence (Figure 1.8). As noted earlier, teeth get a substantial share of attention in fashion magazines and in everyday interactions. The reason? The face is the most exposed part of a person combined with movements of the mouth caused by speaking and by many moods expressed in the face. These readily seen movements accordingly draw notice and attention to the observed person's teeth. Following the eyes' attention to a person's teeth, framed by moving actions of the mouth, people rightfully or wrongly infer far more information about the person observed. Accordingly, teeth considered to look esthetically appealing tend to be accompanied with corresponding inferences, assumptions, stereotypes, and expectations about individuals whose teeth communicate good and positive, bad and negative, or somewhere in between (Table 1.2).

Research methodology

Researchers use observation, survey, and experiment, along with variations of each, to study physical attractiveness phenomenon. Surveys are abundant to contemporary society but have limited application for this research area. A survey might ask people (respondents) directly or indirectly whether another person's physical attractiveness influences their assumptions and expectations about the person, likely behaviors toward the person, and so forth. Such a survey can obtain insightful data depending on the circumstances. When it comes to appearances and particularly physical attractiveness, respondents too often provide less than truthful responses to be in line with societal ideals. For that reason and others, when asked, people routinely and inaccurately self-report that another person's physical attractiveness makes no difference. However, when placed in parallel "candid camera" situations, evidence time after time confirms that "actions speak louder than words" when dealing with physical attractiveness phenomenon.

The dichotomy between what most people say regarding another person's physical attractiveness and what these same people do is well documented. Representing anecdotal data, simply focusing on this aspect expressed in the words and actions of friends often reveals the reality of respective differences. Mass media investigations provide equally strong findings through often-entertaining field experiments; examples include American television programs broadcast nationally as reported by correspondent John Stossel on the ABC News program *20/20*, correspondent Keith Morrison on the NBC News program *Dateline NBC*, and supermodel turned television host Tyra Banks on *The Tyra Banks Show*. The physical attractiveness variable in each of these instances was manipulated either by casting multiple actors considered to possess high or low physical attractiveness or by making-up individual actors accordingly. Research procedures then record with hidden cameras and hidden microphones the reactions and interactions with these actors by members of the public. Despite less stringent scientific research procedures, these mass media investigations yield findings overwhelmingly parallel and supporting of the attitudes and behaviors reported repeatedly in scholarly journal articles investigating the consequences of physical attractiveness.

The importance of facial appearance

Allport observes, "Most modern research has been devoted not to what the face reveals, but what people think it reveals."[12] He describes tendencies to perceive smiling faces as more intelligent and to see faces that are average in size of nose, hair, grooming, set of jaw, and so on, as having more favorable traits than those that deviate from the average. Summarizing an experiment by Brinswick and Reiter, Allport notes, "One finding…is that in general the mouth is the most decisive facial feature in shaping our judgments."[4] Meerloo observes, "Through the face, one feels exposed and vulnerable. One's facial expression can become a subject of anxiety."[13]

Studies suggest that even infants can tell an attractive face when they see one, long before they learn a society's standards for beauty. Results of experiments with two groups of infants were reported by psychologist Judith Langlois and five colleagues at the University of Texas at Austin. One group consisted of infants aged 10–14 weeks with an average age of 2 months and 21 days. Sixty three percent of the infants looked longer at attractive faces than at unattractive faces when shown pairs of slides of white women. The second group consisted of 34 infants whose ages ranged from 6 to 8 months. Seventy one percent of the infants looked longer at attractive faces than at unattractive faces.[14–18]

Any dentist dealing with appearance changes in the face must consider the psychological and the physical implications of the treatment. The consideration must involve not only results and attitudes following treatment but also causes, motivations, and desires that compel the patient to seek esthetic treatment (Figure 1.9A and B).

"The psychological concept of self and body image is totally involved in esthetics,"[19] notes Burns, continuing with the observation that dentofacial deformities have been largely regarded in

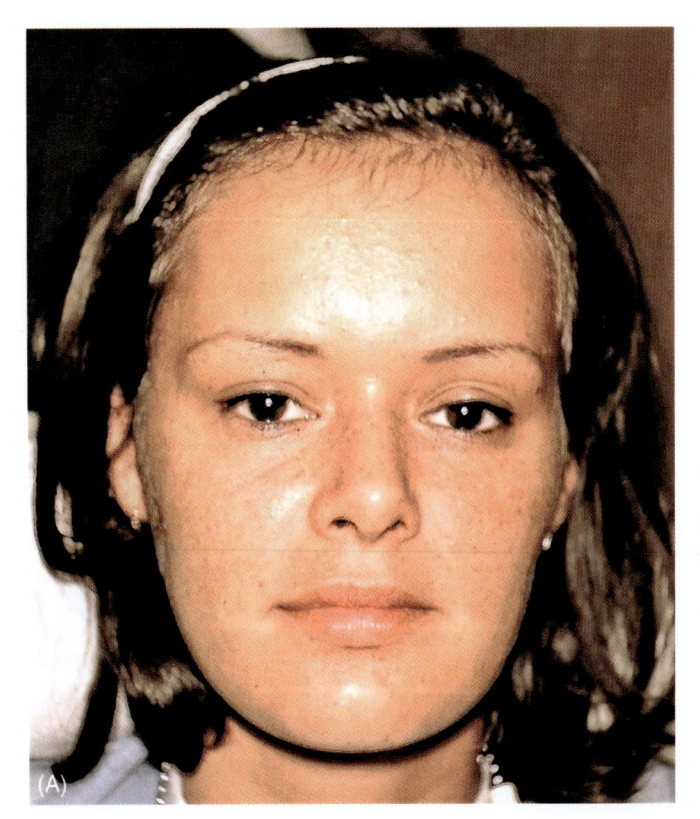

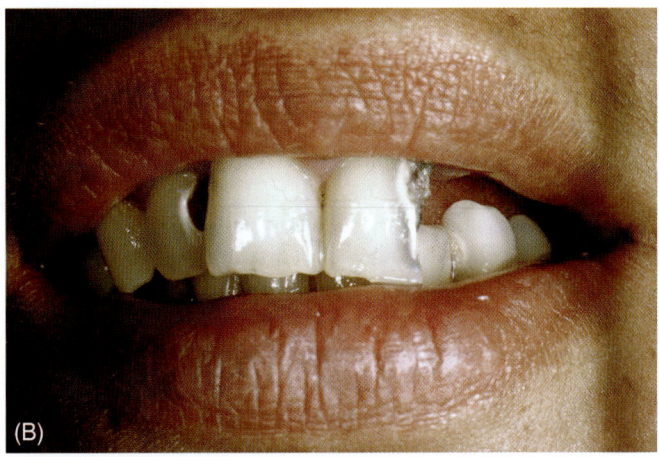

Figure 1.9 (A and B) This girl shows why she chose not to smile. Despite the total breakdown of the oral cavity, her motive in seeking dental treatment was esthetic.

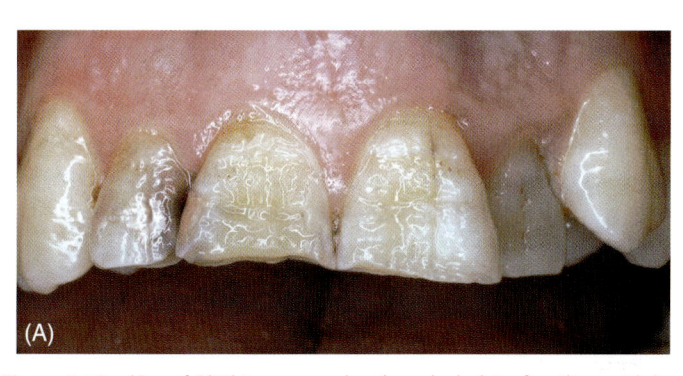

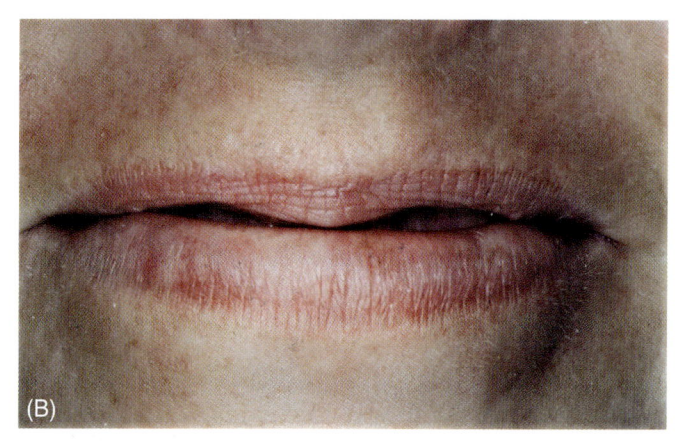

Figure 1.10 (A and B) This woman developed a habit of smiling with her lips together to avoid showing her unsightly maxillary incisors.

terms of diagnosis and treatment, rather than in terms of their psychological ramifications. Burns' consideration of the psychological aspects of esthetic treatment stems from his initial observation that the mouth is the focal point of many emotional conflicts. For example, it is the first source of human contact—a means of alleviating or expressing discomfort or expressing pleasure or displeasure (Figure 1.10A and B).

Functions of teeth

The appearance of a person's teeth communicates much about that person. Therefore, it is not surprising what people actually want to achieve with their teeth and smile. The functions of teeth in the minds of many people include the role of communicating information. Part of the way we communicate is through smiling at one another. Proper functioning of teeth for these people means more than to chew well and pain-free. They believe consciously or subconsciously that the look of their teeth substantially influences the perception of themselves by themselves and by others. Accordingly, the look of another person's teeth can influence the perception of these people. The reality is that the esthetic appearance of a person's teeth does contribute to the person's overall appearance and connects that person to physical attractiveness phenomenon.

Demeaning comments, shunning, and even bullying becomes a way of living for individuals sentenced to visibly missing, crowded, spaced, or protrusive teeth, or other dental anomalies. This is true at least for those individuals without the means for corrective action toward less negative appearances of their teeth. These individuals—male and female, young and old—make ill-fated attempts to avoid those negative reactions. Typical attempts include avoiding all smiling for fear of showing their esthetically unappealing teeth, or concocting a smile that never shows teeth, or using a hand or napkin to cover the mouth while speaking face to face. As well as looking a bit foolish or robotic, their thoughts and actions take a toll on these individuals. The tolls range from avoiding valuable social interactions to missing employment opportunities.

Tolls on a person can be particularly great on those of younger ages, in elementary school through high school. The negative consequences go far beyond affecting only self-image and self-confidence. Their reactions can exert their own toll with damage and costs to others and one's self. Evidence of such reactions makes news reports periodically and too frequently. For example, those bullied can become antisocial and even take up criminal ways, and, in some cases, end either their own life and/or the lives of others.

The mouth can be a particularly significant component of a person's physical attractiveness, which at the same time is rather inseparable from teeth and smile. One of psychology's most revered, Gordon Allport, once observed that people perceive smiling faces to be more intelligent[12] and, citing another research project noted, "…in general the mouth is the most decisive facial feature in shaping our judgments" about a person.[2] Accordingly, actions that include esthetic dentistry likely should be performed at earlier rather than later ages. Consider the 13-year-old girl pictured in Figure 1.7. Before esthetic dental treatment, she reported that kids called her names due to the appearance of her teeth. Professionals would readily interpret these taunts as demeaning with potential negative influences far beyond this girl's early teen years.

An improved self-image leading to increased self-confidence with assistance from esthetic dentistry is not limited to teenage girls. A good smile in these regards can produce improvements in psychological and social well-being for individuals of all ages in all walks of life. Figure 1.4A and B shows the before and after photos of teeth of an internationally accomplished ice skater, mid-20s in age, reported to have gained a new sense of self-confidence after cosmetic dentistry transformed her unpleasing smile into a much more appealing smile.

Personal values

The depth and breadth of a person's physical attractiveness far exceeds first impressions. Hidden and not-so-hidden values drive thoughts and actions that produce significant consequences whereby higher physical attractiveness is overwhelmingly beneficial and lower physical attractiveness is overwhelmingly detrimental. Awareness of this reality provides insight into why and how physical attractiveness can strongly motivate people to value it, retain it, and pursue more of it.

Consider the value of physical attractiveness embraced by Lucy Grealy, a well-educated, best-selling author, known to have many friends, loving family members, sincere romantic relationships, and mass media critical acclaim for her book, *Autobiography of a Face*. In review of a book written by a long-term friend that describes Ms Grealy as a cancer survivor and recipient of 38 operations, *The New York Times* states:

> "Stricken with Ewing's sarcoma at the age of nine, Grealy [who died at age thirty-nine] endured years of radiation and chemotherapy followed by a series of reconstructive operations, most of them unsuccessful. Yet it was the anguish of being perceived as ugly, and of feeling ugly, that she identified as the tragedy of her life. …Grealy came to feel that her suffering as a cancer patient had been minor in comparison."

Values placed on a person's own physical attractiveness vary between individuals. Although the real-life case above might reflect a small, unreasonable, extreme portion of people, it might not. "Beauty was a fantasy, a private wish fraught with shame" for Ms Grealy, who was never able to free herself from "her desire to be beautiful." At various levels, all people throughout their lives hold personal feelings to be more physically attractive. Despite sometimes denial or lack of awareness, evidence overwhelmingly shows that most if not all people value higher levels of physical attractiveness.

As well as valuing others more or less as influenced by their physical attractiveness, it influences one's own value. Researchers for the 2005 Allure State of Beauty National Study that surveyed more than 1700 Americans concluded, "…among the most surprising statistics from the study is that enhancing their [physical] appearance fuels women's confidence." Data from that 2005 survey showed "Ninety-four percent [of the respondents] agree that the more beautiful they feel, the more confident they are." The two factors are interrelated intricately as signaled by the high portion of respondents, 94%, who "say that when they feel more confident, they take more time to look good."

Employment: a closer look

Employment in direct regard to physical attractiveness phenomenon merits a closer look because of the prominent role that gainful work commands throughout nearly every person's life. Two *Newsweek* magazine surveys in 2010 summarized the findings found consistently as reported in scholarly journals. *Newsweek* collected their data from 202 corporate hiring managers in positions ranging from human resource employees to senior-level vice presidents and from 964 members of the public with survey procedures that ensured a nationally representative sample. The subtitle for the reporting article proclaims, "The bottom line? It pays to be good-looking." Their conclusion based on these data: "…paying attention to your looks isn't just about vanity, it's about economic survival [and]…managers are looking beyond wardrobe and evaluating how 'physically attractive' applicants are." Also concluded, these 2010 data "confirm what no qualified (or unqualified) employee wants to admit: that in all elements of the workplace, from hiring to politics to promotions, looks matter, and they matter hard."

Here are some of those specific findings, which highlight how or why looks matter more than you might have imagined.

- **Getting hired**—Among managers, 57% believe that a (physically) "unattractive [but qualified] job candidate will have a harder time getting hired; 68% believe that, once hired, looks will continue to affect the way managers rate job performance." Among members of the public, "63 percent said being physically attractive is beneficial to men who are looking for work, and 72 percent said it was an advantage for women in any job search" (Figure 1.11A–C).
- **Looks above education**—Asked to use a 10-point scale to rate a series of character attributes with 10 being the most important for securing employment, "looks came in third (with a mean score of 7.1), below experience (8.9) and confidence (8.5), but above where a candidate went to school (6.8) and a sense of humor (6.7)."
- **Return on investments**—For individuals considering where or how best to invest their job-hunting resources, 59% of "hiring managers advised spending as much time and money 'making sure they look attractive' as on perfecting a résumé."
- **Lessons learned**—Reverse older or heavier looks, in light of the managers at 84% and 66% respectively stating that, "they believe some bosses would hesitate before hiring a qualified job candidate who looked much older than his or her co-workers" and "they believe some managers would hesitate before hiring a qualified job candidate who was significantly overweight."

For employment decisions, it can be legal to differentiate/discriminate in light of a person's physical attractiveness; that is, if these differentiations are truly based on differences of physical attractiveness and not based on differences of factors prohibited by federal law such as age, sex, race, and so forth. Accordingly, 64% of hiring managers shared these sentiments, stating, "they believe companies should be allowed to hire people based on looks—when a job requires an employee to be the 'face' of a company." It is also important to realize just how much a great smile can be, especially to a person who otherwise might not be judged as attractive. A person can be fat or thin, tall or short, but a winning smile can make the difference in being hired or not.

The business of looking good

Pursuits to look good—whether to retain or to increase physical attractiveness—continue despite downturns and upturns in the broader economy. Proof of collective expenditures can be seen in the somewhat regular mass media reports that highlight annual numbers for sales and services in related industries and professions. Underlying these expenditures, options available to maintain and enhance an individual's physical attractiveness are ever increasing along with continuously evolving wants, demands, innovations, and technological advances.

Providers of products and services to meet the wants of people concerning physical attractiveness range from companies within the cosmetics and beauty sector of world commerce to the professional practitioners regulated through local state licensing requirements. A list of the most notable commerce entities with focus on physical attractiveness begins with major diversified corporations (Unilever, Procter & Gamble, etc.) and continues with major branded companies (Estee Lauder, L'Oreal, etc.). The cosmetic surgery profession likely represents the most visible among professionals regulated by state licensing, with their associations (American Society for Aesthetic Plastic Surgery [ASAPS], American Association of Plastic Surgeons [AAPS], etc.) tabulating and disseminating information about their collective procedures performed.

Suppliers and providers pertinent to the business of looking good are expansive and commonly referred to in summary manner as the beauty industry. A wide array of products and services constitute this industry, sometimes with varying definitions used

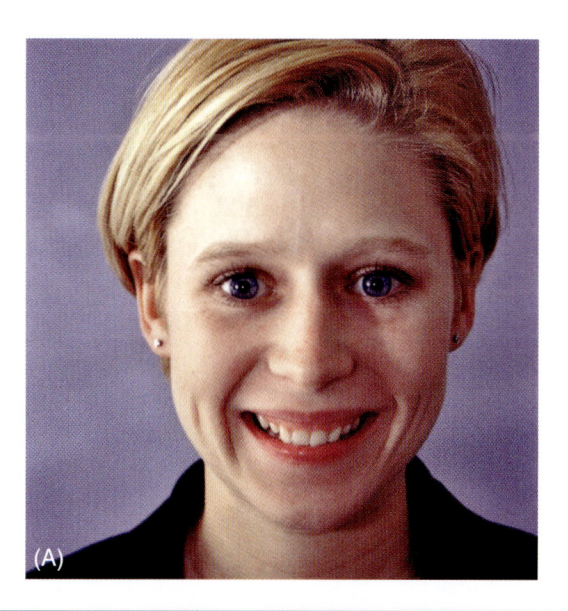

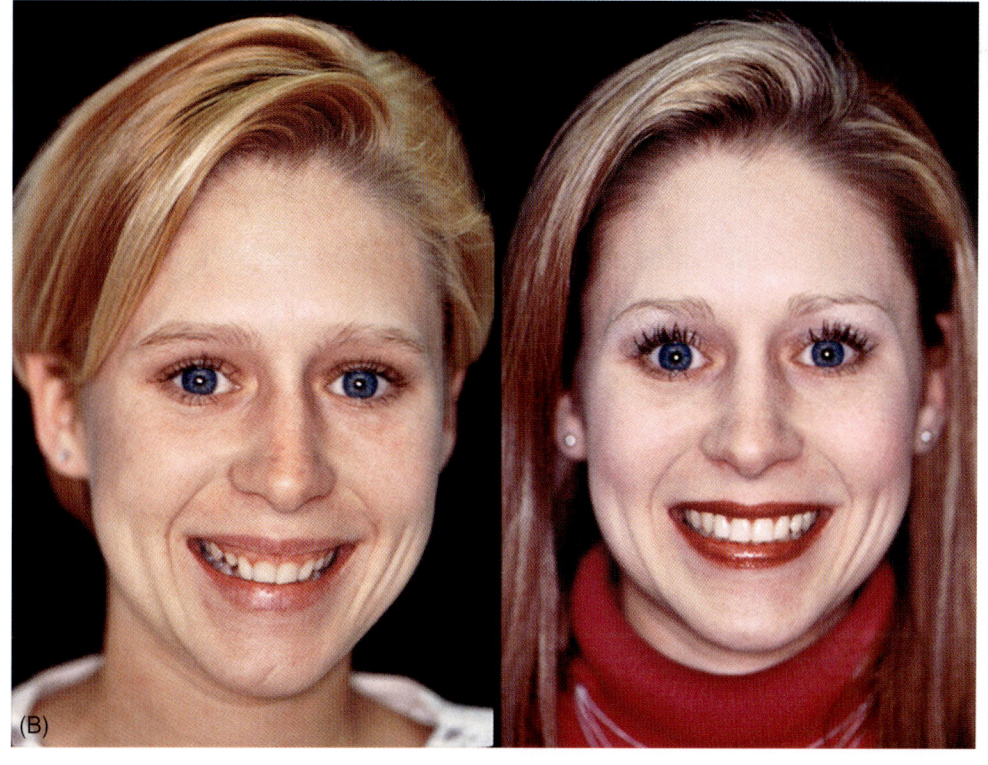

Figure 1.11   (A–C) This young woman refrained from smiling because she was embarrassed by her high lip line that revealed too much of her gums. She said it affected her personality and relationships. She received implants, orthodontics, bleaching, cosmetic contouring, and gum surgery to lengthen her teeth and give her a more attractive medium lip line and overall smile.

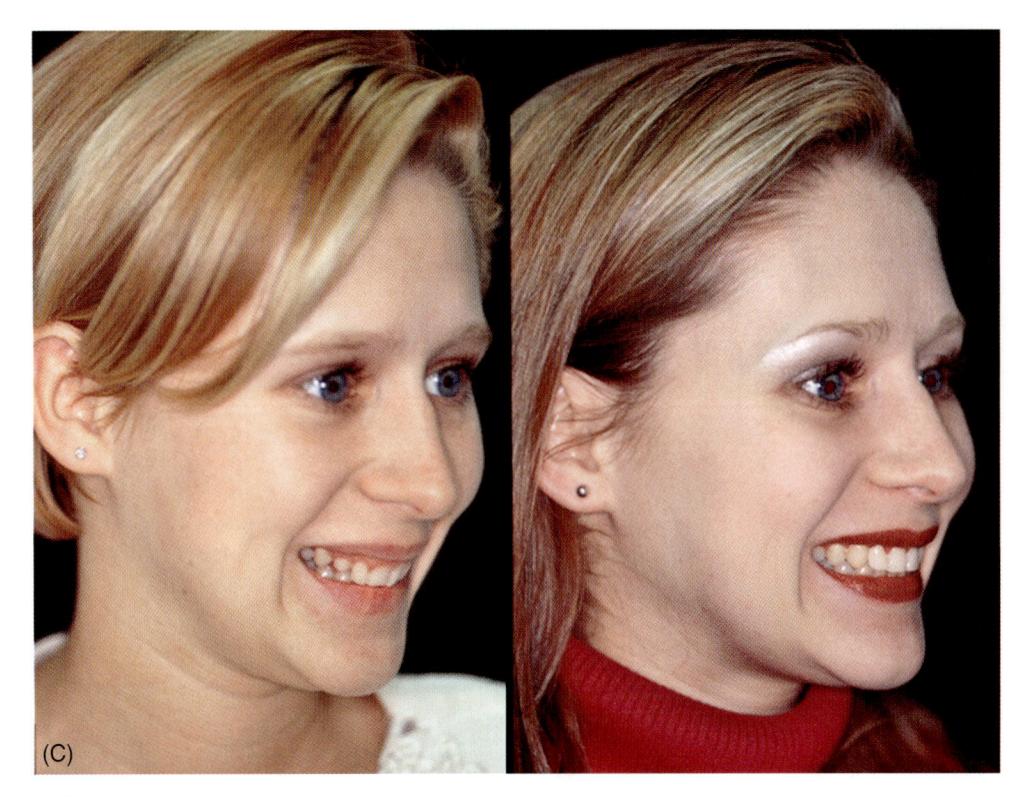

Figure 1.11 (Continued)

to categorize the variety of products and services. Nevertheless, consumer purchases in pursuits to enhance or retain physical attractiveness total large annual sales. For example:

- Personal care products contributed US$236.9 billion in 2013 to the US economy, spanned 3.6 million US jobs held by individuals of diverse backgrounds, and in 2014 accounted for a $5.8 billion export trade surplus (http://www.personalcarecouncil.org/sites/default/files/2016Year InReviewFinal.pdf).
- Hair care services generate nearly $20 billion in annual sales in the United States alone, and $160 billion worldwide (http://www.firstresearch.com/industry-research/Hair-Care-Services.html).
- Retailers focused entirely on cosmetic and beauty products generate $10 billion annual sales and number about 13,000 stores (Figure 1.12A–C).

Cosmetic surgery represents a prominent option for people to enhance or retain their physical attractiveness. It accordingly represents a sizeable portion of consumer purchases that are reasonable to align with the beauty industry moniker. In these regards, the two leading professional organizations for surgeons certified by the American Board of Plastic Surgery who specialize in cosmetic plastic surgery—the American Society of Plastic Surgeons (ASPS) and the American Society for Aesthetic Plastic Surgery (ASAPS)—each with thousands of members, some of whom overlap with membership in both societies, systematically collect statistics from their members about types and numbers of procedures performed annually.

Recent annual statistics from both ASAPS and ASPS, which today have their largest ever memberships, document strong motivation by people to enhance or retain one's own physical attractiveness regardless of personal costs, efforts required, and economic conditions. Late 2010, ASAPS reported "Despite Recession, Overall Plastic Surgery Demand Drops Only 2 Percent From Last Year" based on 2009 statistics, their most recent annual data available from their members at that date. Early 2011, ASPA reported "Plastic Surgery Rebounds Along with Recovering Economy; 13.1 Million Cosmetic Procedures Performed in 2010, up 5%," based on 2010 statistics from their members. Over a longer time span, ASAPS data reveal that cosmetic procedures have increased 147% in number since beginning in 1997 to collect these statistics.

Bottom-line statistics, in one of the worst general economic times in American history, include ASAPS reporting nearly

> Consumers spent nearly $10.5 billion in 2009 for cosmetic surgery procedures (ASAPS data). Breast augmentation was the most frequent surgical procedure, and facial fillers (such as Botox) were the most frequent nonsurgical procedure. Demographically, although people seeking cosmetic procedures remained in the same approximate proportions as reported in earlier years, they increasingly cross differences in race and ethnicity (whose collective minorities represented 22% of all cosmetic procedures with Hispanic/Latino at 9%, African American at 6%, Asians at 4%, and 3% for other non-white people), as well as differences in gender and age.

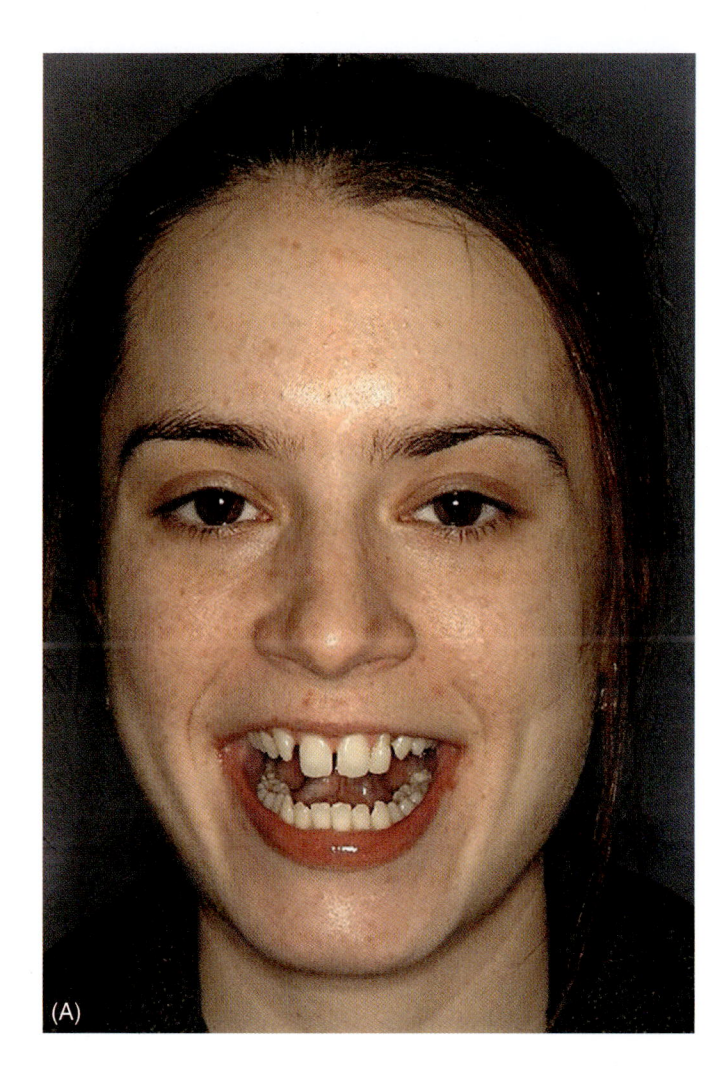

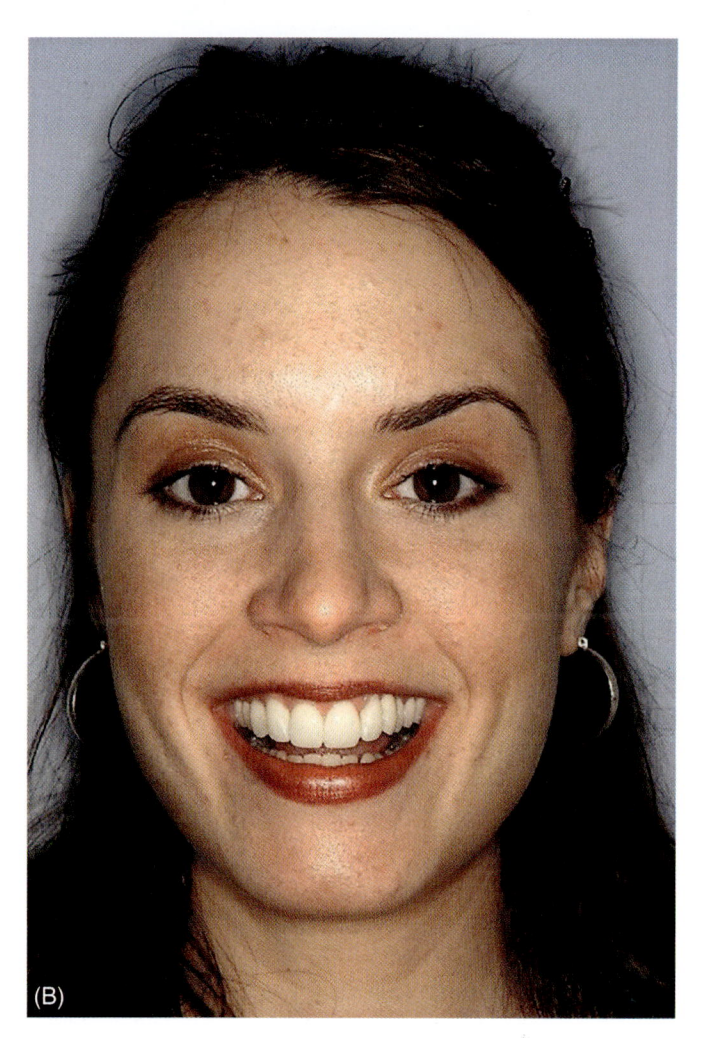

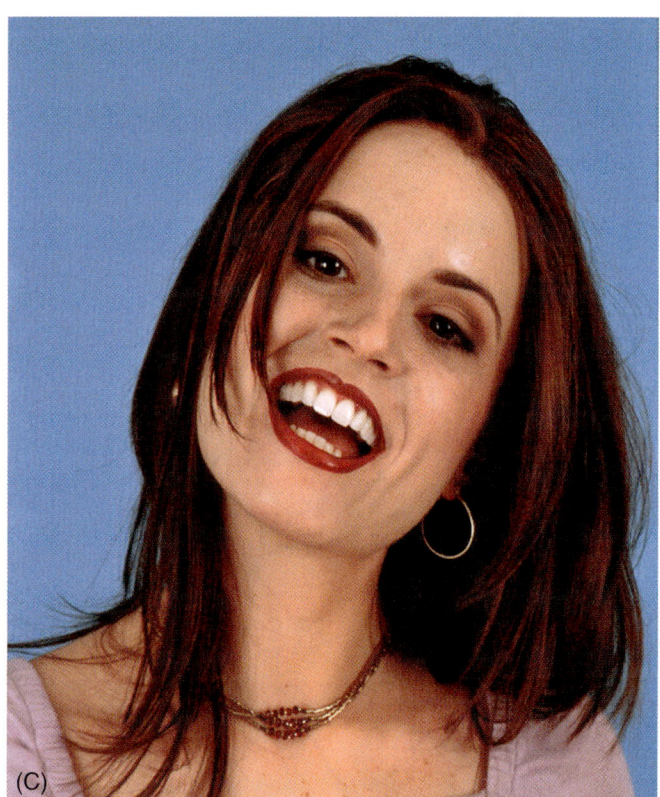

Figure 1.12 **(A–C)** Before and after full face smile photos: this 22-year-old waitress was too embarrassed to smile, which limited her full potential both socially and in reaching her career goals. Porcelain veneers and a resin-bonded fixed bridge were made without reducing the tooth structure. The result of her new smile and full hair and face make-over was a life-changing physical and mental transformation for this young woman.

10 million cosmetic procedures (surgical and nonsurgical) during 2009. That finding is despite economic conditions that delayed and decreased expenditures for most all products and services, with expectations for corresponding growth of purchases to resume as the economic improves. Accordingly, a year later in an improving but still bad overall economy, ASPA reported more than 13 million cosmetic procedures performed during 2010.

Today, people motivated to pursue various physical attractiveness options locate the necessary financial resources in creative ways. No longer do they rely solely on personal savings in pursuit of looking better. Suitable efforts and expenditures directed toward a person's physical attractiveness certainly can be correct, and a wise return on investment given our world in which looking better in nearly all circumstances has benefits throughout life.

Patient response to abnormality

The smile is the baby's most regularly evoked response and eventually signifies pleasure. Thus, any aberration it reveals can naturally be a point of anxiety. Frequently the response to a deformity or aberration can be out of proportion to its severity. Abnormality implies difference, a characteristic undesirable to most people. To diminish differences, they may resort to overt or subtle means of hiding their mouths (Figure 1.7A and B). However, as Rottersman notes, "The response may not be out of all proportion to the stimulus. This is a signal for the doctor to exercise caution, and to attempt to discern what truly underlies the patient's response" (W. Rottersman, personal communication). Understanding the patient's motives requires acute perception on the dentist's part, informed by a thorough examination and history that reveal the patient's actual dental problems.[20] The patient's own assessment of his problems and his reaction to them are of equal importance. The dentist should be alert for a displacement syndrome, in which an anxiety aroused by real and major emotional problems may be transferred to a minor oral deformity. When a patient with a long-standing complaint finally presents for treatment, the dentist must determine what prevented him or her from coming for treatment sooner. A patient who criticizes a former dentist is apt to be hostile, and the dentist should not present a treatment plan before determining what the patient believes treatment can accomplish.

Psychology and technology

For all patient treatments intended to change facial appearances, it is important to consider psychological dimensions as well as the treatment procedure and technology. Esthetic dentistry demands attention to the individual patient's desires, goals, and motivations, as well as physical conditions. Patients interested in esthetic dentistry present any number of scenarios. Every patient is an individual who likely requires individual attention to an extent. As well as actual dental conditions, their reasons for seeking treatment might reflect varying wants, feelings and anxieties, personalities and self-images, and unrelated or unrealistic perspectives, motivations, goals, and expectations. Complicating the reasons are interconnected influences from spouses, coworkers, aging, cultural changes, changes in socioeconomic level, and so forth. Stated succinctly by one dentist, "The reasons why patients seek esthetic treatment are as varied and intricate as the reasons they avoid. …such as orthodontic, cosmetic restorative, cosmetic periodontal, plastic or orthographic surgery, or any combination of these."

> The individual's own feelings about dental esthetics are in some ways the most important. They determine his or her self-image in conjunction with that individual's perception of what and who are important in their lives. As much as possible, the dentist who devotes time to esthetic dentistry then functions as a vehicle of sorts to help patients realize their wants in the realm of feasibilities. Accordingly, practitioners of esthetic dentistry must understand what patients mean with their particular words and take appropriate actions in the context of ethics, good judgment, and technological capabilities.

A patient's own assessment of, reaction to, and perspective of dental issues are important. At the same time, the dentist needs to be alert to potential displacement syndrome whereby the patient transfers attention from unrelated or unrealistic emotions and problems to a minor or uncorrectable dental malady. Relative to other areas, esthetic dentistry may encounter more of these situations with variations. For example, before presenting a treatment plan for patients with a long-standing complaint about a dental issue, it should be determined why the person did not come sooner for treatment. Similarly, before presenting a treatment plan for a patient who might be highly critical of a former dentist or dental treatment, it should be determined what the patient believes treatment now can accomplish. See also Chapter 2 in this volume.

Patient types and dentist alerts

The reasons why patients seek esthetic treatment are as varied and intricate as the reasons they avoid it. How adults feel about and care for their mouth often reflects past, current, and future oral developmental experiences. Adults in their mid-20s may not have developed a sense of the meaning of time in the life cycle. Lack of oral health care may reflect a denial of mortality and normal body degeneration. Between the ages of 35 and 40 adults become reconciled to the fact they are aging and a renewed interest in self-preservation emerges. This interest is often directed toward various types of self-improvement such as orthodontic, cosmetic restorative, cosmetic periodontal, plastic or orthognathic surgery, or any combination of these. Patients sometimes cloak their actual dental needs with peripheral and unrealistic motivations, perceptions, and goals. At least some insight to understanding tangential orientations of these different types of patients might be necessary to complement a thorough examination and history.

Our teeth and mouths are critical to psychological development throughout life. Often, the way we treat our mouths and teeth indicates how we feel about ourselves. If we like ourselves, we work toward good oral health. Once we have reached this goal, our sense of well-being is increased (Figure 1.13A–C).

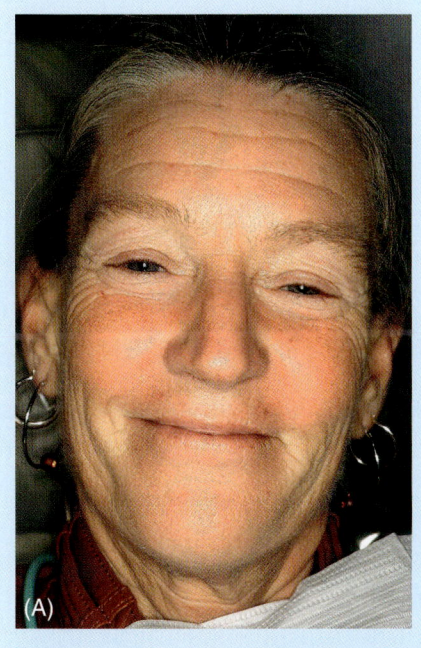

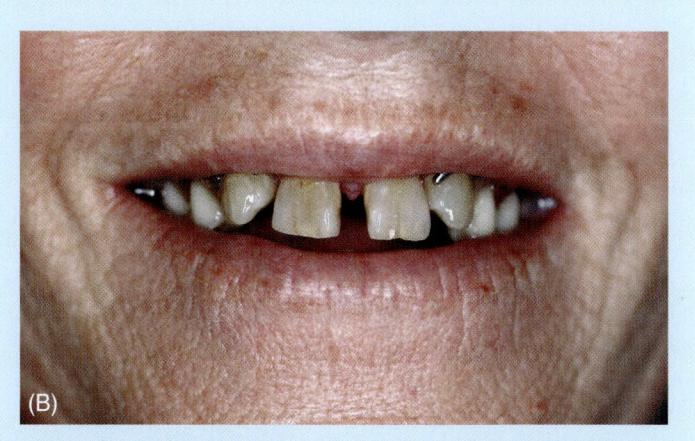

Figure 1.13 (A) This patient chose not to smile which affected her self-image and personality. (B) Since our teeth and mouths are critical factors in psychological development in life, it is not difficult to see why this patient chose not to smile.

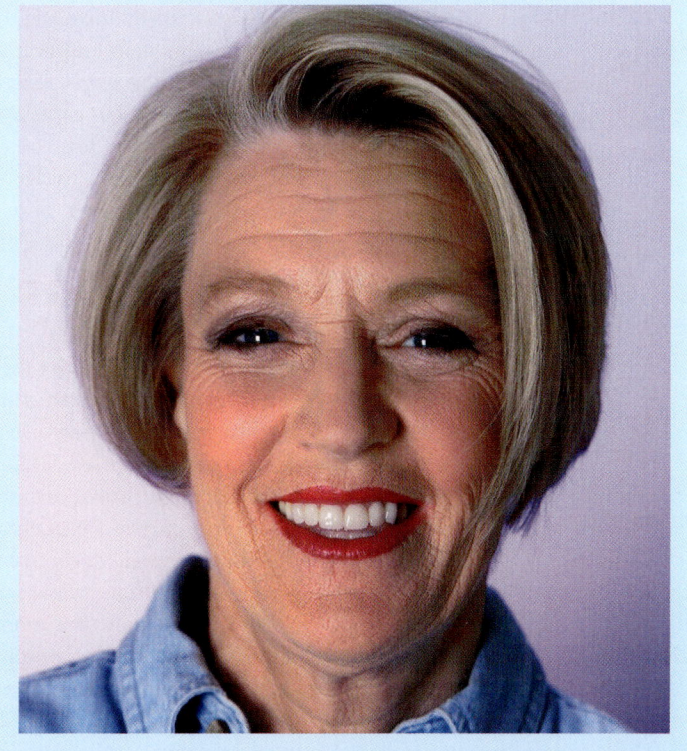

Figure 1.13 (C) The smile was restored with an upper-implant-supported denture and a lower fixed and removable partial denture. Following a complimentary make-over, it is easy to see why this lady has a completely different outlook on life with her new self-image.

Burns, in his discussion of motivations for orthodontic treatment, cites the results of a study by Jarabak who determined five stimuli that may move a patient toward orthodontia. The motives, also applicable to esthetic dentistry, are as follows: (1) social acceptance, (2) fear, (3) intellectual acceptance, (4) personal pride, and (5) biological benefits. (It should be noted that these stimuli pertain only to patients who cooperate in treatment.)[6,19]

A spirit of cooperation and understanding between you and your patient is paramount to successful esthetic treatment. This relationship is a kind of symbiosis in which each contributes to the attitude of the other. The necessity for close observation and response on your part, particularly to nonverbal clues offered by the patient, cannot be overemphasized. The confidence generated by a careful and observant dentist will be perceived by the patient; so, unfortunately, will a lack of confidence. A competent, confident, professional dentist can reinforce the positive side of the ambivalence that patients feel toward persons who can help them but who they fear may hurt them.

Much psychological theory in dental esthetics must be formulated through analogy because of the comparatively recent recognition of the importance of dental esthetics and the consequent lack of a comprehensive database. The most obvious parallel field is plastic surgery. In a pioneering paper published in 1939, Baker and Smith[21] posited a system that categorized 312 patients into three groups based on personality traits as they related to a desire for corrective surgery, the motives for requesting it, and the prognosis for successful treatment.

- Group I—Ideal individuals for successful treatment with well-adjusted personalities, moderate success in life, aware that all life problems cannot be solved by better-looking teeth, and realistically want treatment to improve esthetics and/or for greater comfort. In your own practice, patients who fall into the first group are moderately successful people who want repair of their disfigurements for cosmetic reasons or comfort, not as an answer to all their problems. They do not expect too much from the improvement and they have a realistic visual concept of the outcome. They are ideal subjects for successful treatment.
- Group II—Irksome individuals of two types. The very irksome type are individuals who remain unhappy with results despite the excellent technical outcome achieved through prior treatment, indicating the same will happen with future treatments. Underlying that unhappiness, they continue past dysfunctional thinking about their prior appearance defects causing unrelated life problems outside the oral cavity or they find actual life with better-looking teeth to be not as great as they had earlier unrealistically fantasized. A substantially less irksome type in this Group II category are passive apologetic individuals who are grateful for any and all treatment, even though past results proved technically unsatisfactory as likely will be results of future treatments.
- Group III—Individuals with psychotic personalities for whom treatment outcomes will never be satisfactory in their view, regardless of actual technical results. Their visibly unattractive dental esthetics that existed before treatment served then as a focal point of their life problems and will probably continue always. With these people, any esthetic correction serves only to disrupt the rationalization process. Soon, some other defect is seized upon as the focus for their continuing psychotic delusions. These individuals warrant other professional treatment such as psychological or psychiatric counseling because dental treatment alone likely only disrupts their delusional rationalizations with no significant benefit in the longer term.

As expressed above, patients focused on cosmetic dentistry can be greatly appreciative and/or greatly demanding. Nevertheless, they must all be satisfied with their results. This satisfaction usually means their concept of a natural looking outcome that meets their pretreatment expectations and receives "a thumbs up" approval in the eyes of the patient and the most significant other(s) in the patient's life. Advance measures, pretreatment, by the dentist to improve the likelihood of posttreatment satisfaction include the following:

- Listen well to the wants and perspectives of the patient before embarking on treatment. This "listening" extends to observing well any possible pertinent nonverbal clues exhibited by the patient.
- Discuss well any concerns, questions, expectations, and as much or little detail as appropriate for the individual patient.
- Present treatment options along with their procedures, timelines, advantages, and disadvantages or limitations.
- Be "realistically idealistic," expressing the ideal but realistic scenario while being neither unrealistically optimistic that then builds too high of expectations that cannot be met and will generate dissatisfaction. Nor should you be unreasonably pessimistic. The latter balances lower expectations that results will nearly always meet and exceed and for that reason will nearly always generate substantial satisfaction with positive word-of-mouth evaluative comments to family and friends.
- Trial smile procedures are discussed in detail in Chapter 3.

The dentist–patient relationship should be long term, which by definition concerns posttreatment. Esthetic dentistry offers this opportunity more so than other dental treatments. Patients typically deliberate over this decision longer and with more thought invested than for other dental treatments. This greater investment in the decision process combined with improvement of appearance/physical attractiveness, as well as dental health, sets the stage for a rather special bonding consequence analogous to that between a cosmetic surgeon and a patient. To increase this likelihood, just as there are pretreatment alerts and actions for dentists when delivering esthetic treatments, there are posttreatment alerts and actions. For patients satisfied with their results, reinforcing words and careful direction for maintenance along with additional optional treatments might be well appropriate. This situation certainly poses opportunity for good word-of-mouth comments by the patient to family, friends, and potentially coworkers. Alternatively, the patient might experience confusion posttreatment. Commonly known as buyer's remorse, it is a mental uncertainty or uneasiness about whether the decision, effort, and cost were worth the change or lack of change in appearance. Dentists who perceive such will serve everyone well by explaining fully the situation and maybe at the same time meeting with the most significant other(s) in the patient's life.

Psychology and treatment planning

Esthetic dental treatment can enhance a patient's own intensely personal image of how he or she looks and how he or she would like to look. As Frush observes, "A smile can be attractive, a prime asset to a person's appearance, and it can be a powerful factor in the ego and desirable life experiences of a human being. It cannot be treated with indifference because of its deep emotional significance." Frush notes that in any esthetic treatment there is the need for consideration of a patient's satisfaction with the natural appearance and function of the result. Artificial appearance or failure to satisfy the patient's expectations may damage his or her ego. Frush terms such damage a negative emotional syndrome (J.P. Frush, personal communication).

Frush continues, "The severe emotional trauma resulting from the loss of teeth is well recognized, and dentists, being the closest to this emotional disturbance, normally have a deep desire to help the patient through the experience as best they can. It is of prime importance to understand that a productive and satisfying social experience after treatment depends upon the acceptance of the changed body structure and the eventual establishment of a new body image by the patient as it is. The acceptance of treatment by the patient is made considerably easier when the prosthesis accomplishes two basic esthetic needs: the portrayal of a physiologic norm, and an actual improvement in the attractiveness of the smile and thus all related facial expressions." Facilitating such acceptance requires several things from the dentist: (1) constructive optimism, never exceeding the bounds of fact and candor; (2) specific demonstration of the means and methods to be employed in treatment; and (3) an open discussion of all patient anxieties and the proposed treatment options.

> Healthy teeth are taken for granted; when they are painful, they become a point of exclusive attention. However, such overt stimulus is not necessary for a patient to become obsessively concerned about the appearance or health of the teeth. As an integral component of the body image, teeth can be the focus of feelings ranging from embarrassment to acute anxiety. As noted earlier, teeth may not be the actual cause of the disturbance, but instead the object of displaced anxieties.

All of these anxieties related to dental deformities are influenced by the patient's own view of the dental deformity and the reaction of other people to that deformity. Root notes that, "The first and foremost psychological effect of dentofacial deformity manifests itself in a sense of inferiority. This sense of inferiority is a complex, painful, emotional state characterized by feelings of incompetence, inadequacy, and depression in varying degrees."[22] These feelings of inferiority are a significant part of a patient's self-image, desire for treatment, and expectations of what the treatment can accomplish. Every patient is an individual and requires individual treatment. Generalities almost never apply; they are more useful as guidelines and suggestions than as prescribed courses or methods of treatment.

Predicting patient response

When certain patients appear for treatment, it is wise to proceed with extreme caution, and it is suggested that function alone be used as the criterion for operative intervention. Regardless of the technical success of the procedure, it would only serve to exacerbate, rather than remove, expression of their incipient psychosis. Many times, the restorations look good to you, but the patient still expresses dissatisfaction. This dissatisfaction may be a manifestation of some underlying fear or insecurity rather than a desire for artistic perfection in the restoration. Desire for artistic perfection may be indicative of a patient's underlying problems and may make it impossible for you to treat that person successfully. If we can know enough about the patient's personality to determine the various factors influencing his or her desire for esthetic correction, we would then be better equipped to predict the degree of psychological acceptance of that correction.

> How can these patients be recognized by the busy dentist? Although experience may be the best teacher, the cardinal requirement is to show an interest in the patient's complete makeup. Look at the patient as an integrated human being, not just as another oral cavity. Baker and Smith offer the following questions to help evaluate patients:[21]
>
> 1. What was the patient's personality prior to the disfigurement?
> 2. What was the patient's emotional status when first conscious of his or her disfigurement?
> 3. What part has the disfigurement played in forming the present personality? In other words, is there some limitation in personality development because, for instance, the patient does not smile? What habit patterns have developed?
> 4. What will probably be the emotional effect of the esthetic correction of the defect?

Obviously it will take some time to arrive at the answers. The conclusion should reveal to which group this patient belongs, and in this way you can better predict the patient's acceptance of the esthetic results. Consideration of the emotional status of any patient who seeks esthetic treatment is important. It can help preclude unpleasant reactions toward either the treatment or you in those cases where treatment, though functionally and artistically successful, is unsatisfactory to the patient. Therefore, the patient's entire personal, familial, and social environment must be considered in relation to esthetics.

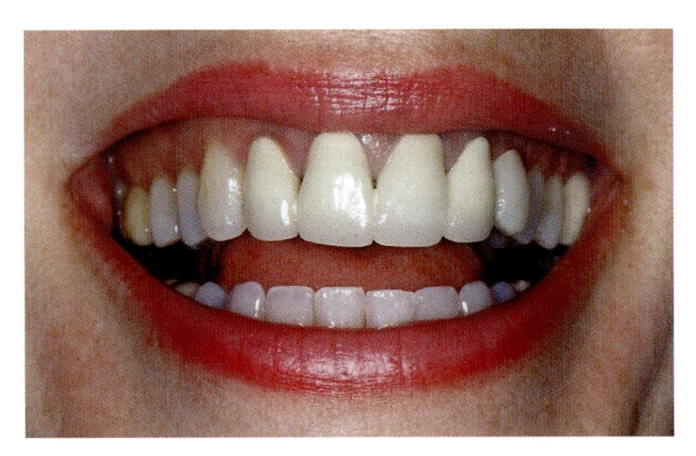

Figure 1.14 **(A)** This patient reached a point in her life where she realized her smile was looking much older than she felt.

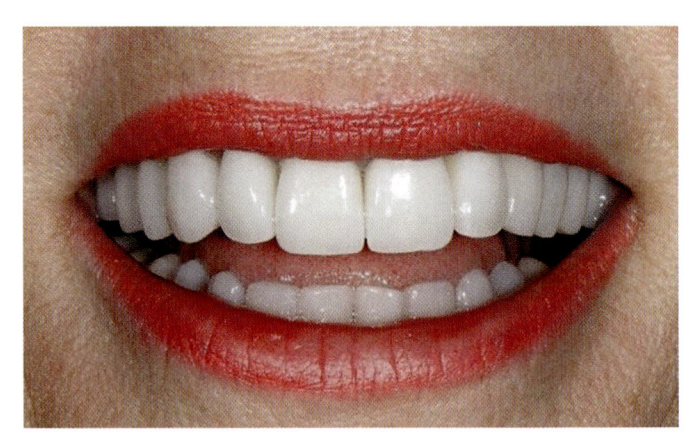

Figure 1.14 **(B)** A new smile make-over helped restore her youthful smile and self-esteem.

"Crossroads"

Well-adjusted individuals go through life, treating esthetic dental problems as tooth-by-tooth decisions. However, many individuals reach a point in their lives where they look in the mirror and realize their smile is looking much older than they feel. Such was the case with the patient in Figure 1.14A and B. Many years ago, the American Dental Association even made a movie about these individuals who reach a "crossroads" in their lives.

And, in those regards, the patient's entire personal, familial, and social environment must be considered in relation to esthetics.

References

1. Aboucaya WA. *The Dento-Labial Smile and the Beauty of the Face* [thesis]. No. 50. Academy of Paris, University of Paris VI; 1973.
2. Anderson JN. The value of teeth. *Br Dent J* 1965;119:98.
3. Guerini V. *A History of Dentistry from the Most Ancient Times Until the End of the Eighteenth Century.* New York: Milford House; 1969.
4. Ai S, Ishikawa T. "Ohaguro" traditional tooth staining custom in Japan. *Int Dent J* 1965;15:426.
5. Goleman D, Goleman TB. Beauty's hidden equation. *Am Health* [now the Time-Warner publication *Health*]. March 1987.
6. Jarabak JR. *Management of an Orthodontic Practice.* St. Louis, MO: CV Mosby; 1956.
7. Goldstein RE. Esthetic dentisty—a health service. *J Dent Res* 1993;3:641–642.
8. Cash TF, Winstead BA, Janda LH. The great American shape up. *Psychol Today* 1986:30–37.
9. Sheets CG. Modern dentistry and the esthetically aware patient. *J Am Dent Assoc* 1987;115:103E–105E.
10. Patzer GL. *Looks: Why They Matter More Than You Ever Imagined.* New York: AMACOM Books; 2008.
11. Wilson PR. Perceptual distortion of height as a function of ascribed academic status. *J Soc Psychol* 1968;74:97–102.
12. Allport GW. Pattern and Growth in Personality. *New York: Holt and Rinehart*; 1961:479.
13. Meerloo JAM. *Communication and Conversation.* New York: International Universities Press; 1958.
14. Langlois JH. Attractive faces get attention of infants. *Atlanta Journal* 1987;May 6:6, 14.
15. Langlois JH. From the eye of the beholder to behavioral reality: the development of social behaviors and social relations as a function of physical attractiveness. In: Herman CP, Zanna MP, Higgins ET, eds. *Physical Appearance, Stigma, and Social Behavior: The Ontario Symposium.* Hillsdale, NJ: Erlbaum; 1986:23–51.
16. Langlois JH, Roggman LA. Attractive faces are only average. *Am Psychol Soc* 1990;1:115–121.
17. Langlois JH, Roggman LS, Casey RJ, et al. Infant preferences for attractive faces: rudiments of a stereotype? *Dev Psychol* 1987;23:363–369.
18. Langlois JH, Roggman LA, Rieser-Danner LA. Infant's differential social responses to attractive and unattractive faces. *Dev Psychol* 1990;26(1):153–159.
19. Burns MH. Use of a personality rating scale in identifying cooperative and non-cooperative orthodontic patients. *Am J Orthod* 1970;57:418.
20. Levinson N. Psychological facets of esthetic dentistry: a developmental perspective. *J Prosthet Dent* 1990;64:486–491.
21. Baker WY, Smith LH. Facial disfigurement and personality. *JAMA* 1939;112:301.
22. Root WR. Face value. *Am J Orthod* 1949;35:697.

Additional resources

American Society of Plastic Surgeons. *Plastic Surgery Rebounds Along with Recovering Economy; 13.1 Million Cosmetic Procedures Performed in 2010, up 5%.* https://www.plasticsurgery.org/news/press-releases/plastic-surgery-rebounds-along-with-recovering-economy (accessed February 13, 2011).

Antonoff SJ. Esthetics for the indigent. *Quintessence Int* 1979;3:33–39.

Baudouin JY, Tiberghien G. Symmetry, averageness and feature size in the facial attractiveness of women. *Act Psychol [Amst]* 2004;117:313–332.

Baumeister RF, Bushman BJ. *Social Psychology & Human Nature.* Belmont: Thomson Wadsworth; 2008.

Berscheid E. America's obsession with beautiful people. *US News & World Report Inc*;1982;Jan 11:60–61.

Brisman AS. Esthetics: a comparison of dentists' and patients' concepts. *J Am Dent Assoc* 1980;3:345–352.

Cahill A. Feminist pleasure and feminine beautification. *Hypathia* 2003;18:42–64.

Christensen GJ. *A Consumer Guide to Dentistry*. St. Louis, MO: CV Mosby; 1995.

Cinotti WR, Grieder A, Springob HK. Psychological aspects of orthodontics. In: *Applied Psychology in Dentistry*. St. Louis, MO: CV Mosby; 1972.

Cropper E. *Concepts of Beauty in Renaissance Art*. Aldershot: Ashgate; 1998.

Cunningham MR. Measuring the physical in physical attractiveness: quasiexperiments on the sociobiology of female facial beauty. *J Pers Soc Psychol* 1986;50:925–935.

Devigus A. The perfect smile. *Int J Esthet Dent* 2014;9:465.

Dunn WJ, Murchison DF, Broome JC. Esthetics: patients' perceptions of dental attractiveness. *J Prosthodont* 1996;5:166–171.

Espeland LE, Stenvik A. Perception of personal dental appearance in young adults: relationship between occlusion, awareness and satisfaction. *Am J Orthod Dentofacial Orthop* 1991;100:234–241.

Ettinger RL. An evaluation of the attitudes of a group of elderly edentulous patients to dentists, dentures, and dentistry. *Dent Pract* 1971;22:85.

Fastlicht S. Tooth mutilations in pre-Columbian Mexico. *J Am Dent Assoc* 1948;36:315.

Fastlichts S. Dental inlays and fillings among the ancient Mayas. *J Hist Med Allied Sci* 1962;17:393.

Fastlichts S. La odontologia en el Mexico prehispanico [Dentistry in pre-Hispanic Mexico]. *J Clin Orthod* 1970;14:588.

First Research. Personal Care Products Manufacturing Industry Profile, 11/1/2010 Quarterly Update. http://www.firstresearch.com/Industry-Research/Personal-Care-Products-Manufacturing.html (accessed February 13, 2011).

Fitz-Patrick CP. Is dental appearance important in business? *Oral Hygiene* 1963;53:52.

Försterling F, Preikschas S, Agthe M. Ability, luck, and looks: an evolutionary look at achievement ascriptions and the sexual attribution bias. *J Pers Soc Psychol* 2007;92(5):775–788.

Gibson R. Smile's power means more than just lip service. *Albuquerque J*. 1. sect B 1977;June 15.

Gibson RM. *The Miracle of Smile Power*. Honolulu: Smile Power Institute; 1977.

Giddon DB. The mouth and the quality of life. *NY J Dent* 1978;48(1):3–10.

Gilbert J. Ethics and esthetics. *J Am Diet Assoc* 1988;117:490.

Goldstein RE. *Change Your Smile*, 4th edn. Chicago, IL: Quintessence; 2009.

Goldstein RE. Communicating esthetics. *NY State Dent J* 1985;51:477–479.

Goldstein RE. Current concepts in esthetic treatment. In: *Proceedings of the Second International Prosthodontic Congress*. St. Louis, MO: Mosby; 1979:310–312.

Goldstein RE. Study of need for esthetics in dentistry. *J Prosthet Dent* 1969;21:589.

Goldstein RE. The difficult patient stress syndrome: part 1. *J Esthet Dent* 1993;5:86–87.

Goldstein RE, Garber DA, Goldstein CE, et al. The changing esthetic dental practice. *J Am Dent Assoc* 1994;125:1447–1457.

Goldstein RE, Lancaster JS. Survey of patient attitudes toward current esthetic procedures. *J Prosthet Dent* 1984;52:775–780.

Goodman RM, Gorlin RJ. *The Face in Genetic Disorders*. St. Louis, MO: CV Mosby; 1970.

Hatfield E, Sprecher S. *Mirror, Mirror*. Albany, NY: State University of NY Press; 1986.

Henderson D, Steffel VL. *McCracken's Removable Partial Prosthodontics*. St. Louis, MO: CV Mosby; 1973.

Hoffmann-Axthelm W. *History of Dentistry*. Chicago, IL: Quintessence; 1981.

Kanner L. *Folklore of the Teeth*. New York: Macmillan; 1928.

Kerns LL, Silveira AM, Derns DG, Regennitter FJ. Esthetic preference of the frontal and profile views of the same smile. *J Esthet Dent* 1997;9:76–85.

Kranz PH. *Dentistry Shows its Biblical Roots*. Atlanta, GA: Alpha Omegan 30; 1985.

Land M. Management of emotional illness in dental practice. *J Am Dent Assoc* 1966;73:63.

Lavine BH. Elizabethan toothache: a case history. *J Am Dent Assoc* 1967;74:1286.

Lee JH. *Dental Aesthetics*. Bristol, CT: John Wright and Son; 1962.

Leinbach MD, Fagot BI. Pretty babies. *Allure* 1992 November;52.

Lenchner NH, Lenchner M. Biologic contours of teeth: therapeutic contours of restorations, Part 1. *Prac Perio Aesth* 1989;1(4):18–23.

Levin RP. Esthetic dentistry in the next decade. *Dent Econ* 1990;80:53–59.

Levinson N. Anorexia and bulimia: eating function gone awry. *J Calif Dent Assoc* 1985;13:18–22.

Levinson N. Oral manifestations of eating disorders: indications for a collaborative treatment approach. In: *Textbook of Eating Disorders*. New York: Plenum Press; 1987:405–411.

Linn L, Goldman IB. Psychiatric observations concerning rhinoplasty. *J Psychosom Med* 1949;11:307.

Lombardi RE. Factors mediating against excellence in dental esthetics. *J Prosthet Dent* 1977;38:243–248.

Lucker GW. Esthetics and a quantitative analysis of facial appearance. In: Lucker GW, Ribbens KA, McNamara JA, eds. *Psychological Aspects of Facial Form*. Ann Arbor, MI: The Center for Growth and Development, University of Michigan; 1981.

Mack MR. Perspective of facial esthetics in dental treatment planning. *J Prosthet Dent* 1996;75:169–176.

Mafi P, Ghazisaeidi MR, Mafi A. Ideal soft tissue facial profile in Iranian females. *J Craniofac Surg* 2005 May;16:508–511.

Maret SM. Attractiveness ratings of photographs of Blacks by Cruzans and Americans. *J Psychol* 1983;115:113–116.

Martins CC, Feitosa NB, Vale MP. Parents' perceptions of oral health conditions depicted in photographs of anterior permanent teeth. *Eur J Paediatr Dent* 2010;11:203–209.

Miller MB. Options: the key to satisfied patients [editorial]. *Pract Periodontics Aesthet Dent* 1996;8:402.

Moskowitz M, Nayyar A. Determinants of dental esthetics: a rationale for smile analysis and treatment. *Compend Contin Educ Dent* 1995;16:1164–1166.

Nash DA. Professional ethics and esthetic dentistry. *J Am Dent Assoc* 1988;117(4):7E–9E.

O'Regan JK, Deweym ME, Slade PD, Lovius BBJ. Self esteem and aesthetics. *Br J Orthod* 1991;18:111–118.

Patzer GL. *The Physical Attractiveness Phenomena*. New York: Plenum Publishing; 1985.

Patzer GL. Measurement of physical attractiveness: truth-of-consensus. *J Esthet Dent* 1994;6:185–188.

Patzer GL. Reality of physical attractiveness. *J Esthet Dent* 1994;6:35–38.

Patzer GL. Self-esteem and physical attractiveness. *J Esthet Dent* 1995;7:274–277.

Patzer GL. Understanding the casual relationship between physical attractiveness and self-esteem. *J Esthet Dent* 1996;8:144–147.

Patzer GL. *The Power and Paradox of Physical Attractiveness*. Boca Raton, FL: Brown Walker Press; 2006.

Patzer GL. *Why Physically Attractive People Are More Successful: The Scientific Explanation, Social Consequences and Ethical Problems*. Lewiston, NY: Edwin Mellen Press; 2007.

Peck S, Peck L, Kataja M. The gingiva smile. *Angle Orthod* 1992;62:90–100.

Pitel ML, Raley-Susman KM, Rubinov A. Preferences of Lay Persons and Dental Professionals Regarding the Recurring Estheitc Dental Proportion. *J Esthet Rest Dent* 2016 2:102-109.

Prinz H. *Dental Chronology*. Philadelphia, PA: Lea & Febiger; 1945.

Qualtrough AJE, Burke FJT. A look at dental esthetics. *Quintessence Int* 1994;25:7–14.

Rhodes G. The evolutionary psychology of facial beauty. *Ann Rev Psychol* 2006;57:199–226.

Rhodes G, Zebrowitz L (eds). *Facial Attractiveness: Evolutionary, Cognitive and Social Perspectives*. Westport, CT: Ablex; 2002.

Rigsbee OH, Sperry TP, BeGole EA. The influence of facial animation on smile characteristics. *Int J Adult Orthodon Orthognath Surg* 1988;3:233–239.

Ring ME. *Dentistry: An Illustrated History*. St. Louis, MO: Mosby; 1985.

Ring ME. Dentisty in ancient Egypt. *Compend Contin Educ Dent* 1986;VIII:386.

Romero J. *Multilaciones Dentarias Prehispanicas De Mexico y Americaen General [Pre-Hispanic dental multilingualism of Mexico and American general]*. Mexico: Instituto Nacional de Antropologia de Historia; 1958.

Rosenthal LE, Pleasure MA, Lefer L. Patient reaction to denture esthetics. *J Dent Med* 1964;19(3):103–110.

Slavkin HC. What's in a tooth? *J Am Dent Assoc* 1997;128:366–369.

Stella L. The archaeology of teeth. *UNIDI Press* 1979;5(19):20–23.

Strauss R, Slome B, Block M, et al. Self-perceived social and functional effects of teeth: dental impact profile. *J Dent Res* 1989;68:384.

Talarico G. Morgante E. The human dimension: esthetic in society and in medicine. *Eur J Esthet Dent* 2014; 8;136–154.

Thornhill R, Grammer K. The body and face of woman: one ornament that signals quality? *Evol Hum Behav* 1999;20:105–120.

Townsend JM, Levy GD. Effect of potential partners' physical attractiveness and socioeconomic status on sexuality and partner selection. *Arch Sex Behav* 1990;19:140–164.

Vallittu PK, Ballittu AS, Lassila VP. Dental aesthetics—a survey of attitudes in different groups of patients. *J Dent* 1996;24:335–338.

Voss R. Problem of treatment according to the patient's wishes. *ZWR* 1971;80:557.

Wagner IV, Carlsson GE, Ekstrand K, et al. A comparative study of assessment of dental appearances by dentists, dental technicians, and laymen using computer aided image manipulation. *J Esthet Dent* 1996;8:199–205.

Woodforde J. *The Strange Story of False Teeth*. London: Routledge and Kegan Paul; 1968.

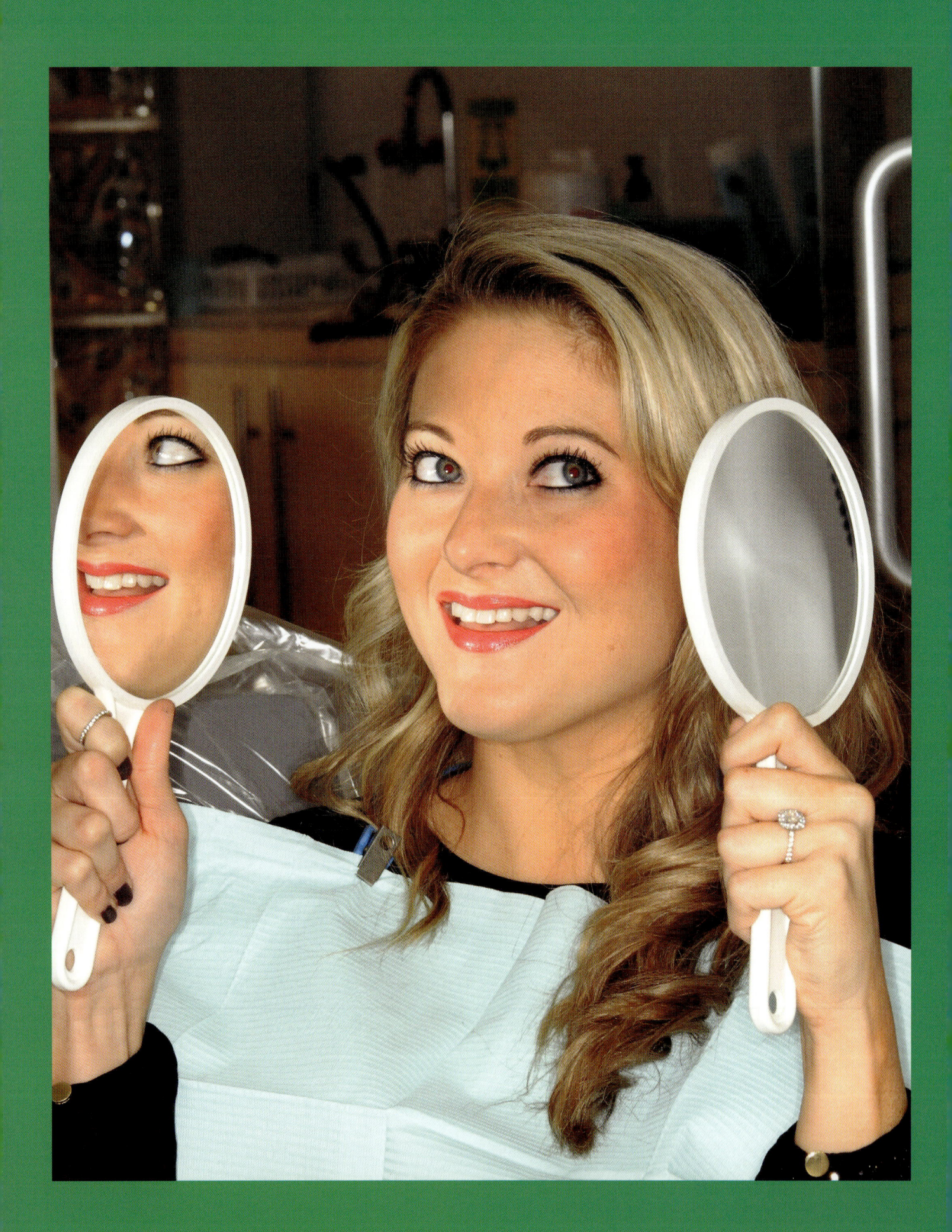

Chapter 2 Successful Management of Common Psychological Challenges

Shirley Brown, DMD, PhD

Chapter Outline

Introduction — 26	If the patient with an eating disorder is a minor — 36
Brief description of psychological terms and concepts — 26	Personality factors in esthetic dentistry — 36
Mood disorders — 27	The anxious patient — 37
Depression — 27	The angry patient — 38
Bipolar disorder — 29	The demanding patient — 38
Obsessive-compulsive disorder — 30	Treating the patient with Narcissistic Personality Disorder — 40
Eating disorders — 31	Life event stress and adjustment disorder — 41
Bulimia nervosa — 31	The dental patient with body dysmorphic disorder — 42
Anorexia nervosa — 34	

I had rarely heard him sounding so emphatic or so perplexed. My friend and colleague, Dr J, is a renowned restorative dentist. He called to refer a patient to my psychotherapy practice:

"I told her I might be able to help her, but that I won't even touch her mouth until she sees you for psychotherapy."

Really? What's the issue?

"Well, she's a lovely 45-year-old, a successful radiologist who, since having a porcelain crown placed on tooth number 5 about a year ago, believes that she is hideous and refuses to be seen in public. She's had to resign from her medical practice. Other than doctors' appointments, she won't leave the house. She even cuts her own hair! She harassed the office of the dentist who made her the crown to such a degree that he had to change the office phone number. Each plastic surgeon she consults tells her she's just aging, which has convinced her of a local conspiracy against her by plastic surgeons. The dentist who treated her is very capable, and a number of terrific dentists have refused to treat her. The thing is, she actually does have some occlusal problems, and I agree the crown could look a little more harmonious. The woman is truly suffering, and I think I could help her. But not until she's had some therapy!"

Ok. Well, thanks for the referral… I'll try to get her scheduled and see what I can do. I'll be in touch.

Introduction

One of the greatest challenges in dental practice is the psychologically difficult patient. We dentists are entertained by sharing our tales of the strange and outrageous, patient "war stories." Patients, for their part, lament the apparent obliviousness of the "typical" dentist, who fills the mouth with instruments and cotton before embarking on provocative topics of conversation. Patient behaviors in the dental chair range from routine to irrational, and dentists' management skills range from naturally talented to insensitive and impatient. Certainly, most dental school applicants emphasize their "people skills" in their application essays. Yet dental education generally lacks formal training in psychology or patient management. This state of affairs leaves many dentists poorly equipped to successfully handle the challenging patient encounter, and many patients wishing for greater mental comfort from their dental experiences. The benefits of closing the often wide gap between patient demand and dentist skills are many, and include reduced stress for all concerned, better treatment plan acceptance, better clinical outcomes, and practice growth through referrals from satisfied patients. Since it can be nearly impossible for patients to evaluate a dentist based on his or her technical proficiency, it is pain management and patient comfort that distinguish the patient-rated "great" dentists from all others. This results in enhanced referral rates as well as reduced risk of malpractice suits.

For the dentist whose practice focuses primarily or largely on esthetic procedures, there are additional, very particular considerations in the area of patient management. This is due to the fact that higher concentrations of certain patient types are more likely to seek esthetic dentistry. These include individuals going through normative life transitions when their physical appearance has greater than usual salience, such as early and middle adulthood, as well as patients with certain pathologies of mood, behavior, and personality, such as depression, eating disorders, and narcissistic personality disorder (NPD). See Table 2.1.

This chapter provides you with detailed background information on each of the most common patient challenges that you are likely to encounter and clear guidelines for improved management of these patients. Case examples will provide "real-life" illustrations and will go beyond the usual sharing of bizarre or frustrating experiences with patients to a more informed and practical understanding from which to enhance the success and satisfaction of esthetic dental practice.

Brief description of psychological terms and concepts

Mood disorders are the most common psychological diagnoses in the general population and thus in dental practice (20.8% in the US adult population).[1] The rate of major depression has been estimated at 19%,[1] the rate of bipolar disorder (BD; formerly manic depressive disorder) is estimated to be 3.9%,[1] the rate of anxiety disorders, such as obsessive-compulsive disorder (OCD), is estimated to be 18.1% of the US population.[1] These three main

Table 2.1 Disorders of Special Concern to Esthetic Dentists

Category	Disorder
Mood disorders	Depression Bipolar disorder (BD) Obsessive-compulsive disorder (OCD)
Eating disorders	Anorexia nervosa (AN) Bulimia nervosa (BN)
Personality types	The anxious patient The angry patient The demanding patient
Narcissistic personality disorder (NPD)	
Life event stress/adjustment disorder	
Body dysmorphic disorder (BDD)	

mood disorders should be clearly understood by the esthetic dentist because of management demands and because psychoactive medications commonly used to treat these syndromes can affect the oral cavity significantly. In addition, body dysmorphic disorder (BDD), which is a less prevalent subcategory of OCD, is particularly important to understand as it presents extreme and special challenges and protocols for the dental practice.

Eating disorders, which include anorexia nervosa (AN) and bulimia nervosa (BN),[2] are of high and increasing prevalence in the general population, estimated at 2.7% in US children and adolescents; AN is estimated at 0.6% in US adults (0.9% female and 0.3% male), and BN at 0.6% in US adults (0.5% female and 0.1% male).[1] Although both of these syndromes present the dentist with specific clinical and management challenges, there is a higher concentration of individuals with BN who seek esthetic dental procedures. This is in part because people whose work places them in the public eye, such as modeling, acting, and television talent, are under higher pressure to maintain thinness and therefore at greater risk of becoming bulimic. Of all the eating disorders, BN results in the greatest degree of damage to oral structures, particularly the anterior esthetic zone of the mouth, for reasons to be described. Mortality rates from medical complications and suicide have been estimated at 4% for AN and 3.9% for BN, the highest of all mental disorders.[3]

Personality disorders are a group of conditions in which the individual's persistent style of thinking, feeling, and behaving deviate significantly from social norms and interfere with personal and professional relationships. These differences stand apart from the symptoms of mood disorders, which can co-occur, and generally respond to long-term psychotherapy but not to psychoactive medications. Of the 10 main personality disorders, NPD stands out as a significant source of management challenge for the dentist. Prevalence rates for the personality disorders cannot be meaningfully estimated due to the difficulty of accurate survey measurement.

Patients with difficult personalities that are not so extreme as to be diagnosed as "disordered" will also be discussed (such as being angry or demanding), as they comprise a large segment of the esthetic dentistry patient population.

Adjustment disorders are diagnosed when individuals lack adequate coping skills to handle specific life events, such as relationship breakups, poor grades, job loss, illness, and aging. This diagnosis is rendered when there is a specific event that causes marked distress that interferes with social and/or occupational functioning, in excess of what would normally be expected. It has been criticized as being too vague a diagnostic category, yet clinicians do find it to be useful and the dentist is likely to encounter it. Some patients will be reacting within normal limits to stressful life events, and others will react pathologically. Both subcategories will potentially require extra management care to optimize dental treatment success.

Mood disorders

Depression

> #### Case example: Depression
>
> Steve, a patient who had an esthetic reconstruction 2 years previously, arrives for his recall visit. On his medical update form, Steve indicates that since his last recall he is now taking a new medication, the antidepressant Zoloft (sertraline). His oral examination reveals poor oral hygiene, gingival inflammation, and incipient marginal caries around several of his all-ceramic crowns. When gently queried by his dentist, Steve discloses that in the past year he had experienced a major depressive episode that included a suicide attempt. He had been hospitalized, successfully stabilized, and is now doing much better in regular weekly psychotherapy and antidepressant therapy. Steve admits that his mouth is constantly quite dry and his gums bleed when he brushes his teeth. He admits to having ceased all flossing during his illness, but is ready to "get back on track with everything."

> #### Case example: Undiagnosed depression
>
> Susan arrives for her new patient visit after having made and canceled three previous appointments. She makes little eye contact and interacts only minimally with the front desk staff. The receptionist alerts the dentist to her unusual behavior. Susan mentions to the hygienist conducting the oral exam that her reason for seeking treatment is to improve the esthetics of her smile, in the hope that looking better would help her feel better. Her oral exam reveals poor oral hygiene, and all of her incisors are chipped, discolored, and evidence severe occlusal wear. The hygienist passes all of this information on to the dentist, so that when he begins his consultation he is suspicious that Susan might have a psychological problem, perhaps depression. Indeed, since he is aware of the typical signs of the disorder, the dentist is able to include specific questions in the interview while reviewing Susan's medical history, and thereby learn that Susan is feeling blue and weepy, having trouble sleeping, and does not have her usual energy. This had been her condition for the past 2 months.

These two patients exemplify some of the major challenges facing the dentist when dealing with patients with depression, a highly prevalent mood disorder. In the case of Steve, the challenge is primarily clinical management of his present mental and dental status coupled with enhanced oral disease prevention. For Susan, the challenges include detecting the possibility of undiagnosed depression, successful referral for mental health treatment, and staging of esthetic dental rehabilitation to minimize treatment failure and maximize the positive effects of improved dental esthetics on her overall health and well-being.

Elements of successful dental treatment of behaviorally challenging patients include careful screening and assessment, psychiatric consultation or referral, and clear communication, particularly in the area of treatment planning. The extra time and effort can be more than offset by enhanced patient comfort and compliance, and thus greater treatment success and dentist satisfaction. It is also very effective to foster close communication among all members of the dental team—from receptionist to hygienist to assistant to dentist—since patients often reveal important information to staff members, who can alert and guide the dentist to a possible management problem early enough in the process that critical adjustments can be made and conflicts or errors prevented.

Box 2.1 lists the diagnostic criteria for major depression in the current *Diagnostic and Statistical Manual* used in psychiatry and psychology (*DSM-5*).[2] It is helpful for dentists and their treatment teams to be familiar with these criteria when evaluating new and returning patients for esthetic treatment. It is also advisable that medical history forms used in esthetic dental practice include specific questions that can gently yet clearly elicit signs that a patient may be suffering with depression, whether previously diagnosed or not.[4,5] Alternatively, you may prefer to administer a brief, validated depression questionnaire such as the Beck Depression Inventory (BDI).[6] Although Steve was forthcoming about his depression history, many patients unfortunately feel too stigmatized to offer such details voluntarily. Specific questions and validated questionnaires are no guarantee, but they do increase the probability of disclosure significantly. Box 2.2 lists suggested depression-related questions for inclusion on medical history forms.

Our patient Steve illustrates some of the most important management considerations when dealing with a history of depression. First and foremost, you and your staff should approach a patient like Steve in a manner that is respectful, concerned, and competent. He should be made to feel comfortable with having disclosed details of his illness, since only with such disclosure can he be treated safely and effectively. He should be reassured that his dental needs can be addressed, after some preliminary data gathering, and that his psychiatric history will be kept confidential. It will be necessary for the dentist to obtain the patient's written consent to communicate with the psychiatric treatment team, in this case consisting of his psychiatrist and psychotherapist. This consent must be given by the patient to all of the doctors who wish to communicate with each other, and is a standard aspect of psychotherapy practice.

Once consent for release of information has been obtained, the dentist should speak to the patient's prescribing psychiatrist

> **Box 2.1 Diagnostic criteria for major depressive disorder.**
>
> Five (or more) of the following symptoms have been present during the same 2-week period and represent a change from previous functioning.
>
> 1. Depressed mood most of the day, nearly every day, as indicated by either subjective report (e.g., feels sad or empty) or observation made by others (e.g., appears tearful). Note: in children and adolescents, can be irritable mood.
> 2. Markedly diminished interest or pleasure in all, or almost all, activities most of the day, nearly every day (as indicated by either subjective account or observation made by others).
> 3. Significant weight loss when not dieting or weight gain (e.g., a change of more than 5% of body weight in a month), or decrease or increase in appetite nearly every day. Note: in children, consider failure to make expected weight gains.
> 4. Insomnia or hypersomnia nearly every day.
> 5. Psychomotor agitation or retardation nearly every day (observable by others, not merely subjective feelings of restlessness or being slowed down).
> 6. Fatigue or loss of energy nearly every day.
> 7. Feelings of worthlessness or excessive or inappropriate guilt (which may be delusional) nearly every day (not merely self-reproach or guilt about being sick).
> 8. Diminished ability to think or concentrate, or indecisiveness, nearly every day (either by subjective account or as observed by others).
> 9. Recurrent thoughts of death (not just fear of dying), recurrent suicidal ideation without a specific plan, or a suicide attempt or a specific plan for committing suicide.

> **Box 2.2 Depression - related questions for inclusion on medical history forms.**
>
> Since your last dental visit, have you been bothered by any of the following?
>
> - Attention problems or difficulty focusing
> - Feeling hopeless or helpless
> - Crying spells
> - Increased appetite
> - Decreased appetite
> - Inadequate sleep or insomnia
> - Excessive sleepiness
> - Lack of energy
> - Loss of interest or pleasure in your usual activities
> - Persistent sadness or low mood
> - Increased irritability
> - Increased worry about your health
> - Suicidal thoughts

about his antidepressant therapy and document medical approval for dental treatment. Possible interactions of the antidepressant medication with agents and medications that may be used in dental treatment, including local anesthetics, vasoconstrictors, antibiotics, and analgesics, should be discussed, and medical permission documented, particularly if he has any other medical conditions, like cardiac disease. *This is vitally important* because antidepressant medications can interact adversely with epinephrine, codeine, benzodiazepines, and erythromycin, and can cause orthostatic hypotension. These concerns are particularly important in patients with preexisting cardiac disease, in whom the risk of atrial fibrillation and ventricular tachycardia may be increased.[7] While these interactions are less frequent with newer antidepressants, such as Wellbutrin (bupropion), and selective serotonin reuptake inhibitors (SSRIs)—the category of antidepressants to which Zoloft (sertraline) belongs—they continue to be a concern with older categories of antidepressants still in use, such as tricyclic antidepressants (TCAs) and monoamine oxidase inhibitors (MAOIs).[7]

It may be advisable for you to consult with the patient's psychotherapist at this stage as well, gaining any suggestions for ways to be more responsive to his needs, to establish a collaborative professional relationship, and to partner with the therapist in staging the treatment to maximize its positive impact on his self-esteem and emotional stability. Once he has been medically cleared for treatment, and you have attained a fuller understanding of his psychiatric history and current status, you may proceed with the dental treatment plan.

Steve's oral examination findings were consistent with the typical presentation of depressed individuals: due to low mood, oral hygiene is often neglected, leading to gingival inflammation and periodontal disease. Xerostomia is a common side effect of most antidepressant medications (Figure 2.1).[7,8] Individuals often use sugar-sweetened candy and beverages to stimulate salivation, and it is not unusual for the quality of their diets to deteriorate while experiencing major depression. These factors combine to increase the caries rate in patients with major depression.[7,8]

Therefore, treatment planning should focus on treating and preventing periodontal disease, through subgingival scaling and root planning, restoring the dentition through caries elimination, and enhanced emphasis on in-office oral hygiene therapy and improved home care. More frequent recalls and topical fluoride applications have been strongly recommended.[8] The dentist should not hesitate to recommend an improved, less cariogenic diet to both the patient and the medical treatment team. Artificial saliva products and sugar-free candies and gum to stimulate salivation can be very helpful in reducing the effects of xerostomia.[7,8]

Susan, the other new patient profiled above, certainly seemed to be an excellent candidate for esthetic restoration, based on

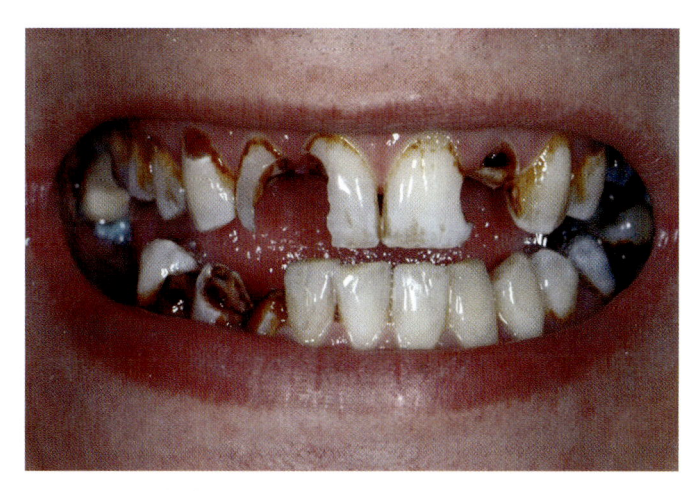

Figure 2.1 Individuals with mood disorders may present with rampant caries, due to poor oral hygiene and xerostomia from some psychoactive medications.

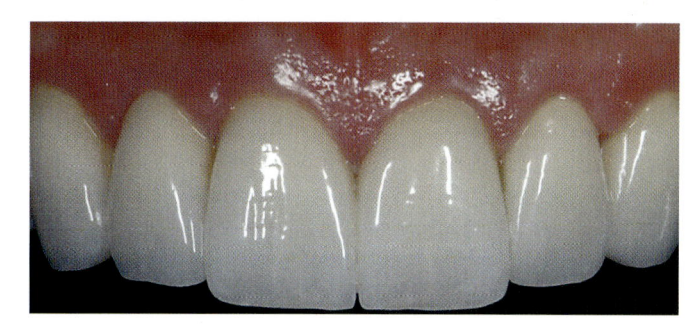

Figure 2.2 Dental restoration can enhance optimism and self-esteem in patients with a history of mood disorder.

her oral examination. However, her behavior and medical history suggested that she might be suffering from an as yet undiagnosed major depressive episode. The best way for you to approach a patient like Susan would be to establish rapport with her as well as possible in the initial visit by carefully reviewing her medical and dental histories and gently inquiring as to whether she had considered that she might be suffering with depression. You should be prepared to give her contact information for several well-regarded psychiatrists and psychotherapists in the community. The best-case scenario is that you have accurately detected a case of depression and that the patient will follow up with psychiatric treatment.

Whether or not this occurs, the dental treatment plan should begin with scrupulously clear communication between you and the patient. You should use photos of esthetic smiles to elicit a sense of what she expects as an esthetic result, and ascertain whether or not her expectations are reasonable. If they are not, some extra time spent illustrating what she *can* expect will help to prevent disappointment and difficulties at the end of the active treatment phase. Once you and the patient have worked out an agreement on the esthetic goals, you should prepare a detailed treatment plan—including such details as a description of what she will experience with her temporary restorations, how long appointments should take, the projected interval of time between appointments, and the realistic appearance of the final restorations.[4,5] The patient should then be asked to sign a statement indicating that she has understood and agrees to the treatment plan. In this way, important details are discussed in advance, consent to the treatment plan is as fully informed as possible, and treatment can proceed in an atmosphere of enhanced trust.

Successful behavioral management might require the patient's visits to be shortened to accommodate her emotional state. She may also require extra encouragement and reassurance. Clinical dental management should include intensive oral hygiene instruction and frequent oral prophylaxis with topical fluoride application, particularly if the patient commences pharmacotherapy with antidepressant medication, putting her at risk of xerostomia and caries. As Susan's depression ameliorates, and as Steve continues to enjoy emotional stability through psychiatric care, the improvement in their smiles is likely to contribute significantly to their emotional health. It is well documented that renewed dental health, especially when dental esthetics have been improved, can contribute to a depressed patient's recovery and long-term emotional stability through enhanced self-esteem and confidence (Figure 2.2).[4,5,7,8]

Bipolar disorder

Case example: Bipolar disorder

A patient, who at his last visit disclosed a history of depression, seems to be euphoric. He arrives late, explaining that he was delayed because he had to stop and write down ideas for a novel that is sure to win a Pulitzer or Nobel Prize. He charmingly offers to "make it up" to the office staff by buying everyone dinner after work. He speaks so rapidly and loudly that it is hard to understand him, and he bounces from one unrelated topic to another.

This is an unlikely scenario, but if it were to occur, your best course of action would be to urge the patient to seek emergency psychiatric care for bipolar disorder (BD). Individuals experiencing a manic episode, as illustrated above, often experience a very rapid mood swing back to deep depression, and self-destructive—even suicidal—behaviors are not uncommon. The scenario is unlikely, since a manic, euphoric patient is probably not going to be thinking about visiting his dentist! The diagnostic criteria for BD are extremely complex, and therefore beyond the scope of this chapter. The interested reader is advised to consult the *DSM-5*.[2]

You are much more likely to encounter a patient with BD who has been previously diagnosed and whose mood has been stabilized by psychiatric treatment. As with depression, you should obtain the patient's written consent to consult with the psychiatric treatment team, to review the patient's current mental status, medications, and any risk of adverse interactions with local anesthetics and other medications commonly used in dental treatment, as well as possible considerations for dental treatment timing and staging.

Patient management should be guided by the awareness that, despite psychiatric treatment, the patient with BD may still suffer rapid mood changes that may affect oral hygiene, commitment to treatment, and ability to tolerate extensive dental procedures.[9,10] As with unipolar depression, it is advisable for you to do your utmost to make sure the patient's expectations of the final result are realistic, to provide a detailed treatment plan, and to have the patient sign an agreement based on the aforementioned criteria. This patient will likely require a little extra patience and encouragement, and possibly shorter appointments. The patient with established BD is likely to be taking an antidepressant as well as a mood stabilizer, such as lithium or lamotrigine, all of which may cause chronic xerostomia. A dry mouth management protocol may be required.

Whereas the patient with BD going through a depressive phase will often present with poor oral hygiene, those having just experienced a manic phase of the disorder may show evidence of overly vigorous flossing and brushing, such as notched gingival lesions and excessive cervical tooth abrasion.[9] Once again, thorough and frequent oral prophylaxis and oral hygiene instruction are of paramount importance, along with use of topical fluorides and dietary counseling.

As with the depressed patient, a relatively small investment in time, effort, and information gathering promotes successful relationships and treatment of the esthetic dental patient with BD. The opportunity to enhance the self-esteem and psychological well-being of such patients can be particularly satisfying for the esthetic dental team.

Obsessive-compulsive disorder

> ### Case example: Obsessive-compulsive disorder
> Jerry had been a highly particular patient from his very first visit, but his behavior really raised alarms when he failed to show up for his recall appointment, especially when he disclosed the reason for his "no-show." He had chosen to be treated in this practice based on its reputation not only for high-quality esthetic dentistry, but even more for its adherence to strict sterilization guidelines. Office sterility was, according to Jerry, always his greatest concern. After his previous dentist retired it had taken him a while to find another office he could trust to be as clean as he needed it to be. Jerry was willing to drive from his home over an hour away from the practice.
>
> Another concern of Jerry's was radiation exposure. He refused most dental radiographs, except when a tooth was symptomatic or to check an endodontic procedure, and insisted on being fully swathed in lead aprons. Jerry also elected to have his procedures done without local anesthetic. He explained that the discomfort was less aversive than his concern about possible needle contamination. The dental team members were willing to comply with these limitations and were careful to document in the patient's chart whenever he declined a recommendation.
>
> Jerry was otherwise a patient who was easy to accommodate: he paid his bills on time, complied with treatment, and reliably arrived early for his appointments, always providing adequate notice when he needed to change his appointment schedule.

> When he failed to arrive for his recall, the dentist and his staff were concerned, since it was so extraordinary, and their concerns were only heightened when they learned his reason: "You see, after I drove to the appointment and parked my car, I remembered that the hygienist had just returned from her maternity leave. I became afraid that if someone didn't pick up after their dog and I unknowingly stepped in it, I could pass the germs on to the hygienist, who might then pass them on to her new baby and make her sick. I just couldn't come in. So I drove all the way back home. I'm so sorry!"

At this point, the dentist decided to contact a psychologist to whom he often referred, who confirmed that Jerry was most likely suffering with a type of anxiety disorder known as obsessive-compulsive disorder (OCD), the diagnostic criteria of which are found in Table 2.2. The dentist's role, in this instance, was to

Table 2.2 Diagnostic Criteria for Obsessive Compulsive Disorder (OCD)

Must exhibit obsessions or compulsions	The obsessions and/or compulsions cause marked distress, are time-consuming (take more than 1 h per day), or interfere substantially with the person's normal routine, occupational or academic functioning, or usual social activities or relationships.
	The content of the obsessions or compulsions should not be restricted to any other major Axis I psychiatric disorder, such as an obsession with food in the context of an eating disorder.
Obsessions	Recurrent and persistent thoughts, impulses, or images experienced, at some time during the disturbance, as intrusive and inappropriate and cause marked anxiety or distress.
	These thoughts, impulses, or images are not simply excessive worries about real life problems.
	There is some effort by the affected person to ignore or suppress such thoughts, impulses, or images, or to neutralize them with some other thought or action.
	At some time, the affected person recognizes that the obsessions are a product of his or her own mind rather than inserted into his or her own mind from some outside source.
Compulsions	Repetitive activities (e.g., hand washing, ordering, checking) or mental acts (e.g., praying, counting, repeating words silently).
	The person feels driven to perform these in response to an obsession or according to rules that must be applied rigidly.
	These behaviors or mental acts are performed in order to prevent or reduce distress, or prevent some dreaded event or situation.
	However, they are either clearly excessive or not connected in a realistic way with what they are designed to neutralize or prevent.

speak with Jerry about this possibility, gently encourage him to obtain professional help, and offer several good referral options for psychologists and psychiatrists. Jerry selected one of the psychologists on the dentist's list, an international expert who happened to have her research center and practice in the area.

This case illustrates the relative ease with which a demanding patient can be accommodated, and the importance of building rapport and trust between the patient and the dental team. Without such trust, it would have been much less likely that the dentist would have felt comfortable discussing the suspected problem with Jerry, and even less likely that Jerry would have acted on the recommendation. When he returned for his recall after successful stabilization of his OCD, he was extremely grateful to the dental team for their sensitivity and help, and was able to proceed with esthetic dental treatment.

Eating disorders

Case example: Bulimia nervosa

At age 23, Jenna had secretly suffered with severe bulimia for 10 years when she made what turned out to be a fateful dental appointment. Years later, looking back on how she began her recovery from bulimia, it would seem ironic that she would credit her dentist with responsibility for helping her to take the first steps toward a more normal life. And yet she now realized that the effects of so many years of multiple daily vomiting episodes had produced a distinctive and characteristic pattern of damage in her mouth. Being gently yet firmly confronted with it by her new dentist, she could no longer continue denying that she had a severe problem and needed help.

Her recovery began when a friend remarked that her front teeth looked a little strange. She realized she had convinced herself that no one noticed her teeth, but that this was clearly a distortion of reality. Her embarrassment prompted two reactions: first, and characteristically, a new round of intense binging and purging, but second, and more importantly, a decision to find an excellent dentist, one who practiced far enough away from where she lived that he would not be likely to know her parents or any of her friends. She made an appointment for an examination. Filling out the medical history form raised her concerns about detection somewhat, since they included specific questions about recent weight fluctuations and eating habits. She hesitated over these, and then decided to answer them as truthfully as she could without divulging just how severe her eating problems were.

Fortunately, her dentist was well informed as to the characteristic presentation of individuals with bulimia. Indeed, the suspicions raised by his new patient's appearance and history were confirmed by even a cursory look at her face and mouth. The first thing he noticed about her was how tense her facial musculature appeared, especially her upper lip. This was a facial posture that had become natural to her, as the need to hide her worsening anterior dentition had progressed over the years of binging and purging.

The dentist also noticed the puffiness of her cheeks and the squarish appearance of her lower face that were the results of parotid swelling, findings that he knew were common in patients who habitually induced vomiting. He was also able to glance at her hands, where he saw the characteristic callus on the knuckle that had been raised by being scraped against her front teeth countless times during purging by stimulating the palate with her index finger to induce vomiting.

The dentist knew that bulimia is an extremely secretive disorder, one that sufferers were deeply ashamed to admit to and that he would have to approach his new patient with sensitivity and care. He was prepared with a bulimia hotline number, eating disorder treatment and support websites, and names of local treatment centers and therapists whom he trusted. So he explored the subject with her using a recommended approach:

"It's my job to understand problems that you're having with your mouth but that may influence your overall health as well. I'm here to help you beyond just repairing your teeth. The changes in your teeth are ones I usually see in people who vomit very often, and your responses to some of the questions on the medical history form are ones that I usually see in people who have an eating problem. Have you been having a problem with binging and purging?"

The preceding case study illustrates the vital role that the informed dental team can play in the diagnosis and treatment of individuals with eating disorders like bulimia nervosa (BN). There is also wide agreement that, due to the often severe damage to the dental anterior esthetic zone inflicted by frequent vomiting, as well as the prevalence of this syndrome in young women and other individuals highly concerned about their appearance, the esthetic dental team is more likely than others to encounter increased numbers of eating-disordered individuals seeking their services. The diagnostic criteria for anorexia nervosa (AN) and BN are listed in Table 2.3. Both anorexia and bulimia are extremely serious psychological disorders that can end in death as a result of severe physical complications or suicide.

Bulimia nervosa

In contrast to someone with anorexia, who will present with obvious emaciation, the new dental patient with BN will not likely be identified based on weight, since individuals with BN typically appear to be of normal or average weight. This greatly increases the likelihood that dentists will encounter new patients with *undiagnosed* BN. The informed dental team can play a crucial role in the detection, referral for treatment, and case management (i.e., secondary prevention) of BN.[11–15] As illustrated by the case study earlier in this section, this is because individuals with BN, who due to intense shame about their disorder often remain untreated for years and even decades, usually display a distinct pattern of oral and physical findings that are pathognomonic of BN. The dentist and team who are equipped with knowledge about these findings may therefore be the first to detect BN, presenting a unique opportunity and responsibility to diagnose, refer, and help manage the medical and psychological treatment of these patients.

Table 2.3 Diagnostic Criteria for Anorexia Nervosa (AN) and Bulimia Nervosa (BN)

Anorexia nervosa	Refusal to maintain body weight at or above a minimally normal weight for age and height (e.g., weight loss leading to maintenance of body weight less than 85% of that expected; or failure to make expected weight gain during period of growth, leading to body weight less than 85% of that expected).
	Intense fear of gaining weight or becoming fat, even though underweight.
	Disturbance in the way in which one's body weight or shape is experienced, undue influence of body shape on self-evaluation, or denial of the seriousness of the current low body weight.
Bulimia nervosa	Recurrent episodes of binge eating. An episode of binge eating is characterized by both of the following: 1. Eating, in a discrete period of time (e.g., within any 2 h period), an amount of food that is definitely larger than most people would eat during a similar period of time and under similar circumstances. 2. A sense of lack of control over eating during the episode (e.g., a feeling that one cannot stop eating or control what or how much one is eating).
	Recurrent inappropriate compensatory behavior to prevent weight gain, such as self-induced vomiting; misuse of laxatives, diuretics, enemas, or other medications; fasting; or excessive exercise.
	The binge eating and inappropriate compensatory behaviors both occur, on average, at least once a week for 3 months.
	Self-evaluation is unduly influenced by body shape and weight.
	The disturbance does not occur exclusively during episodes of AN.

An esthetic dentistry practice is likely to encounter a higher number of individuals with BN because there is high overlap between individuals at elevated risk of becoming affected by bulimia and the patient population of an active esthetic dentistry practice. High-risk populations for BN include:

- girls and young women
- middle-aged women
- gay men and sexually conflicted younger men and boys
- certain athletes—gymnasts, wrestlers, jockeys
- dancers, especially classical ballet
- fashion models
- people in the public eye—actors, TV talent
- people of relatively high socioeconomic status
- people in high-pressure professional positions, especially female chief executive officers.

Therefore, it is essential for the esthetic practice to be equipped to detect, communicate, refer, and help manage the patient with BN and to stage esthetic reconstruction to produce the most positive influence on the patient's recovery and the greatest longevity of the dental restorations. Detection can best begin by embedding specific questions in the new patient medical history form (see below). A positive response to any of these questions should raise the suspicion of the member of the team administering and reading the form; these positive responses should be flagged for the dentist at the first visit.

Suggested questions for patient medical history form:

- Do you spend a lot of time worrying about your weight and wishing you were thinner?
- Does your weight often fluctuate by more than 5 lb (2.25 kg)?
- Have you ever tried to make yourself vomit after eating too much?
- Have you ever used laxatives to lose weight?
- Do you go on diets frequently?
- Do you exercise specifically to make up for extra calories?
- Have you developed chronic painless swelling below your ear(s)?

As you move on to the oral exam, you should assess the appearance and symmetry of the patient's face, since people with BN frequently present with swelling of one or both parotid glands (Figure 2.3). The presence and extent of parotid swelling correlate with the duration and frequency of daily vomiting. It is not unusual for parotid swelling and the resulting squarish appearance of the lower face to be the patient's presenting complaint. As in the case of Jenna described above, many people with bulimia develop a tight lip posture when they speak and smile, a habitual way of attempting to hide the damage to their front teeth. In addition, people who vomit frequently may present with significant eye puffiness.

You might also attempt to visualize the patient's index and middle finger knuckles for calluses (Russell's sign; Figure 2.4). These can develop from the repeated action of scraping the knuckles against the upper teeth, in the process of using the fingers to induce the gag reflex in the soft palate to induce vomiting after a high-calorie binge.

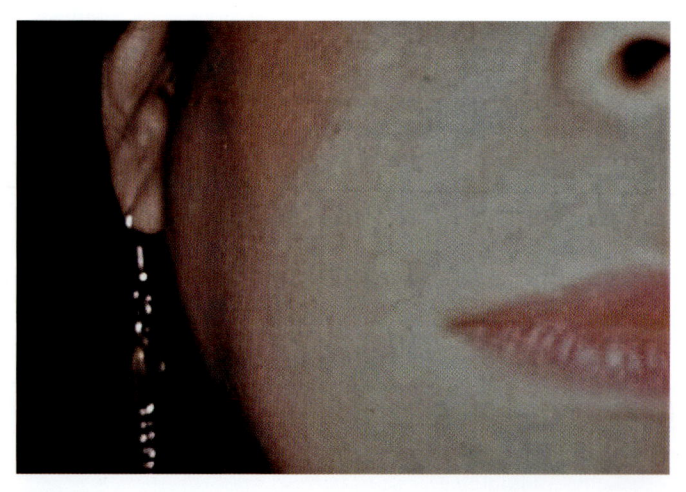

Figure 2.3 Parotid gland enlargement in bulimia nervosa.

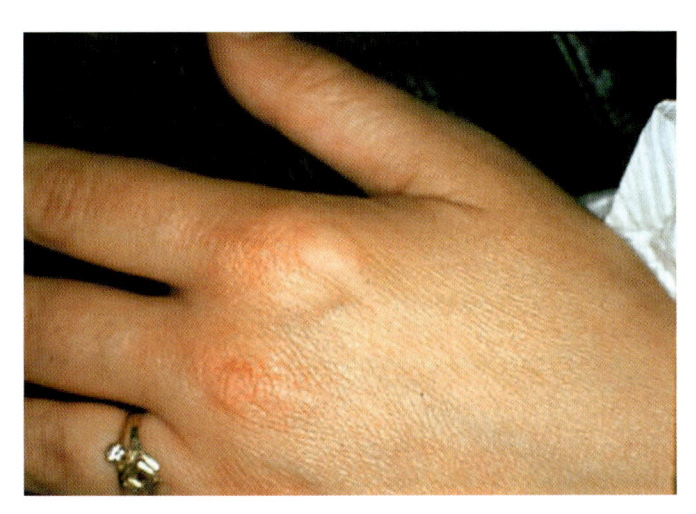

Figure 2.4 Russell's sign: knuckle calluses resulting from induced vomiting in eating disordered patient.

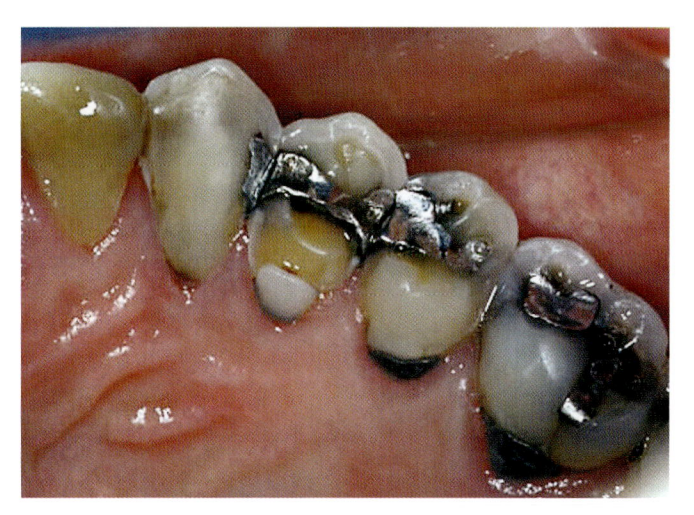

Figure 2.6 Palatal enamel erosion and "amalgam islands" from frequent vomiting in BN.

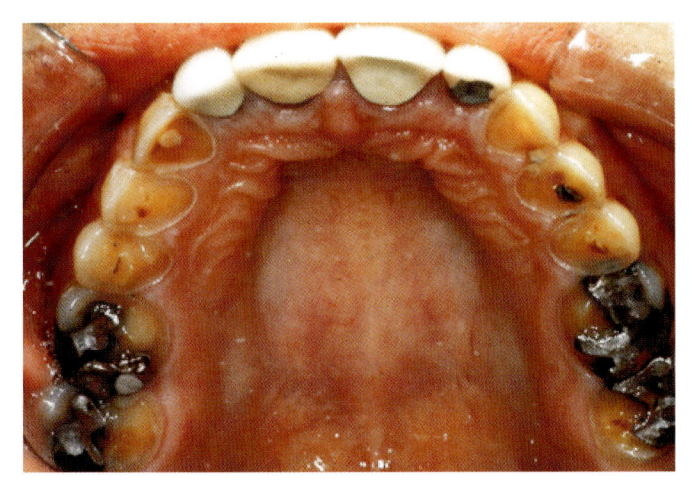

Figure 2.5 Typical glassy erosion—perimylolysis—seen in bulimic individuals. Note lingual erosion of cuspids and bicuspids, with narrow enamel band at gingival margins.

The most common and most damaging finding in the mouths of people with BN, particularly after at least 2–3 years of multiple daily vomiting episodes that repeatedly bathe the teeth in corrosive stomach acids, is a unique pattern of dental erosion. Known as *perimylolysis*, this erosion typically occurs on the palatal surfaces of the upper anterior teeth, with thinning and notching of the incisal edges of the upper and lower anterior teeth, and posterior amalgam or composite restorations that appear as raised islands, where the enamel has eroded around them, along with smooth, glassy loss of contour on unrestored teeth.[11,13,14] In the early stages of the disorder, the erosion will be milder and appear as glassy smoothing of normal anatomy. When advanced, this erosion often causes thermal sensitivity, another common presenting complaint (Figures 2.5 and 2.6).

Self-induced vomiting may cause visible traumatic lesions on the soft palate and upper pharynx. Xerostomia is also a frequent finding, the result of poor nutrition and dehydration. Many individuals with BN seem to be fastidious about their oral hygiene, so the caries rate may not be increased. However, where there is extensive cervical erosion after many years of vomiting, exposed dentin surfaces can become carious. Furthermore, many patients with BN experience periods of depression, during which time they may neglect their hygiene and experience increased caries, particularly if they tend to binge on cariogenic foods.[16] (See Chapter 22 in this volume, entitled Abfraction, Abrasion, Attrition, and Erosion.)

Any combination of positive answers to screening questions and positive physical and oral findings should raise serious suspicions that the new patient is presenting with a case of undiagnosed BN. At this point, many dentists might experience uncertainty about how to proceed. It is an unfortunate, if understandable, fact that most dentists do not feel equipped to confront their patient with these concerns.[13,15] Given the high likelihood of encountering patients with undiagnosed BN in an esthetic dentistry practice seeking to improve their oral health and especially a damaged smile, it is incumbent on you to gain confidence in your ability to speak with these patients about their bulimia and establish a safe environment. See the suggested script used by Jenna's dentist in the previous case example of BN.

Naturally, many individuals who have been hiding their bulimia for a long time will initially deny their problem. They may even have learned to attribute the erosion to high consumption of lemons or to chronic acid reflux from gastroesophageal reflux disease (GERD). It is also the case that some new patients will have experienced weight change and body size preoccupation—and indicate such on their medical history form—without suffering from an eating disorder. You and your team should be very aware, therefore, that enamel erosion from habitual lemon or acidic soft drink consumption occurs primarily on the *facial* and *cervical* surfaces of the teeth, and erosion from GERD occurs primarily on the *occlusal* surfaces in the *posterior* region of the mouth where the acidic refluxed material pools. Only long-term, repeated vomiting produces the particular erosion pattern of perimylolysis: *mostly on the palatal surfaces, mostly on the anterior teeth*, where the stomach acids are propelled during vomiting, and where the rasping thrust of the tongue's action accelerates the erosion.

Alone, or especially in combination with any of the other common signs of bulimia—that is, parotid enlargement, palatal lesions, knuckle callus, and positive responses to the medical intake questions—this erosive pattern of perimylolysis is pathognomonic for BN and should immediately signal you to step into the vital role of secondary prevention of this potentially life-threatening syndrome.[11,13,15]

The patient who denies the problem—and this is expected—should nevertheless be offered the names and contact information of local treatment centers and therapists who specialize in eating disorders. It is also very helpful to provide a list of online resources, such as informational and supportive websites and hotlines, for people struggling with eating disorders. Many practitioners fear that if they persist in this way, they may lose the patient. Actually, this can be accomplished in a nonconfrontational yet concerned manner that the patient is much more likely to experience as caring and vitally helpful, even if he or she continues to deny the problem. With the goal of retaining the patient while encouraging him or her to seek medical and psychological care, it is recommended that you schedule the patient for an initial oral prophylaxis and treatment planning appointment at this time, while also letting the patient know that you intend to follow up regarding your concerns.

At subsequent appointments, the subject of BN should be raised again in a concerned manner, and the patient should be told that you recommend only palliative care until the teeth are no longer vulnerable to ongoing erosion, since this will significantly compromise the process and prognosis of the restorations. While palliative therapy is occurring, you will have more opportunities to encourage the patient to seek therapy and the prospect of a beautiful, definitive esthetic reconstruction can be highly motivating. Nevertheless, if the patient continues to deny the problem and refuses to seek therapy, you will have to decide at this point whether or not to proceed with definitive care, given that an acceptable prognosis for dental treatment depends on cessation of the vomiting habit. Many practitioners elect to proceed with treatment, at least placing temporary restorations, in an effort to continue to engage and motivate the patient with improved function and appearance. If you do elect to proceed, you should thoroughly document your efforts to get the patient into therapy for the BN, and that your recommendation to delay definitive care was overridden by the patient.

If, as hoped, the patient does admit to her problem and does follow through with treatment, you should remain actively engaged in the therapeutic process through coordinating care with the medical/psychological/nutritional team. Nutritional interventions are among the central features of rehabilitation for patients with eating disorders. It is not unusual for the medical team to prescribe simple carbohydrates, since these provide a ready source of calories without producing the sense of stomach fullness that can be aversive to people with eating disorders. If the dental team is involved in coordinating care, it is appropriate to recommend to the medical team that non-sweet foods, such as cheese, be consumed at the same time to buffer salivary acidity and reduce the deleterious effect of simple sugars on the teeth. The promise of a beautiful smile can be a powerful motivator for commitment to therapy and recovery from BN if definitive esthetic rehabilitation is timed optimally in the patient's course of therapy. A useful worksheet for dental treatment planning of the patient with a diagnosed eating disorder is found in Table 2.4.

Throughout dental treatment, whether palliative or definitive, as long as the patient continues to induce vomiting—even when the frequency of vomiting has been significantly reduced—the patient should be advised not to brush the teeth immediately after vomiting, as this accelerates enamel erosion. Rinsing immediately with water is the best measure, followed, if possible, by a 0.05% sodium fluoride rinse to neutralize acids and protect tooth surfaces and restoration margins.[11]

Anorexia nervosa

People with AN are easy to recognize, since they usually appear emaciated, and they will likely present for dental treatment during or following psychiatric and medical stabilization. Therefore, it is unusual for the dental team to be in a position of detecting a case of AN. Nevertheless, it is important that you and your team be knowledgeable about the disorder to deliver safe, appropriate, and timely treatment. It is also important because some patients have a history of cycling from AN to BN and back again numerous times during the course of their illness, so that they may present with signs of both disorders over time. Significant medical problems are associated with both AN and BN. These may include dehydration, hypothermia, electrolyte abnormalities, abnormal cardiac function, gastrointestinal complications, endocrine disturbances, osteoporosis, amenorrhea, and infertility. This incomplete list highlights the urgency of pretreatment consultation with the patient's medical team. The patient's physician should be consulted regarding any current medical issues that could be exacerbated by dental treatment. If the patient is not felt to be medically stable, all dental treatment other than acute palliation should be delayed.[11]

Common oral manifestations of AN result largely from malnutrition, and include soft tissue lesions such as glossitis, angular cheilitis, candidiasis, and mucosal ulceration. Elevated caries rates are sometimes seen when the individual neglects oral hygiene, which is common, and when highly cariogenic, sugar-rich foods are prescribed to bring about rapid weight gain during medical stabilization.[12]

You should consult with the treatment team members—internist or family physician, psychiatrist, psychotherapist, and, possibly, nutritionist—to optimize the timing of esthetic dental reconstruction, such that the patient is medically and psychologically stable enough to tolerate dental treatment. Since it is common for patients with AN to be treated for concurrent depression and/or anxiety, the psychiatrist should be consulted regarding the patient's medications and possible interactions and precautions. The psychotherapist can provide any special guidelines for making the patient more comfortable during treatment. For example, some patients recovering from AN feel anxious when *any* references—even flattering ones—are made to their appearance or their health. In such cases, it is a simple matter for the dental team to be informed, so that in their interactions with the patient they will attempt to omit such well-meaning but unwelcome comments. Once the patient has been medically

Table 2.4 Worksheet for the New Dental Patient With a Diagnosed Eating Disorder

Name						
Birth date						
I. History						
A. Type of disorder						
B. History of disorder						
1) Age at onset						
2) Current status	Active		Inactive			
3) Frequency of episodes at most active stage						
4) Periods of abstinence						
5) Precipitating factors						
II. Past medical/dental treatment for disorder						
A. Medical treatment						
B. Psychological treatment	In-patient:		Out-patient:			
C. Dental history						
1) Initial detection of oral/dental problems						
2) Preventive measures						
3) Restorative therapy						
4) Frequency of preventive/treatment appointments						
III. Current status						
A. General health quality	Date of most recent physical exam:					
B. Under active medical care?	Yes		No			
Under active psychological care?	Yes		No			
C. Medications and dosages						
D. Disorder under control?	Yes		No		For how long?	
E. Examination findings						
Head and neck						
Lymph nodes	+	−	Intraoral			
Skin	+	−	Occlusion	+	−	
Symmetry	+	−	Lips	+	−	
Temporomandibular joint	+	−	Mucosae	+	−	
Parotid swelling	+	−	Gingiva	+	−	
Commissures	+	−	Palate	+	−	
			Throat	+	−	
			Tongue	+	−	
Dentition						
Enamel erosion						
Location	Upper anterior:		Palatal	Incisal	Cervical	
	Lower anterior:		Lingual	Incisal	Cervical	
	Upper posterior:		Premolar	Molar	Occlusal	Cervical
	lower posterior:		Premolar	Molar	Occlusal	Cervical

(Continued)

Table 2.4 (Continued)

Name					
Extent		Mild	Moderate	Severe	
Symptomatic		No	Cold	Hot	Sweet
IV. Patient concerns					
Esthetic					
Comfort					
Parotid swelling					
Nutrition					
Other					
V. Treatment options					
A. Medical/psychological referral/continuation					
B. Eating disorder treatment referral/continuation					
C. Support group referral/continuation					
D. Dental therapy					
1) Emergency					
2) Palliative					
3) Preventive					
4) Definitive					
VI. Patient questions/comments:					

Adapted by a worksheet provided by Dr Robert Cowan, University of Missouri School of Dentistry.

cleared, treatment should be able to proceed without significant difficulty. The standard guidelines of regular oral prophylaxis, topical fluoride application, thorough oral hygiene instruction, and emphasis on good home care apply to the anorexic patient. These patients often suffer with xerostomia, both from their antidepressant medications as well as dehydration caused by their poor nutrition.[13,14] In such cases, artificial salivas and a dry mouth protocol are helpful, and the patient's nutritionist can be enlisted to support and reinforce it.

If the patient with an eating disorder is a minor

Given that the average age of onset of eating disorders has been shifting from the late teens to the earlier teens, it is likely that some of the patients with eating disorders encountered in the practice will be minors. Each state in the USA has its own statutes delineating the age at which patient–doctor communication is protected by privacy laws, and it is often younger than the legal age for other privileges, like alcohol consumption. Other countries will also have their own specific laws about this. In the Commonwealth of Pennsylvania, for example, the legal drinking age is 21, yet the age at which doctor–patient communication becomes protected is 14. You should become acquainted with your own state's or country's statutes. If the new patient with a suspected eating disorder is a minor, you must approach the patient's parent(s). This can be especially challenging in close communities where the patient's parents may be friends, acquaintances, or colleagues of yours. Nevertheless, you have a responsibility to sensitively approach the parent with your findings and concerns, and urge medical and psychological care.

Eating disorders are serious psychological illnesses that can and do result in death from physical complications and suicide. They rarely resolve without treatment, and early detection vastly improves prognoses. The dental team is in a unique position to detect and refer for life-saving treatment, with the additional role of providing a powerful motivator for recovery in the form of a beautiful new smile.

Personality factors in esthetic dentistry

Case example: Narcissistic personality disorder

The patient was a well-known actress. She intended to have extremely white porcelain veneers fabricated for all of her teeth. She arrived in the office after having conducted a wide search to locate "the world's best" esthetic dentist. She expressed conviction that her new dentist was, indeed, "a genius," where all dentists she had seen

> previously were "incompetent hacks." After treatment planning and discussion about the optimal shade for her full-mouth veneers (i.e., more natural, not bright white), although she refused to be persuaded, a full-day appointment was scheduled for tooth preparation, impressions, and temporization. A half hour after her appointment time, when she still hadn't shown up, the receptionist contacted her assistant by cell phone and was told that since her plastic surgeon had had an unexpected cancellation that morning, she had decided to have a breast augmentation and lift instead. She demanded to be treated in the dental office the next day, offering no apology for breaking the full-day appointment without even the consideration of an explanatory phone call. For a steeply increased fee, she was rescheduled for the next day. Immediately after being seated in the dental operatory, she lifted her shirt to a roomful of team members, revealing her bra-less self and asking: "How do you think they turned out?"

"Personality" has been defined as "the sum total of all the behavioral and mental characteristics by means of which an individual is recognized as being unique" (*World English Dictionary*), or "the essential character of a person" (Dictionary.com). In addition, "personality arises from within the individual and remains fairly consistent throughout life" (About.com). Everyone has a personality, some traits of which can manifest in a dental patient as being "difficult" or "challenging." In some cases, these difficulties or challenges are so extreme as to be clinically pathological, as illustrated in the above case example. This is an admittedly extreme—but actual—example of the behavior of a patient who has a diagnosable case of narcissistic personality disorder (NPD), the diagnostic criteria for which are found in Table 2.5.

In discussing personality, we are now shifting from psychological problems that can be successfully treated with medications and psychotherapy, many of which have a partial basis in neurochemical imbalances (such as depression, OCD, and eating disorders), to those that are very different in a number of important ways. Whereas many people with mood disorders and eating disorders often seek psychological and psychopharmacological treatments, people with personalities that are difficult or clinically disordered rarely seek psychological treatment, with the exception of the anxious personality type. This is because they most often perceive any problems they have in their personal or professional lives as external to them, not their "fault." Sometimes these "difficult" traits even have benefits, as noted in the adage "The squeaky wheel gets the grease," where the behaviors that make them difficult nevertheless compel others to comply with their wishes and demands. Furthermore, some personality traits that cause problems in relationships can confer advantages in certain careers. One need look no further than many successful politicians for a clear example of this phenomenon.

The earlier focus of this chapter was on teaching the dental team to detect serious psychological problems and then facilitating referral for psychiatric care, or dealing appropriately with a previously diagnosed disorder through consultation and collaboration with psychological professionals. In contrast with all of the previous disorders, personality disorders should *not* be assessed or discussed with the patient by the dental team. The focus with challenging personality traits and personality disorders is for the reader to gain the ability to interact skillfully and with minimal frustration for all concerned while providing excellent esthetic dental care.

The anxious patient

For most people, it is impossible to conceive of dental treatment without anxiety. It remains the most pervasive reaction to dental care, unfortunately, despite enormous advances in pain control, patient comfort, and dentists' management skills. Some patients are able to adequately manage their anxiety in the dental chair. However, many others are unable to cope with the anticipation and experience of some inevitable discomfort, and act out their anxiety through expressions of fear and dread, physical tension

Table 2.5 Diagnostic Criteria for Narcissistic Personality Disorder (NPD)

A. Significant impairments in personality functioning manifested by:
  1. Impairments in self functioning (a or b):
      a. Identity: excessive reference to others for self-definition and self-esteem regulation; exaggerated self-appraisal may be inflated or deflated, or vacillate between extremes; emotional regulation mirrors fluctuations in self-esteem.
      b. Self-direction: goal-setting is based on gaining approval from others; personal standards are unreasonably high in order to see oneself as exceptional, or too low based on a sense of entitlement; often unaware of own motivations.
  And
  2. Impairments in interpersonal functioning (a or b):
      a. Empathy: impaired ability to recognize or identify with the feelings and needs of others; excessively attuned to reactions of others, but only if perceived as relevant to self; over- or underestimate of own effect on others.
      b. Intimacy: relationships largely superficial and exist to serve self-esteem regulation; mutuality constrained by little genuine interest in others' experiences and predominance of a need for personal gain.
B. Pathological personality traits in the following domain: Antagonism, characterized by:
  1. Grandiosity: feelings of entitlement, either overt or covert; self-centeredness; firmly holding to the belief that one is better than others; condescending toward others.
  2. Attention seeking: excessive attempts to attract and be the focus of the attention of others; admiration-seeking.
C. The impairments in personality functioning and the individual's personality trait expression are relatively stable across time and consistent across situations.
D. The impairments in personality functioning and the individual's personality trait expression are not better understood as normative for the individual's developmental stage or sociocultural environment.
E. The impairments in personality functioning and the individual's personality trait expression are not solely due to the direct physiological effects of a substance (e.g., a drug of abuse, medication) or a general medical condition (e.g., severe head trauma).

while in the dental chair ("white knuckling"), and flinching at the slightest touch, to name just a few of the challenging behaviors that are all too familiar to every practicing dentist and hygienist.[16]

Some patients will have a diagnosed anxiety mood disorder, such as generalized anxiety disorder (GAD) or panic disorder, while others suffer from characteristic high anxiety as a personality style. Patients with an anxiety mood disorder will often be under psychiatric care for their mood problem, and will be taking medications such as antidepressants and anxiolytics (e.g., benzodiazepines). The medical history form should reveal these medication regimens, and as with all patients undergoing psychiatric care, you should, after assuring the patient of confidentiality and obtaining consent, consult with the patient's psychiatrist and psychotherapist to clear them for treatment and obtain guidance on possible drug interactions and specific management strategies. As always, you should generate a detailed treatment plan that is carefully reviewed with the patient until there is consensus on *realistic* goals and outcomes, and obtain the patient's signature of informed consent to this treatment plan.

Although the reasons for patient anxiety may appear to be self-evident, *the tremendous value in talking to the patient about his or her anxiety cannot be over-emphasized*. And while many dentists may not consider themselves to be strongly empathetic and may believe that it is impossible to learn empathy, the simple sentence "I notice you seem to be very anxious. Would you like to talk about it?" is really very easy to learn and deliver sincerely, no matter one's empathy level. Simply asking the question signals the patient that the dentist is aware and concerned, which makes the anxious patient begin to feel a bit safer and more open to relaxing or at least coping better. More often than not, the patient will reveal that he or she wants more information about the procedure.

With a small allocation of extra time to answer the patient's questions about what to expect, you can provide the patient with better mental preparation and greater ability to accept and brace for some unavoidable discomfort. Some patients appreciate being offered a hand mirror for observing the procedure, which gives those who want it a perceived measure of control that modulates their anxiety. Even the smallest attention on your part to the patient's anxiety provides the thing he or she seeks most: *validation* of his or her concerns. Simple validation—even when there is no possible modification in the procedure to improve actual patient comfort—can greatly mitigate the effects of patient anxiety and facilitate smoother and more successful treatment.

Many fine esthetic practices have found that offering relaxing, spa-derived amenities, such as personalized music systems, foot massage, and soothing aromatic oils in the operatory are both relaxing to patients and profitable to the practice. A number of noted dentists have also been motivated to learn and offer hypnosis to their anxious patients, to excellent effect. These special efforts require a small investment in time and resources relative to the large benefits in enhanced patient comfort, satisfaction, and subsequent referral rates.

The angry patient

As is the case with anxiety, the angry dental patient may be reacting to a situation, or be angry by disposition or personality. Situational anger triggers might include the perception of being poorly treated by your staff, harboring lingering resentment about a previous dentist's treatment, belief that your fees are excessive,[17] and even resentment of the patient's own dental condition that requires treatment and expense! There are also myriad reasons for patient anger which are entirely unrelated to the dental experience. Each patient presents for treatment with a distinctive array of personality traits, life pressures, and conflicts that they may proceed to express when they are in the vulnerable position of dental patient, often with significant verbal and nonverbal hostility to the dental team (Figure 2.7).

Whether the patient's anger is dispositional or situational, your focus should be on improved communication with the patient. Again, this does not require becoming the patient's psychotherapist. *Always* attempt to avoid responding to an angry patient with defensiveness, counter-argument, or confrontation, no matter the provocation, but rather maintain a posture of open curiosity and professionalism. A leading question, such as "You seem to be upset. Would you like to talk about it?" can defuse the patient's anger by giving him or her the chance to express the cause of his feelings, and give you a corresponding opportunity to take responsibility and ameliorate the problem (if, for example, the patient feels mistreated by the staff), or at least to express genuine sympathy or empathy, and thereby validating the patient's feelings. Again, the value of simple *validation*, even in the absence of a remedy, cannot be over-emphasized as a way to reduce tensions and facilitate the treatment process.[5]

If, after you have made such a sincere effort at communication, the patient persists with his or her hostile stance, you should strongly reconsider whether to continue with treatment or refer the patient to another office. The dental team is in no way required to withstand continued hostile behavior from a patient, particularly following sincere attempts to explore, mitigate, and validate the patient's complaints.

The demanding patient

This is the category of challenging patients who are considered to be demanding because they attempt to dictate elements of the treatment plan or the sequencing of treatment for reasons that are *not* related to financial constraints. These patients may, for example, demand that a tooth be restored with a bonded onlay when the dentist recommends a full crown, or that an anterior tooth be restored with esthetic bonding rather than a porcelain veneer, in both cases due to a strong preference for what they perceive as a more conservative treatment or because of suspicion that the dentist's recommendation is driven by profit over clinical necessity.[5,17] Another patient may demand that an esthetic reconstruction be done in phases, rather than more comprehensively. There are many more examples of demanding patients that experienced dentists can relate.

You are, by definition, being called on to improve the patient's appearance, with which the patient is, by definition, dissatisfied,

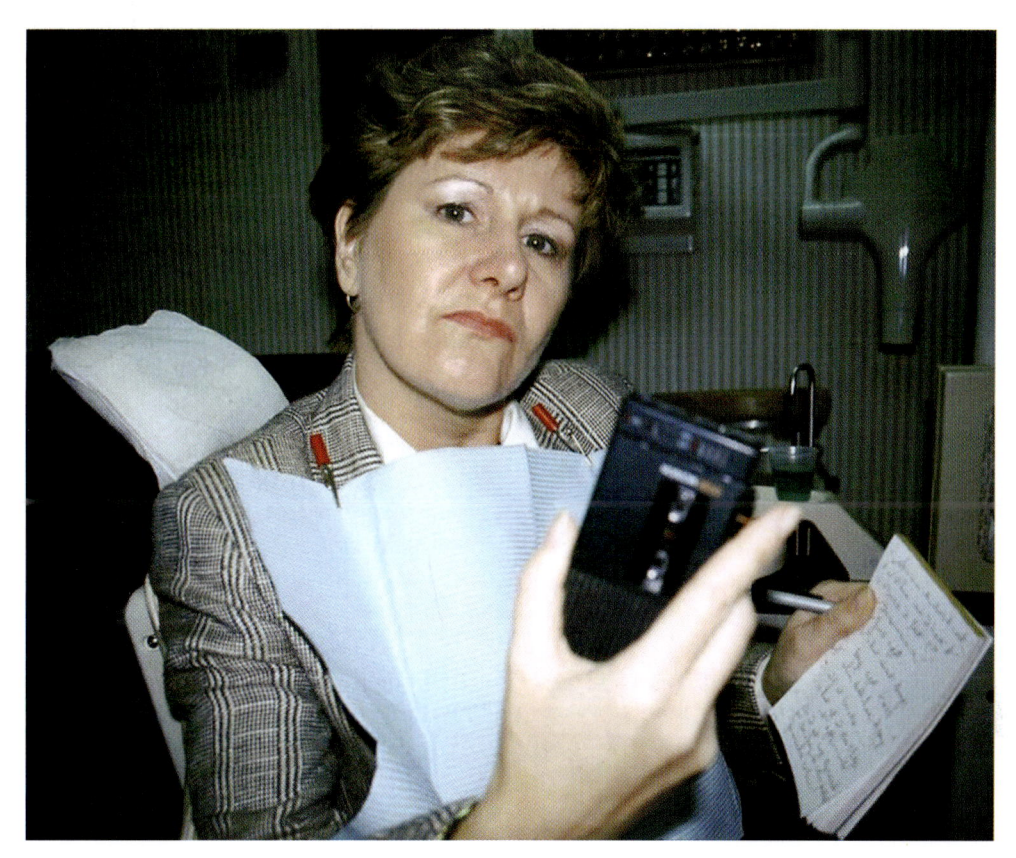

Figure 2.7 Angry patient preparing to record conversations with the dental team, due to previous dental experiences that have made her distrustful.

sometimes mildly, often extremely. Appearance is powerfully related to self-esteem, confidence, and social and professional success.[18–21] It follows, then, that patients seeking esthetic dental treatment will often present with demands, driven by trepidation about treatment outcome, but also by unsatisfying or unsuccessful previous dental experiences, or those of friends or relatives. This reality reinforces the urgent need, highlighted repeatedly throughout this chapter, for you to routinely spend extra time with patients at the very beginning of the relationship, in order to elicit—as thoroughly as possible—a sense of the hopes, fears, past negative experiences, and any other agenda that the patient may harbor, before commencing treatment. In addition to improving the congruence between the patient's esthetic goals and what you feel is realistically possible, this dialogue will afford the patient an opportunity to air any issues and particular demands, and you an opportunity either to modify the patient's demands through information and reassurance, or to assess your capacity to meet these demands (Figure 2.8).

You should make vigorous efforts not to ignore or dismiss such patient demands, because this is most likely to escalate their intensity and increase the possibility of anger, frustration, stress, and compromised treatment outcomes. Where you assess that the demand does not compromise the case, such as when it is an issue of sequencing, it is sometimes advisable to simply comply with the patient's request. However, when you feel that the special demands cannot be met without compromising treatment quality or treatment philosophy, you are entitled and advised

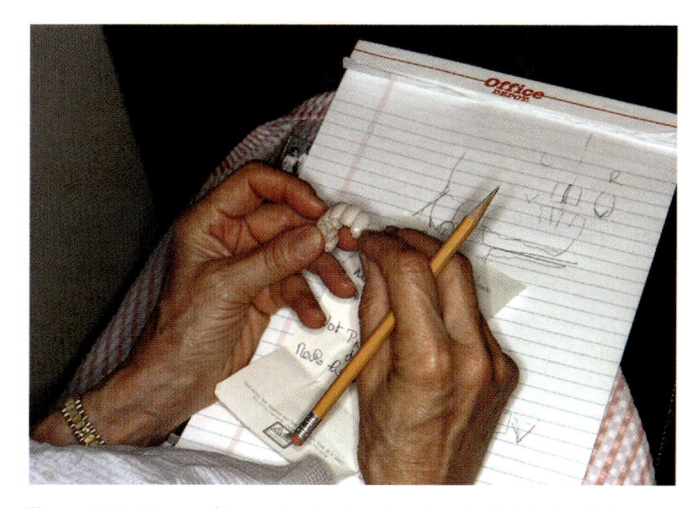

Figure 2.8 Demanding patient using drawing to dictate tooth form.

to strongly consider suggesting that the patient seek treatment elsewhere.

It is more likely that this extended assessment time will yield improved rapport and congruence between you and your prospective patient, and eventual treatment success. As ever, the treatment plan should be as detailed as possible with respect to the sequence and length of appointments, the appearance and maintenance of temporary restorations, the estimated total treatment time, and the appearance of the final result. Obtaining the patient's signed informed consent to treatment is especially necessary for this type of patient.

Treating the patient with Narcissistic Personality Disorder

The foregoing discussion has focused on describing the major personality types that are likely to present for esthetic dental care, and relatively common-sense strategies for improved management that require little extra effort for you and your team to implement, in the service of greater patient retention and satisfaction.

But what about the extremely challenging behavior exhibited by the patient in the case study at the beginning of this section? This question highlights an important consideration in esthetic dental practice: it is *vital* that you be self-aware enough to know your style and strengths with regard to interacting with highly challenging patients. If your honest self-assessment reveals that you would prefer not to treat patients with very challenging personality disorders, you should direct your screening efforts and policies to minimize acquiring such individuals as patients. By contrast, if you feel undaunted and well-equipped by temperament to serve even the very challenging patient personalities, you then need to consider how best to do so while minimizing conflicts and suboptimal outcomes.

How, then, might you approach treating the patient with a personality that is so extreme as to constitute a personality disorder—most commonly NPD—the typical attitudes and behaviors of which go well beyond what is considered within normal limits for demands and challenges on the part of dental patients? (Note: while NPD is just one of numerous recognized personality disorders, the others are less common and of lower concern to the dentist.) And if you prefer not to treat patients with NPD, how can they be screened during the first or second visit, before a commitment to working together has been made?

A critical feature often seen in a new patient with NPD is that the individual has previously visited one or more dentists and describes them in highly disparaging terms, usually coupled with giving you—the prospective new dentist—excessive, lavish praise and certitude, describing you as "of the very highest caliber, highly recommended, the best dentist." This behavior should immediately raise your suspicion and alert you to future challenges should you decide to accept the individual as a patient. Such information can often be elicited by any member of the team during the initial assessment by including in written or verbal form an assessment item such as: "Please tell us a little about your previous dental experiences." (Figure 2.9A and B).

An esthetic dentistry practice is more likely to attract such patients, as a review of the diagnostic criteria for NPD reveals, especially the grandiosity, preoccupation with beauty and success, and sense of entitlement. For this reason, accepting such patients into treatment is a decision that should be made after careful and clear consideration of your personal resources and tolerance for behavioral challenge, against the preference for serving as many patients as possible for a thriving practice. This is a decision that you should feel empowered to make on a case-by-case basis, taking into account such factors as your team's current level of patience and tolerance as well as the current health of your practice.

It is completely appropriate for you to refuse treatment and refer the patient elsewhere, indicating to the person that the team feels the practice is not a good fit for his particular needs. This may be awkward, but not nearly as uncomfortable as accepting such patients when you and your team are not up to the challenge.

Some patients with NPD will not be successfully screened, or you may simply decide to accept the individual as a patient, despite the probability of numerous challenges. In such cases, the following is a list of helpful strategies for reaching an agreeable and realistic treatment plan:

- Listen carefully to the patient during the initial interview, and note any extreme or possibly unrealistic demands or expectations, especially with regard to the esthetic goals.
- Schedule extra treatment planning time to review the patient's goals and expectations, with photographs if possible, and work toward congruence between patient goals and clinical realities.
- Develop and present a highly detailed treatment plan, and obtain the patient's signature of understanding and consent for the treatment plan, as well as office policies and fees for missed and broken appointments.
- Establish a clear understanding and agreement regarding the cost of treatment and schedule of payments; that is, agree with the patient in advance on when payments will be made and when treatment will be paid in full. The patient should sign the fee and payment agreement, which should be a standardized office form so that the patient does not feel singled out.
- Understand that it is likely the patient will at some point test the limits established earlier, and work out a consistent approach to dealing with this patient with the entire office team that is firm but flexible (when possible).
- Some dentists have a policy of raising fees for patients they anticipate will be behaviorally challenging. This solves the problem in two ways: (1) the patient may balk at the high cost and turn elsewhere, which saves you from the aggravation, or (2) if the patient accepts the higher fee, you will feel compensated for the extra time and management effort, and thus less stressed. There is no contraindication to this policy.

It is important for you to understand that every patient has a personality, and these span a spectrum from "normal" to disordered, with many shades between the extremes. This means that many people will present with personality challenges, some even characteristically "narcissistic." In fact, the very focus of esthetic dentistry on appearance inherently attracts some degree of self-focus. It is possible to characterize many patients who seek esthetic dentistry as "self-absorbed," maybe even somewhat grandiose and entitled, even if they do not meet the criteria for NPD. The dentist who attempts to screen out all such patients is likely to have a failing esthetic practice! Thus, it is best for you and your team to cultivate your own faculties of patience,

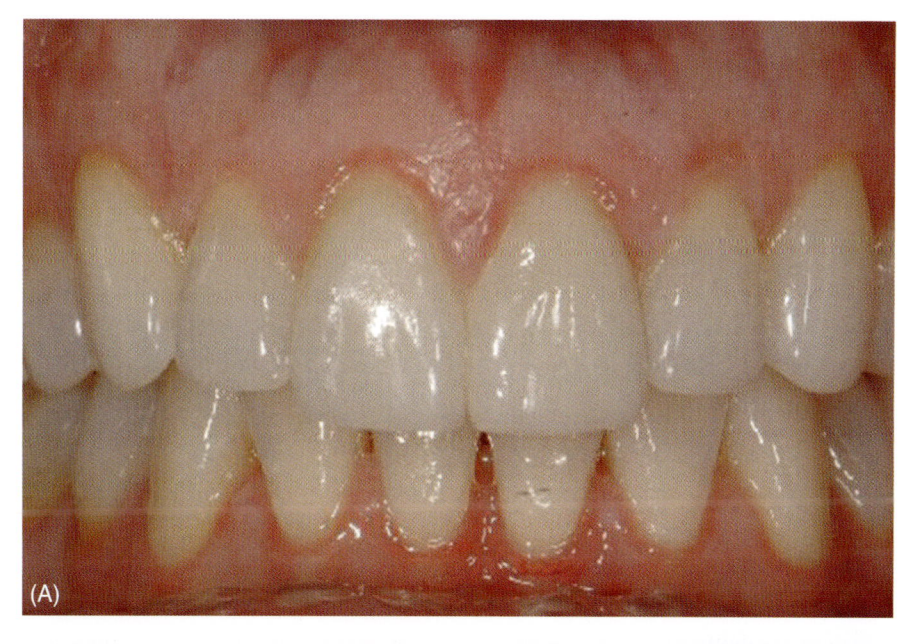

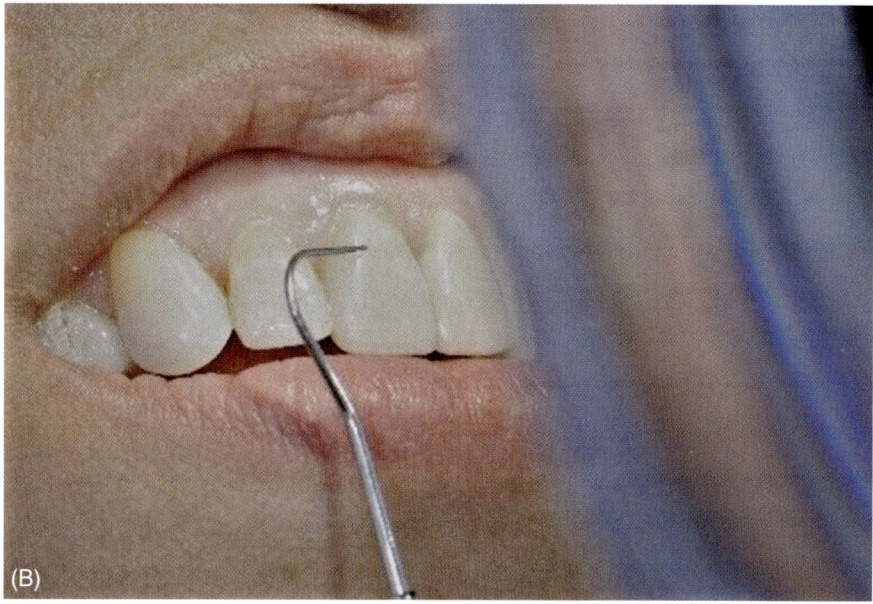

Figure 2.9 **(A)** This patient presented with slight discoloration on her central incisors. Two porcelain veneers were bonded in place after she signed the release form stating she "loved the results." **(B)** This photo captures one of many tiny complaints as she returned every 7–10 days for 3 months with her explorer. She was diagnosed with Body Dysmorphic Disorder and was successfully treated psychiatrically.

compassion, humor, creativity, emotional intelligence, and flexibility, and enjoy the many benefits in personal and professional satisfaction for being facile at managing the vast and varied range of patient personalities.

Life event stress and adjustment disorder

Just as every patient has a personality, so each person experiences life event stresses. Some of these will be unexpected—such as the death of a loved one, job loss, infertility, and divorce. Even planned and happy changes, such as wedding engagements, births, and job promotions, create stress in the individual, because they cause a disruption of homeostasis, which human physiology prefers.

There are also normative transitions that create life event stress. Adolescence is rife with such challenges, as is applying to college and graduate schools, job-hunting, pregnancy, parenting, children leaving home, parental aging, menopause, and retirement.

Most often, people experience heightened stress during such times of loss or transition, followed by adaptation and a return to their baseline functioning. When stressed individuals *do not* return to baseline after a reasonable period of reaction and poor coping, they may be diagnosed with an adjustment disorder (for diagnostic criteria, see Box 2.3). Adjustment disorders may engender either depressed or anxious moods or even both. If the patient is being treated with antidepressant or anxiolytic

> **Box 2.3 Diagnostic criteria for adjustment disorder.**
>
> The development of emotional or behavioral symptoms in response to an identifiable stressor(s) occurs within 3 months of the onset of the stressor(s). These symptoms or behaviors are clinically significant, as evidenced by either of the following:
> - marked distress in excess of what is expected from exposure to the stressor
> - significant impairment in social or occupational (academic) functioning.

> **Box 2.4 Diagnostic criteria for body dysmorphic disorder.**
>
> - Preoccupation with an imagined defect in appearance. If a slight physical anomaly is present, the person's concern is markedly excessive.
> - At some point during the course of the disorder, the individual has performed repetitive behaviors (e.g., mirror checking, excessive grooming, skin picking, reassurance seeking), or mental acts (e.g., comparing his or her appearance with that of others) in response to the appearance concerns.
> - The preoccupation causes clinically significant distress or impairment in social, occupational, or other important areas of functioning.
> - The preoccupation is not better accounted for by another mental disorder (e.g., dissatisfaction with body shape and size in AN).

medications, the dentist should follow the procedure detailed earlier: consent, consultation with the psychiatrist for medical clearance and clarification of any treatment precautions, and consultation with the psychotherapist for specific helpful management recommendations.

During times of transition and heightened stress—whether expected or not—many people will experience a wish to improve their appearance as a means of feeling better. Therefore, you are more likely than others to encounter new and existing patients experiencing life event stress and adjustment problems, from adolescents to younger adults, or, particularly in older adults, as part of an overall "makeover" that may include new diet and exercise regimens as well as cosmetic surgery.

Successful treatment of these patients requires sensitivity, sympathy, empathy, compassion, diplomacy, and possibly a little extra listening time. Knowing about and understanding the difficulties faced by people going through these life stage issues can be very helpful. To be successful, consider taking some time to educate yourself about these subjects, train your staff to be attuned to developments in patients' lives in order to pass on any important developments to you and any other clinicians in the office, and possibly include questions regarding any recent stresses in the medical history and update forms.

Catering to patients going through specific transitions, such as by spending extra time asking about the changes the patient is experiencing and following up thoughtfully at each visit, or offering to coordinate esthetic dental care with other specialists the patient may be seeing, can give patients going through difficult times the feeling of being understood and validated.

The dental patient with body dysmorphic disorder

Returning, finally, to the real-life vignette that introduced this chapter, my friend, the eminent dentist Dr J, was completely correct in assessing his new patient as having a problem so severe that he should not agree to treat her before she underwent successful psychological care. Dr J was aware of the unique challenges of patients with body dysmorphic disorder (BDD) seeking esthetic dentistry, and his new patient raised several significant red flags. She had a cosmetic defect that was minor, but her reaction to it was excessive, and her preoccupation with it was so chronically distressing that she was unable to function professionally. She harbored the delusional belief that since the crown was inserted she had become hideously ugly. She had seen numerous other dentists and cosmetic surgeons before Dr J, some of whom had found her unreasonable and somewhat menacing. This patient clearly had a delusional variant of BDD, the diagnostic criteria of which appear in Box 2.4.

BDD is a form of anxiety disorder that is classified as a subtype of OCD. It is appropriate for this chapter on management of challenging esthetic dental patients to begin and end with BDD, because while this syndrome is not highly prevalent in the population, studies have demonstrated that it is over-represented in the offices of cosmetic surgeons and esthetic dentistry practices.[22,23] Furthermore and most significantly, *patients with BDD should not be treated for their defect, whether real or perceived, unless and until they have been psychologically stabilized.*[22,23]

This recommendation is made to safeguard both patient and practitioner. Studies have shown that for most patients, treating the "defect" can intensify the preoccupation, or simply divert it to a new focus.[22,23] The patient in the case example had in fact presented to her previous dentist with excessive concern about the appearance of her premolar, but he failed to detect the BDD, and went on to crown the tooth. This resulted in a severe intensification of her psychological illness. Fortunately, although the patient became extremely debilitated and nonfunctional, she did not attempt suicide. This is a very real concern, since completed suicide in BDD occurs at an elevated rate. The rate of suicide attempt among patients with BDD has been estimated at 27.5%, and the rate of suicidal ideation has been estimated at 78%.[24]

Treating the "defect" also produced extreme duress for the treating dentist and his practice for months afterward, as the patient sought follow-up correction in a harassing manner that required drastic action in the form of changing phone numbers. In fact, the dentist was fortunate that no other protective measures were required, since it is a matter of record that individuals with BDD have stalked and attacked their cosmetic surgeons.[22] It is also an unfortunate fact that there are frequent lawsuits against cosmetic surgeons but there are no definite statistics regarding the proportion of individuals with BDD who bring lawsuits against their dentists.

It is *urgent* for the dental team to carefully assess the patient they suspect may have BDD before embarking on treatment. Although there is no single question that can disclose BDD, it is always recommended that any new patient be asked an open question about their chief complaint and their reason(s) for seeking treatment. Some "red flag" behaviors and responses that should raise suspicions during the initial interview include:

- excessive concern about a minor or imperceptible dental defect
- highly specific concern about the defect, often accompanied by diagrams and photos
- admitting to spending 1 hour or longer per day thinking about the defect and looking in the mirror, as well as chronic repeated mirror checking
- high dissatisfaction with previous treatment/dentist
- history of "doctor shopping"
- highly unrealistic expectations of treatment, such as belief that correcting the defect will yield professional or romantic success
- "camouflaging" behavior, such as habitually covering the mouth with a hand, scarf, or other item.

A number of other psychiatric disorders commonly co-occur with BDD, including depression, OCD, social phobia, and eating disorders. A history of drug and alcohol abuse is not uncommon, and, as mentioned, suicidal ideation is a frequent issue. Inquiring in the initial interview or medical history as to any history of these common comorbidities can help determine whether the patient indeed suffers with BDD.

Once you have further confirmed a suspicion of BDD, you should privately and sensitively inform the patient that you feel it is not in the patient's best interest to proceed with dental treatment at this time.[22-24] This discussion should be handled in a kind and considerate yet straightforward manner, attempting to avoid offending the patient, but also resisting any attempts by the patient to persuade you to treat. This is another excellent example of the great value of keeping an identified list of trusted local psychiatrists and psychotherapists whose contact information can be given to the patient immediately, greatly facilitating referral and acceptance of vitally needed psychiatric care. Cognitive behavior therapy (CBT) has been shown to be effective in treating patients with BDD, as have antidepressant medications, particularly SSRIs (Figure 2.10A–D).[22,23]

After the patient has been successfully stabilized psychologically, it may be possible for esthetic dental treatment to proceed. To Dr J's credit, he correctly assessed his patient, correctly deferred dental treatment and instead referred her for immediate psychological care. She was successfully treated with a

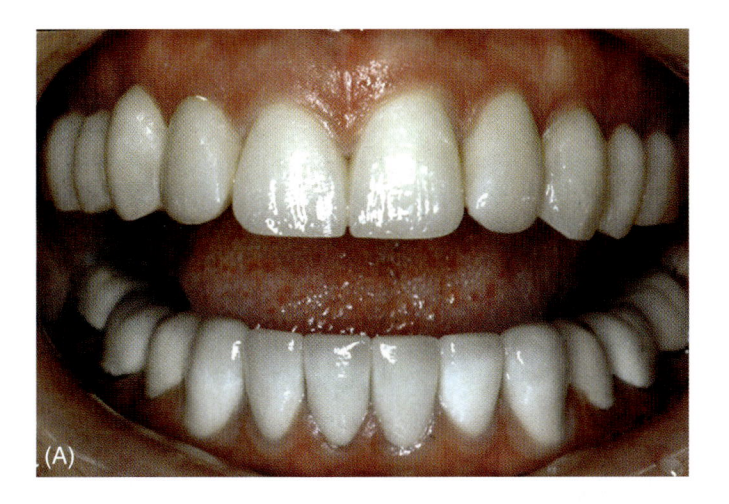

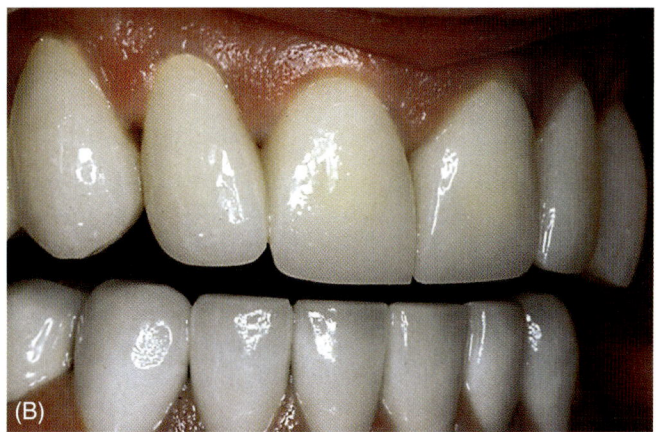

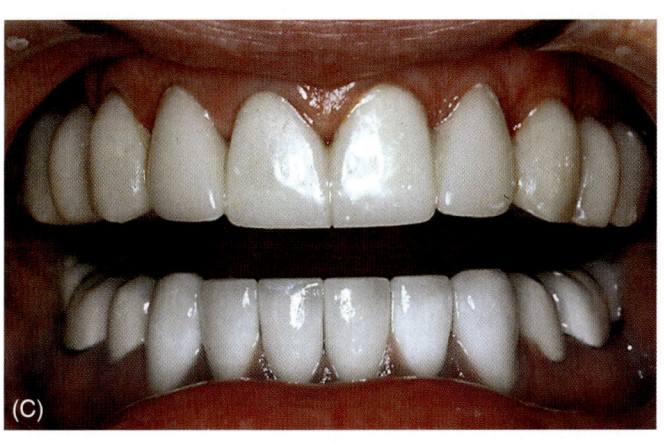

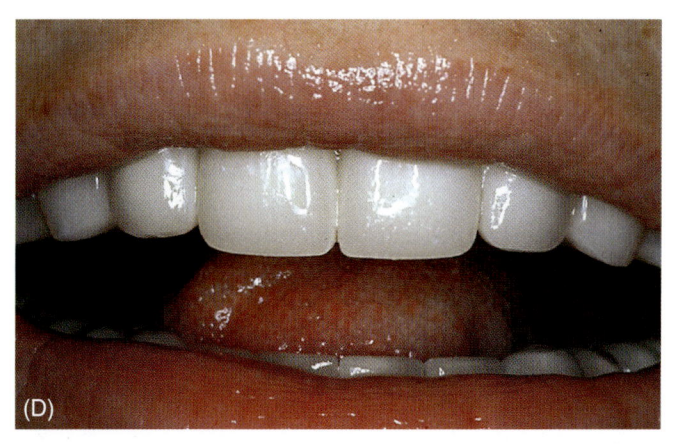

Figure 2.10 **(A–D)** Patient with body dysmorphic disorder (BDD) who required four different provisional bridges to wear on different occasions.

combination of psychotherapy and antidepressant therapy, after which Dr J was able to improve the patient's occlusion and dental esthetics to her satisfaction. He did this in close consultation with her treatment team for proper timing and staging of care, exemplifying the effectiveness of a team approach to care, with the dentist providing critical input and receiving needed guidance for a successful and stable outcome for this highly challenging patient.

Conclusion

You do not need to become a trained psychologist to become skillful at managing patients with mental illness and behavioral challenges. Teamwork, with your own staff and the patient's other medical providers, enhanced communication with patients, and the other basic guidelines described in this chapter can empower you and any motivated dentist to greatly improve your ability to not just tolerate the challenging patient, but experience personal gratification in handling such challenging cases. This is my hope. During our collaboration in treating the very difficult patient with BDD, my friend and colleague Dr J mentioned that it was important to his own sense of professional competence and value to be able to: (in his words): "help any patient in need of dental treatment, even one who is so mentally ill." With motivation and openness to some of the approaches described in this chapter, this enhanced personal competence is certainly within your reach.

References

1. National Institutes of Mental Health. *Statistics* 2015. http://www.nimh.nih.gov/health/statistics/prevalence/any-mood-disorder-among-adults.shtml (accessed September 20, 2017).
2. American Psychiatric Association. *Diagnostic and Statistical Manual of Mental Disorders*, 5th edn. Washington, DC: American Psychiatric Association; 2013.
3. Crow SJ, Peterson CB, Swanson SA, et al. Increased mortality in bulimia nervosa and other eating disorders. *Am J Psychiatry* 2009;166:1342–1346.
4. Goldstein RE, Golden R. Treating difficult and challenging patients, Part 1. *Contemp Esthet Restor Pract* 2003;7(5):20–23.
5. Goldstein RE, Golden R. Treating difficult and challenging patients, Part 2. *Contemp Esthet Restor Pract* 2003;7(8):16–19.
6. Beck AT, Ward CH, Mendelson M, et al. An inventory for measuring depression. *Arch Gen Psychiatry* 1961;4(6):561–571.
7. Keene JK, Galasko GT, Land MF. Antidepressant use in psychiatry and medicine: importance for dental practice. *J Am Dent Assoc* 2003;134:71–79.
8. Friedlander AH, Mahler ME. Major depressive disorder: psychopathology, medical management and dental implications. *J Am Dent Assoc* 2001;132:629–638.
9. Clark DB. Dental care for the patient with bipolar disorder. *J Can Dent Assoc* 2003;69:20–24.
10. Friedlander AH, Friedlander IK, Marder SR. Bipolar I disorder: psychopathology, medical management and dental implications. *J Am Dental Assoc* 2002;133:1209–1217.
11. Brown S, Bonifazi D. An overview of anorexia and bulimia nervosa, and the impact of eating disorders on the oral cavity. *Compendium* 1993;14(22):1594–1608.
12. Faine MP. Recognition and management of eating disorders in the dental office. *Dent Clin North Am* 2003;47:395–410.
13. DeBate RD, Tedesco LA, Kerschbaum WE. Knowledge of oral and physical manifestations of anorexia and bulimia nervosa among dentists and dental hygienists. *J Dent Educ* 2005;69(3):346–354.
14. DeMoor RJG. Eating-disorder-induced dental complications: a case report. *J Oral Rehabil* 2004;31:725–732.
15. DeBate RD, Tedesco LA. Increasing dentists' capacity for secondary prevention of eating disorders: identification of training, network, and professional contingencies. *J Dental Educ* 2006; 70(10):1066–1075.
16. Emodi-Perlman A, Yoffe T, Rosenberg N, et al. Prevalence of psychologic, dental, and temporomandibular signs and symptoms among chronic eating disorders patients: a comparative control study. *J Orofac Pain* 2007;22(3):201–208.
17. Bodner S. Stress management in the difficult patient encounter. *Dental Clin North Am* 2008;52:579–603.
18. Jacobsen A. Psychological aspects of dentofacial esthetics and orthognathic surgery. *Angle Orthod* 1984;54:18–35.
19. Davis LG, Ashworth PD, Spriggs LS. Psychological effects of aesthetic dental treatment. *J Dent* 1998;26:547–554.
20. Morley J. The role of cosmetic dentistry in restoring a youthful appearance. *J Am Dental Assoc* 1999;130:1166–1172.
21. Hofel L, Lange M, Jacobsen T. Beauty and the teeth: perception of tooth color and its influence on the overall judgment of facial attractiveness. *Int J Periodont Restor Dent* 2007;27:349–357.
22. Scott SE, Newton TJ. Body dysmorphic disorder and aesthetic dentistry. *Dental Update* 2011;38:112–118.
23. Naini FB, Gill DS. Body dysmorphic disorder: a growing problem? *Prim Dental Care* 2008;15(2):62–64.
24. Phillips KA, Coles ME, Menard W, et al. Suicidal ideation and suicide attempts in body dysmorphic disorder. *J Clin Psychiatry* 2005;66:717–725.

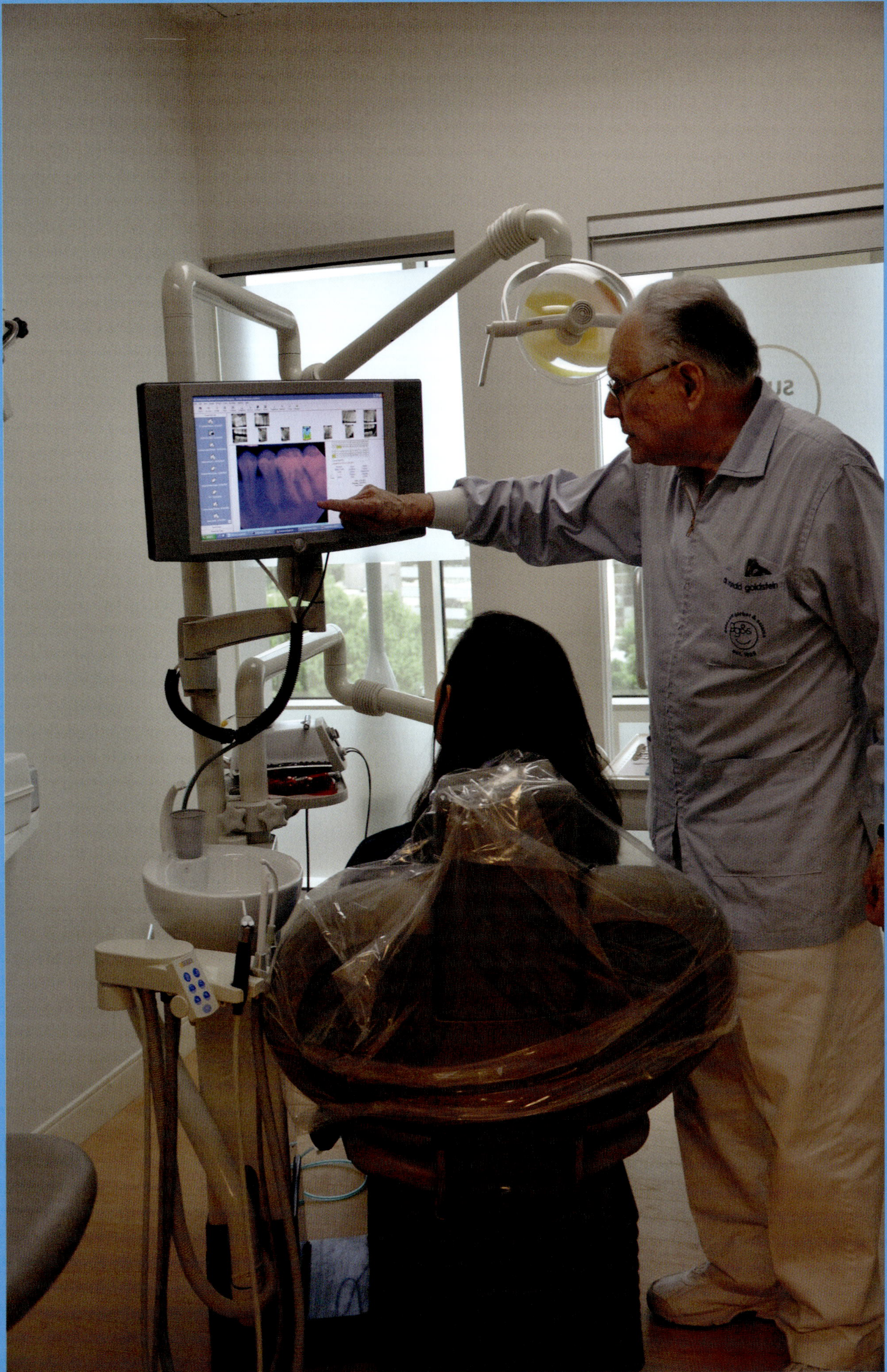

Chapter 3 Esthetic Treatment Planning: Patient and Practice Management Skills in Esthetic Treatment Planning

Ronald E. Goldstein, DDS and Maurice A. Salama, DMD

Chapter Outline

Mutual agreement and informed consent	48	Preparation of a preliminary treatment plan	70
Before the initial visit	48	The role of the treatment coordinator	70
Understanding your patient's personality	48	The Second appointment	70
Educational materials	49	Consulting a specialist	70
Provide a self-smile analysis	49	The final patient presentation	74
The initial visit	51	Problem patients: when not to treat … but refer	77
Important questions to ask	51	The perfectionist	77
Who examines the patient first: dentist or hygienist?	52	The poor communicator	77
What to look for	52	High expectations/limited budget	78
The role of the hygienist	53	The "wrinkle patient"	78
The clinical examination	55	The uncooperative patient	78
Patient examination	55	How to treat problem patients … and keep your staff sane	78
Esthetic evaluation chart	56	Continuous communication	79
Transillumination	56	Cost of treatment	79
Technology and an integrated digital system	67	Training and technical skill	80
Preparation for the second visit	67	Time and complexity of procedure	80
Review of radiographs	67	Artistic skill/patient requirements	80
Evaluation of diagnostic models	67	Overhead	80
Review of medical and dental histories	67	Warranty	81

There is no way to overemphasize the importance of comprehensive treatment planning. Achieving success in esthetic dentistry requires both time and attention to a thorough diagnosis followed by either a single best or alternate treatment plans. The patient who presents with what he or she perceives as a simple problem is still entitled to an expert diagnosis and forecast of any potential problems and ideas for present or future treatment. I have practiced this philosophy for over 50 years and have found that patients appreciate this service regardless of whether they chose to accept an ideal or compromised treatment plan.

Ronald E. Goldstein's Esthetics in Dentistry, Third Edition. Edited by Ronald E. Goldstein, Stephen J. Chu, Ernesto A. Lee, and Christian F.J. Stappert.
© 2018 John Wiley & Sons, Inc. Published 2018 by John Wiley & Sons, Inc.

The objective has and should be to let our patients know how they can not only look their best but also hopefully keep their teeth in good health for a lifetime.

Most esthetically motivated patients who first appear for consultation are eager to begin corrective treatment. Nevertheless, their enthusiasm and, at times, their self-diagnosis should not alter or influence your esthetic diagnosis. Failure to attend to this caution could lead to treatment failure.

Mutual agreement and informed consent

Although the functional aspect of every case should be the dentist's primary consideration, esthetics may well be the patient's *main* concern. Therefore, assurance must be given that success in esthetics is based on a careful and accurate complete diagnosis. In fact, ethically and legally, the dentist is obliged to inform the patient of various treatment alternatives. The standard of care diagnosis and treatment planning today is such that every patient needs to be considered from an interdisciplinary perspective. Regardless of whether or not you plan on referring your patients for specialty consultation, we have an obligation to either get that specialist opinion from others or take on the responsibility ourselves. The authoritarian concept that there is only one way to treat a problem and the old maxim "the doctor knows best" are both outdated. Once the treatment alternatives have been explained, the patient has the ultimate responsibility for making the decision to accept treatment. However, unless the patient's final decision for treatment is within the dentist's ethical and legal bounds, he or she should not be accepted for therapy into that particular practice.

> It is essential that the patient make an informed decision, after receiving from the dentist and staff a thorough explanation of his or her condition and the ramifications of treatment, including the advantages and disadvantages of each treatment alternative. Since this may take a considerable amount of time, much of it can and should be provided by a knowledgeable and experienced staff member. At the same time, the patient should be given printed or even video material for further consideration at home. There are numerous patient education short videos that can be easily attached to email or put on USB drives for the patient to review with his or her spouse, friend, relative, or significant other.

This is the new digital age of "informed consent." Printed information, whether reprints of various popular magazine articles or handouts especially prepared in the dental office, should support and give credibility to the treatment plan proposed. Presenting alternative treatment plans will also allow the patient to choose (usually with your advice) among alternative plans rather than alternative doctors. The dentist who gives the patient a one-choice solution to a complex esthetic problem may also be telling the patient, "Choose between me and my one plan, or find yourself another dentist." The wise dental consumer may elect to obtain a second opinion, to see whether other alternatives are available. New digital treatment planning tools and software are available today that are patient friendly, such as XCPT software, Consult-Pro, CASEY, and, on the implant side, Materialise and Kodak.

Before the initial visit

A patient's perception of the dental practice begins even before his or her first visit. It begins with the telephone call to schedule an appointment. The manner in which the potential new patient is handled by the receptionist, what is said and the tone over the telephone, helps to establish the desired image. If the potential new patient is not treated with professionalism, it may give the impression that the dental practice behaves this way as a whole. It is imperative that this screening is performed to correctly schedule the appropriate time and dentist.

Understanding your patient's personality

Esthetic treatment entails attention to pathology and function; it also requires attention to the patient's attitudes. These attitudes reflect the patient's self-image, which is the sum of appearance, personality, and position in the social milieu, as well as interrelationships with family, friends, business associates, and casual acquaintances.

Successful esthetic dentistry requires skills that involve more than the ability to diagnose and correct functional and pathologic irregularities. Each patient is an individual with a unique problem or concern and should be evaluated as a personality while considering the problem/solution diagnosis. The dentist who is able to master the art of understanding personalities and how to relate to each type will achieve greater treatment planning acceptance. Levin[1] identifies four personality types and suggests the proper response to each of these types.

1. **Driven**: bottom-line person, focuses on results, decides quickly, time-conservation oriented, highly organized, likes details in condensed form, businesslike person, assertive, dislikes small talk. Respond to this personality in a quick, efficient manner, and maximize use of appointment time.

2. **Expressive**: loves to have a good time, cheerleader type, wants to feel good, highly emotional, makes decisions quickly, dislikes details or paperwork, often disorganized and irresponsible, likes to share personal life. Respond to this personality by discussing the benefits of treatment through photographs and stories; engage in small talk, and sound excited.

3. **Amiable**: attracted by people with similar interests, reacts poorly to pressure or motivation, emotional, slow in making decisions, fears consequences, slow to change, a follower more than a leader. Manage this personality type by presenting information over a period of several visits.

4. **Analytical**: requires endless detail and information, technologic mind, highly exacting and emotional. Hardest of the four to reach a decision. Handle this personality type by providing additional information in the form of written, objective materials when suggesting a form of treatment.

The dentist and staff should master the identification of these four personality types. Understanding them and how to relate to each will enhance the doctor–patient relationship as well as the doctor–staff relationship. Interpersonal skills are just as important as technical skills. As Levin says, "After all, we are not just technicians; we are doctors to people."[1] Basically, a personal, communicative relationship between dentist and patient is required.

Educational materials

The dentist's first priority should be to start educating the patient about the techniques and philosophy of the esthetic dental practice. The more understanding that patients have regarding their dental problems and potential solutions, the easier and more effective the first and future meetings will be.

A consumer book like *Change Your Smile*[2] can be of immense value. It is important to have copies of the book (Figure 3.1A) in the reception area and to give or loan a copy of the book for new patients prior to their first visit or certainly prior to discussing various treatment plans. In addition to broadening their understanding of esthetic dentistry, the book helps to prepare them to anticipate realistic fee scales for the various esthetic procedures, each of which is discussed in detail including fee range, advantages, disadvantages, results of treatment, maintenance required by the patient, and realistic esthetic results. This book explains the differences in esthetic dentistry treatment. For example some treatments require payment in advance and insurance rarely covers the costs of such treatments. It is best to give or loan a copy to each new patient before the first visit. Copies can be purchased from the publisher and given to each patient. When purchased in bulk it can be an economical marketing tool for the dental office. This book explains procedures and fees, even for those who are not referred specifically for cosmetic dentistry (Figure 3.1B).

Provide a self-smile analysis

A self-smile analysis, or comparable index, should be explained and made available to the patient before their first visit (Figure 3.2). The importance of such a self-evaluation cannot be overstated. Through this self-analysis, you can begin to recognize and understand the problems uppermost in the patient's

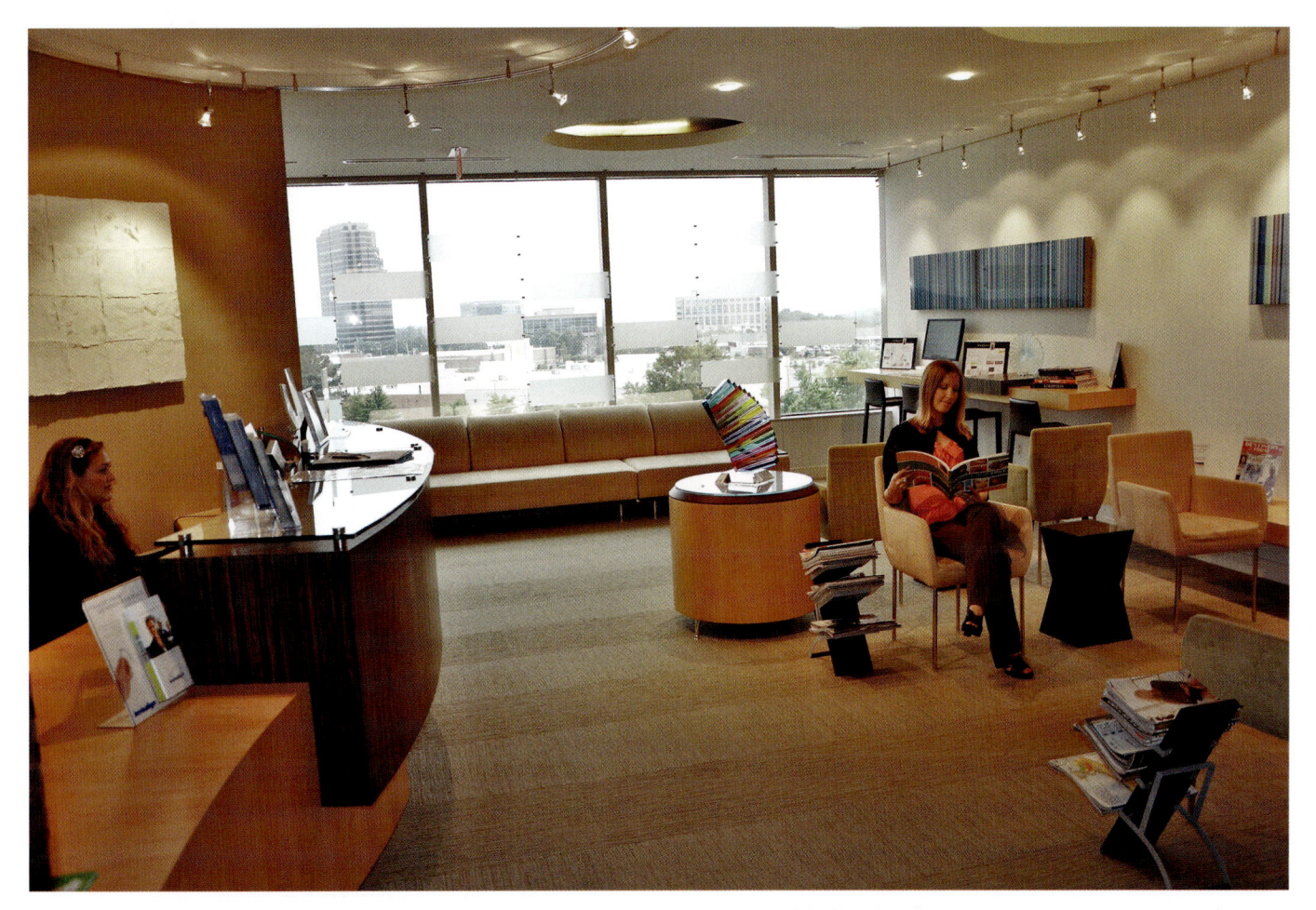

Figure 3.1 **(A)** Although it is best for new patients to receive and read *Change Your Smile* before their first appointment, it is important to have copies in your reception room to reeducate your existing patients.

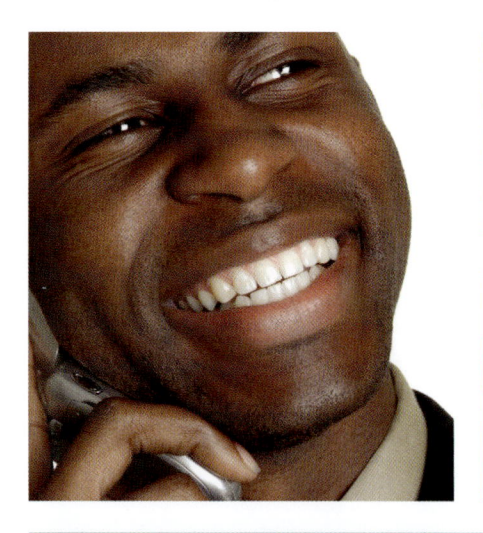

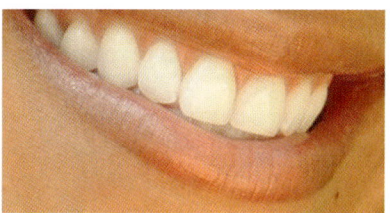

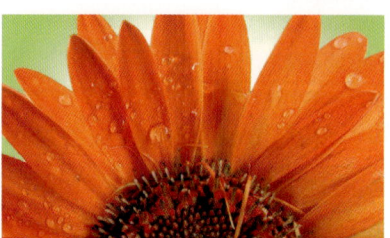

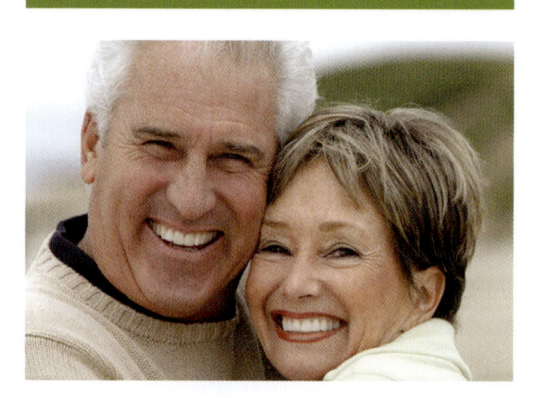

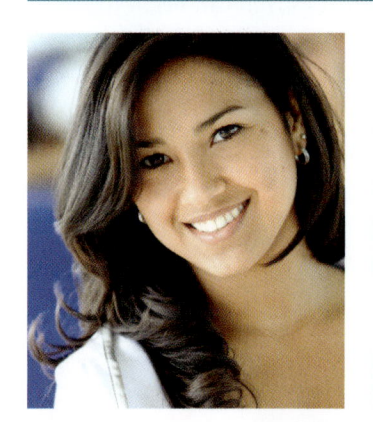

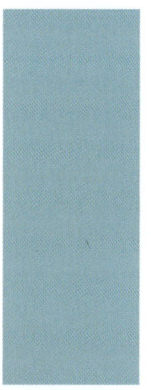

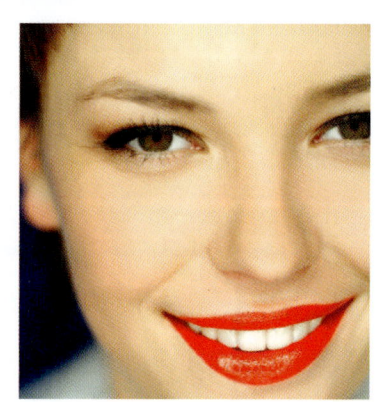

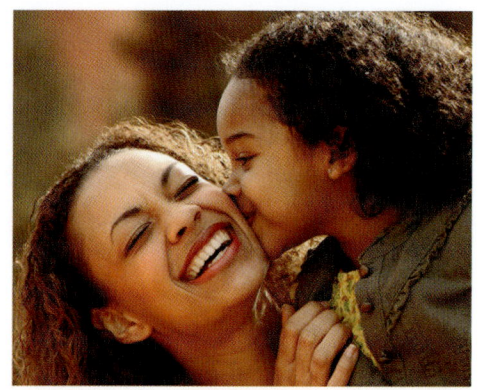

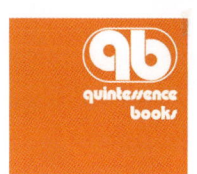

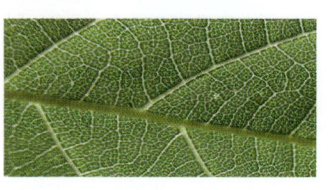

Figure 3.1 (B) A major advantage of having patients review *Change your Smile*[2] before presenting your treatment plan is for them to view realistic fee ranges, advantages, disadvantages, treatment results, and required maintenance for most all esthetic treatments. From *Change Your Smile*, 4th edn. Ronald E. Goldstein, DDS. Reproduced with permission of Quintessence Publishing Co Inc., Chicago.

mind concerning his or her appearance, particularly as he or she is affected by the face, mouth, and smile. It also serves as a documented and convenient starting point for a specific discussion of esthetic treatment that will be workable for the dentist and satisfying to the patient. The self-smile analysis provides a means by which the dentist can avoid two common errors: the beliefs that patients care little about their smiles and that they are willing to accept any recommended course of treatment. Experience indicates that if you accept at face value a patient's remarks such as "If it's good and it lasts, I really do not care what it looks like" or "You are the doctor," you may soon have a dissatisfied patient. Memories can be short, and patients may easily forget the condition of their mouth before treatment, choosing instead to concentrate on anything, however trivial, that they regard as an imperfection. Such reactions illustrate again the depth and breadth of consideration, somatic and psychological, involved in esthetic treatment, and they point to the practical and esthetic value of the self-smile analysis.

SMILE ANALYSIS

Yes No TEETH

☐ ☐ 1. In a slight smile, with teeth parted, do the tips of your teeth show?
☐ ☐ 2. Are the lengths of your central incisors in good proportion with your other front teeth?
☐ ☐ 3. Are the widths of your central incisors in good proportion with your other front teeth?
☐ ☐ 4. Do you have a space (or spaces) between your front teeth?
☐ ☐ 5. Do your front teeth stick out?
☐ ☐ 6. Are your front teeth crowded or overlapping?
☐ ☐ 7. When you smile broadly, are your teeth all the same light color?
☐ ☐ 8. If your front teeth contain tooth-colored fillings, do they match the shade of your teeth?
☐ ☐ 9. Is one of your front teeth darker than the others?
☐ ☐ 10. Are your six lower front teeth straight and even in length?
☐ ☐ 11. Are your back teeth free of stains and discolorations from unsightly restorations?
☐ ☐ 12. Do your restorations—fillings, porcelain veneers, and crowns—look natural?
☐ ☐ 13. Do any of your teeth have visible cracks, chips, or fractures?
☐ ☐ 14. Do you have any missing teeth that you have not replaced?

GUMS

☐ ☐ 15. When you smile broadly, do your gums show?
☐ ☐ 16. Are your gums red and swollen?
☐ ☐ 17. Have your gums receded from the necks of your teeth?
☐ ☐ 18. Do the curvatures of your gums create half-moon shapes around each tooth?

BREATH

☐ ☐ 19. Is your mouth free of decay and gum disease, which can cause bad breath?

FACE

☐ ☐ 20. Do your cheeks and lip area have a sunken-in appearance?
☐ ☐ 21. Does the midline of your teeth align with the midline of your face?
☐ ☐ 22. Do your teeth complement your facial shape?
☐ ☐ 23. Is the shape of your teeth appropriately masculine or feminine for your overall look?

Figure 3.2 The advantage of having your patients complete a self-smile analysis like this one is to help them visualize and communicate to you all potential problems before treatment planning is initiated. From *Change Your Smile*, 4th edn. Ronald E. Goldstein, DDS. Reproduced with permission of Quintessence Publishing Co Inc. Chicago.

There are several ways to get a self-smile analysis form accessible to your patients:

1. Email a copy of your selected version to each new patient, or make it available to download from your practice website.
2. Include it in an information package you mail to new patients.
3. Provide *Change Your Smile*[2] and have them use the self-smile analysis form (p. 4; Figure 3.2).

The advantage of this last method is that *Change Your Smile* contains so much more additional information. It will provide your new patient with treatment alternative summary sheets that will give them more insight into their esthetic problem.

The initial visit

The dentist–patient relationship is the necessary foundation for any satisfactory course of treatment. It must be encouraged and developed from the beginning and is most important in esthetic dentistry. The patient must feel at ease. To this end, a neat, well-ordered, attractive, and comfortable reception area is an obvious prerequisite (see Chapter 5 on marketing). The first visit, which may or may not involve a functional procedure, is the best time to intensify the communication process. The patient's first impression, if positive, will serve as reinforcement for subsequent treatment. If negative, it can be harmful to the atmosphere of candor and trust essential to successful esthetic treatment.

Important questions to ask

Why are they here?

There is no more important information than why the patient came to see you. This is not to be confused with your patient's major complaint. Rather, why are they at your office instead of another? And why did they leave another office (or offices) for yours? Frequently, this information can reveal valuable insight into your patient, his or her fears, needs, desires, and expectations. These may not necessarily be related to a specific dental condition.

Who referred your new patient?

This information can be quite helpful in determining what concerns your new patient has regarding his or her dental needs. One basic problem is that many individuals choose not to disclose this information, not wanting to prejudice you in rendering your opinion. The fear is that you may "slant" your treatment plan based upon the referring patient rather than offer completely objective analysis.

Reasons for patients prefer not to disclose referral source include the following.

1. There is less chance that the dentist can estimate their financial status, which may or may not be the same as that of the referring patient.
2. The patient wants an objective, unbiased opinion.
3. They fear that you might disclose their condition or treatment to the referring patient and they don't want this information disclosed

Therefore, always respect your new patient's right of privacy, especially at first. Often, the referral source will later become known, usually through casual conversation.

Who examines the patient first: dentist or hygienist?

There is always the question of who should see the patient first—you or your hygienist. There are advantages and disadvantages to each being the first contact. (See Figure 3.3 for a typical flow of patient contacts in a practice for comprehensive dental treatment.) Even if the patient wishes an appointment only for a prophylaxis, it may be important for you to see and meet the patient first. Not only is it valuable for you to identify your new patient's primary concerns, it is also quite helpful for you to examine the patient before your hygienist alters the appearance of the mouth (Figure 3.4A). One definite advantage of this is to be able, if necessary, to place the patient in a soft tissue management program before a prophylaxis is scheduled. This can also emphasize to the patient just how essential it is to have healthy tissue before any esthetic treatment is planned (Figure 3.4B). Observe calculus, stains, and baseline oral disease in order to be of maximum help to your patient. Also, be sure to take *photographic records before a prophylaxis removes stains or other visible evidence* of just how your patient performs oral care.

What to look for

Prehygiene: look at the patient and observe the following:

1. **Stains**: what types and severity?
2. **Calculus**: how much and the length of time since the last prophylaxis.
3. **Plaque**: most patients attempt to brush their teeth as well as possible before a dental appointment, so if your patient has a great deal of plaque present it should give you a good idea of how the patient's oral hygiene is lacking.
4. **Habits**: a hygiene appointment could erase valuable evidence left by any harmful habits the patients may have. Examples are heavy smokers or coffee drinkers whose stains would be eliminated after prophylaxis. Therefore, make sure you examine any new patient before a hygiene appointment.

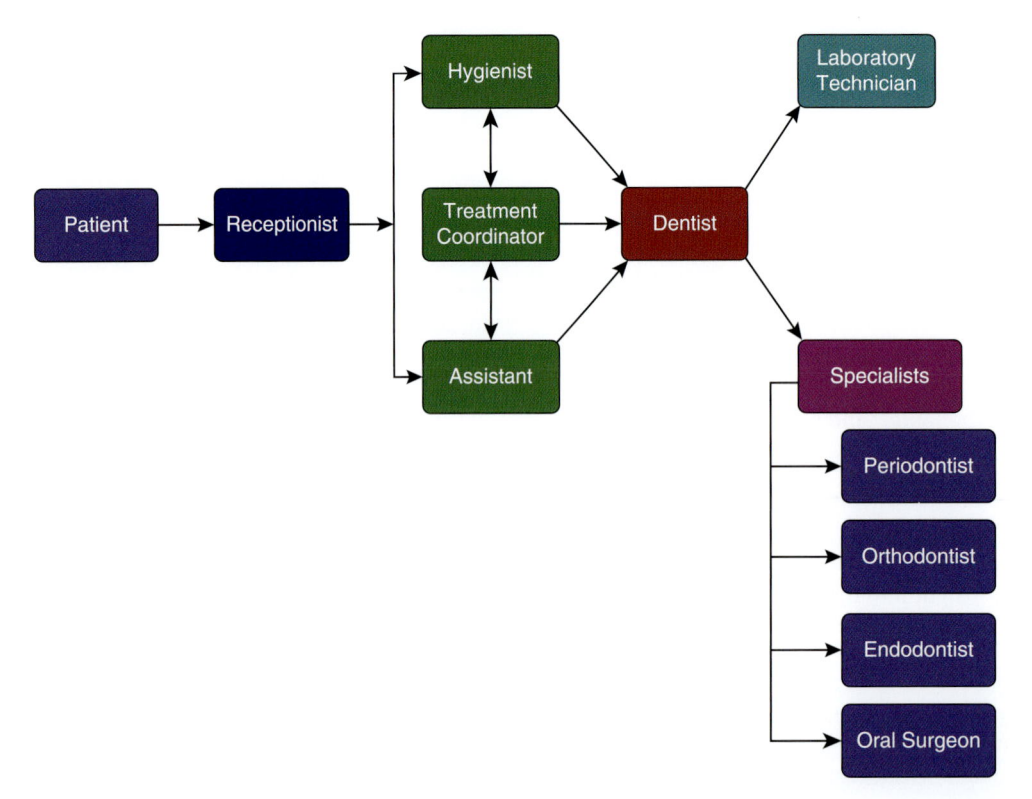

Figure 3.3 Typical sequence of patient office contacts.

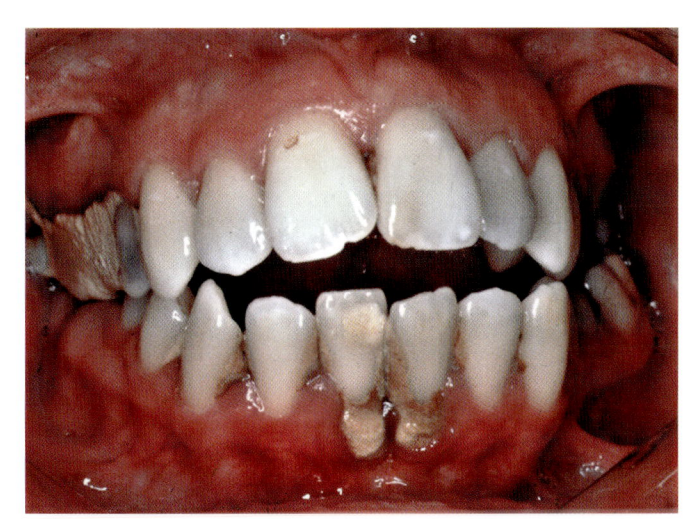

Figure 3.4 (A) A sense of inferiority can create a depression that occasionally causes patients to become desperate about their self-image. In this case, the 28-year old woman was so ashamed of her appearance that she balked at even opening her mouth.

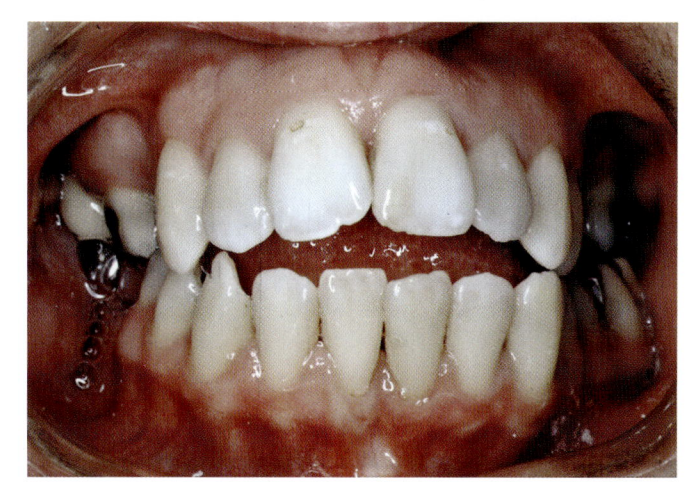

Figure 3.4 (B) The first step was soft tissue management to eliminate inflammation.

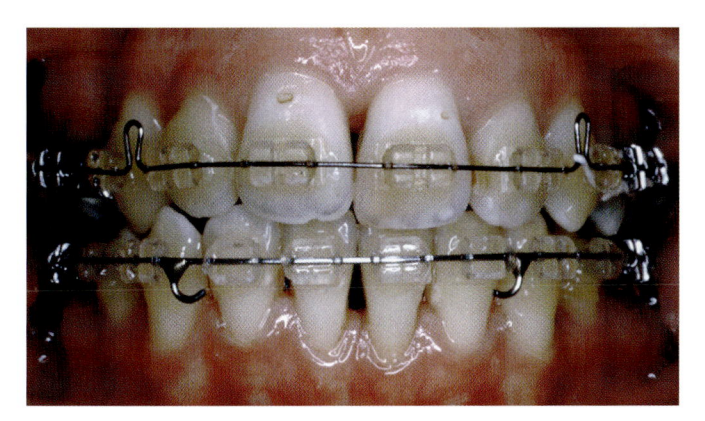

Figure 3.4 (C) Orthodontic treatment corrected the open bite.

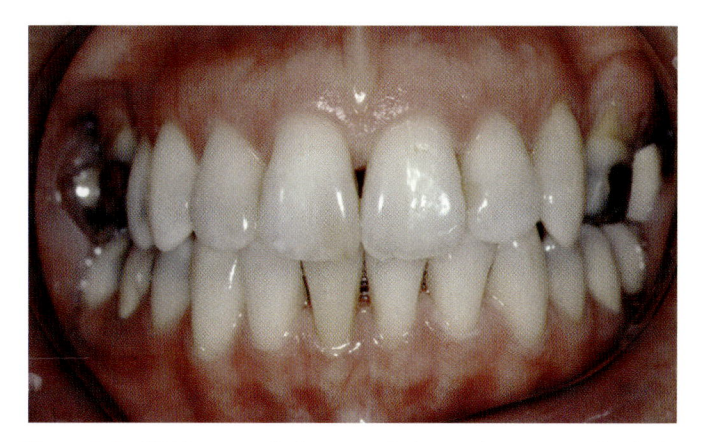

Figure 3.4 (D) The reward of an extended consultation period to help overcome a fear of dentistry is the acceptance of combined therapy to achieve an esthetic result.

5. **Attitude**: another reason to meet the patient before the hygiene appointment is to get a better idea of the patient's personality. After a 30- to 50-minute hygiene appointment, the patient may be stressed, out of time, or even non-communicative.

Remember, you can uncover important information during this initial interview, and it is imperative to ascertain that you have sufficient information to develop a comprehensive treatment plan. The more difficult the esthetic problem, the more time is required for patient information gathering. Failure to obtain even one critical piece of patient information can make the difference between esthetic success and failure. Sources of this essential information may include the receptionist, dental assistant, hygienist, dental laboratory technician, and treatment coordinator. Although we assume that all of the above individuals have contact with the patient, valuable information can also be gained by involving your laboratory technician with the patient's esthetic concerns. In most cases, the laboratory technician will be able to tell you whether the technical problems involved can be easily overcome. This information is also essential before finalizing your patient's treatment plan because, for example, your fee

and that of the technician can vary considerably based on the technical requirements involved (Figure 3.4C and D).

The role of the hygienist

The hygienist may be the second, third, or fourth member of the treatment team the patient meets. However, the hygienist usually is the first who actually performs treatment and therefore must be fully proficient in hygienic techniques and subtle investigation while maintaining a reassuring manner. Often the hygienist will develop a special relationship with your patient. This rapport can result in learning crucial information that can make your treatment a success or warn you of possible failure. The hygienist must be both inquisitive and observant enough to help discover potentially harmful habits and bring them to the attention of both the patient and you. Such habits include lip, cheek, or nail biting, chewing ice or other foreign objects, or grinding of teeth. As the teeth are being cleaned, the patient's desires in regard to esthetic treatment can and should be determined. Preliminary observations can be made concerning obvious discolorations,

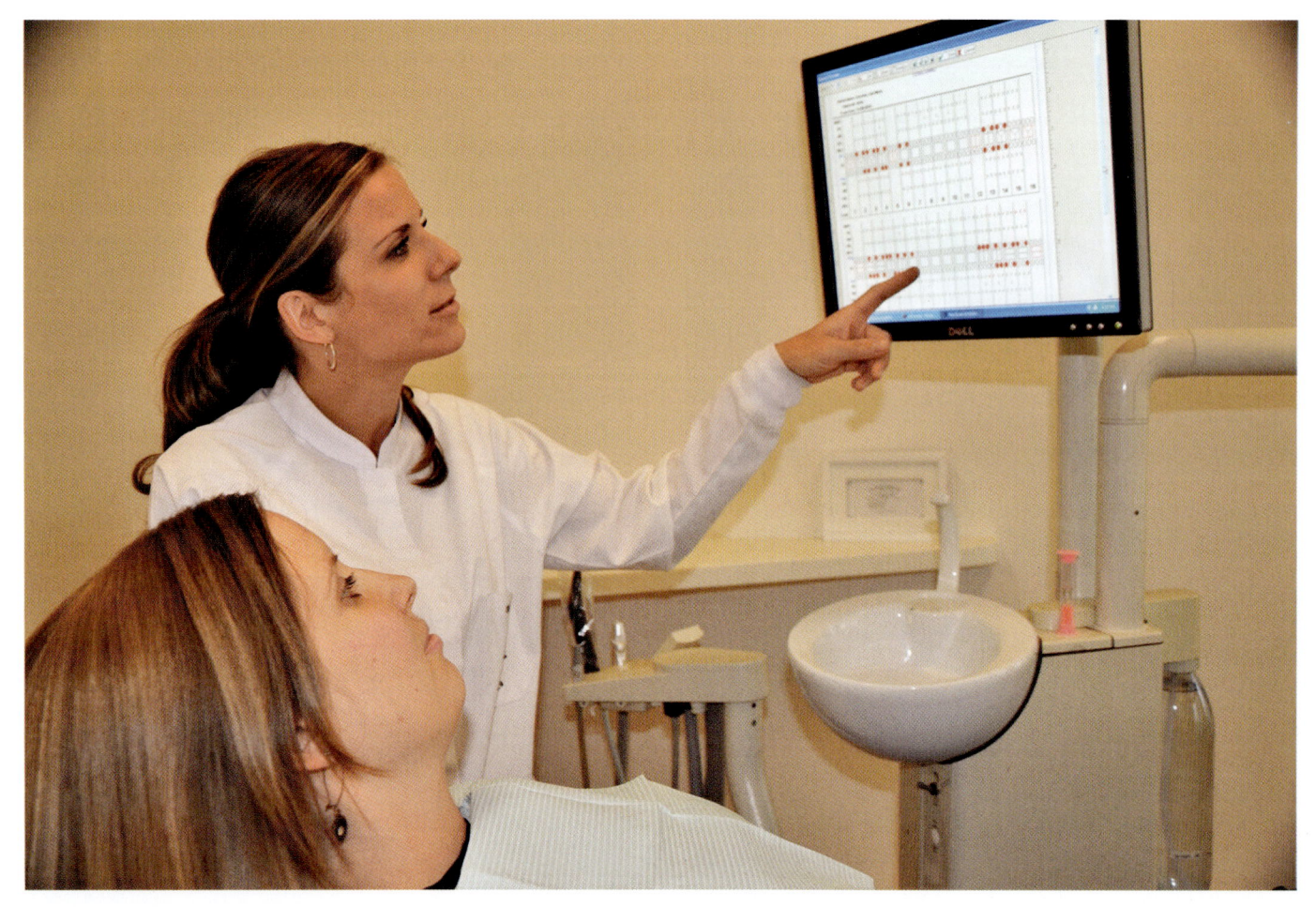

Figure 3.5 **(A)** The rapport between hygienist and patient often can help uncover a patient's interest in esthetic dentistry.

necessary restoration, ill-fitting crowns, and so on. The approach can be in the form of a question, such as, "Does this concern you? If so, the doctor may be able to correct it." The possibility and applicability of esthetic treatment should be of central concern, but the concern should not manifest itself at this time as direct recommendations or specific advice to the patient. The hygienist must be alert to cues that indicate a patient's interest in esthetic dentistry. A patient who covers his or her mouth when laughing is making a wordless, vitally important statement. Lips pulled tightly over the teeth, constricted cheeks, or a tongue pressed against a diastema are subconscious signals from the patient. Directly or indirectly, they express a patient's concern for his or her appearance. The hygienist should communicate these observations to the dentist in private. Our office has found it extremely useful to have intraoral cameras available for the hygienist to utilize for each patient. I especially like to walk into the operatory to do my periodic examination only to find several pictures already up on the monitor. This means the hygienist has already informed and shown areas to the patient that she would like me to check. Even if I feel the specific problem may not need treatment at present, patients appreciate the hygienist always looking out for possible problem areas that might be a future concern (Figure 3.5A).

At the initial visit, the patient may see the dentist for a comparatively brief time. This depends upon the patient's ability and desire to spend up to several more hours for the "second visit" at the same appointment. If the patient is from out of town, it is usually advisable to plan both first and second visits at the same appointment to reduce the patient's travel time and costs. This may also be a reason to send the out-of-town patient a copy of *Change Your Smile*[2] (Figure 3.1B) in advance of the appointment since the final diagnosis may well be presented in one day.

Good rapport must be established while convincing the patient that only after a thorough study of radiographs and other diagnostic aids will treatment alternatives be suggested. In addition to a medical and dental history, thorough charting of both periodontal and general tooth conditions, diagnostic models, occlusal analysis, and digital color photographs are taken at this visit (Diagnodent, Kavo, USA). Normally, specific suggestions should be postponed until the second visit. At that time, you should examine and discuss treatment alternatives as well as the patient's own esthetic evaluation as it is revealed in the self-smile analysis unless the patient has previously completed this self-examination.

The clinical examination

Every new patient receives a clinical examination. For the patient who is primarily interested in cosmetic dentistry, an esthetic clinical evaluation is mandated. This patient may have already received a prophylaxis, radiographs, examinations, and treatment plans from several other offices. Therefore, the initial appointment with you may be specifically for an esthetic evaluation, and more time should be reserved to listen to the patient's problem and desires. The remainder of the appointment is focused on the non-esthetic but functional clinical analysis.

Patient examination

Although the entire stomatognathic system should be evaluated, there are three main components of any clinical examination:

- facial analysis
- evaluation of the teeth, occlusion, and arch arrangement
- determination of the periodontal status.

Note: for more advanced cases, 3D cone beam computed tomography (CBCT) may be performed as part of this examination. The order in which you perform these specific functions is not important, just as long as you spend sufficient time on each one. At Goldstein, Garber, and Salama, we do the facial analysis first.

Teeth and arch examination

Regardless of which chart you use, a tooth-by-tooth examination is essential to verify functional as well as esthetic limitations for the desired treatment. As basic as it may sound, there is no substitute for an extremely sharp explorer. Although some schools may be moving away from explorer use, I find it extremely helpful in verifying restoration margins and particularly subgingival crown margins.

> It is virtually impossible to visually determine the soundness of each individual tooth. Saliva, plaque, and food deposits can too easily fill a defective margin and make it appear "perfect." The absence of stain around a leaking or defective margin may make it easy to overlook the necessity of including that tooth in your treatment plan. Therefore, each surface of each tooth should receive a thorough evaluation. Magnifying lenses of 2.5 diopter or greater are extremely valuable tools in being able to properly detect defective restorations as well as other defects.

There are two technologies that I have found indispensable. Both the chairside microscope and intraoral camera provide essential views for precise tooth surface exams. The microscope can provide a brilliant and clear extreme close up of tooth restoration defects. Microcracks can be so clearly seen and photographed while the patient discovers them on the chairside monitor and sees them through the stereoscopic lens. Then there is the use of the intraoral camera which will not only support your findings but also may reveal to you other deformities not seen by either the naked eye or with the aid of magnifying loops. The intraoral camera also has the ability to easily transilluminate and photographically record hidden microcracks that could easily alter your treatment plan. This photographic or video examination of the mouth can also make you aware of potential pit and fissure problems or hidden surface caries that could be overlooked in your visual examination or even missed with the explorer. I also consistently make use of a hand-held laser caries detection device (Diagnodent) to evaluate any suspicious pits and fissures (Figure 3.5B). Finally, an intraoral camera provides

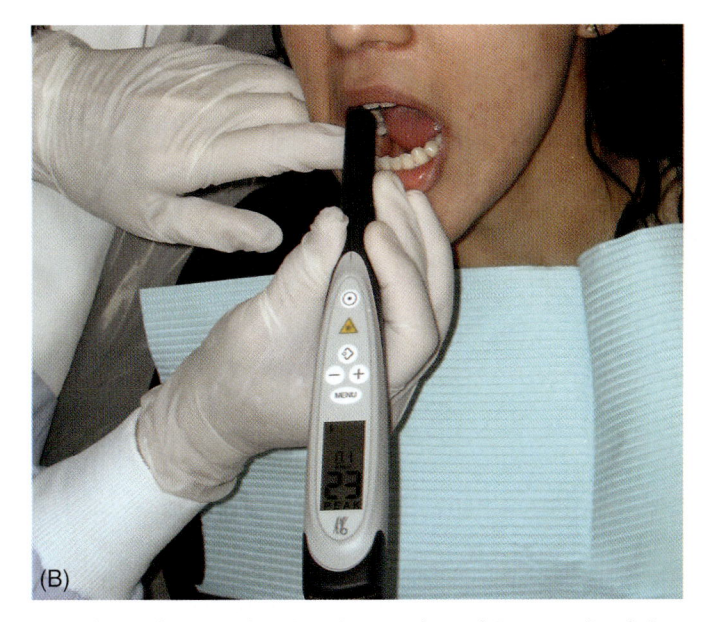

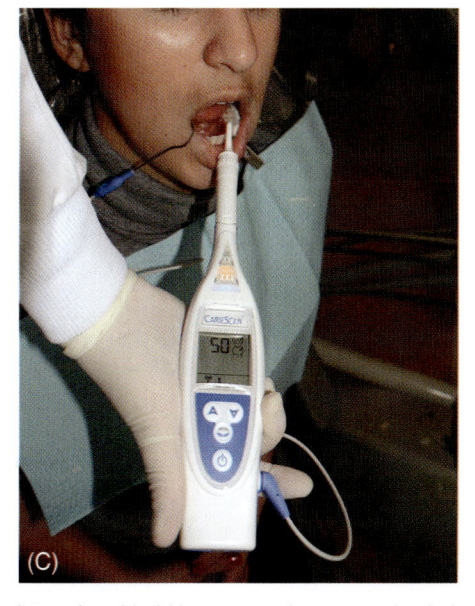

Figure 3.5 **(B and C)** Both Diagnodent (Kavo) in panel B and Cariescan (Ivoclar) in panel C are hand-held laser caries devices used to help evaluate any suspicious pits and fissures.

for easier and more accurate communication with your patient so that he or she can more readily understand the reasons for your treatment recommendations. Pay particular attention to cervical and incisal erosion as well as any large, defective restorations.

At what point do you suggest crowning versus the more conservative treatment of bonding, veneers, or porcelain inlays or onlays? Esthetically and functionally, it may be much better to conserve the labial (or lingual) enamel rather than reduce it to place a crown. This is one instance where patients should be given a choice after being informed of the advantages and disadvantages of each treatment option. Frequently, informed patients will opt for the more costly but more conservative procedure.

Arch alignment

Arch integrity should be evaluated both vertically and horizontally. Although orthodontics can correct most arch deformities, restorative treatment frequently can provide an acceptable esthetic and functional compromise. Determine the plane of occlusion and analyze just how discrepancies will affect the ability of your ceramist to create occlusal harmony. Slight irregularities in tooth-to-tooth position can make such a difference in the final arrangement that it always pays to take adequate study casts and then double-check your initial visual analysis to ensure that you can achieve the occlusal and incisal plane you wish. I have estimated that approximately 50% of my new patients over the years have had orthodontic consultations prior to arriving at a treatment plan. Years ago I coined the phrase "compromise orthodontics" whereby the teeth are moved into a better but not perfect position. This can allow a better restorative result than if the teeth were left in their original position. Now, with Invisalign so many more adults are accepting orthodontic treatment than ever before because the technique eliminates visible brackets of any kind, which can be a turn off for many adult patients.

Periodontal evaluation

Evaluation of bone support, tissue recession, tooth mobility, bleeding points, and periodontal pockets all have tremendous influence on your ability to achieve an esthetic as well as functional result (Figure 3.5C). Presence or absence of appropriate ridge tissue also can change the treatment approach. A major reason for predestined esthetic failure is a failure to realize the negative factors involved.

If your patient has a periodontal condition that you feel will not heal with routine prophylaxis treatment, you may first wish to institute soft tissue management procedures. This is especially important if the final treatment plan could vary, depending on how successful the soft tissue management therapy will be. In fact, spending extensive time establishing your patient's entire treatment plan at this time could be counterproductive. What may appear to be the best plan of action now could be considerably altered depending on not only your therapy, but also on how well the patient follows your homecare program. The patient's periodontal condition may well need to be reanalyzed after soft tissue management with you or your hygienist. Therefore, a consultation with the periodontist can either be at or after the initial appointment or after any disease control. One advantage in having the periodontist see the patient in this state is because he or she will be viewing the patient with the tissue in the best condition possible without a surgical or other periodontal therapy. But failure to achieve a successful esthetic and functional periodontal condition that serves as the framework for the teeth can make or break the final result.

Facial analysis

The first step in facial evaluation is to make sure you are viewing your patient at an appropriate angle. Have your patient stand or sit up in the chair with his or her gaze parallel to the floor. Then you can more easily tell if a part of the face is out of proportion. Later, computer imaging can confirm this for you. Note any facial deformities or parts of the face that stand out disproportionately (Figure 3.6).

Next view your patient's profile at rest, smiling, and with lips closed. This view can also reveal potential esthetic problems depending upon what will eventually be planned for the patient. Also, by you viewing the profile it allows the patient to also voice any problems that he or she may want corrected. The problem may be nondental such as a nose or chin that the patient may not be happy with which can prompt you to offer possible solutions and an eventual consultation with either a plastic or oral surgeon.

Visualize your intended changes, such as increasing the interincisal distance, or shortening, widening, or narrowing the teeth. Then confirm your ideas via computer imaging. Try to see how your patient's appearance could be improved. To do this you need to visualize an ideal facial form and identify what is lacking to make that face ideal. You may not be able to accomplish this—nor does every patient wish to be "perfect"—but for those who do, your careful evaluation can be extremely helpful. The more you do this the better you will become at helping your patients see what is needed to improve their appearance. A video camera and monitor also allow both you and your patient to see the face in two-dimensional silhouette form. By recording your patient while speaking various facial positions can be seen, thus making it easier to identify the extent of any esthetic problems.

Esthetic evaluation chart

To accurately diagnose a patient's problems and then create the best esthetic treatment plan, an esthetic evaluation chart is helpful. It can be a simple one-page form as developed by Goldstein (Figure 3.7) or a more elaborate version. The comprehensive charts developed by Levine, Oquendo, and Dawson incorporate both esthetics and function in their evaluation criteria. There are a number of excellent esthetic evaluation forms and several of the best are presented in Appendices A, B, and C at the end of Volume 1. All critical areas of the teeth, mouth, and face are displayed in an easy-to-understand diagrammatic fashion. Whether you use one of these charts or develop one of your own, they can be valuable diagnostic tools in your treatment planning.

Transillumination

Large tooth fractures can usually be observed clinically, but most enamel microcracks are rarely seen unless the affected teeth are either transilluminated (Figure 3.8A and B) or viewed with an

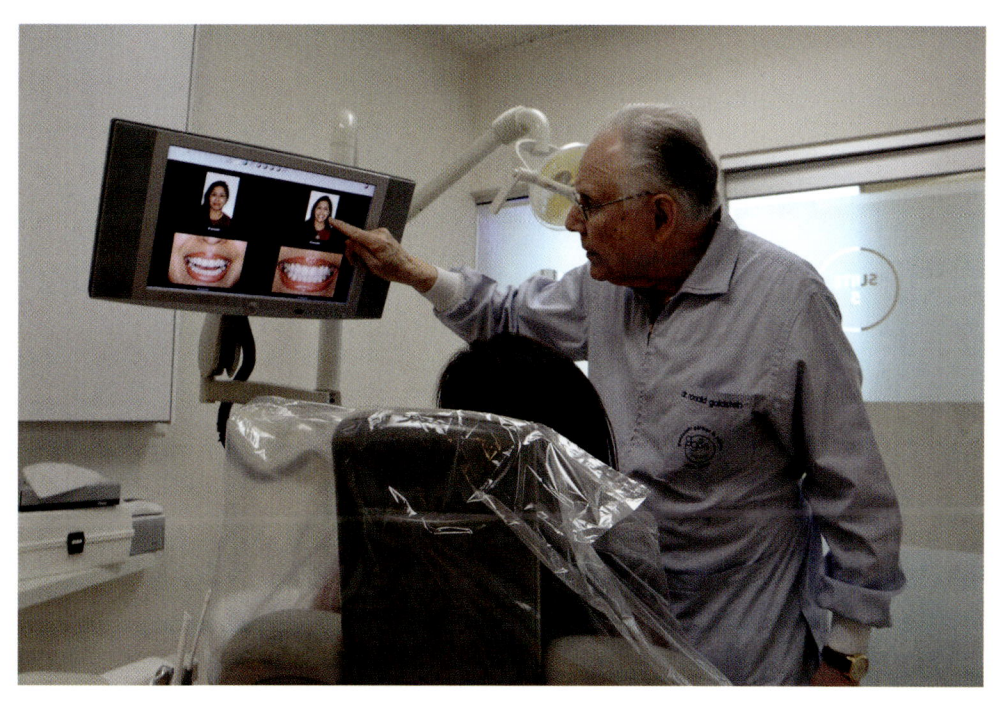

Figure 3.6 Facial evaluations should be made both in person, face to face, and recorded photographically. The digital photograph provides the two-dimensional silhouette from which it is easier to determine facial deformities.

intraoral camera. Therefore, you should allow sufficient examination time to transilluminate or view each tooth and record whether there are vertical, horizontal, or diagonal, or if no microcracks are present. This will help you predict the probability of future problems.

The presence of microcracks does not mean it is necessary to bond, laminate, or otherwise restore the tooth. The greatest percentage of teeth with vertical microcracks are not restored and rarely offer problems. However, teeth with horizontal or diagonal microcracks, usually the result of substantial or unusual trauma, may warrant repair. At the very least, bonding over the microcrack, if sensitive, can be useful in reducing discomfort and help to seal the defect and hold the tooth together. Another reason for detecting microcracks is to alert the patient to the fact that these tooth defects are present. Also, advise the patient that these microcracks stain more easily than solid enamel so some dietary change may need to be suggested. For instance, heavy smokers and coffee drinkers need to know that they may have new motivation to quit or seriously reduce some of the main causes of stain.

The intraoral camera

The simplest high-tech method of documenting the presence of microcracks is the use of an intraoral camera. It allows you to show patients their microcracks enlarged on a TV monitor, and also to record the finding on either a photograph or video. Thus, the patient involved in an accident claim has tangible evidence to provide insurance companies with proof of damaged teeth.

An intraoral camera provides instant visualization of the patient's teeth in real time. It is a powerful communication tool that helps you and your patient focus on "how to treat" instead of "why treat?" In today's high-tech society, patients relate to live video images in a way they seldom do to a sketch or X-ray. Since an intraoral camera also has the ability to store the images it records, the pictures are available later to both you and your patient, to demonstrate the before- and after-treatment images (Figure 3.9A–F).

> With the capability to see and record conditions such as the presence of enamel cracks, the intraoral camera has become one of the most valuable diagnostic aids in the dental operatory. It is the best tool to allow you to reveal which teeth and/or restorations are defective. In addition to showing your patient exactly why you are suggesting restorative therapy during the treatment planning stage, you can use the camera as a continuous communicator and educator during treatment. For example, you can point out actual caries under an old filling you are replacing. Since very few patients have ever seen real "decay," you are also reinforcing your credibility as an honest practitioner performing necessary procedures.

A major use of the intraoral camera in esthetic dentistry is in showing patients defective restorations. This is especially useful when discussing how defective Class II restorations might affect the color of the proposed porcelain laminates. To achieve ideal esthetics when making porcelain laminates, the teeth should be uniform in color. Thus, an old amalgam restoration that has darkly stained a part of the tooth can influence the color of the final laminate. The intraoral camera will provide convincing evidence that the offending restoration should be changed prior to laminate construction. Another reason to use some of the intraoral camera is that by recording what you find after removing an old restoration you are acknowledging any pathology present and also any potential future problem as a

Clinical Examination of Conditions Present

A Color
- Discoloration _____
- Unsightly restorations _____
- De-calcification_____ Hypercalcification _____
- Caries _____
- Stains_____
- Other _____

B Size and shape
- Large teeth_____Small teeth _____
- Faulty restorations _____
- Attrition_____ Abrasion_____ Erosion _____
- Other anomalies of tooth form, size or number _____

C Arrangement
- Missing teeth_____Crossbite _____
- Chipped or fractured teeth_____Open bite _____
- Uneven incisors_____Excessive overbite _____
- Excessive uniformity_____Spaced incisors _____
- Protrusion maxillary teeth_____Crowded incisors _____
- Protrusion mandibular teeth_____Closed vertical dimension _____
- Smile line _____
- Undererupted and extruded teeth _____

D Periodontal
- High lip line _____ Low lip line _____
- Inflamed gingiva_____Receding gingiva _____
- Hypertrophic gingiva_____Calculus _____
- Plaque_____Cleft _____
- Advanced bone loss _____
- Gingivitis _____
- Periodontitis_____
- Other _____

E Other abnormalities _____

Treatment Indicated for Esthetic Improvement
- Subject needs some_____no_____elective _____
- Cosmetic contouring _____
- Orthodontia_____major_____minor _____
- Operative_____
- Prosthodontia _____
- Bridgework_____
- Periodontia_____SGC_____GPY_____GTY _____
- Other _____

Figure 3.7 Original esthetic evaluation chart. (Goldstein, R. Esthetics in Dentistry, 1st edition, 1976.) Although there are many newer forms available (see Appendices A–C), many of the conditions listed here are still quite relevant.

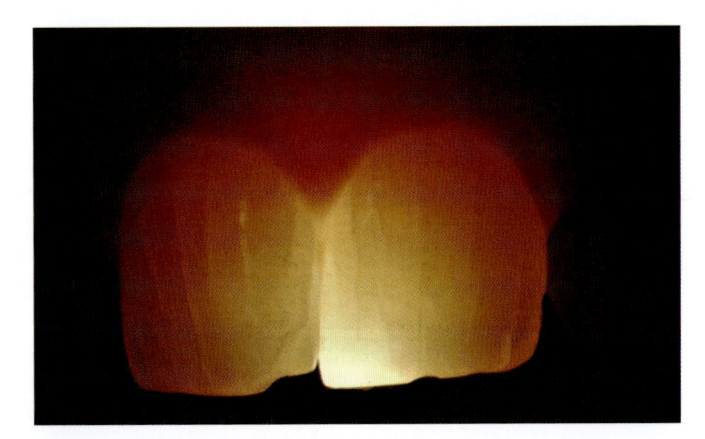

Figure 3.8 (A) Using an intraoral transilluminator is an excellent method of diagnosing microcracks. The intraoral camera can also record these microcracks.

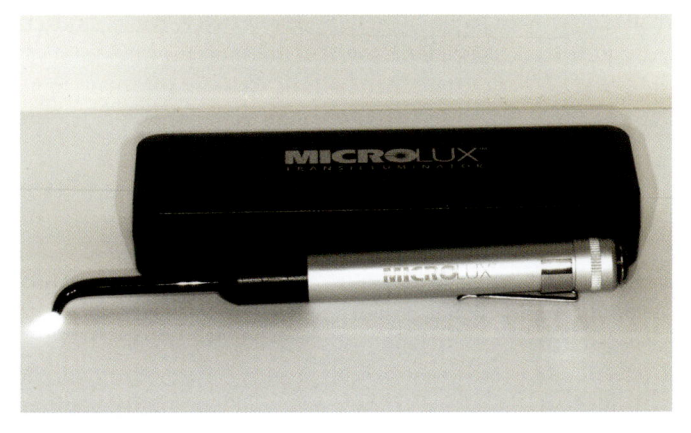

Figure 3.8 (B) Transillumination is easily accomplished using one the many Microlux (AdDent) tips. One of the most useful ones is a vertical tip that can help visibility and measure post preparations.

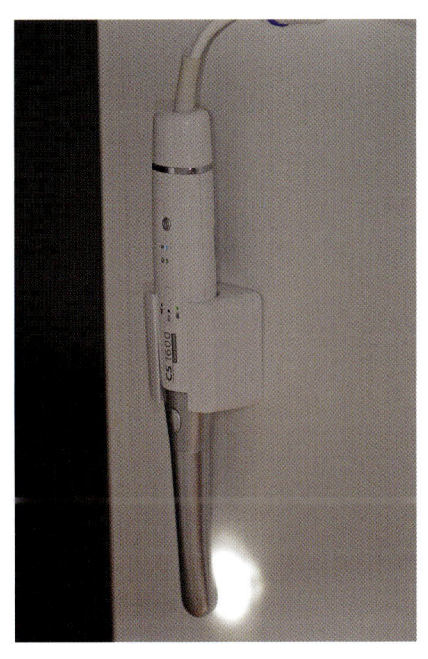

Figure 3.9 **(A)** This Kodak 1600 intraoral camera has auto focus which can either be wireless or wired, and it makes it easy for both dentist and hygienist to quickly record a patient's condition including potential caries identification technology.

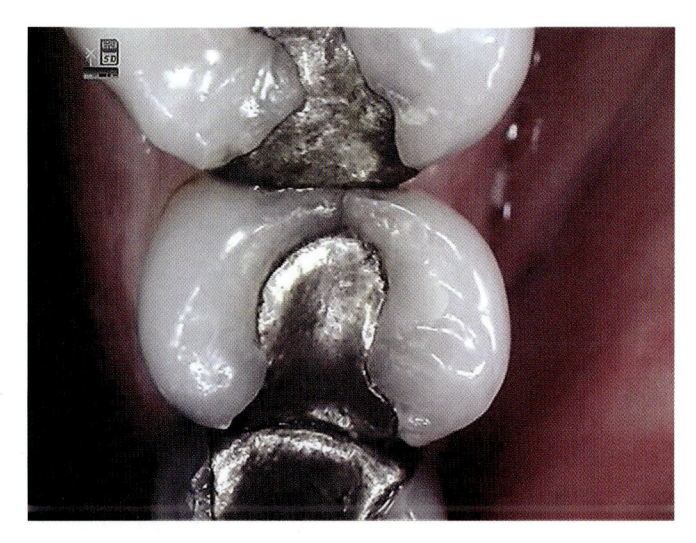

Figure 3.9 **(B)** One of the major uses of the intraoral camera is to record and show your patient severe microcracks that may result in catastrophic tooth fracture. Such an example is seen in the bicuspid photograph.

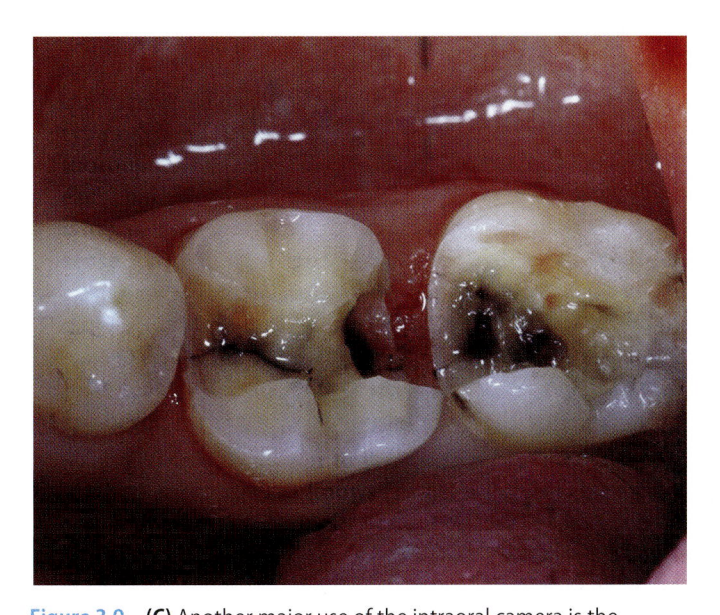

Figure 3.9 **(C)** Another major use of the intraoral camera is the important recording of deep microcracks along the pulpal floor. This recording will be helpful in showing your patient that the tooth was damaged prior to your restorative treatment.

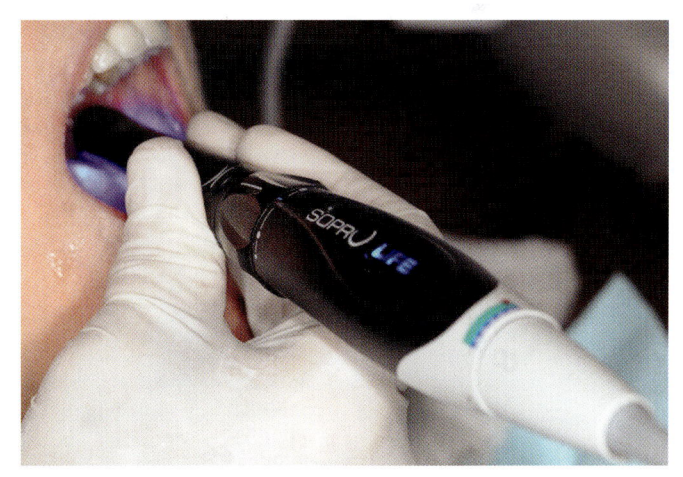

Figure 3.9 **(D)** The SOPROLIFE intraoral camera not only provides visual evidence of what you see, but also quickly converts to a light-induced fluorescence evaluator to help distinguish carious from noncarious tooth structure.

result of an existing microcrack on the pulpal floor, deep decay, or other hidden problem.

The extraoral camera

Digital photography has virtually transformed diagnosis to the point that there is little excuse today for not adding digital photographs to your diagnostic records. For every new patient our dental assistant takes a complete series of extraoral photos, uploads them to the patient's photo chart, and when I come in to see the patient for the first time the photos are already on the chairside monitor. This makes it much easier to show the patient potential problems as well as having the patient point out areas of his or her concern. We train our assistants to take good digital photos before we even see a new patient, which really helps both the patient and me look at the various photos in two dimensions. When you view your patient in the dental chair, you are seeing the patient in 3D. However, Pincus (personal communication) pointed out that when you look at a photo, you are then looking at the image in 2D which is much better to help you see silhouette form and easier to detect esthetic defects. (See Chapter 7 on practical clinical photography for instruction on views to capture.)

There are also times when you would be smart to record your patients' comments and pictures using a video camera. This can be especially important if the patient is complaining of "botched

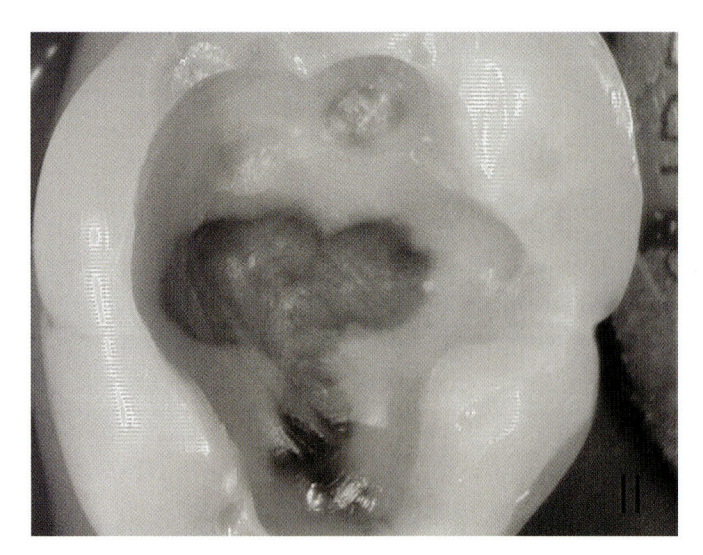

Figure 3.9 **(E)** This photo was taken after caries was thought to be removed under a defective amalgam restoration.

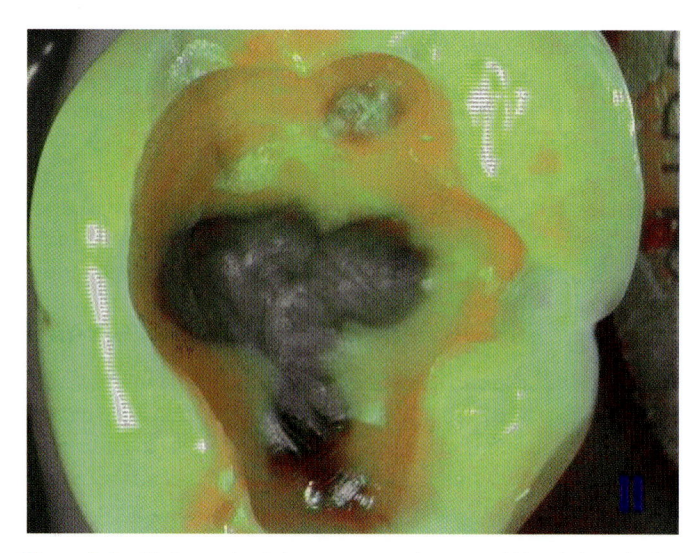

Figure 3.9 **(F)** A simple click converts to the special blue light, which reveals in red where caries was still present.

dentistry" or is so unhappy with the previous dentist that a lawsuit could be occur in the future. The better records you have of the patient's actual condition and what the patient is unhappy with the less likely you will be misquoted or misunderstood. Furthermore, your own words cannot be misconstrued by the patient. Acquiring a good, high-definition video camera is unnecessary today because a cell phone can take high-definition video with ease, so it makes little sense to not have your potentially difficult patients recorded.

A dual form of recording information will capture simultaneously the pretreatment full face and smile of the patient as well as the conversation relative to his or her perceived condition or problem. However, a panoramic film or even a CT scan may not be able to give you the detail you need for a complete diagnosis. Both an audio and video recording are extremely helpful if there is any future question about the exact condition with which the patient originally presented. Viewing the 2D full-face aspect on a TV monitor makes it easier for both you and your patient to accurately see the silhouette form. This is also true when recording the patient's right and left profiles, and close-up smiling and speaking. Most patients are amazed by what is revealed in these views. They become acutely aware that this is what everyone else sees and can be more motivated to make sure these views can eventually present them in the most flattering way possible. The result is greater potential for a more comprehensive treatment plan (Figure 3.10).

X-Rays

Although the typical full-mouth radiographic series is indispensable to patient examination, there are times when some patients will object to even digital radiation regardless that it may be 90% less than with traditional radiation techniques. In these cases, it is extremely valuable to have technology like a CBCT scan or panographic radiograph. Digital radiographs are also used to take multiple views at different angles of problem areas, and the fact that it is instantaneous can save time in diagnostic procedures. This technology is also helpful when fitting inlays, onlays, crowns, posts, and virtually all other fixed prostheses where try-in adjustments are usually necessary to obtain perfection in fit (Figure 3.11A). Patients will not object to further radiographs when they realize how little radiation the process involves. This means you can continue to fit your prosthesis and repeatedly check the margin with additional X-rays until it is perfect. A major enhanced advantage of digital radiographs is the ability to communicate information to your patient, even in color. Many patients have difficulty in seeing a problem using the typical grey scale of the X-ray (Figure 3.11B).

Occlusal analysis

Evaluating occlusion of your new patient is essential to both function and esthetic treatment planning. The simplest way to initially observe the occlusion is through accurate diagnostic casts mounted on an adjustable articulator. When this step is combined with a clinical evaluation it becomes easier to determine if orthodontic therapy needs to be a part of your treatment plan. This analysis also will help you explain why orthodontics may be an important final step in the treatment plan. You will definitely need to have clear records of your recommendations and if the patient refuses to even consider orthodontics this fact definitely must be documented and even initialed in the chart. I have had many cases of unhappy patients with compromised restorative treatments whereby the patient stated orthodontics was not offered as part of the treatment plan only to find after consulting with the previous dentist that orthodontics was indeed mentioned but not written down in the patient's chart. Consequently, regardless of a patient's preconceived notion that they would not consider orthodontics, after insisting on a joint consultation with the orthodontist, about half of these patients elect to have either ideal or compromised orthodontic treatment.

Periodontal charting

No part of the esthetic examination is more important than ascertaining the condition of your patient's supporting bone structure. The most perfect restoration in the world will fail if placed in a tooth with a weak supporting structure. Therefore, functionally, esthetically, and legally you are required to thoroughly examine

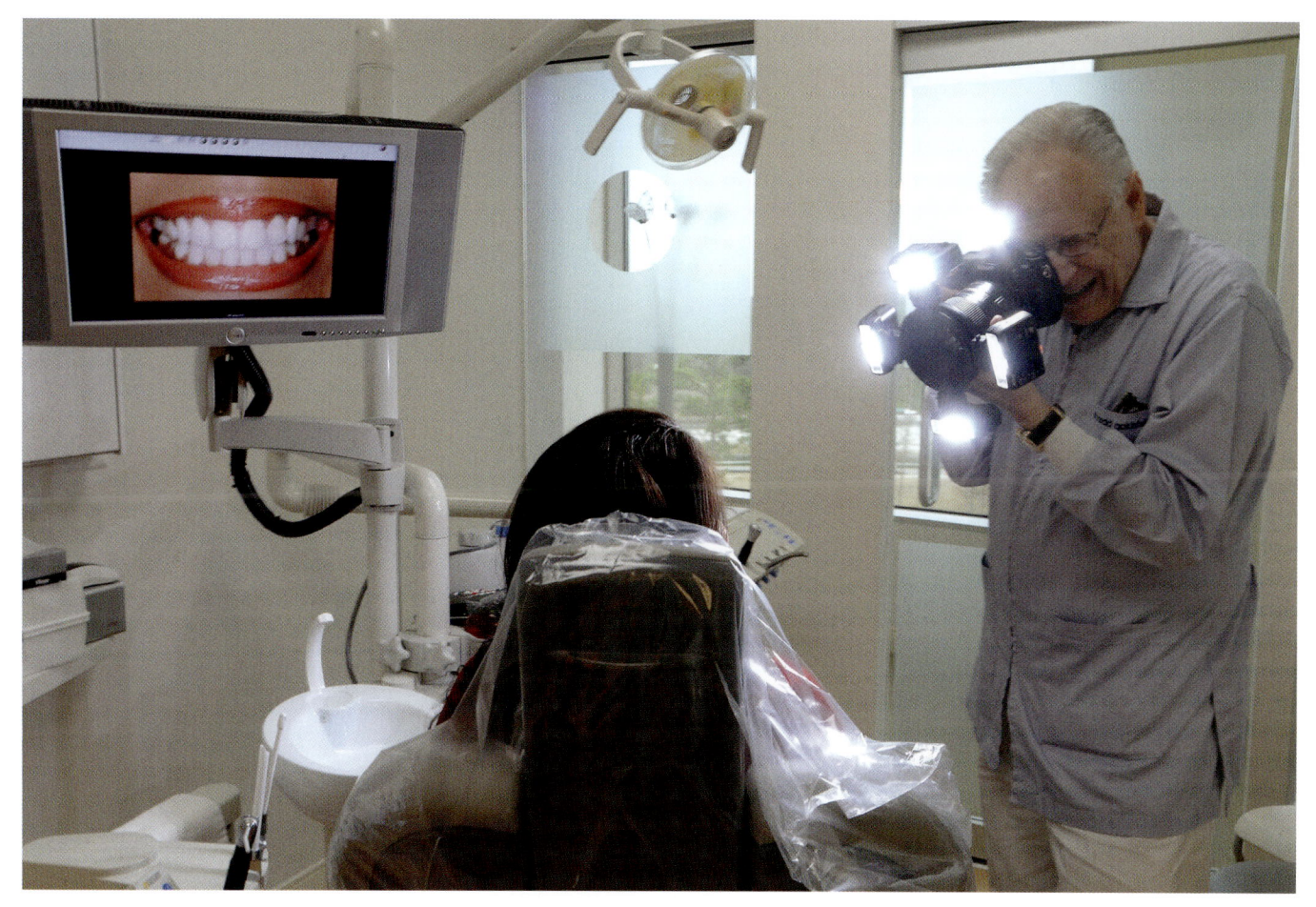

Figure 3.10 Although there are a multitude of extraoral cameras that can be used for patient photographs, a Nikon D300 with four flashes is able to provide excellent digital images.

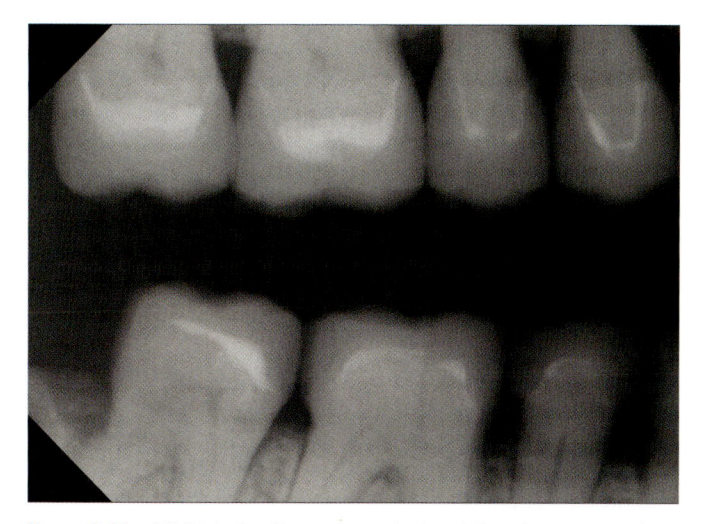

Figure 3.11 **(A)** Digital radiographs make it quick and easy to verify the interproximal fit of your prosthetic restorations before final seating.

full-mouth radiographs as well as probe teeth in six locations. This can be done with a traditional periodontal probe or an accurate 0.5-mm-increment thin colored probe (Figure 3.11C and D) (Goldstein ColorVue Probe, Hu-Friedy), where the data can be recorded electronically using a voice-activated system. One major advantage in producing a color, 8 × 10 in (20 × 25 cm) easy-to-comprehend chart to give to the patient is to make him or her feel more responsible for any diagnosed periodontal problems (Figure 3.12). It is far better to give your patients tangible evidence of their periodontal problems rather than merely verbally informing them of your findings. Voice activation makes it easy and quick for your hygienist to perform this periodontal charting on virtually every patient and also enables you to provide periodic progress charts when necessary.

Computer imaging

Used first in 1986 by plastic surgeons and the beauty industry, the computer makes it possible to digitally alter the pictures of a patient's teeth and face, and to produce a picture of how they might look after cosmetic treatment (Figure 3.13). This visual prediction of potential treatment solutions to esthetic problems offers an unparalleled method of letting you and the patient look at how your intended esthetic correction will not only change your patient's smile, but also, in many cases, his or her entire face. It also accomplishes the following:

- It lets you do a better job of treatment planning by allowing you to visualize a possible result, which can then be studied to determine its esthetic effect.

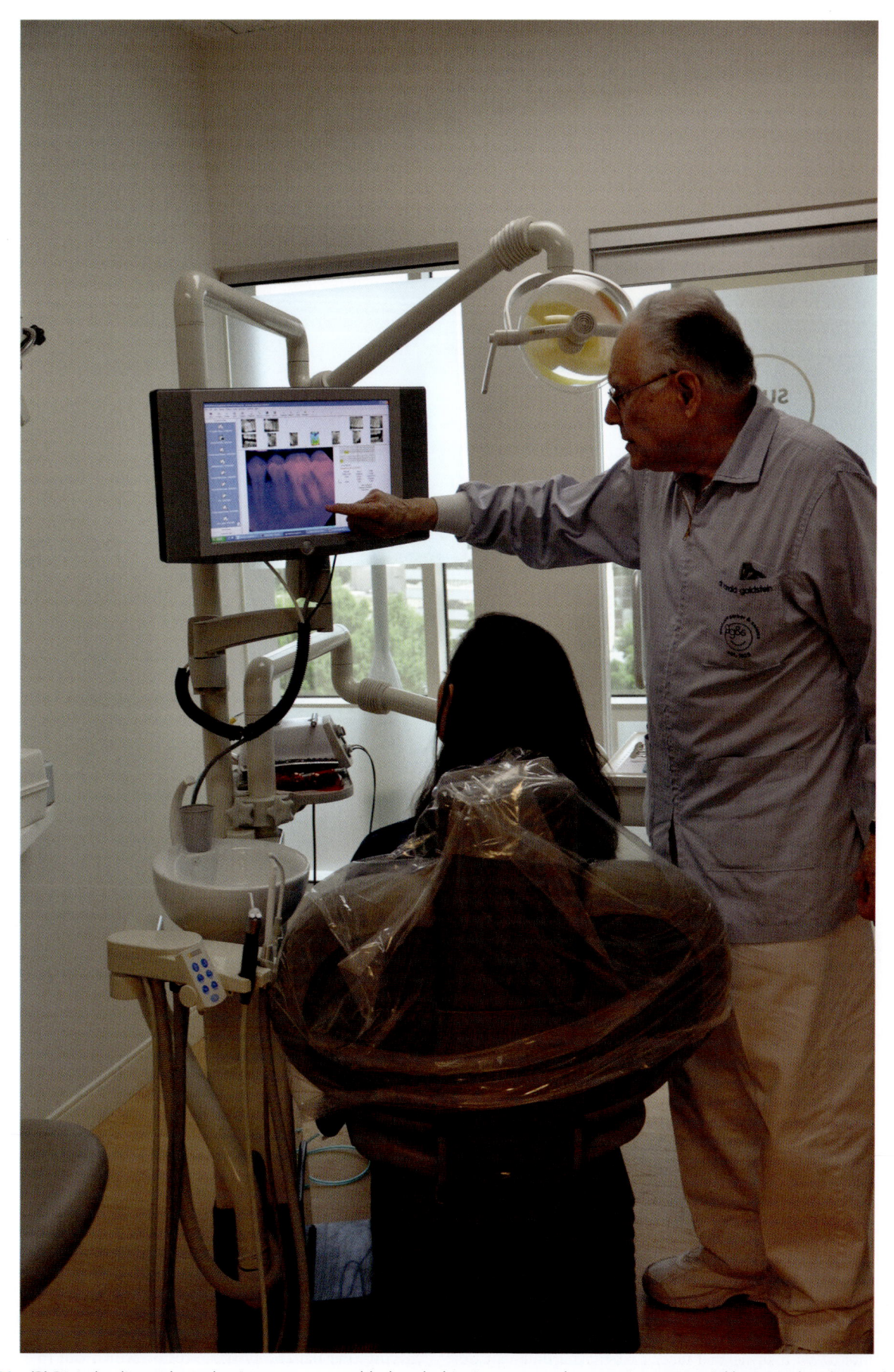

Figure 3.11 **(B)** Digital radiography makes it easy to convert black and white images to color so patients can quickly see and understand what the dentist is describing.

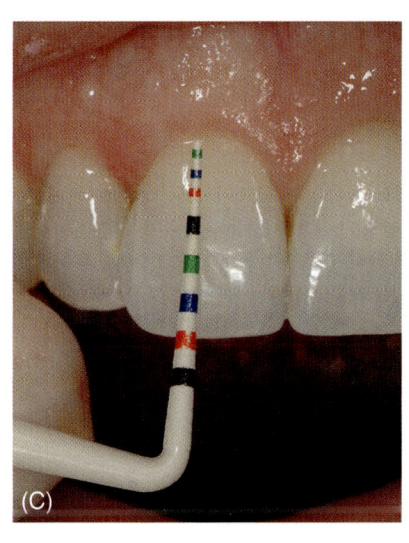

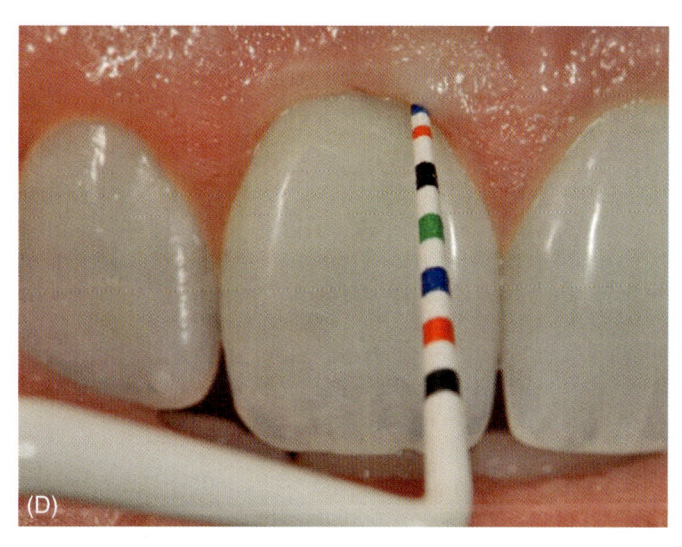

Figure 3.11 **(C and D)** The Goldstein ColorVue Probe is more comfortable than the metal probe and more precise since it measures in 0.5 mm increments up to 3 mm.

- The patient is able to view your intended correction and make suggestions on how he or she would like to see it modified.
- Based on feedback from the patient, further computer imaging allows you to show patients how they can look with any number of additional or different esthetic changes and improvements. You are therefore limited only by your creative ability.
- It increases patient motivation by demonstrating the positive aspects of an improved appearance and enhanced self-image, and reducing patient uncertainty and anxiety.
- It helps to establish the fact that your office employs state-of-the-art diagnostic and communicative tools and techniques, making a positive statement about the type of dentistry you practice. The real value in enabling a patient to see proposed changes is ensuring that both dentist and patient envision the same result. If, for any reason, they do not have the same expectations, this is the proper time to make any changes regarding results. Certainly, unmet expectations after your treatment can require either redoing or altering the correction; or even worse, they may establish a defensive position with the patient, which frequently causes a wider communication gap. At the very least, one can avoid discovery after the fact, which is expensive. Retreatment of the patient is usually done at a loss for the dental office. It does not take too many losses of this type to realize that esthetic imaging can be a valuable asset when a major esthetic correction is being planned.

There is a legitimate question raised when turning to the decision of who is to perform the imaging. Obviously, many dentists like to make their own computer changes while others prefer to have a computer imaging therapist assist in providing this service. In our office, we chose to have a talented dental assistant train to be able to make the necessary computer enhancements to both smile and face. This assistant is capable of understanding our intended changes, plus she is artistically qualified and has excellent ability to communicate with the patient. This last fact also saves the doctors considerable "explanation" time. However, the imaging therapist can be a hygienist or another person knowledgeable about dental procedures. The patient must be made to clearly understand that the image produced by the computer is only an approximation of intended results you feel he or she can reasonably attain. If you plan to give a copy of the computerized image to the patient, remember to always print, in color, a disclaimer clause on the copy. This clause may read as follows:

> This picture is for purposes of illustration only. It does not represent a guarantee of any kind.

The following is a good example of just how important computer imaging can be: a 26-year-old professional athlete was concerned about his crowded teeth (Figure 3.14A). Clinical examination revealed a high lip line with gingival tissue covering the cervical third of the teeth. This combination resulted in a disproportional smile/tooth relationship to the full face. The patient's previous dentist stressed the ideal solution of orthodontics but did not give him any alternative. The patient felt there must be an alternative, such as crowning. When verbally discussing the various options for improving his appearance, the patient could visualize how straight the teeth would look, but he had difficulty understanding the need for cosmetic periodontal therapy. Computer imaging was used to show the patient what could be expected of cosmetic periodontal surgery plus 10 porcelain veneers (Figure 3.14B, right-hand panel). When he saw the intended result through computer imaging, his immediate question was, "How fast can the treatment be accomplished?" Following cosmetic periodontal surgery, 10 porcelain veneers were inserted to achieve the look in Figure 3.14C. Computer imaging played a major role in convincing this patient of the importance of both procedures to obtain maximum esthetic results.

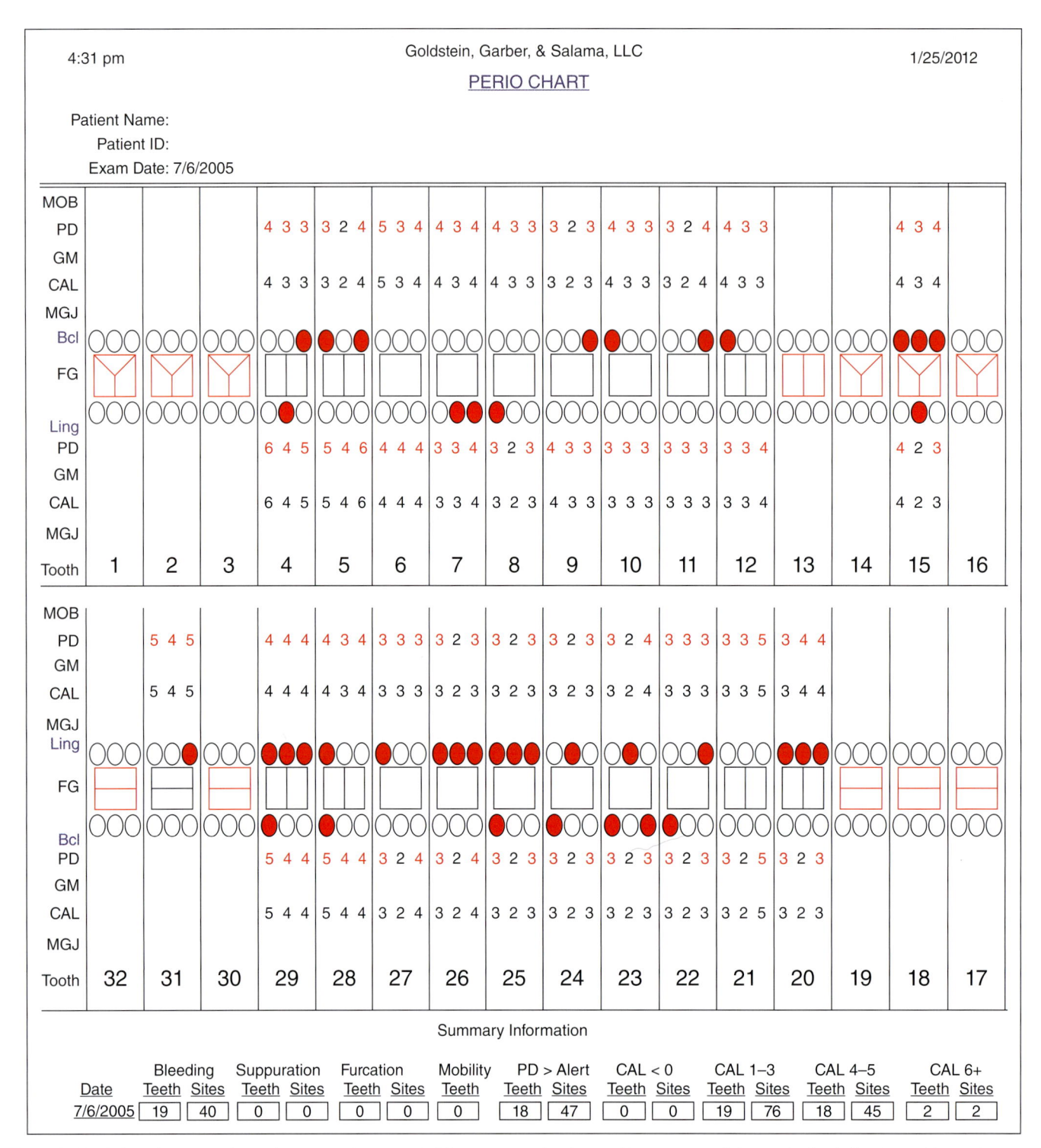

Figure 3.12 A digital perio-probing chart is another essential diagnostic tool to be used in treatment. It is easy for both dentist and hygienist to read and compare results.

The major advantages of computer imaging are outlined below.

- Computer imaging demonstrates to the patient 2D views of their teeth and smile that they would not normally see (Figure 3.15).
- It provides full-face frontal and profile views that can help you and your patient visualize the effects of proposed changes to the teeth and gingival tissues on the face.
- It may indicate what not to do, and highlight undesirable results. Not infrequently, certain intraoral changes can have a detrimental effect, instead of the desired one, by being too perfect or too imperfect. Equally damaging is making teeth too light or too dark. Although not guaranteeing a perfect shade, the computer can help illustrate to the patient an acceptable, approximate shade range. A critical consideration for imaging occurs when orthodontic treatment achieves occlusal success

Chapter 3 Esthetic Treatment Planning

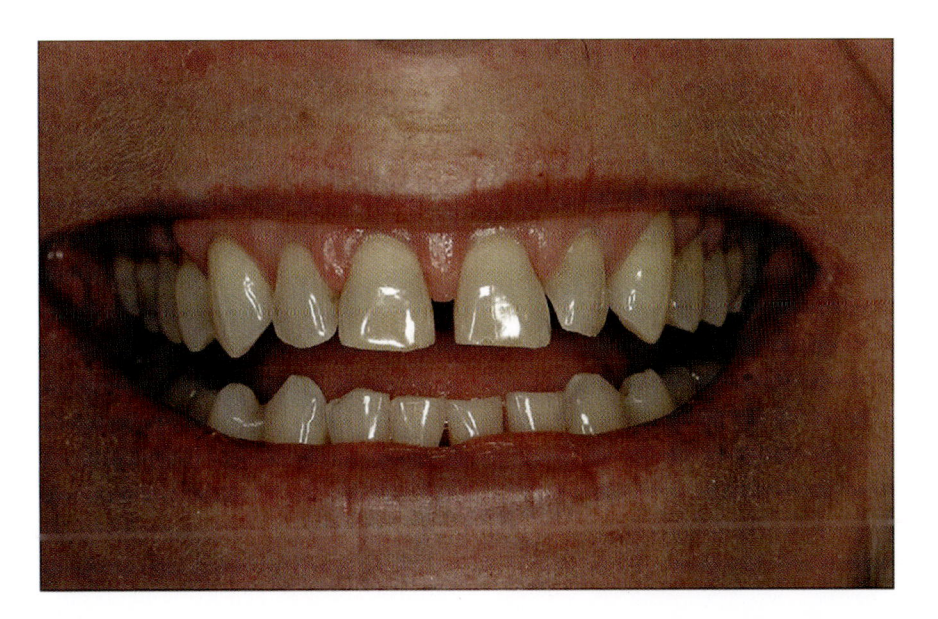

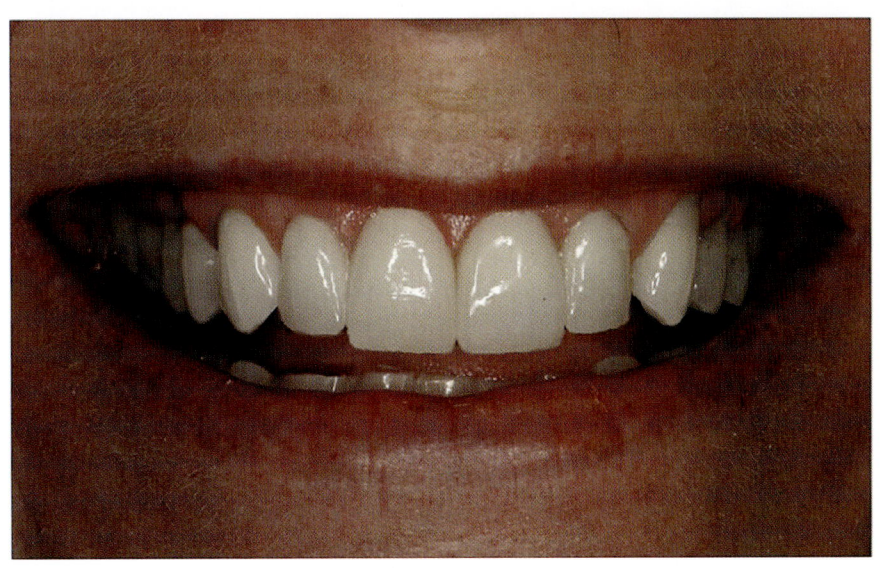

Figure 3.13 Although there are many ways of showing a patient the results of treatment, esthetic imaging is an excellent method of demonstrating potential results of diastema closure. A disclaimer should always appear on the photos stating: "This photo is for illustration only and does not represent a guarantee of any kind."

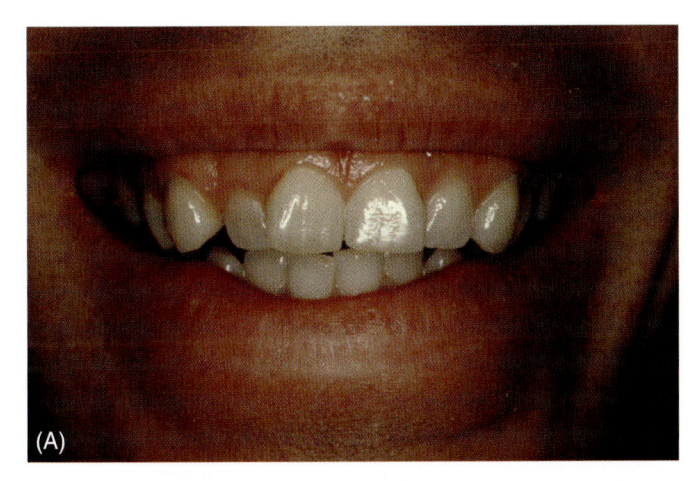

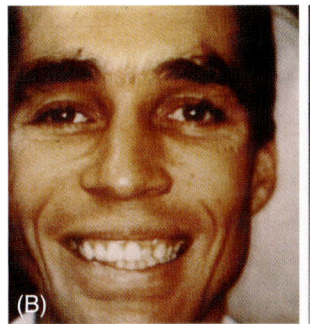

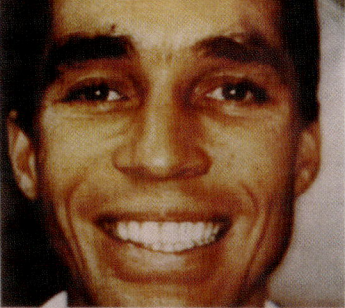

Figure 3.14 **(A and B)** Although crowded teeth caused this international tennis star to seek esthetic treatment, computer imaging indicated the need for cosmetic periodontal-gingival raising therapy for improved facial proportion. Imaging also gave him a much desired alternative to orthodontic therapy by demonstrating the proposed results using porcelain veneer restorations.

only to destroy facial balance. For example, moving anterior teeth lingually either with orthodontics or through prosthetic means may make for occlusal success, but it may cause more prominence to the patient's nose. Your patient may like his or her nose as it is. Making the proposed change could produce an esthetic disaster from the patient's point of view.

- When restorative treatment consists of bonding, veneers, or crowns, imaging can be invaluable during the try-in phase when the patient or dentist is not absolutely certain of the optimal length or width of the new restoration. Rather than blindly removing existing porcelain incisal edges on the restoration, which could ruin your esthetic result, it is easier to image your patient and make the changes on the screen. You and your patient can then come to a mutual agreement on what looks best.

- Another critical area where computer imaging can make a significant difference is in the communication between the dentist and the off-site laboratory technician. That communication is most often in the form of models, impressions, and written notes. If an actual picture reflecting what you and your patient expect is given to the laboratory technician, the probability of a successful result is greatly improved.

Trial smile

The trial smile is the very best method for both patient and dental team, including the laboratory when necessary, to view proposed esthetic changes. This extra step is essential to avoid esthetic failure. There have been many times when a patient did not initially like our plan and we were fortunate to make the necessary changes in the trial smile to obtain patient approval. Once you have that approval take alginate impressions so both you and the laboratory will have the model to use as a guide for the final restorations.

Although the subject of trial smile is dealt with extensively in Chapter 42 on temporization it should be noted here that a next or even substitute step may be a trial smile. No doubt a patient can more easily grasp the effect of lengthening the teeth with a mock-up direct composite resin applied to his or her own teeth. Nevertheless,

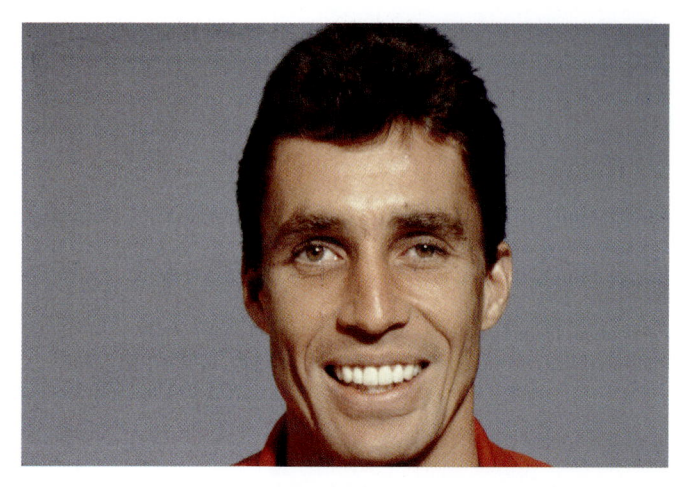

Figure 3.14 (C) The final smile would not have been possible had this patient not been motivated to undergo both periodontal and restorative therapy after seeing the potential results via computer imaging.

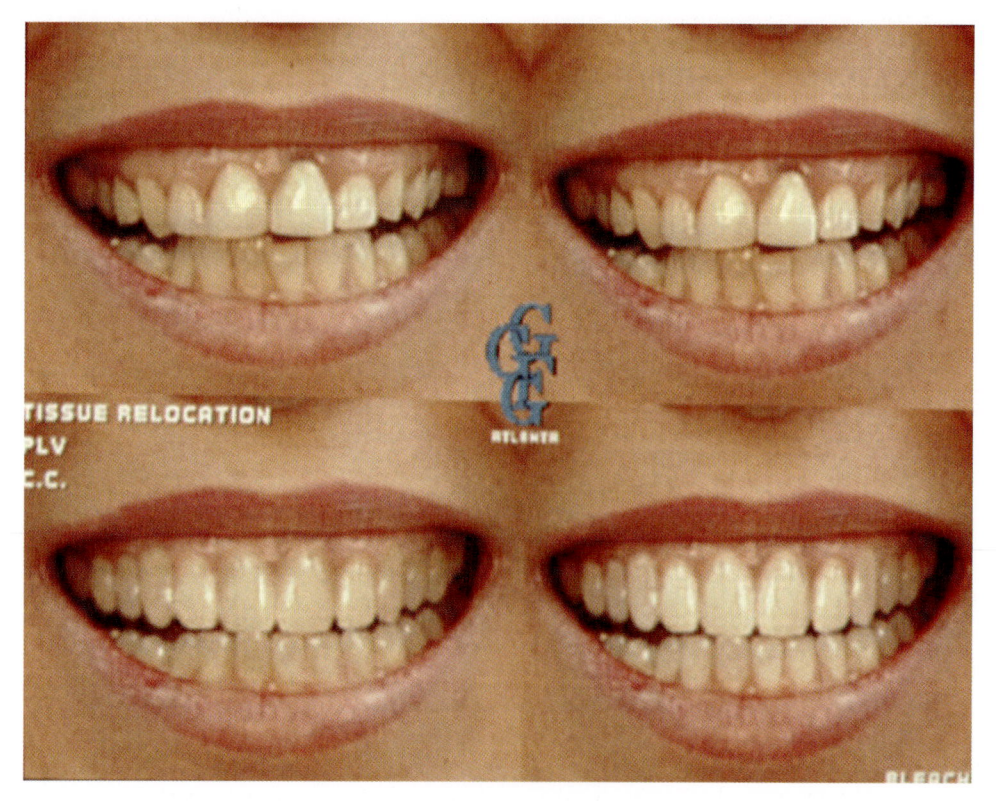

Figure 3.15 This computer imaging printout shows the importance of taking a lateral view since this aspect as seen by others is seldom observed by the patient.

looking at a 2D effect is of advantage as well. So an esthetic imaging photo of before and after plus an extraoral photo of the patient's own teeth being altered by mock-up composite (or tooth-colored wax) can help the patient make a more educated decision.

Technology and an integrated digital system

Dentistry is fast heading toward a paperless office where every conceivable record can and will be computerized. The patient's file, including all diagnostic and treatment records, can already be stored, displayed, printed, and transported electronically. One of the major advantages of this trend is that it enables you to accumulate vast amounts of knowledge about your patients and retrieve the information faster than by looking through pages of records to find, for instance, what cement you used many years ago to seat a particular crown.

State-of-the-art diagnostic procedures are now controlled by an integrated workstation. The advantage of this clinical and management-oriented system is the ability to add and retrieve information quickly and easily from multiple, flexible locations within the office. Records, X-rays, and reports are not misplaced. A patient's last X-ray and the next day's schedule should be at your fingertips while you are on the phone determining how and when to treat the patient. You may even have workstations at home for on-call situations involving any patient in your practice. This is especially valuable for multidoctor and multilocation practices. Fast and comprehensive specialty and referral consultations are easily made using modems. Third-party reimbursement is certainly faster if claims are submitted electronically, and procedure approvals can be higher with the ability to submit more in-depth documentation.

Various components of typical integrated system include:

- practice/business management system
- extraoral camera and video, with memory and printer
- intraoral camera
- digital radiography
- occlusal analysis
- voice-activated periodontal and general oral diagnostics
- caries detection analysis
- patient education and interactive video system
- esthetic imaging system
- CBCT and 3D treatment planning software.

The voice-activated charting component is actually the core of the system from a clinical perspective because it generates the basic information of the electronic chart. In addition, temporomandibular joint analysis and esthetic evaluation can be incorporated into this integrated system. The video recordings become a form of informed consent. While recording face and smile, you also capture the patient's voice stating that he or she understands what a particular procedure is and why it is being done. For the esthetic practice, this can prove to be a definite advantage, especially if a patient presents a problem after treatment.

Photographic records need to be the rule rather than the exception. Recreating the circumstances of a restorative procedure takes only seconds if they are stored in the system. Three-dimensional diagnostic models and even their occlusion are possible when the principles of computer-aided design/computer-aided manufacturing (CAD/CAM) are integrated into the system.

The first visit frequently ends with the recording of the patient's images. The actual computer imaging correction often occurs after the patient leaves, either by or in consultation with the dentist. You may also consider using Digital Smile Design in treatment planning for your patient, (see Chapter 4).

Preparation for the second visit

Review of radiographs

Preliminary reading of radiographs should reveal obvious caries, periodontal disease, and evidence of abscess or other pathology. Any teeth to be considered for crowning should be examined on the radiograph to see if the pulps are large or receded, because their condition can alter treatment expectations. Teeth that have deep caries or thickened apices may sometimes require root canal therapy. It is essential to determine and treat any necessary endodontic treatment before inserting esthetic crowns. Performing an endodontic procedure on a newly cemented porcelain crown is not a pleasant task, especially given the possibility of lingual surface fracture. Therefore, interim treatment crowning for an extended period may be indicated before you insert the final restorations.

Evaluation of diagnostic models

Diagnostic models are an essential part of the treatment planning procedure. However, they must be accurate and well-made, and contain as much detail as possible. Arch relationships and tooth form, size, and arrangement should be studied. It may be necessary to consult a specialist with the diagnostic models before the patient's second visit. Several questions should be asked when reviewing the models:

1. Is repositioning needed for a proper esthetic result?
2. Can restorative dentistry alone achieve esthetic balance?
3. Are periodontal or other surgical procedures necessary for a successful restorative result?
4. Do wear facets indicate a loss of vertical dimension or any other occlusal problem? It might be necessary to wax-up an intended restoration as well as various alternatives to help the patient choose the best one. A wax-up is an important diagnostic and visual aid and enhances diagnosis and communication between the patient and dentist.

Review of medical and dental histories

The dentist should be aware of any systemic physical or mental disease. Using a history chart similar to that in Figure 3.16A and B, the dentist can learn if a patient has any of the various medical ailments that could compromise a successful esthetic result. It is

MEDICAL STATUS FORM

Name: _____ Birth date _____
Address: _____ Sex ___M ___F
_____
Phones: home: _____
          work: _____   Cell: _____
          email: _____

The dentistry you receive has an important interrelationship with the health problems that you may have, or medications you are taking. It is imperative that you provide the following information to help us treat you as effectively and safely as possible.
Please initial that you read this paragraph: _____

Are you under a physician's care now?	( )yes ( )no	If yes, please explain: Dr. Name: Address: Telephone Number: Date of last physical exam:
Have you ever been hospitalized or had a major operation in the past five years?	( )yes ( )no	If yes, please explain:
Have you ever had a serious head or neck injury?	( )yes ( )no	If yes, please explain:
Are you taking any prescription or non-prescription medications, pills, herbal supplements, aspirin, ibuprophen, vitamin E or drugs?	( )yes ( )no	If yes, please list and explain: _____ _____ _____ _____
Are you taking or have you taken bisphosphonate for osteoporosis: such as Actonel, Boniva, Fosamax, Zometa or Aredia?	( )yes ( )no	If yes, please explain:
Have you ever been advised to take pre-medication for dental visits?	( )yes ( )no	If yes, please explain:
Have you ever had a lesion biopsied or removed from the mouth or lips?	( )yes ( )no	If yes, please explain:
Are you on a special diet?	( )yes ( )no	If yes, please explain:
Do you smoke or use tobacco?	( )yes ( )no	If yes, how much? How long?
Do you use controlled substances?	( )yes ( )no	If yes, please explain:
Do you consume alcohol?	( )yes ( )no	If yes, please explain:
Has anyone told you that you snore?	( )yes ( )no	

WOMEN: Are you pregnant or trying to get pregnant?   ( ) Yes   ( ) No
          Taking oral contraceptives?   ( ) Yes   ( ) No
          Nursing?   ( ) Yes   ( ) No

DA/RDH Initials: _____
Dr. Initials: _____

Figure 3.16 **(A)** Medical history form (page 1).

important to know, for example, if the patient can tolerate sitting for extended periods during try-ins or difficult staining procedures. As an alternative, can and should conscious sedation be utilized? It is obvious that not every patient can undergo cosmetic restorative treatment. The patient's history can show if there are systemic diseases that can cause problems, particularly in combined therapy cases where orthodontics, periodontics, and full-mouth reconstruction are performed. An esthetic result that will last for any length of time is difficult to achieve if there is continual periodontal breakdown due to preexisting disease.

Are you allergic to any of the following:

☐ Aspirin ☐ Penicillin ☐ Tetracycline ☐ Erythromycin ☐ Codeine

☐ Acrylic ☐ Metal ☐ Sulfa ☐ Local Anesthetics ☐ Latex

☐ Other: _____ ☐ No Known Allergies

Do you have, or have you had, any of the following?

AIDS/HIV Positive	☐ yes ☐ no	Implants-Hip/Breast/knee/tooth	☐ yes ☐ no
Allergies	☐ yes ☐ no	HPV (Human Papilloma Virus)	☐ yes ☐ no
Alzheimer's Disease	☐ yes ☐ no	High Blood Pressure	☐ yes ☐ no
Anaphylaxis	☐ yes ☐ no	Hives or Rash	☐ yes ☐ no
Anemia	☐ yes ☐ no	Hypoglycemia	☐ yes ☐ no
Angina/Chest Pains	☐ yes ☐ no	Irregular Heartbeat	☐ yes ☐ no
Arthritis/Gout	☐ yes ☐ no	Kidney Problems	☐ yes ☐ no
Artificial Heart Valve	☐ yes ☐ no	Leukemia	☐ yes ☐ no
Artificial Joint	☐ yes ☐ no	Liver Disease	☐ yes ☐ no
Asthma	☐ yes ☐ no	Low Blood Pressure	☐ yes ☐ no
Blood Disease	☐ yes ☐ no	Lung Disease	☐ yes ☐ no
Blood Transfusion	☐ yes ☐ no	Mitral Valve Prolapse	☐ yes ☐ no
Bruise Easily	☐ yes ☐ no	Osteoporosis	☐ yes ☐ no
Cancer	☐ yes ☐ no	Periodontal "gum" Disease	☐ yes ☐ no
Chemotherapy	☐ yes ☐ no	Psychiatric Care	☐ yes ☐ no
Celiac Disease	☐ yes ☐ no	Radiation Treatments	☐ yes ☐ no
Congenital Heart Disorder	☐ yes ☐ no	Recent Weight Loss	☐ yes ☐ no
Convulsions	☐ yes ☐ no	Renal Dialysis	☐ yes ☐ no
Cortisone Medicine	☐ yes ☐ no	Rheumatic Fever	☐ yes ☐ no
Diabetes	☐ yes ☐ no	Rheumatism	☐ yes ☐ no
Drug Addiction	☐ yes ☐ no	Scarlet Fever	☐ yes ☐ no
Eating Disorder (Bulimia and/or Anorexia)	☐ yes ☐ no	Stomach/Intestinal Disease/Ulcers	☐ yes ☐ no
Emphysema	☐ yes ☐ no	Shortness of Breath	☐ yes ☐ no
Epilepsy or Seizures	☐ yes ☐ no	Sickle Cell Disease	☐ yes ☐ no
Excessive Bleeding	☐ yes ☐ no	Sinus Trouble	☐ yes ☐ no
Excessive Thirst	☐ yes ☐ no	Special Diet	☐ yes ☐ no
Fainting Spells/Dizziness	☐ yes ☐ no	Spina Bifida	☐ yes ☐ no
Frequent Cough	☐ yes ☐ no	Shingles/Herpes/Cold sores/Fever blisters	☐ yes ☐ no
Frequent Diarrhea	☐ yes ☐ no	Stroke	☐ yes ☐ no
Fequent Headaches	☐ yes ☐ no	Swelling of Limbs	☐ yes ☐ no
Glaucoma	☐ yes ☐ no	Thyroid Condition	☐ yes ☐ no
Heart Attack/Failure	☐ yes ☐ no	Tonsilitis	☐ yes ☐ no
Heart Murmur	☐ yes ☐ no	Tuberculosis	☐ yes ☐ no
Heart Pace Maker	☐ yes ☐ no	Tumors or Growths	☐ yes ☐ no
Heart Trouble/Disease	☐ yes ☐ no	Venereal Disease	☐ yes ☐ no
Hemophilia	☐ yes ☐ no	Yellow Jaundice	☐ yes ☐ no
Hepatitis A, B, C, D, or E	☐ yes ☐ no	Contact Lenses	☐ yes ☐ no

Have you ever had any serious illness not listed above? ( ) Yes   ( ) No
If yes, please explain: _____
To the best of my knowledge, the questions on this form have been accurately answered. I understand that providing incorrect information can be dangerous to my (or patient's) health. It is my responsibility to inform the dental office of any changes in medical status.

Signature of patient, parent or guardian _____ date _____

DA/RDH Initials: _____
Dr. Initials: _____

Figure 3.16 (B) Medical history form (page 2).

The dental history can indicate the patient's familiarity with dentistry. From this, the dentist can judge how much time should be allowed for the second visit or if subsequent visits will be necessary before the final presentation. Frequently, the patient with little knowledge of dentistry will require several visits before a successful case presentation can be made. The patient's "dental IQ" indicates his or her opinion of dentists and dentistry. *The patient who is extremely critical of previous dentists may soon be critical of the current dentist.*

Preparation of a preliminary treatment plan

A preliminary treatment plan should definitely be formulated and it is also prudent to use an organized form on which to place these clinical recommendations (Figure 3.17). Although it may be revised considerably, different alternatives should be considered before the second appointment. A quadrant-by-quadrant outline of functional necessities with a separate list of esthetic options will suffice. One major consideration will be to determine what modifications may be necessary and I have found that Fradeani's Laboratory Checklist to be invaluable (Appendix C). Although the diagnosis and treatment planning phase for the treatment of esthetic dental problems can occupy a considerable amount of time, the presentation of the findings can often be better handled by a treatment coordinator skilled in the art of patient communication than by the dentist.

The role of the treatment coordinator

The ideal dental treatment coordinator is skilled in all the phases of dental practice including insurance and patient accounts, and has a good rapport with people. The treatment coordinator's job begins either when the patient telephones for information as a new patient or upon the patient's initial meeting with the dentist. The treatment coordinator needs a full and clear understanding of all phases of treatment to enable him or her to present the treatment plan to the patient in an easy-to-understand format (Figures 3.18A). After the treatment coordinator has presented a plan that is mutually acceptable to the doctor and the patient, the next step is to have your patient sign the treatment plan which should include your financial arrangements. Only then should your patient be scheduled for treatment (Figure 3.18B).

With the increasing use of auxiliary personnel, a dental treatment coordinator can be the backbone of the treatment team's communication process, providing support to the dentist, dental assistants, hygienist, receptionist, bookkeeper, and office manager alike. Your dental treatment coordinator should spend about half of the average workday dealing with treatment planning. Another third of the day will be devoted to necessary paperwork including insurance and accident cases. That leaves the balance of the day for patient problems—fees, miscommunications, and explanations of complicated dental procedures that the patient may not completely understand.

All lines of professional communication help to provide a smooth and effective treatment process for the patient. The treatment coordinator should maintain the credibility of the dentist and staff and reinforce the entire staff's dedication to ensuring the patient's faith in treatment already begun. It involves organizing and streamlining all aspects associated with patient treatment. This also requires checking the insurance and personal information that the patient provides.

Although payment for esthetic dentistry is always arranged in advance, if the treatment plan extends over considerable time a payment plan may need to be developed and explained fully to the patient. Some dentists do not want to talk about money with patients while others are perfectly comfortable doing so. If you are uncomfortable discussing fees with patients, you may too often end up giving away a good portion of your time, or working for a lower fee than you would normally charge. Therefore, for the financial health of your practice, make sure the treatment coordinator discusses fees and methods of payment with the patient.

The second appointment

In many instances, one appointment is all that is needed to diagnose, image, plan treatment, and make financial arrangements with your patient. However, more complex patient problems will usually require a second appointment.

A completed self-smile analysis form (see Figure 3.2) should be discussed with the patient before reviewing the radiographs with the dentist. With a thorough analysis, useful conclusions can be made about the patient's attitude toward his or her esthetic problems. The smile analysis provides information helpful to understanding the patients' attitudes, which should never be ignored. Patients may ask the impossible or make statements that point to more profound wishes and attitudes. Hear not only what a patient says but also what he or she means. If the planned esthetic treatment is simple, present the final treatment plan soon after the self-smile analysis has been discussed. For the patient with a difficult tooth problem (repositioning or periodontal involvement), consultation with a specialist should be arranged.

Consulting a specialist

Too often a dentist, anxious to begin treatment, fails to stress the importance of the patient consulting with a specialist. So many more patients will opt for full or minor orthodontics now if the procedure can be accomplished without brackets. Fortunately, invisible means of repositioning teeth through a series of transparent matrices, such as Clear Correct or Invisalign, have solved this problem. I also suggest using the term "repositioning" instead of "orthodontics," as it can elicit a more receptive patient response. Dentists often do not emphasize the functional objectives of tooth repositioning, and consequently may not motivate patients to seek orthodontic treatment that might be highly beneficial to their periodontal health. It is often a more conservative treatment option.

In most instances when there are difficult spaces to restore, even a minor orthodontic intervention can make a tremendous difference in the final result. It is important to let the patient know what options he or she has and the degree of excellence

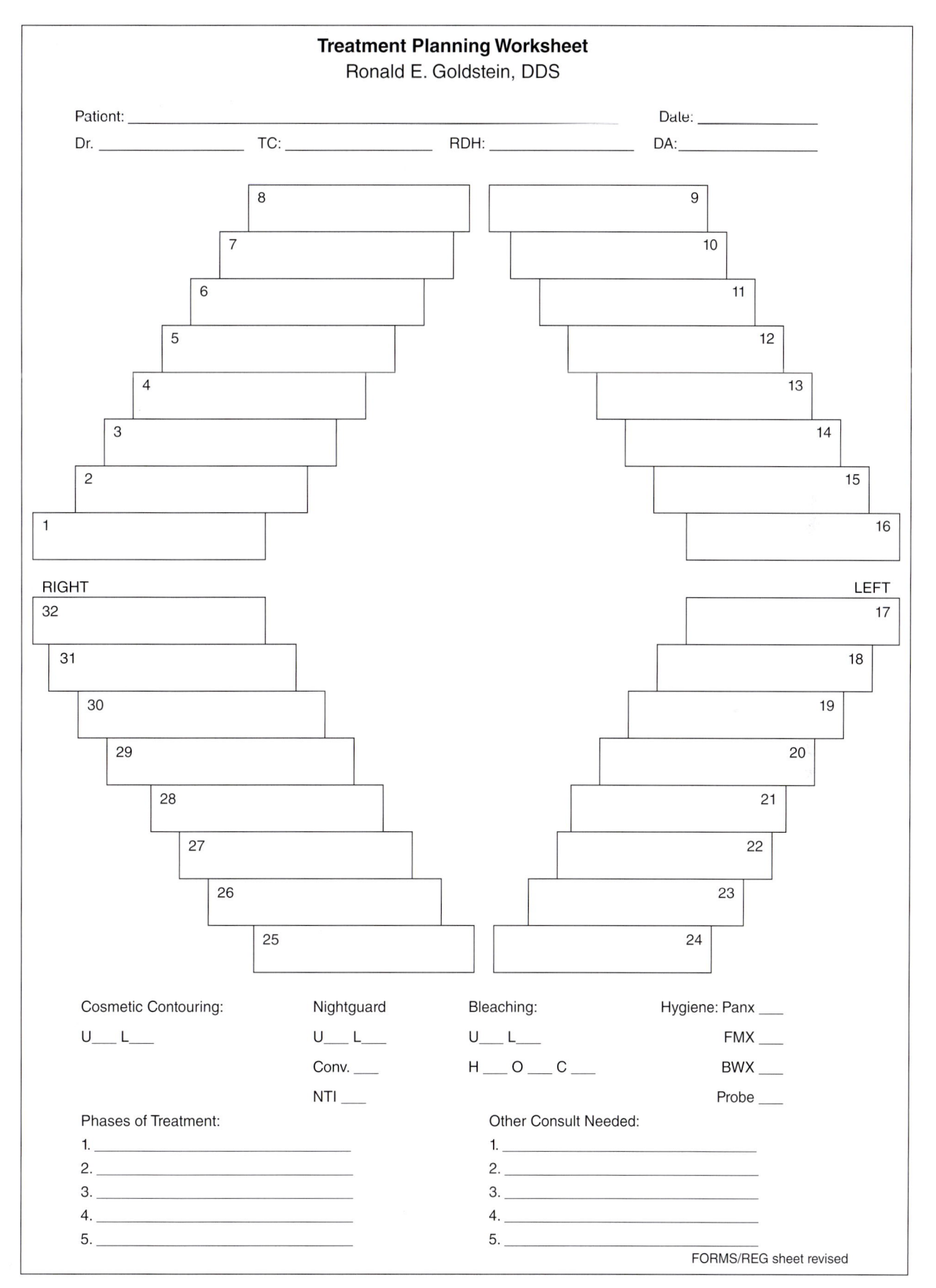

Treatment Planning Worksheet
Ronald E. Goldstein, DDS

Patient: _____ Date: _____
Dr. _____ TC: _____ RDH: _____ DA: _____

RIGHT — teeth 1–16 (upper), 17–32 (lower) — LEFT

Cosmetic Contouring:
U ___ L ___

Nightguard
U ___ L ___
Conv. ___
NTI ___

Bleaching:
U ___ L ___
H ___ O ___ C ___

Hygiene: Panx ___
FMX ___
BWX ___
Probe ___

Phases of Treatment:
1. _____
2. _____
3. _____
4. _____
5. _____

Other Consult Needed:
1. _____
2. _____
3. _____
4. _____
5. _____

FORMS/REG sheet revised

Figure 3.17 There are many digital diagnostic and treatment forms but this simple chart allows easy listing of proposed treatment for each tooth.

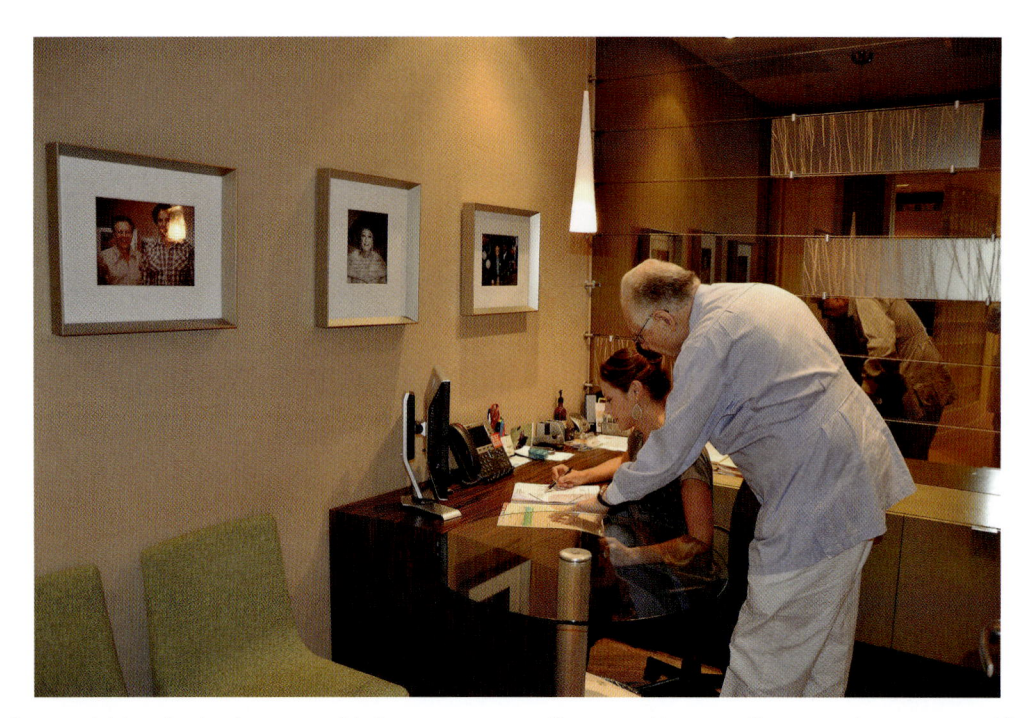

Figure 3.18 **(A)** It is essential that the dentist meets with the treatment coordinator, making sure all aspects of treatment and fees are correct before presenting the final treatment plan to the patient.

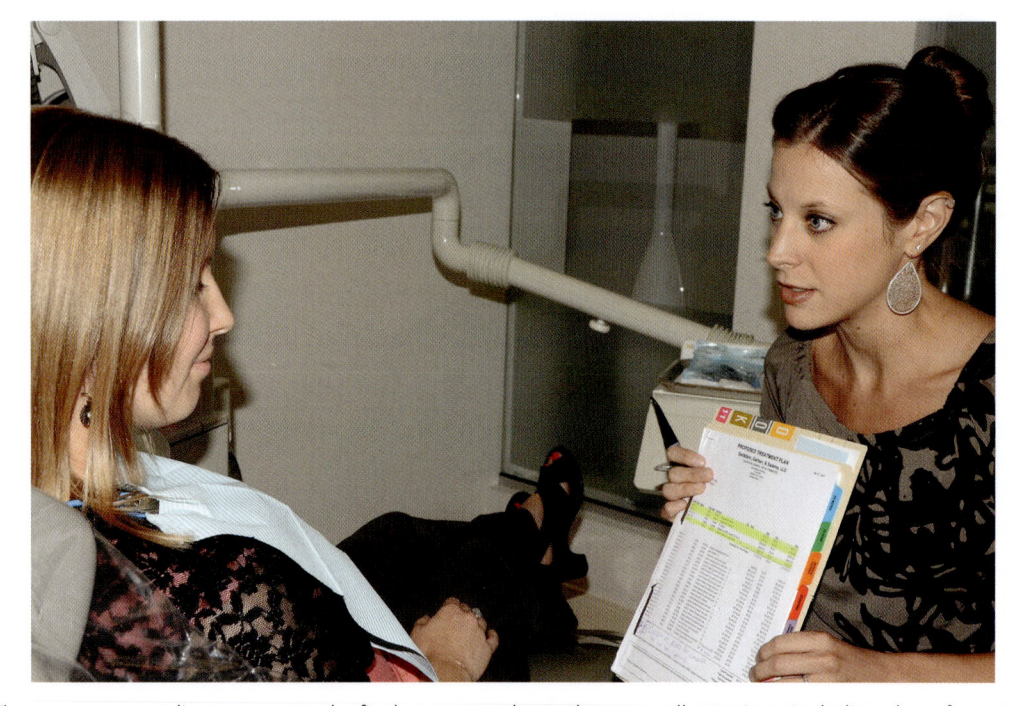

Figure 3.18 **(B)** The treatment coordinator presents the final treatment plan and answers all questions, including about financial arrangements, before the patient signs the treatment form.

that could be obtained with or without orthodontic treatment. A "compromised" esthetic result can be achieved with limited conservative orthodontics.

The next most important specialty to consider is periodontics. The control and correction of bone loss that could complicate the diagnosis or compromise the treatment results are obvious reasons to refer to a periodontist. In addition, the patient's soft tissue needs to be observed during maximum smiling. Could tissue repositioning help create a more favorable tooth size relative to the patient's face or smile? Would ridge augmentation help make a more realistic result? These, plus other questions regarding where and what type of margins to create, are typical problems that could be successfully solved with the aid of a periodontist skilled in cosmetic surgical techniques. Thickening of the

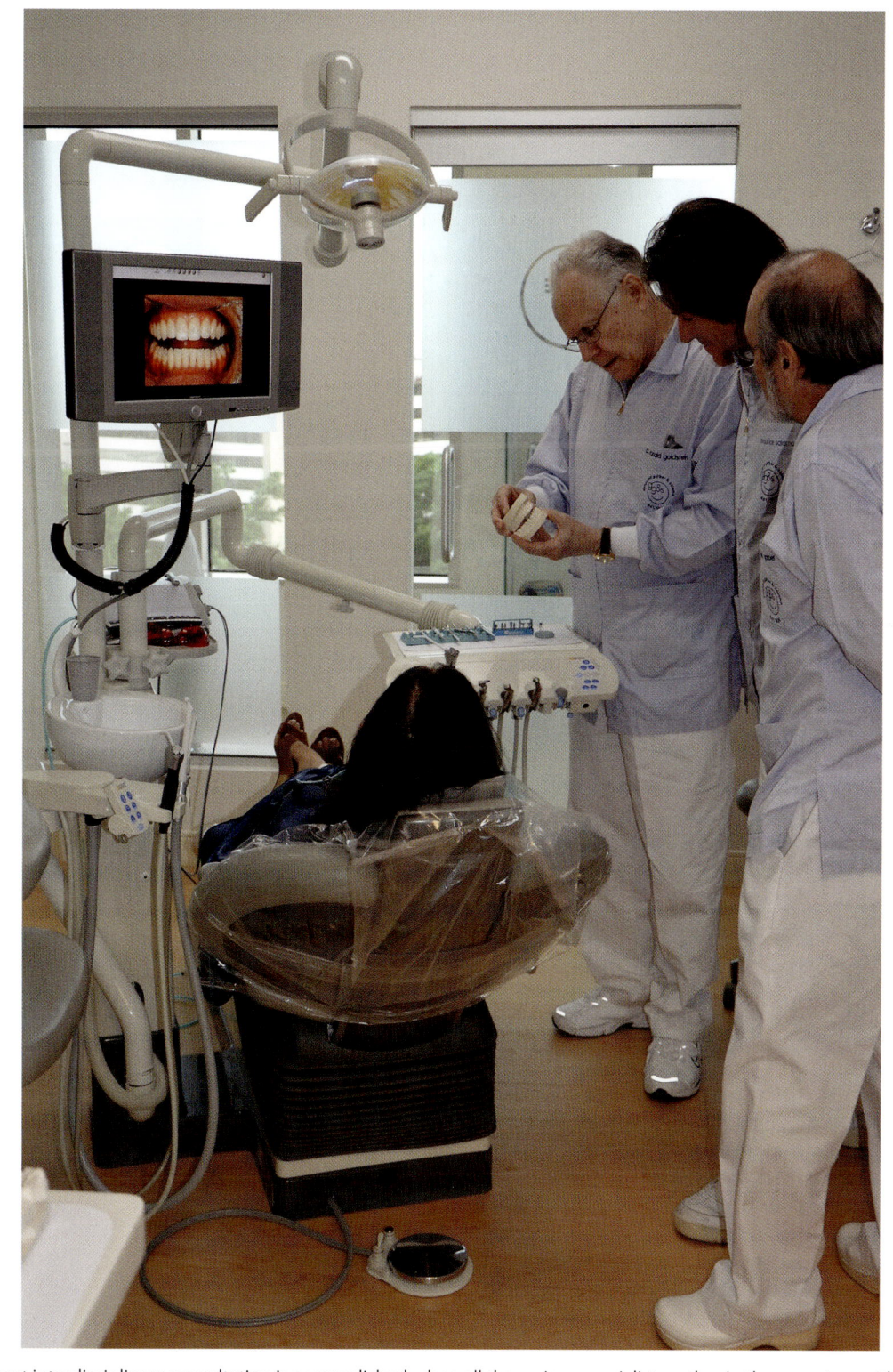

Figure 3.19 The best interdisciplinary consultation is accomplished when all the various specialists gather in the operatory with the patient to discuss a comprehensive treatment approach. This often must take place late in the afternoon or after hours so that all can attend.

periodontal gingival biotype to preserve marginal soft tissue levels and color is critical when performing all forms of cosmetic restorative dentistry. Connective tissue crafting is often requested.

A major problem with specialist consultation is communication between the general dentist and specialists. The typical method is referring and then expecting a letter in return. What this misses is "group thinking," which can be extremely beneficial especially in complex cases. I have always tried to get the various specialists in the operatory together with me so that interdisciplinary thinking among all of us can arrive at the ideal and even compromised plan. Although the various specialists happen to be in our office now, many years ago I would arrange the patient's appointments at

> If the above is not feasible then I suggest creating a high-tech network with your main referral sources so that you can both discuss and review the patient's records at the same time. Video conferencing and eventually simultaneous holographic consultation will be routine in both medical and dental practices. Digital photos, radiographs, and Skype can work just as well today.

5:00 pm and have the various specialists come to my office to first review the records, X-rays, mounted models, and photographs and then all of us see the patient at the same time. This procedure always resulted in an appreciative patient as well as clear sequence of therapy and detailed treatment planning (Figure 3.19).

When there are questionable areas regarding periapical pathology, such as in teeth with deep, old restorations or periapical thickening, an endodontic consultation is in order. Previously placed ill-fitting crowns or endodontically questionable teeth could also seriously compromise the esthetic result unless you treat these areas, if necessary, before you begin.

Finally, oral surgery must be considered when facial deformities could also complicate maximum esthetic results. This may involve scheduling a consultation with a plastic surgeon as well, if needed. The best way to communicate the advantages of obtaining specialty consultations is to let your patient know that you work with an excellent team consisting of orthodontists, periodontists, plastic surgeons, endodontists, and oral surgeons, and that your interest is in obtaining the best possible result based on their desires or preconceived images. You also need to stress that you are treating him or her as a whole person, not just treating the teeth. Finally, make sure you help your patient visualize the various options available. Eventually holographic group consultations will be possible and economically feasible especially when it is impractical to have all the specialists in one place at the same time.

The final patient presentation

The final case presentation should be a carefully prepared, easily understood treatment plan. Visual aids, before-and-after photographs, slides, models, intra- and extraoral video and computer imaging, and examples of the procedures should be used to assist in communicating the possibilities and limitations of esthetic treatment. Many patients would also like to see your treatment results on other patients if possible. There are four basic methods for helping patients visualize your suggested solutions for their individual esthetic problems.

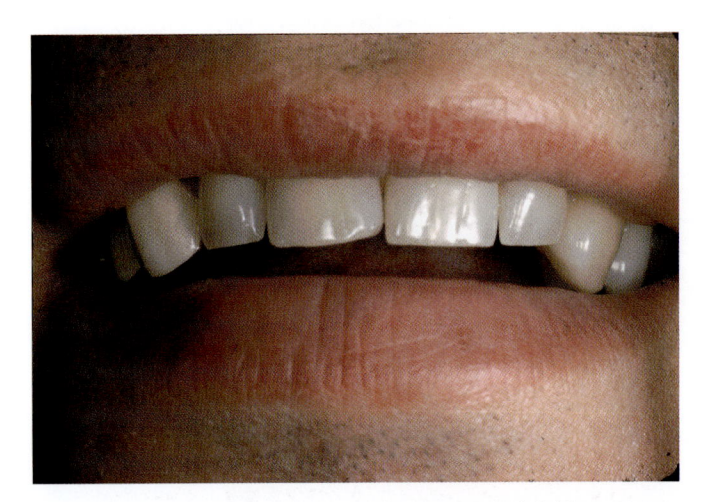

Figure 3.20 (A) Even with computer imaging it is helpful for patients to be able to see how changes will affect their speaking ability and the appearance of their lip line. This patient was unhappy with his smile and wanted longer teeth.

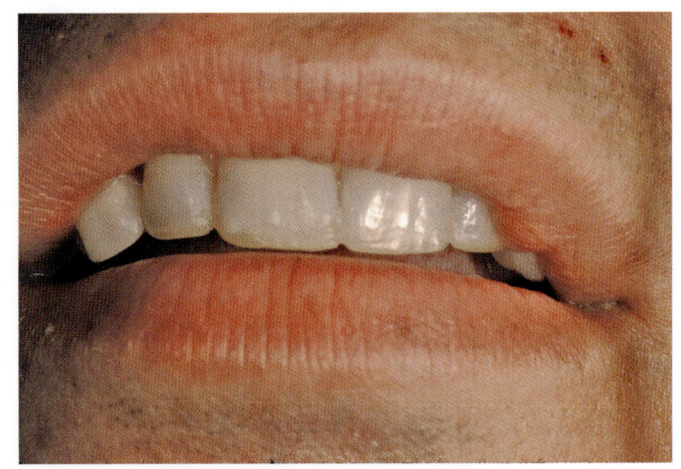

Figure 3.20 (B) Tooth-colored wax applied to the central incisors showed the patient how the final restorations would correct his problem.

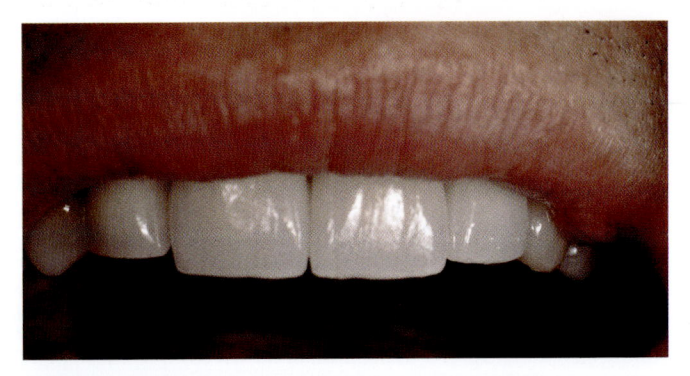

Figure 3.20 (C) Visualizing the improvement motivated this patient to obtain esthetic correction with fixed ceramic restorations.

1. **Soft, tooth-colored wax or composite resin applied directly in the mouth**: the advantages to this technique (Figure 3.20A–C) are as follows:
    - it is the least costly for the patient
    - it is the quickest method
    - it is especially useful in space or diastema problems.
2. **A waxed study model**: when the potential solution to an esthetic problem requires extensive tooth preparation, this method can be effective for those patients who are used to visualizing plans, such as an architectural blueprint (Figure 3.21). The waxed model is also important from a diagnostic standpoint when your patient has a space problem. By preparing the teeth, then waxing them, you can determine if there is too much or too little space for normal-sized tooth

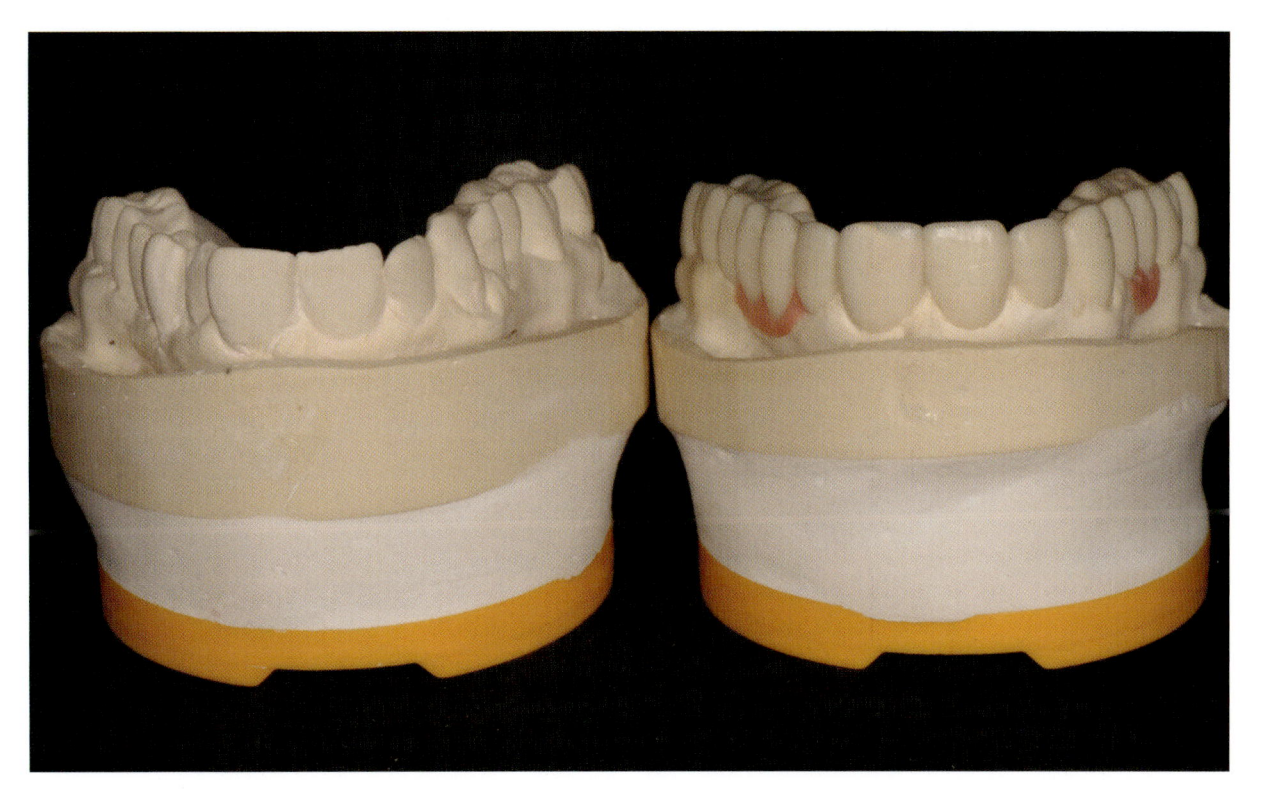

Figure 3.21 Creating waxed models of the available choices helps the patient understand the treatment options and enhances the dentist's diagnostic ability.

replacement. This allows you to adjust the treatment plan as necessary to make certain you can create an adequate esthetic restoration.

3. **Esthetic imaging**: as previously stated, esthetic imaging may be the best method to help your patient visualize your intended corrections (see Figure 3.13). The printouts and the image on the monitor can be effective communication tools. This method also allows you to easily alter your treatment plan to reflect various compromises. Rarely will it be necessary for your patient to return for further imaging if you have thought of possible options in advance. It is also effective to show your patient the various choices, since most people will opt for the best look, provided they can find a way to afford the correction. For patients with complex problems, the combination of computer imaging and waxed diagnostic models will be the best choice for complete visualization.

4. **Trial smile**: by far, a trial smile is the very best method of assuring that your patient will be happy with your final result. There are several methods of accomplishing this procedure; most of them require a good wax-up of the intended result. Next, a silicone matrix can be made of the wax-up which can then be applied directly in the mouth with either acrylic or composite resin. Also, consider using Snap-On Smile (DenMat) for a longer lasting trial smile (Figure 3.22A–E). The same procedure can be done by making the final restoration in the laboratory instead of directly in the patient's mouth. It all depends on the size and position of the teeth. Naturally not all restorative or orthodontic problems can be translated into a trial smile over the natural teeth. In these cases, either direct bonding or esthetic imaging may suffice. Trial smile may indeed have to wait until the temporary stage in certain instances and this will be covered in Chapter 42 on esthetic temporization.

CBCT and 3D planning software

The role of the CBCT unit and 3D planning software has been established as an indispensable part of ideal diagnostic evaluations and treatment planning. The ability to see the relationship of the patient's bone, soft tissue, and vital anatomy in relation to their existing or planned implants, grafting, and restoration is critical to avoiding error.

Today, we have the ability to interact with digital and optical files simultaneously and use Dual Scan protocols, stitching the model images to the CBCT images of the patient and allowing for optimal treatment planning accuracy for surgeon and restorative dentist.

The ability to evaluate pathology of the jaws and teeth as well as the quality and quantity of bone available for implant placement allows us to execute our treatment with safety, precision, and esthetics in mind.

Often, we can plan the cases on these 3D software applications using simulated implant libraries and transfer this information into surgical guides for the implant surgeon to mimic what was planned digitally. Additionally, this information can be used to create stereolithographic models of the patient's jaws for further evaluation.

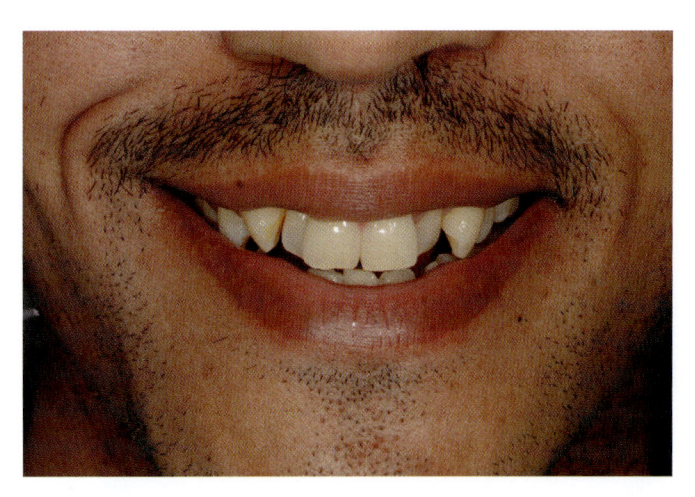

Figure 3.22 **(A)** This patient had an extremely difficult malocclusion requiring orthodontic therapy.

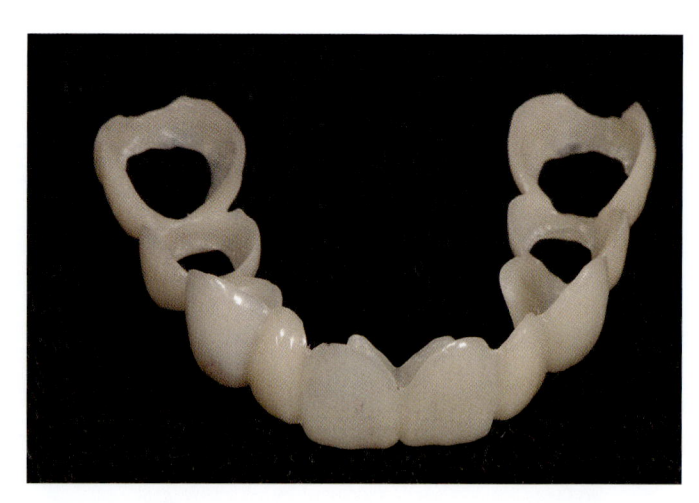

Figure 3.22 **(B)** A removable appliance (Snap-On Smile) was made to create a realistic trial smile that he could wear and visualize the result of his treatment outcome.

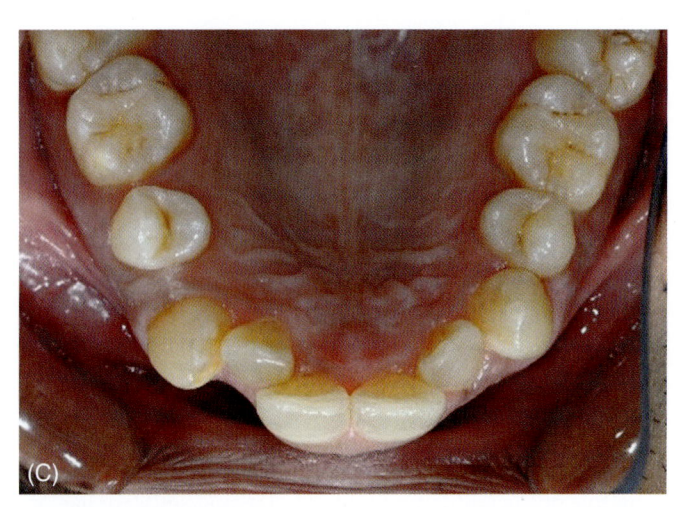

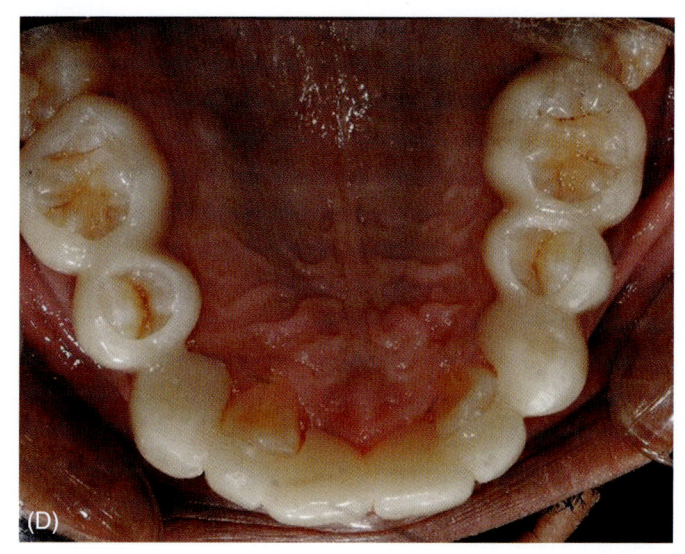

Figure 3.22 **(C and D)** Note in this occlusal photo how the appliance attaches to the teeth.

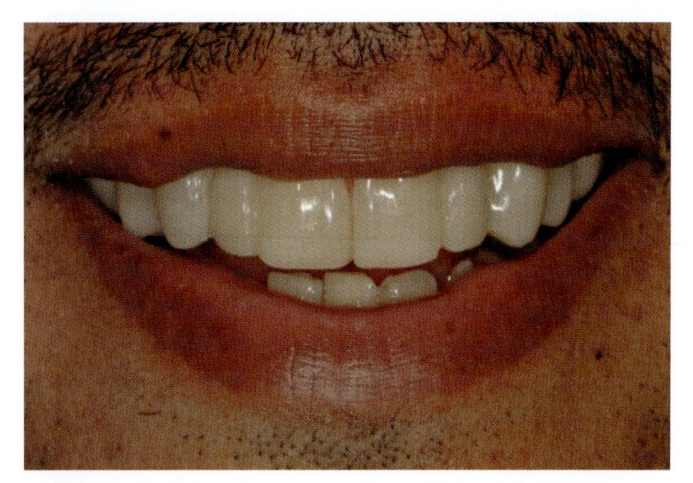

Figure 3.22 **(E)** The patient was pleased with his trial smile which allowed him to experience the reaction of family and friends to his new look.

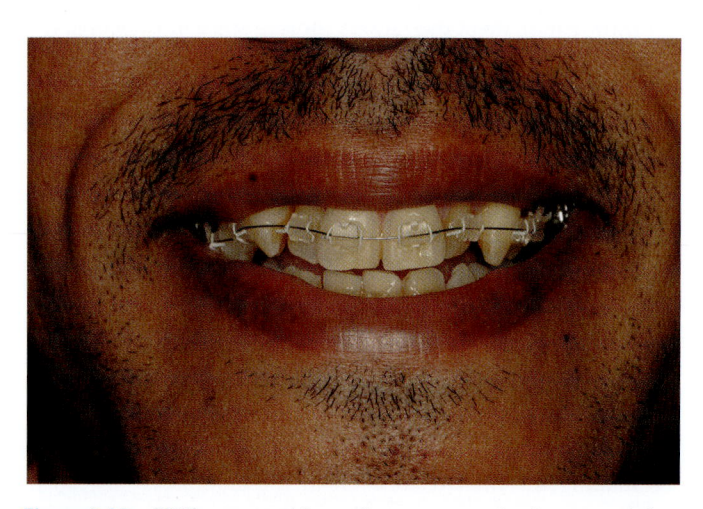

Figure 3.22 **(F)** The removable appliance was motivating enough for the patient to undergo orthodontic therapy 3 years later.

From a restorative perspective, abutments can be selected from these libraries and a provisional restoration can be designed and fabricated based upon these 3D plans using 3D printing technologies.

The future is upon us and looks bright indeed regarding the implementation of all these new digital technologies.

Problem patients: when not to treat … but refer

It is impossible for any one dentist, regardless of how capable he or she is, to satisfy every patient's esthetic needs. Most new patients are on their best behavior during the initial interview session. That is why it takes a skillful dentist and staff, as well as extra time, to ascertain what kind of patient is presenting to your office. Your goal is to determine who should be the patient you refer to another colleague. There is an entire chapter devoted to this subject, Chapter 2, which you and your clinical personnel should read and digest for a better understanding of patients and how to manage them. Nevertheless, to help with your decision of whether or not to treat certain patients, the following patient-type categories can be incorporated into your treatment philosophy.

The purpose of classifying potential problem patients here is not to dissuade you from treating them. Rather, it is to make you and your staff more aware of the potential consequences of treating certain types of patients. You and your staff should now be able to recognize better a potential problem before it happens. The treatment sequence outlined in Figure 3.3 is extremely important in this regard. The chain of people who can give you information as to the patient's personality is the receptionist, the assistant/hygienist, and then the treatment coordinator. Be sure to use the input from these key staff members before you elect to take up a patient's esthetic treatment. Should you decide to treat a problem patient, be sure to adjust your fees accordingly.

> Remember, it is not enough to just cover the cost of treatment of such patients. If you elect to dedicate the extra time, effort, and above all, stress (not only yours but also that of your staff and perhaps even your family), you are entitled to a reasonable profit for doing so. Your staff and family expect and deserve it as well. The greater is the difficulty, time, and effort required, the greater is the multiple of one's routine fee. In the past 54 years many of the perceived "difficult" patients who elected not to proceed with my proposed treatment due to the increased fee have gone elsewhere for treatment—only to come back years later, still not happy. Now they will have to spend even more money to have their treatment redone. Incidentally, if you misjudged the patient the first time by referring when, perhaps, they might have been a perfectly acceptable patient, do not make the mistake of underestimating the amount of time, stress, and costs involved in redoing that patient's case.

The perfectionist

This patient has the highest standard of esthetic excellence. Unless you are willing to spend an inordinate amount of diagnostic and treatment time with this patient, you are much better off, emotionally and financially, making an early decision to refer this patient. Deciding to treat this type of patient may mean charging two, three, or even four times your normal fee in order to cover the extra time, stress, laboratory and office costs, and extended warranty for this patient. Offices that elect to do this should also consider the probability of having to redo the treatment several times in an attempt to satisfy this patient's esthetic and functional demands. Will it be worth it and can your office afford this type of expense? Too often, dentists find that treating these patients costs them so much they would have paid another dentist double the amount after they have failed in their attempts to satisfy the patient. Although many of us may enjoy a challenge, the question is, can your office afford the risk of taking on such a challenge?

The poor communicator

These are the patients who cannot communicate what they want because they do not themselves know what they want. They may show you a picture of exactly what they desire, but when they eventually see it in their mouth they may be terribly disappointed. Even study models with wax-ups may look good to these patients, but that approval may be of no benefit when the final restoration is in their mouth. What can be most frustrating is to show this type of patient a computer image of his or her enhanced smile, which may be enthusiastically received but, amazingly, not appreciated when tried in. The problem is, these people really do not know what they want when it comes to their own appearance. Typically, they have difficulty making up their minds in other areas of their lives as well. They may be constantly redecorating their homes, apartments, or offices. They may be frequently frustrated with their hairstyles and constantly changing their barber or hairstylist in an attempt to find that "perfect" style. The real problem here is identifying these types of patients before agreeing to treat them. This is one of the hardest categories to identify because, at first glance, these people seem so easy to please. You may be tempted to proceed with treatment too hastily only to find that you, in fact, are now treating the type of patient you may have wished you had referred. One important clue to help you recognize this patient type is that he or she presents to you in the middle of treatment from another office. Frequently, that dentist may have redone their treatment many times before the patient sought another opinion. If this is the situation, carefully analyze the treatment with which the patient presents. Has it been done poorly? Is it esthetically inferior? Frequently, the patient will state "I hear you're the best." Although we all like to think we can do something better, "better" may, however, be just another failure to this problem patient. And the sad situation is that few, if any, practitioners may be able to satisfy this patient. Frequently, the root of the problem is psychological. The patient may not truly know what he or she wants. Other times he or she is looking for your esthetic dentistry to solve a problem that only a psychologist or psychiatrist can solve.

High expectations/limited budget

There is nothing wrong with patients who are limited in the amount of money they can invest in their dental treatment. In fact, this may make up the majority of your patients. However, proceed cautiously with the budget-conscious patient who has extremely high esthetic expectations. Rather than having a dissatisfied patient, you are much better off explaining that because they may not be able to afford the ideal or recommended treatment due to the great amount of time, cost, and so on involved, they need to compromise. If this is the case you will need extensive documentation and informed consent forms signed before beginning any therapy.

The "wrinkle patient"

These patients are afraid of looking old. They expect esthetic dentistry to make them look young again, expecting you to get rid of their wrinkles by "plumping out" the restorations. Unfortunately, your dentistry may not be able to accomplish this esthetically, which can make for patient dissatisfaction.

The other type of patient in this category is the one who claims that wrinkles appeared after the esthetic treatment. This is one of the situations where the before full-face photograph is essential. It is advised that these photographs be taken with and without makeup. Ask the patient to remove all makeup, thus allowing you to more accurately see facial characteristics, which will help you in your diagnosis and treatment. Then point out every wrinkle and/or other facial deformities that are not likely to change. However, be quick to point out to this type of patient that you work with an excellent team which includes a plastic surgeon, and that, following your dental treatment, the plastic surgeon may be able to improve that condition if they desire. Follow this suggestion with a recommendation for a consultation with a plastic or oral surgeon during your diagnostic stage—never after your treatment is complete. Make sure to document the recommendation so that you will not be taking responsibility for something you cannot control.

The uncooperative patient

This is another potential problem patient that can be overlooked if your diagnostic time is too short. Frequently, this patient presents with poor dentistry or no restorative dentistry at all. Hygiene is either nonexistent or inadequate at best. They will vociferously complain about a previous dentist and staff. The major problem with these patients is they will not accept responsibility for any of their problems or faults. A typical response of a patient with extremely worn teeth may be, "I never grind my teeth," and he or she may become agitated at you for even suggesting it. Or, "I brush my teeth six times a day," despite the extensive presence of plaque indicating less than adequate homecare. These patients are frequently so abusive to everyone in your office, including you, that your staff will agree that no fee you may charge is worth the aggravation of treating this type of patient. This is certainly one time when a consultation with your staff about accepting this patient for treatment in your practice would be extremely beneficial. If you do decide to accept this patient, you should consider substantially increasing your fee. A doubling, tripling, or more might be appropriate.

How to treat problem patients ... and keep your staff sane

There are several precautions to take if you elect to treat problem patients.

1. **Be prepared to spend much more time in diagnosis.** The best way to handle patients who have difficulty communicating what they want is to schedule several diagnostic sessions. Use different approaches to attempt to understand what your patient visualizes as a final result. It is essential for your patient to understand that this is "their" problem, and you will try to help correct it. The only time you can accomplish this is during the diagnostic stage. This diagnostic phase must be considered as a period of discovery not only of the intraoral condition but also of the patient's psychological and visual concept of self-image. If your patient refuses to admit a problem, it would be wise for you to avoid accepting any treatment liability. If you proceed with treating such a problem patient, *it is essential that you and the patient sign a limited treatment liability agreement* which outlines exactly the specific treatment and specific time period of treatment, including posttreatment care.

2. **You should never proceed with your treatment plan until both you and your patient have a thorough understanding of what your treatment will be.** Make sure your treatment coordinator has your patient sign a consent form, following an oral presentation of recommended treatment, that all options were presented and that the patient understands the options and agrees with the treatment. Next, follow up with a detailed treatment letter listing any exceptions or potential problems that could be encountered.

3. **When treating problem patients, consider treatment in phases or sequential therapy.** The advantage of treating problem patients in phases is that you never proceed to the next phase until the patient is pleased with the current phase of treatment. The following is an example of how this may occur.

    - **First phase**: diagnosis and treatment planning. This may consist of soft tissue management, all diagnostic tests and records, specialist referrals, and appropriate endodontic and periodontic therapy. Salivary diagnostics and genetic testing for periodontal disease and susceptibility may also be considered.

    - **Second phase**: treatment splinting and/or bleaching. This is the time to redo and alter, as necessary, treatment crowns or bridges until your patient is esthetically pleased and signs your release to proceed to phase 3. If a problem patient says, "I like them just the way they are except I want this tooth built out a little more," you should not proceed to the next phase of treatment. Make the necessary changes and let the patient live with the changed restoration for at least another week to make sure no other exceptions arise. The patient must be pleased with the appearance of the treatment splints; otherwise he or she may well be dissatisfied with the final restoration, stating, "I thought it would be different!" It also means using a capable laboratory to make well-shaded and proportioned acrylic temporaries, which becomes the trial smile.

- **Third phase**: placement of final restorations. Your treatment should virtually duplicate the temporaries. Take either a very good alginate or, even better, a vinyl polysiloxane impression to accurately record just how your patient wishes to look. When all is done, the patient should be satisfied with the esthetic treatment you have painstakingly performed.

4. **Make sure your fee is adjusted appropriately.** You should apportion your fee to the various phases after determining your expenses and desired profit in each phase of treatment. The fact that your increased fee may be considerably higher than that of other colleagues should play no role in setting your fee. Your attitude should be, if the patient does not understand your special abilities and the extra effort you will expend in helping to solve his or her problem, you are better off letting another dentist suffer the consequences, including the financial loss, in dealing with this type of problem patient. In the final analysis, you should thoroughly consider all of the problems associated with each patient, whether a difficult clinical or emotional issue, or both. In some cases an astute staff member may sense that you cannot satisfy a particular patient. In all cases, be upfront and honest about your decision that this patient may be better treated by another dentist. Issues of patient abandonment do not apply if you decide to not treat during the diagnostic phase and before any treatment has begun.

5. **Pay particular attention to your treatment warranty and make sure the patient knows exactly what work and how long the guarantee covers.**

Continuous communication

Treatment planning is not complete until the patient makes a final decision about accepting treatment. However, follow-through by the treatment coordinator is necessary throughout your patient's treatment. Any proposed changes to your treatment plan must involve your treatment coordinator. In fact, if your proposed changes affect your fee, then be certain to have the new case fee verified with the patient by the treatment coordinator prior to your beginning the altered treatment procedures.

How esthetic procedures differ from ordinary dental procedures should be explained. The patient must understand that esthetic dentistry may be time-consuming and, unlike routine procedures, does not always produce immediate results. Differences such as time involved for extra try-ins, treatment plans that require chairside carving and shaping of temporaries, staining of porcelain at the chair side, and the dentist's time and expertise should all be discussed. The patient must be convinced and satisfied that any additional time necessary for better esthetic results is worth the investment.

Dentists should be aware that patients are often completely unfamiliar with esthetic dentistry and are reluctant or unable to ask the important and relevant questions about the procedures. The limitations of esthetic dentistry should also be explained to the patient. While esthetic treatment can produce dramatic improvements, it cannot do everything. If compromise is necessary, say so. It becomes the dentist's responsibility, therefore, to see that all doubts and questions are cleared away during the final case presentation. You must be careful not to impose your own esthetic notions on the patient. Superior knowledge and training make dentists the arbiters of what is practical and workable; they do not give him or her any precedence in matters of esthetic preference.

Esthetic treatment demands personal communication between patient and dentist that must continue throughout treatment. Be an acute observer, a precise listener, and an understanding interpreter. Always remember that good communication can make it possible to change an insecure frown into an assured smile.

Cost of treatment

One of the biggest stumbling blocks to offering quality esthetic dentistry is the mistaken belief that your patients will be reluctant to pay for it. One of my former patients was a bricklayer dissatisfied with his smile. He came to the appointment rather poorly dressed and not well-groomed. I spent a considerable amount of time trying to educate him as to why the best esthetic dentistry might cost more. I gave him three alternative choices for different qualities of esthetic treatment and thoroughly explained the differences among the three. He eventually chose the best and most costly quality dental service. My father believed I had spent too much time with someone who did not appear to be interested in such a high-quality procedure. However, this taught me (and my father) never to judge someone by first appearance.

This is not to say you should spend the same amount of time with every patient. It becomes obvious that not everyone will be receptive to learning the differences between quality and average treatment. In the final analysis, it will be up to you to determine if the patient who is not interested in understanding the differences will be the patient you wish to treat. Generally, these patients are shoppers who will base their decision on price only.

The different classifications of patients will have different motivations and expectations for esthetic dentistry. Some are influenced more by the life expectancy of the restoration while others care more about the esthetic result.

> Almost every patient wants to know, "How much is it going to cost?," even before visiting the dental office. In fact, some patients, the price shoppers, will call to request prices before deciding to make an appointment. These people are usually driven primarily by price, and yet still may have a high esthetic dental need. Probably the most difficult task most dentists face is answering the fee question. Your fee should reflect the quality of care your office provides and should not be presented with apology. If the patient views the treatment as a need and is aware of the benefits of that treatment, he or she will usually consent to the proposed treatment plan, provided finances are not a problem. I also recommend that your potential patients read, Change Your Smile,[2] specifically the postscripts on page 54 regarding fees.

The patient will usually feel more at ease with a third party, the treatment coordinator, and thus more comfortable voicing questions about fees at this time. If necessary, a compromise or a different treatment alternative can be introduced when there is genuine dissatisfaction or a problem with a patient's ability to pay. If this situation occurs, it is often helpful for the treatment coordinator to suggest, "Let me speak with the doctor and see if some compromise treatment can be arranged." You may then choose to alter the terms, the total fee, or suggest alternative treatment plans. The amount of a fee is not as important as how your patient perceives it. A company president may reject even moderately priced dentistry, whereas the president's secretary may accept the same treatment plan and fee if he or she realizes the need and finds a way to prioritize the expense. One of the most important components of any case presentation is showing your patients the difference between ordinary and exceptional esthetic dentistry. For instance, show the difference between a regular porcelain crown and one of inlaid porcelain. Show the difference in an extracted tooth that has routine bonding versus one with characterized bonding. Always have two types of laminates: one with opaque monochromatic porcelain and one with color and artifacts built in. And, remember, not every patient wants or appreciates the difference. Patient feedback helps you know who your patient is and how to approach your esthetic dentistry treatment plan to gain acceptance.

Many dentists have little awareness of the factors upon which they should base their fees for esthetic dentistry. Therefore, they feel inadequate or unable to properly define and, unfortunately, even defend their fees. One thing should be made clear from the outset. Most patient insurance policies do *not* appropriately cover fees for esthetic dentistry. So how should fees be determined? The following are key factors that should be considered when you establish your fees for esthetic dentistry.

Training and technical skill

This consists not only of your educational background but also the amount of time and money you invest in brief and/or extensive courses, web-based distance learning, educational videos, reading books, magazines, and newsletters (including the volumes of information you receive from dental suppliers and manufacturers). Do not forget all those dental meetings you have attended—not only the cost of the meeting but the cost of lost income and the time away from your family and personal life. The website www.dentalxp.com is an excellent adjunct site to any education you may be receiving. Practitioners with more experience and higher level of skill should charge higher fees than someone just graduating from school. Fees should reflect your training, years of experience, and technical skill.

Time and complexity of procedure

The amount of time necessary for a procedure is just part of the fee formula. Consider the extra time you may need to spend with certain demanding patients. How much extra time will you allow for patients who ask a lot of questions? Time should cover diagnosing, planning, accomplishing the procedure, redoing, repairs, and postoperative visits. Is a crown just a crown? Is it just as difficult to do a crown on a right central incisor as it is to do one on a bicuspid? Or how about a "hidden" second molar? Laminating or crowning a single tooth to match an adjacent tooth is many times more difficult a procedure to accomplish than if you crown or laminate two or four teeth. More advanced clinical and laboratory skills are needed for the former. Is it not considerably easier to match a maxillary first or second molar to another one than to perfectly match one central incisor to another? In fact, if you are treating a single tooth, your cost per tooth is considerably more than that for doing six or eight teeth. Consequently, there is a significant difference in your cost, depending upon which procedure you are doing.

Artistic skill/patient requirements

Patients vary. Some truly do not care what your result looks like, just as long as it fits. Others may not seem to care—until he or she goes home and looks closely in the mirror. *Always give a patient a mirror and have him or her hold it at arm's length because that is the perspective from which other people will observe.* However, if your office has a good lighted area to place a nice wall-mounted mirror then this will suffice (Figure 3.23). The patient who holds the mirror very close requires something different of us; he or she is usually the perfectionist and you may need to adjust your fee accordingly. Another important consideration is your artistic ability. It is accepted, often expected, in every profession and culture to pay more for the best. We pay more for the best sculptures, artwork, photographs, ceramics, jewelry, and all types of other things that require artistic skill. We refer to our profession as "the art and science of dentistry." The science is well understood, but the art has been ignored for too long. You deserve to be compensated based in part on your artistic skill.

Overhead

Your overhead is based on so many factors, including where you are geographically, rent, upkeep, materials, and most of all staff salons. Laboratory fees, if any, must be considered, as well as the quality of the laboratory, the materials, and the equipment that you use. Does your office employ the latest in high-tech equipment? All of these things benefit the patient but cost money. If your office is a state-of-the-art facility, then it should be

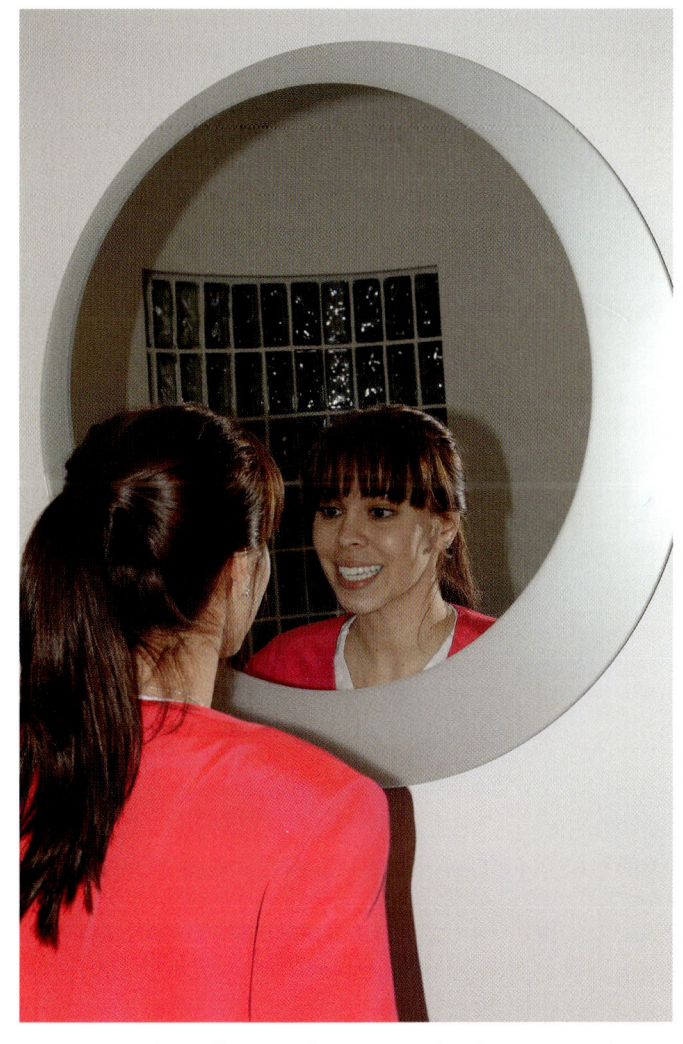

Figure 3.23 This wall-mounted mirror is perfect for patients to be able to see their smile and face the way others will be looking at them.

differentiated from the offices that appear outdated and are, in fact, furnished with antiquated equipment.

Warranty

What do you guarantee? Are you giving a minimal or extended warranty? Is it 3 months, 6 months, or 1 year? For how many months will you render free aftercare and for how many years will you provide service at a reduced fee and at what percent discount? Are your patients told to wear a protective appliance? Do they or will they wear it? They may have accidents, caries, periodontal conditions, tooth loss, or root fracture; are you guaranteeing your treatment against all those things? You prescribe home care; are they going to do all that you expect? Your warranty must point out the circumstances under which you will guarantee your dental treatment. Are you guaranteeing that if your patient bites into a candied apple your laminate will not break? If eating habits are expected to change after you insert your ceramic crowns or laminates, then this, too, must be stressed and put into your warranty. The best car manufacturer may not honor its warranty if the owner does not fulfill the agreement—changing oil and allowing the dealer to perform necessary maintenance. Are you prepared to honor your warranty for patients who do not come in for routine prophylaxis and clinical examination? Certainly, damage caused by neglect can be costly. A well-constructed warranty and fee structure can help to protect you against patient-neglect situations.

References

1. Levin RP. Patient personality assessment improves case presentation. *Dent Econ* 1988;78(9):49–50,52,54–55.
2. Goldstein RE. *Change Your Smile*, 4th edn. Chicago, IL: Quintessence; 2009.

Additional resources

Baratieri LN. *Inspiration People, Teeth and Restorations*, 1st edn. New Malden, UK: Quintessence; 2012.

Brezavscek M, Lamott U, Att W. Treatment planning and dental rehabilitation of periodontally compromised partially edentulous patient: a case report-Part 1. *Int J Esthet Dent* 2014;9:402–410.

Chiche GJ, Pinault A. *Esthetics of Anterior Fixed Prosthodontics*, 1st edn. Chicago, IL: Quintessence; 1994.

Chiche GJ, Aoshima H. Functional versus aesthetic articulation of maxillary anterior restorations. *Pract Periodont Aesthet Dent* 1997;9:335–342.

Chiche J, Aoshima H. *Smile Design*, 1st edn. Carol Stream, IL: Quintessence; 2004.

Coachman C, Salama M, Garber D, et al. Prosthetic gingival reconstruction in the fixed partial restoration. Part 1: introduction to artificial gingiva as an alternative therapy. *Int J Periodont Restor Dent* 2009;29:471–477.

Coachman C, Salama M, Garber D, et al. Prosthetic gingival reconstruction in the fixed partial restoration. Part 3: laboratory procedures and maintenance. *Int J Periodont Restor Dent* 2010;30:19–29.

Coachman C, Van Dooren E, Gurel G, et al. Smile design: from digital treatment planning to clinical reality. In: Cohen M, ed. *Interdisciplinary Treatment Planning: Principles, Design, Implementation*, Vol 2. Chicago, IL: Quintessence; 2012.

Cohen M, ed. *Interdisciplinary Treatment Planning: Principles, Design, Implementation, Vol 1*. Chicago, IL: Quintessence; 2008.

Cohen M, ed. *Interdisciplinary Treatment Planning: Principles, Design, Implementation, Vol 2*. Chicago, IL: Quintessence; 2012.

Feraru, M. Musella, V. Bichacho, N. Individualizing a smile makeover. *J Cosmet Dent* 2016;32:109–119.

Ferencz J, Silva N, Navarro J. *High Strength Ceramics*, 1st edn. Hanover Park, IL: Quintessence; 2014.

Fradeani M. *Esthetic Rehabilitation in Fixed Prosthodontics. Esthetic Analysis: A Systematic Approach to Prosthetic Treatment, Vol 1.* Chicago, IL: Quintessence; 2004:35–61.

Fradeani, M. *Esthetic Analysis: A Systematic Approach to Esthetic, Biologic, and Functional Integration, Vol 1*, 1st edn. Hanover Park, IL: Quintessence; 2004.

Fradeani M, Barducci G. *Prosthetic Treatment: A Systematic Approach to Esthetic, Biologic, and Functional Integration, Vol 2*, 1st edn. Hanover Park, IL: Quintessence; 2008.

Gurel G. *The Science and Art of Porcelain Laminate Veneers*, 1st edn. Berlin: Quintessence; 2003.

Kano P, Dooren EV, Xavier C, et al. State of the art, the anatomical shell technique: mimicking nature. In: Durante S, ed. *Quintessence of Dental Technology, Vol 37*, 1st edn. Chicago, IL: Quintessence; 2014:95–112.

Kim, J. *The Master Ceramist*, 1st edn. New York, NY: Jason J. Kim Oral Design New York Center; 2009.

Kois JC. Successful dental treatment: getting the best possible results. *Dear Doctor* 2012;5:46–58.

Kois JC, Spear FM. Periodontal prosthesis: creating successful restorations. *J Am Dent Assoc* 1992;123:108–15.

Kois JC, Hartrick N. Functional occlusion: science-driven management. *J Cosmet Dent* 2007;23:54–55.

Kois JC. Diagnostically driven interdisciplinary treatment planning. In: Cohen M, ed. *Interdisciplinary Treatment Planning: Principles, Design, Implementation*. Chicago, IL: Quintessence; 2008:189–212.

Magne P, Belser U, eds. *Bonded—A Biometric Approach*. Chicago, IL: Quintessence; 2002:270–273,358–363.

Romano R. *The Art of the Smile*, 1st edn. New Malden, UK: Quintessence; 2005.

Romano R. *The Art of Detailing*, 1st edn. New Malden, UK: Quintessence; 2013.

Salama M, Coachman C, Garber D, et al. Prosthetic gingival reconstruction in the fixed partial restoration. Part 2: diagnosis and treatment planning. *Int J Periodont Restor Dent* 2009;29:573–581.

Spear, FM. Treatment planning materials, tooth reduction, and margin placement for anterior indirect esthetic restorations. *Inside Dent* 2008;4:4–13.

Spear, FM. Achieving the harmony between esthetics and function. Presented at: *The XIV Italian Academy of Prosthetic Dentistry International Congress*; November 9, 1995; Bologna, Italy.

Spear FM, Kokich VG, Mathews DP. Interdisciplinary management of anterior dental esthetics. *J Am Dent Assoc* 2006;137; 160–169.

Sulikowski A, Yoshida A. Suface texture: a systematic approach for accurate and effective communication. *Quintessence Dent Technol* 2003;26:10–19.

Tarnow D, Chu S, Kim J. *Aesthetic Restorative Dentistry Principles and Practice*, 1st edn. Mahawah, NJ: Montage Media Corporation; 2008.

Terry D, Geller W. *Esthetic and Restorative Dentistry Material Selection and Technique*, 2nd edn. Hanover Park, IL: Quintessence; 2013.

Viana PC, Correia A, Neves M, et al. Soft tissue waxup and mock-up as key factors in treatment plan: case presentation. *Eur J Esthet Dent* 2012;7:310–323.

Wilkins RG, Kois JC. Using a system of diagnosis and treatment planning to reduce stress. *Compend Contin Educ Dent* 2000;21: 485–491.

1.2mm 3.5mm 3.5mm 1.5mm

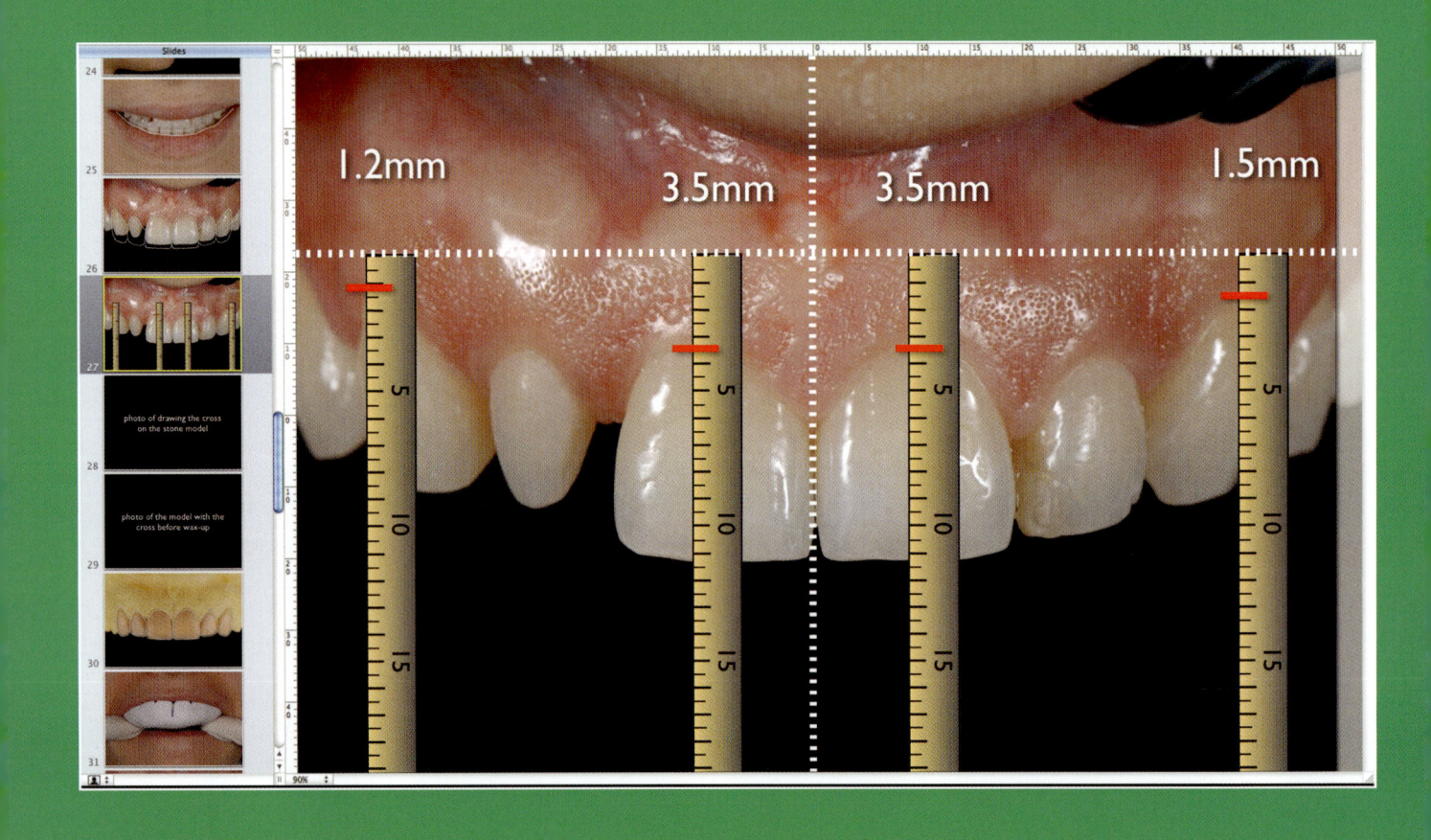

Chapter 4 Digital Smile Design: A Digital Tool for Esthetic Evaluation, Team Communication, and Patient Management

Christian Coachman, DDS, CDT, Marcelo Calamita, DDS, MS, PhD, and Andrea Ricci, DDS

Chapter Outline

Advantages of Digital Smile Design	86	Patient understanding and marketing tool	86
Accurate esthetic analysis	86	Dynamic and effective treatment planning presentation	87
Increased communication among the interdisciplinary team	86	Educational tool	87
Feedback at each phase of treatment	86	Digital Smile Design workflow	87

Excellence will never be achieved by chance, but by using a consistent systematic approach for diagnosis, communication, treatment planning, and, eventually, execution. The incorporation of protocols and checklists[1-7] for quality control and information management will guarantee that every critical point is performed effectively, double checked, and communicated correctly.

In order to obtain predictable and consistent treatment outcomes, the design of the restorative treatment should be clearly defined at an earlier stage. This data must guide the succeeding phases of the rehabilitation,[8] scientifically integrating all of the patient's needs and desires and the functional, structural, and biological specifics into the esthetic treatment design. It works as a frame of reference for the treatment that will be performed.[9,10]

However, many of these pieces of information may not be taken into consideration if their real meaning is not transferred in an adequate way to the design of the restorations.

The Digital Smile Design (DSD) is a practical multiuse clinical tool with relevant advantages: it can strengthen esthetic diagnostic abilities, improve the communication between team members, create predictable systems throughout the treatment phases, enhance the patient's education and motivation, and increase the effectiveness of case presentation. It is an effective digital treatment protocol which utilizes 2D clinical and lab images of the patient and the proposed treatment plan including planes of reference, facial and dental midlines, incisal edge position, lip dynamics, basic tooth arrangement, and the incisal plane.

Digitally drawing reference lines and shapes over the patient's photo, following a predetermined sequence, allows the team to better evaluate the esthetic relation between the teeth, the gingiva, the smile, and the face. DSD is an extraordinary multipurpose tool that can be utilized by all team members to better understand, visualize, and implement the treatment plan. As the use of the DSD can make the diagnosis more effective and the treatment planning more consistent, the effort required to implement it will be rewarded, making the treatment sequence more logical and straightforward, saving time and materials and reducing the costs during the treatment.

Advantages of Digital Smile Design

Accurate esthetic analysis

The DSD allows a careful esthetic analysis of the patient's facial and dental features and a gradual discovery of many critical factors that might have been overlooked during the clinical, photographic, or study models evaluation. The drawing of reference lines and shapes over extra- and intraoral digital photographs performed in presentation software such as Keynote (Apple iWork) or MS Powerpoint (Microsoft Office), following a predetermined sequence, will enhance the diagnostic vision. It also helps the team to assess and understand limitations and risk factors such as asymmetries, disharmonies, and violations of esthetic principles, adding critical data to the process of treatment planning.[1] Choosing the appropriate technique is easier once the problem has been identified and the solution clearly visualized.

Increased communication among the interdisciplinary team

The main goal of the DSD protocol is to simplify communication, transferring key information from the patient's face to the working cast, and to the final restoration.

The DSD protocol provides effective communication between the interdisciplinary team members, including the dental technician. Team members can identify and highlight discrepancies in soft- or hard-tissue morphology, discussing over high-quality images on the computer screen the best possible solutions for the case. Every team member can add information directly on the slides, in writing or using voice-over, simplifying the process even more. All team members can access this information whenever necessary—"in the cloud"— changing or adding new elements during the diagnostic and treatment phases.

Traditionally, the dental technician has implemented the smile design with the restorative wax-up. He or she creates shapes and arrangements in accordance with restricted information, following instructions and guidelines provided by the dentist in writing or by phone. In many cases the technician is not given enough information to utilize his or her skills to their maximum potential and the opportunity to produce a restoration that will truly satisfy the patient is missed.

When the treatment coordinator or another member of the restorative team who has developed a personal relationship with the patient takes the responsibility for the smile design, the results are likely to be superior. This individual has the ability to communicate the patient's personal preferences and/or morphopsychological features to the laboratory technician, providing information which can elevate the quality of the restoration from one that is adequate to one that is viewed by the patient as exceptional.[7,8,11]

With this valuable information in hand and from the 2D DSD, the dental technician will be able to develop a 3D wax-up more efficiently, focusing on developing anatomical features within the parameters provided, such as planes of reference, facial and dental midlines, recommended incisal edge position, lip dynamics, basic tooth arrangement, and the incisal plane.

Transferring this information from the wax-up to the "test-drive" phase is achieved through a mock-up or a provisional restoration.[4,6,12] The design of the definitive esthetic restorations should be developed and tested as soon as possible, guiding the treatment sequence to a predetermined esthetic result. Efficient treatment planning results in the entire treatment team being able to better identify the challenges they will face and will help expedite the time to initiate and ultimately complete treatment.[8]

Feedback at each phase of treatment

The DSD allows a precise reevaluation of the results obtained in every phase of the treatment. The sequence of the treatment is organized on the slides with the photos, videos, reports, graphics, and drawings, making this analysis simple and effective. At any time any team member can access the slide presentation and check what was done until that moment. With the Digital Ruler, with which drawings and reference lines are created, it is possible to perform simple comparisons between the before and after pictures, determining if they are in accordance with the original planning, or if any other adjunctive procedures are necessary to improve the outcome. The dental technician also gains feedback related to tooth shape, arrangement, and color so that final refinements can be made. This constant double-checking of information ensures that a higher-quality product will be delivered from the laboratory and also provides a great learning tool for the entire interdisciplinary team.

This process also becomes a very useful library of treatment procedures that can be used in many different ways. Going back to "old" cases and understanding visually how they were performed is effective as a learning experience.

Patient understanding and marketing tool

The DSD is an important marketing tool to motivate the patient, making him or her understand the issues and treatment options, compare before and after pictures, and value all the work that was done. Moreover, the fact of creating slides about the treatments performed generates a personal library of clinical cases that can be shared with other patients and colleagues, and the most appropriate cases can be further transformed into interesting slideshows of one's work.

Dynamic and effective treatment planning presentation

The DSD makes the treatment planning presentation more effective and clear because it allows patients to see and better understand the combined multiple factors that are responsible for their oral-facial issues. The case presentation will be more effective and dynamic for these patients since the problem list will be superimposed over their own photographs, increasing the understanding, trust, and acceptance of the proposed plan. The clinician can express the severity of the case, introduce strategies in treatment, discuss the prognosis, and make case management recommendations.[1] It also can be used for medico-legal purposes, registering the improvements that were achieved and the reasons for each one of the decisions made during the treatment.

Educational tool

The DSD can increase the impact of the presentations because it adds visual elements into the slides that will improve the educational aspects of the lecture. The audience can understand better the issues that were previously highlighted and the presenter can minimize the use of the laser pointer.

Digital Smile Design workflow

The DSD protocol is performed by the authors using Keynote; however, other similar software such as MS PowerPoint can also be used with minor adjustments in the technique. Keynote allows simple manipulation of the digital images and the addition of lines, shapes, drawings, and measurements over the clinical and laboratory images. The main steps of the DSD are described and illustrated below.

In order to begin the process, three basic photos are necessary: full-face at rest, full-face with wide smile and teeth apart, and retracted photo of the upper arch with teeth apart. A short video is also recommended capturing the following lip positions: at rest, wide smile, stretched from a frontal view, 45°, and profile. On this video a few basic questions can be asked of the patient to explain their main concerns, needs, and expectations. Then, the photos and videos are downloaded and inserted on the slide presentation (Figure 4.1).

1. **The cross**: two lines must be placed on the center of the slide, forming a cross (Figure 4.2). The full-face photo with the teeth apart should be positioned behind the cross.

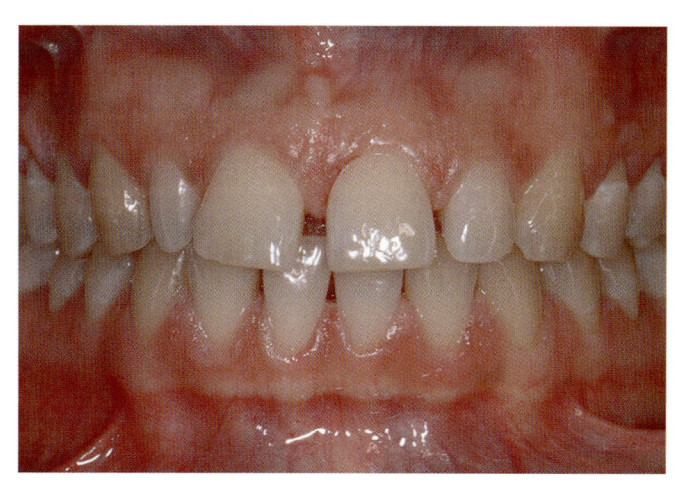

Figure 4.1 Pre-operation photo.

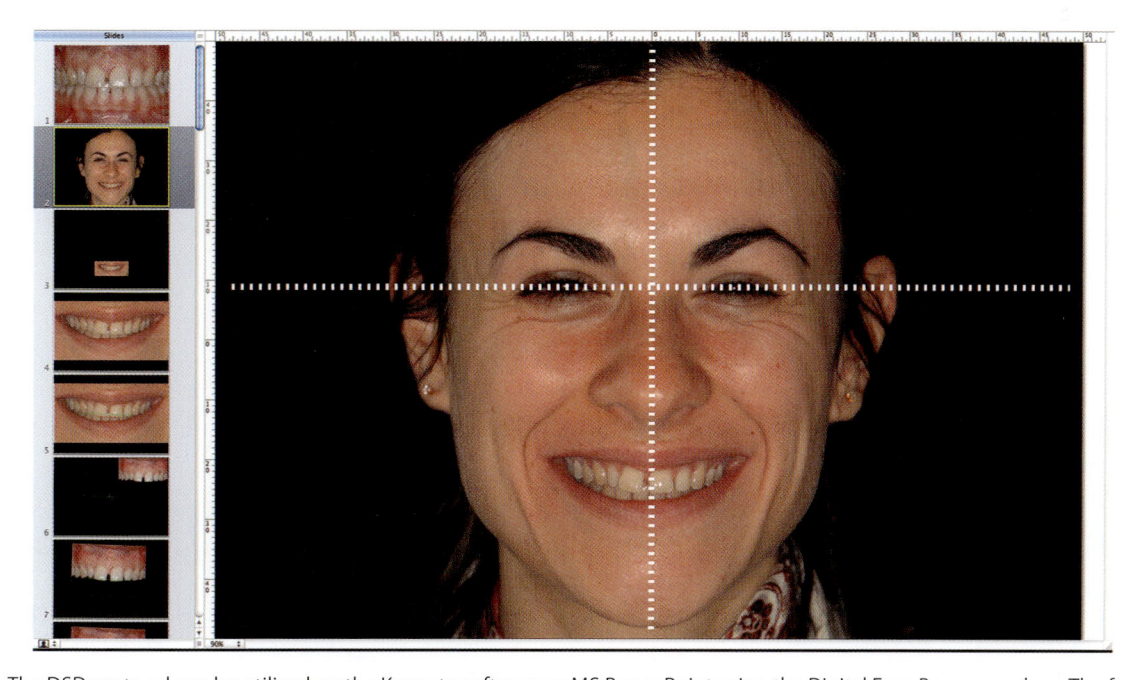

Figure 4.2 The DSD protocol can be utilized on the Keynote software or MS PowerPoint using the Digital Face Bow procedure. The face photo is placed on the slide to start the DSD sequence and is adjusted behind the two white dotted lines (the cross), determining visually the ideal facial midline and horizontal reference.

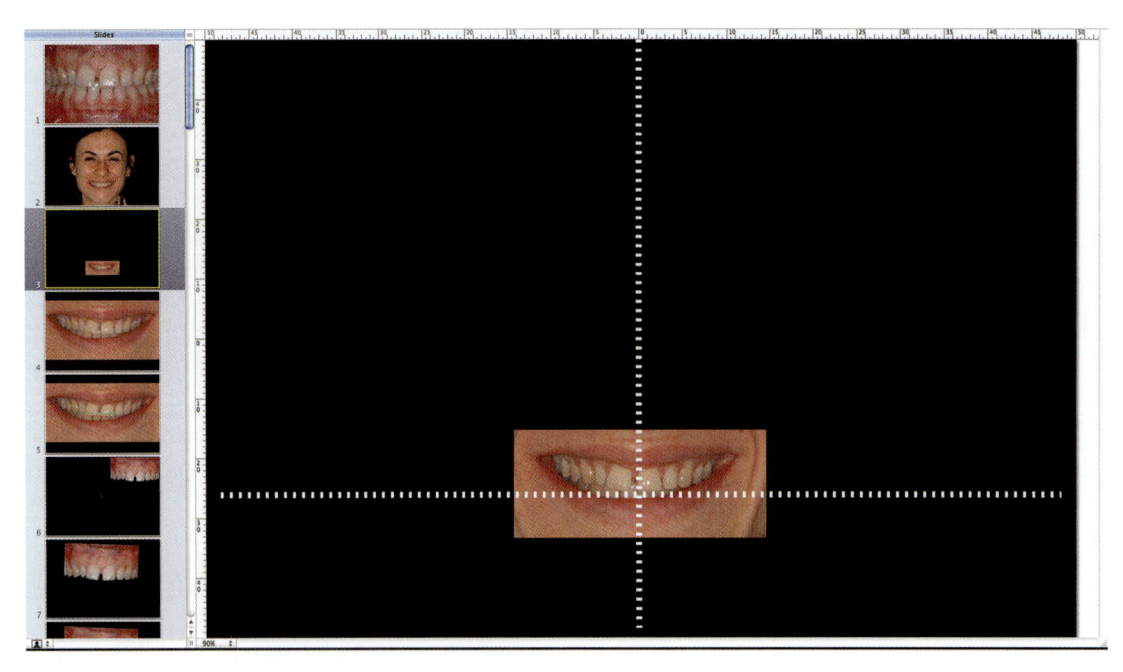

Figure 4.3 The horizontal line is moved to the mouth area and the face photo is cropped showing only the overall smile.

2. **Digital facebow**: relating the full-face smile image to the horizontal reference line is the most important step in the smile design process. The interpupillary line should be the first reference to establish the horizontal plane, but it should not be the only one. It is also necessary to analyze the face as a whole and then determine the best horizontal reference that creates harmony. After determining the horizontal reference line, it is time to outline the facial midline according to facial features like the glabella, nose, and chin (Figure 4.2).

3. **Smile analysis**: dragging the horizontal line over the mouth will allow an initial evaluation between the relation of the facial lines and the smile. It is possible to evaluate midline and occlusal plane shifting and/or canting (Figure 4.3).

4. **Smile Simulation**: simulations can be done to fix incisal edge position, canting, shifting, tooth proportion, and soft tissue architecture (Figure 4.4).

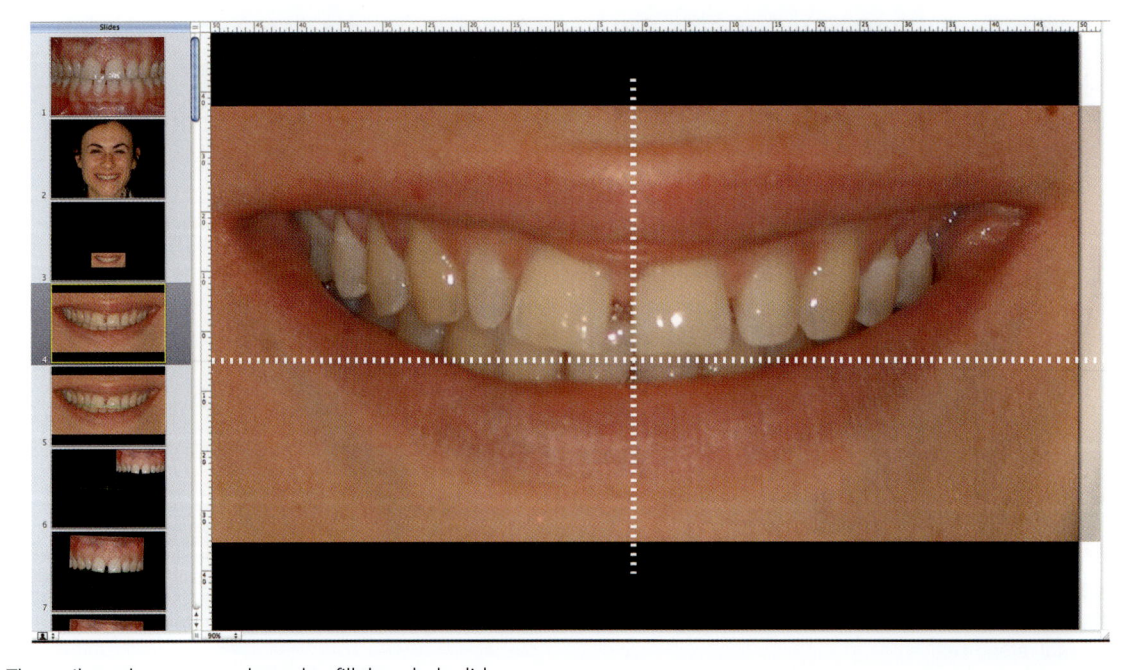

Figure 4.4 The smile and cross are enlarged to fill the whole slide.

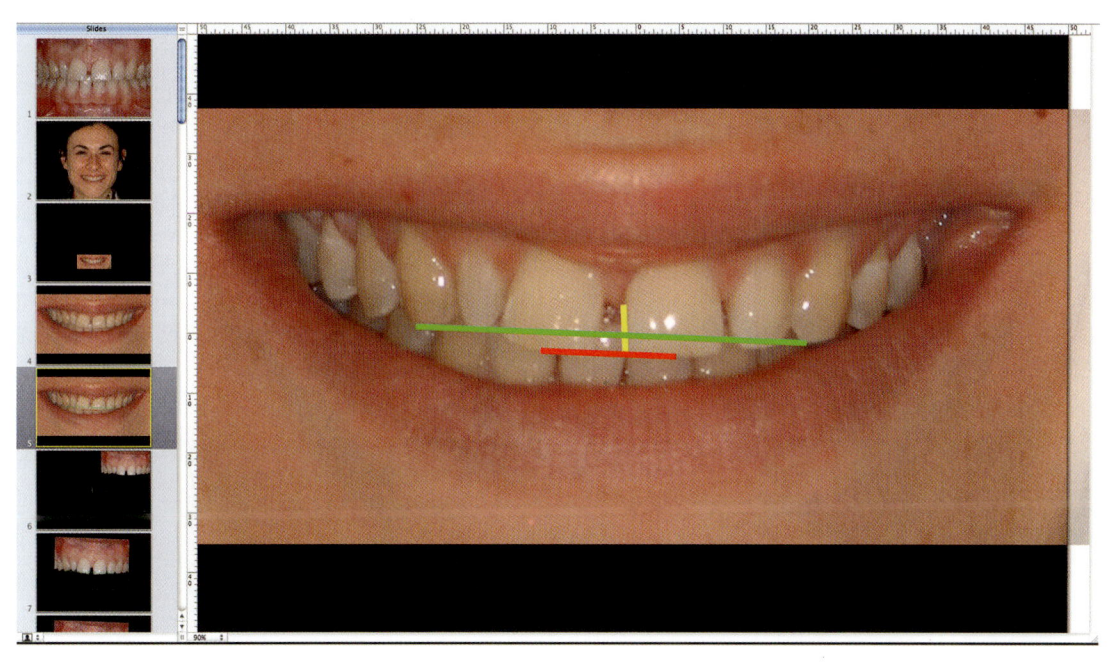

Figure 4.5 Three transferring lines are created. Green line: cuspid tips. Red line: incisal edge of the centrals. Yellow line: mesial of the central incisor.

5. **Transference from the face to intraoral**: in order to analyze the intraoral photo in accordance to the facial references one needs to transfer the cross to the retracted photo using three transferring lines drawn over the smile photo (Figure 4.5):

   Line 1: from the cusp tip of one canine to the tip of the contralateral canine.
   Line 2: from the middle of the incisal edge of one central to the middle of the incisal edge of the other central.
   Line 3: over the dental midline, from the tip of the papilla to the incisal embrasure.

   Thus, four features on the photo should be calibrated: size, canting, incisal edge position, and midline position. Line 1 guides the two first aspects (size and canting); line 2 guides the incisal edge position, and line 3 guides the midline position (Figure 4.6).

6. **Measuring tooth proportion**: measuring the width/length proportion of the central by placing a rectangle over the

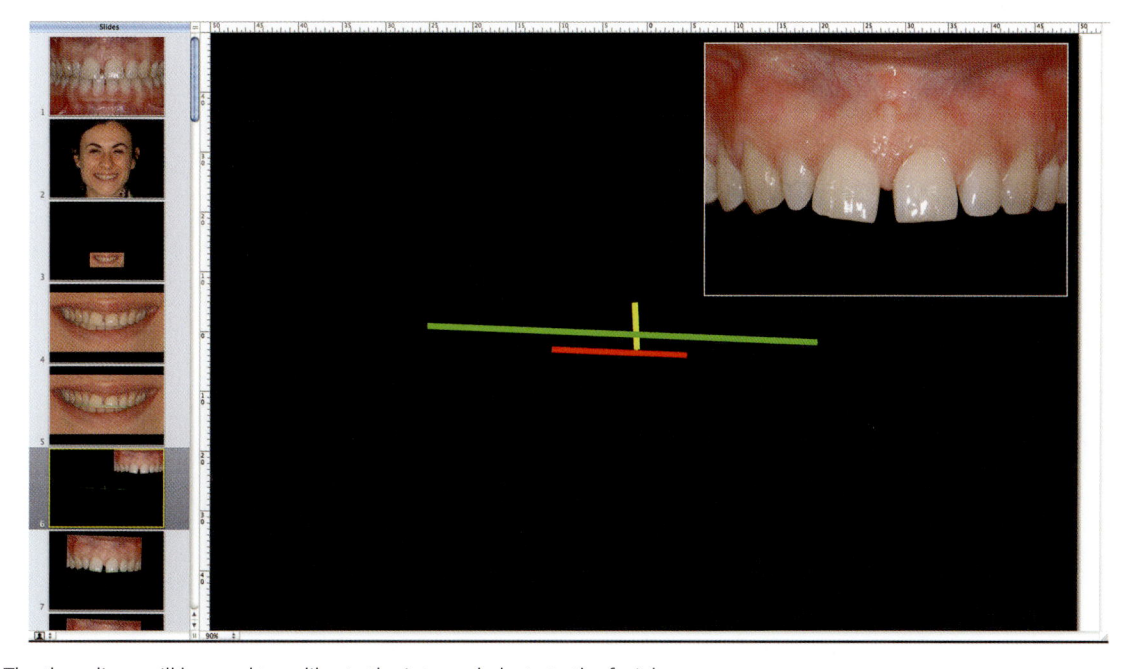

Figure 4.6 The three lines will be used to calibrate the intraoral photo to the facial cross.

edges of the central (Figure 4.7) is an effective way to start understanding what needs to be performed when it comes to redesigning a smile. The other analysis that should be performed is to compare the actual proportion of the patient's central in relation to ideal proportions according to the literature[2-8] (Figure 4.8).

7. **Tooth outline**: from this point on, all the drawings may be customized, depending on the case, on what you want to visualize and what you want to communicate with the team, technician, and the patient. One can draw the teeth outlines over the photo or copy and paste a pre-made outline from a personal library. The selection of the shape of the teeth will depend on other factors such as: the morphopsychological interview, patient's desires, facial features, and esthetic expectations[11,13] (Figures 4.9 and 4.10).

8. **White and pink esthetic evaluation**: after having all the lines and drawings performed according to the facial lines and the smile line, one can have a clear understanding about all the esthetic issues involving the upper arch such as tooth proportion, interdental relationship, relationship between the teeth and the smile line, discrepancy between facial and dental midline, midline and occlusal plane canting, soft

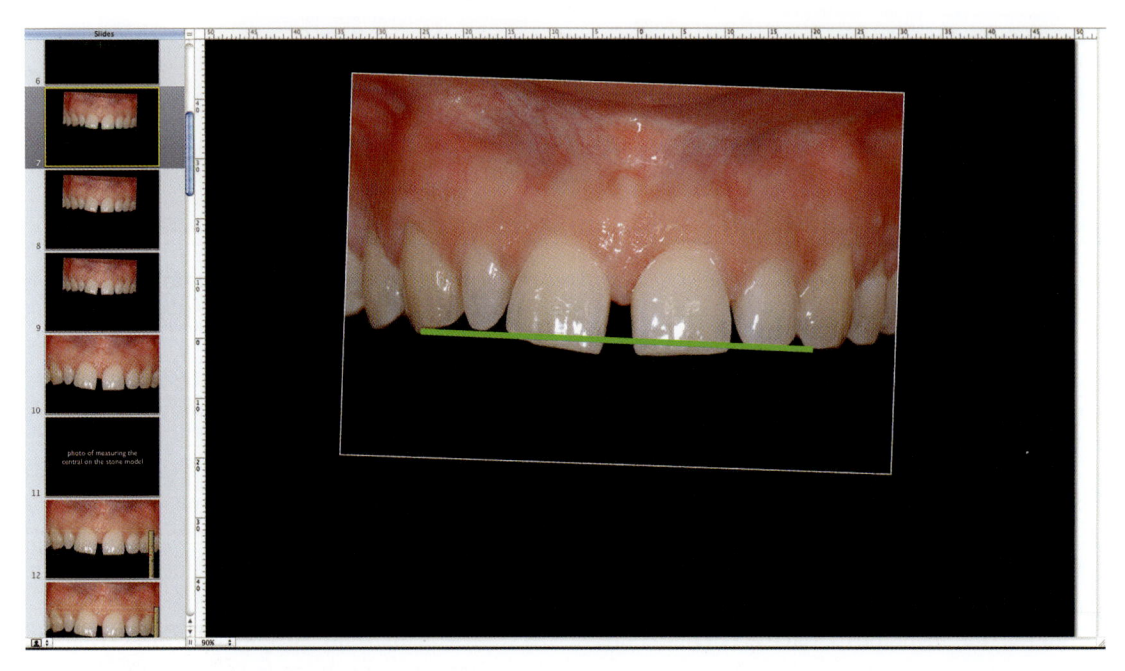

Figure 4.7 The first step to calibrate the intraoral photo is to adjust the size and inclination of the photo so that the cusp tips are touching the ends of the green line, exactly as performed on the facial photo.

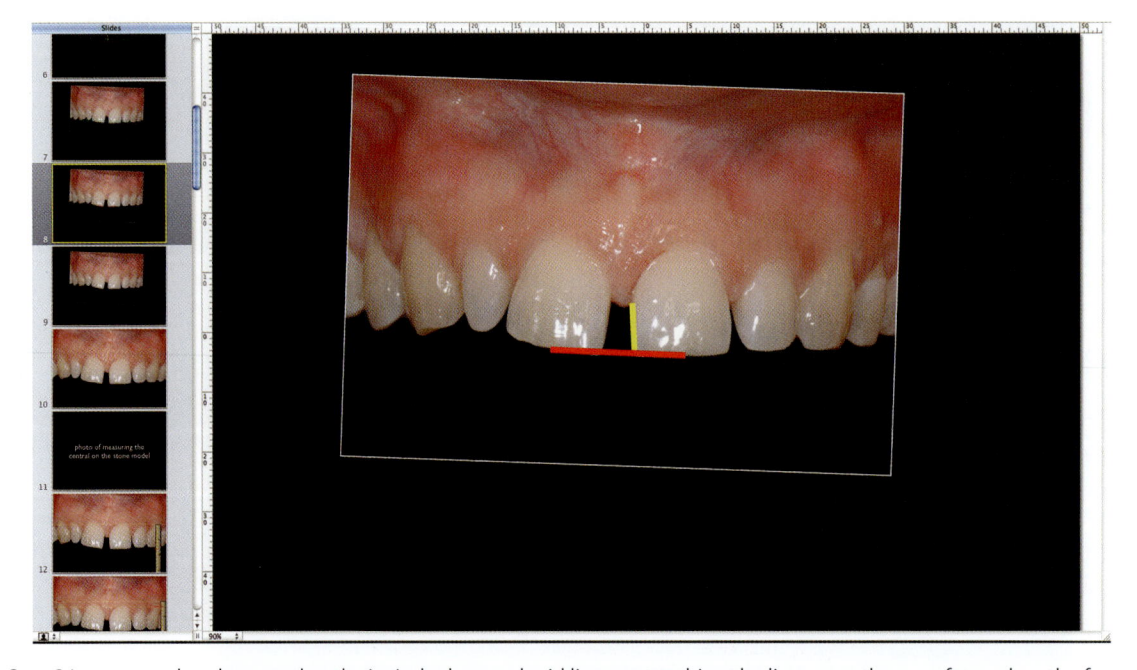

Figure 4.8 Step 2 is to move the photo so that the incisal edges and mid line are touching the lines, exactly as performed on the face photo.

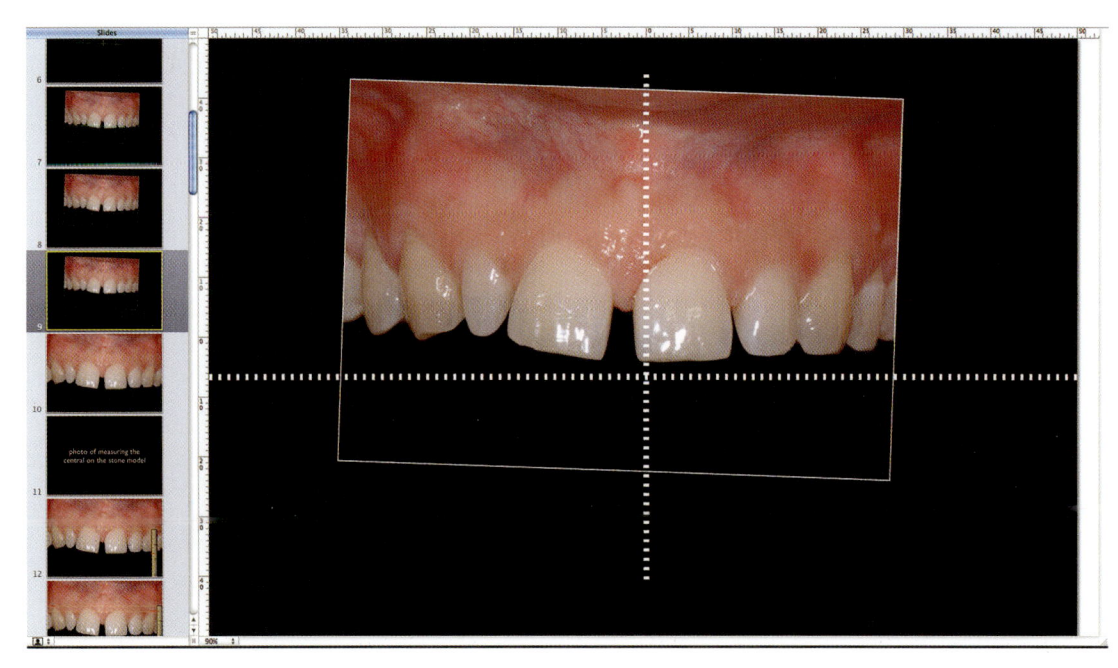

Figure 4.9 The dotted white lines are reintroduced into the slide and now the intraoral photo is calibrated with the facial cross.

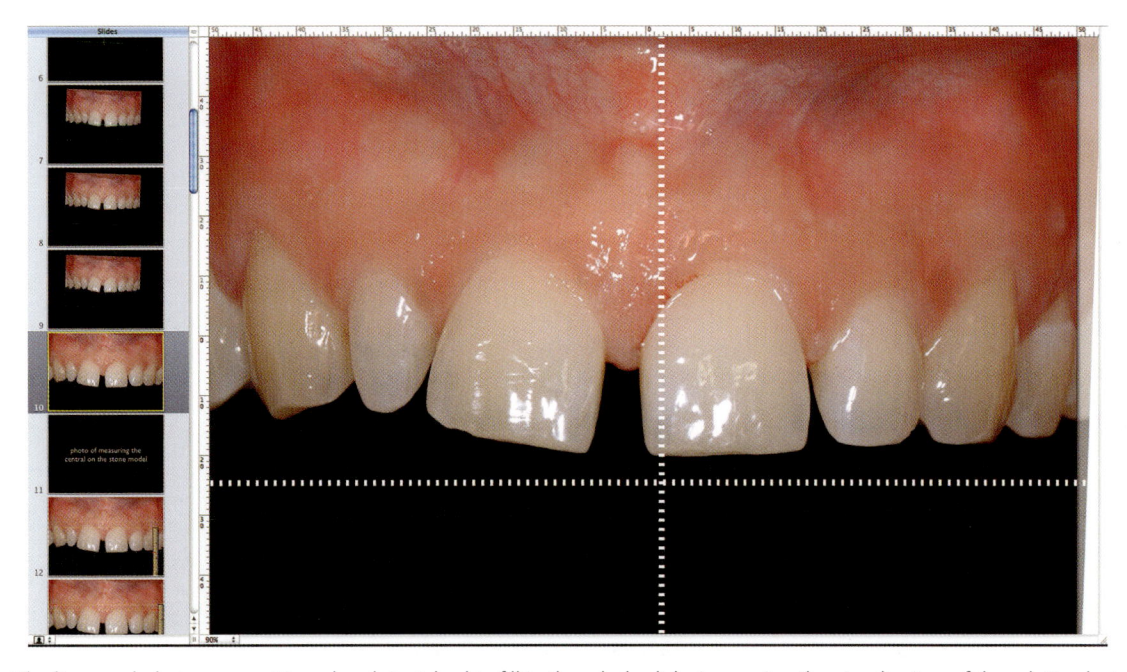

Figure 4.10 The lines and photo are positioned and stretched to fill in the whole slide, improving the visualization of the relation between teeth, soft tissues, and the facial cross.

tissue disharmony, relationship between soft tissue and teeth, papillae heights, gingival margin levels, incisal edge design, tooth axis, and so on (Figure 4.11).

9. **Digital Ruler calibration over the intraoral photo**: after all the lines are placed and drawings made, one can proceed with the calibration of the Digital Ruler over the intraoral photo by measuring the real length of one central incisor on the model (Figure 4.12) and transferring this measure to the computer (Figure 4.13). Once the Digital Ruler is calibrated one can start making any kind of measurements over the anterior area of the image (Figure 4.14).

10. **Transferring the cross from digital to the model**: the first step is to digitally move the horizontal line over the intraoral photo and place it above the gingival margin of the six anterior teeth. With the Digital Ruler the distance is measured between the horizontal line and the gingival margin of each tooth and these sizes are written down on the slide (Figure 4.15). These measurements are transferred to the

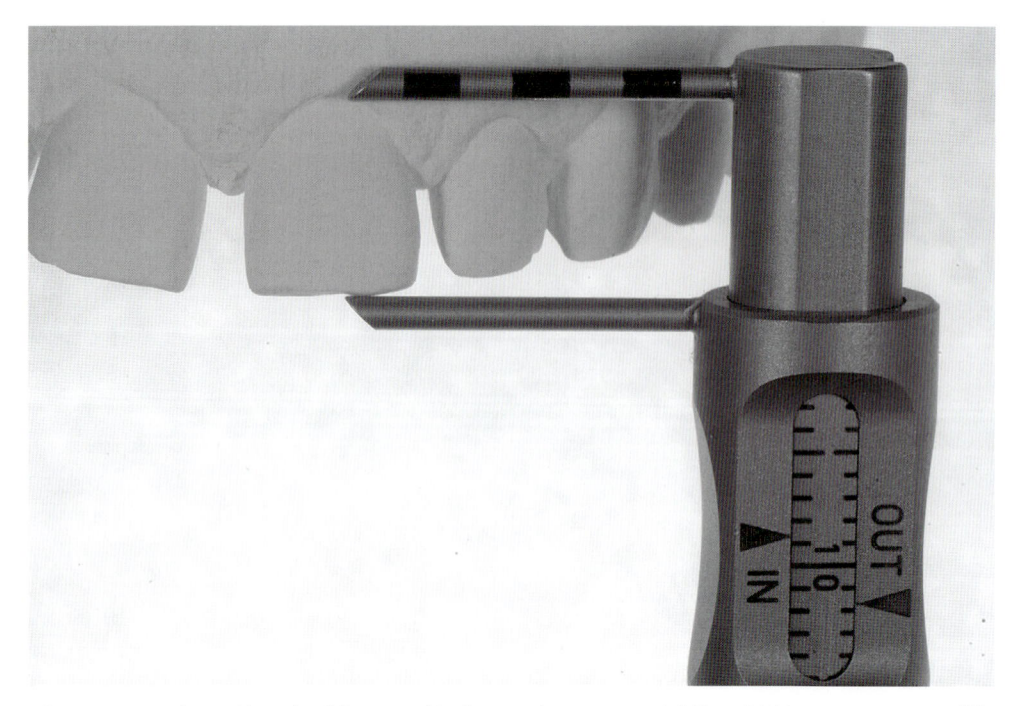

Figure 4.11 With a caliper measure the real length of the central incisor on the stone model (8 mm). This measurement will be used to calibrate the Digital Ruler.

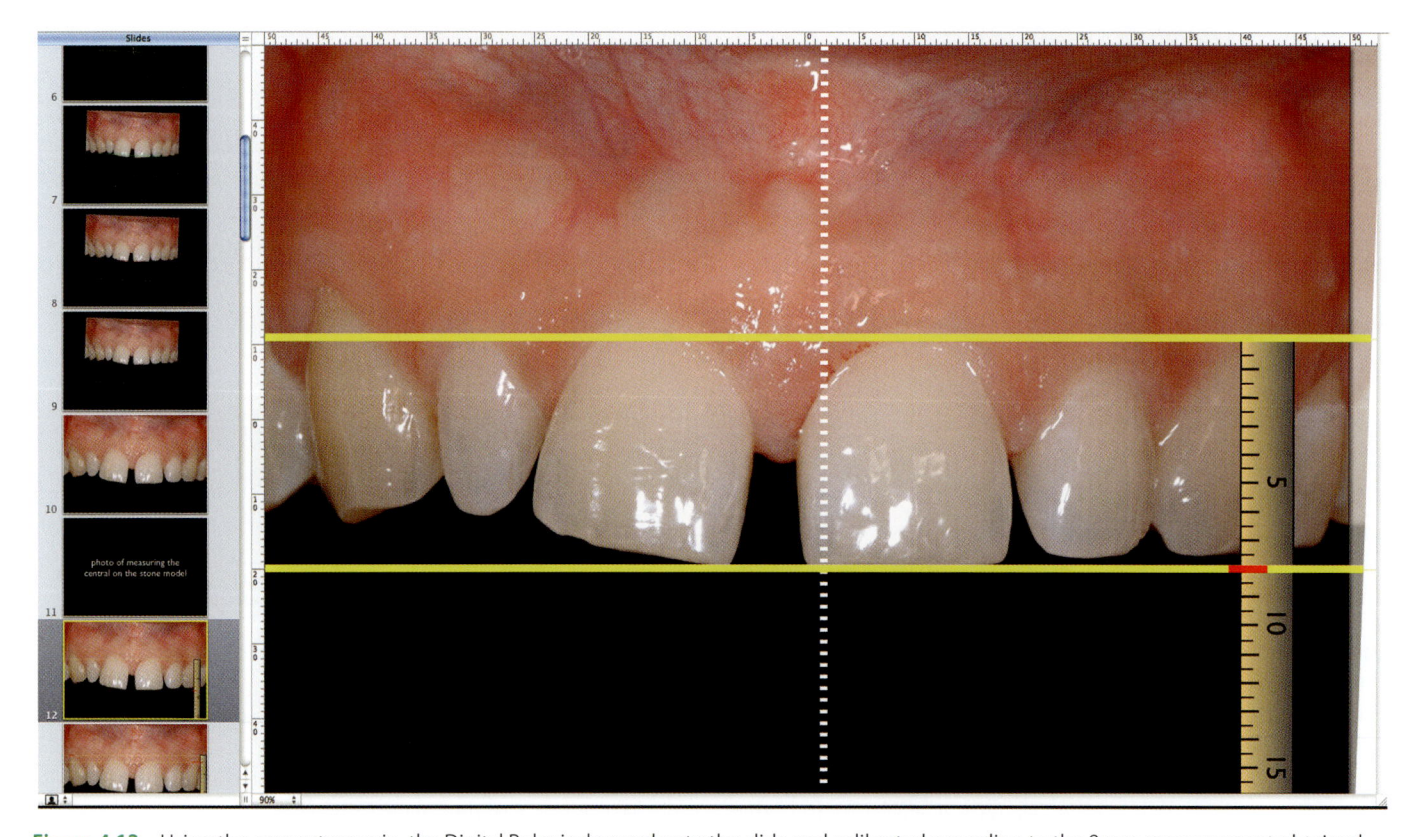

Figure 4.12 Using the computer again, the Digital Ruler is dragged onto the slide and calibrated according to the 8 mm measurement obtained. The zero on the ruler is placed on one of the yellow horizontal lines and then the ruler is stretched or reduced until the #8 reaches the other yellow line.

Chapter 4 Digital Smile Design

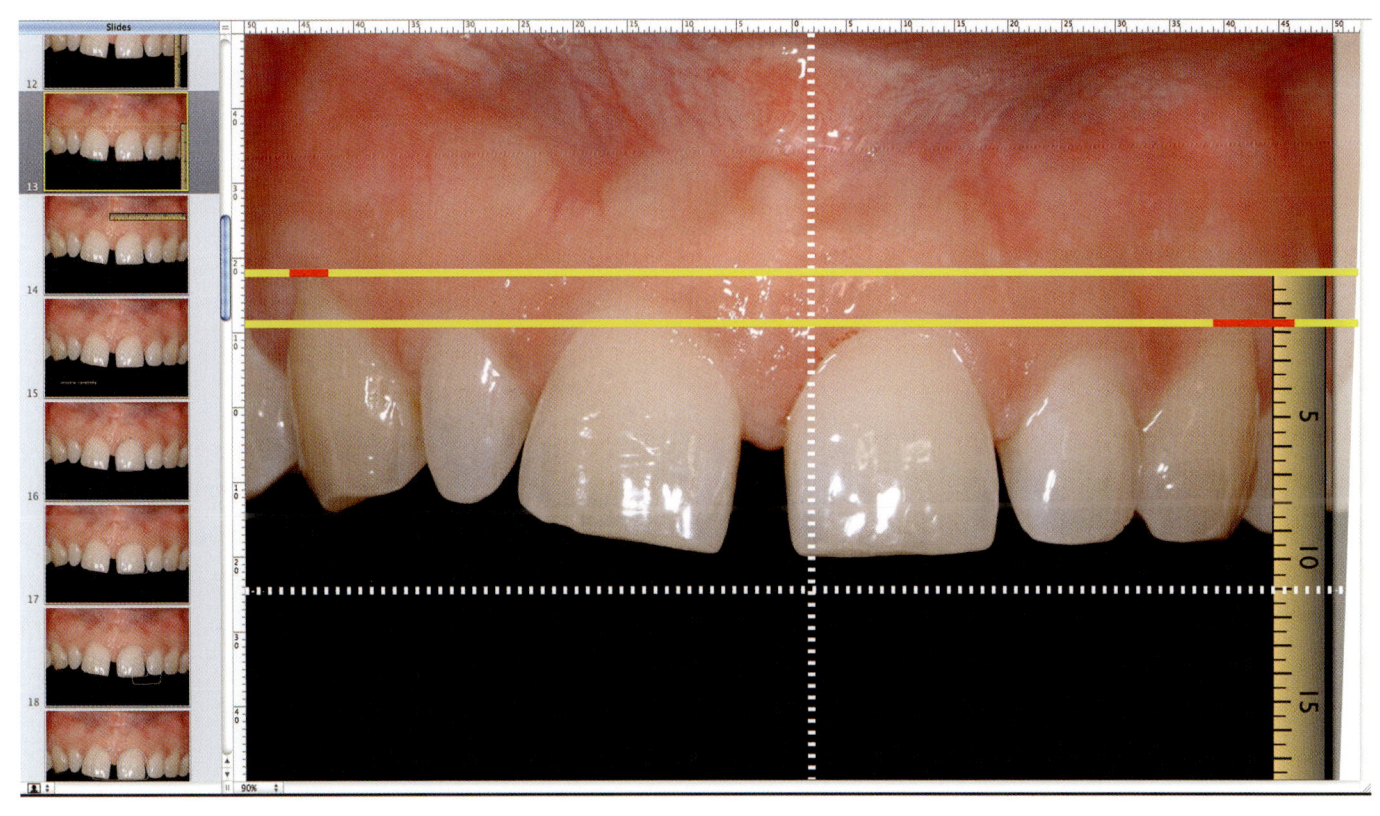

Figure 4.13 After calibration, measurements can be performed on top of the photo on the anterior area. For example, the discrepancy between the heights of the cervical of the cuspids is 1.7 mm.

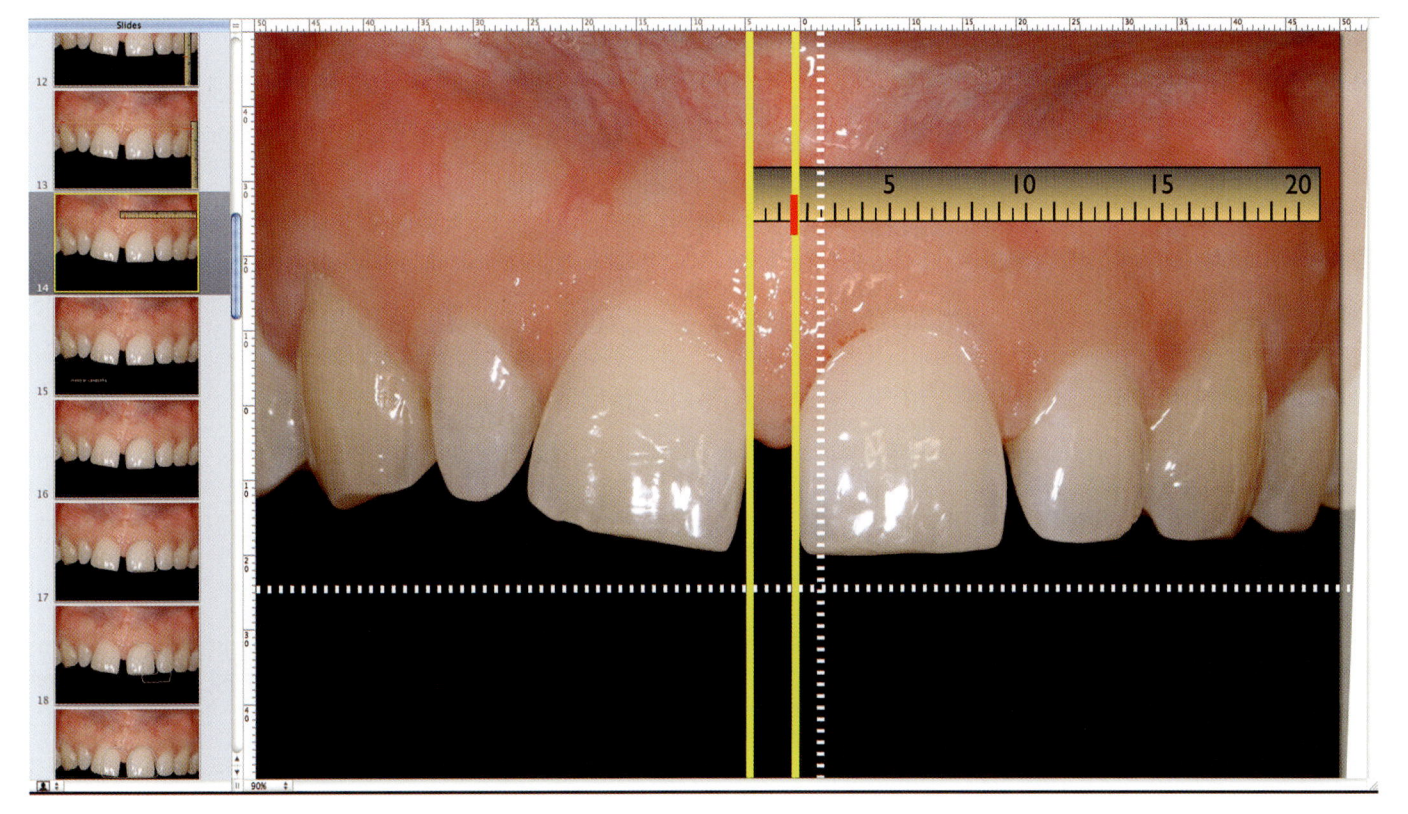

Figure 4.14 Measure the diastema, 1.5 mm.

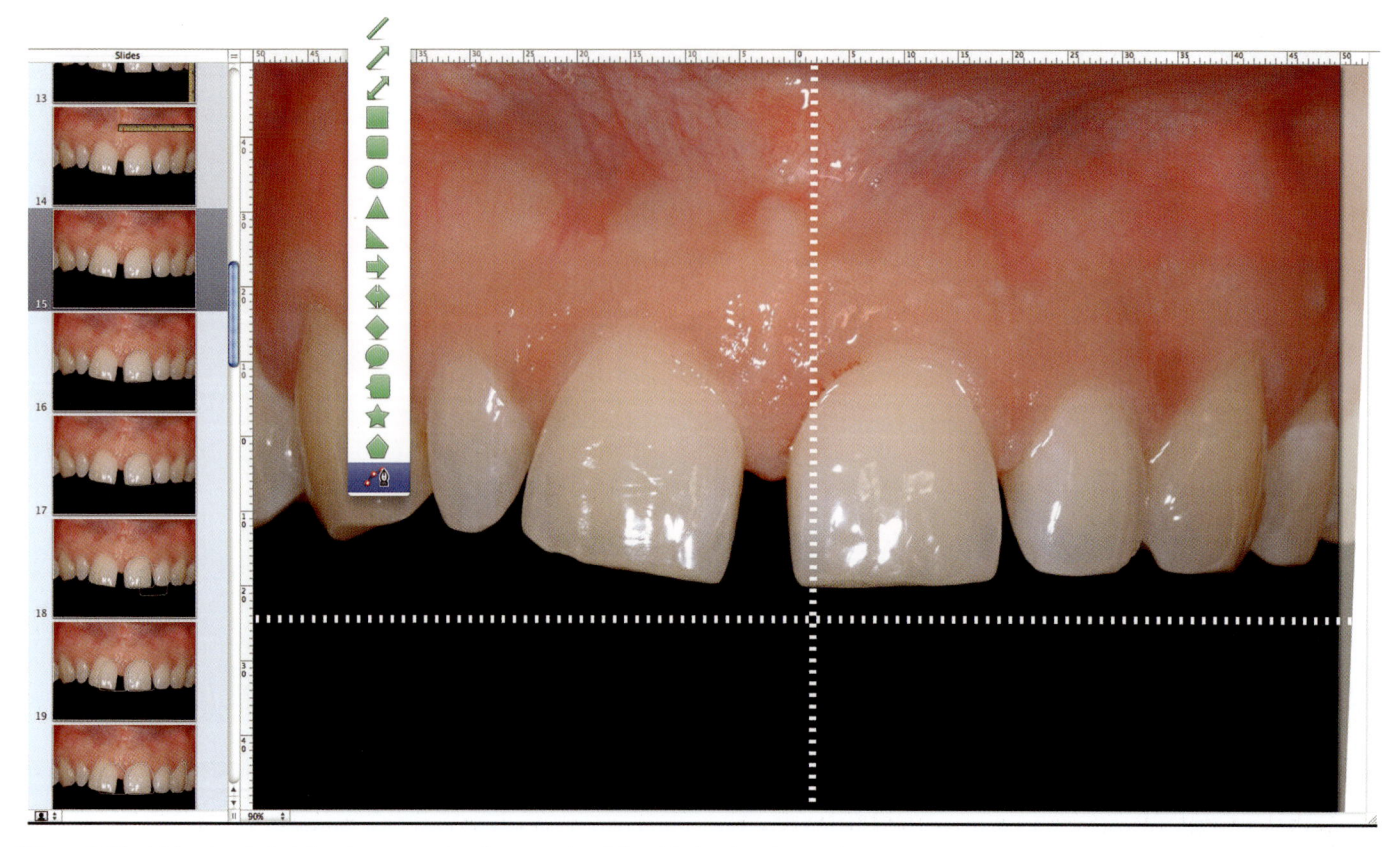

Figure 4.15 Make the digital drawings over the photo on the slide with the drawing tool.

model with the aid of a caliper, marking on the model with a pencil the same exact distances above the gingival margins that are shown on the computer and connecting the dots that creates a horizontal line above the teeth. The next step is to transfer the vertical midline, perpendicular to the horizontal line. One should measure the distance between the dental midline and the facial midline at the incisal edge level on the computer and then transfer this mark to the model with the caliper (Figure 4.16). After drawing the cross on the model (Figure 4.17) it is possible to transfer the information digitally planned, such as crown lengthening, incisal edge reduction, root coverage, and so on. At this point all the information necessary to the technician to develop a precise and useful wax-up is on the slides and on the model, guiding him or her to best perform this procedure (Figure 4.18).

The guided diagnostic wax-up is integrated with the patient's facial features and emotional needs. It is an important reference for the following surgical, orthodontic, and restorative procedures. Several guides can be produced over this wax-up to control the procedures as surgical stents, orthodontic guides, implant guides, crown lengthening guides, tooth preparation guides, and so on. The next important step is to evaluate the precision of the DSD and the wax-up performing a "test drive" (Figure 4.19). It can be a mock-up or a provisional, depending on the case. After the patient's approval of the "test drive," one can plan and adapt all the following procedures to achieve the desired result. The tooth preparation should be minimally invasive allowing just enough clearance to create proper ceramic restorations (Figure 4.20). The fabrication of the final restorations should be a controlled process with very little final adjustments (Figure 4.21), and the final result should be completely integrated, exceeding the patient's expectations (Figures 4.22 and 4.23).

The DSD is a practical multiuse tool with clinically relevant advantages: it can strengthen esthetic diagnostic abilities, improve the communication between team members, create predictable systems throughout the treatment phases, enhance the patient's education and motivation, and increase the effectiveness of case presentation. The drawing of reference lines and shapes over the patient's photo, following a predetermined sequence, allows the team to better evaluate the esthetic relation between the teeth, the gingiva, the smile, and the face.[14]

Chapter 4 Digital Smile Design

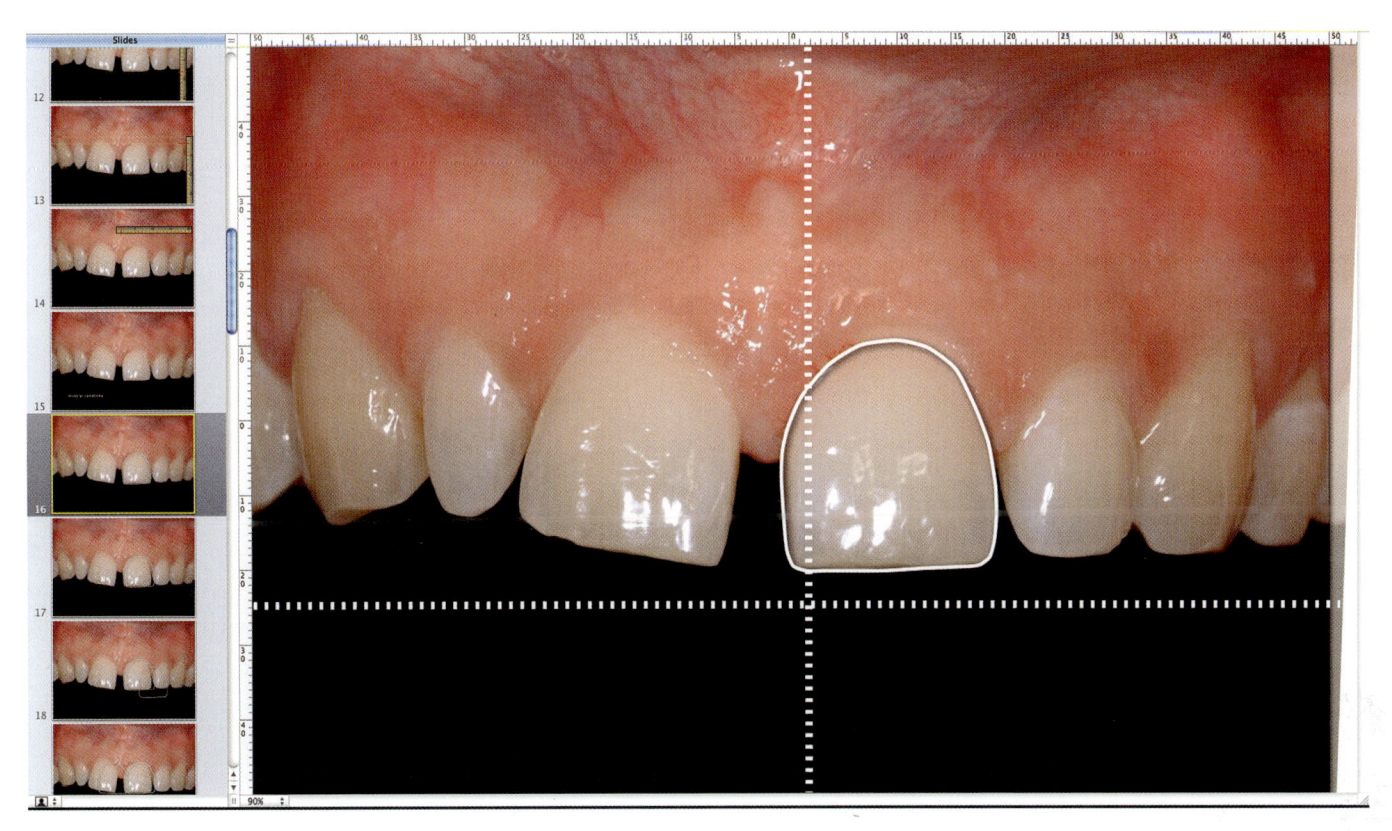

Figure 4.16 Draw the central incisor.

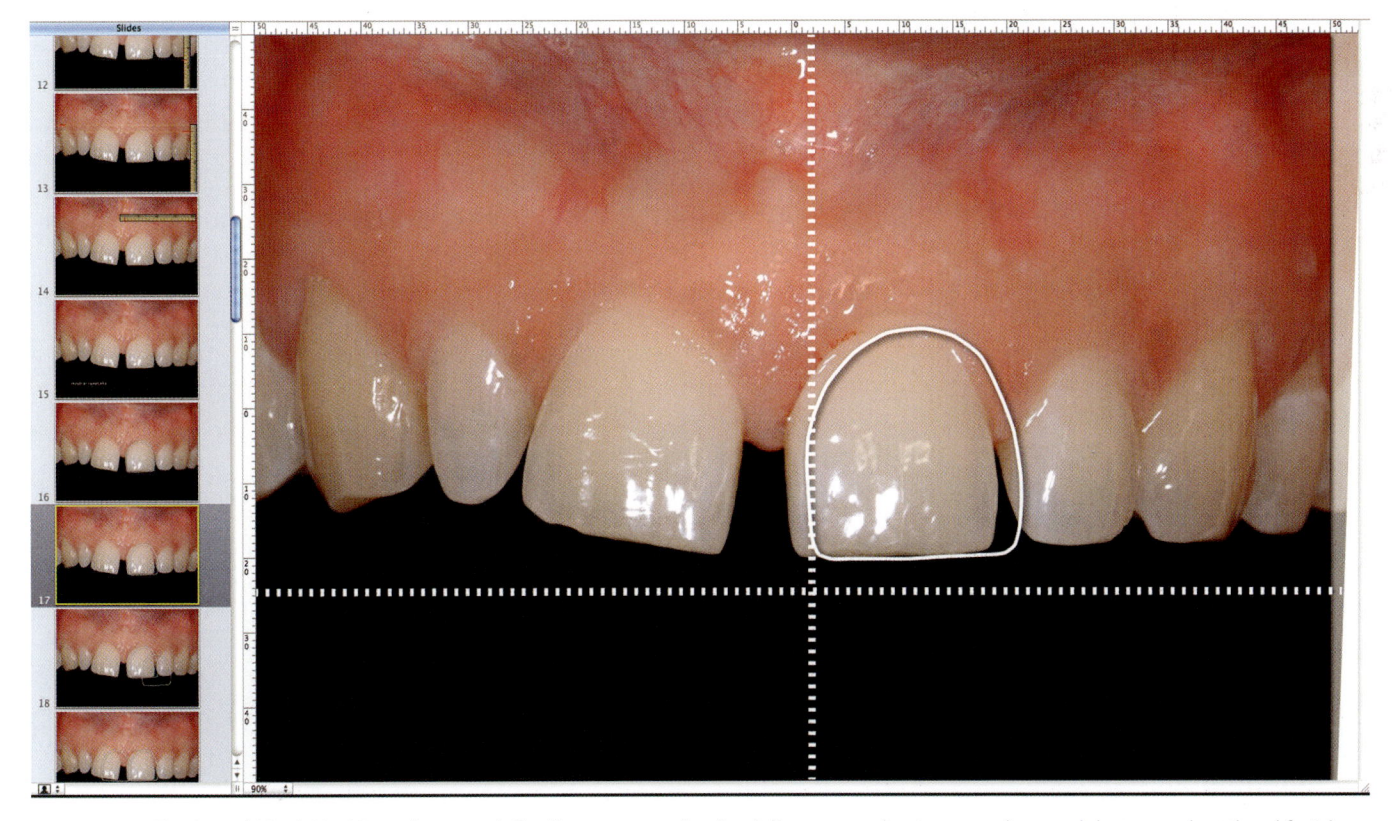

Figure 4.17 The Digital Mock-Up. Move the central distally to remove the distal diastema and to improve the match between dental and facial midline.

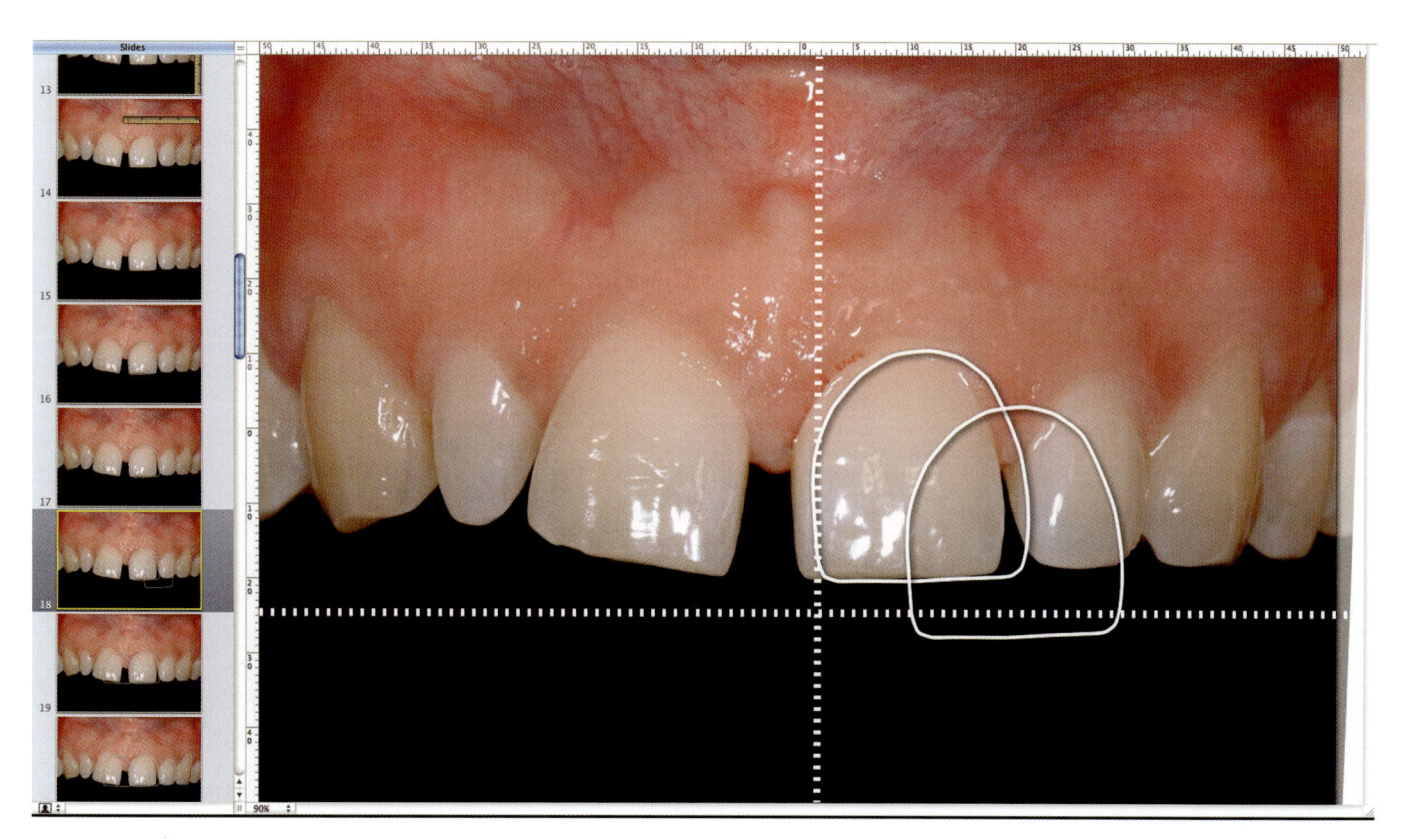

Figure 4.18 Duplicate the drawing of the central.

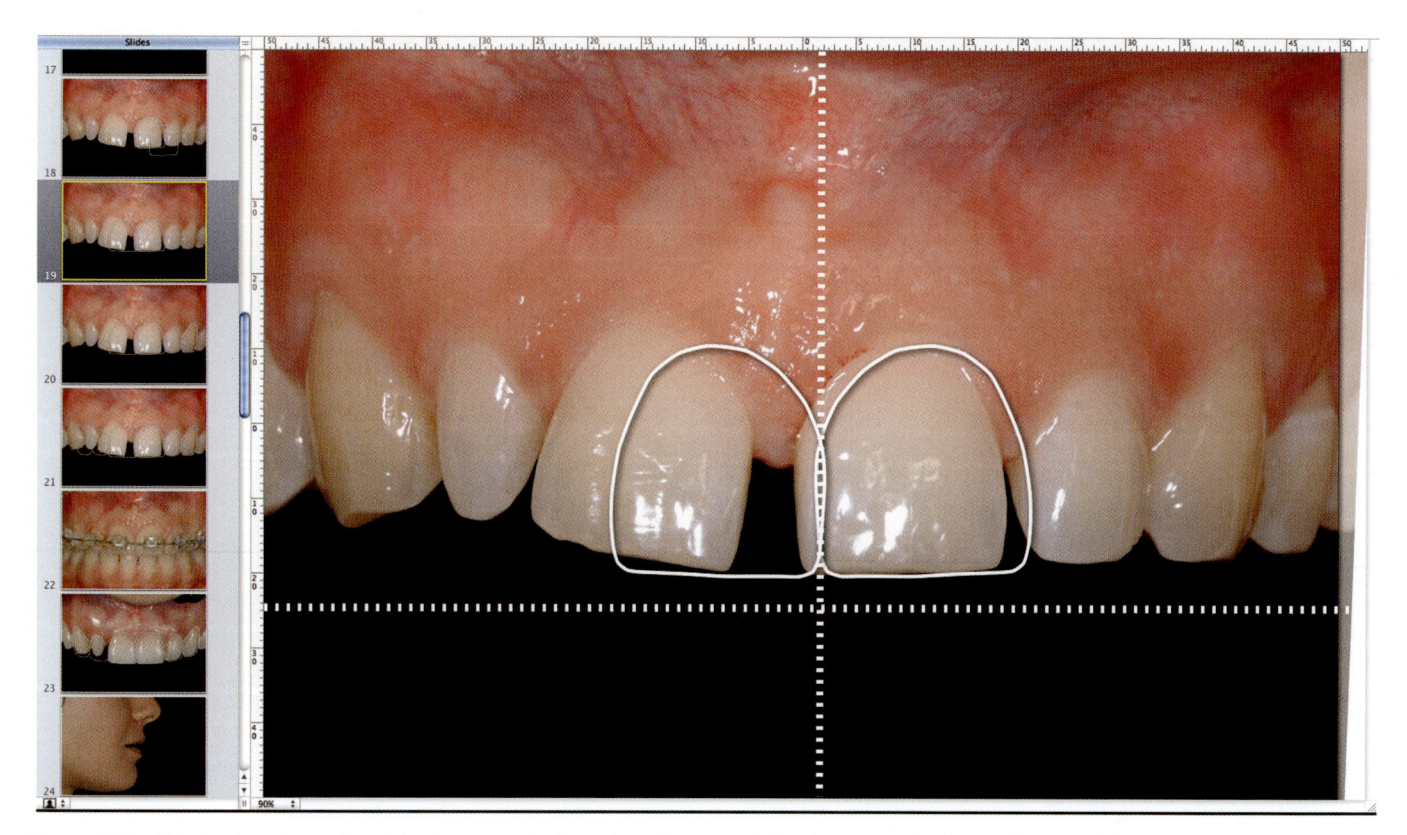

Figure 4.19 Flip the drawing and position it symmetrically to the other central. One can immediately visualize the difference between the actual and ideal position of the right central.

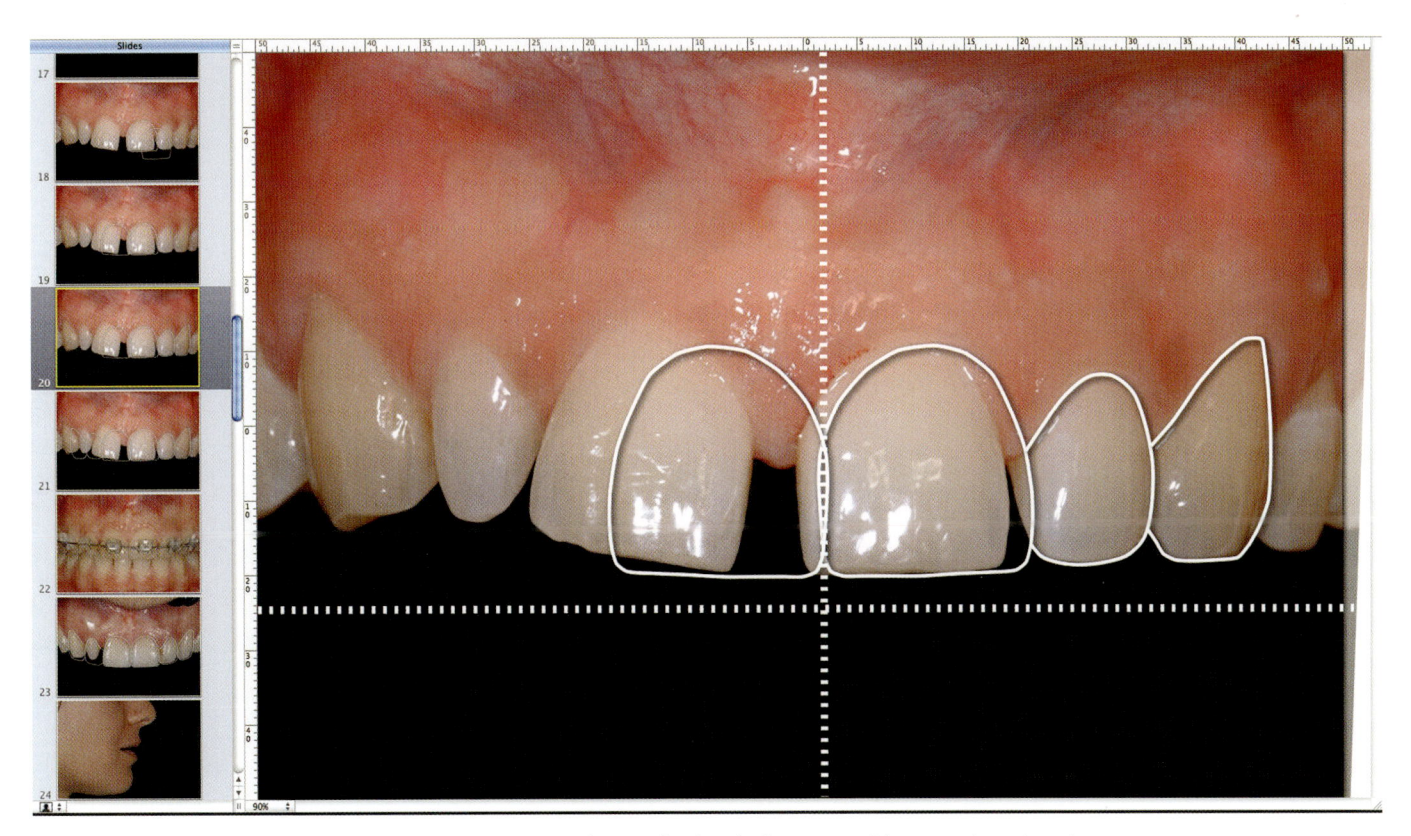

Figure 4.20 Draw the left lateral and cuspid to serve as a reference for the ideal position of the contralateral teeth.

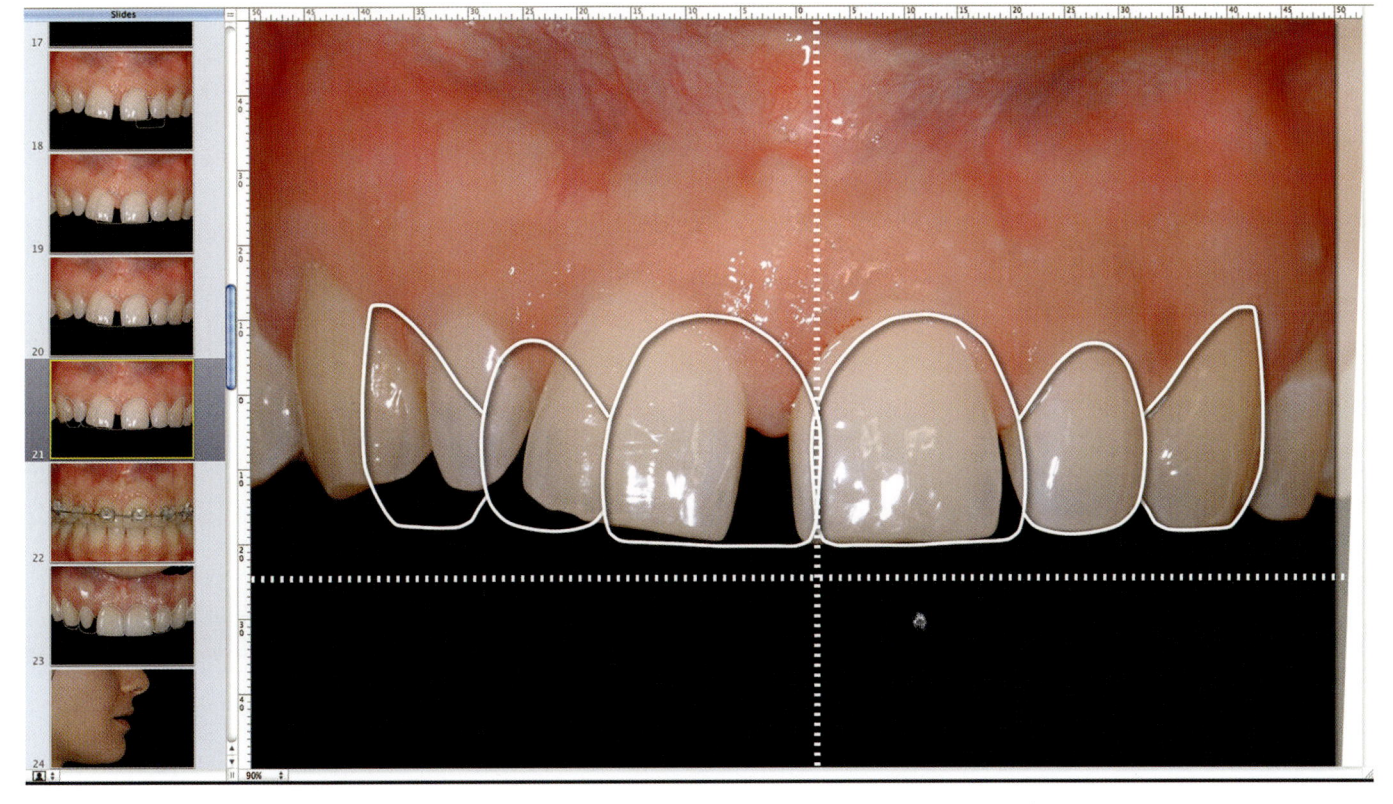

Figure 4.21 Flip and position the lateral and cuspid drawings symmetically in order to visualize the discrepancy between actual and ideal position of the six anterior teeth. This can demonstrate to the orthodontist the movements required as well as showing the patient the necessity of orthodontics to allow for minimally invasive preparations for veneers.

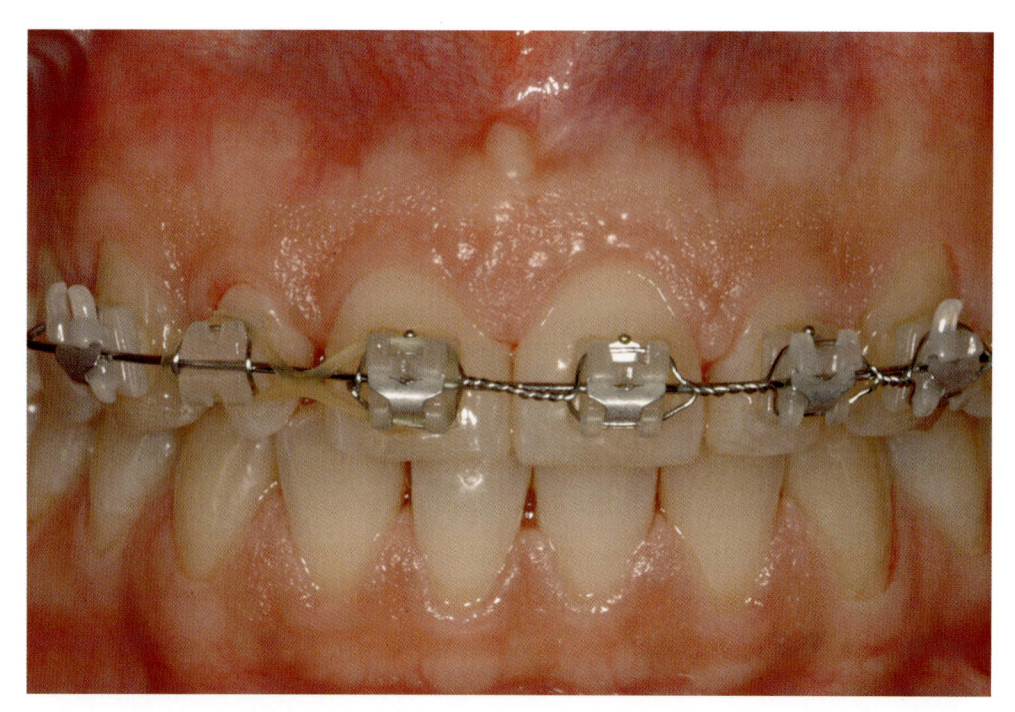

Figure 4.22 Situation after orthodontics.

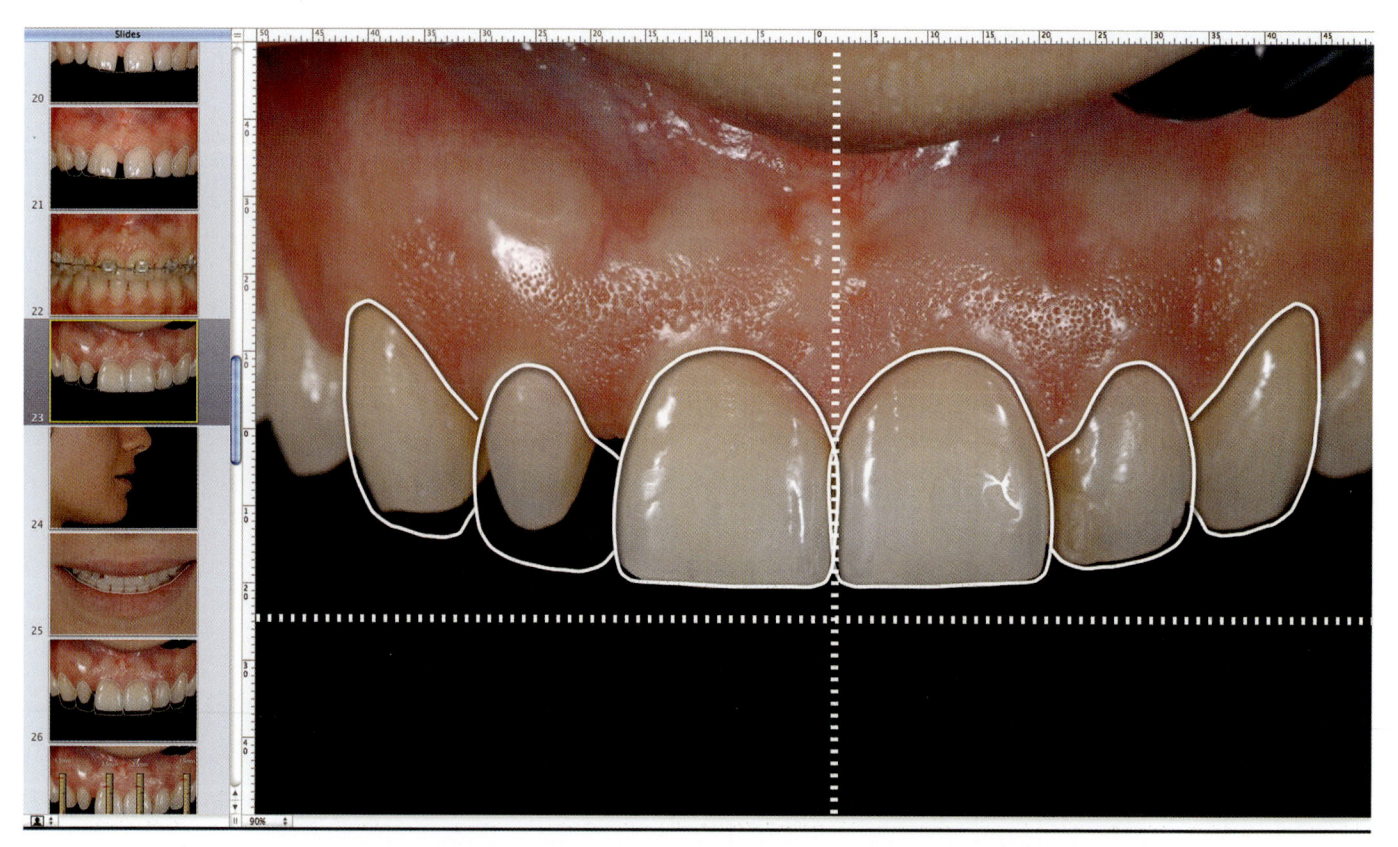

Figure 4.23 **(A)** The effectiveness of ortho treatment can be visualized by superimposing the digital planning drawings over the post treatment photo. This helps demonstrate any further corrections needed.

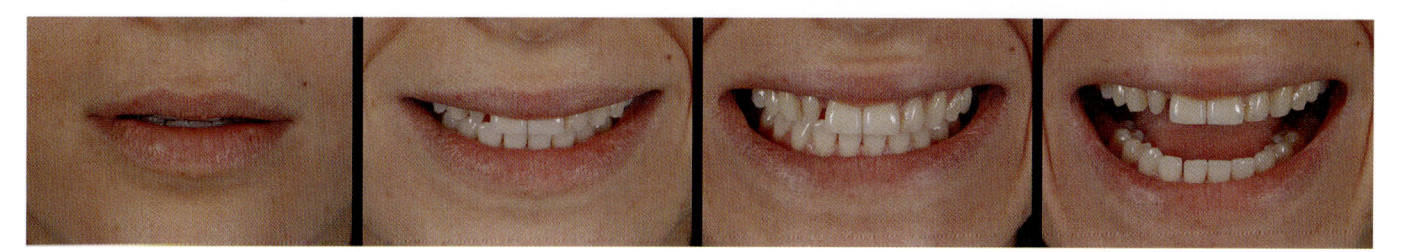

Figure 4.23 **(B)** Planning the restorative procedures. Photo protocol for smile analysis after ortho.

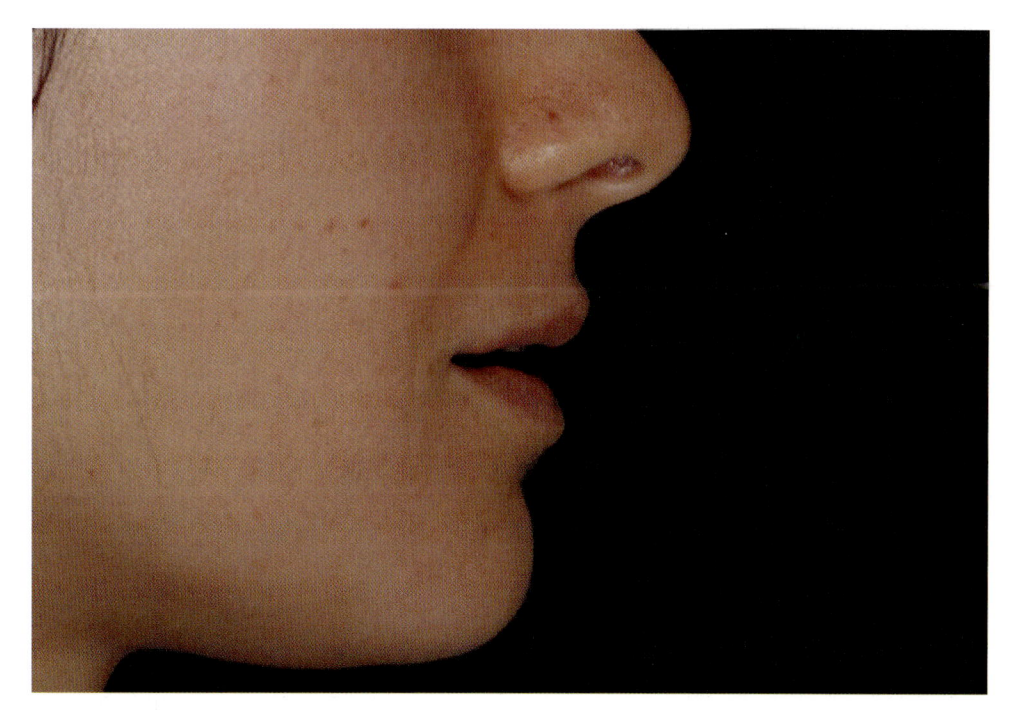

Figure 4.24 The profile photo is also important to help analyze the buccal/palatal position of the centrals in relation with the lips.

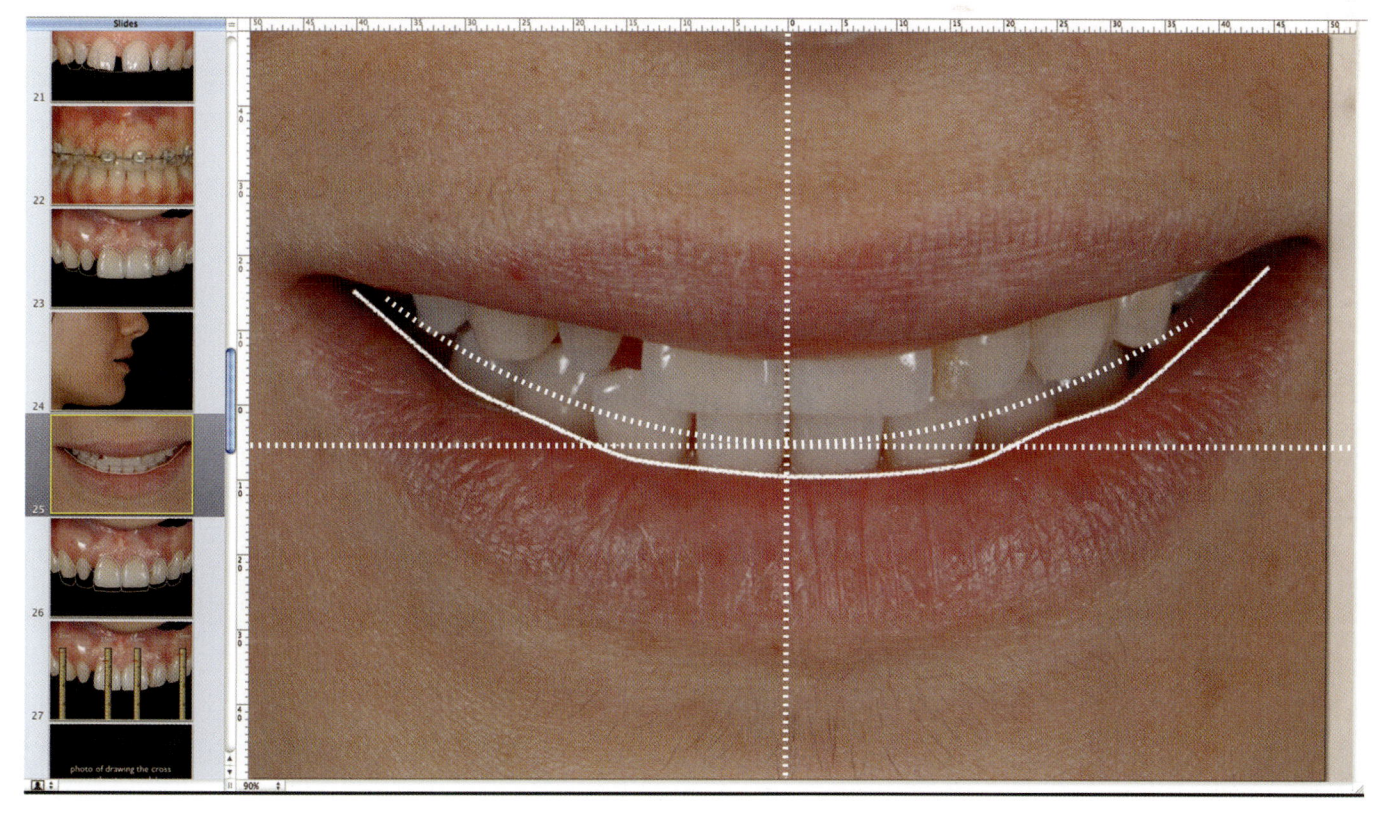

Figure 4.25 Digital planning for the restorative procedures. Analyzing the relation between the length of the anteriors and the lips. The first guess about how much one can lengthen the anteriors (curved dotted line).

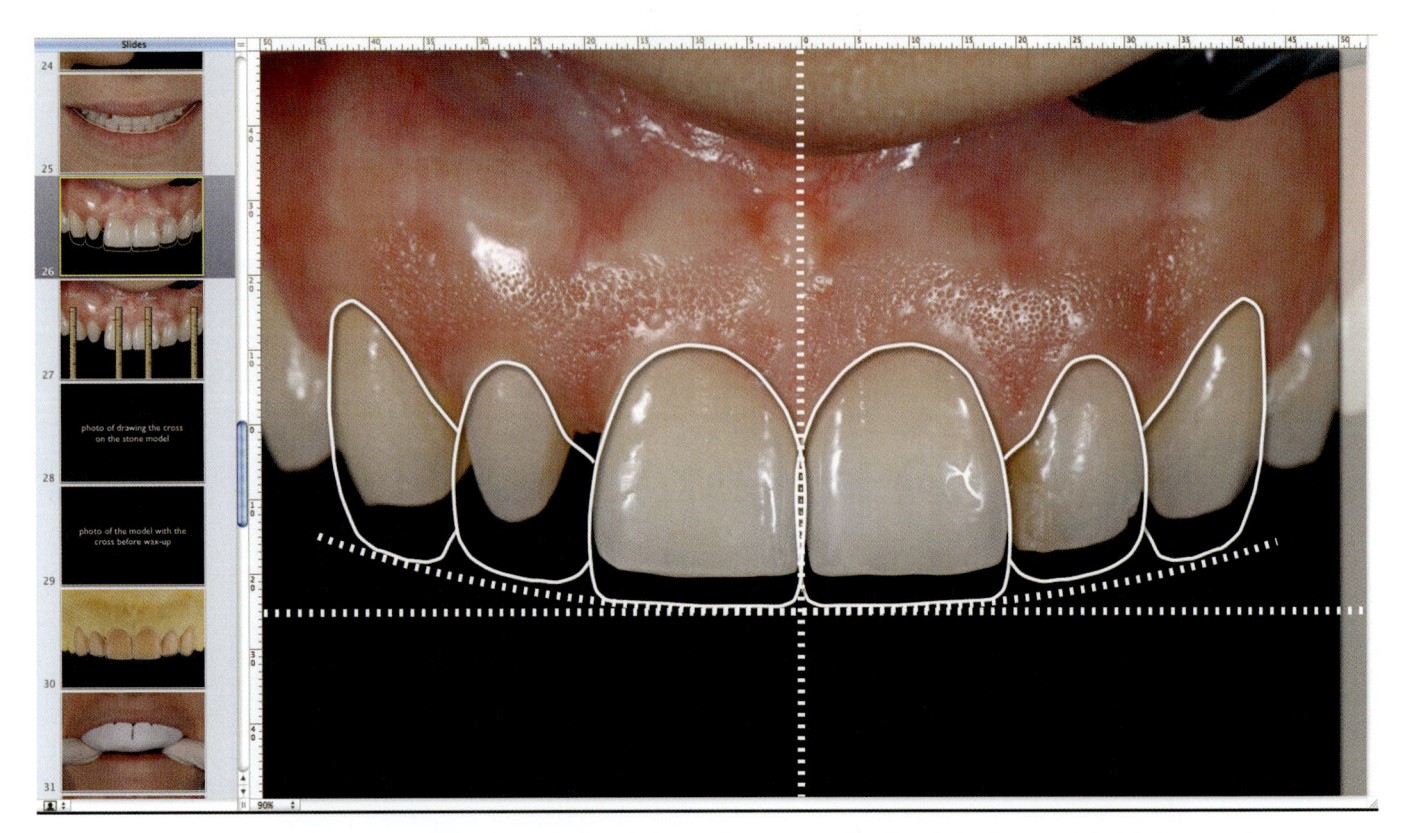

Figure 4.26 **(A)** Digital Mock-Up, giving an idea about ideal tooth design. One can visualize the relation between ideal design, actual tooth position, and soft tissues.

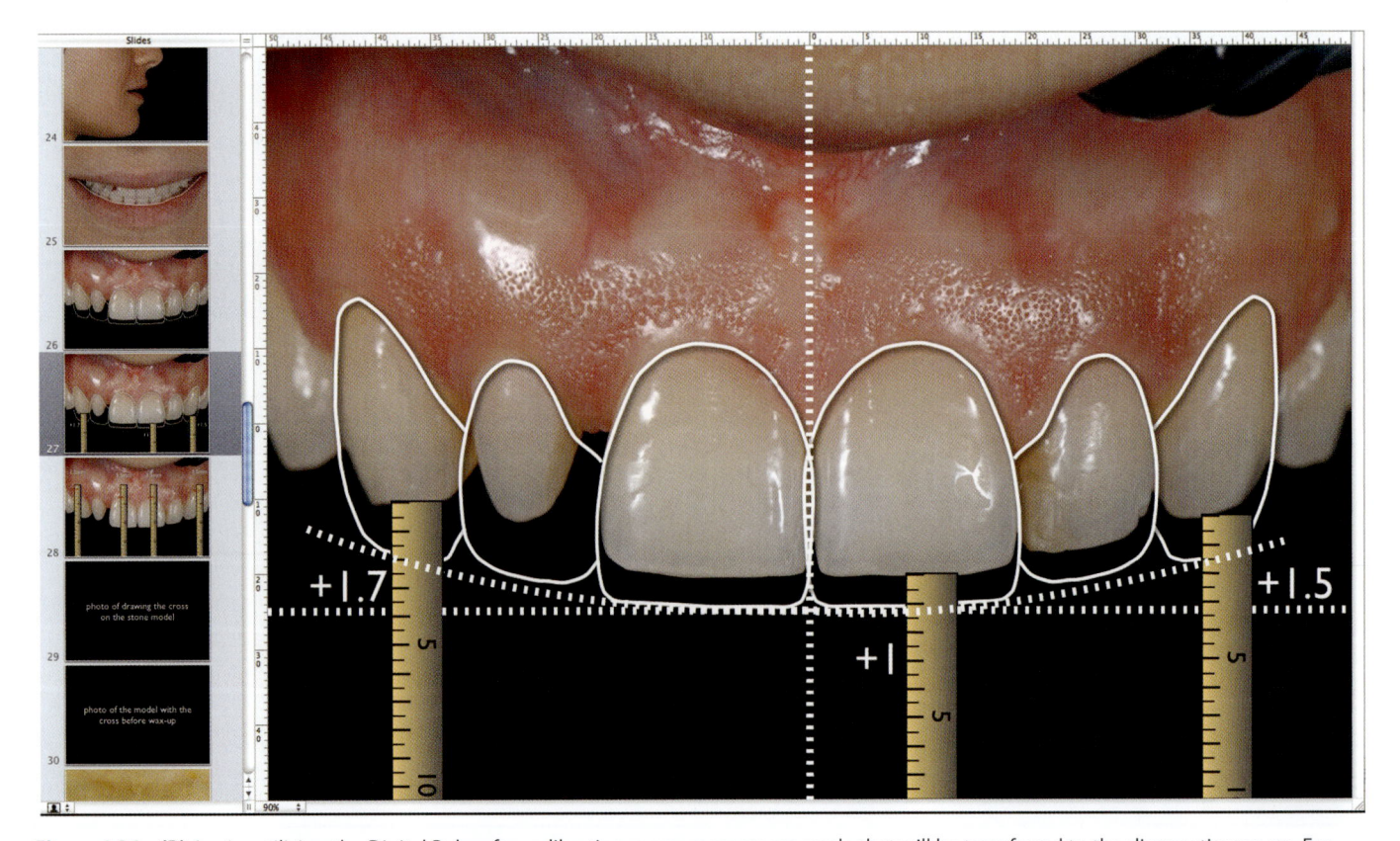

Figure 4.26 **(B)** Again, utilizing the Digital Ruler after calibration measurements are made that will be transferred to the diagnostic wax-up. For example, the amount of lengthening: 1.7 mm on right cuspid, 1 mm on left central, and 1.5 mm on left cuspid.

Chapter 4 Digital Smile Design

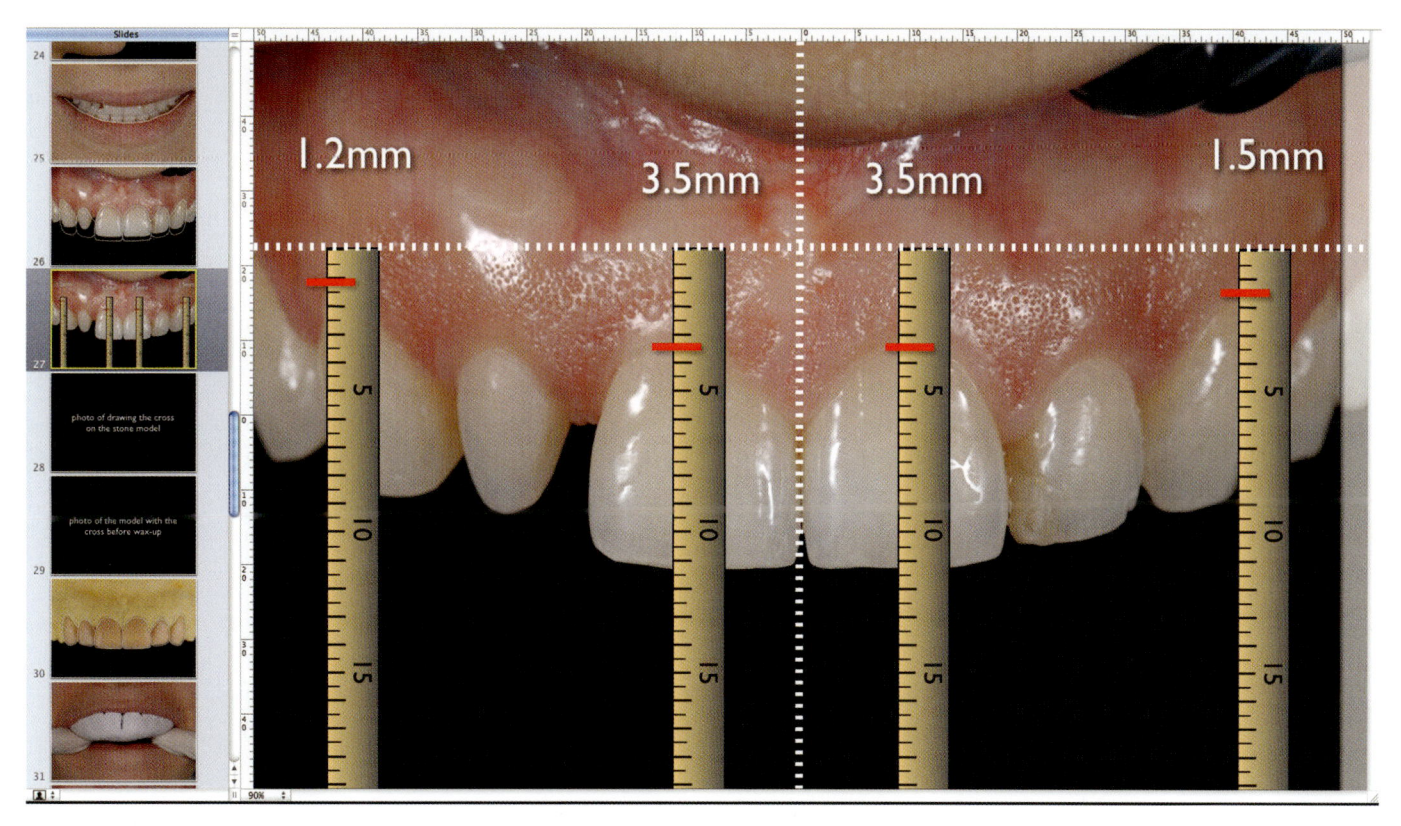

Figure 4.27 One of the main steps of the DSD technique, transferring the cross from the computer to the model to allow for a diagnostic wax-up that is integrated with the patient's face. The horizontal dotted line is placed above the teeth and the distances from the line to the cervical of the centrals and cuspids are measured.

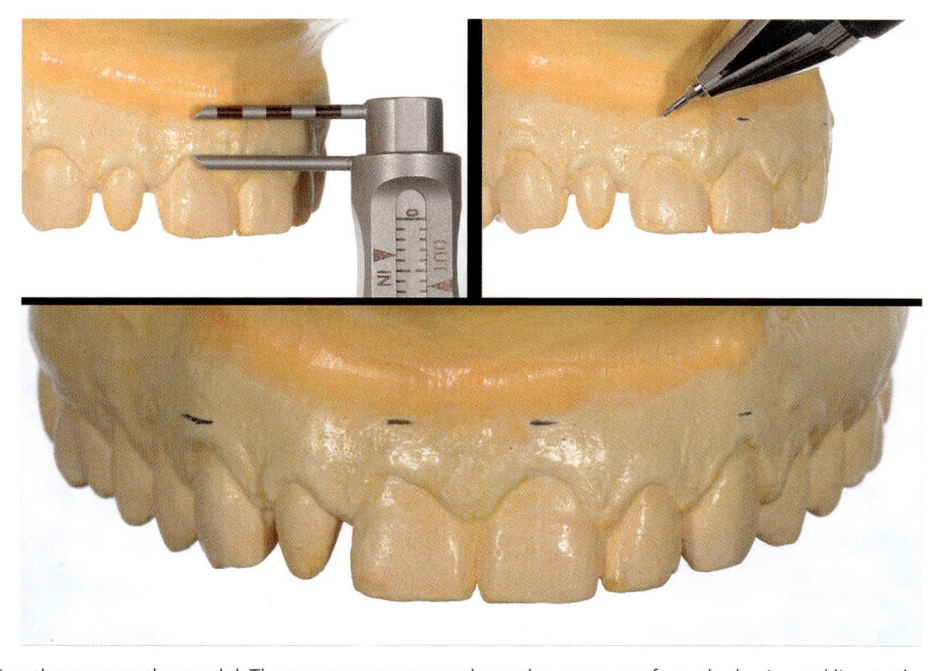

Figure 4.28 Transferring the cross to the model. The measurements made on the computer from the horizontal line to the cervical of the teeth are marked on the model by using a caliper. Then the four marks are connected creating the horizontal reference on the model.

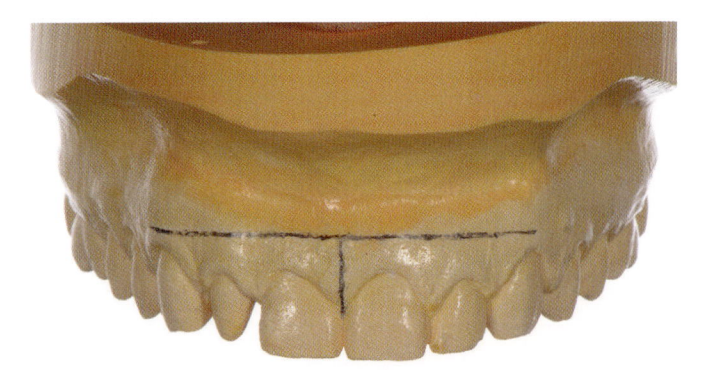

Figure 4.29 The vertical line can also be transferred from digital to the model. Now the model has the references for the wax-up to be developed without missing the midline and the occlusal plane.

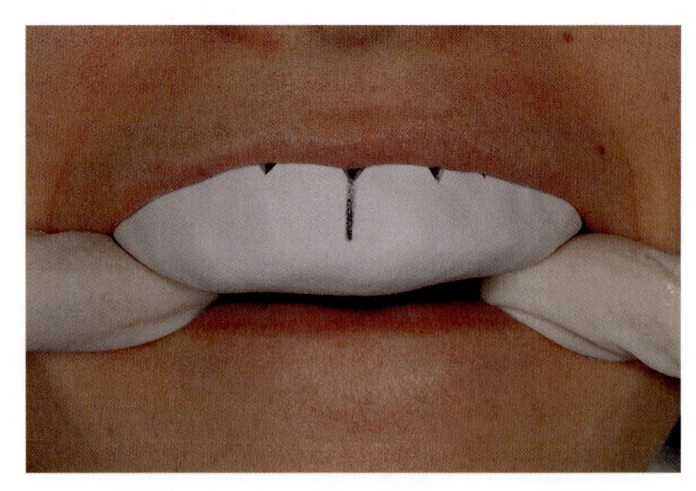

Figure 4.31 The wax-up is transferred to the mouth to create a mock-up by utilizing a silicone index (Matrix Form 60-Anaxdent).

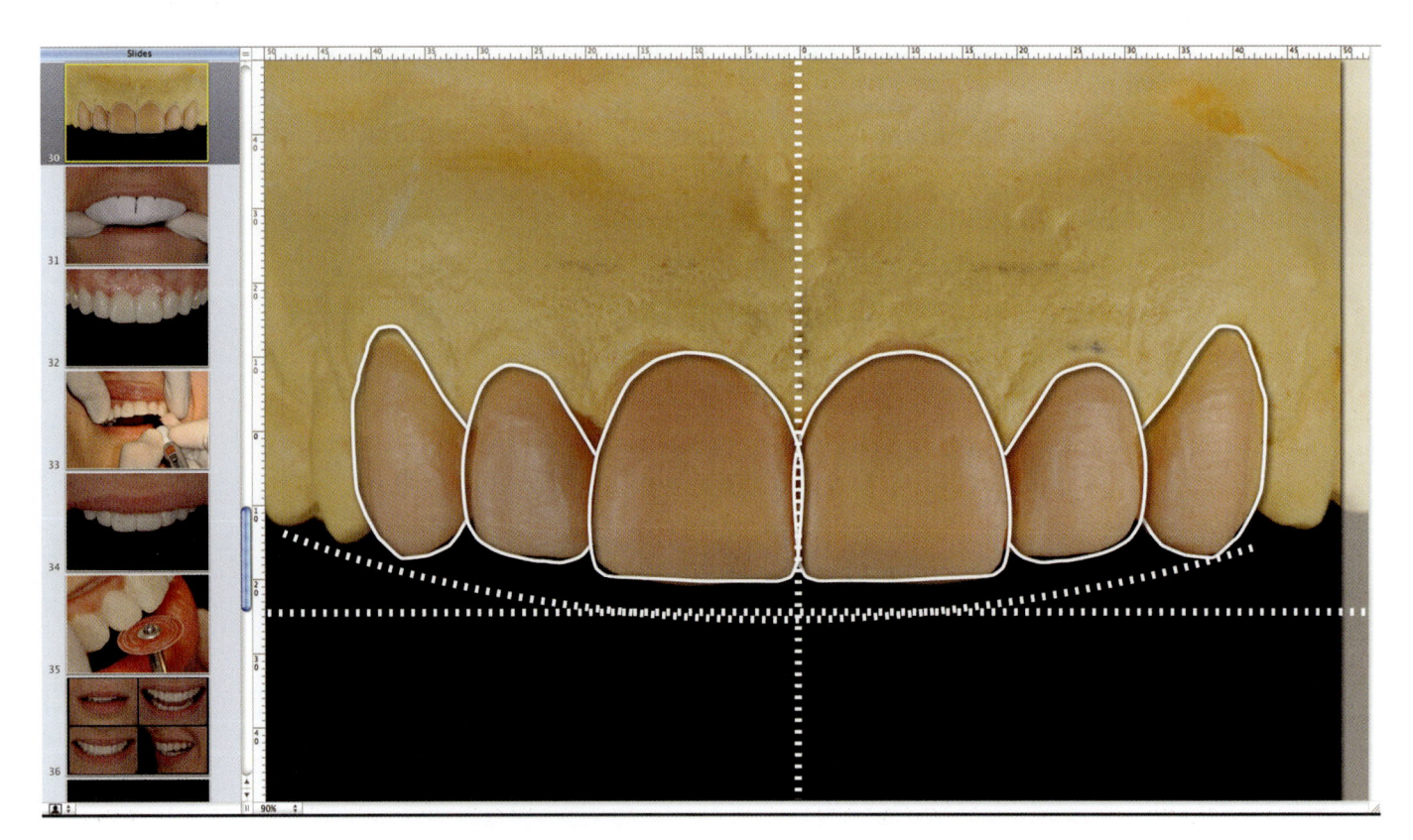

Figure 4.30 Guided diagnostic wax-up, guided by the digital planning and in harmony with the facial cross.

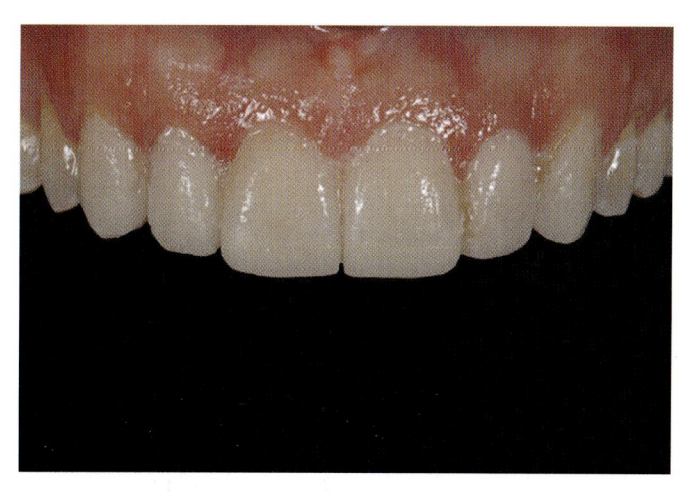

Figure 4.32 The mock-up made with a bis-acryl type of material.

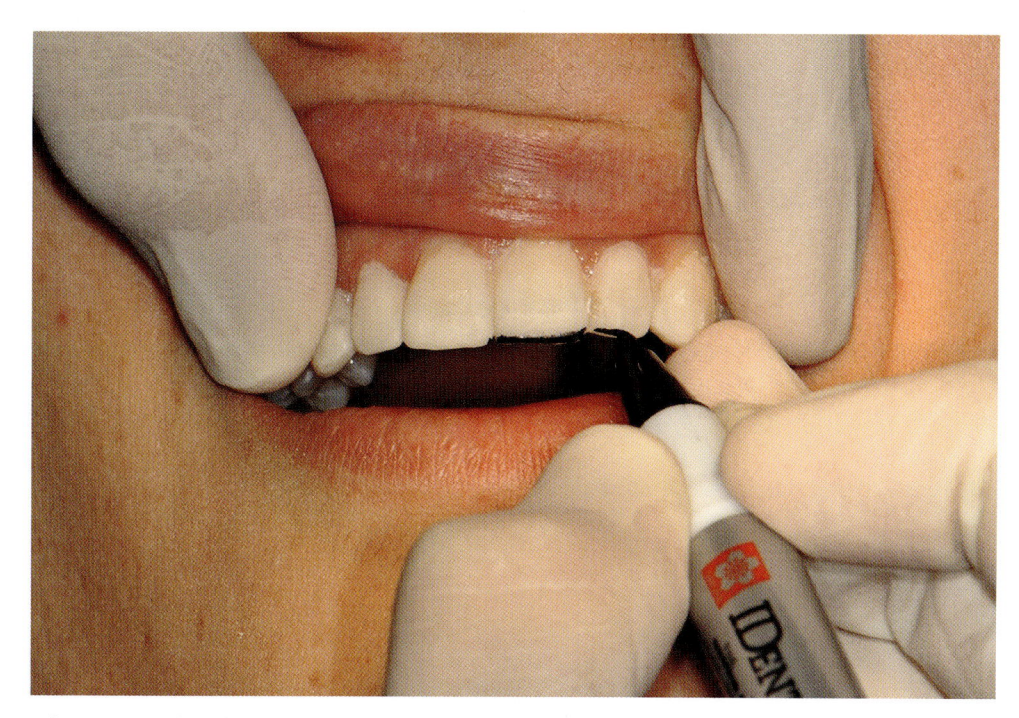

Figure 4.33 If the mock-up seems a little long, a permanent black marker can be used to create the illusion of shorter teeth before actually shortening them.

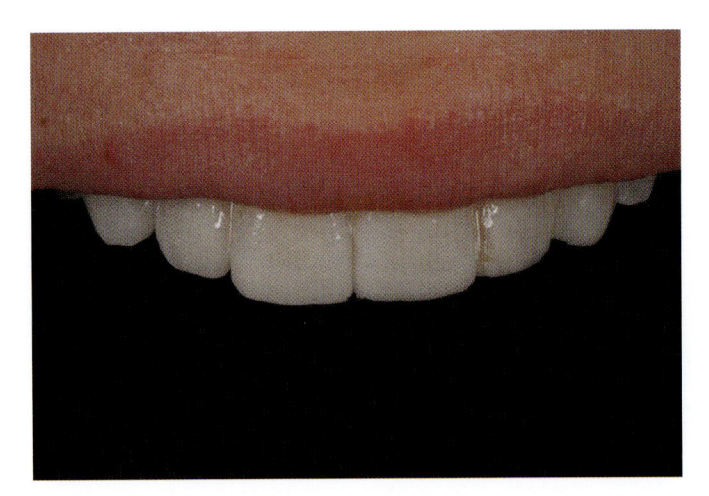

Figure 4.34 The smile with the simulation of shorter teeth on the left side.

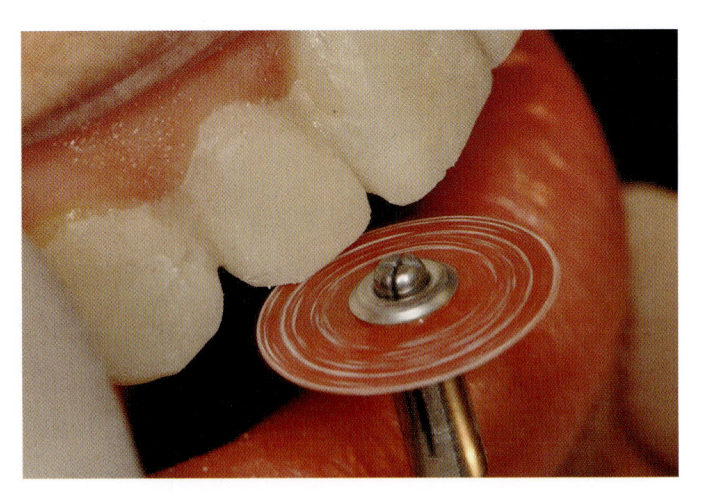

Figure 4.35 Shortening the mock-up with a sand disk.

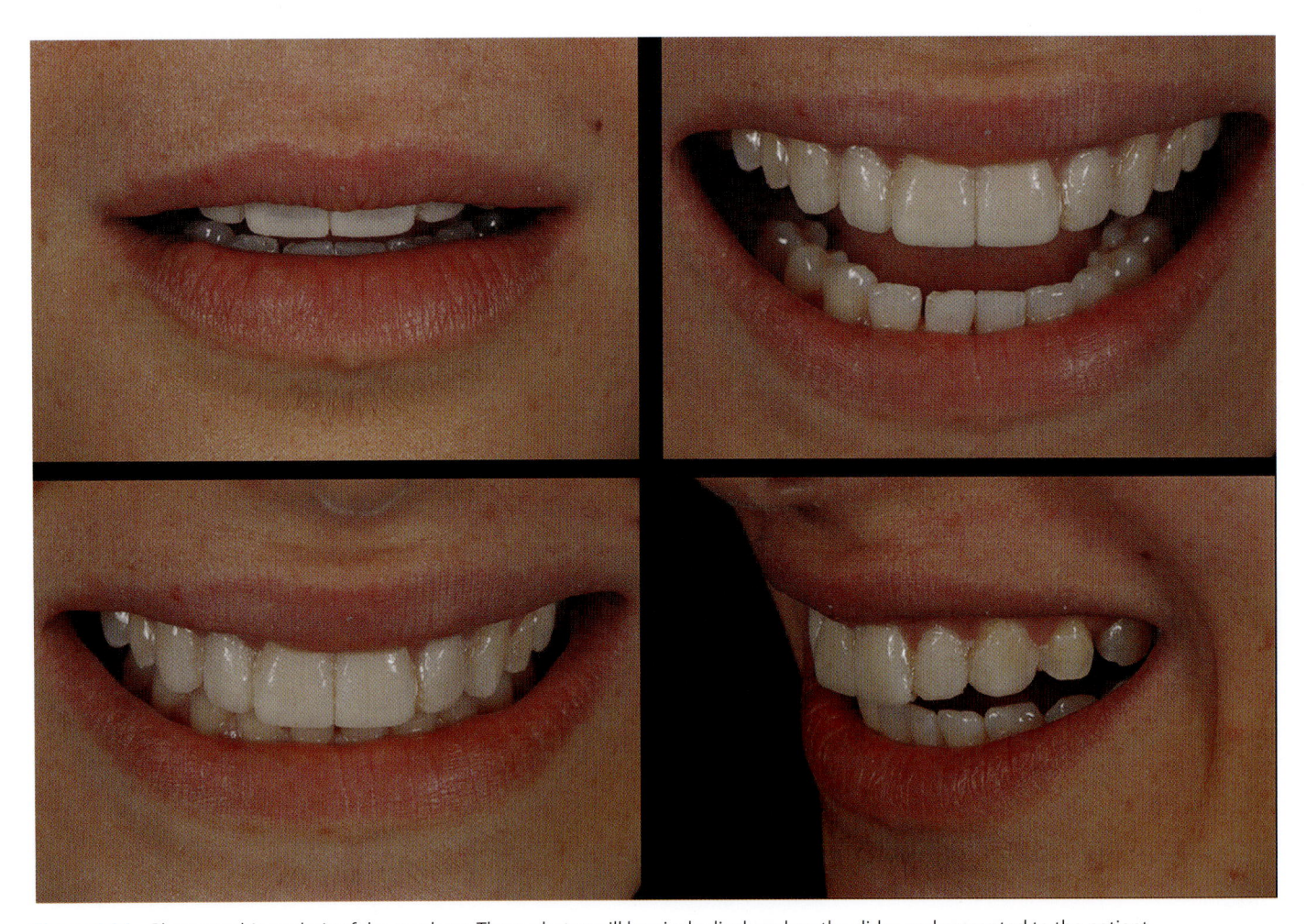

Figure 4.36 Photographic analysis of the mock-up. These photos will be nicely displayed on the slides and presented to the patient.

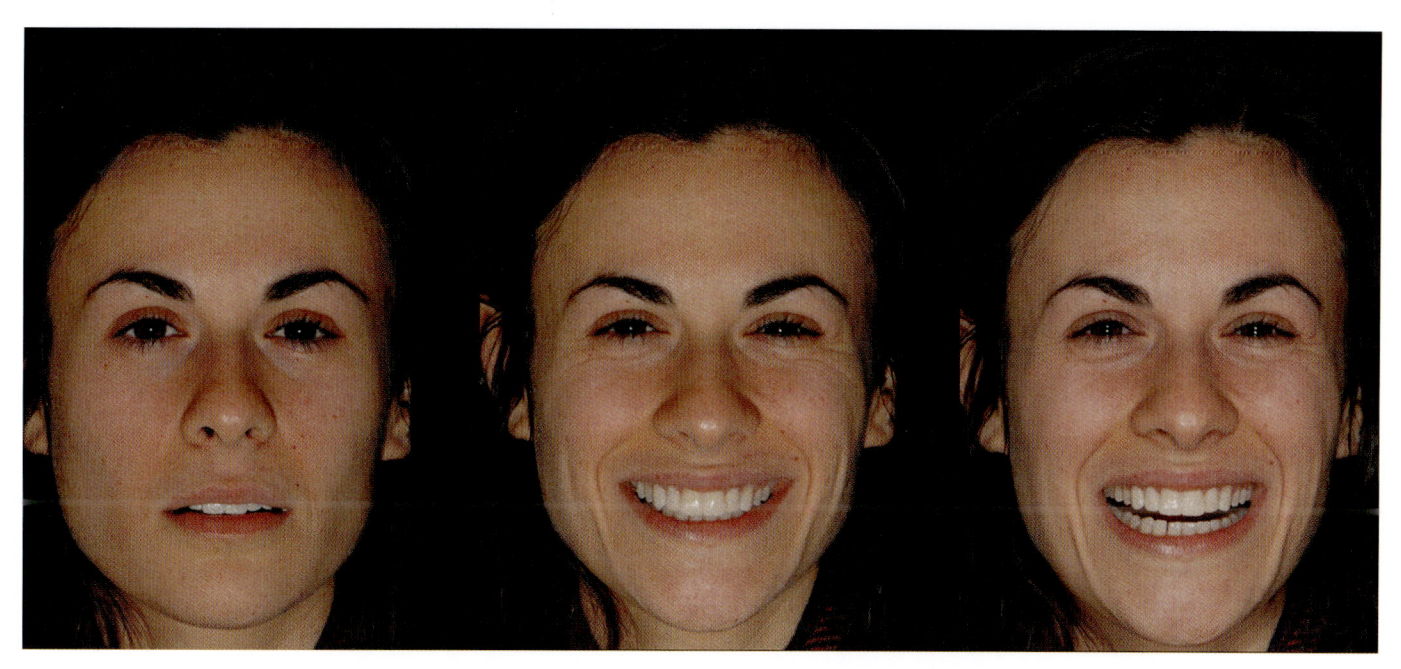

Figure 4.37 The smile design should always be presented to the patient by images and videos rather than by the mirror.

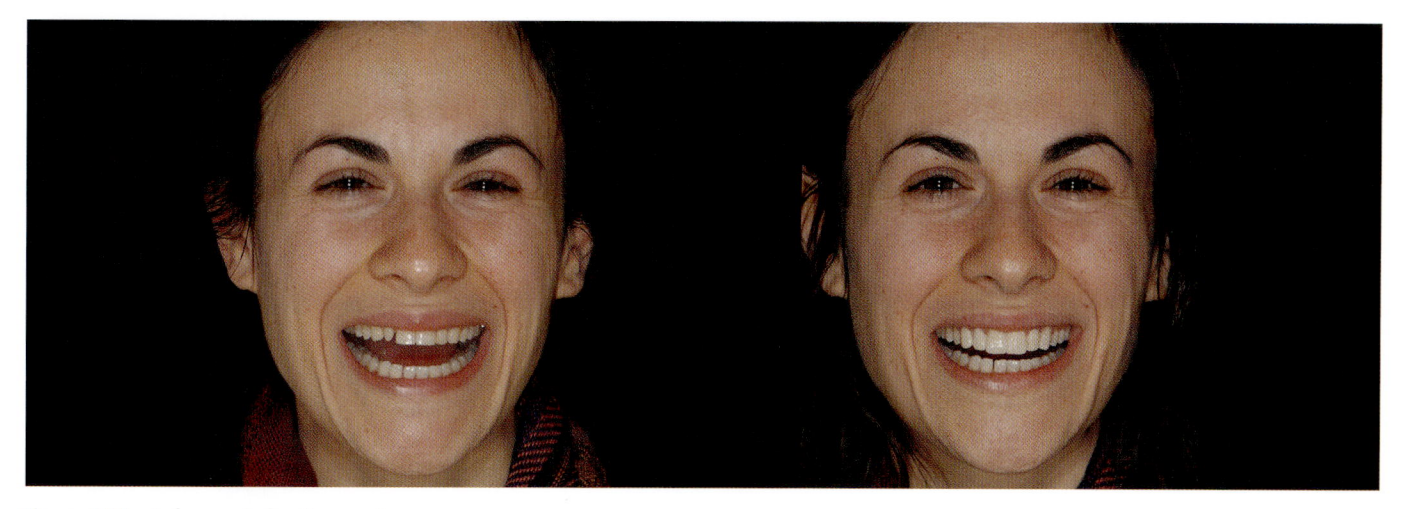

Figure 4.38 Before and after the mock-up.

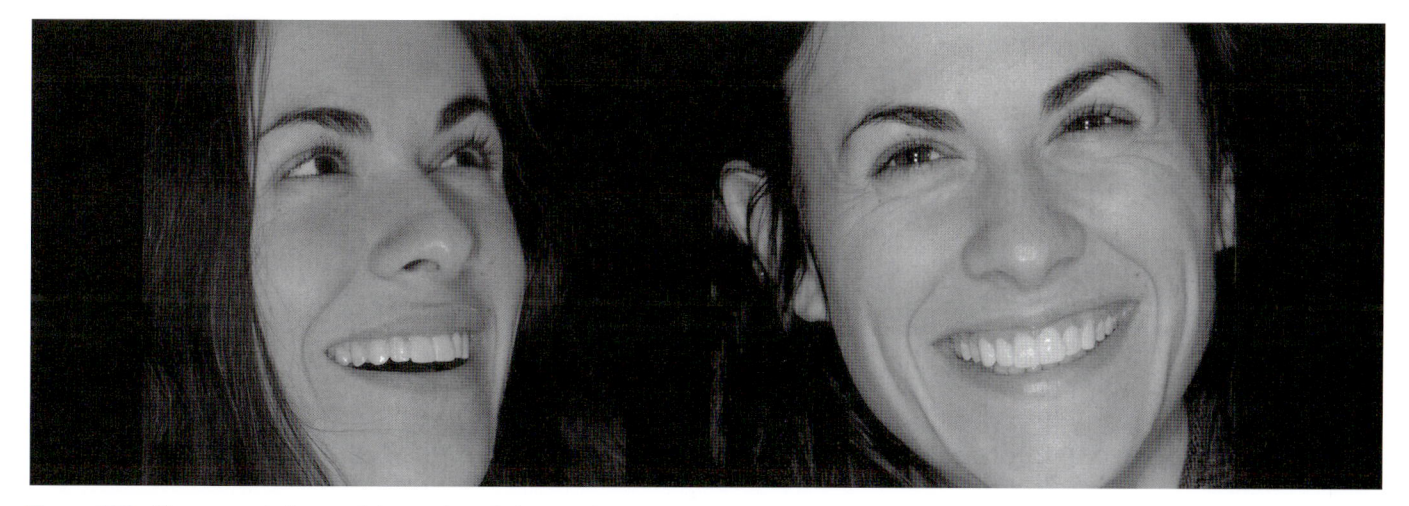

Figure 4.39 These casual photos of the mock-up help stimulate, motivate, and engage the patient.

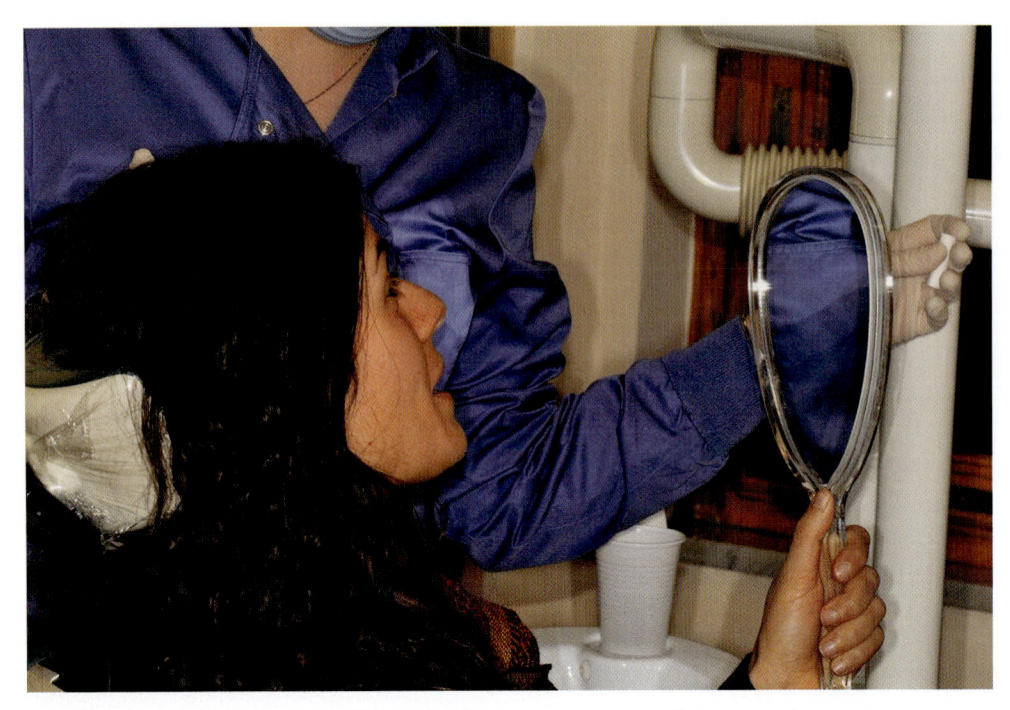

Figure 4.40 Presenting the smile design with just the mirror is not effective in presenting all the possibilities to the patient.

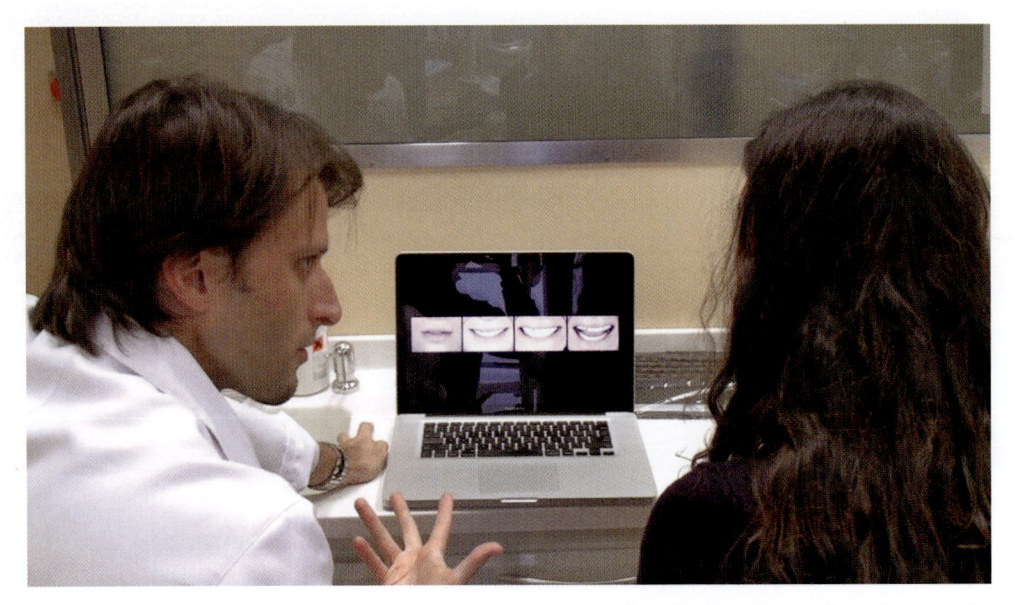

Figure 4.41 The photos and videos allow the patient to see the changed smile from all angles in order to fully understand the integration of the smile design to their face.

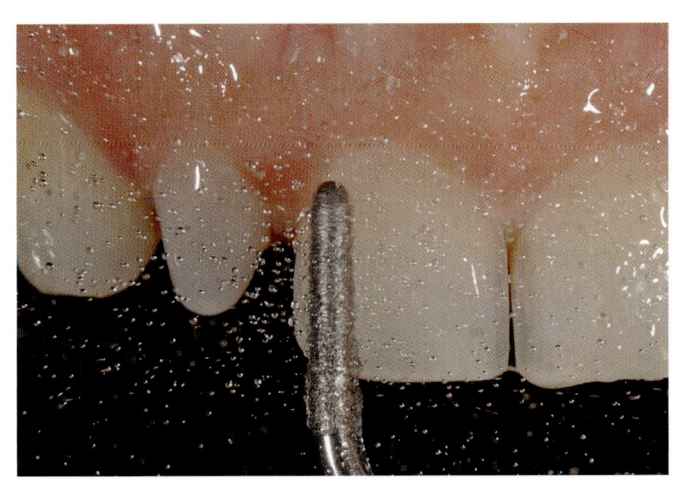

Figure 4.42 After the smile design project is approved by the team and the patient, the clinical procedures can be planned as tooth preparation. The tooth preparation will be as minimally invasive as possible if one knows exactly the final ideal forms.

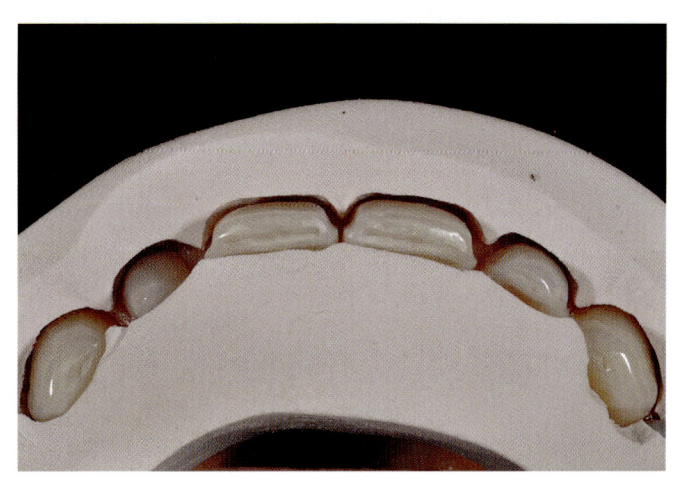

Figure 4.44 A very important analysis is done when comparing the preps with the silicone index that shows the ideal buccal position according to the mock-up.

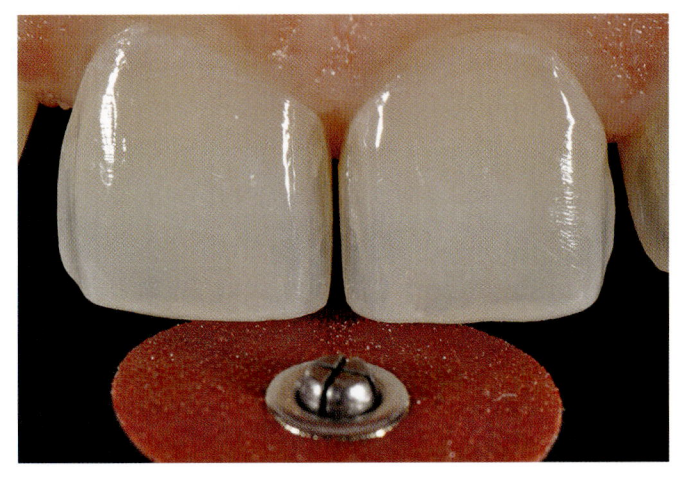

Figure 4.43 Finishing the tooth preparation. One can notice an almost prepless situation.

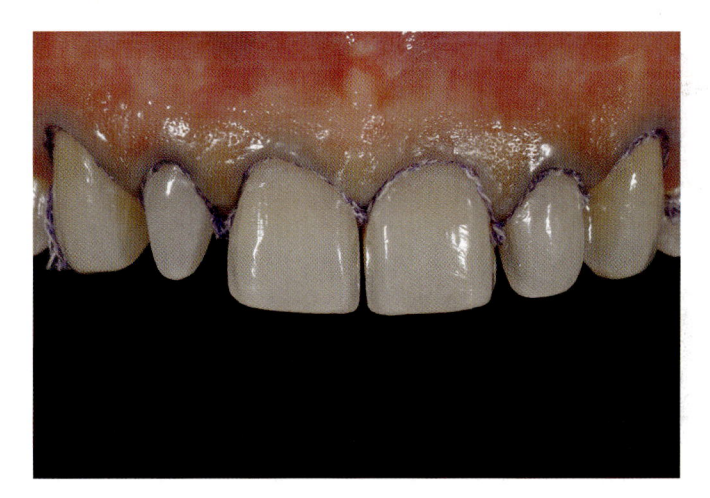

Figure 4.45 Impression.

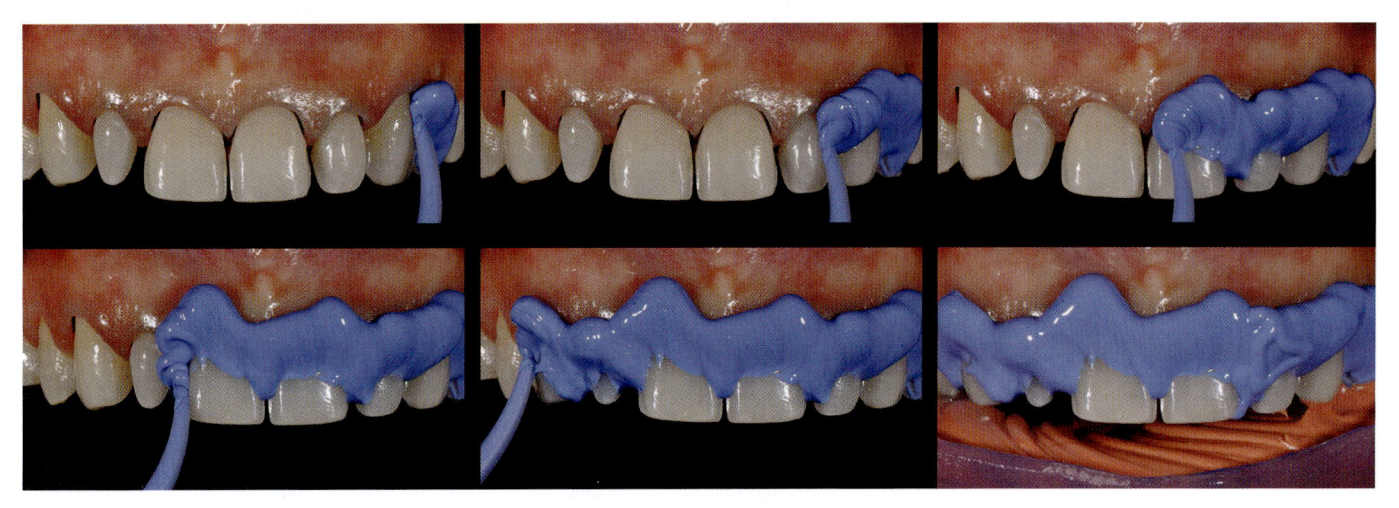

Figure 4.46 Impression.

108 Principles of Esthetics

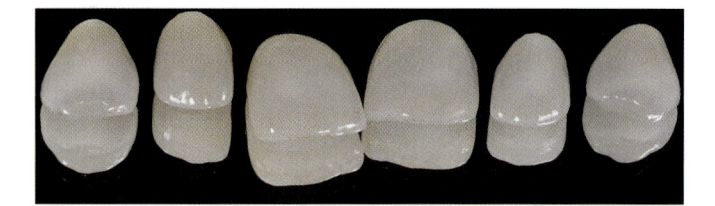

Figure 4.47 Monolithic ceramic veneers (Emax LT BL4).

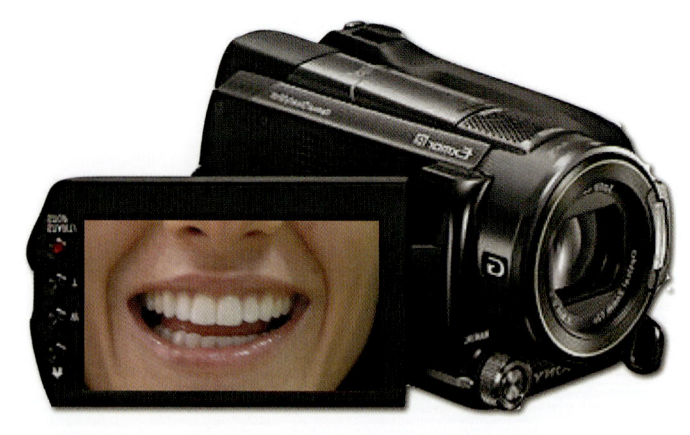

Figure 4.50 A video of the try-in allows the dentist and the patient to evaluate in all the details the integration between the veneers, the smile, and the face, allowing for final adjustments before final cementation.

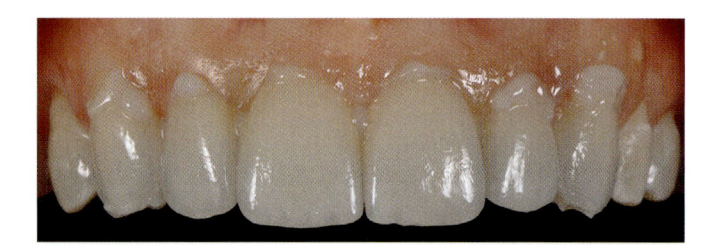

Figure 4.48 The veneers in position with try-in paste (Variolink Try-in paste).

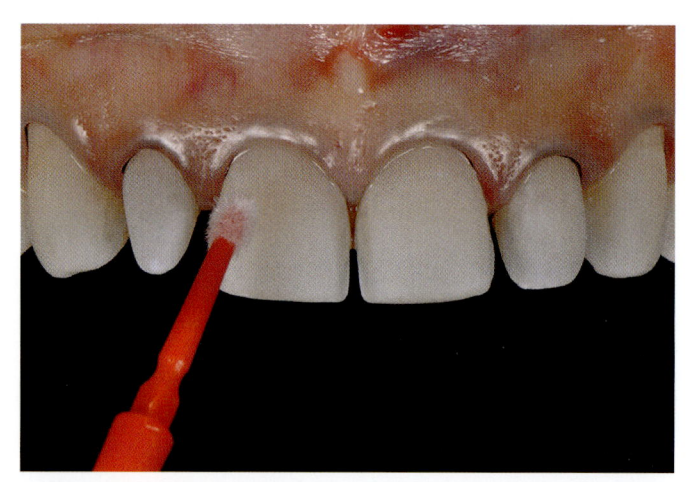

Figure 4.51 Bonding procedures.

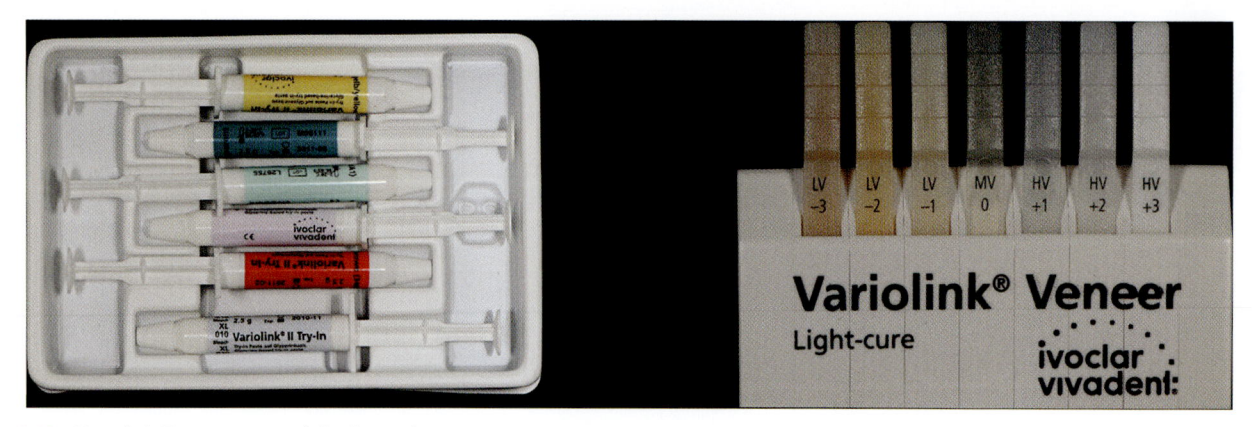

Figure 4.49 Variolink Try-in paste and shade guide.

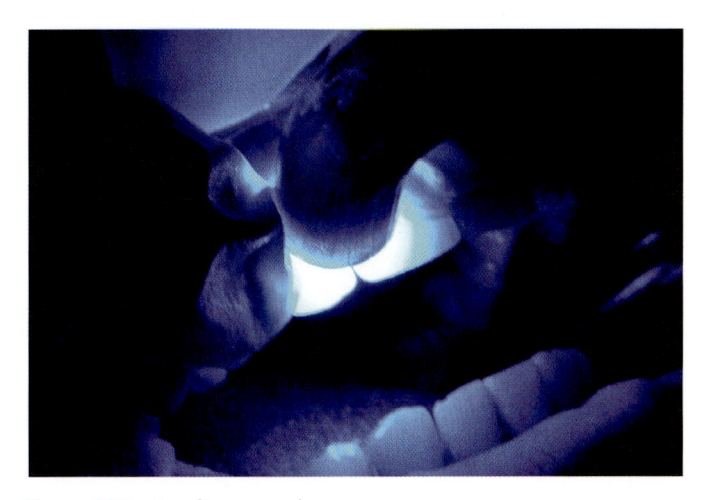

Figure 4.52 Bonding procedures.

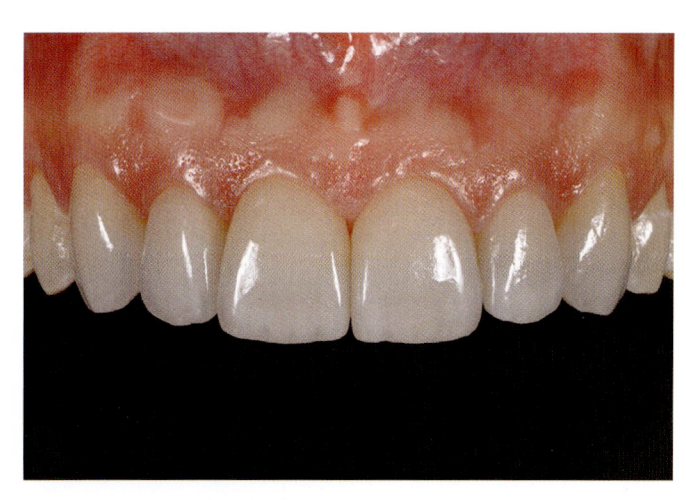

Figure 4.53 Immediately after cementation showing a very good soft tissue condition.

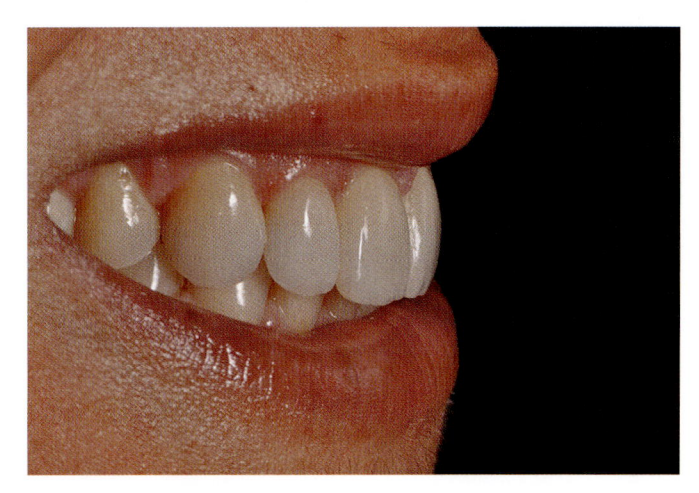

Figure 4.54 Smile integration.

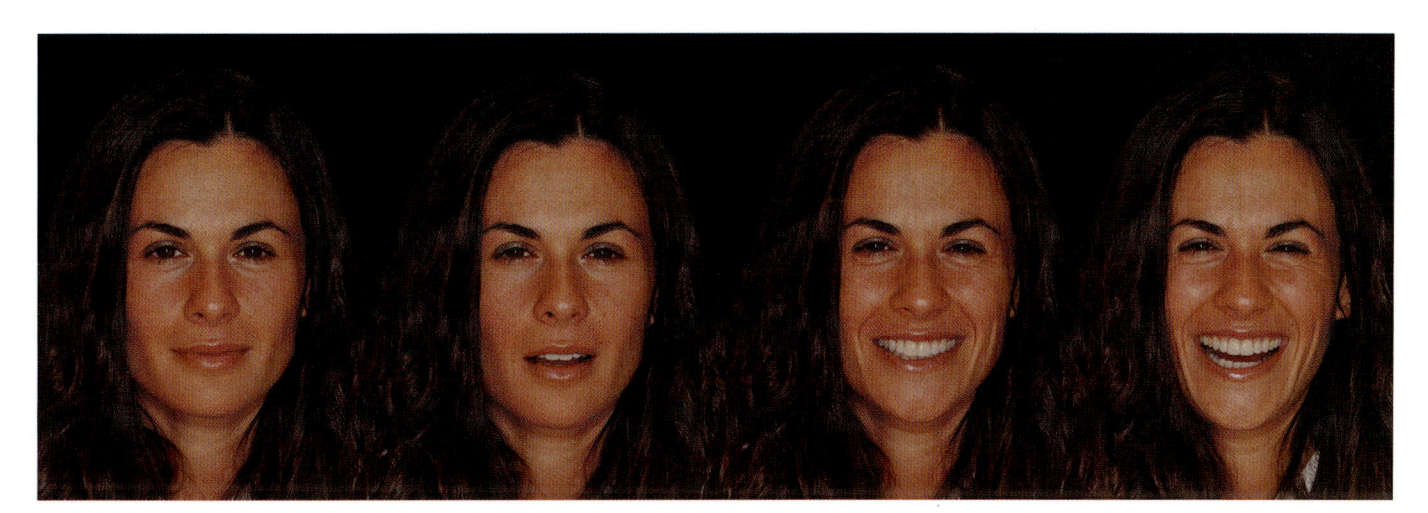

Figure 4.55 Final face photos.

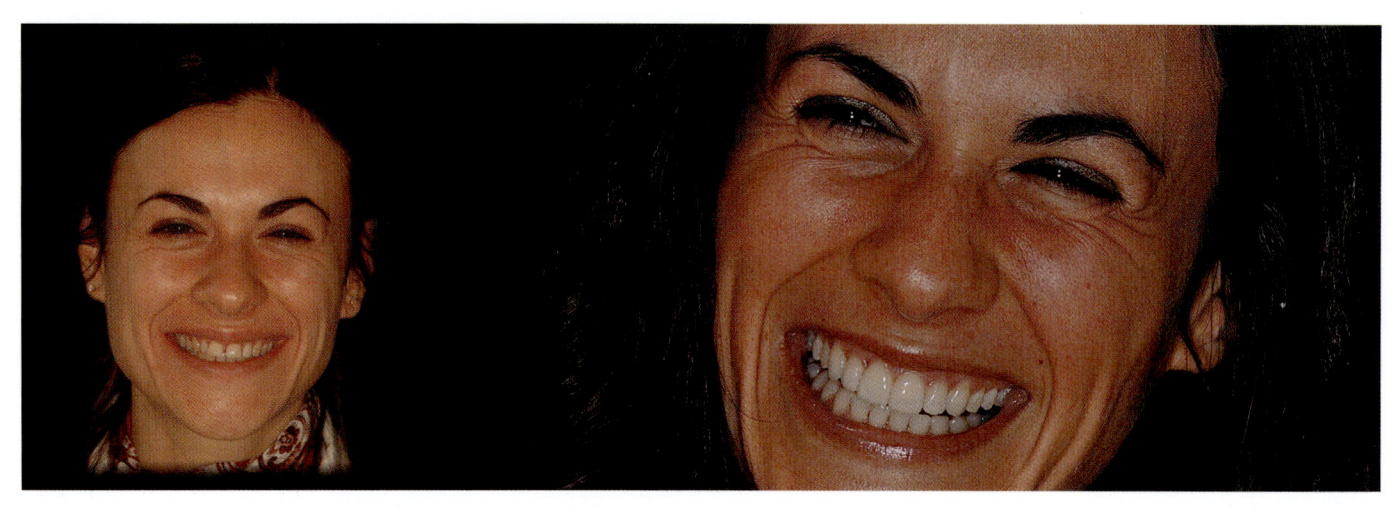

Figure 4.56 It is important to present the patient with a before and after comparison slide to demonstrate the overall value and improvement to his or her smile.

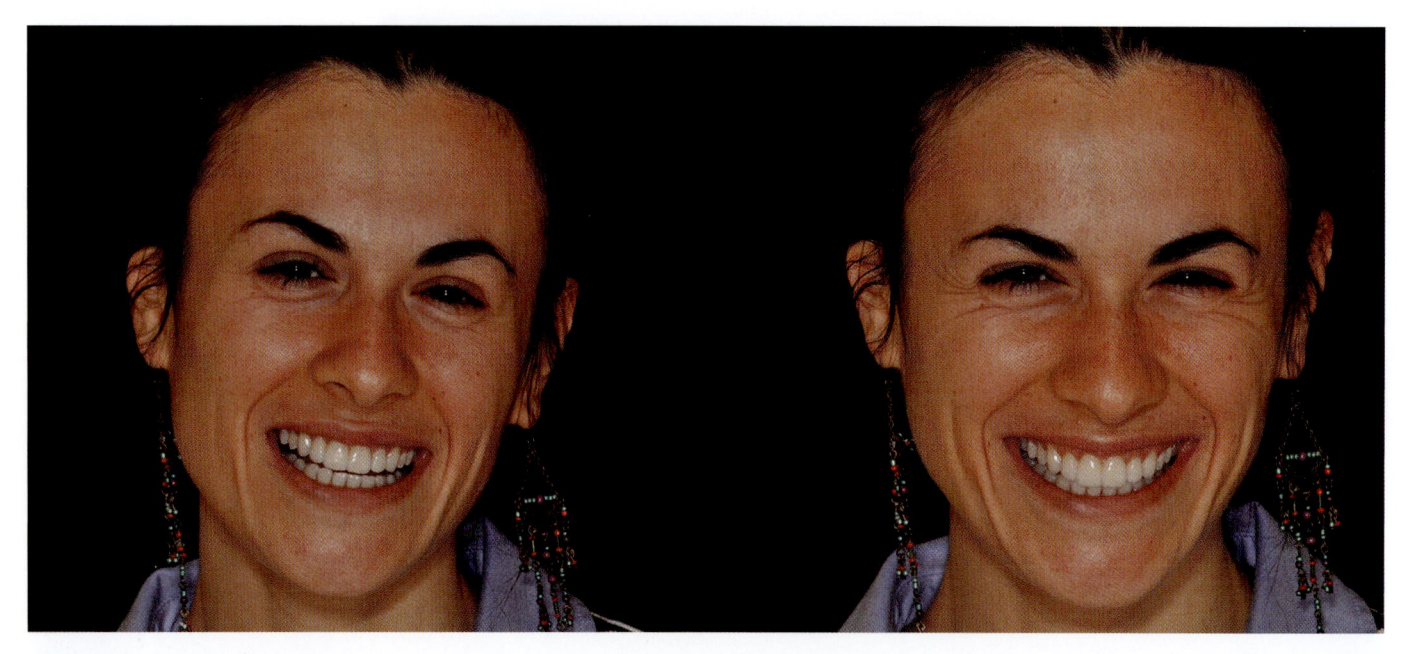

Figure 4.57 Post-op after 1 year.

References

1. Coachman C, Van Dooren E, Gürel G, et al. Smile design: from digital treatment planning to clinical reality. In: Cohen M, ed. *Interdisciplinary Treatment Planning. Vol. II: Comprehensive Case Studies*. Hanover Park, IL: Quintessence; 2011.
2. Goldstein RE. *Esthetics in Dentistry: Principles, Communication, Treatment Methods*. Ontario, ON: B. C. Decker; 1998.
3. Chiche GJ, Pinault A. *Esthetics of Anterior Fixed Prosthodontics*. Hanover Park, IL: Quintessence; 1996.
4. Magne P, Belser U. *Bonded Porcelain Restorations in the Anterior Dentition: A Biomimetic Approach*. Carol Stream, IL: Quintessence; 2002.
5. Fradeani M. *Esthetic Rehabilitation in Fixed Prosthodontics: Esthetic Analysis: A Systematic Approach to Prosthetic Treatment*. Carol Stream, IL: Quintessence; 2004.
6. Gürel G. *The Science and Art of Porcelain Laminate Veneers*. Berlin: Quintessence; 2003.
7. Rufenacht CR. *Fundamentals of Esthetics*. Carol Stream, IL: Quintessence; 1990.
8. Dawson PE. *Functional Occlusion: From TMJ to Smile Design*. St Louis, MO: Mosby; 2007.
9. Spear FM. The maxillary central incisor edge: a key to esthetic and functional treatment planning. *Compend Contin Educ Dent* 1999;20(6):512–516.
10. Kois JC. Diagnostically driven interdisciplinary treatment planning. *Seattle Study Club J* 2002;6(4):28–34.
11. Paolucci B. Visagism and dentistry. In: Hallawell P, ed. *Integrated Visagism: Identity, Style, and Beauty*. São Paulo: Senac; 2009:243–250.
12. Gürel G, Bichacho N. Permanent diagnostic provisional restorations for predictable results when redesigning smiles. *Pract Proced Aesthet Dent* 2006;18(5):281–286.
13. Paolucci B, Gürel G, Coachman C, et al. *Visagism: the Art of Smile Design Customization*. São Paulo: VM Cultural; 2011.
14. Coachman C, Calamita MA. Digital smile design. *Quintessence Dent Technol* 2012;35:103–111.

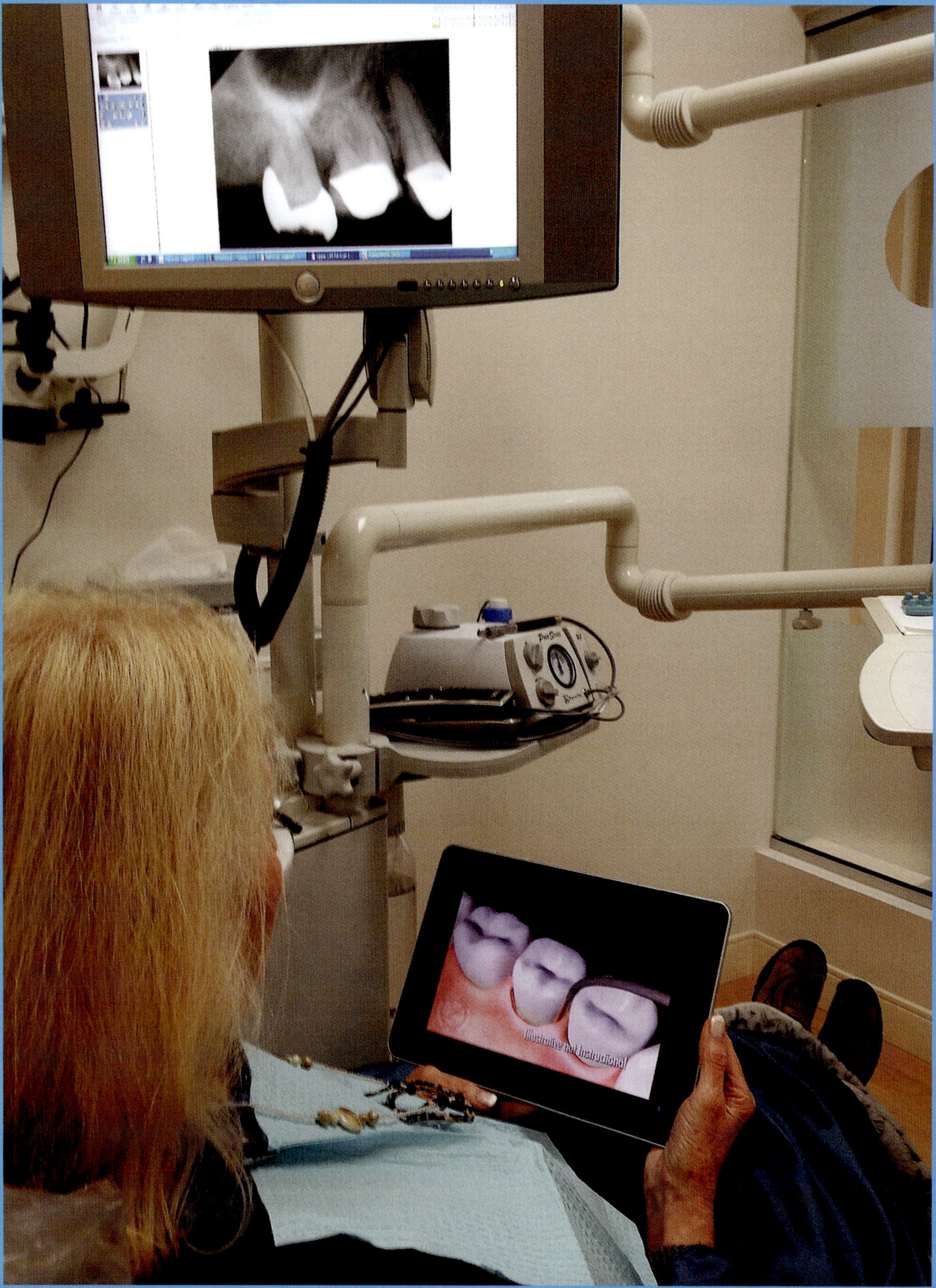
Illustrative not Instructional

Chapter 5 Esthetics in Dentistry Marketing

Roger P. Levin, DDS and Ronald E. Goldstein, DDS

Chapter Outline

What is dental marketing?	113	Advertising	125
Creating a brand	114	Telephone and online directories	125
Developing a marketing plan	114	Television commercials	125
What is internal marketing?	115	Radio	128
Internal marketing strategies	115	Outdoor billboard advertising	128
Critical components to successful marketing	115	Direct mail	128
What is external marketing?	122	Online group discount shopping services	128
External marketing strategies	124	Public relations	128

Why is marketing such an important strategy for cosmetic dentistry? Consider these facts:

- There are more than 77 million baby boomers in the United States.[1]
- Millions of people have watched TV makeover shows.
- Nearly 14 million cosmetic surgery procedures were performed in 2016.[2]
- Eighty percent of people are not happy with their smiles.[3]
- More than $16 billion is spent annually on smile enhancements in the United States.[4]

[1] From US Department of Labor report, "Aging Baby Boomers in a New Workforce Development System," Available at: http://www.doleta.gov/Seniors/other_docs/AgingBoomers.pdf.
[2] American Society for Aesthetic Plastic Surgery. Available at: https://www.surgery.org/sites/default/files/ASAPS-Stats2016.pdf.
[3] American Academy of Periodontology. Available at: http://www.perio.org/consumer/smile.htm.
[4] The Doctor Weighs In. Available at: https://thedoctorweighsin.com/the-multi-billion-dollar-demand-for-cosmetic-dentistry/.

For the foreseeable future, cosmetic dentistry will be a vibrant industry with a growing patient base, especially with more and more baby boomers and members of generation X trying to hold on to their youthful appearance. However, this does not mean that every cosmetic practice will automatically experience significant growth. To fully realize esthetic production, practices must become very proactive in their marketing initiatives. To achieve the highest level of success, esthetic practices need to promote their services through internal and external marketing. These two systems are necessary to attract new patients, retain current patients, boost esthetic case acceptance, and drive practice growth. With the right mix of internal and marketing strategies, a practice is well positioned to continually increase esthetic treatment and production.

What is dental marketing?

Marketing is the process whereby a business promotes a product or service to its customers. In the case of dental practices, the service being provided is dental care and treatment.

Unfortunately, marketing has often been a hit-or-miss proposition for many dental practices. This should not come as a surprise for a number of reasons:

1. Marketing can be an inexact science. In the business world, even a well-executed marketing campaign can fall flat due to poor timing, bad luck, or unforeseen circumstances.
2. Dentists receive little training on how to market their practices. Dentists learn dentistry at dental school—not how to market and manage a practice.
3. For much of the profession's history, dentists did not have to do much marketing, except for investing in attractive signage and a Yellow Pages advertisement. The marketplace has changed over time. The Internet and social media have brought a new dimension to marketing practices.
4. Marketing a dental practice and its services is very different from promoting other types of businesses. As a unique profession, dentistry requires specialized marketing techniques.
5. As the main provider of patient care and the practice leader, dentists are already extremely busy. Taking on additional marketing activities can present a significant challenge.

Like other business owners, dentists today need to engage in marketing to reach the highest levels of success. Unfortunately, marketing and dentistry have had an uneasy relationship. In past years, marketing was viewed as unethical and problematic by the majority of dentists. The rationale for this thinking was that dentistry, as a health-care profession, should not be soiled by the world of advertising. After all, this was dentistry—not something that could be packaged and sold like a used car on a late-night TV commercial. This hands-off approach to marketing essentially prevented practitioners from promoting themselves. Beginning approximately 15–20 years ago, attitudes started to change as more in the health-care industry, including hospitals and medical doctors, embraced high-impact marketing vehicles such as newspapers, radio, the Internet, and television.

Today, dental practices should model the best businesses and implement effective internal and external marketing programs. In the current marketplace, practices need to convey relevant information on specific services or opportunities to current and potential patients to market effectively. Educating patients through marketing activities benefits both the patient and the practice.

Creating a brand

A strong brand establishes positive and attractive qualities about your practice in the minds of current and potential patients. Those favorable impressions created by your brand can lead to increased case acceptance, more patient referrals, and, ultimately, greater profitability. Your brand drives your practice image. An effective brand should reflect the type of services performed in the practice. As practices add cosmetic services, many dentists fail to update their brands. The doctor may think of his or her practice as a modern cosmetic practice, but patients still perceive it as a typical general practice. As dentists begin the process of developing a brand, they need to ask the following questions to determine the practice's competitive advantages:

- What are the strengths of the practice?
- Why should patients come to this practice rather than another?
- What sets it apart from the other practices in the area?
- Do the team and the doctor currently have the necessary skills to successfully rebrand the practice?
- Are the practice's hours of operation different from other area practices? Does the practice offer more or less convenience to patients?
- What intangibles (special awards, community services, etc.) does the practice possess that will help in developing its brand?

Answering these questions will help dentists begin the process of determining the practice's brand. These differentiators will help the doctor select what elements are needed to develop the right brand for the practice.

Developing a marketing plan

The first step in designing a marketing plan is to identify the goals of the practice. One practice's goal may be to build a strong practice of 2000 active patients with an average patient production that leads to a $1.8 million per year gross revenue. Another practice may have a goal of providing primarily high-end cosmetic dentistry.

In the past 25 years, we have noted numerous practices that have launched marketing plans with a goal of simply "growing the practice." Unfortunately, that is not an effective goal because it is not specific. Details matter in marketing, just like they do in dentistry. Vague goals result in ineffective marketing strategies. Align your marketing plan with defined goals.

The following questions can help doctors develop specific marketing goals:

- Does the practice need more new patients? If so, how many per month?
- What is the average production per patient? Per new patient?
- Does the practice need more referrals? If so, how many per month?
- Does the practice have a sufficient number of new patients and referrals but need to enhance the case acceptance rate? If so, how much?
- What percentage of patients who contact the office actually make appointments?
- What cosmetic services are being utilized by current and new patients?
- What kind of cosmetic practice does the doctor want to create?

What is internal marketing?

Internal marketing refers to marketing activities that target current patients, motivating them to remain active in the practice, learn about all of the services offered, and refer others. The following recommendations are all part of a practice's internal marketing:

- Build a strong brand.
- Educate every patient about all services.
- Train the team to ask for referrals.
- Provide superior customer service.
- Stay in contact with patients to build and strengthen relationships.
- Reactivate inactive patients.

What is the most effective kind of internal marketing for the practice? Different patients respond to different types of marketing. Unfortunately, many practices take a scattershot approach to marketing rather than implementing a well-designed series of strategies that retain and attract patients. To be successful in building the patient base, internal marketing should be *ongoing*, *consistent*, and *positive*. As more dentists incorporate elective procedures into their practices, internal marketing becomes increasingly important to practice success. Whitening, porcelain laminate veneers, dental implants, and even removable appliances are all examples of services that many people desire but do not necessarily need. A practice focused on these types of value-added elective dental services is positioning itself for increased production and profit by successfully attracting the right type of patients through internal marketing. Properly implemented, internal marketing enables the practice to identify and attract new patients through specific strategies that result in referrals from existing patients. One such strategy is using appropriate scripting to ask satisfied patients to refer friends and family during checkout. In addition to bringing in more new patients, internal marketing helps the practice identify more treatment opportunities and increase case acceptance rates for active patients.

Internal marketing strategies

Internal marketing is often the most effective way for dentists to grow their practices and increase production. With their networks of family, friends, neighbors, and coworkers, current patients are an excellent source for new patient referrals. These patients know the practice and are more than happy to refer others if they have experienced superior care and exceptional customer service. By using internal marketing, dentists can generate more patient referrals, drive growth, and take their production to a higher level.

Internal marketing results in word-of-mouth advertising, which may be the most powerful form of advertising because other people (i.e., patients)—not the team or the doctor—are recommending the practice. This occurs when the level of patient care and customer service continually exceed expectations. When patients are extremely satisfied with the treatment and service, most will gladly recommend the practice to their friends and family, especially when the office asks them to do so.

Critical components to successful marketing

- Facility
- Doctor and team appearance
- Customer service
- Patient education
- Case presentation
- Patient referrals
- Patient communication

Facility

Appearance matters, especially for an esthetic practice. Patients are unlikely to accept treatment designed to make their teeth look significantly better if the office atmosphere is unattractive. Although this is true for any type of dental practice, it is especially important for practices that are promoting esthetic dentistry. An attractive office helps make patients feel comfortable during the cosmetic exam and instills confidence that the practice understands the importance of presentation. Improving the office's appearance is an effective method to add value to the practice. Patients must feel that they are in an esthetically pleasing environment, which reflects the ability of the doctor and team to provide excellent cosmetic dentistry. To achieve superior customer service, dentists and their team members need to view their practices through the eyes of their patients. How does the practice look from the outside? Is the building inviting? Is it landscaped and maintained well? Is the carpeting in the reception area in good shape? Is the furniture attractive and comfortable? Is it free and clear of clutter?

Walk through the entire office as if you were a patient and make notes about areas that need to be addressed. In addition, consider hiring an interior decorator or designer. The money spent on an interior designer is minor compared to the benefit gained by creating an attractive office that reflects your esthetic philosophy (Figure 5.1A–G).

> Remember, cosmetic dentistry is about esthetic beauty, so the office's appearance should reflect that, too!

Doctor and team appearance

Everyone in the practice should present a professional appearance. Uniforms or designated clothing should be attractive, clean, and up to date. As a health-care provider specializing in esthetics, a cosmetic practice must maintain high standards when it comes to dress and apparel. Patients have certain expectations regarding the doctor's and team's appearance, which should be professional and attractive (Figure 5.2A and B).

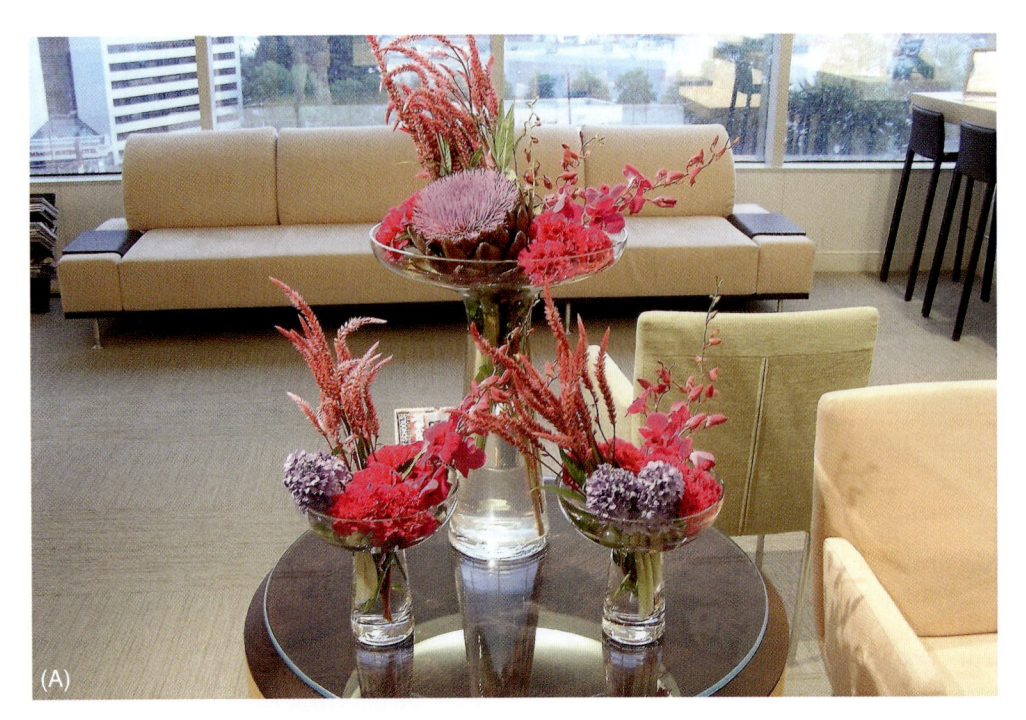

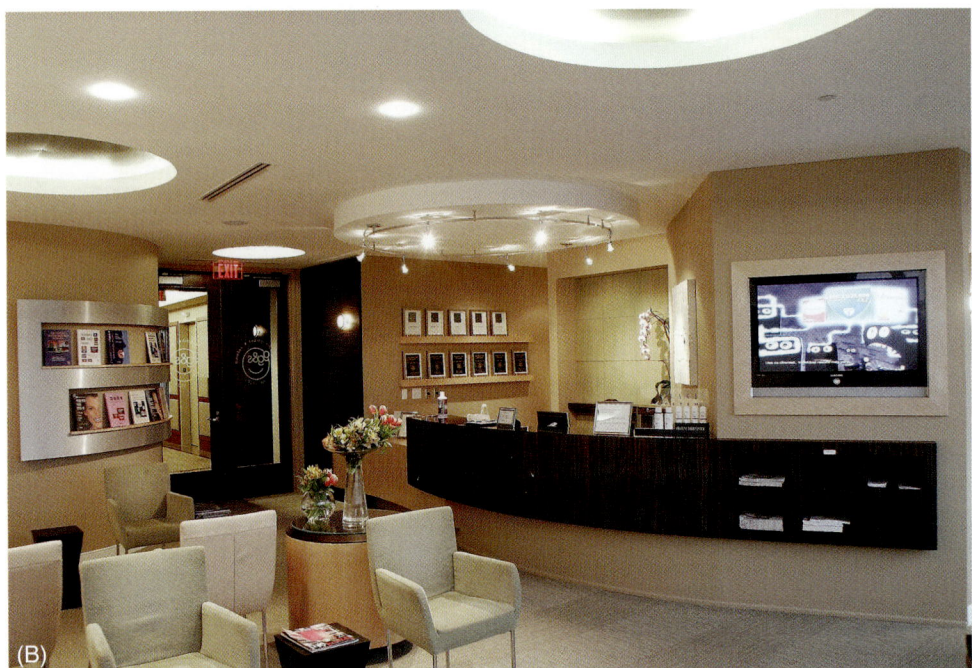

Figure 5.1 **(A and B)** Esthetically pleasing décor enhances the patient's perception of the dentist's esthetic taste. The presence of colorful flowers and other art décor around the office may also help to enhance your patient's confidence in your esthetic judgment.

In addition, the team should be seen as a showcase for the dentist's cosmetic skills. Consider offering staff members free or discounted cosmetic treatment, thus making them walking advertisements for the procedures the doctor wishes to promote. When patients walk in and are met by a sea of shining, beautiful smiles, the impression is quite dramatic. Even patients who have never considered cosmetic enhancement may start thinking about how much they would like a nice, bright smile after seeing the team's new and improved smiles. The issue of dress and appearance turns out to be more important than it might seem because patients decide whether to move forward with the treatment based on their perceptions of the dentist. If those impressions are negative, patients will turn down the treatment. They judge everything, including hair, nails, clothing, and posture. A neat, professional appearance is mandatory for every member of the team.

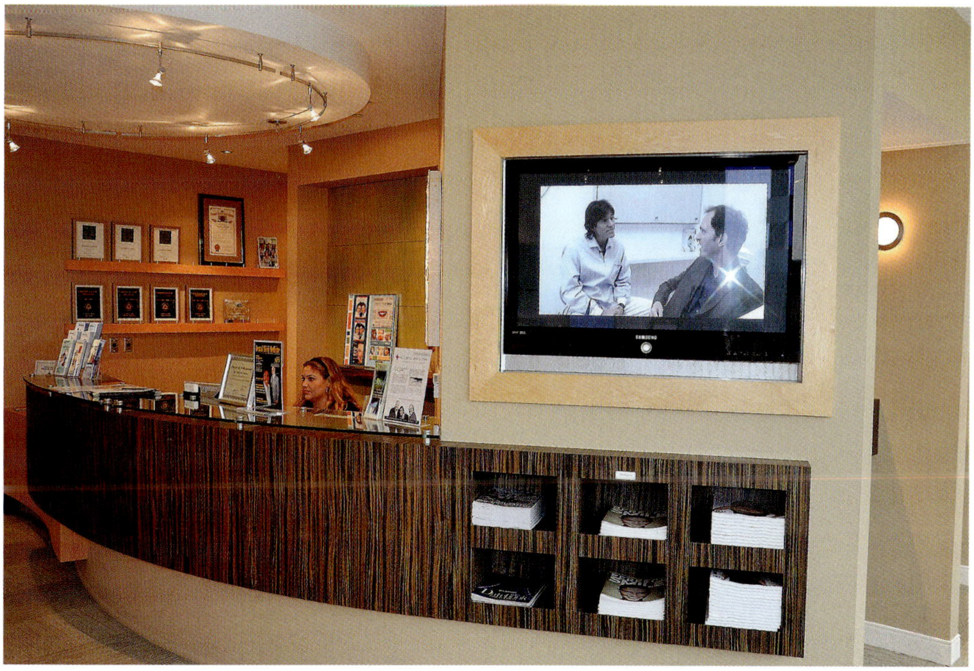

Figure 5.1 **(C)** For your reception area, in addition to news or entertainment videos, consider more personal educational programs with you as the teacher.

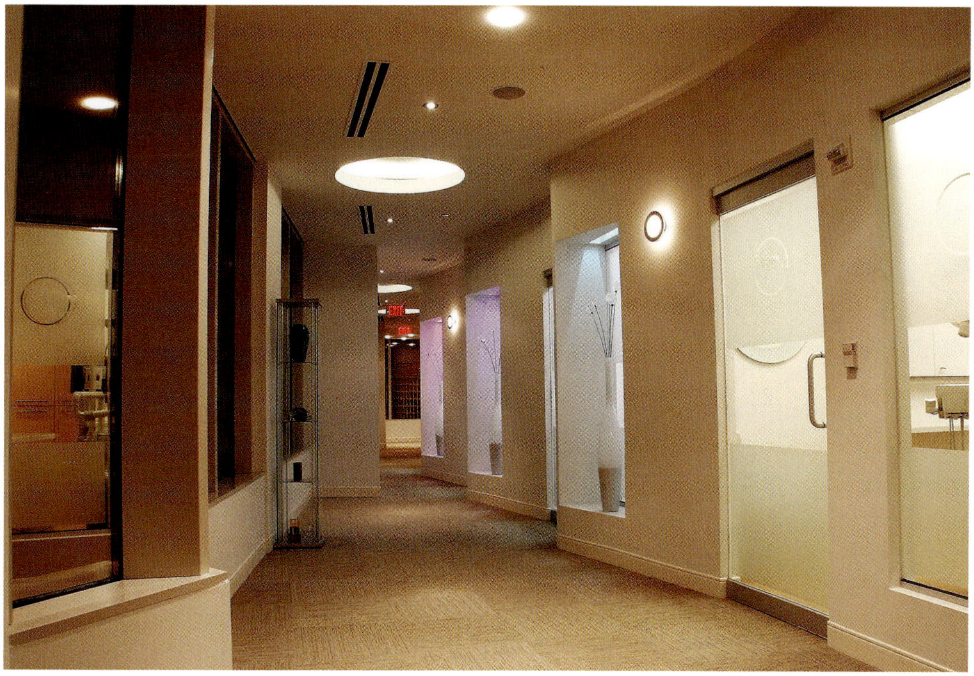

Figure 5.1 **(D)** Whenever possible, the entrance to patient treatment rooms should also be an attractive, pleasing, and comforting experience.

Customer service

Superior customer service occurs when every single process and system have been designed with one purpose in mind—to exceed patient expectations at every step of the way. This means that every team member has been trained with appropriate scripting, coaching, and mentoring to "wow" patients during their appointments, to create value for all practice services and procedures, and to view every interaction as an opportunity to build and strengthen a long-term practice–patient relationship.

Excellent customer service is the cornerstone of effective internal marketing. Patients love to be seen promptly, have their questions answered courteously and enthusiastically, and be treated like VIPs. Surpassing patient expectations can be difficult, but achieving the wow factor leaves an impression that stays with patients for a long time. By providing superior customer

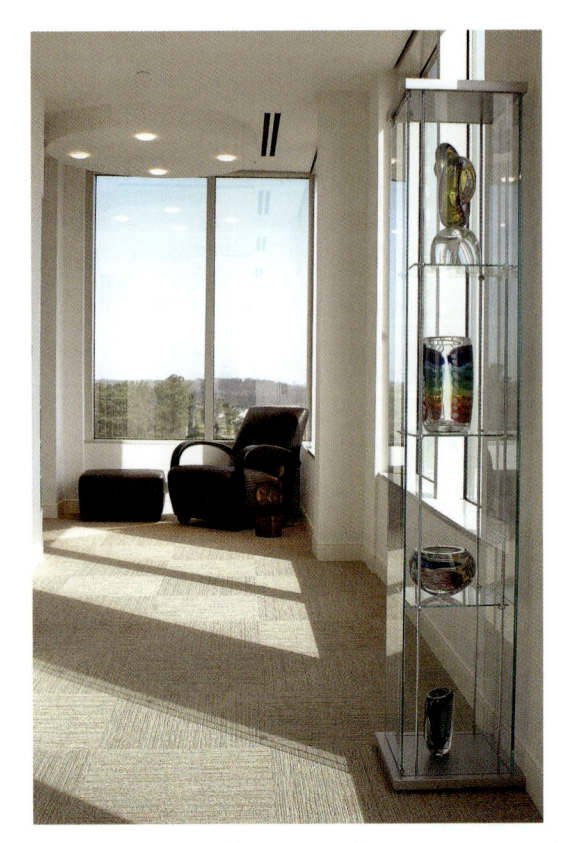

Figure 5.1 **(E)** This dental office uses art glass so patients can relate to the doctors' esthetic taste.

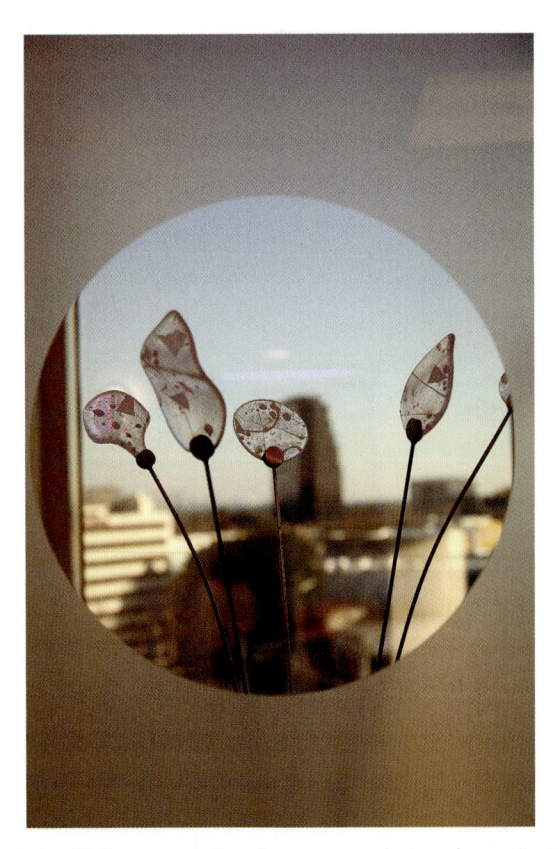

Figure 5.1 **(F)** Custom art glass flowers were designed so patients sitting in the dental chair can see the different colored petals.

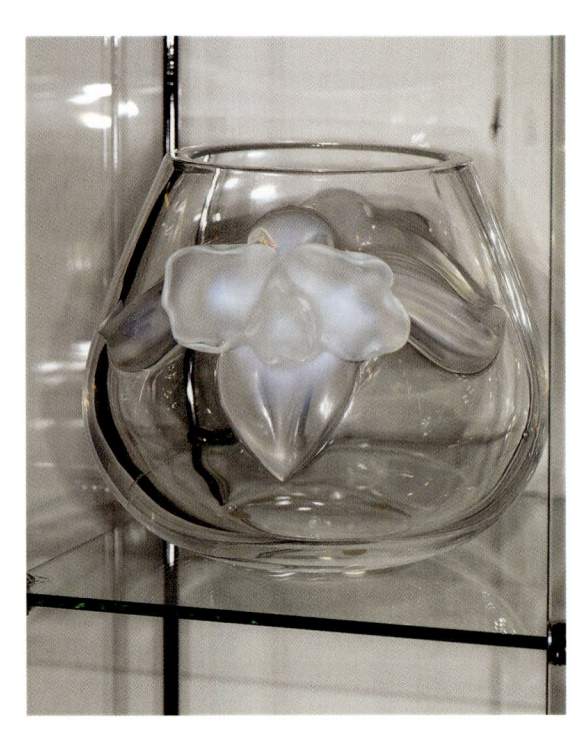

Figure 5.1 **(G)** This unique Lalique crystal bowl has a double meaning. In addition to its beauty, the fluorescence in this bowl can help patients visualize the artistry and fluorescence that will be used in creating their ceramic restorations.

service, dentists will motivate more patients to recommend their practice, which leads to more new patients and increased production (Figure 5.3A).

What are some essential features of customer service that can be applied to every patient? The following factors can help practices achieve outstanding customer service:

- All patients should be greeted enthusiastically as they enter the office. A clear script should be used to welcome patients. The scheduling coordinator should let patients know how delighted the practice is to see them.

- Make beverages available to patients. Coffee, tea, and bottled water create a warm, home-like environment. People are more comfortable when they feel that their needs are being met. A comfortable patient is more likely to be open-minded, interested in what the dentist has to say, and more willing to consider different options (Figure 5.3B).

- Patients should be escorted everywhere in the office. Each team member who comes in contact with patients has a *moment of truth*—a point of contact that should always be used to enhance the practice–patient relationship. Say hello, smile, ask a personal question, and escort patients when the opportunity exists and thank them for visiting the office.

- Smiling is critical for practices determined to expand their cosmetic production. A smile conveys to the patient that the practice is glad to see them. Due to the pace of today's dental practices, dentists and team members can sometimes forget to smile. Remember, nothing welcomes patients as much as a smiling face.

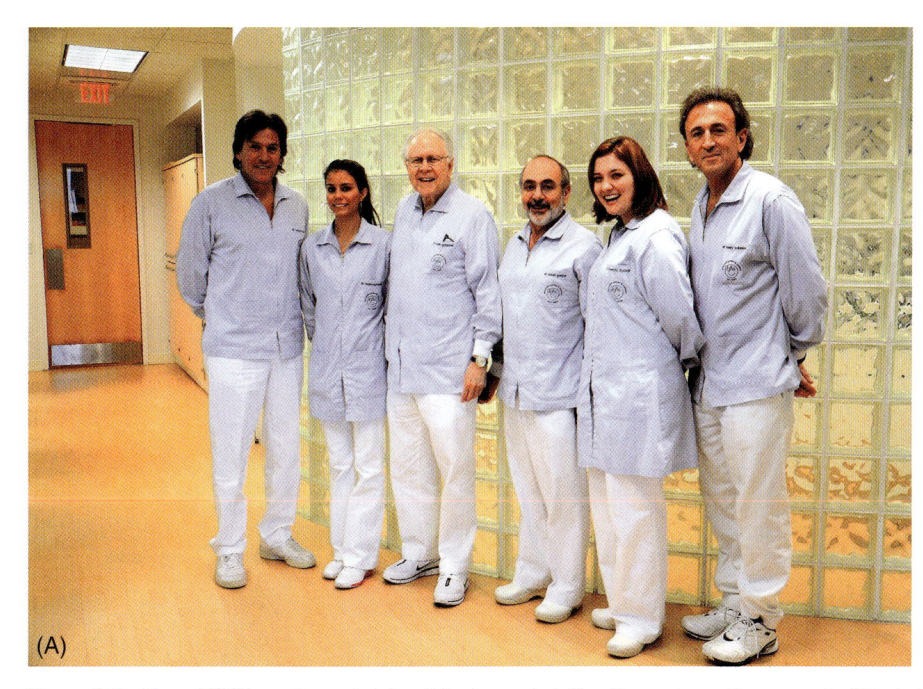

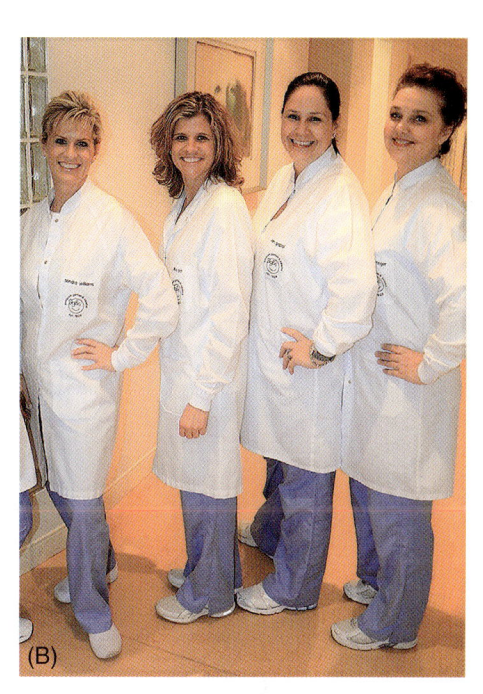

Figure 5.2 **(A and B)** The color and style of doctor and staff uniforms is another aspect of the total office image. (A and B) Two examples of physician's uniforms and staff uniforms

- Every time a patient visits the practice, learn at least one new thing about them. It is important that this type of information be kept in their files, so it can be referred to before the next visit. This enables the dentist and the team to strike up a conversation in a more personal way.
- Compliment patients. Who doesn't love to receive compliments? If the team is trained to provide superior customer service, they will put smiles on patients' faces and brighten their day. People like to go to a place where they are treated courteously in a positive, welcoming environment.
- Thank every patient for visiting the office. The doctor, assistant or hygienist, and front desk staff should always end conversations by thanking the patient. Let the person know that he or she is appreciated. This results in patients feeling extremely positive about the office and looking forward to their return visits.

Patient education

Practices should use a variety of patient education tools to emphasize the benefits of cosmetic dentistry, including:

- cosmetic brochures
- posters
- before-and-after photographs and digital software
- newsletters, e-newsletters, and website updates
- patient testimonials

These devices demonstrate to patients the practice's commitment to cosmetic dentistry. Even more than simple awareness, such tools define the practice as a center for cosmetic dentistry where patients can expect to receive professional,

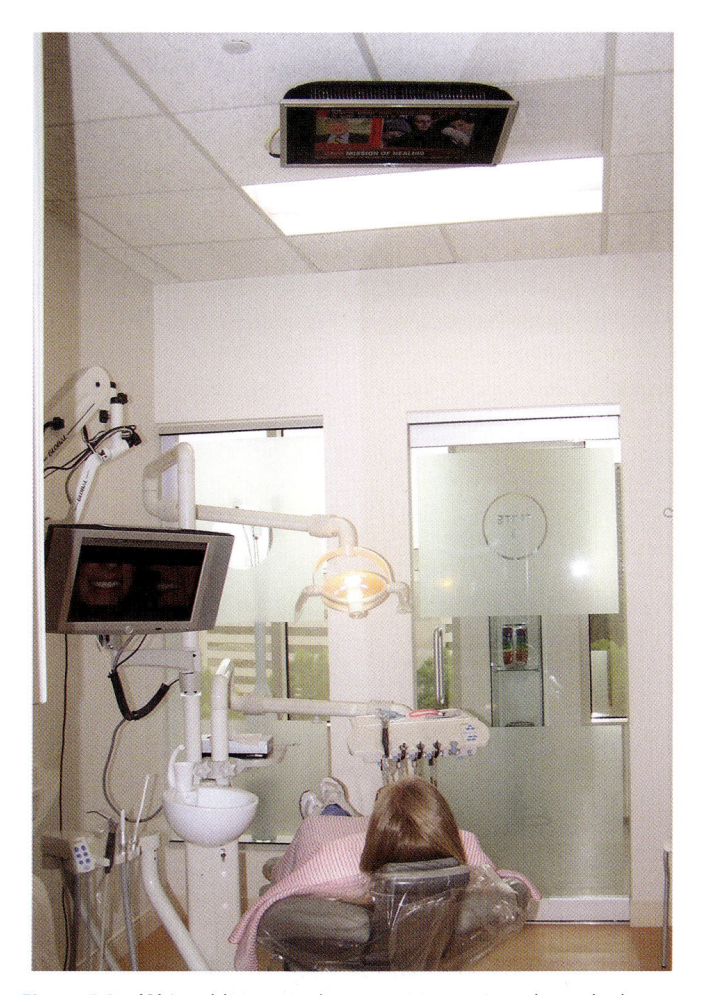

Figure 5.3 **(A)** In addition to other amenities, patients have the luxury of watching their favorite program on the ceiling HD television, both while waiting and during treatment.

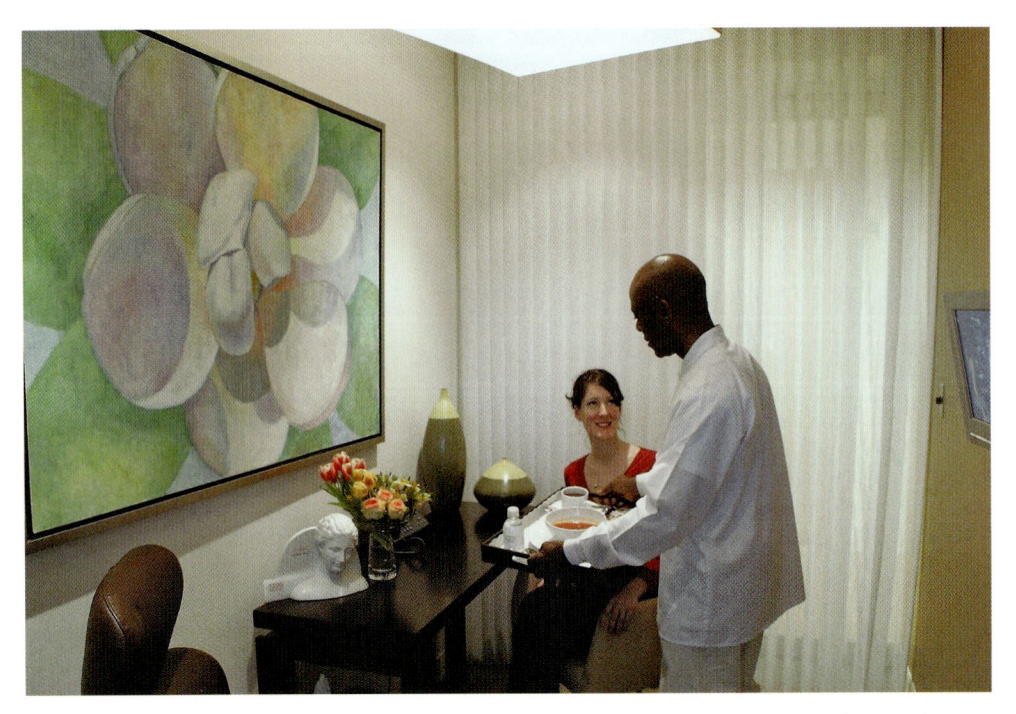

Figure 5.3 (B) This office has a comfort room for patients who have extended treatment visits. While waiting for the laboratory to complete her restorations, this patient is being served lunch by one of the office's most valuable team members.

state-of-the-art care. Many patients still do not think of their dentist as a cosmetic dentist. Fortunately, every dentist has the power to change that perception. In today's world, where consumers are becoming more aware of health and beauty options, practices can take advantage of this growing trend. Many current patients would be interested in smile enhancement if—and only if—they become aware that these services are offered. When offices combine a strong practice culture, along with excellent patient education tools, the practice is on the road to developing a powerful brand. However, efforts at patient education can fall flat if patients don't experience a high level of customer service from team members (Figure 5.4A).

Patient education is critical to gaining the case acceptance needed to increase cosmetic procedures performed in the practice. However, unlike need-based dentistry, where patients are often in pain and accept treatment as a way to relieve that pain, patient education for esthetic services is a much more comprehensive process (Figure 5.4B).

The more informed patients are of the services offered, the greater the opportunities for increasing case acceptance. Many practices have also incorporated a program of giving their new patients copies of the consumer book *Change Your Smile*[1] not only to educate the patient but also to encourage more referrals.

Case presentation

Accepting treatment for esthetic dentistry is usually much more of an emotional decision than other types of traditional services. Patients will not make a decision to accept a cosmetic case based on need—they are not usually experiencing pain—but rather on the emotional feelings they get when thinking of how much better they will look and feel after a cosmetic procedure is performed. It is more of a heartfelt decision on the patient's part.

The dentist's job is not to be overwhelmingly clinical during case presentation, but rather emphasize the many emotional benefits the cosmetic procedure provides. Taking time to tell patients how good they will look and feel about their smile is an effective way to increase case acceptance. Most patients are willing to learn all the ways their smile can be enhanced, especially since many patients are completely unaware of all the options available now. Motivated patients will find a way to pay the fee involved for the procedure, if the value and benefits are clearly explained. This type of presentation creates greater case acceptance that ultimately leads to increased practice profitability (Figure 5.5A). The key to showing patients the benefits of cosmetic dentistry begins with a case presentation that is both motivating and exciting. Patients want to see themselves transformed. Begin a conversation about cosmetic dentistry by asking patients questions such as:

- Are you happy with your smile?
- Is there anything about your smile that you don't like?
- Have you ever thought about whitening?
- Do you know you could have a smile like this? (Use appropriate visual aid here.)

These "conversation starters" are a great way to get patients to think about cosmetic dentistry. In addition, you may wish to consider offering a complimentary cosmetic exam to attract new patients. During the cosmetic exam, each anterior tooth should be scored against a shade guide. Patients are given an understanding of the shade guide in advance and then scored, so that they know exactly what their shade is versus what it *could* be.

There has been a shift in the consciousness of Americans based on the hundreds of millions of dollars spent on television

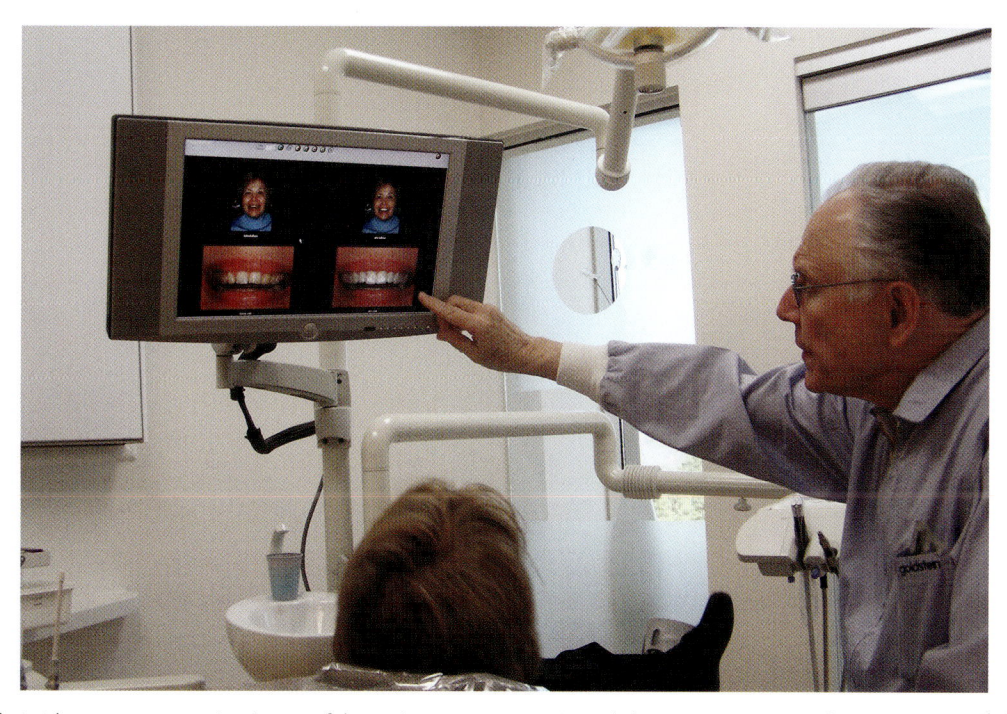

Figure 5.4 **(A)** A chairside computer monitor is one of the easiest ways to consistently keep your patients informed. It is also helpful for demonstrating both intra- and extra-oral pictures to your patients throughout their treatment.

advertising for over-the-counter whitening products and the success of "makeover" reality shows. The message is out—you can't have a beautiful face without a beautiful smile. The result of this heightened consciousness is that more Americans are interested in cosmetic dentistry. Why wait for patients to raise the issue of cosmetic dentistry? Offering a complimentary cosmetic exam opens a dialogue with patients. Many will be unaware of all the different types of elective services currently available. By educating patients about their current cosmetic condition against the standard of a shade guide, practices create a sense of comparison for patients, which often leads to diagnosis and the presentation of treatment options (Figure 5.5B).

Cosmetic dentistry has the power to transform not only smiles but lives. And that is something most patients will be excited about, if the message is presented in the right way.

Patient referrals

One of the strongest internal marketing strategies is to actually ask patients for referrals. The staff interacts with patients at every step of the treatment process, with countless opportunities to encourage referrals. Training the dental team to ask for referrals can lead to a dramatic increase in new patients. Scripting will help the staff consistently deliver a strong marketing message. When patients remark how pleased they are with the practice, team members should be trained to respond appropriately. For instance, the script could direct staff to thank patients at the end of treatment and say, "We love having patients like you. Please tell your friends about us." Patients are often thrilled to refer their friends and family. Anyone who refers a patient should receive a personal thank-you call from the dentist and the office manager. At their next appointment, referring patients should receive a

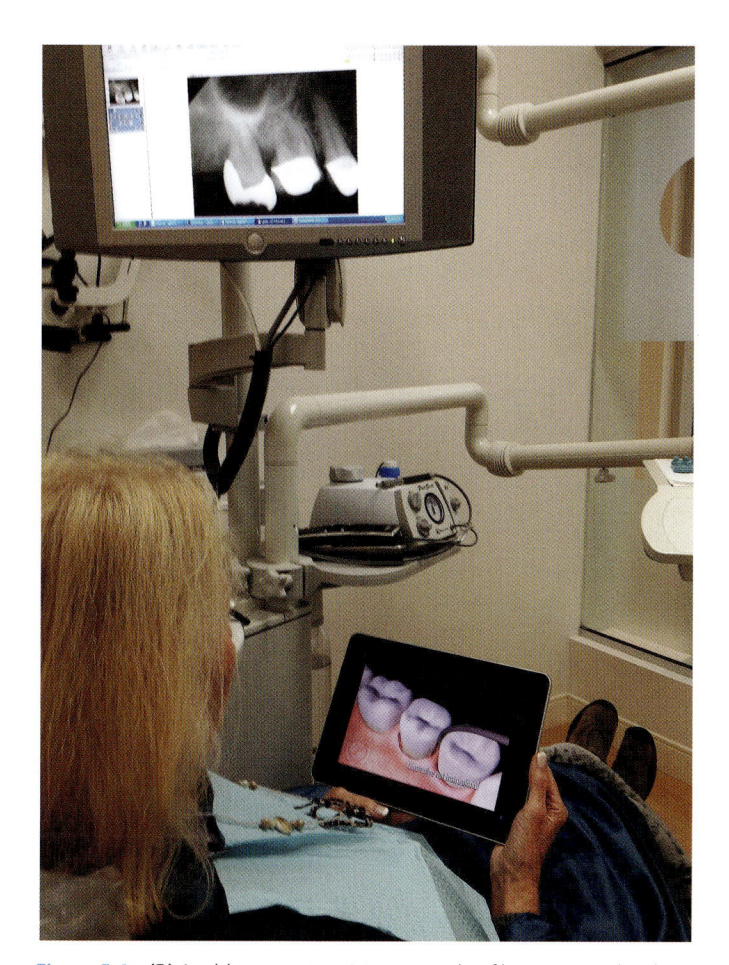

Figure 5.4 **(B)** A tablet computer is an example of how new technology can be used to easily educate your patients while in the chair. This patient is viewing a video of a proposed laser-assisted new attachment procedure (LANAP) to help better understand the treatment.

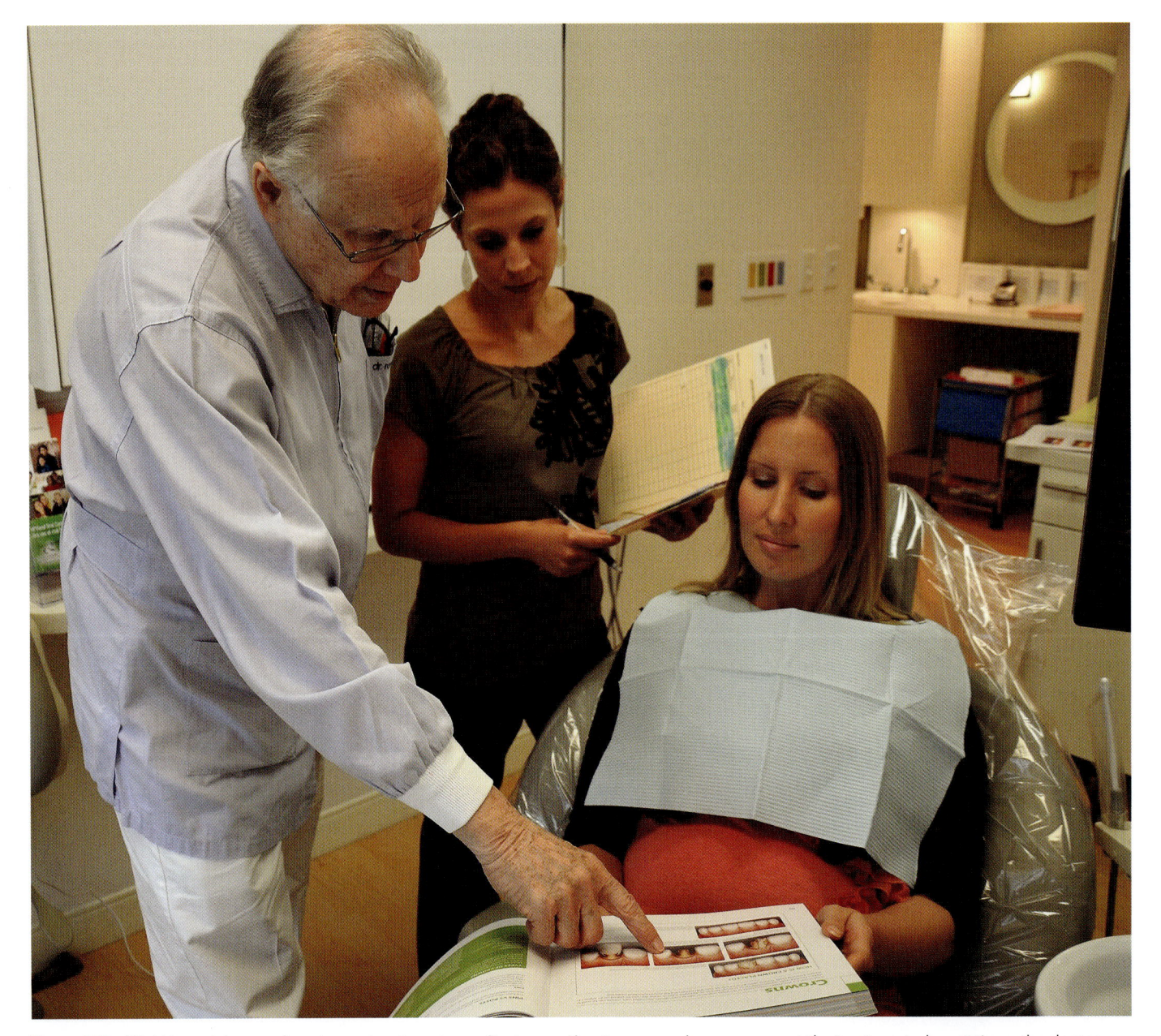

Figure 5.5 **(A)** Although in most instances a treatment coordinator or other team member can present the treatment plan, at times the doctor may be called upon for more detailed explanation.

thank you from at least four staff members, including front desk personnel, the assistant, the hygienist, and the doctor. Recognition and appreciation are very meaningful to all patients. To increase patient awareness, make sure the office displays signs that say, "we appreciate referrals," or "the greatest compliment you can pay our practice is to send a friend or refer a friend." If signs aren't obvious and the scripting isn't effective, people will not likely think of referring others to the practice (Figure 5.6A and B).

Patient communication

When patients refer their friends, these potential new patients will want to find out more information about the practice. That means having a professional, state-of-the-art website where people can learn more about the practice, the services offered, and the doctor's professional background. The website should be easy to navigate and highlight the quality care provided to patients, including a full list of cosmetic services.

What is external marketing?

With external marketing, the practice is communicating with people outside of the office who may not be familiar with the practice. Therein lies the challenge. The main goals of external marketing are to

- create awareness
- build a positive reputation
- attract new patients.

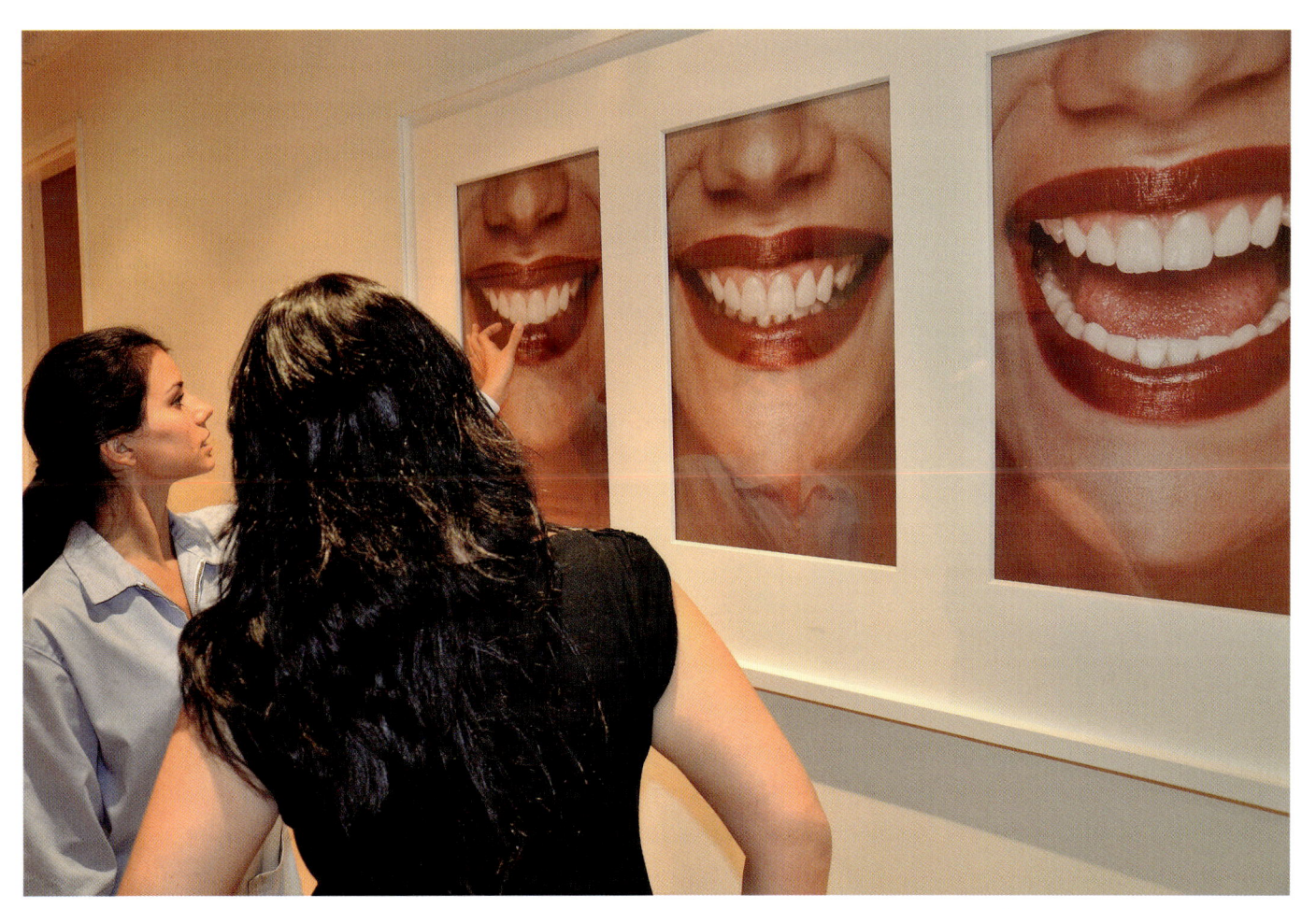

Figure 5.5 **(B)** Internal marketing should always be considered when planning for office décor. These colorful photographs from a renowned Brazilian photographer and artist help to show the ingredients of a beautiful smile. Reproduced with permission of Dudú Medeiros.

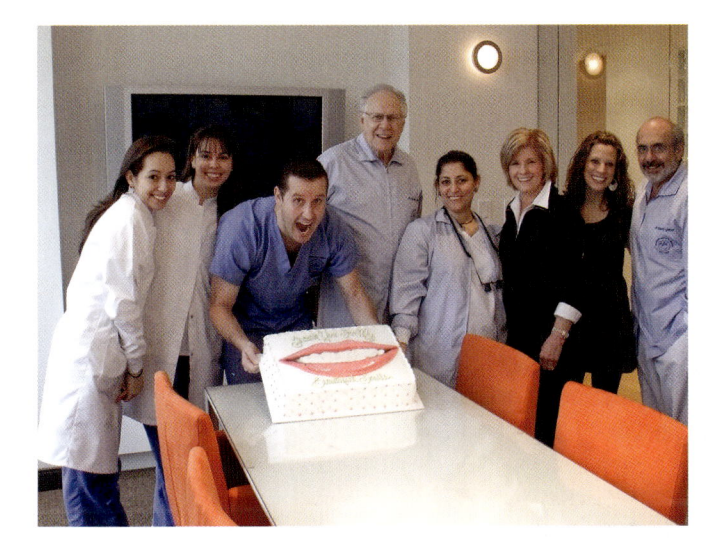

Figure 5.6 **(A)** The ultimate success of any marketing program is satisfied patients who are willing to refer their family and friends. This cake presented to the dental team is evidence of that satisfaction.

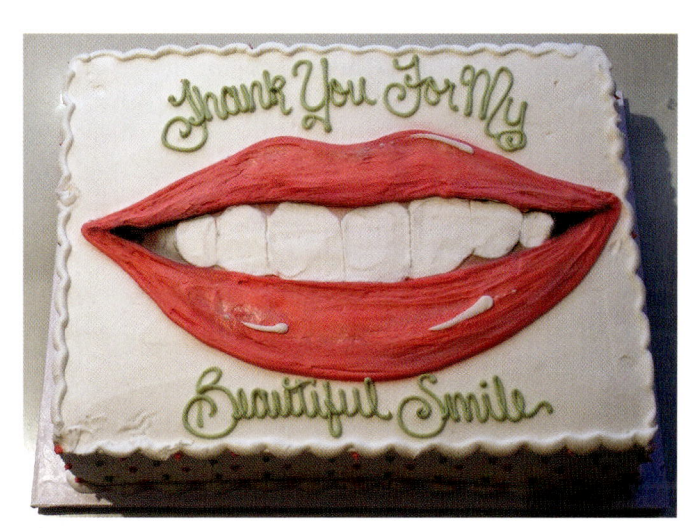

Figure 5.6 **(B)** The design of the cake was the creation of the patient.

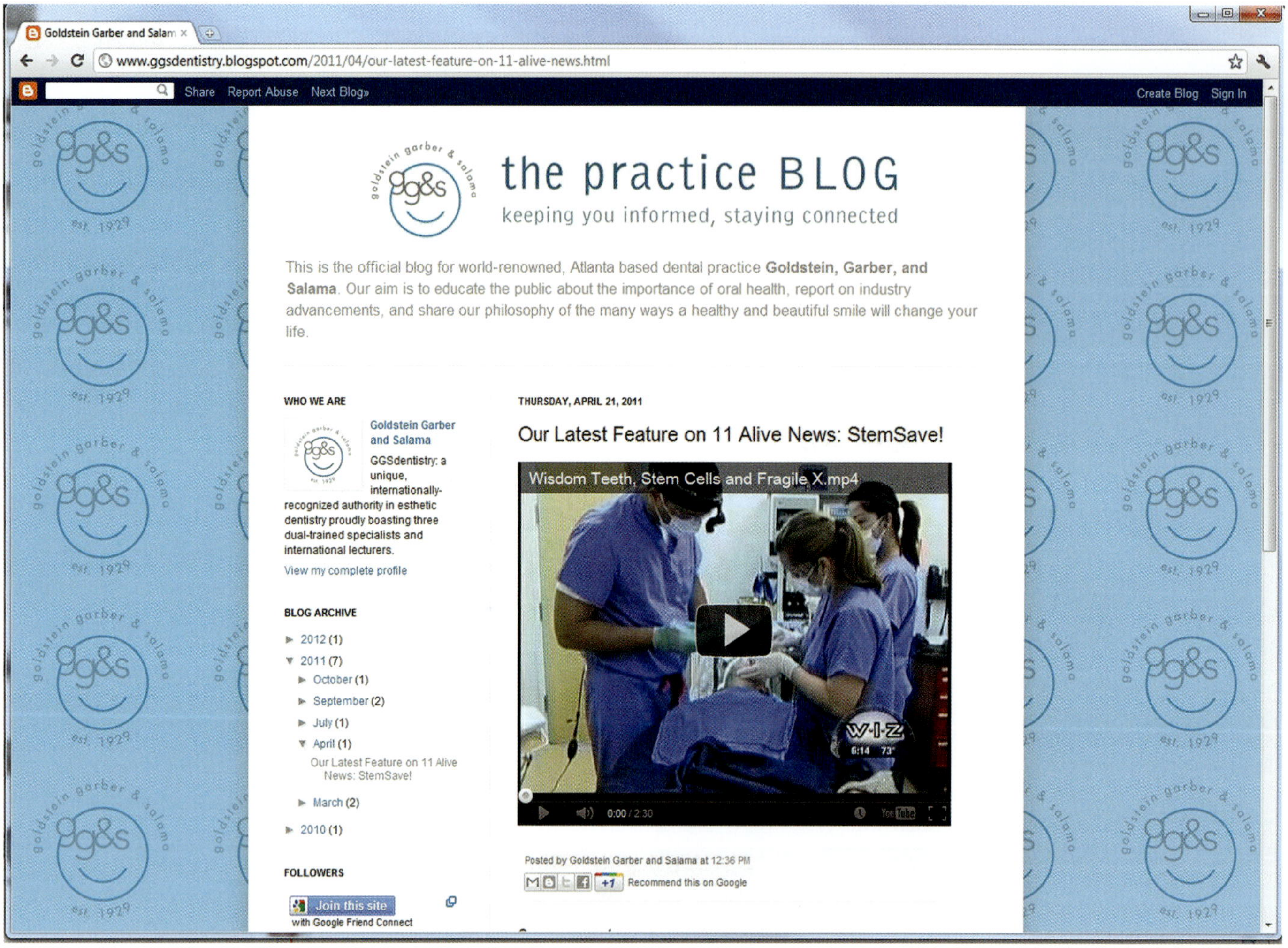

Figure 5.7 **(A)** A good example of external and internal marketing is seen in this blog which was a website posting of a news clip of the practice's work with StemSave.

The two main forms of external marketing are advertising (e.g., newspaper ads, or online) and public relations. Advertising, whether in print, on the web, or by other media, can be more expensive than other forms of marketing. Of course, having a quality website is one of the most effective forms of external marketing. The practice's website is the place that new patients and potential patients will first visit. They will want to see what kinds of services are offered, where the practice is located, what patients are saying about the office, and so forth.

Public relations focuses on building the practice's reputation in the area through activities such as working with schools and local nonprofit groups. Many dentists allow tours of their offices, give presentations on good oral health at schools, and sponsor local sports teams. Some dentists write a weekly or monthly column on oral health matters for the community newspaper. Positive outreach builds goodwill with local residents and businesses. Remember, marketing—both internal and external—should be reflective of the practice's brand and image in the community (Figure 5.7A and B). A good internal marketing program will help drive external marketing success. To reach the highest levels of success, marketing must be consistent and ongoing. A hit-or-miss approach will usually lead to haphazard results. Successful practices use a variety of approaches to retain current patients and attract new patients.

External marketing strategies

How do practices attract more new patients? How much should offices invest in external marketing? What strategies—direct mail, telephone directory ads, websites, radio and television advertising, and billboards—will yield the best results? The answer is that it depends on the practice goals, budget, current patient base, location, and other factors such as demographics of the target market. External marketing, when developed as a part of an overall marketing plan, can be extremely effective. However, many external marketing efforts should be approached with caution because they can be costly and fail to generate the desired results. Yet, some newer developments in external marketing, such as social media, offer promising results for a minimal expense.

What should be the focus of community marketing and advertising campaigns? Clearly, conveying the competitive edge

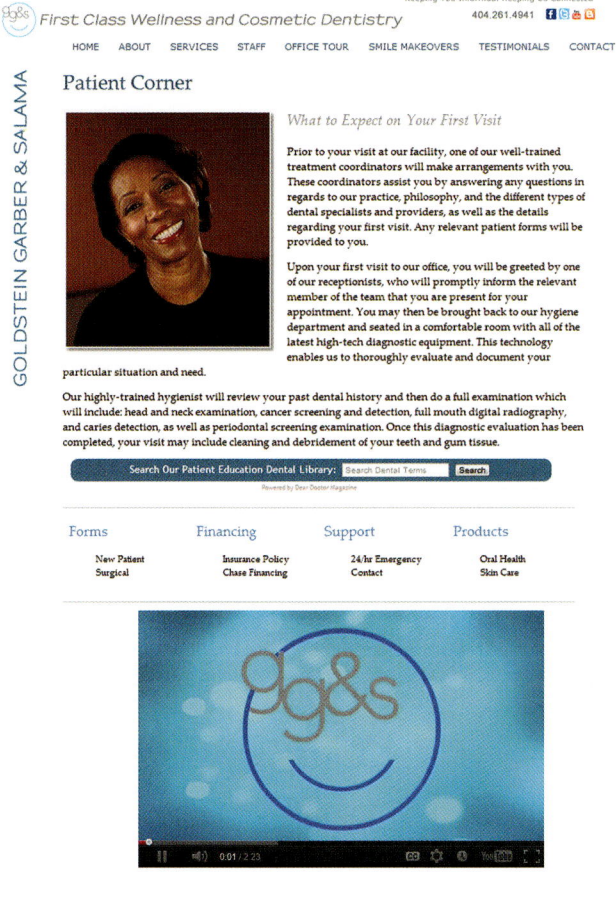

Figure 5.7 (B) The website should be easy to navigate and have a section for new patients and what they can expect on their first visit.

of the practice should be the primary message. There is a greater chance for positive feedback by including information about advanced technology and unique services. As a rule, advertising focused on specific esthetic services and the associated benefits is usually far more powerful than announcement-style advertising. Patients are frequently attracted by the services mentioned rather than by general information on the practice itself.

The external marketing strategies to consider include the following:

- Advertising:
  - website
  - telephone and online directories
  - television
  - radio
  - outdoor billboard advertising
  - direct mail
  - magazines/newspapers (Figure 5.8)
  - group discount shopping services.
- Public relations:
  - community relations
  - social media.

Advertising

Website and internet security

Today, your website is the first place where many new patients are introduced to your practice. Websites are a necessity, not a luxury, for most types of businesses. But simply having a website does not mean that the office will automatically derive benefits from it.

Business website design has grown increasingly more intricate and sophisticated and today's users and patients expect a well-designed interactive website. Work with professionals to design and maintain an excellent website. Update it frequently to keep it fresh. What good is a website if people don't come to visit?

The website should be easy to navigate and highlight the quality care provided to patients. It should have a section for new patients that details what they can expect on their first appointment. The website should include the following:

- dentist's biographical sketch including professional background
- what to expect on the first appointment (printable forms, description of the consultation process)
- directions to the office, hours of operation, and contact information
- virtual tour of the office
- services/procedures offered
- before-and-after treatment photos
- e-newsletter sign-up (Figure 5.9)
- contact information.

Many dentists wonder if their practice's website needs all of the latest technical security features. The answer is—absolutely yes! These days, an unsecured website is dangerous for patients, the practice, and possibly other doctors as well. For example, suppose someone hacks a practice's website. The hacker could potentially obtain sensitive patient information such as names, addresses, Social Security numbers, and perhaps even financial information. The hacker might also be able to access correspondence and treatment information that is going back and forth to other practices. Most of this activity is easily stopped through good online security.

Telephone and online directories

Today, people look for products and services much differently than 10 years ago. Although newspaper and magazine ads have their place, newer forms of media such as online directories and ads can have a much greater ability to bring patients to the practice for a lower cost.

Television commercials

Television commercials can make a powerful impression with potential patients. Unfortunately, it is also extremely expensive to produce a commercial and buy air time. Although cable TV can offer lower rates, the time slots available usually deliver fewer viewers. Something to keep in mind with commercials is that

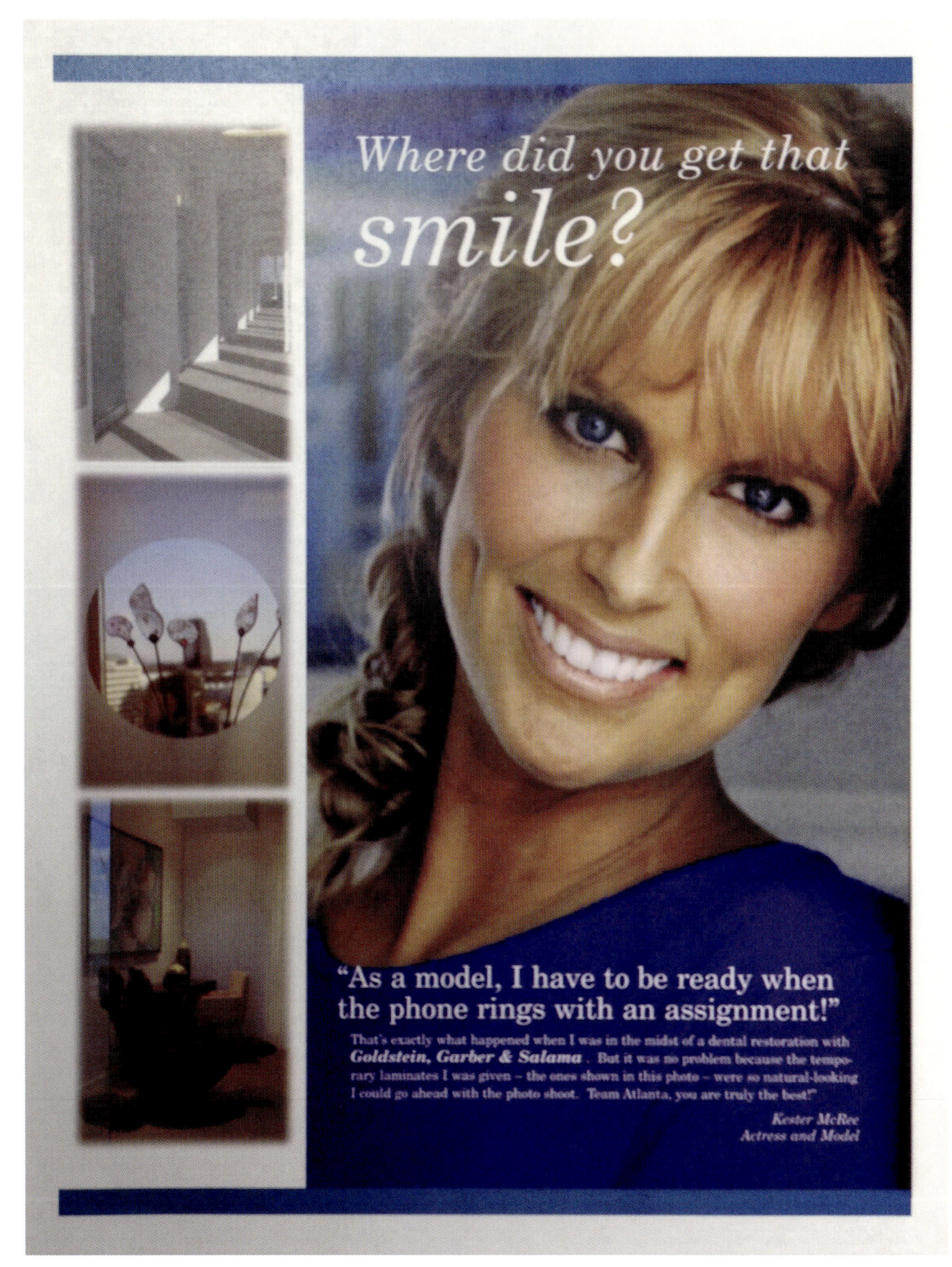

Figure 5.8 Local magazine ads can target marketing to specific geographic areas close to your practice location.

GOLDSTEIN GARBER & SALAMA

We believe in spreading
HOPE + ♥

As cosmetic dentists, our lives revolve around our patients and the joy that their vibrant smiles bring to their lives every day. You've heard about the social effects that having an unattractive smile can have on a person but what about those who are struggling to find a reason to smile at all?

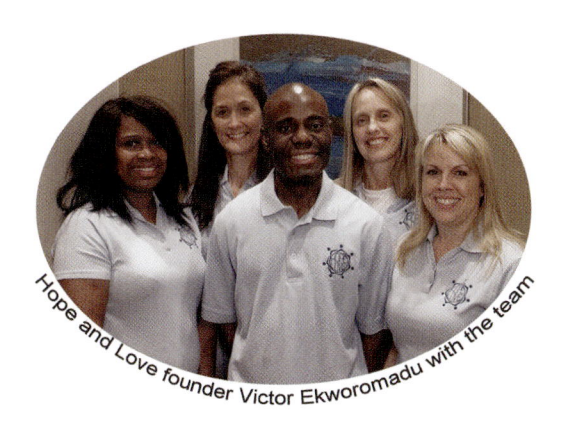

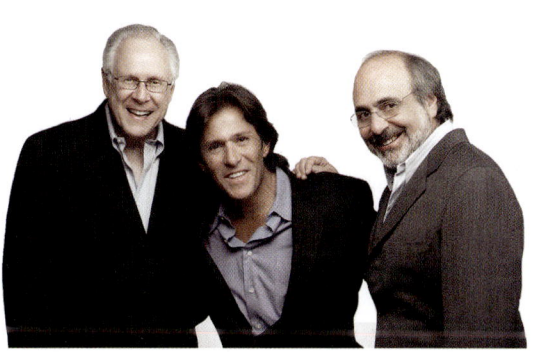

first class wellness and cosmetic dentists

The employees of Atlanta's Goldstein Garber and Salama are active volunteers at Hope and Love for Familes of Georgia, Inc., a non-profit organization founded in 2003 to offer emergency and temporary assistance to needy families that are unable to make ends meet.

As you can imagine, the needs this year are even greater than ever because of the current economic situation. We want to encourage and help these people get back on their feet so they can take care of their families, contribute to society, and be less dependent on the government.

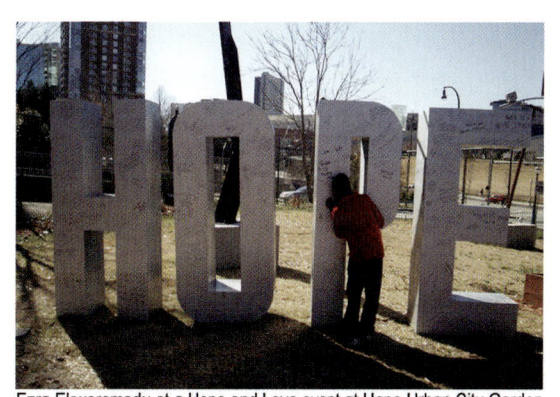

Hope and Love founder Victor Ekworomadu with the team

> *"Success is not truly realized until we reach out and make a difference in the lives of the less fortunate."*

Hope and Love helps families with food, clothing, school supplies, and household itmes, occassionally temporary rent and utilities. If you have made a 2012 resolution to give back or join your community, this is the perfect opportuniy. For more information visit www.hopelove.org or call 770.649.9650.

Ezra Ekworomadu at a Hope and Love event at Hope Urban City Garden

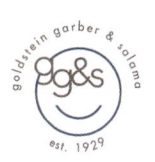

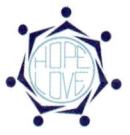

600 Galleria Parkway | Ste 800 | Atlanta, GA 30339 | 404.261.4941 | www.goldsteingarber.com

Figure 5.9 This office newsletter demonstrates that this practice is involved with local charity in the community.

viewers will be able to tell a quality commercial from a poorly produced one. If skilled professionals create it, the quality will show on the screen. Conversely, if the commercial was produced inexpensively, its limited production value will be obvious and could reflect poorly on the practice.

Radio

Although less expensive than television advertising, radio ads are only effective if the right people are listening. Too often, the only attractive rates are for time slots that have few listeners. Usually drive-time hours have many listeners but costs can be prohibitive. Keep in mind that radio is not the powerhouse it once was. With so many outlets for entertainment, far fewer people listen to radio than they did 20 or 30 years ago. The good side of this, however, is that rates can be affordable in many instances.

Outdoor billboard advertising

Billboard advertising has limited effectiveness and can be a significant expense. Only the people who happen to drive by the billboard have the chance of seeing it. Even then—how many will actually notice it? Unless the practice has created an extraordinary ad that will captivate drivers and passersby, outdoor advertising may not be the best choice of where to put the office's marketing efforts.

Direct mail

Direct mail can be effective. One study found that 66% of direct mail is opened, 82% is read for a minute or more. Further, 56% of people who responded to direct mail went online or visited the physical store and 62% who responded made a purchase. Some 84% or more said that personalization made them more likely to open direct mail.[5] Although the web continues to chip away at direct mail, these statistics show that it is far from dead. One thing to keep in mind about direct mail advertising is that a 2% open rate is considered very successful. That means most direct mail goes unread. However, that shouldn't dissuade a practice from using direct mail. There are times when direct mail is a good way to reach patients. As with any published work, make certain that what the practice sends out is professionally designed and written. The effectiveness of direct mail will be blunted by spelling mistakes or amateurishly designed pieces. When the practice is ready to mail its piece, the office should purchase an up-to-date mailing list to reach its targeted audience, whether it is by age, income, zip code, or other parameters.

Online group discount shopping services

In the past few years, we have seen an influx of online group discount shopping services such as Groupon and Living Social. Dental practices who sign up with these online shopping sites offer discounted services to attract new patients. If enough people sign up for the deal, the deal is on. The dental practice shares the revenue with the discount shopping service. The hope is that these bargain hunters will become active patients. Indicators show that the results are mixed. It is too early to conclude the true effectiveness of this type of marketing. A number of practices have found that people coming to the practice through one of these deals are only coming for their one-time discounted service. Some practices have successfully "wowed" the bargain hunter and retained them as a patient.

When considering whether to try offering this type of deal, determine whether your practice can schedule all the people who bought your deal in a timely fashion without undermining the customer service you provide to existing patients. Keep in mind that those who visit the practice with coupons in hand may be sitting in the waiting room with your patients. If they engage in a discussion, are you comfortable with your patient knowing he/she is paying substantially less for the same service? It is also important to make sure that engaging in a deal with a group shopping discount service does not violate the ethics code of your state dental association.

Public relations

Community relations

Many practices make the mistake of dashing off a "press release" to the local newspaper and expecting it to just show up in print. In truth, newspapers are deluged with press releases that are often nothing more than advertisements. A majority of the time, any press release sent to a newspaper is quickly discarded. To stand a chance of being printed, press releases should be newsworthy and should not contain language straight out of a practice's brochure.

An even better approach to getting public relations (PR) would be writing for the local community newspaper. Many smaller papers are looking for interesting content from local business people. Writing a short monthly column on oral health care for either the print or online version of a local publication is an excellent way to build the practice's brand and position the office as the leading dental care provider in the area. Another suggestion is to appear on a local radio or TV station as an oral health expert when the need arises. Getting involved in your community is also an excellent PR strategy. Sponsoring recreation league and high school teams, participating in community health fairs, and speaking at area schools are a few examples of building a strong reputation as a caring member of the community (Figure 5.9).

Social media

More and more businesses are using social media, such as Facebook, YouTube, Twitter, and LinkedIn, to strengthen customer relationships and generate customer loyalty. Social media has emerged as another powerful tool to reach current and potential patients, but that does not make it an appropriate marketing channel for all dental practices. Social media can be

---

[5] Forbes. Available at: https://www.forbes.com/sites/forbesagencycouncil/2017/01/10/five-ways-to-spice-up-your-direct-mail-marketing-in-2017/#5c1592f34d3e.

an incredibly useful method to reach patients, but it has to be evaluated to determine its effectiveness. Survey your patients to find out if they use social media and how often they do so. Practices that decide to utilize social media platforms should ensure that all of their marketing efforts are integrated and support one another.

If the practice decides to integrate social media in its marketing, there has to be someone in the practice—the office manager, the marketing coordinator, or another team member—to monitor traffic, update content, and respond to questions. This requires a time commitment, but the benefits can be positive in terms of outstanding patient retention.

> Another avenue to consider is search engine ranking—when a "keyword" is typed in, where does your practice rank? Also, looking at positive patient feedback from sites that rate medical practices, many people check the patient reviews before going to a practice.

Reference

1. Goldstein RE. *Change Your Smile*, 4th edn. Chicago, IL: Quintessence; 2009.

Additional resources

ADA Council on Dental Practice. *Your Dental Team as a Marketing Resource*. Chicago, IL: ADA Council on Dental Practice; 1997.

ADA Council on Dental Practice. *The Power of Internal Marketing*. Chicago, IL: ADA Council on Dental Practice; 2004.

Berkowitz EN. *Essentials of Healthcare Marketing*. Burlington, MA: Jones & Bartlett Publishers; 1996.

Dzierzak J. The cosmetic practice: building from the ground up. *J Colo Dent Assoc* 1993;72(1):11–13.

Leebov W. *Customer Service for Professionals in Health Care*. Bloomington, IN: iUniverse; 2003.

Levin RP. Advanced marketing strategies to build the esthetic dental practice. *Alpha Omegan* 1994;87(4):13–16.

Levin RP. Want to increase cosmetic dentistry? Targeted internal marketing is your secret weapon. *Compendium* 2007;28(12):674–675.

Levin RP. *Dental Practice Marketing—9 Strategies for Internal Marketing*. https://www.dentalcompare.com/Featured-Articles/1863-9-Strategies-for-Internal-Marketing/ (accessed October 4, 2017).

Orent T. *10 Secrets to a Cosmetic Practice Explosion*. Framingham, MA: Gems Publishing; 1998.

Rooney K. Consumer-driven healthcare marketing: using the web to get up close and personal. *J Healthc Manag* 2009;54:241–251.

Swerdlick M. *Prime Positioning*. American Marketing Association; September 1, 2007.

Overcontouring of crowns

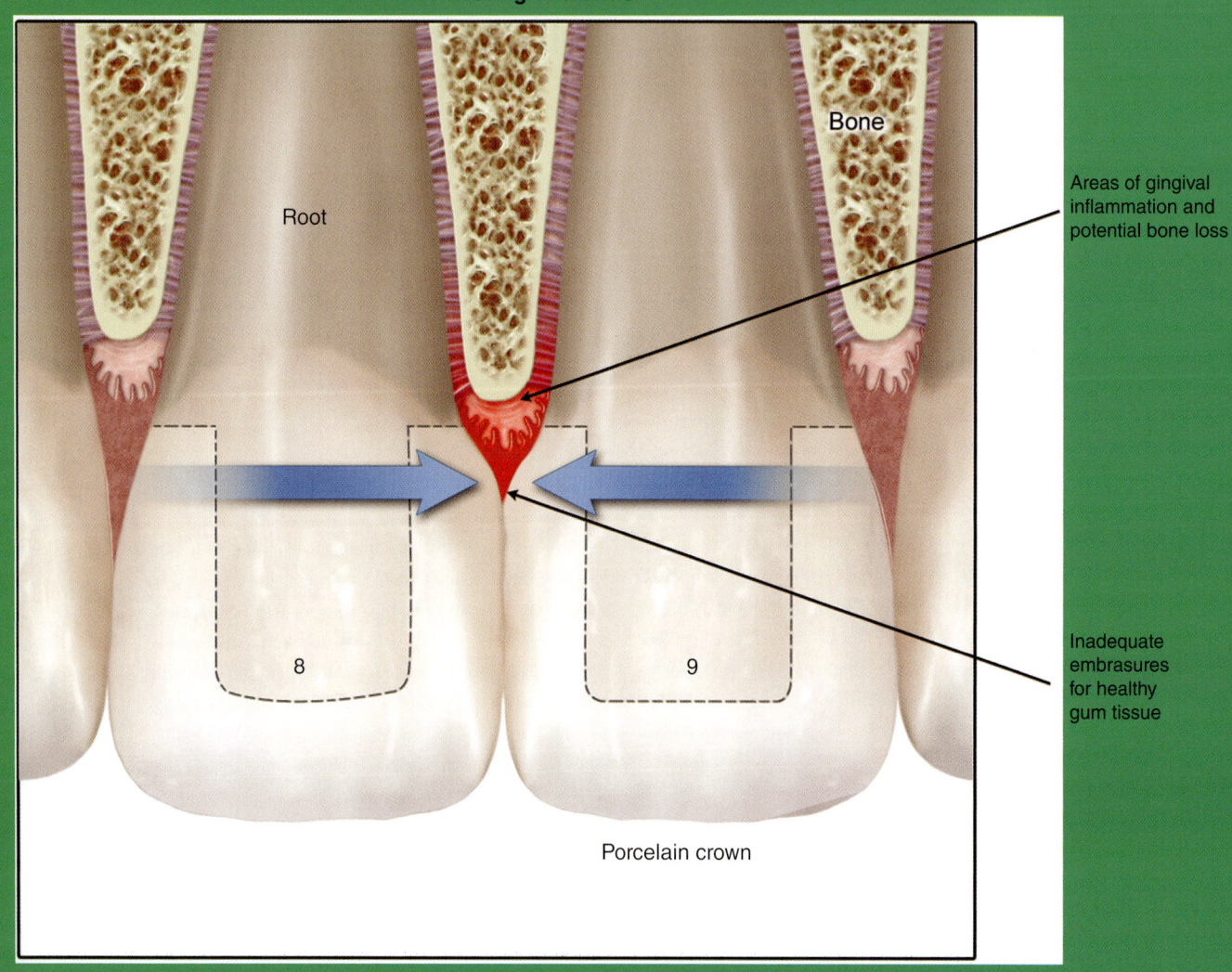

Root

Bone

Areas of gingival inflammation and potential bone loss

Inadequate embrasures for healthy gum tissue

8　9

Porcelain crown

Chapter 6 Legal Considerations

Edwin J. Zinman, DDS, JD

Chapter Outline

Dentist's legal obligation to update skills and practices	132	Orthodontic root resorption	144
Informed consent	132	Misinformed consent	144
Disclosure of potential risks and complications	132	Who has responsibility for informed consent?	144
Disclosure of alternative treatments	132	Patient's right of privacy and confidentiality	145
Patient's commitment to follow-up care	133	Doctor–patient relationship	145
Consent forms and signatures	133	Nonconsent or consent for less invasive procedures	145
Negligent customary practice	133	Dentist's right to refuse treatment	145
Guarantee or warranty	137	Patient abandonment claims	145
Patient esthetic perceptions	137	Right of a patient to choose a dentist	146
"I'm sorry" legal protection	138	Refunds	147
Prognosis and longevity	138	Examples of esthetic malpractice cases	147
Try-in appointment	138	Case 1: overcontoured crowns	147
Complete dental records and documentation	139	Case 2: overbuilt laminates	148
Chart documentation	141	Case 3: external root resorption with bleaching	148
Electronic records	142	Case 4: excessive laser sculpting	149
Complete dental records	142	Telephone or e-mail consultation	150
Standards of care versus reasonable patient standards	143	Federal requirements and product warnings	150
Nonnegligent risks and obligations to treat	144	Botox	151
Bleaching precautions	144	Jury trials	151

Although it would be helpful to be able to identify a suit-prone patient and refuse treatment, this is not the reality. It is this author's experience that virtually all plaintiffs in dental negligence litigation have not previously sued a health-care professional or anyone else. Consequently, the best means to avoid malpractice suits is to adhere to the basic principles of quality care and to communicate realistic expectations to the patient. A dentist's ethical[1] and legal obligation is to always protect the patient's best interest.[2] Tort laws with potential threat of litigation spur dentists to practice safely.

To prove malpractice, a plaintiff patient must first establish the applicable standard of care. Second, the patient must prove that the defendant dentist violated this standard of care with resultant damages or injury. In a malpractice suit, each side presents expert testimony. Expert witnesses may rely on and/or consider external evidence of the standard of care, such as clinical practice guidelines which the various dental specialties or dental organizations promulgate.[3-5]

Dentist's legal obligation to update skills and practices

Dentists have a legal obligation to remain current through continuing education and update their armamentarium with currently accepted or proven technological advances. It might be said that a practicing dentist who graduated 20 years ago but failed to take continuing education courses possesses 1 year's experience repeated 20 times. Advances in adhesive chemistry and resin technology have expanded esthetic dentistry capabilities. Composite restorations have become an accepted material for Class III, IV, and V restorations in anterior teeth but remain questionable as a standard restoration for occlusal and proximal areas of posterior teeth with strong occlusal loading.[6] Conservative restoration preparation decreases marginal degradation and fracture associated with composites. Composite restorations are not recommended for molar teeth in which the cavity preparation exceeds two-thirds of the distance between the buccal and lingual cusps.

New high-tech devices such as Diagnodent (Kavo) help the dentist to discover if an occlusal stain is just a stain or caries. If the technology reveals there is a carious lesion present, simply sealing to entomb the decay is advisable or eliminate incipient decay with an air abrasion or burs before sealing; otherwise caries may continue to develop underneath the sealant.[7] Furthermore, if any part of the sealant breaks off or if the bond becomes detached, the caries may develop at a much more rapid rate, leading to endodontic disease.

Informed consent

Dentists have a professional and legal responsibility to provide each patient with sufficient information that enables the patient to make an informed choice decision whether to agree to a proposed treatment that poses significant potential complications. The process of the dentist providing this information and documenting the patient's agreement to the proposed treatment is known as *informed consent*. Informed consent may be oral or written, but a written consent form is more credible to a jury. Written documentation of informed consent also avoids the perils of a conflict between dentist and patient regarding who said what and when.

Any unconsented procedure performed on a patient constitutes battery, which may subject the dentist to punitive damages for unauthorized touching. Consent may be explicit—that is, the patient stating "I accept"—or implied by the patient's tacit approval of the dentist's treatment plan following the dentist's explanation of proposed therapy.

The purpose of informed consent is not simply to satisfy legal requirements, rather the informed consent process should aid the patient to understand why a particular treatment plan is recommended and the essential elements of proposed treatment.

Procedures that pose virtually no risk or significant adverse effects do not require informed consent; for example, repair of a chipped composite in a nonmarginal area. Dentists should not rely on consent obtained by the referring dentist. It is the treating dentist's responsibility to obtain adequate informed consent.

Informed consent, a legal doctrine, requires the dentist to provide adequate disclosure of benefits versus risks of procedures and reasonable alternative therapies.[8,9] This is so the patient is fully advised of the nature of the suggested treatment and inherent nonnegligent potential complications. Although the procedure may be performed with the highest degree of dental practice and care, the dentist may still be found negligent for inadequate disclosure of inherently unavoidable potential risks of treatment, which are known to the dentist but which the lay patient does not know or suspect. Although a patient consents to a treatment, that consent is voidable if their decision was made without adequate information regarding reasonable risks or complications.

Disclosure of potential risks and complications

Informed consent includes advising a patient of the pros and cons of proposed treatment and treatment alternative benefits and risks. It is permissible to inform the patient of the dentist's recommended treatment among various treatment options. Ultimately the patient decides among various proposed treatment options or can refuse all.

The principal potential complications and risk of proposed treatment should be disclosed to the patient. In some states, practitioners are not liable for failing to disclose potential risks or complications if the community practice was to not disclose these risks or complications.[10]

Many courts reject the proposition that the scope of disclosure obligations is determined exclusively by community practice. Instead, a patient has a right to be informed of available options and the complications of each option, regardless of community disclosure practices.[9]

This "objective" standard has been adopted in a majority of states in the United States.[11-15] In these states, a court will determine whether a particular disclosure should have been made based on the court's own assessment of whether the information might have affected the patient's willingness to undergo the procedure. Sufficient information to allow an informed choice must be disclosed. However, disclosure of an extremely remote risk is not required. It is not required to give a lengthy discourse on all conceivable complications if the potential is very remote. When in doubt, a dentist should disclose a particular treatment risk. Consent to negligent care is legally voidable.[16]

Disclosure of alternative treatments

Disclosure should be made of alternative procedures and likely results of these alternative procedures. Reasonable alternative procedures should be disclosed even if the dentist does not perform them. The patient should understand why the dentist has recommended a particular treatment in preference to potential alternatives. For instance, if your patient has crowded teeth but states he or she does not want orthodontic treatment, you are still obligated to state the reasons that orthodontic treatment would be the ideal preferred treatment plan as the best way to correct the malalignment. State the advantages of orthodontic treatment such as less expense over patient's lifetime, less invasive treatment, and likely elimination of root canal risks resulting from esthetic restoration preparations.

A patient should not be asked to consent to negligent care nor should the dentist provide it if the esthetic compromise exceeds the reasonable functional capabilities of restorative materials. Bleaching or bonding vital teeth is an accepted treatment for stained teeth. The esthetic utilizations of porcelain laminates include covering tetracycline staining and recreating physiological contours of teeth.[17]

Failure to offer the alternatives of bonding, bleaching, or porcelain laminates instead of full coverage crowning, if feasible, violates the doctrine of informed consent. This is because complete crowning can result in greater potential endodontic or periodontal complications.[18] Orthodontic option should be provided for diastema closure as an alternative to cosmetic restorations.

To avoid any misunderstanding, the dentist should orally describe to the patient the pros and cons of bonding. Written consent forms are strong evidence that the patient was fully advised and understood the benefits as well as the risks of bonding compared to alternative restorative procedures. In addition to a chart entry that the patient was fully advised by the dentist concerning bonding, Form 6.1 is offered as a suggested informed consent guideline form for bonding.

Informed consent requires disclosure of reasonable alternatives, which necessarily includes less invasive and reduced-risk procedures.[19,20] A reasonable dentist should always attempt to provide thin veneers in enamel. Thick veneers prepared into sensitive dentin risks endodontic complications unless tooth position contraindicates thin or no-prep veneer. Form 6.2 is an informed consent form for alteration of existing restorations. Form 6.3 is an informed consent form for approval of existing restorations.

Patient's commitment to follow-up care

The patient should be clearly advised of required follow-up care. The patient should know what subsequent actions are needed to maximize the likelihood of a successful outcome. Before authorizing a procedure, the patient should commit to performing the "required follow-up care" and acknowledge potential compromised esthetics and durability resulting from inadequate follow-up. Patient should initial the section of the informed consent form regarding the patient's obligation to achieve long-term success.

Consent forms and signatures

The state of the art in esthetic dentistry is constantly changing and improving, thus dentists should consult with a knowledgeable lawyer in their state before adopting an informed consent form. Laws vary from state to state. These forms should be reviewed periodically to assure that they reflect current laws and current practice standards.

Do not simply hand the informed consent form to the patient and ask the patient to sign. Instead, the dentist should explain to the patient in layperson's terms the material on the form. The patient should be encouraged to ask any questions and seek clarification about proposed treatment and alternative treatments. Answers should be given in understandable lay language and explained with diagrams and photos. These photos should be part of the patient's dental record with dates to document when these photos were shown and explanations given. If the patient refuses to listen or read about the possible complications and risks and alternative treatments, stating they "trust the dentist's judgment" this should be clearly noted in the patient's record. The form should note that the patient was offered the opportunity to be advised of the alternatives, benefits, complications (ABCs) but declined to be informed of these options. The patient should sign the consent form with a notation that the *patient refused to participate in the informed consent process*. The patient's signature should be witnessed by at least one person other than the dentist. The executed consent form is an integral part of the patient's record. The patient may initial each paragraph or section of the consent form, but the patient's signature on the document suffices for agreement to the whole document (see Form 6.4).

Informed consent alternatives, benefits, complications (ABCs):

- diagnosis in nontechnical terms
- recommended treatment
- alternative treatment options: clinical condition may require modification of treatment plan
- benefits of treatment (results and patient satisfaction are not guaranteed)
- potential risks and complications
- required follow-up and self-care for successful results.

Negligent customary practice

A negligent custom is not consonant with reasonable and prudent care, which the standard of practice requires. Many negligent customs, although widely practiced, are nonetheless unreasonable and therefore substandard. In other words, average customary care is below the average of reasonable care if it is not reasonable and prudent. Examples include the use of contraindicated cold sterilizing solutions to disinfect instruments[21] and unnecessary exposure of the patient to a higher dose of X-rays because newer types of X-ray, such as digital methods, are not used.[22–25] Other examples include failure to use a rubber dam for nonsurgical endodontics, omission of charting of periodontal pockets, and/or clinical attachment loss. Caries risk assessment should be included in a comprehensive exam to assess the risk of future recurrent caries causing failure, which may otherwise compromise the esthetic durability benefits of new restorations.[26,27]

A majority of dentists do not practice impression disinfection,[28] despite the US Centers for Disease Control and Prevention (CDC) recommendation. In the United States, Occupational Safety and Health Administration (OSHA) guidelines are designed to protect employees from the risk of infection transmissions by instituting controls that prevent contact with

INFORMED CONSENT TO BONDING: BENEFITS AND LIMITATIONS FOR PATIENT INFORMATION

A. <u>Introduction</u>
Bonding pros and cons are discussed in this form, so you may understand and appreciate the benefits as well as the limitations of bonding.

Bonding is a dental procedure which bonds plastic dental restorative materials to your teeth. Plastic bonding may last for several years but is less strong than the more durable or longer lasting restorations such as porcelain laminates or crowns (caps).

Most patients are gratified by the immediate improvement in their smile and appearance, which bonding accomplishes usually without local anesthesia. Initially, tooth surfaces which are to be "bonded" to the plastic material are prepared by etching or roughing the surfaces with a chemical. This is similar to wallpapering by first applying a chemical to prepare the wall before application of the wallpaper.

Bonding materials are applied in layers to the teeth until the desired esthetic results occurs. The bonding material is hardened by a curing process with high intensity light shielded from the patient's eyes. If the patient is esthetically displeased, bonding material may be added, removed, or recontoured to improve esthetics.

B. <u>Alternatives</u>
   1. Crowning of teeth
      Although individuals experiences may differ markedly from statistical averages, the average bonding life expectancy before repair or replacement is required is approximately 5 to 8 years. Porcelain crowns, which require the grinding of natural tooth structure, local anesthesia, and impressions, last on the average 10 years, but may last up to 15 years. Esthetic life ranges between 5 to 15 years. Chipping or fracturing can occur with any dental material at any time after placement. However, bonding can be repaired more easily by the application of additional bonding material to the fracture site whereas crowns may require total replacement to achieve a comparable esthetic result.
   2. Other Dental Materials
      Porcelain veneers are porcelain shells, which, after some minor tooth reduction, are cemented to the outside surface of teeth. Esthetic life ranges between 5 to 12 years.
   3. Nontreatment
      Bonding is designed primarily for esthetic reconstruction in selected areas of the patient's mouth. Patients may also elect treatment for tooth fracture or replacement of existing restorations that are decaying or breaking down and likely to cause future decay problems. Many patients choose bonding for psychological reasons since an improved appearance may benefit the patient socially or aid career advancement.

C. <u>Risk of Bonding</u>
   1. Staining can occur with smoking and excessive amounts of coffee and tea.
   2. Durability varies but is approximately five to eight years before replacement is required.
   3. Chipping or fracturing may necessitate periodic repair or replacement.

D. <u>Consent</u>
   I have read the above informed consent document, which has legal significance. All of my questions concerning bonding have been answered by the doctor or I have no questions. I hereby consent to bonding for esthetic reasons and/or treatment of dental decay, if any exists.

Date_____ Patient_____ Witness_____

Form 6-1 Informed consent for Bonding.

blood-borne pathogens. CDC provides similar infection control guidelines for blood-borne infections, which reasonably clinicians should follow carefully.[29] Impressions should be disinfected before being sent to the dental lab for prostheses although this is honored in the breach more than the observance.[30]

Composite restorations can potentially cause pulpal irritation with the acid-etch technique if the acid reaches dentin when the dentinal tubules become exposed during the procedure. Children or adults with extremely large pulp chambers are prime candidates for pulpitis. Therefore, in these instances, exposed dentin may require protection before the etchant is applied. Not all practitioners recognize or appreciate the risk of pulpal irritation resulting from microleakage or chemical irritation from poorly cured resins, but careful clinicians do.[31]

The philosophy of "extension for prevention," originally advocated by GV Black, is no longer necessary, especially utilizing conservative composite resin Class II restoration with proper home care. Moreover, no current credible evidence exists that subgingival margins prevent decay. Although subgingival margins are used in patients with a high or medium

Informed Consent Statement

Altering of Existing Restorations

Patient's Name (printed):

_____

I understand that any time existing porcelain restorations are altered, the porcelain could chip and/or fracture. However it is my desire that Dr. _____ refinish and/or reshape the porcelain in/on my teeth in an attempt to help me obtain the functional and/or esthetic shapes I desire. In the event chipping or fracture occurs, I will not hold _____, his staff or Legal Name of Practice liable; and it will be my personal responsibility to pay for replacement or repair as necessary.

I have also had the opportunity to ask and receive answers to all my questions regarding this treatment.

I have read the above and have discussed with Dr. _____ and/or also his dental assistant the risks and treatment options available to me. I understand that dentistry is not an exact science and no guarantees can be made to me regarding this treatment. I hereby give my permission to proceed with alteration of my teeth and/or restorations.

Signed _____ Date _____

Witness / Dental Assistant _____ Date _____

Name and Address of Practice

Telephone and email address

forms/REG informed consent re altering existing restorations

Form 6-2 Informed consent altering of existing restorations.

Informed Consent Statement Regarding

Approval of Provisional Restorations ("Temporaries")

Patient name _____

Doctor _____

Dental assistant _____

This will serve to confirm that I have had the opportunity to evaluate the shape, form, size, and color of the temporary restorations that have been fabricated, and I approve of these provisional restorations and agree to proceed with fabrication of final restorations.

_____

Patient   date

_____

Parent or guardian if patient is a minor   date

_____

Witness   date

Name and Address of Practice

Telephone and email

forms/REG informed consent re temporaries

Form 6-3 Informed consent approval of provisional restorations.

---

lip line for esthetic purposes, subgingival margins can cause inflammation by shifting plaque subgingivally. However, many dentists continue to place porcelain laminates up to 0.5 mm subgingivally, although esthetics can be accomplished with porcelain margins ending at, rather than below, the free margin of the labial gingiva.[32] Excessively deep subgingival margins risk biologic width invasion that may require crown-lengthening surgery to correct.[33] This practice, however, must be balanced

> **ESTHETIC CONSENT TO SILVER FILLING AMALGAM REPLACEMENT WITH COMPOSITE RESIN**
>
> I consent to the removal and replacement of my existing silver amalgam fillings in teeth number_____, _____, and _____, with new restorations consisting of _____.
> restoration name
>
> Doctor _____ has informed me of the following:
> name
>
> 1. My existing amalgam fillings are sound and well functioning. If not replaced, my present amalgams will likely last a number of years.
> 2. Current scientific evidence has established the biologic safety of amalgams. Therefore, there is no necessity to replace my present amalgams for any medical or dental health reasons. I have been provided and read American Dental Association literature concerning amalgam safety.
> 3. Proposed new restorations are designed to esthetically resemble adjacent natural tooth structures. An ideal or perfect match is not guaranteed nor likely. Natural aging of adjacent tooth structure can darken or yellow over the years compared to the newly placed ceramic restorations, which may necessitate periodic replacement.
> 4. Replacement restorations are durable but not permanent. Plastic composite fillings may last approximately three to five years. Crowns or caps last on average between 10 and 15 years. Durability predictions represent statistical averages. Each individual's restorative longevity may vary depending upon a variety of factors, including, but not limited to each patient's intake of coffee, tobacco, and tea; oral hygiene, and frequency of professional maintenance visits.
> *5. Replacement risks include, but are not limited to, root canal therapy in a small percentage of cases, pulp (nerve) exposure, cusp or enamel fracture and presence of deep stains from the older amalgam restoration being replaced.
> 6. Doctor has personally explained the risks and esthetic benefits of amalgam replacement, as well as the reasonable alternative of doing nothing with my present amalgams. Doctor has answered any of my questions concerning amalgam replacement.
> 7. I understand the above and consent to amalgam replacement solely for esthetic reasons.
>
> Date _____ Patient _____ Witness _____

Form 6-4 Consent form for replacement of amalgams.

against the risk of ending a margin at or just beneath the gingival margin where potential gingival shrinkage may allow a dark porcelain fused to metal margin to show. Porcelain veneers bonded to enamel can be durable for more than 16 years.[34] Compared to enamel bonding, dentin bonding lacks long-term durability and thus has reduced longevity. Consequently, porcelain veneer preparations, particularly in the gingival third, should avoid sensitive dentin exposure.

Another example of negligent customary substandard practice is prophylactic amalgam removal to prevent or treat systemic diseases. The mercury used in properly constructed dental amalgam restorations has not been established as a cause of any systemic diseases except in the few rare cases of mercury allergy confirmed by dermatological testing. The amalgam contains elemental mercury rather than the more toxic methyl (organic) mercury. Nine grams of mercury would have to be swallowed before the patient would suffer an acute toxic reaction. The amount of mercury vapor released from amalgam fillings in released air is far less than the accepted medically permissible dosage. The threshold limit value is 0.05 mg/m^3 of air for 8 hours a day for a total of 40 hours per week. Removal of existing amalgams contributes temporarily, but significantly, to mercury vapor in expired air; consequently, the possible exposure effects of amalgam removal, if any, prior to unnecessary replacement, mitigates against its prophylactic removal. Background mercury exposure also occurs daily from the environment and from ingested fluids.

The incidence of mercury allergy is rare, as evidenced by a Swedish study that identified only 82 cases in Sweden's entire health insurance program during a 12-year period for an incidence of 0.0012%.[31,35] If suspected, a dermatologist can verify allergy to common dental metals and also conduct blood and urine mercury testing. The American Dental Association (ADA) Mercury Testing Service recommends a thorough review of mercury hygiene habits if testing reveals levels above 50 µg of mercury per liter of urine. Prophylactic amalgam removal and replacement with composites or other restorative materials for systemic disease prevention is not scientifically justifiable. Amalgam replacement is indicated only if an existing restoration is dentally unsound or the patient requests replacement for esthetic reasons and preparations remain conservative without excessive stress-bearing occlusion. ADA Principles of Ethics and Code of Professional Conduct, revised April 2012, provides in pertinent part as follows:[36]

5.4.1 Dental Amalgam and other restorative Materials: Based on current scientific data, the ADA has determined that the removal of amalgam restorations from the non-allergic patient for the alleged purpose of removing toxic

> **Informed Consent Statement Regarding**
>
> **Approval of Restorations**
>
> I approve of the color, shade, glaze, shape and size of the porcelain laminate(s) and/or crown(s) that have been fabricated for my teeth and wish to have them permanently cemented in my mouth. I approve of the restorations in every way. I understand that after they are cemented it will be impossible or difficult to change them without removal of tooth structure, damage to the restoration(s), discomfort, and additional expense. I have discussed this with Dr. John Smith and have had all my questions answered to my satisfaction prior to cementing the restorations.
>
> _____
> Patient's name printed
>
> _____
> Patient's signature   date
>
> _____
> Witness   date
>
> Name of Practice
> Address of Practice
> Telephone
> Email
>
> forms/REG approval of restorations

Form 6-5 Informed consent for approval of restorations.

substances from the body, when such treatment is performed solely at the recommendation or suggestion of the dentist, is improper and unethical.

A patient consent to amalgam replacement for esthetic reasons is justified, but a systemic rationale is scientifically unjustifiable therapy. For replacement of amalgam fillings, the patient must sign a special consent form regarding amalgam replacement (see Form 6.4).

Guarantee or warranty

Esthetic dentistry is particularly vulnerable to claims of broken promises since patient expectation may not equate with dental realization, particularly if the dentist promises more than can reasonably be delivered. Dentist's statements such as "You will be as beautiful as a star" are tantamount to giving the patient a guarantee or warranty that the esthetic result will match the esthetics of a "Hollywood" smile.

The law does not require that the esthetic result match or meet the subjective and capricious esthetic standard of an *unreasonable patient* demanding esthetic perfection. The law measures an objective standard of satisfactory esthetics as judged by a *reasonable person* regardless of a patient's particular whim or perfectionistic desire. Nevertheless, *a dentist who foolishly guarantees a particular cosmetic result must satisfy the subjective esthetic whim of the patient*. Warranty, if proven, voids the usual rule of negligence law that a dentist is not a guarantor of a particular cosmetic result.[37,38]

To avoid a claim of warranty, a dentist should promise to do his or her best, even if the best may not ultimately satisfy the patient's arbitrary esthetic desire. No dentist using synthetic materials can exactly duplicate a natural tooth or cause it to age esthetically identical to the adjacent or opposing unrestored teeth. The patient should be provided a reasonable time to view the final restorations intraorally. The patient should sign the approval of restorations form prior to final cementation. See Form 6.5.

Patient esthetic perceptions

Dental esthetics is associated with a person's self-confidence. A patient's overall physical attractiveness may be correlated with career and social success.[39] Patients perceive factors that detract from an esthetic smile. However, patients are generally less critical esthetically than dentists.[40]

Some patient esthetic standards of acceptance follow:[40,41]

- A 3.0 mm maxillary midline deviation is near the threshold of esthetic acceptance. When made aware of midline deviations, patients prefer those that are coincident with each arch and the facial midline.
- Patients accept a discrepancy in gingival heights between central incisors of up to 2.0 mm, but prefer an absence of gingival height discrepancy. A 3.0 mm open embrasure (black triangle) between the maxillary central incisors is noticeable to patients. Unilateral alterations are more critical to patients than bilateral alterations.
- Gingival display esthetics is related intimately to the shape and position of the lips that frame the teeth and gingival tissues. Patients prefer no gingival display, with the upper lip height at the gingival margin of the maxillary central incisors. Patients nevertheless tolerate a range from 4.0 mm

of maxillary central incisor coverage to 3.6 mm of maxillary gingival display.

- Patients prefer smile arcs that are consonant with the contour of the lower lip rather than a "reverse" or "flat" appearance. Smile arc has a greater impact on esthetics than do buccal corridors. A flat smile arc decreases attractiveness ratings, regardless of the buccal corridors. Patients favor small or absent buccal corridors rather than broad toothy smiles. Extraction of premolars does not appear to predictably affect patients' perceptions of buccal corridors or dental esthetics. Thus, the number of teeth displayed is an important determinant in achieving dental attractiveness.

Patients have varying degrees of sensitivity to dental esthetics but with less critical requirements than dentists. Dentist's esthetics goals should conform to the patient's esthetic perceptions with pretreatment discussion in accordance with informed consent rather than blindly adhering to a dentist's ideal esthetics concept.

"I'm sorry" legal protection

Thirty-seven states in the United States have enacted "I'm sorry" laws that disallow health-care providers' apologies or statements of compassion as evidence of negligence or liability in malpractice cases. "I'm sorry" laws protect a dentist's statement conveying sympathy or compassion related to pain or suffering so that it cannot be used as evidence of admitting liability in a dental malpractice suit. These laws allow and encourage dentists to state to patients that they are sorry for an unwanted event or bad outcome without fear that these words will be construed in court as self-incrimination. The law does not apply to a statement of admitting negligence or fault that is part of or made in addition to a statement of feeling sorry for a negative outcome. In 2013, Pennsylvania was the most recent state to add "I'm sorry" legislation. Pennsylvania, Florida, and Nevada laws have mandates for written disclosures of adverse events/bad outcomes to patients and their families. Colorado is exceptional in that it also makes "admission of fault" inadmissible in the court of law. Under the Federal Rules of Evidence apologies are ordinarily admissible in civil court to prove liability. The language and scope of "I'm sorry" laws vary from state to state.[42] Thus, it is a good idea to investigate your own applicable law.

An upfront apology or expression of sympathy can relieve anger and frustration. This reduces the level of emotion and paves the way for an expedient resolution rather than lengthy and costly litigation. Patients do not usually sue because they are greedy, but instead because they want to know what went wrong and are seeking acknowledgment of the dentist's error. "I'm sorry" laws facilitate the continuation of the dentist–patient relationship following an adverse event. Concealing a mistake is a major genesis of litigation, particularly when a subsequent treating dentist reveals what the prior dentist previously concealed.

The American Medical Association Code of Medical Ethics, which sets forth the standards of professional conduct, states that when a patient suffers significant medical complications that may have resulted from the physician's mistake or judgment, the physician is ethically required to disclose to the patient all the facts necessary to ensure understanding of what has occurred. These guidelines also state that a physician's concern about legal liability that might result from full disclosure should not affect the physician's candid disclosure to the patient.[43–45]

The ADA Principles of Ethics and Code of Professional Conduct, revised April 2012, provide in pertinent parts as follows:[36]

> Section 5 Principle: Veracity ("Truthfulness"). The dentist has a duty to communicate truthfully.
>
> Dentist shall not represent the care being rendered to their patients in a false or misleading manner.
>
> Section 5.A. Representation of Care.
>
> This principle expresses the concept that professionals have a duty to be honest and trustworthy in their dealings with people. Under this principle, the dentist's primary obligations include respecting the position of trust inherent in the dentist-patient relationship, communicating truthfully and without deception, and maintaining intellectual integrity.

Prognosis and longevity

Prognostications on crown longevity should be based on average crown life expectancy rather than wishful optimism. Porcelain crown studies indicate a useful, functional life of 10 years.[46] However, esthetic longevity is less than functional longevity due to yellowing or darkening of adjacent and opposing teeth due to age and/or gingival recession over time. Esthetic crown life can range from 5 to 10 years.[47] Accordingly, the patient should be advised of this esthetic replacement expectation.

Porcelain fractures occur for many reasons, ranging from inadequate restorative preparation to extreme bruxism. If a fracture occurs, bonding repairs may be considered. Composites have a useful life of 3–8 years,[47] and so the patient should be advised.[32] Otherwise, the disappointed patient may sue, claiming a lack of informed consent and/or being warranted or promised a permanent restoration built to last an esthetic lifetime. Many dentists take advantage of the summary pages in *Change Your Smile*[47] after each esthetic treatment option outlining the advantages and disadvantages, range of restoration life expectancy, cost ranges, and maintenance required. If you give or lend this book to your patient, make a note in the chart which pages you advised the patient to read.

Try-in appointment

Consent should be obtained not only initially but also at the try-in appointment. Inquire in advance if the patient is trying to esthetically please someone else. Request that this person also be present at the try-in. Otherwise, the patient may leave appearing satisfied but quickly change his or her mind after a trusted friend or spouse criticizes the esthetics. At completion of the try-in, record in the patient's chart the patient's approval of fit, comfort,

Date	Service
3/31/2015	HX: NCR-pt has had a cold
	DX: Try-in lower partial
	TX: Tried in lower framework w/ wax bite rims. Bite adjusted in wax. Wax-up of teeth adjusted. Pt. approves shape and color of teeth and stated, "These look great. I really like them." Pt. advised teeth will be processed as he approved.
	AX: None
	CX: None
	RX: None
	FX: Rel /L partial; photos made of try-in

I accept the cosmetics, contour and position of the teeth as they appear today at the try-in visit.

Date _____ Patient _____ Witness _____ Patient signature

HX: Health history
DX: Disposition—reason for this appointment
TX: Treatment narrative
AX: Anesthetic used
CX: Complications, problems, etc.
RX: Prescriptions given
FX: Follow-up—next appointment

Form 6-6 Try-in approval form.

and esthetics. Although not legally required, for difficult patients the chart entry may be initialed and witnessed on the chart itself or on a separate form (Form 6.6).

With the availability of newer materials, temporaries should not be esthetically inferior restorations. Although not as critical as the final try-in approval, the patient should see and approve the temporaries before leaving the office to avoid surprise or embarrassment when the patient views temporaries at home with their family. Whenever possible, the new concept of trial smile should be implemented. This will also help to ensure there will be less chance of misunderstanding about what you and your patient envisioned esthetically. See Chapter 3 for more information.

Complete dental records and documentation

Records "remember," but patients and dentists may forget. A patient-approved treatment plan should be signed and documented in the chart (Form 6.7). A patient follow-up letter constitutes additional documentation verifying the patient's consent to both the specific procedures and the costs of those procedures (Form 6.8). Such a letter is a permanent addendum to the patient's record, which may be introduced into evidence at trial as corroborating evidence. Juries trust written documentary evidence more than oral testimony since a short pen is more credible than a long memory, particularly if the record was made before any threat of litigation occurred. Therefore, avoid statements in the confirming letter to the patient that may imply any esthetic guarantee. For example, do not write a letter stating, "Following treatment, you will look 100% better and undoubtedly will get the sales position for which you recently interviewed." Instead, write "I will try my best to improve your smile and hope that you obtain the employment position you are seeking." The latter is a safe statement since the law obligates a dentist to always use the dentist's best clinical judgment in diagnosis and treatment.

Written records documenting clinical findings, diagnosis, treatment plan, and prognosis are the minimum that a dentist is obligated to maintain. Informed consent does not absolutely require written verification in the chart but is more credible than oral consent alone. The following statement documents that informed consent was provided if later disputed by the patient: "Patient advised on usual bonding risks including fracture, chipping and staining, and preventive maintenance measures." Video informed consent is admissible in court as part of the dentist's records (Form 6.9).

Dental records serve the following functions:

1. They document the course of the patient's dental disease and treatment (dental history, differential and final diagnosis, treatment plan, and treatment provided).

2. They document all communication among the treating dentist and other concurrent health-care providers, consultants, subsequent treating practitioners, and third-party carriers.

3. They serve as an official document in dental/legal matters (lawsuits), and, if properly maintained, will demonstrate a sound plan of dental planning and management.

Phase	Date Plan	Appt	Provider	Service		Tth	Surf	Fee	Ins.	Pat.
1	03/10/14		RG1	0925B	Lab Fee-#3&30			$1,650.00	$0.00	$1,650.00
1	03/10/14		RG1	D2392	Resin- 2 surf., post-permanent	2	DO	$782.00	$0.00	$782.00
1	03/10/14		RG1	D2740	Crown-porcelain/ceramic substr.	3		$3,295.00	$0.00	$3,295.00
1	03/10/14		RG1	D2950	Core buildup, includ any pins	3		$504.00	$0.00	$504.00
1	03/10/14		RG1	D2799	Crown-Provisional	3		$750.00	$0.00	$750.00
1	03/10/14		RG1	D2393	Resin-3 surf., post. permanent	4	MDB	$866.00	$0.00	$866.00
1	03/10/14		RG1	D2393	Resin-3 surf., post. permanent	28	MDB	$866.00	$0.00	$866.00
1	03/10/14		RG1	D2740	Crown-porcelain/ceramic substr.	30		$3,295.00	$0.00	$3,295.00
1	03/10/14		RG1	D2950	Core buildup, includ any pins	30		$504.00	$0.00	$504.00
1	03/10/14		RG1	D2799	Crown-Provisional	30		$750.00	$0.00	$750.00
					Subtotal For This Phase:			$13,262.00	$0.00	$13,262.00
2	03/10/14		RG1	0925B	Lab Fee-#19			$825.00	$0.00	$825.00
2	03/10/14		RG1	D2393	Resin-3 surf., post. permanent	12	MDB	$866.00	$0.00	$866.00
2	03/10/14		RG1	D2393	Resin-3 surf., post. permanent	15	DOB	$866.00	$0.00	$866.00
2	03/10/14		RG1	D2393	Resin-3 surf., post. permanent	18	BOL	$866.00	$0.00	$866.00
2	03/10/14		RG1	D2740	Crown-porcelain/ceramic substr.	19		$3,295.00	$0.00	$3,295.00
2	03/10/14		RG1	D2950	Core buildup, includ any pins	19		$504.00	$0.00	$504.00
2	03/10/14		RG1	D2799	Crown-Provisional	19		$750.00	$0.00	$750.00
2	03/10/14		RG1	D2393	Resin-3 surf., post. permanent	20	MDB	$866.00	$0.00	$866.00
					Subtotal For This Phase:			$8,838.00	$0.00	$8,838.00
3	03/10/14		RG1	D9940	Occlusal guard			$985.00	$0.00	$985.00
					Subtotal For This Phase:			$985.00	$0.00	$985.00
					Subtotal:			$23,085.00	$0.00	$23,085.00

Disclaimer: I realize that this is the proposed treatment plan and it may be revised due to clinical factors that may change as we progress. _____

Total Proposed: $23,085.00
Total Completed: $0.00
Total Accepted: $0.00
Proposed Insurance: $0.00

I agree to pay 2 weeks In advance If treatment is over $3500. If treatment Is under $3500 I agree to pay for services as rendered. X_____

I understand and accept the treatment plan as proposed herein. I have had all of my questions answered and wish to begin treatment. Payment is due before services are rendered.

Patient or Guarantor's Signature _____ Date_____

Current Dental Terminology (CDT) © American Dental Association (ADA). All rights reserved

Form 6-7 Treatment plan approval form. Note the box in which the patient signs to acknowledge the cost of treatment and how it will be paid for.

4. The demonstrate conformity with peer review evaluation standards.
5. Photographic records documentation: with the advent of digital photography, there is little reason for not taking adequate close-up digital photographs of the patients' condition during the first appointment. This provides an excellent record of exactly how the patient appeared before any treatment is planned. Viewing these photos with the patient is more helpful than giving the patient a mirror to describe the patient's pretreatment esthetic dissatisfaction. Some patients

Date

Dear Patient:

It was a pleasure meeting you last week. As a follow-up to your initial consultation, I am enclosing a copy of the "Estimated Dental Treatment," which Dr. Ronald Goldstein recommended. Listed below is your treatment schedule.

First Appointment: The bleaching technician will perform an office bleach in your lower anteriors. A custom follow-up home bleaching appliance will be fabricated and instructions provided for further bleaching at home. During the first visit, which lasts approximately two hours, Dr. Smith will check the bleaching color achieved.

Second Appointment: All the upper teeth will be prepared for crowns (#2 through #15). A set of new temporaries or treatment splint will be constructed during this all-day visit, which includes initial cosmetic contouring or reshaping of the new crowns. Should endodontics (root canals) be required, the referred specialist or endodontist will advise you of such additional endodontic fee.

Third Appointment: Approximately two weeks later, a metal try-in appointment lasts about 2 1/2 hours in which the crowns' metal substructure are fit checked and then returned to the dental laboratory for porcelain baking. Final seating (cementing) visit is scheduled in two weeks.

Fourth Appointment: Final crowns are fitted and cemented in place. Cosmetic contouring on the lower anteriors is finalized and impressions for a nightguard taken. Please allow a full day for this appointment.

Follow-up Visit: Following the initial completion of your dental treatment, additional short visits are scheduled for any minor adjustments and to finalize the occlusion (bite) and check health of surrounding gum tissue.

If I can be of further assistance, please do not hesitate to call me.

Sincerely,

Form 6-8 Example of patient follow-up letter after initial consultation.

Name of Practice
Address of Practice

PERIODONTAL VIDEO INFORMED CONSENT

CERTIFICATION: I have viewed the video entitled "Periodontal Diagnosis and Treatment, Version 4.1." This video has aided my understanding of periodontal diagnosis and periodontal therapy.

John Smith, DDS, has encouraged me to ask any questions before proceeding, which I have done. Dr. Smith has answered any and all of my questions.

I agree to periodontal treatment with full and complete understanding of my options of nonsurgical, surgical care, and/or referral to a periodontist and elect;

_____ Non-surgical periodontal therapy only with Dr. Smith and staff

_____ Periodontal surgery by Dr. _____

_____ Non-surgical periodontal therapy, and after reevaluation, surgery as necessary by Dr. Smith

Date_____ Patient_____ Witness_____

Form 6-9 Video consent form.

---

may have very short memories of how they previously appeared. Pretreatment photos can save a great deal of mid- or posttreatment discussion of what the dentist may or may not have restoratively changed compared with pretreatment clinical appearances.

Chart documentation

Although patients may forget, a dental record remembers. If a dentist forgets, the dentist's records help remember. Erroneous entries should have a line drawn through the error and a corrected entry written above or below, indicating a later entry. Never block out or white out an entry so that it cannot be read, to avoid suspicion of falsified records. Entries can be made in ink, or pencil. If a pencil is used, avoid erasures which may suggest record alterations.

Spoliation is the legal tort name for altered, destroyed, or substituted dental records. In the United States, only Alabama, Alaska, Florida, Indiana, Kansas, Louisiana, Montana, New Mexico, Ohio, and West Virginia explicitly recognize an independent tort action for spoliation.[48] Nevertheless, the other states may issue evidentiary, monetary, or state board discipline for acts of spoliation.[49] Record spoliation adversely affects credibility and thus should be avoided. In Valdez v. Worth, D.DS., spoliation evidence included (a) spilled cola on the dentist's chart precluding expert questioned document examination, (b) destroyed models due to alleged mud on models from a flood, (c) defendant dentist's hygienist testified certain chart entries were added after her treatment, and (d) chart times were contrary to the plaintiff's phone records. The $641,441 crown and veneer award reflected a "pattern of prevarication" of an untruthful defendant.[50,51]

> **Example of chart documentation of informed consent**
>
> Date: 3/4/2015. Patient read pages concerning bonding in *Change Your Smile* (pp. 138, 145–150).[47] Patient fully understands pros and cons of partial coverage bonding and alternative of complete coverage crowning. Patient told doctor "You have answered all of my questions about bonding. I agree to bonding my upper six front teeth."
>
> Signature at the end of chart entry by patient and witness is optimal but not mandatory. If patient does not sign, the assistant should initial to confirm what doctor told patient.

Electronic records

The Health Information Technology for Economic and Clinical Health Act of 2009 authorizes grants to promote "meaningful use" of electronic health records (EHRs). EHR systems permit computerized provider-order entry of medications to flag potential drug interactions, allergic reactions, errors, and safety alerts with respect to doses. EHRs have the potential to reduce injuries and malpractice claims.

Implementing new information systems may initially elevate, rather than decrease malpractice risks. Risk of error potentially increases during the implementation as dentists transfer from an existing familiar system to a new electronic format. Studies have documented increases in computer-related errors from incorrectly entering clinical data into the electronic record.[52] Effective training can minimize the incidence of such errors. Dentists have a duty to minimize such risks during the transition period from paper to electronic records.

EHRs hold considerable promise for preventing harmful errors and associated malpractice claims. EHRs promote complete documentation and timely access to patient information, facilitating sound treatment planning, decreasing transcription errors, and improving communication among treaters.[9,53] EHRs record all time stamps of computer data entries, called metadata. Metadata provide a permanent electronic footprint which can be used to track entry change activity. Under federal law, metadata are discoverable in civil trials.[54,55] State law, which governs most malpractice litigation, varies as to the discoverability and admissibility at trial of metadata.[56] Metadata can be used to authenticate the EHR and/or to verify that an EHR was modified at the time of treatment rather than belatedly. If the record was modified at a questionable time to deliberately alter records, metadata may prove record falsification.[54,55]

Some EHR systems prompt clinicians to document reasons for overriding clinically significant alerts. As the use of EHRS grows, failure to adopt an EHR system may constitute a deviation from the standard of care. Once a critical mass of providers adopts EHRs, other may need to follow. As the use of EHRs becomes commonplace, the legal standard of care will follow suit. Latecomers to the EHR standard may be subject to liability.

Complete dental records

A complete dental record should include the following:

- dental history to date
- medical history with current updates:
    - name and phone number of the patient's physician(s) and date of last medical examination
    - systemic diseases such as bleeding disorders, diabetes, hepatitis, rheumatic fever, and HIV
    - current drugs and dosages, length of time taken, and recent changes
    - allergies and drug sensitivities
    - cardiac abnormalities, current blood pressure, and pulse rate;
- chief complaints
- clinical examination findings
- diagnosis (including differential, if uncertain)
- treatment plan:
    - all signed consent forms and/or video consent, photographs shown to the patient during treatment explanations;
- present and/or future referrals
- progress notes
- completion notes
- cancelled or missed appointments and stated reasons
- emergency treatment
- patient concerns, dissatisfactions, and planned follow-up including potential referrals
- prescriptions (pharmacy and dental laboratory)
- financial records and ledger
- diagnostic quality radiographs.[3]

Standards of care versus reasonable patient standards

State laws vary regarding the duty of informed consent. Although each state requires that the patient be advised of the material risks of treatment, the variations among the states concern whether adequate disclosure pertains to what a reasonable patient may justifiably want to know, or what a reasonable dentist should disclose in accordance with standard of care practice.

In a lawsuit in those states that rely upon what a reasonable dentist should disclose, the duty of disclosure requires expert dentist testimony regarding the standard of practice concerning such material disclosures. On the other hand, in those states that determine informed consent from the perspective of the reasonable patient standard, it is for the jury to determine what a reasonable patient would wish to know irrespective of the customary practice of disclosure.[8] Thus, in states such as California or Wisconsin, where no expert testimony is mandated, the state would permit the jury to determine what a reasonable patient

Clinical case: Unnecessary crowning

In another example (Figure 6.1A–C), a patient alleged unnecessary crowning since he was not offered the alternative of bonding or bleaching.[59] These options should have been provided since treatment was done purely for esthetic rather than restorative reasons. Thus, even if the crowns were well constructed, the patient in such a case could still claim that he already suffered and would likely suffer future repetitive trauma from necessary crown removal, repreparation, and

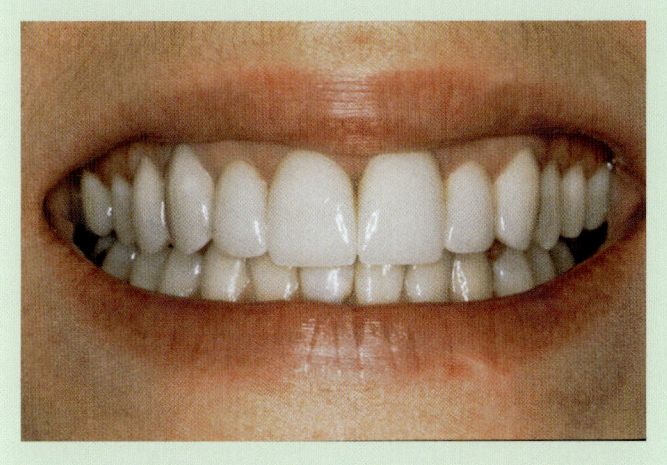

Figure 6.1 (A) This 29-year-old man wanted esthetic treatment to lighten his natural tooth structure to match the two previously crowned left central and lateral incisors.

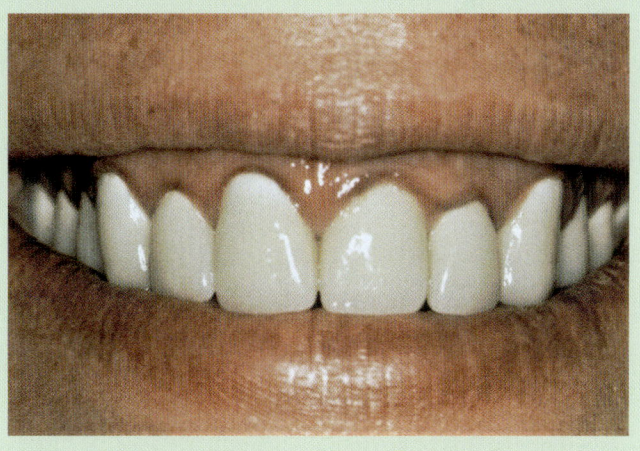

Figure 6.1 (B) After several more conservative consultations, including bonding, bleaching, and periodontal therapy, he chose a dentist who elected to crown all of his teeth. Note the extensive presence of periodontal disease.

replacement. Such replacement may be necessitated once every 10–15 years due to material wear but also every 5–10 years due to esthetic changes. Simple bonding or porcelain laminating with little or no tooth reduction represents a reasonable and preferred alternative in this case (Figure 6.1A–C). This case resulted in a jury verdict for $120,000, an expensive lesson for the dentist involved.

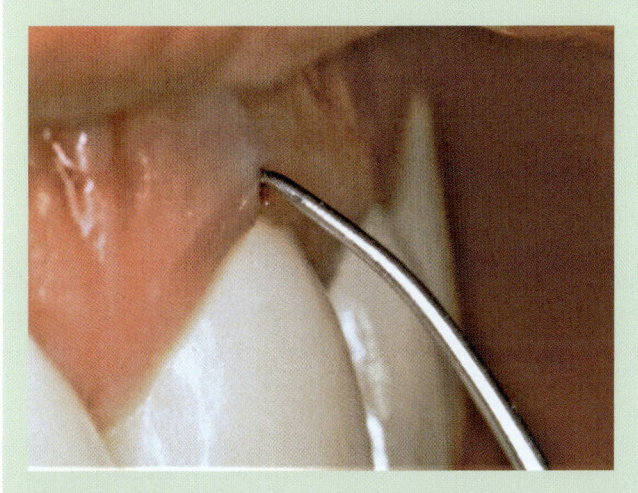

Figure 6.1 (C) Unesthetic crowning. Note open margin.

would expect the dentist to advise irrespective of how many or how few dentists do so.[8,37,57,58]

For instance, internal bleaching of nonvital teeth occasionally results in external root resorption. In the states requiring expert testimony, the patient would lose the suit unless an expert witness testified that the standard of practice among reasonably careful dentists is to advise the patient of the statistically small but recognized risk of external root resorption.

Nonnegligent risks and obligation to treat

Although a nonnegligent risk may occur despite the best of care, a dentist is nonetheless legally obligated to reasonably prevent, reduce, and subsequently minimize the risk once it becomes clinically apparent. Because external root resorption is known to be an associated risk of bleaching, the dentist should take periodic diagnostic-quality periapical radiographs to check for early root resorption and take appropriate action to arrest the condition if and when it first appears (see Figure 6.5). Calcium hydroxide therapy may remineralize bleach-associated external root resorption or arrest its progress if treated early. Also, a rubber dam can help prevent bleach injury to exposed root dentin.[60]

Bleaching precautions

- Use of rubber dam when using high-concentration bleaching solution to reduce gingival and pulpal irritation.[61]
- Minimum necessary bleaching times and temperatures to preserve pulpal vitality.[61]
- Avoidance of abrasive bleaching techniques that expose dentin, particularly in cervical areas where the enamel is thinnest. Be aware that the enamel does not actually meet the cementum in 10% of teeth.[62]
- Avoidance of cervical area bleaching of nonvital teeth. If bleaching is required, place a base over the endodontic fill to the level of the epithelial attachment, followed by placement of a calcium hydroxide paste into the canal for several days after bleaching.[63]

Orthodontic root resorption

Root resorption resulting from orthodontic treatment is another example of a nonnegligent risk of treatment being changed from merely a duty of informed consent disclosure to that of active intervention. Root shortening and its associated risk of premature loosening or loss of teeth occurs predictably with teeth that have already undergone some degree of root resorption prior to orthodontic therapy or in teeth with existing blunted roots. During orthodontic treatment, periodically the dentist should radiographically monitor the patient for development of any progressive root resorption. Once discovered, orthodontic treatment can be halted, a rest period of 3 months from active movement initiated, or the degree of attempted correction of the occlusion compromised to prevent or minimize any additional root resorption. On the other hand, Invisalign orthodontics virtually eliminate root resorption risks. Monitoring delayed eruption of permanent cuspids includes panorex and/or cone beam computed tomography (CBCT) to diagnose if ectopic canines are causing root resorption collision of adjacent laterals.

Misinformed consent

Misinformed consent is misrepresentation of treatment risks. For instance, advising a patient that full mouth extractions for implants are necessary since teeth will soon be lost anyway is a false and misleading representation if the remaining teeth are reasonably sound in tooth structure and periodontal support. Natural teeth have a longer longevity than implants.[64] Similarly, recommending prophylactic endodontics for restorative treatment is contraindicated in the absence of endodontic pathosis. However, if you anticipate likely pulp exposure, be sure to warn the patient before restoration preparation. Many clinically well-documented oral implant systems may be abandoned for the potential benefit of new, but untested devices. Some oral implant systems are introduced clinically without adequate clinical research. Implant informed consent forms should include the risk of failure, non-osseointegration, and implant segment fractures such as the screw or implant body. Advise that if the implant requires removal, a new implant replacement may be considered.

Who has responsibility for informed consent?

It is the responsibility of the dentist to obtain informed consent. An assistant may give the consent form to the patient and ask the patient to review the form. However, the dentist must personally review the relevant information with the patient and offer to answer any patient questions. Assistants may supplement information with patient discussion but not substitute entirely for the dentist's diagnosis of the informed consent's ABCs. Thus, informed discussion is a nondelegable duty, because only the dentist is licensed and possesses the educational training to respond to the patient's questions.

If the patient is a competent adult, it is enough to proceed with the patient alone. Complications arise, however, when the patient is a child, mentally incompetent, or not fluent in the dentist's own language. For patients who are minors, consent should be obtained from a parent or guardian. Generally, individuals younger than 18 years are considered minors, although, consent age law varies from state to state. Prudent practice for a teenage patient is to obtain consent from both the patient and the parent or guardian. If a family member is present during the informed consent discussion, note the name on the chart and have the family witness also sign the informed consent form as an additional witness. If the patient does not speak or understand English, or the dentist's native language, an assistant or family member who speaks this language can act as an interpreter. Consent forms translated into the patient's own language are preferable. A suggested introduction for an informed consent form is given below.

"I want you to understand not only what I plan to do, but also what follow-up care will be necessary. After I finish the explanation, I will ask you to sign a document which indicates that you agree to the proposed treatment. Sign the form only if you are comfortable with the recommended treatment and understand the alternatives, benefits and potential complications. Before signing, please feel free to ask me any questions that you have about the treatment procedure."

Patient's right of privacy and confidentiality

Dentists may use patient photos for teaching, research, or promotional materials and advertising. The Federal Health Insurance Portability and Accountability Act requires the patient's written authorization for photos to be used for any of these purposes. The patient's right of privacy and confidentiality of the dentist–patient relationship is violated unless the patient consents to disclosure and publication of patient photos.[65]

Doctor–patient relationship

Would you rather be liked or respected by patients? The typical dentist's answer to this question is "I want both! I want to be both liked and respected. In fact, I want to be loved and respected." But there are times that the patient will make a request that places you in a position of making a tough choice between being liked and respected.

Practice principles are paramount. Do not compromise the standard of care or dental care ethics. Patients who respect you as a dentist with principles will usually like the dentist for taking a firm stand. In turn, they will refer patients who appreciate a dentist who refuses to compromise quality. A patient should not be offered treatment choices that are negligently designed. On the other hand, the dentist should refuse a patient's request for negligent treatment. The patient must then respect the dentist's refusal to compromise the dentist's principles.

If patients do not respect the dentist's judgment, they will be less compliant with recommendations. A positive doctor–patient relationship is an integral part of treatment. Patients who like you will be more likely to return for recommended tests and follow your treatment recommendations. Anonymous dentist rating websites encourage disgruntled patients to post their displeasure of dentists they dislike. Patients are less likely to sue dentists whom they like. Patients who like you build rapport and trust your judgment.

Dentists should strive to base treatment planning on evidence-based science and not primarily on what is the most profitable treatment plan. When patients demand quick fixes that compromise the dentist's best judgment, the dentist should not succumb to patient-dictated substandard treatment options. The entire dental team should be educated to explain to patients why your recommended course of treatment, maintenance, and at-home regimen is the preferred option for achieving not only esthetics but also optimal dental health.

Nonconsent or consent for less invasive procedures

To avoid a patient's claim that treatment was unconsented and/or consent was given for a less invasive procedure, follow these suggested steps:

- Ask the patient to explain what procedure is being performed that day.
- Provide a mirror and ask the patient to point to which of their own teeth are being restored.
- Show the patient that their informed consent forms match exactly what the patient stated and pointed out regarding which specific teeth are being restored.
- Use demonstrative models or photos to show how the patient will appear after teeth preparation both with and without temporization.
- Ask the patient if they have any questions and answer each in lay language.
- Document in the chart: time out[66] was provided and staff witnessed.

Dentist's right to refuse treatment

A dentist has the legal right to refuse to treat anyone, except for reasons of race, religion, disability, or abandonment in midtreatment.[67] A demanding patient may attempt to convince you to treat, despite your misgivings, by appealing to your vanity. Despite the patient's praise, the patient's needs may be unique, special, or so demanding that the patient would be better served by a dentist who can spare the additional time necessary to satisfy the patient's exceptional esthetic demands. Although it might temporarily feed one's ego to hear a patient's flattery and confidence in your skills, you may be sorry when their unrealistic esthetic expectations are unmet.

Accordingly, be suspect of the patient whose dental history includes complaints that other well-qualified dentists failed to satisfy the patient's esthetic needs. Notwithstanding your exceptional reputation, skills, and experience, you will likely not succeed if other competent dentists have failed.

Patient abandonment claims

Collective dental wisdom teaches that a patient may not be satisfied with esthetic dentistry if a payment balance is still owing. Therefore, it is sound practice management and legally permissible to demand payment in full initially or before completion. However, a dentist cannot avoid completion, once begun, even though a balance is due, without risking a lawsuit for patient abandonment.

Reasonable temporization and periodic restorative maintenance until the balance is paid may represent a prudent measure to prevent a lawsuit for abandonment if the patient has temporary financial difficulties but wishes to continue treatment.

Right of a patient to choose a dentist

A patient has the right to decide on a dentist of his or her own choice. This right usually involves selecting the best available dentist skilled in cosmetic procedures. However, insurance companies and managed care plans will generally attempt to provide, instead, the most economical choice. The following case demonstrates that courts allow patients to exercise their right to select a dentist.

A 19-year-old woman was a front-seat passenger in a vehicle that was struck broadside when it turned in front of another vehicle (Figure 6.2A–F). The jury found both drivers were

Figure 6.2 **(A)** This 19-year-old accident victim presented with emergency splinting material previously applied by her attending oral surgeon.

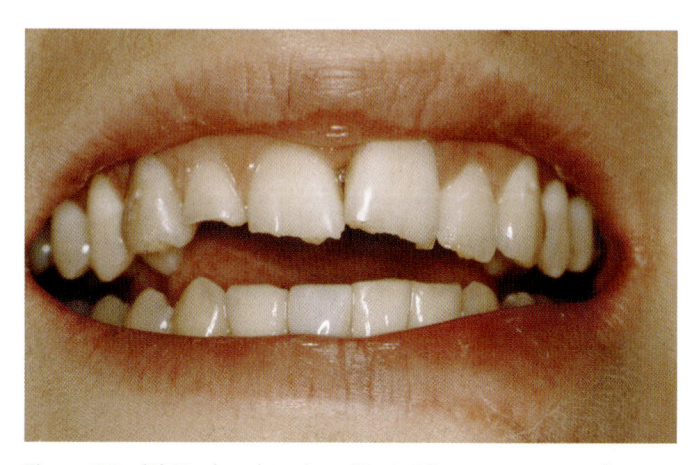

Figure 6.2 **(B)** Displaced teeth and incisal fractures are seen after splinting material was removed.

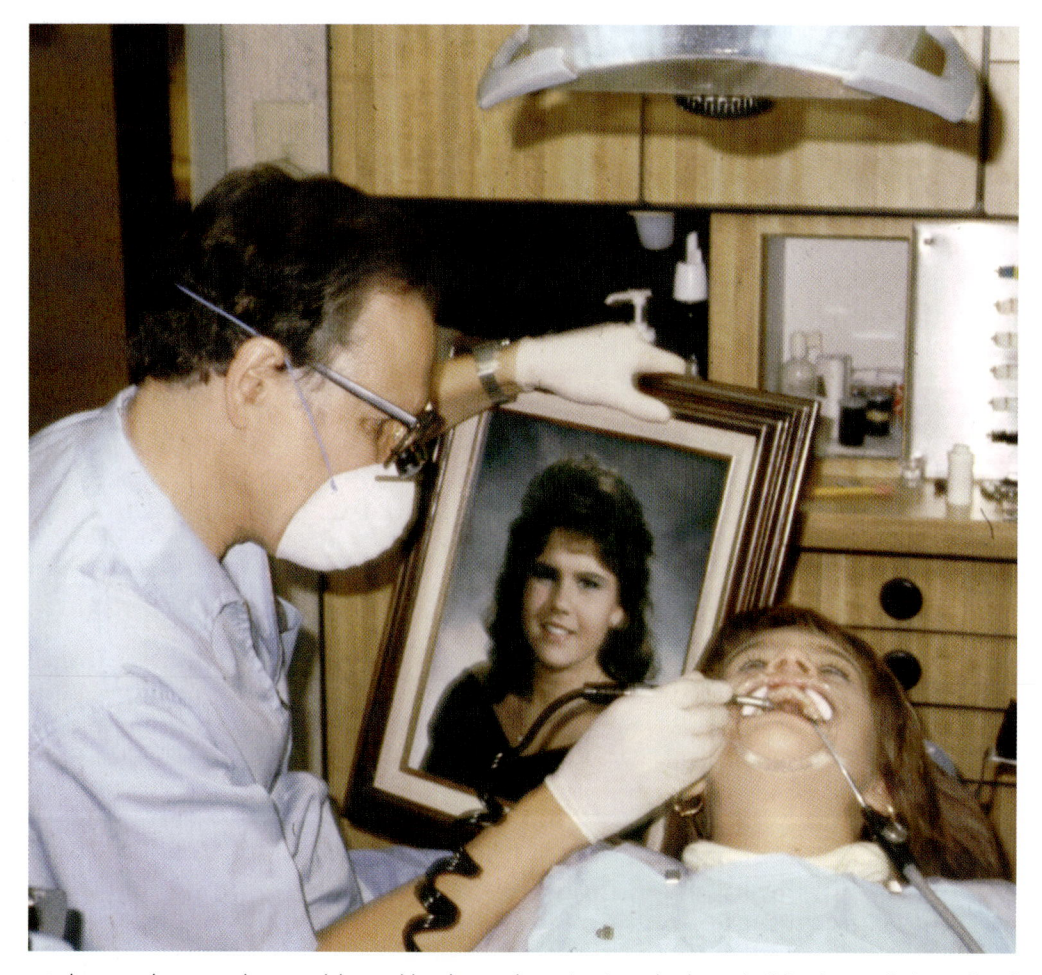

Figure 6.2 **(C)** A recent photograph was used as a model to mold and carve the patient's teeth when rebuilding her teeth during first direct bonding stage.

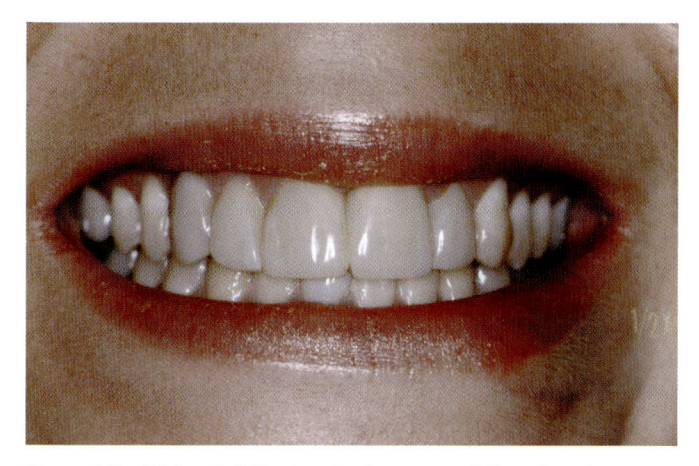

Figure 6.2 **(D)** Result following the first stage of direct bonding.

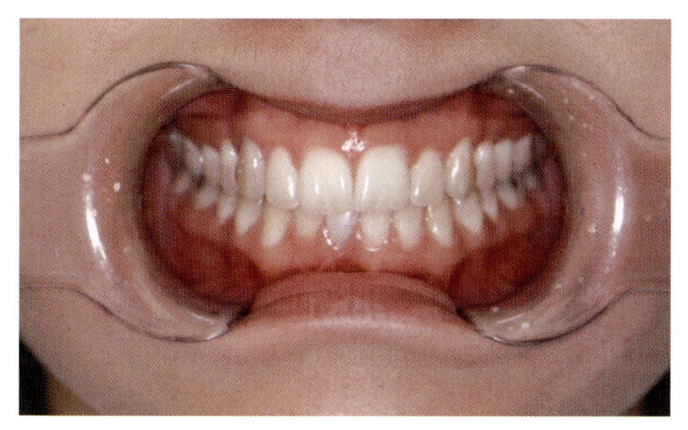

Figure 6.2 **(E)** Patient's orthodontist provided a photograph of the patient following his successful orthodontic treatment only 10 months prior to the accident.

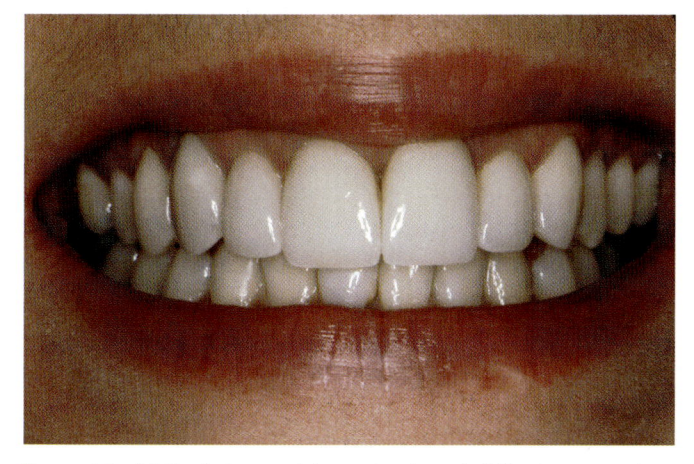

Figure 6.2 **(F)** Final picture of the patient's smile following second-stage treatment with porcelain laminate veneers.

responsible for the collision and compensated the passenger victim for her pain, suffering, and hospital and medical expenses associated with her injuries. The jury's verdict of $90,000 also compensated her for future costs associated with maintenance of her restored teeth, including periodic replacement of laminate veneers over her lifetime.

The following were legal implications from this case:

- it admitted into evidence the plaintiff's orthodontic post-treatment photographs to prove the virtually ideal esthetic condition of the patient's teeth before the accident
- it recognized the value of conservative dental treatment such as the use of porcelain laminates
- it confirmed the right of the accident victim to choose a dentist with greater expertise and higher fees than the lesser-skilled dentists in her insurance plan
- it awarded a sufficient amount of compensation to periodically re-treat or maintain restored teeth for the victim's lifetime.

Refunds

Maloccurrence does not alone prove malpractice.[37] An unsatisfactory result may on occasion occur despite the best of care. On the other hand, an untoward complication or bad result may be caused by the dentist's negligent error or omission. For example, overcontoured restorations and/or with open or submargins violate the standard of care and should be returned to the lab to be remade rather than using them in cementation. It is good patient relations to redo or correct unesthetic restorations without additional charge to a patient. For instance, chipping or fractures occurring within 1 or 2 years of completion should be considered for remake without charge. If the dentist concludes that a patient likely will not be satisfied, esthetically or otherwise, a refund is not an admission of fault. Rather, it is an admission of mutual frustration. Both dentist and patient would be better served with selection of a new dentist. A dentist is entitled to a fee for reasonable esthetic attempts to satisfy a patient. A refund and releasing the patient to another dentist might be the better choice and less expensive in the long run if you feel this patient will never be satisfied and will be constantly asking for more retreatments.

Settlement offers are usually inadmissible in court,[68] whereas admissions of fault are admissible. To avoid the appearance of an admission of guilty negligence, the dentist may write on the refund check "Refund settlement" or draft a release (Form 6.10), which the patient should sign at the time of refund. A recent California case held that unless with a refund the dentist also advises the patient of the applicable statute of limitations, the statute of limitations may be tolled.[69]

Examples of esthetic malpractice cases

Case 1: overcontoured crowns

A 45-year-old woman wanted to improve her smile. Neither bonding nor orthodontics was offered as alternatives to crowning. Overcontoured crowns contributed to periodontal disease. Her appearance after the necessary periodontal surgery was unesthetic due to the continued existence of the original crowns and the newly exposed crown margins and roots (Figure 6.3A and B). See also Figure 6.3C and D.

RELEASE OF ALL CLAIMS

_____, in consideration of $ _____, hereby acknowledges as received, does release _____, DDS, his agents, and/or employees, and all other persons or corporations of and from any and every claim, right, liability, and/or causes of action of whatever kind or nature the undersigned has, or may hereafter have, whether known or unknown, arising out of, or in any way connected with, the dental care and treatment of _____, including any act or omission of _____, DDS, his agents and/or employeees.

It is likely that future harm or injury may occur. This release is intended to cover and does cover all present and any and all further claims against _____, DDS, his agents, corporations, and/ or employees, who are finally and forever compromised, settled, and discharged.

The undersigned acknowledges that _____, DDS, denies any liability but has agreed to the terms of the release to buy peace and resolve all differences between dentist and the undersigned patient.

Date _____

Patient' signature _____

Witness _____

Form 6-10 Release of all Future Claims with refund settlement check.

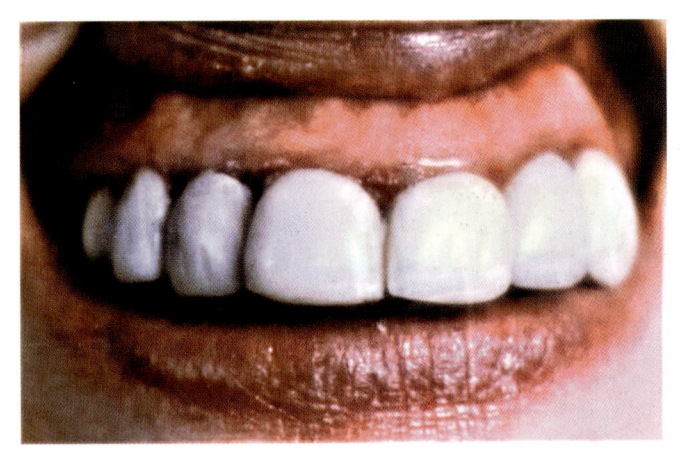

Figure 6.3 **(A)** Crowns prior to periodontal surgery.

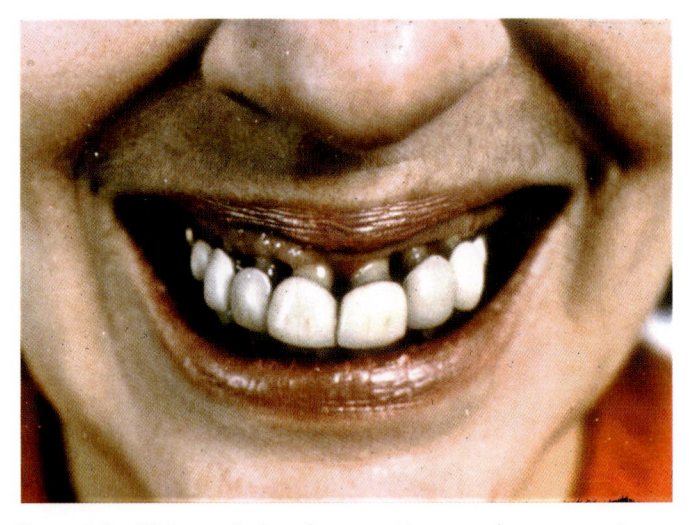

Figure 6.3 **(B)** Postperiodontal surgery. Note grossly open margins.

Case 2: overbuilt laminates

A young model sought to improve her smile. The dentist suggested porcelain laminates to improve the shape and color of her teeth (Figure 6.4A). Unfortunately, the dentist overbuilt the laminates with a resulting bulky look that destroyed her original smile's attractiveness (Figure 6.4B). A new dentist reconstructed porcelain laminates that provided the esthetics that the woman sought. Dentists have an obligation to provide esthetic enhancement to their patients upon request if reasonably attainable. At the very least, patients should not be restored in an esthetically inferior way or appear worse than when first presented.

Case 3: external root resorption with bleaching

Figure 6.5 is a California case in which the dentist was unaware of the risk of external root resorption associated with bleaching endodontically treated teeth and failed to disclose such a risk to the patient despite the literature discussing such risks. The manufacturer of the bleaching agent was also a defendant in the lawsuit for inadequately disclosing root resorption risks in the product information provided with its product. Root resorption is usually avoidable by retaining endodontic root obturation fill to the cement–enamel junction.

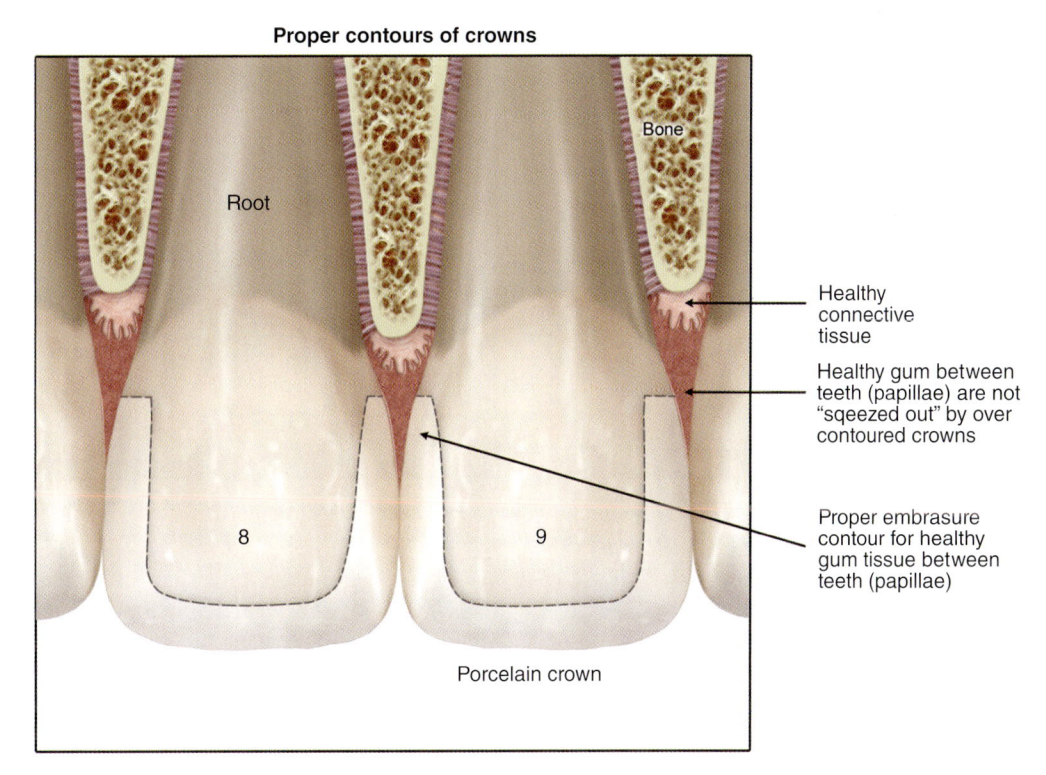

Figure 6.3 **(C)** Proper contours of crowns.

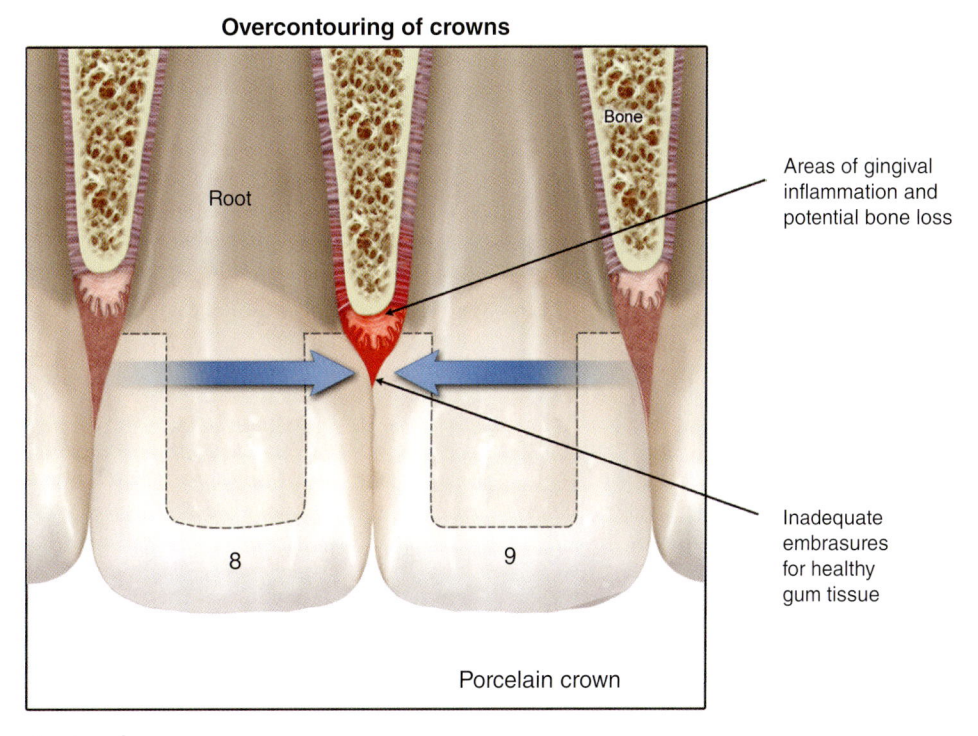

Figure 6.3 **(D)** Overcontouring of crowns.

Case 4: excessive laser sculpting

Biologic width invasion causation commonly is caused from direct invasion with restorative marginal placement into the epithelial or connective tissue attachment.[33,70] On the other hand, if gingival tissues are laser sculpted excessively, subsequent gingival healing re-establishes the former biological width causing biologic width invasion with resultant gingival inflammation. A California general dentist advertised that she strived for perfection in performing her cosmetic dentistry. The patient's chief complaint was her discolored tooth #9 and a gummy smile. Figure 6.6A is preoperative photo.

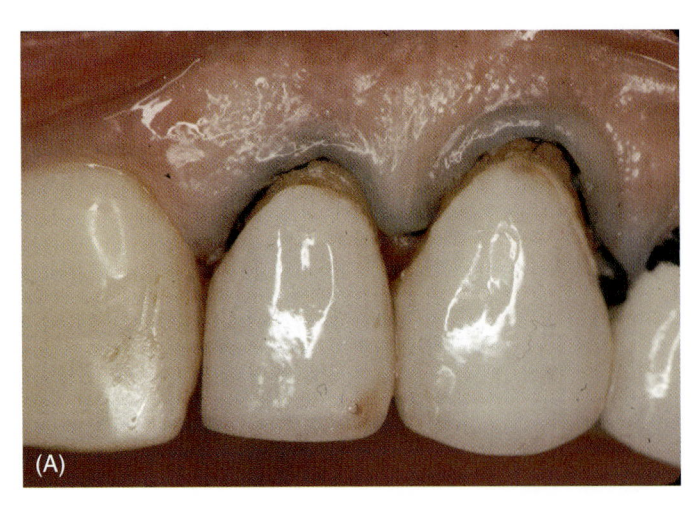

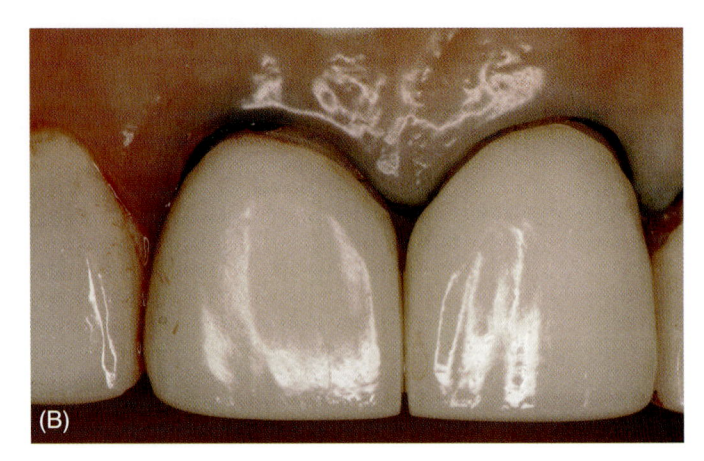

Figure 6.4 (A and B) Cotton displacement cord packed into the gingival sulcus to illustrate defective margins.

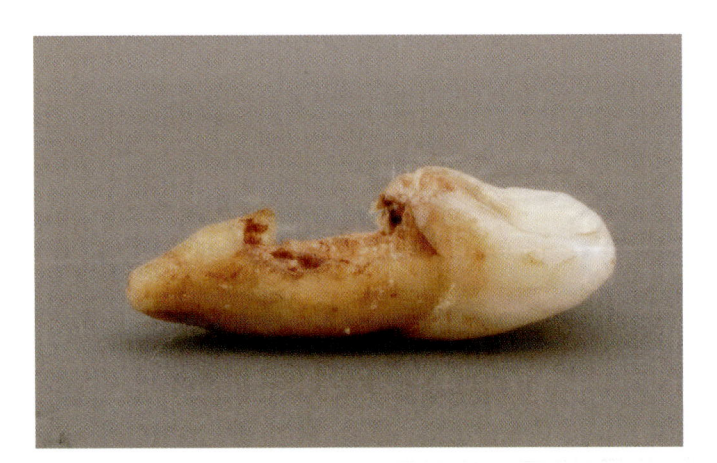

Figure 6.5 Postbleaching external root resorption.

The defendant dentist claimed she performed laser sculpting with minimal gingival reduction during the preparation of veneers from #5 to #12. Twenty-three restorations were prepared and temporized in 2 h 40 min under intravenous sedation to achieve an improved smile. Figure 6.6B demonstrates biological width adjacent to porcelain, rather than epithelial and connective tissue attached to root surfaces, causing iatrogenic gingivitis. Resultant gingival inflammation and ulceration required crown lengthening surgery to re-establish a healthy gingival complex.

A judgment of $641,441 was satisfied,[50] which included fees for future veneer replacements for lower anteriors since the option of noninvasive bleaching and Invisalign was not offered. Instead, the dentist only recommended and performed invasive mandibular anterior veneers.

Telephone or e-mail consultation

Offering advice without conducting an examination increases the risk of an erroneous diagnostic or treatment decision. Courts have held that telephone communications between a dentist and a patient can be sufficient to establish a dentist–patient relationship necessary for malpractice liability. It may even constitute negligence to e-mail advice to a patient who was never examined rather than be examined in person. E-mails may create a written documented record of negligent advice. On the other hand, e-mails may help prevent adverse events by allowing a patient to express clinically significant concerns that the patient does not believe warrant an office visit so that the dentist may offer suggested home care, specialist referral, or stat reappointment.

E-mails that are answered with boilerplate language from staff members, or otherwise unresponsive to patients' concerns, are likely to provoke patient dissatisfaction. Failing to respond to patient e-mails within a reasonable period of time could constitute a violation of the standard of care. Conversely, dentists who are highly responsive to patient e-mails may strengthen the dentist–patient relationship. Research has linked a propensity to sue with patients' satisfaction with their dentists and the dentist's communication skills. Dentists should establish a protocol for e-mails before initiating an e-mail relationship. Also, dentists should notify patients of these guidelines and obtain informed consent for the use of electronic communications.

Federal requirements and product warnings

Under federal law, the OSHA requires manufacturers to supply material safety data sheets concerning their products. If not given with the product at the time of sale, it must be available from the manufacturer upon request.

The Hazard Communication Standard (HCS) requires chemical manufacturers, distributors, or importers to provide Safety Data Sheets (SDSs) (formerly known as Material Safety Data Sheets or MSDSs) to communicate the hazards of hazardous chemical products.

Product liability suits require that the patient who is injured prove a product defect. Once proven, the product manufacturer is strictly liable even in the absence of any proven negligent design or manufacturing process. Product design defect includes failure of the manufacturer to warn of likely injury risks associated with product use.

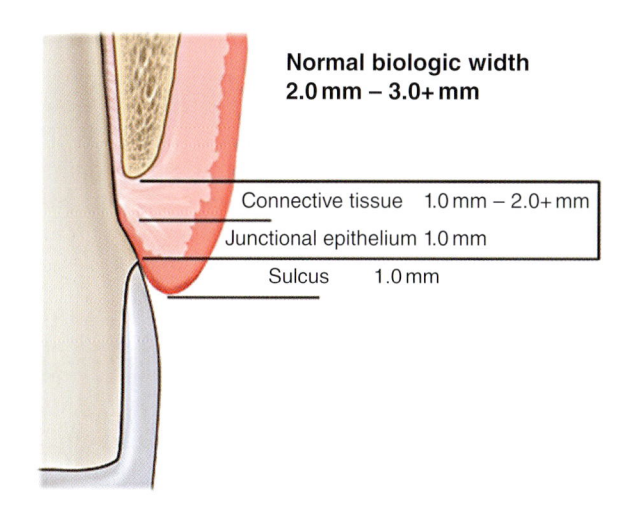

Figure 6.6 **(A)** Normal biological width.

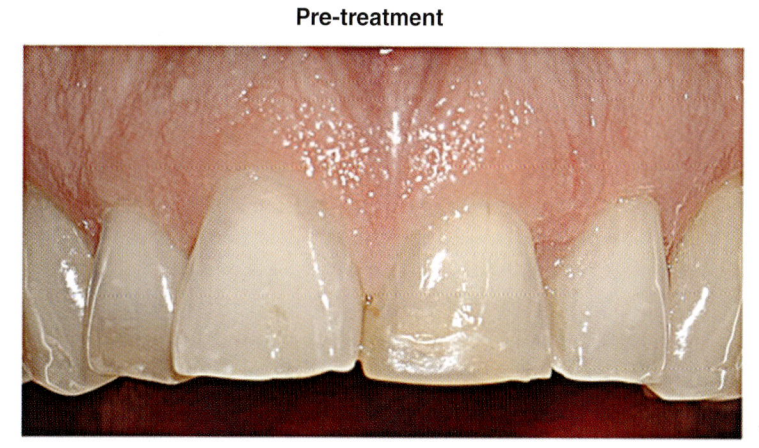

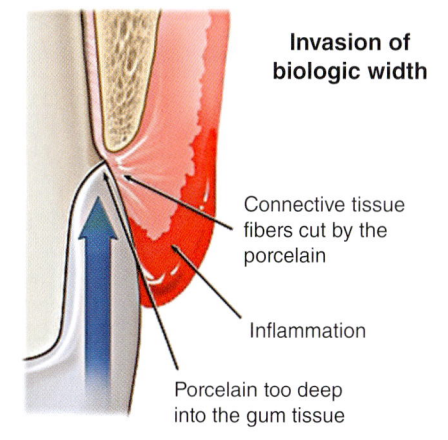

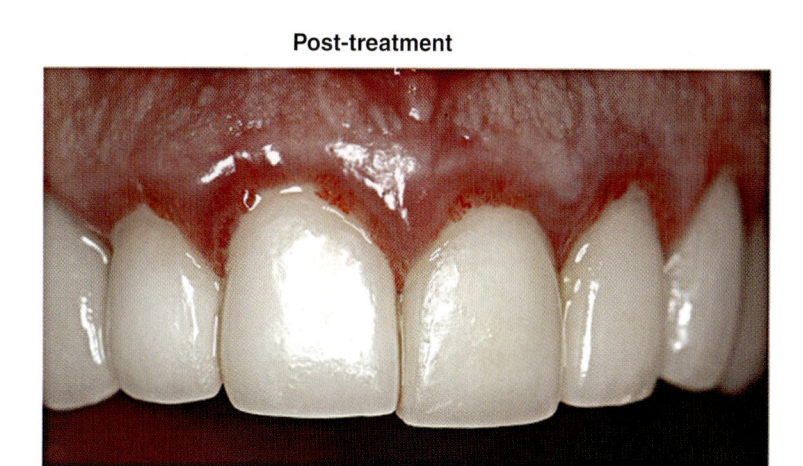

Figure 6.6 **(B)** Gingival inflammation of biologic width invasion resulting from failure to wait for laser sculpting to heal before veneer preparations.

Botox

Approximately 21 states allow dentists to use Botox. Many states require at least 16 hours of training to use Botox. A Massachusetts dentist was disciplined for unauthorized use of Botox and inadequate sterilization procedures.[71] Under the Massachusetts board's rules, only certified oral and maxillofacial surgeons who have been trained in the use of Botox and dermal fillers can use Botox for the treatment of "disease, disfigurement, or dysfunction." Dentists who provide Botox should possess adequate training and comply with their respective state dental board requirements for Botox training and administration.

Jury trials

Esthetics may be in the eye of the beholder. However, in a civil trial, both the dentist and patient are beholden to the jury. A reasonably careful dentist has little to fear and much to appreciate with juries who are generally fair minded in rendering a verdict. The runaway verdict is mostly mythical and rare since judges and appellate courts reduce or reverse such verdicts exercising their sound judicial wisdom. A fair trial requires expert witnesses who are not biased or disregard contrary evidence-based research.[57]

Conclusion

Here is a summary of malpractice prophylaxis meaures.

1. Suggest that your patient read your cosmetic dentistry literature, which provides a list of the limitations as well as advantages of the proposed esthetic treatment. An excellent example of this would be a specific chapter in *Change Your Smile*[47] that the patient acknowledged having read, and had all his or her questions answered. The note might read as follows: "Patient read and discussed Chapter X in *Change Your Smile* with the doctor. All patient questions answered and patient consented to treatment of teeth # ___ and #___ with _____ (restoration)".

2. Educate your patients about their esthetic problems as well as any potential complications that may occur during treatment. Give alternatives or choices of treatment for each problem explaining risks and benefits of each alternative. Communicate verbally the limitations of each proposed treatment. Consider supplementing this verbal consent with a written consent form.

3. Forecast an accurate range of restoration life expectancy, both esthetically and functionally.

4. Following the consultation, write a treatment plan letter to the patient confirming your findings and plans.

5. Do not promise to satisfy the patient's esthetic demands. Rather, state you will work hard to do your best in an attempt to please the patient, although there are no guarantees of success.

6. Provide good-looking and well-fitting temporaries to fulfil your patient's esthetic desires. Make sure the color, form, fit, and tissue compatibility are acceptable.

7. Obtain and record the patient's approval at the try-in appointment before placing any final restoration. Ask questions at the try-in stage, such as "Do you see anything else you wish to be changed before we place the final glaze or polish?"

8. Determine if there is anyone else whose opinion the patient values, and, if so, include that person at the try-in appointment. It is most helpful and a valuable source of psychological reinforcement to have the patient's spouse, family member, or friend present at this appointment to offer suggestions and aid the dentist in obtaining the final approval.

9. Observe gingival healing following your treatment. At the postoperative examination verify removal of all cement, absence of overhangs, and that all surrounding gingival tissues are healthy. If not, continue to see the patient until tissue health is restored. Correct all deficiencies. Re-emphasize oral hygiene measures necessary to maintain the esthetic restorations. Record your recommendations legibly in the patient's chart.

10. If the patient fails to return, telephone to make sure there is no problem. Most patient dissatisfaction can be eliminated or eased with good communication between the dentist and the patient, even in instances of evident dental negligence. Patients are more likely to sue an uncaring dentist than a perceived friend.

11. If the patient expresses dissatisfaction, suggest that he or she return to the office to attempt to solve the problem. If the patient refuses, again be helpful in letting the patient know that you have done your best, would be happy to refer him or her to another dentist for further treatment or consultation, and would be willing to discuss the matter with any other dentist of the patient's choice, or consider paying for another dentist's corrective care upon receipt of a treatment estimate. Your general liability policy, usually included with the professional liability policy, typically pays $5000 or more for any "accident" under the medical benefits portion of the policy. This can be applied to the corrective care fee of another healthcare provider.

12. Plan a potentially difficult patient's treatment plan in stages. For example, the first stage is the temporization phase, and you should quote a fee for just this service. This fee will take into consideration approximately how many hours it may take to satisfy your patient's reasonable esthetic demands for temporaries. If initial esthetic success is unattainable, the patient has the option of being referred elsewhere. The patient's only obligation is the fee charged for performing stage one, already paid in advance.

13. Legal abandonment does not result if the patient is notified of the termination of the dentist–patient relationship, is given ample opportunity to find another dentist, and the termination does not jeopardize the patient's dental health. Thus if both the dentist and patient agree that the final restorations will be completed with another dentist, no legal abandonment occurs. Offer to transfer patient models and records to the new dentist and to care for the patient's emergencies for 30 days until the transfer is complete.

The only guarantee for esthetic dentistry is to do your best rather than guarantee or warrant a specific esthetic result. Keeping current with continuing education courses in esthetic dentistry optimizes the outcome for successful esthetic restorations and surrounding tissues.

References

1. American Dental Association principles of ethics and code of professional conduct. Section 4. Revised April 2012. See also *J Am Dent Assoc* 2007;3:393–394.
2. Am.Jur 2d, Physicians and Surgeons §110.
3. Tomasi C, Wennstrom JL, Berglundh T. Longevity of teeth and implants—a systematic review. *J Oral Rehabil* 2008;35(suppl 1):23–32.
4. Comprehensive periodontal therapy: a statement by the American Academy of Periodontology. 2011 Jul. National Guideline Clearinghouse: 008726.
5. The 2010 Guidelines of the Academy of Osseointegration for the Provision of Dental Implants and Associated Patient Care.
6. Heymann H, Swift E, Ritter A. *Sturdevant's Art and Science of Operative Dentistry*. St Louis, MO: Mosby; 2014:e66.
7. Soncini JA, Maserejian NN, Trachtenberg F, et al. The longevity of amalgam versus compomer/composite restorations in posterior primary and permanent teeth: findings from the New England Children's Amalgam Trial. *J Am Dent Assoc* 2007;138(6):763–772.
8. California Book of Approved Jury Instruction. (2015) 535.
9. McQuitty v Spangler 406 Md. 744, 962 A.2d 370 (2008).
10. Ramos v. Pyatti, 534 N.E.2d 472 (Ill.App. 1989); Roybal v. Bell, 778 P.2d 18 (Wyo. 1989).
11. Beal v. Hamilton, 712 S.W.2d 873 (Tx 1986).
12. Kashkin v. Mt Sinai Medical Center, 538 NYS.2d686 (Sup.Ct.1989).
13. Largey v Rothman, 540 A.2d 504 (N.J. 1988).
14. Nelson v. Patrick, 326 S.E.2d 54 (Pa. 1984).
15. Gibson G, Jurasic M, Wehler C, et al. Longitudinal outcomes of using a fluoride performance measure of adults at high risk of experiencing caries. *J Am Dent Assoc* 2014;145(5):443–451.
16. *Knight v. Jewett* (1992) 3 Cal.4th 296, 312. (dicta)
17. Chen JH, Shi CX, Wang M, et al. Clinical evaluation of 546 tetracycline-stained teeth treated with porcelain laminate veneers. *J Dent* 2005;33(1):3–8.
18. Spear F. Esthetic correction of anterior dental malalignment: conventional versus instant (restorative) orthodontics. *J Esthet Restor Dent* 2004:16:149–164.
19. Ritz v. Florida Patient's Compensation Fund, 436 S.2d 987 (Fla. 1983).
20. Christensen GC. Thick or thin veneers. *J Am Dent Assoc* 2008;139:1541–1543.
21. Dental Products Report (December 1985). U.S. government halts sporicidin sales. *ADA News* 1992;23:1.

22. Givol N, Rosen E, Taicher S, Tsesis I. Risk management in endodontics. *J Endod* 2010;36(6):982–984.
23. Sfikas PM. Informed consent: how performing a less invasive procedure led to claim of battery. *J Am Dent Assoc* 2006;137(6):722.
24. Tyndall DA, Price JB, Tetradis S, et al. Position statement of the American Academy of Oral and Maxillofacial Radiology on selection criteria for the use of radiology in dental implantology with emphasis on cone beam computed tomography. *Oral Maxillofacial Radiol* 2012;113(6):817–826.
25. Zinman EJ, Masters D. Implant informed consent, an animated video. Available on request to Edwin J. Zinman.
26. Cochrane NJ, Cai F, Hug NL, et al. New approaches to enhanced remineralization of tooth enamel. *J Dent Res* 2010;89(11):1187–1197.
27. Riley JL III, Gordan VV, Ajmo CT, et al. Dentists' use of caries risk assessment and individualized caries prevention for their adult patients: findings from the Dental Practice-Based Research Network. *Community Dent Oral Epidemiol* 2011;39(6):564–573.
28. Almortadi N, Chadwick RG. Disinfection of dental impressions – compliance to accepted standards. *Br Dent J* 2010;209:607–611.
29. CDC. *Summary of Infection Prevention in Dental Setting: Basic Expectations for Safe Care.* https://www.cdc.gov/oralhealth/infectioncontrol/pdf/safe-care2.pdf (accessed November 9, 2017).
30. Matalon S, Eini A, Gorfil C, et al. Do dental impression materials play a role in cross contamination? *Quintessence Int* 2011;42:e124–e130.
31. Ingle JI, Bakland LK, Baumgartner JC. *Endodontics*, 6th edn. Shelton, CT: People's Medical Publishing House; 2008:1076.
32. Goldstein R, Garber D, Schwartz C, Goldstein C. Patient management of esthetic restorations. *J Am Dent Assoc* 1992;123:61.
33. Newman MG, Takei HH, Klokkevold PR, Carranza FA. *Clinical Periodontology*, 11th edn. St Louis, MO: WB Saunders; 2011:610–611.
34. Layton D, Walton T. An up to 16-year prospective study of 304 porcelain veneers. *Int J Prosthodont* 2007;20(4):389–396.
35. Williams v. Sprint/United Mgmt. Co., 230 F.R.D.640 (Kan. 2005).
36. American Dental Association: principles of ethics and code of professional conduct. Section 5. Revised April 2012.
37. California Book of Approved Jury Instructions. 2018. Instruction 505. See also American Jurisprudence Proof of Facts, 3d. August 2015.
38. Huffman v. Lindquist, 37 Cal.2d 465 June 1951. 234 P.2d 34; 29 A.L.R.2d 485.
39. Wilson R. Restorative dentistry. *J Am Dent Assoc* 1985;111:551.
40. Witt M, Flores-Mir C. Laypeople's preferences regarding frontal dentofacial esthetics: periodontal factors. *J Am Dent Assoc* 2011;142(8):925–937.
41. Witt M, Flores-Mir C. Laypeople's preferences regarding frontal dentofacial esthetics: tooth-related factors. *J Am Dent Assoc* 2011;142(6):635–645.
42. Kowalczyk L. Massachusetts Hospitals Urged to Apologize, Settle. Boston Globe. A1. May 28, 2012.
43. AMA Code of Medical Ethics. Opinion 8.082—Withholding Information from Patients. 2012.
44. AMA Code of Medical Ethics. Opinion 8.12—Patient Information. 2012.
45. AMA Code of Medical Ethics. Opinion 8.121—Ethical Responsibility to Study and Prevent Error and Harm. 2012.
46. Land MF, Hopp CD. Survival rates of all-ceramic systems differ by clinical indication and fabrication method. *J Evid Based Dent Pract* 2010;10(1):37–38.
47. Goldstein R. *Change Your Smile*, 4th edn. Chicago, IL: Quintessence; 2009.
48. Silha R. Methods for reducing patient exposure involved with Kodak Ektaspeed dental x-ray film. *Dent Radiogr Photogr* 1980;54:80.
49. California Business and Professions Code. (2018) Sect. 1680 (s)
50. Ingrid Valdez v Sherri Worth, D.D.S. 2012. Orange County Superior Court. No.: 30-2010-00348533. See also photos in Eggleston, DW. Case of the Month: Gummy Smile, Biologic Width and Laser Surgery: A patient study. Orange County Dental Society Impression. Page 29, April 2012.
51. Perkes C. Celebrity dentist loses malpractice case. *Orange County Register*, May 30, 2012. http://www.ocregister.com/articles/worth-356376-valdez-documents.html (accessed October 4, 2017).
52. Mangalmurti SS, Murtagh L, Mello MM. Medical malpractice liability in the age of electronic health records. *N Engl J Med* 2010;363(21):2060–2067.
53. Classen PC, Bate DW. Finding the meaning in meaningful use. *N Eng J Med* 2011;365(11):855–858.
54. Miller AR, Tucker CE. *Electronic discovery and electronic medical records: does the threat of litigation affect firm decisions to adopt technology?* Washington, DC: Federal Trade Commission; 2009.
55. Quinn MA, Kats AM, Kleinman K, et al. The relationship between electronic health records and malpractice claims. *Arch Intern Med* 2012;172(15):1187–1189.
56. White SC, Pharoh MJ. *Oral Radiology*. St Louis, MO: Mosby Elsevier;2009:78.
57. Jackler, R.K. Testimony by otolaryngologists in defense of tobacco companies 2009-2014. *Laryngoscope* 2015;125(12):2722–2729.
58. Jandre v Bullis; 2010 Wi.App136.
59. The Americans with Disabilities Act, Public Law 101–336; Americans with Disabilities Act Title III Regulations, 28 CFR Part 36, "Nondiscrimination on the basis of disability by public accommodations and in commercial facilities," U.S. Department of Justice, Office of the Attorney General; and Americans with Disabilities Act Title I Regulations, 29 CFR part 1630, "Equal Employment Opportunity for Individuals with Disabilities," U.S. Equal Employment Opportunity Commission.
60. Nixon PJ, Gahan M, Robinson S, Chan MF. Conservative aesthetic techniques for discoloured teeth: 1. The use of bleaching. *Dent Update* 2007:34(2):98–100, 103–104, 107.
61. Kihn PW. Vital tooth whitening. *Dent Clin North Am* 2007;51(2):319–331, viii.
62. Blanchard SB, Derderian GM, Averitt TR, et al. Cervical enamel projections and associated pouch-like opening in mandibular furcations. *J Periodontol* 2012;83(2):198–203.
63. Plotino G, Buono L, Grande NM, et al. Nonvital tooth bleaching: a review of the literature and clinical procedures. *J Endod* 2008;34(4):394–407.
64. Tomasi C, Wennstrom JL, Berglundh T. Longevity of teeth and implants - a systematic review. *J Oral Rehabil* 2008;35(suppl s1):23.
65. HIPAA Administrative Simplification Regulation. (2009) 44 Code Fed Reg Part 160 and 164(A)(E).
66. Joint Commission Guidelines: Guidelines for Implementation of the Universal Protocol for Prevention of Wrong site, Wrong Procedure and Wrong Person surgery. 2012.
67. Tellez M, Gray SL, Gray S, et al. JADA Continuing education: sealants and dental caries: dentists' perspectives on evidence-based recommendations. *J Am Dent Assoc* 2011;142(9):1033–1040.
68. Federal Rule of Evidence (2012) 408.
69. Coastal Surgical Institute vs. Blevins (2015) 232 Cal. App. 4th 1321.
70. Hemptom TJ, Dominici JT. Contemporary crown-lengthening therapy: a review. *J Am Dent Assoc* 2010;141:647–655.
71. Massachusetts Board of Registration v Helaine Smith. August 30, 2011.

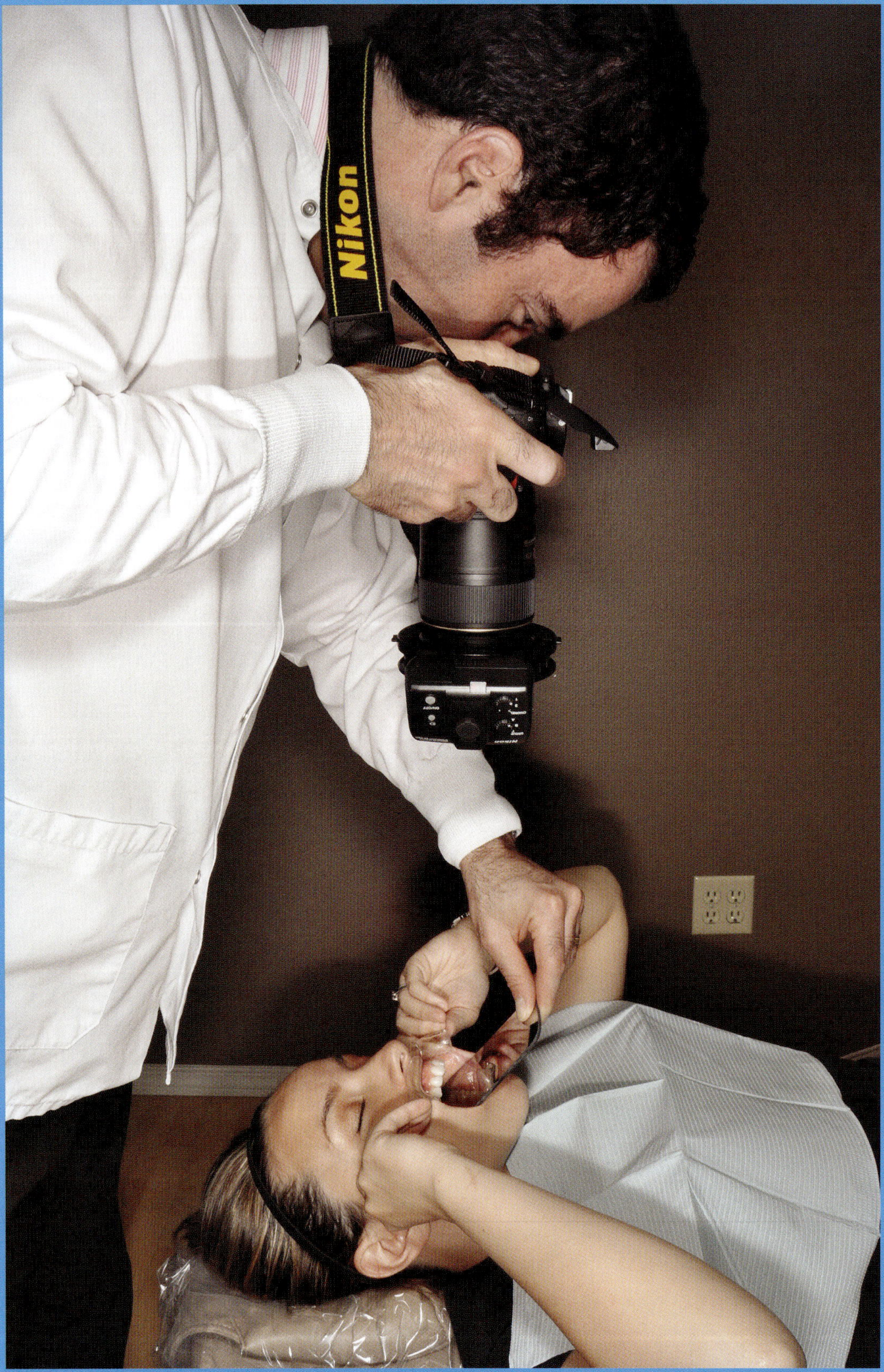
Nikon

Chapter 7
Practical Clinical Photography

Glenn D. Krieger, DDS, MS

Chapter Outline

Why take clinical images at all?	156	Retractors	171
When to take images	157	Composition of images	171
Clinical applications for images	157	Full-face smile	171
Case documentation	157	Full-face repose	173
Laboratory communication	157	Full-face profile	173
Patient education	158	Close-up smile	173
Dental education	158	Close-up repose	174
How to select a camera	158	Retracted closed	175
Important features in choosing an SLR camera	159	Retracted open	176
Setting up the SLR camera	163	Left and right lateral	176
ISO	164	Maxillary arch	178
Image types	164	Mandibular arch	178
Through the lens versus aperture priority	165	Image storage and presentation	179
Understanding lighting	166	Importing images	179
f-stop and flash settings	166	Saving images	179
Create a quick-reference settings checklist	168	Presenting images	180
Other necessary equipment	169	Video	180
Mirrors	169	Video camera recorders (camcorders)	181

For years, dentists have struggled to find effective ways to communicate with patients about treatment. Many dentists have fumbled with an articulator while discussing treatment needs with a wide-eyed patient. Bracket tray covers have served as canvases for the charcoal drawings of clinicians trying to explain a procedure to a disengaged patient. The most technologically savvy dentists would project a slide on a viewer in a somewhat scary approximation to a family vacation gone wrong. No matter the medium used, dentists have continuously encountered difficulty helping patients better understand their current conditions and dental needs.

Clinical photography helped to close the communication gap; however, film and slides were not without their problems. The time necessary for the developing process often delayed the treatment planning phase, and errors in taking pictures didn't show up until the processed images were viewed at a later date. Often, faulty shots were not able to be retaken because treatment may have already been finished by the time the images were

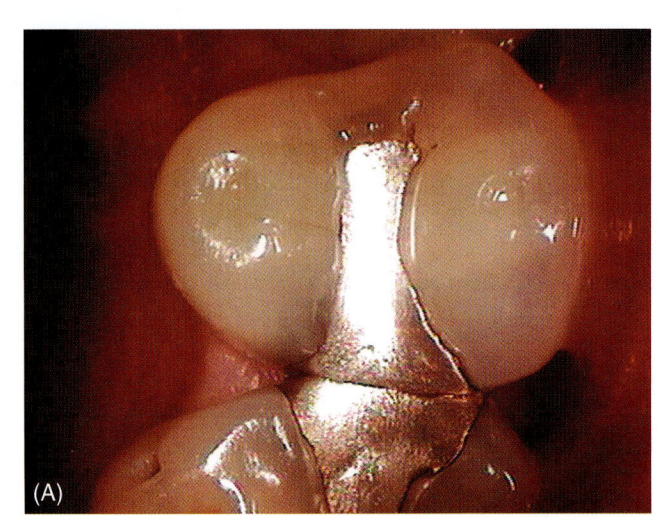

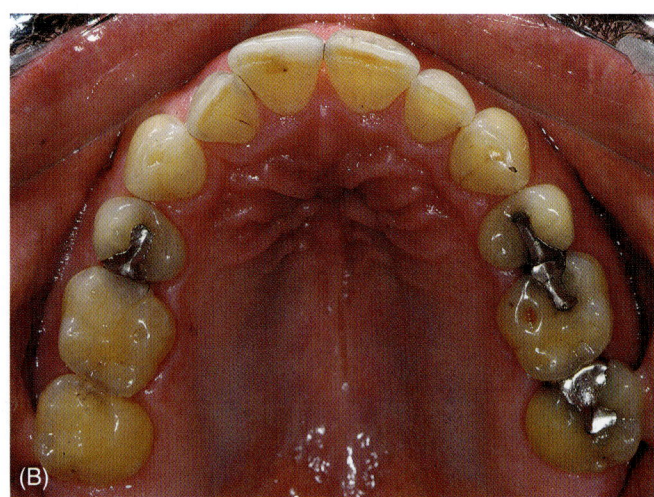

Figure 7.1 **(A and B)** Notice the different fields of view of the same teeth when viewed through a wand-like camera (A) versus a single-lens reflex (SLR) camera. Wand-like cameras, though simple to use, may detract from a patient's ability to understand how one tooth fits into the bigger picture.

returned from the lab. The clinician got one chance to master lighting and composition while photographing clinical procedures. Too dark or too light, out of focus or damaged film, the images of surgical procedures or restorative techniques could not be retaken. Although film cameras had drawbacks, until recently they were the only choices that dentistry had. One could choose the speed of the film and slide versus prints and could even choose a brand that suited their color preferences; however, the applications were limited. Dentists often had to convert slides to prints to communicate with the patients. Printed 8 × 10 blowups of clinical images, superimposed with tracing paper, were often the best way to demonstrate proposed outcomes. The return on investment for the time spent getting images ready for presentation often wasn't worth it. That is, until the advent of digital photography.

Early digital cameras for clinical use were large and expensive pieces of equipment whose quality rarely rivaled that of film. First-generation digital cameras were fickle, and their images were almost always recognizable as being taken with a digital camera. Color saturation was often far off, and the screens on the back of the camera almost required superhuman vision to discern the subject matter being photographed. However, these digital behemoths did afford one major luxury that even the finest film camera could not match: they allowed instantaneous viewing and processing of an image. Finally, a clinician could capture an image and retake it if any aspect didn't meet expectations. Images could be transferred quickly and easily from the camera to a computer and quickly printed out for patient viewing or to accompany a laboratory prescription. Sure, the images were of lower resolution, and the cost of such technology made it a difficult leap for the average dentist, but even with its limitations early digital photography showed promise of a new world of communication for the dentist with patients, technicians, insurance companies, and colleagues.

Of course, "wand-like" digital cameras had been around, but these limited-field cameras, often with "fish eye" lenses, were limited in their application. Although excellent for tooth-by-tooth demonstrations for patients and insurance documentation, the small fields of view (Figure 7.1A and B) hampered dentist's abilities to discuss comprehensive treatment plans or collaborate for interdisciplinary treatment planning. The new generation of digital "35 mm-like" cameras allowed full arches and portrait images to be captured without distortion and in their entirety, albeit with odd colorations, touchy mechanics, and a "digitized" look and feel. Thankfully, subsequent generations of digital cameras improved upon the early models. They became more rugged and less expensive, offered higher resolution, and began to rival, and ultimately surpass, the quality found in traditional films. Suddenly, dentists found a predictable, cost-effective, instantaneous way to document cases and present treatment options to patients, and a whole new world opened up to them.

Why take clinical images at all?

Whether collaborating between colleagues or presenting treatment options to a patient, a well-composed set of clinical images is the most valuable tool in the dentist's office. Nonetheless, there are numerous reasons why one would want to capture images in other situations as well. Clinical images are the best way to document any condition or treatment. One can observe a hard- or soft-tissue lesion and follow it over time through the proper use of images. In addition, one can take images throughout the course of treatment to teach other dentists how to perform a procedure. Another good reason to capture images is to provide a solid means of legal documentation of every case. Time and again, clinicians have found themselves in cases that could have been easily dismissed had preoperative images been available. Of course, practicing defensively is not a fun way to run a clinical practice; however, if the images are already being used for other purposes, isn't an ancillary use as legal protection a nice benefit?

When to take images

Imagine a patient who requires a considerable amount of dentistry involving several specialists and a treatment plan that could take years to complete. Of course, in a case like this, one would consider taking a comprehensive set of images before treatment planning and presenting the case to the patient. However, at what other times should images be taken, and why?

The aforementioned case is an obvious situation where images could help a dentist and patient agree upon a treatment plan and for collaborating dentists to agree upon a treatment sequence and roles. Unfortunately, even in extensive interdisciplinary cases, many dentists take that first set of images and stop there. They view the images as simply "a means to an end." In other words, the images are seen as a way to increase case acceptance and design a treatment plan, but not more than that. Often, clinicians learn best by looking at cases that have been treated, including steps along the way, to objectively evaluate how to best treat future cases. Any dentist who has looked at their cases after completion can affirm that it is a humbling experience, but one that leads to phenomenal clinical growth. Ultimately, it is up to the dentist's discretion when to take images; however, when in doubt, consider capturing images. One can always ignore images that have been taken, but can never go back in time to document a case that wasn't photographed.

Clinical applications for images

One can obviously use images as a part of the diagnostic workflow or as a part of the treatment planning process; however, there are numerous applications aside from those already mentioned. Included are case documentation, laboratory communication, patient education, and dental education.

Case documentation

Case documentation is an excellent reason to take images. Documenting a patient's initial presentation is a great way to be able to reference back to the beginning of a case at any time. If one has questions about the patient's initial tooth position or lip support related to the overall esthetics of the case, one need to only look back at the original images. Furthermore, documenting initial presentations in cases where there may be unrealistic patient expectations can assist dentists in avoiding difficult misunderstandings later in treatment. There is no substitute for color images of the original condition when it comes to referencing the initial presentation of the patient. Another aspect of case documentation is the photographic documentation of undiagnosed conditions. For instance, soft tissue pathology or "odd" presentations of any kind may be followed for extended periods of time through the judicious use of serial images.

Laboratory communication

Images play a vital role in the successful outcome of any esthetic case, but not for the reasons that most clinicians think. Although shade match is by far the most thought-of reason for taking images, other reasons for taking images include representation of form, shape, surface texture, and other aspects of the hard and soft tissue worth presenting to the laboratory technician (Figure 7.2).

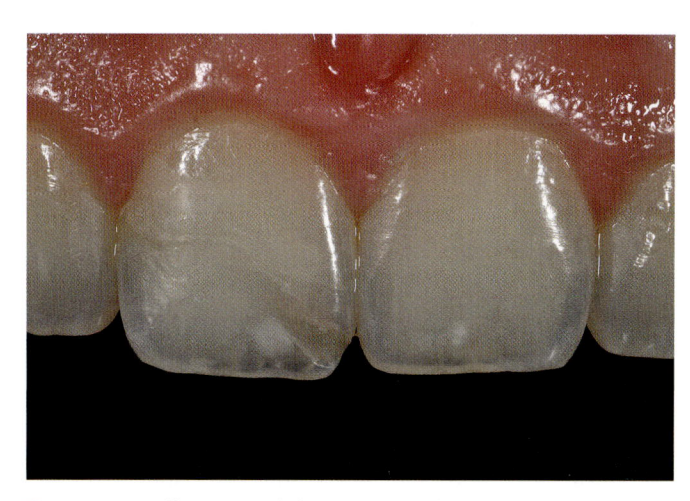

Figure 7.2 Well-composed clinical images allow exceptional communication between all members of the team. Nuances including tooth shape, form, translucency, color, and texture can be well represented in a properly composed image.

In terms of shade matching, there is an extremely broad topic. Although high-quality digital single-lens reflex (SLR) cameras can do an adequate job of capturing basic esthetic information without having to make many adjustments or accommodations, shade is an altogether different situation. Currently, there is no camera capable of capturing "perfect" color without having to create custom settings using a white balance-like card. Although not a difficult concept to understand or implement, it does require a basic working knowledge of the concepts related to color and how the camera views it. It is not the intention of this chapter to delve into all of the aspects related to the workflow of color management; however, there are many resources available today that can assist clinicians in a number of different methods to attain accurate color of their images. Simply recognize that no matter what is claimed by those manufacturing or selling cameras for clinical use, there is no such thing as a camera that will capture perfect color directly "out of the box."

Nonetheless, it is worth recognizing that for most situations perfect color accuracy plays a relatively small role in the overall needs analysis when considering the implementation of a clinical photography protocol. Of greater importance is the need for color *consistency* throughout a series of images and proper lighting. Of course, it would be ideal if every single image ever taken had the same level of color accuracy; however, as mentioned earlier, attaining this goal does require some investment of time and energy. If one is taking a set of images to show a patient their current condition, the need for perfect color is far less important than a case where shade is being communicated to a laboratory for veneer fabrication, and, even then, color plays only one part in a larger equation. Of importance in every image is proper lighting management and composition because without these, perfect color is virtually useless.

Patient education

There is nothing that can motivate a patient toward accepting ideal dental care better than a well-composed set of clinical images demonstrating failing dentistry or dental pathology. Of even more importance is the fact that "seeing is believing" and patients who visualize their dental problems are more likely to accept responsibility for their dental care. Clinicians who utilize a stepwise approach to case presentation which includes digital case presentation will generally find that patients become their partners throughout treatment. Gone are the questions like "What treatment are we doing today?" or "Why are we doing this treatment?" The dentist can feel more comfortable in knowing that patient decisions about treatment are made with a deeper understanding of the current condition and potential treatment options.

Although intraoral cameras are ideal for documenting single-tooth issues such as cracks, decay, and failing restorations, many dental offices do not own one. Digital SLR cameras, used properly, can produce extremely high-resolution pictures of a single tooth in place of intraoral cameras. One need to only set the image up as if it were an occlusal image (discussed later in this chapter) and zoom in on the single tooth (Figure 7.3). An alternative is to crop an existing occlusal image to the desired composition (Figure 7.4). Although not practical for use in all single-tooth applications, it is a fantastic technique when an intraoral camera isn't available.

Dental education

It has been said that "photography is the language of dentistry." Without images, it would be impossible for dental colleagues to discuss a case or come to proper treatment planning decisions. Collaboration between specialties would be based solely on opinions and conjecture, and it would be very difficult to visualize the proposed outcome.

Without photographic documentation of the treatment rendered, it would be extremely difficult for dentists to learn new techniques or applications of materials. Learning would be hindered and the dissemination of information slowed. It is for this reason that most dentists should develop the habit of photographing the steps involved in treatment so that they can, in turn, present their cases to colleagues at study clubs or larger meetings. Without images, there can be no presentation, and the habit of routinely documenting techniques through photographic means is one that must be learned and honed through practice. Of no lessor importance is the value of simply taking images and seeing them enlarged on screens for presentation. There are very few other methods for learning that allow dentists the ability to see their crown preparations or cemented veneers enlarged 30 times. Photographing one's cases causes clinical growth which is further amplified when one starts to present cases to others.

How to select a camera

There are two general categories of cameras available for dental use: single-lens reflex (SLR) and "point-and-shoot" (Figure 7.5A and B). Each type offers advantages and limitations for clinical use. SLRs are characterized by a moving mirror system that permits the photographer to see exactly what will be captured by the film or digital imaging system. Although non-SLR cameras have been touted as being considerably easier to use than SLRs, in

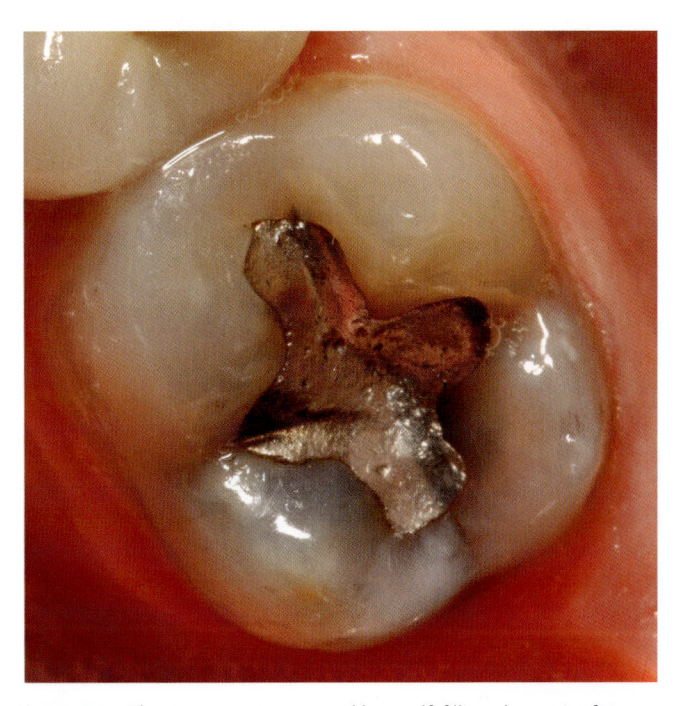

Figure 7.3 This image was captured by itself, filling the entire frame, rather than capturing it as part of a full arch and "zooming in." Notice the detail in terms of sharpness and color as compared to Figure 7.4.

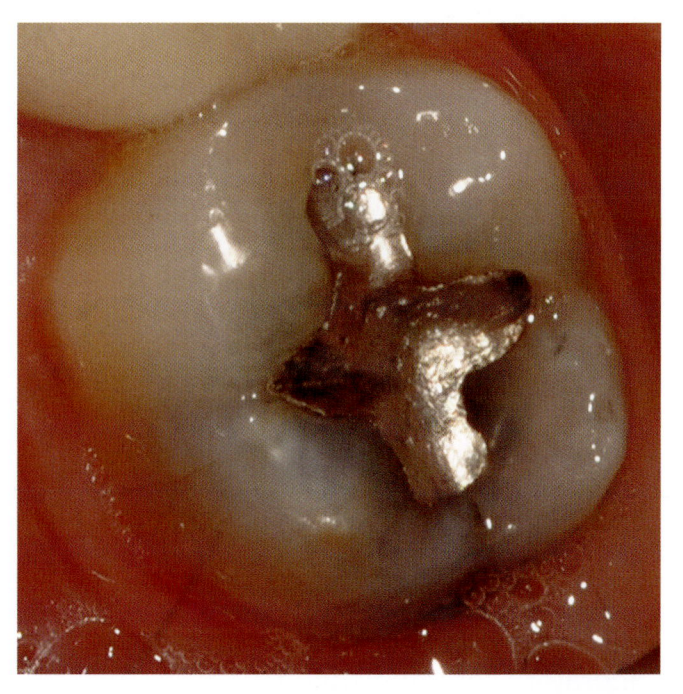

Figure 7.4 This tooth was cropped from an image of the full arch. Aside from loss of detail, capturing a full arch from roughly 60 cm away often makes it difficult to see issues such as saliva, which can block vital components of the image.

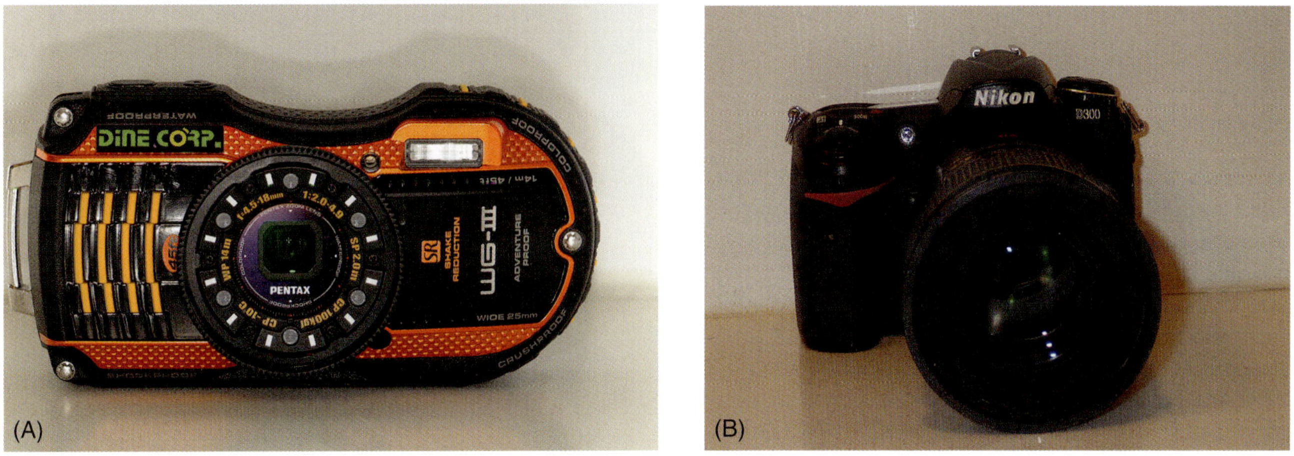

Figure 7.5 Examples of standard "point-and-shoot" (A) and single-lens reflex (SLR) (B) cameras. It can often be difficult to differentiate between the two; however, almost all point-and-shoot cameras do not allow for lenses to be removed and exchanged for other ones.

fact, for dentistry they are not. To capture appropriate images for clinical photography one must be able to control the depth of field, f-stop, flash settings, and, in some cases, shutter speed, features that are almost always absent in non-SLR cameras. Although point-and-shoot cameras can be picked up and quickly utilized, almost no point-and-shoot camera has "macro capability." What this means is that images captured from shorter distances (such as standard dental images) are unable to be brought into focus by the camera. For a camera to capture clear, visible images from close distances, it must have either macro capability or specialized adapters.

Another downside of point-and-shoot cameras is that one cannot change lenses. The standard lens in restorative dentistry has generally been one between 85 mm and 105 mm with some specialists using 60 mm, with all lenses having macro capability. Choosing a single lens for the clinical setting is all that is necessary; however, getting lenses of these types for a point-and-shoot camera is something that simply cannot be done. In SLR cameras, because the macro capability is a function of the lens, not the camera body, one can connect a lens of the proper magnification with macro capability. In short, although a point-and-shoot camera may seem appealing for clinical photography due to its purported ease of use and lower cost, most dentists find an SLR to be far easier to use once they understand the basic setup and use. Because SLR cameras are considered the standard in clinical photography, all discussions from this point forward will center on SLR cameras only.

Important features in choosing an SLR camera

When buying an SLR camera for clinical use, there are a number of features that one should look for. They include cost, screen size, lenses, resolution, functions, size/weight, and flash systems.

Cost

There are a variety of options available when looking at digital cameras in today's marketplace. The consumer-level cameras simply don't have enough features or compatibility to succeed in the dental clinic. As a result, the SLR market for dentists can be broken down into two particular groups: professional and prosumer camera bodies. The professional line is simply something that most dentists do not need to consider. Professional camera bodies are extremely expensive and have considerably more features than any dentist will use in clinic. For instance, shooting 20 frames per second is not something most dentists are ever going to have to worry about. In addition, video capability is something that most dentists won't use and, as a result, is something that doesn't need to be a part of an appropriate clinical camera system. The prosumer line of cameras by any manufacturer is the "sweet spot" for any dentist looking to get started with clinical photography. Camera bodies generally range from US$750 to $1500 with lenses costing an additional $500 to $950 and flash systems anywhere from $250 to $500. If one truly understands what is needed for capturing images, the cost/benefit can be fairly evaluated. Generally, the least expensive SLRs aren't appropriate for dental photography, and the most expensive generally are overkill. By evaluating the features of each particular model, one can determine which camera is truly best for them, rather than taking the advice of a salesman and ending up with a camera that sits on the shelf, unused.

Screen size

The size of the screen on the back of the camera is one of the less important features for clinical photography although many advertising dollars are spent by camera companies to convince you that screen size is of the utmost importance. The only factors one needs to really take into consideration when looking at screen size is "can it be easily viewed while I am capturing images?" The smaller the screen, the harder it is to view an image after capture. Older digital SLRs had screens as small as 4 cm. However, the images they captured were excellent, and if one was able to discern the quality of the image on the screen after capture, a bigger screen would make no difference. The majority of today's digital SLR cameras have screens that are big enough for most clinicians to view images (6–8 cm), so screen size simply isn't as important as it was in earlier generations of digital cameras. However, if one has a difficult time viewing details on the screen, a camera with a larger screen should be considered. To avoid any problems, one should always consider capturing images and viewing them on a screen before buying a camera.

Lenses

It is the opinion of most professional photographers that lenses should be of the same manufacturer as the camera body. There are a number of reasons for this. It is commonly believed that camera manufacturers create lenses to specifically match the camera bodies that they have produced. Although other companies can make duplicate lenses (Figure 7.6A and B), the original research and development has come from the camera company, and, as such, most professional photographers believe in matching their "glass" to the camera manufacturer. A second reason why this is not a bad idea is in the event that something should malfunction, it is always easier to take a camera system that is all of one manufacturer to a certified dealer of that manufacturer and allow them to fix it. Any person who has ever suffered a computer crash and heard the hardware manufacturer say that it is the software and the software manufacturer saying that it is the hardware can understand the value of one company being responsible for both the lens and the camera body. In the long run, this will probably save you a lot of trouble.

Lenses come in a variety of shapes and sizes. The lens for dental use is generally between 60 and 105 mm (Figure 7.7A–C). This is the standard in the industry for the last 30–40 years because it allows the image to have a composition that fits perfectly for dental images that are of the proper composition.

Lenses that are bigger (i.e., 200 or 300 mm) do not allow a wide enough field to capture full-face images in a standard dental setting and lenses that are smaller (i.e., 35 or 55 mm) are often too wide to allow us good close-up images of patients' teeth. As previously mentioned, all lenses for dental use must have macro capability. This allows the clinician to capture an appropriate image from very close. Any dentist who has ever attempted to capture an image without macro capability understands the difficulty in trying to focus an image that is too close for the lens to handle.

Resolution

Resolution, or the amount of information in an image, is a generally misunderstood concept. Years ago, some of the first digital cameras had images that contained 1–2 megapixels whereas cameras of today have more than 20 times that amount. To understand what this means, one must first understand how a picture is composed, from a digital perspective. The basic building block of any digital image is the pixel. A pixel is a square of color that makes up a part of a greater image. A 1 mega (million) pixel image has 1 million squares of color that make up the image. It's easier to understand if one thinks of a digital image as if it were a painting from the famed era of pointilism, where the numerous dots that of paint that make up an image look very different depending on the distance from which the painting is viewed. When viewed up close, all one sees is simply dots of color; however, when viewed from far away the image becomes a masterpiece. This is exactly what occurs in photography with

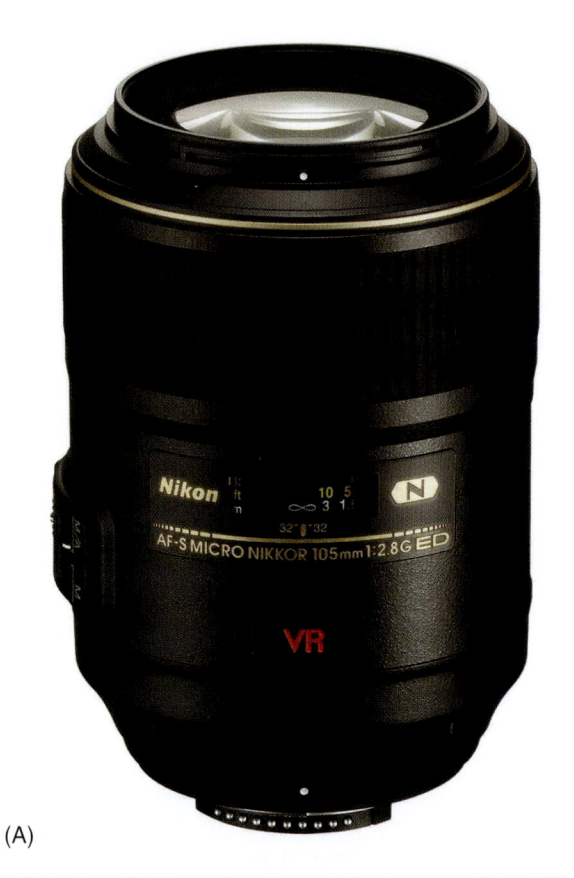

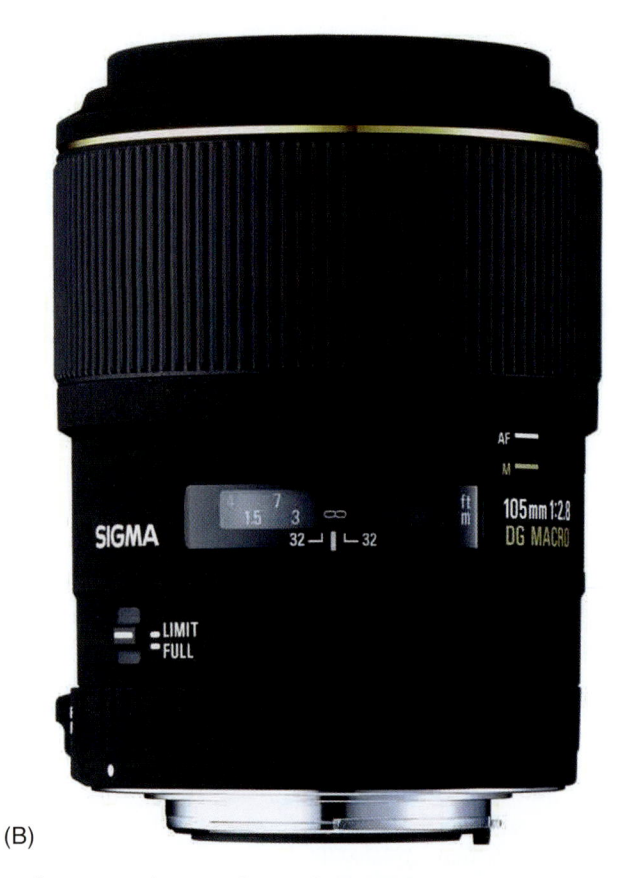

(A)   (B)

Figure 7.6 (A and B) Examples of two similar lenses made by different manufacturers. In this case, they are both 105 mm macro lenses.

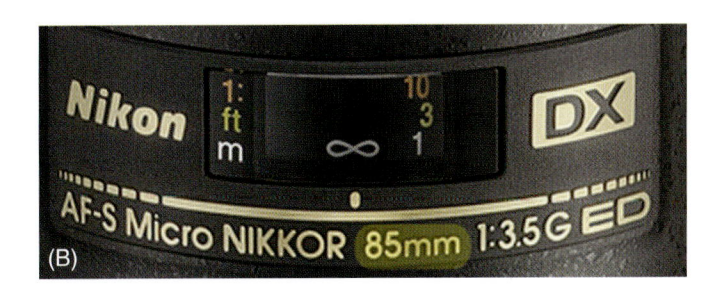

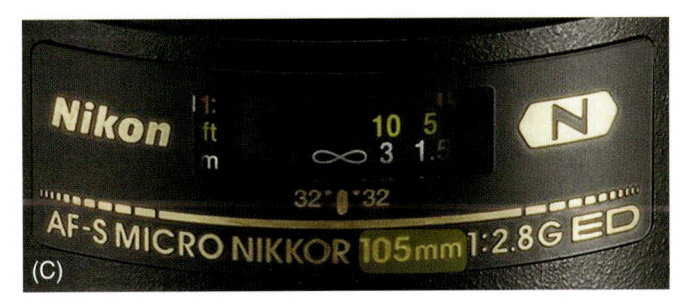

Figure 7.7 One can differentiate lenses by looking on the body of the lens for a proper marking. In this case, three different lenses (A, 60 mm, B, 85 mm, and C, 105 mm) are shown in a close-up view with their markings highlighted in yellow. Note that lenses with a range (i.e., 18–200 mm) are not appropriate for dental use.

pixels. A 1 million pixel image means that there are 1 million squares of color making up the entire image. If one were to enlarge the image to see each individual pixel, one would simply see a blurry square of color, but when seen in normal viewing on a screen, the million pixels appear to be a standard image (Figure 7.8A–E).

It is important to note that the more pixels in an image, the greater the resolution of the image. If an image needs to be enlarged to a much bigger size, there must be much more information present to be able to fill in the new, larger "canvas," and an image that does not have enough pixels to fill the screen will look blurry and "pixelized" (Figure 7.9). Due to the higher resolution of modern digital SLR cameras, this really isn't a concern for anyone looking to capture exceptional clinical images, and one should not necessarily believe that the more pixels, the better the image. If one were going to take an image and enlarge it to fit the size of a billboard, of course, the more pixels the better. However, for dental applications, it is rare that one will ever need that much information in an image. To put this into perspective, let us look at today's traditional monitors, the common output source for most of our images in dentistry.

If one has ever tried to set the properties on a clinical monitor, one would see several different settings appear. The computer might ask you if you wanted 764×620, or 1024×768, or 1600×1200, and so forth (Figure 7.10). The computer is asking how many pixels wide by how many pixels tall the user wants to display for the settings on the monitor. As previously mentioned, the more pixels, the more information, and the crisper the image. So a monitor that is set at 1600×1200 will allow much greater resolution than a monitor set at 600×400 (Figure 7.11A and B). The monitor that is set by 600×400 is only displaying 240,000 pixels. The monitor that is set at 1600×1200 is demonstrating 1.92 million (mega) pixels. If one sets their monitor to the highest resolution of 1600×1200 (a nice mid-level resolution for many monitors), one needs less than 2 million pixels to show a crystal-clear image that can look no better on that monitor. Does it matter if the camera that captured the image can display 6 or 14 million pixels? Not for this particular application because the most that this monitor can show is 1.92 million pixels. As a result, one might believe that more pixels means better screen resolution, but this is untrue, because most modern SLR cameras capture more than 10 megapixels per image.

However, if one is thinking of going to print media such as a publication or large posters, or if one needs to crop the image a great deal, the more resolution the better. That doesn't mean that one should buy a 16 megapixel camera over a 12 megapixel camera simply for printing purposes. Even for cameras that shoot only 3, 4, or 5 megapixels there are software programs available today that will allow lesser pixel images to be enlarged for "bigger" applications. In short, one should not get hung up on the resolution of a camera. This should not be a concern in today's SLR market. Most cameras available will provide more than adequate resolution for any dental use.

Functions

Today's SLR cameras offer a wide array of functions for the user to enjoy. However, many of the functions that separate one model from another are generally unused in dental photography. For instance, some cameras will allow the user to capture 20 images per second, something that no dental photographer will ever use. Other models will allow high-definition video capture, something that most novice clinical photographers can easily do without practice. Understanding the "essential" functions that a camera must possess is important for anyone thinking of buying a camera for clinical photography. Many camera manufacturers differ in the way they approach the features of the cameras, so it is important that users try out each system to see which one fits them best.

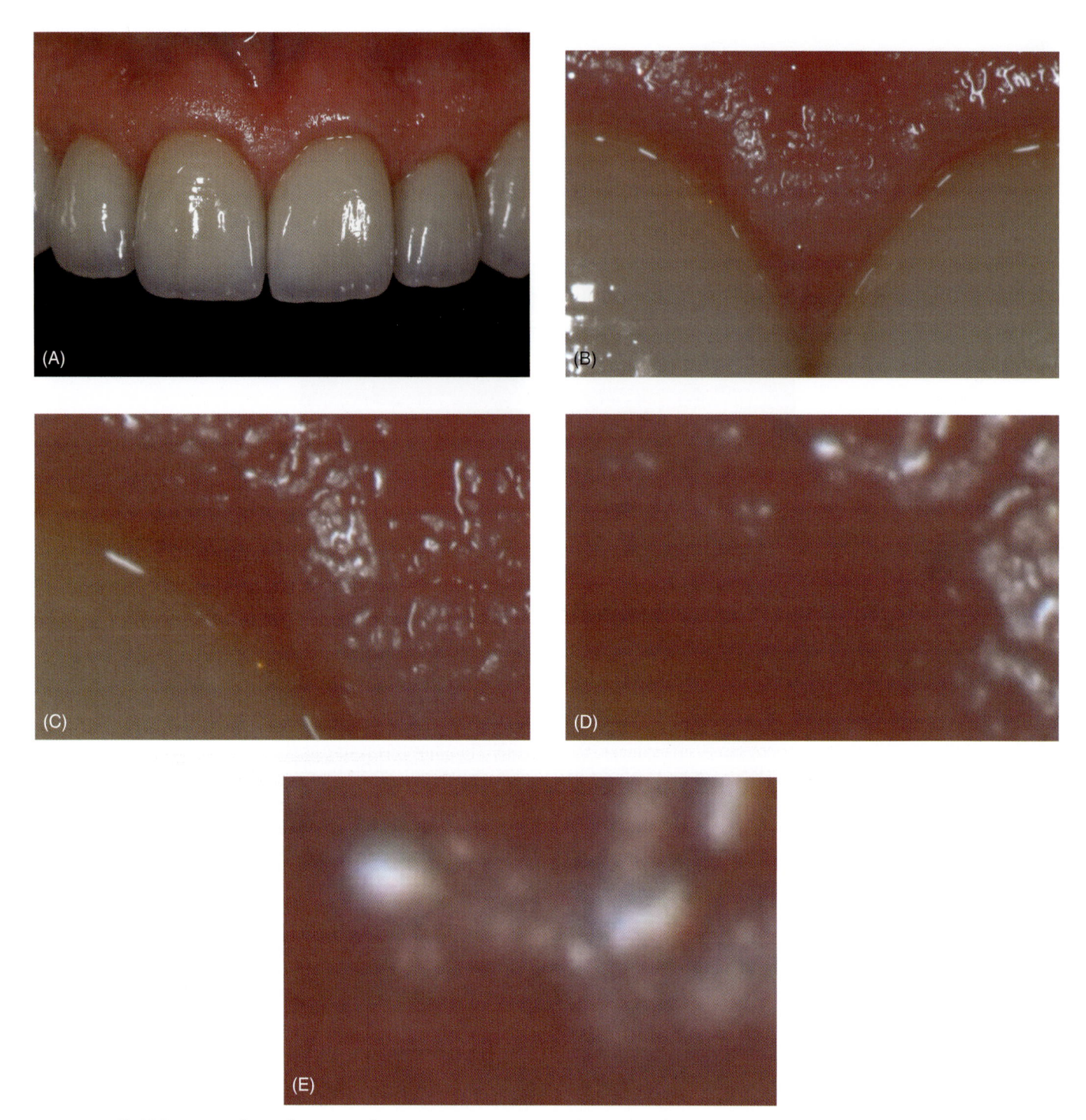

Figure 7.8 **(A–E)** Starting with a well-composed image, consecutive images demonstrate how pixels can become more apparent as one repeatedly zooms in. In the final image, particularly in the light areas, one can see the individual pixels very clearly.

One of the major features that virtually every SLR has is the ability to view the histogram. Discussion of the histogram will come later in this chapter; however, one can consider it a vital tool in evaluating the lighting of a captured image. Some cameras display the histogram as a small tool in the corner of the screen, whereas others allow a full screen overlay. Just like the image itself, the larger the histogram displayed, the easier it is to see and evaluate. This should be a consideration when looking at different camera models. Another component of every camera system is the ability to access and change camera settings. Some cameras make it extremely easy and others are more difficult. One should certainly evaluate a number of systems to determine which one makes them feel comfortable with its daily use.

Size/weight

Cameras come in many different sizes and weights. There isn't much to say on the subject other than one should find a camera that fits their hands comfortably. Although some camera bodies

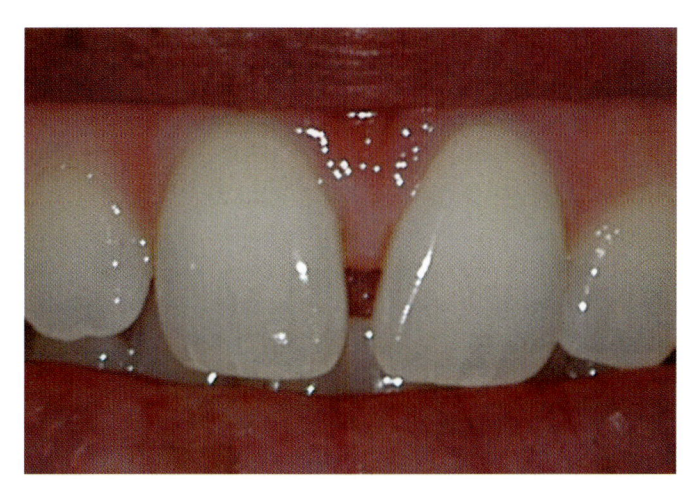

Figure 7.9 When one crops an image too much and then expands it to fit a larger area, the amount of pixels in the image may be less than the display requires. In cases such as this, the image is said to be "pixelized."

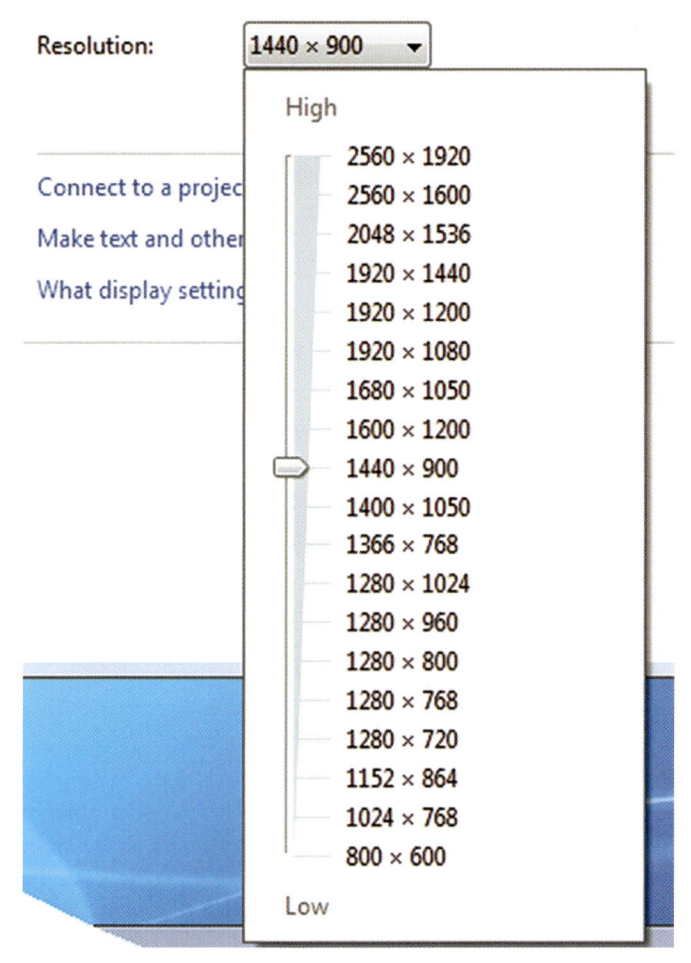

Figure 7.10 An example of different monitor resolution options offered in Microsoft Windows.

are heavier than others, before selecting based solely on the body's weight one should definitely attach the matching lens and flash first. Some camera companies produce a lighter camera, but heavier flash systems or lenses, making the overall weight greater.

If one is buying a camera to be used primarily by the staff, one should keep in mind that a camera system that feels good in the doctor's hands may not feel the same to the staff. One should certainly let the staff members pick up and handle the cameras before purchase if they will be the ones shooting most of the images.

Flashes

Flashes come in a variety of shapes and sizes. The two primary types of flashes for use in dentistry and macro photography are "point flashes" and "ring flashes" (Figure 7.12A–C). A point flash, as its name would imply, is a flash that has a single point of light to be focused in an area. Traditional older camera systems used single-point flashes that could be rotated around the lens for different directional lighting capability. With only one point of light, many shadows were produced, often obscuring vital parts of the subject. Most modern systems have solved this problem by containing at least two point flashes allowing for better lighting and more effective control of the shadows.

Ring flashes have a continuous circle of light around the lens which allows even lighting on the subject. The advantage of a ring light is its even light; however, this can also be a disadvantage. Dentists and technicians need to see appropriate shadows to truly understand the contours and shapes of teeth. Ring flashes, particularly when used from short distances, tend to "wash out" most shadows thereby creating a very "flat" surface texture. Double-point flashes do not have this problem. They provide an even light but at the same time allow a dentist to view surface texture and shapes in a way that ring flashes simply do not. There are attachments that allow users to mount flashes on a very wide or narrow mount to allow different lighting setups and angles. If one is looking to experiment with different lighting scenarios, these attachments are generally inexpensive and are worth trying; however, one should first try to use their flash system as described by the manufacturer (Figure 7.13). Another consideration in today's technological world is whether the flash is wired or electronically controlled. There are flash systems available today that send an infrared pulse to an external flash to allow it to fire without the use of any wires. Although not a major consideration, it is worth thinking about if you are concerned about wires getting in the way.

Every flash system, regardless of manufacturer, point or ring, and wired or unwired, should allow adjustment of the intensity of the flash power. This will be discussed later in this chapter and is one of the major reasons for choosing SLR cameras over other camera types. The flash should allow adjustable power settings of at least full power and a quarter of full power. Of course, the more settings, the better, but it isn't necessary.

Setting up the SLR camera

Setting up an SLR camera can seem like a daunting task; however, if one realizes that there aren't really a tremendous number of settings that we need to be worried about, it becomes much easier. The settings that one needs to consider include ISO, flash settings, image type, image quality, image size, and display mode, some of which will be discussed further here.

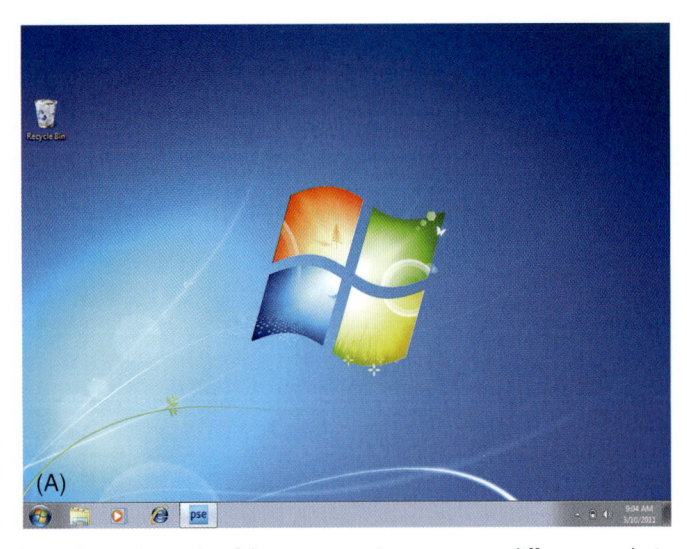

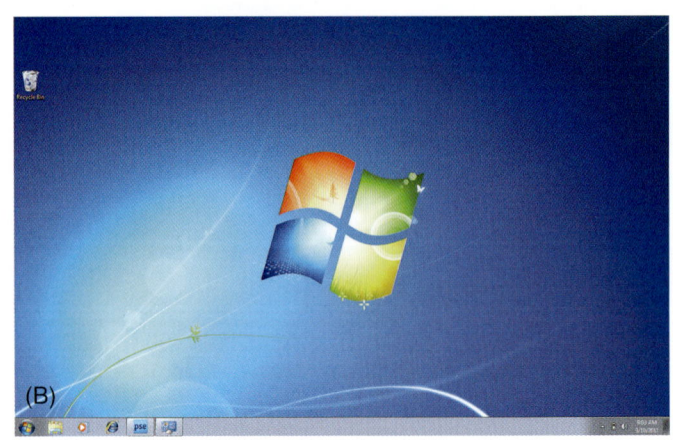

Figure 7.11 Example of the same monitor set to two different resolutions. **(A)** It is set to 1024 × 768 and **(B)** it is set to 1440 × 990. Notice how some icons become smaller (B) because their set number of pixels making up the icons take up less space on the screen with more pixels.

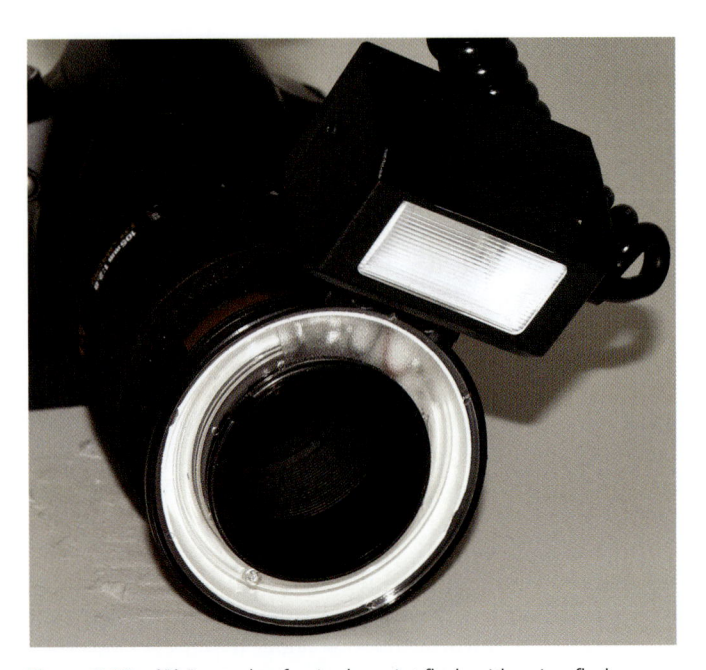

Figure 7.12 **(A)** Example of a single-point flash with a ring flash.

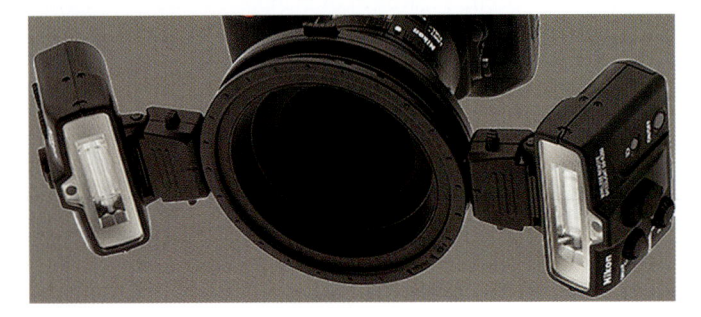

Figure 7.12 **(B)** Example of a double-point flash.

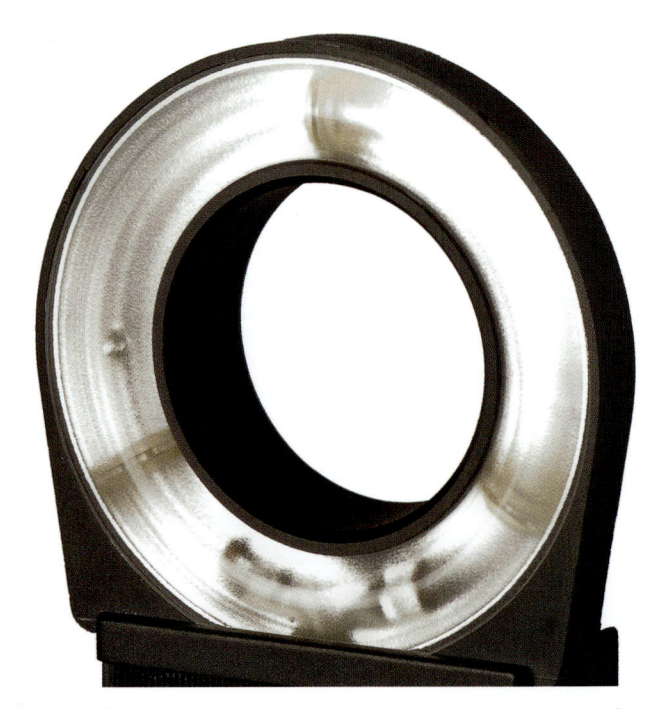

Figure 7.12 **(C)** Example of a ring flash alone. Many dentists confuse their double-point flashes with ring flashes. To be a true "ring" flash, it must be an uninterrupted circle of flash.

one might shoot ISO 3200 in a dark room such as a sporting event or a concert, ISO 100 would be perfect for shooting a bright sunny day in the park or indoors with an extremely strong flash. For dentistry, the ideal ISO is 200. This allows a proper balance between flash and lighting for a well-lit image.

Image types

There are generally three choices of image type on most SLR cameras. They are RAW, TIFF, and JPEG. A good way to compare the differences in these three image files is to think of three options of preparing a pizza. The first option is homemade from

ISO

ISO refers to the camera sensor's sensitivity to light. The higher the number, the greater the sensitivity. For instance, an ISO of 100 is far less sensitive to light than an ISO of 3200. Although

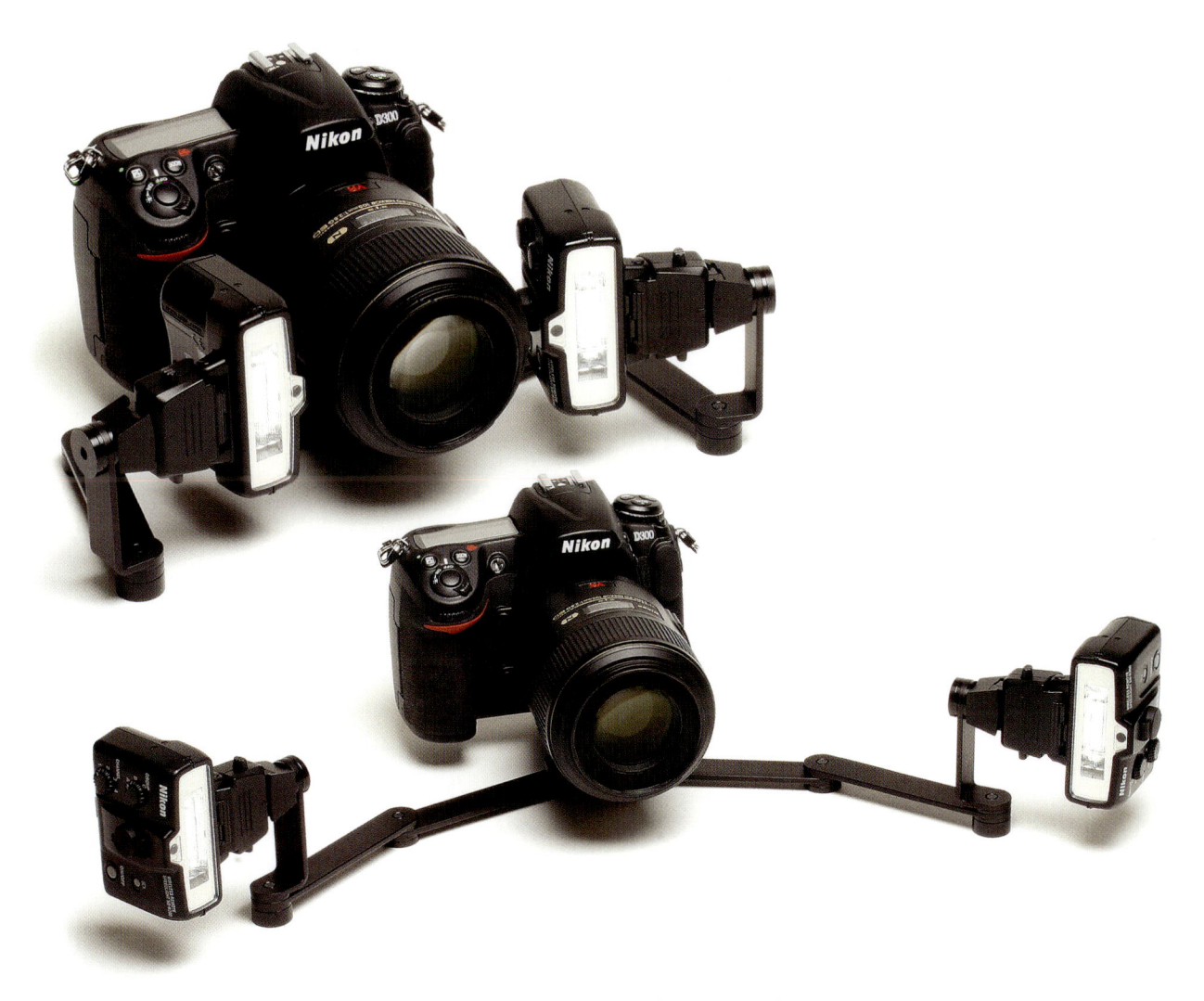

Figure 7.13 An example of a camera attachment which allows multiple positions for the macro flash. Moving the flash away from the lens makes it more difficult to control lighting, but it rewards the photographer with better shadows and highlights for diagnostic purposes.

scratch which produces the best quality but is the most time-consuming and difficult. This is like the RAW image which gives the photographer full control over every aspect of the image but requires a tremendous amount of time and expertise, which is not what most dentists need for everyday clinical practice. The second pizza option is one with premade commercial crust and sauce and with options to choose cheese and toppings. This is comparable to the TIFF image which requires less time and management than a RAW image, but still offers a good-quality image. Unfortunately many cameras manufactured today do not include TIFF as an option. The third option is the quickest and easiest: order a pizza to be delivered. This is equivalent to the JPEG image which is suitable for dentists in everyday use and requires less space on the hard drive. The JPEG with a large/fine setting gives the dentist enough information to display any image on a monitor or screen. If one wants to use the images for commerial publication or enlarge to poster size, JPEG files present a bit of a challenge. However, there are software programs that can convert JPEGs for publication or enlargement. For most dentists, a JPEG image is fine.

Through the lens versus aperture priority

Through the lens (TTL) is a setting available on almost any SLR digital camera. It was designed to allow the camera's metering system to make most of the decisions related to settings rather than leaving it to the photographer. TTL does work beautifully in many settings; however, the extreme images of dentistry which include only two to three colors (white, black, and pink) from 15 cm away is something that confounds most TTL systems. Camera manufacturers have consistently produced better and better systems for helping photographers; however, none of them are yet to match the photographer's ability with manual settings for the dental arena. As a result, the best setting on any SLR camera for dental photography is "aperture priority." To better understand what aperture priority is, one must first understand the end goal when capturing images.

One of the main advantages of an SLR camera over a point-and-shoot camera is the ability to instantly view the histogram. A histogram is a diagrammatic representation of how light entering a camera is processed by tone. The easiest way to think

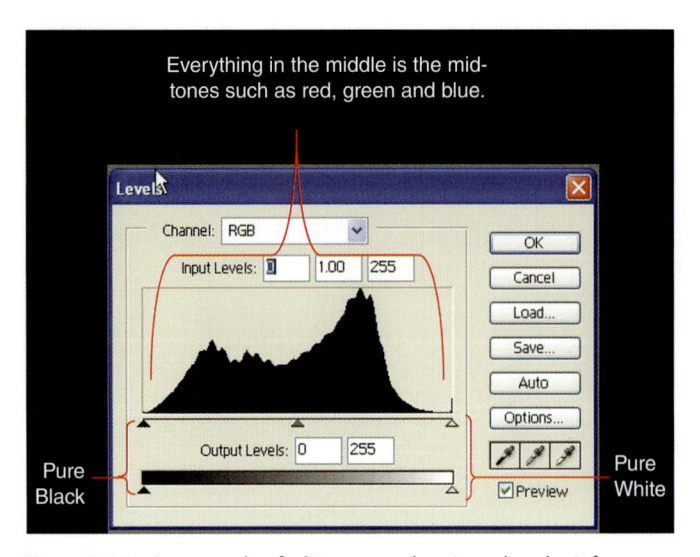

Figure 7.14 An example of a histogram showing what the information means.

of the histogram is as follows: imagine one were to visit an orchard that produced both yellow and red apples. There are millions of apples in the orchard; however, this individual is charged with the task of diagramming the exact makeup of the orchard based on the apples that are produced. Imagine further that there were 255 empty barrels lined up in a row and on the left-most barrel one placed the reddest apple from this orchard, and on the right-most barrel was placed the most yellow apple in the orchard. Every other apple in the orchard can then be graded using that left-most and right-most apples as your guide. If an apple had an equal amount of red and yellow in it, it would go in the middle barrel. Anything with slightly more red would go to the left, anything with slightly more yellow would go to the right, and so on. At the end of the day, one could count the number of apples in each barrel and chart them on a graph with the *x*-axis being the color of the apples in each barrel and the *y*-axis being the number of apples in each barrel. This would allow one the opportunity to look at a graph and immediately understand the makeup of the orchard in terms of red versus yellow apples.

A histogram is exactly the same thing as the orchard; however, instead of using red and yellow apples as the guide, the camera is using absolute black and absolute white as references, with black on the left and white on the right and all the other color combinations in between, based on lightness versus darkness (Figure 7.14).

If an image is slightly darker, meaning it has more dark pixels, the biggest broadest peak will be slightly left of center. If an image is lighter, containing more light pixels, the biggest peak will be slightly to the right of the middle. The darker an image gets, the more the biggest and broadest peak will swing to the left. The lighter an image, the more it will swing to the right. A histogram will allow a photographer the opportunity to instantly view the tonal makeup of an image by simply using that tool (Figure 7.15A–C). What does a histogram have to do with the quality of one's images? If one can master the tonal control of an image, the lighting will be perfect every time, so understanding the histogram is a key to capturing proper lighting. Although

it may seem like a daunting task, over time, understanding a histogram will be simple. If one looks at a histogram, one can tell what is in the image. For instance, notice the picture of the molar in Figure 7.16A. If one was to look at all the pixels making up this image, one could see that the general makeup of this image would be composed of cream or lighter pixels. Of course there is some blue and some brown and some gray, but the general makeup of this image is on the lighter side. It is not bright white (like the reflections on the tooth which are, in fact, bright white), but it is lighter. By looking at the histogram (Figure 7.16B), one can notice that the biggest and broadest peak is to the right side, not to the left. This is exactly what one would expect. In looking at another non-dental image, one can see a perfect balance between light and dark. In this particular image, one can notice all of the darker trees which represent the darker pixels on the left side as well as the whiter pixels that make up the snow represented on the histogram on the right side. If one understands the makeup of a histogram, one understands exactly the lighting makeup of that image.

One should attempt to shoot all clinical images with the biggest, broadest peak centered in the middle of the histogram. This means that the image has even lighting that is spread out through the entire spectrum and will meet the needs of any application for that image. If one has to err, one should err to the left, or darker side (Figure 7.17A and B). If one needs to edit the image, much more can be done with an image that is slightly darker than one that is slightly lighter. The next question then is how does one control the lighting in an image? This is done through the f-stop or aperture.

Understanding lighting

f-stop and flash settings

All SLR lenses have apertures that allow more or less light into the camera. By changing f-stop settings, one can make these apertures bigger or smaller. The bigger the aperture, the more light is allowed into the camera, and the image will appear brighter. The smaller the aperture, the less light is let into the camera and the image will appear darker. One of the more counterintuitive components of the entire camera flash system is the relationship of f-stops to aperture size. A higher f-stop (i.e., 32) actually causes the aperture to be smaller, thereby letting in less light and making the image darker. An f-stop that is lower (i.e., 3.5) will make the aperture larger thereby allowing more light. It is counterintuitive for most people because we think higher numbers allow more light and lower numbers allow less light. However, that is the exact opposite from the truth. The reason is because the f-stop represents an inverse number. An easy way to think about f-stops and the amount of light they allow is to consider it as if it were sunscreen.

If one were to go out into bright sunlight and was afraid of burning, one would put on a high SPF sunscreen (i.e., 50). If one were to go into a slightly darker, cloudy day, one might use a lower SPF (i.e., 8). Remember that one should treat their f-stop in the same way. When more light is present, the higher of an

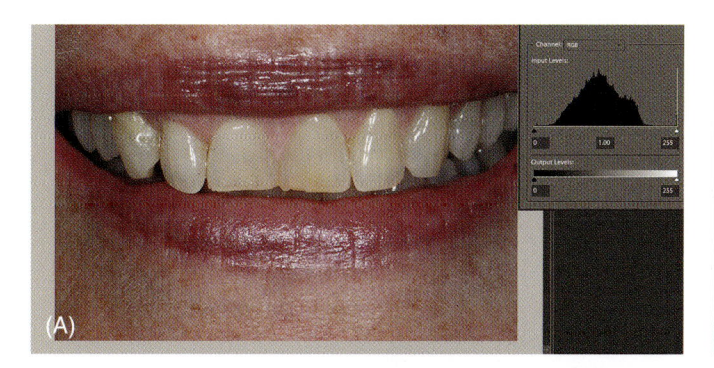

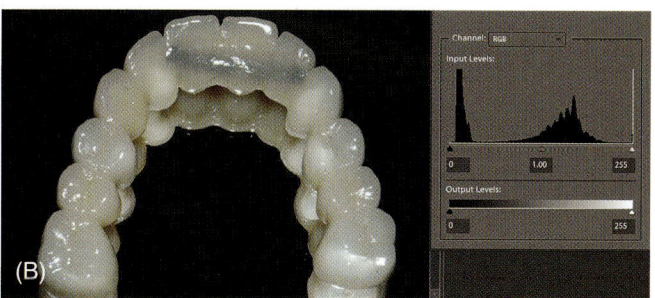

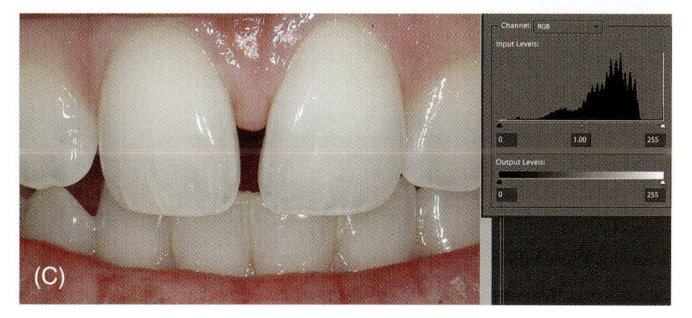

Figure 7.15 (A–C) Examples of different images and their corresponding histograms. Examine the images and note what colors within the images create each of the peaks. Every single pixel is properly represented by its histogram.

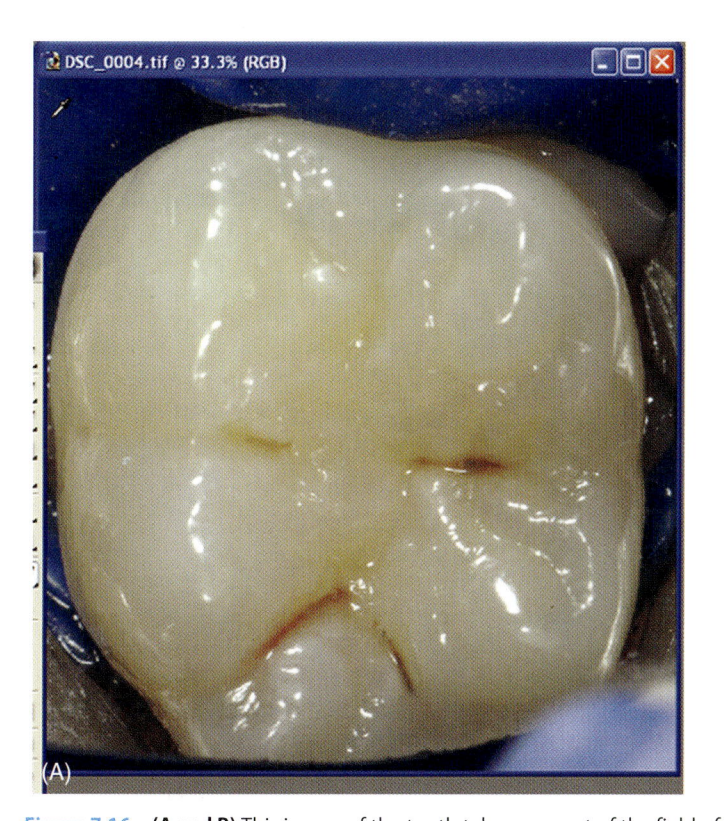

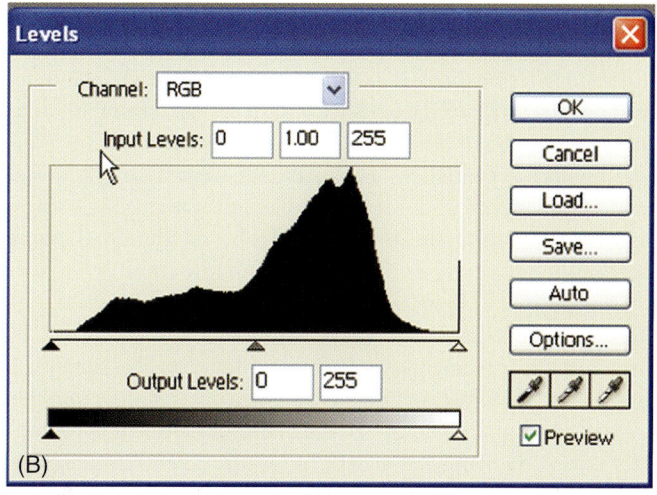

Figure 7.16 (A and B) This image of the tooth takes up most of the field of view. The tooth is not pure white, but rather an "off white." Notice how the largest and broadest peak in the histogram is found in an area that is representative of this tonal makeup. The skinny peak on the right side of the histogram represents the light reflecting off of the tooth.

f-stop one should use. The lower the amount of light available, the lower the f-stop should be. It takes a little bit of time to understand this concept, but once mastered will allow ideal control over lighting every time.

Another component to mastering ideal lighting is understanding flash settings. Once again, this is an area that almost no point-and-shoot cameras allow, but it is critical for perfect images every time. An effective flash system for dental photography

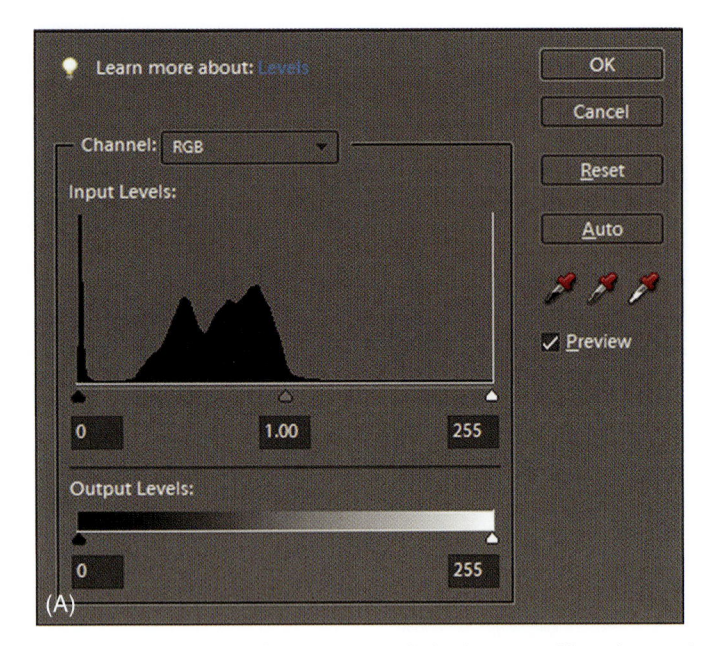

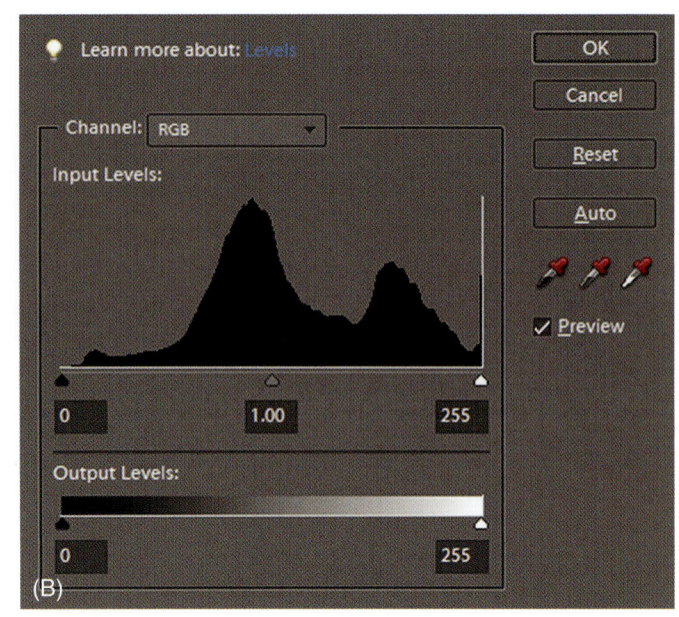

Figure 7.17 Examples of histograms with the largest and broadest peak centered (**A**) and to the left (darker side) of midline (**B**).

should allow at least three settings: M(1/1), 1/4, and 1/32. This allows the clinician to manipulate the lighting through the flash. Obviously the higher the setting, the more light the flash will supply. The reason why the amount of lighting matters is, because it will work with the f-stop to allow ideal depth of field. A greater depth of field means that more of the image will be in focus. A smaller depth of field means that only a short distance of the image is in focus.

The key to f-stops is the following: the higher the f-stop, the greater the depth of field. The lower the f-stop, the smaller the depth of field. Because of this, a clinician wants to shoot as high an f-stop as possible in almost all dental settings so that as much of the image is in focus as possible. It reduces the chance of an out-of-focus image and allows viewers to see everything in focus rather than some of it in focus and some of it out of focus. How does one achieve this? By using a higher flash setting, it forces one to use a higher f-stop setting (to let in less light). By using a higher f-stop setting, the depth of field is better, thereby allowing more of the image to be in focus (Figure 7.18A and B).

Consider the following: to achieve a centered histogram, one might be able to shoot an image with 1/1 (the most flash). By throwing out a tremendous amount of light on the subject, it would force the clinician to turn the f-stop up as high as possible to let in less light. In doing so, the depth of field will automatically adjust, allowing the dentist to capture a central incisor all the way back to a second molar in focus at the same time with a beautiful histogram. However, one could also capture a broad, centered histogram with a lesser amount of light (i.e., 1/32) and a very low f-stop (i.e., 3.5) allowing a beautiful histogram with very little depth of field. The histogram is an excellent tool for allowing one to understand the lighting, but understanding f-stops and flash settings allows a clinician the opportunity to fine tune the depth of field, which is one of the most important features. The whole concept of histograms, f-stops, and depth of field can be daunting to someone who is not used to it. However, realize that there is a way to capture the ideal lighting every time while taking into account all of these important factors.

Create a quick-reference settings checklist

It is very helpful and efficient to create a quick-reference sheet of settings for the clinic (Figure 7.19). This is easy and should only take about 30 minutes. Start by placing fresh batteries into a camera, seating a patient in a chair, and shooting an image of their face with a full flash and a medium-range f-stop such as 14. Look at the histogram and evaluate where the broadest peak falls relative to the center of the screen. If the histogram is to the right of center, one has an image that is too bright. As a result, one must turn up the f-stop to the next number and reshoot the image. If the image is still too bright, turn the f-stop up again continuing this process until the histogram is centered.

If the histogram is too dark, or to the left, one could turn the f-stop down continuously until the histogram was finally in center. If there are fresh batteries in the camera, one can write down the flash setting and f-stop for the full-face image and use that setting for every other full-face image taken in the practice. Generally speaking, the overwhelming majority of patients will fit into this flash setting. However, should there be an anomaly and one needs to make an adjustment, it is as simple as turning the f-stop up or down one stop to accommodate the histogram that did not fit the proper criteria. If a clinician goes one step further and shoots every one of their possible images with an ideal histogram, recording the f-stop and flash setting, this valuable quick-reference sheet can be used for every image in the dental setting. One need not "reinvent the wheel" every time an image needs to be taken. It is a good idea to create a reference list

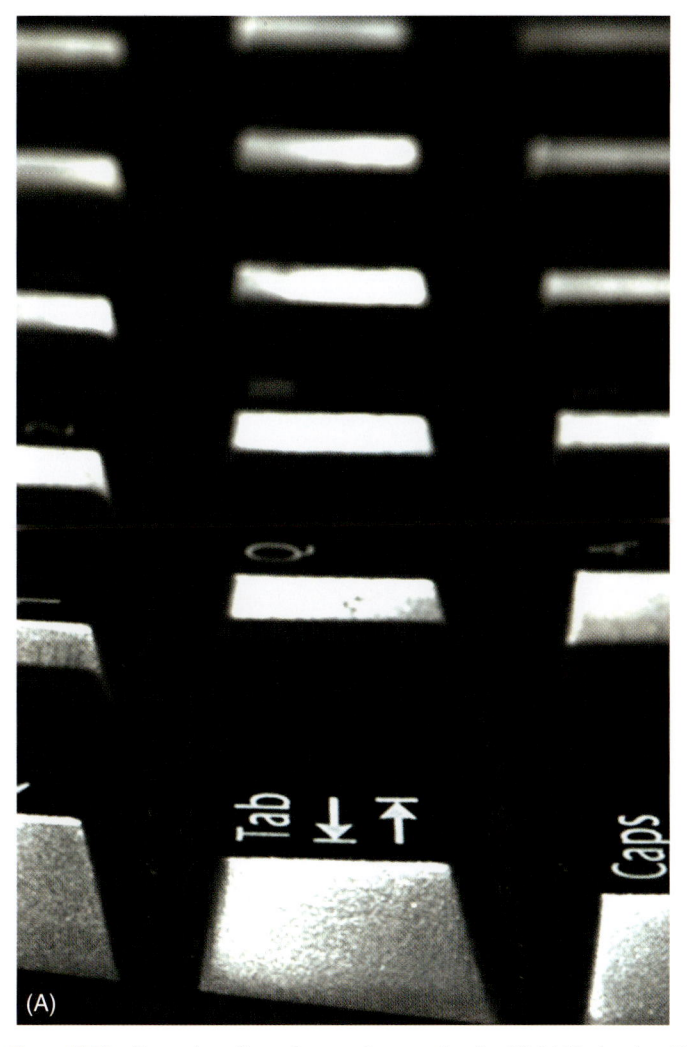

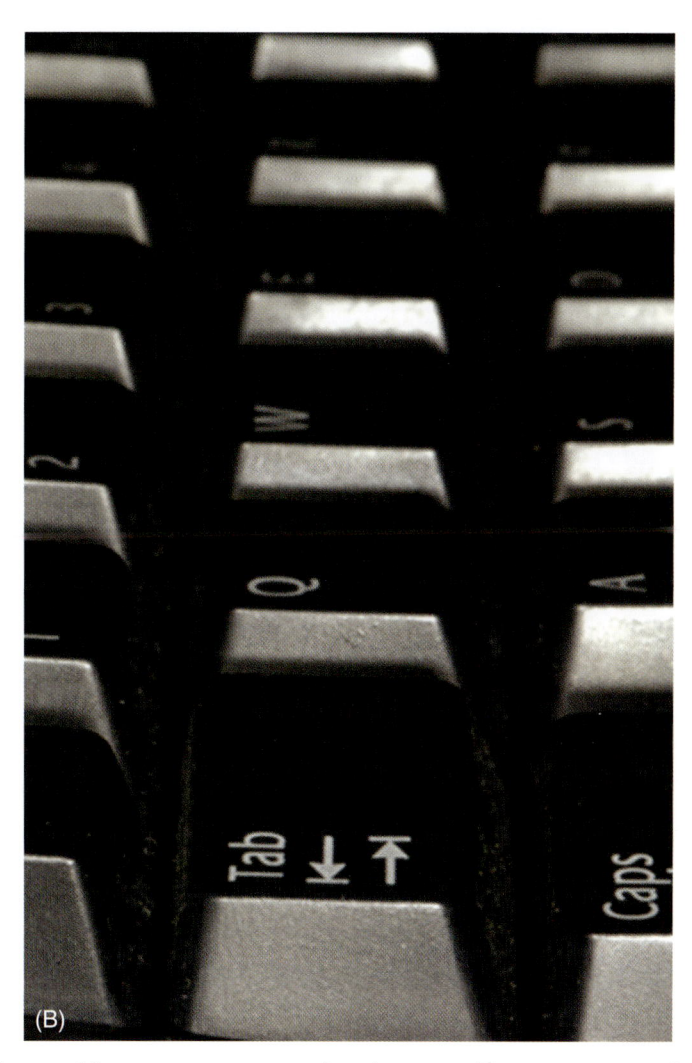

Figure 7.18 Examples of how f-stop relates to depth of field. Notice the difference of focus as one moves away from the camera. Images were captured with a very low f-stop (**A**) and with a very high f-stop (**B**), allowing a much greater depth of field in the latter where many more keys are in focus..

of appropriate camera settings for each image, print it on bright-colored paper, and laminate it. Then the dentist need only glance at this sheet for each image, set the camera, and take the image. This particular setup will work almost every time for every image regardless of the patient variability. If the images are not producing well using these settings, it is probably because the batteries in the flash are beginning to weaken and they should be changed. Although understanding histograms, depth of field, and f-stops can be somewhat challenging to most clinicians, once mastered, the dentist will never have to worry about lighting again, and the advantages of aperture priority over TTL will become apparent.

Other necessary equipment

There are two basic pieces of equipment, aside from the camera, that clinicians need to capture an ideal set of images: mirrors and retractors.

Mirrors

To capture a full arch or lateral image, one cannot fit the camera in a patient's mouth. Nor can one retract the lips to the point where an ideal image can be captured without the use of mirrors or retractors. Mirrors come in a variety of shapes and sizes as well as different coatings. The three most common coatings available today are chromium, titanium, and rhodium. All three offer advantages and disadvantages with rhodium being the most commonly and longest used mirrors of the three.

Mirrors come in a variety of shapes and sizes. Some are designed for lateral arch images, others for maxillary or mandibular arches, and others for lingual or palatal shots. Regardless of the application, one of the most common mistakes for novice photographers is to use a mirror that is too small (Figure 7.20A and B). Because newer clinical photographers are afraid of causing discomfort to the patient, smaller mirrors are generally chosen which do not allow the entire subject matter to be

Approximate Starting Points for Flash and f-stops

Type of Image	Flash setting	f-stop	Magnification
Full Face (smile, repose or profile)	M	14	~1:10
Smile or Repose (close up)	¼	25	1:3
Retracted (Closed or Open)	¼	32	1:2.5
Max or Mand Occlusal	¼	25	1:3
Maxillary Front 6	¼	45	1:1.8
Mandibular Front 6	¼	40	1:1.6
Lateral arch	¼	36	1:2.25
Max 6 Occl	¼	36	1:2
Mand 6 Occl	¼	36	1:1.8
2 Centrals (Characterization)	1/32	32	1:1
2 Centrals (Normal)	1/32	29	1:1
Single tooth (mirror)	¼	57	1:1

Figure 7.19 Keep a quick-reference checklist of correct camera settings to control lighting. It is important to note that different camera and flash combinations can cause many of the settings to differ from the ones in this example; however, once determined, the settings themselves will differ very little from patient to patient.

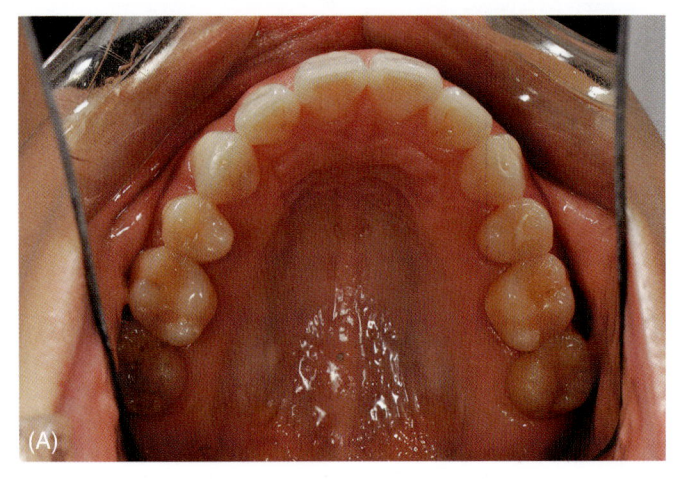

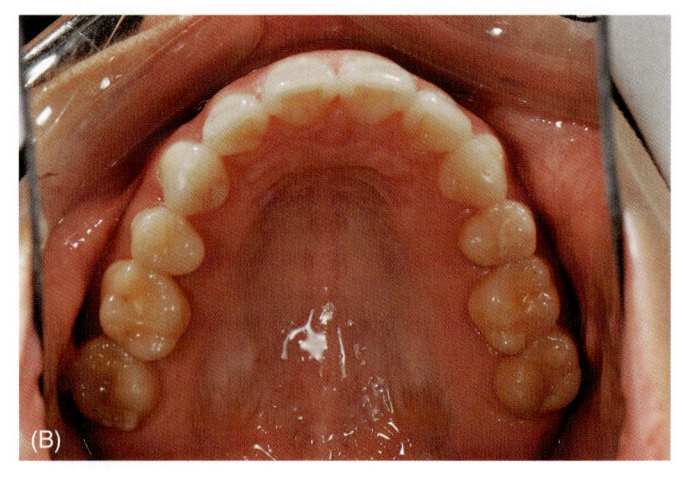

Figure 7.20 A common mistake for the clinician is to choose too small a mirror, thinking that it will be more comfortable for the patient. Notice the difference between (A) and (B), based solely on the use of a larger mirror in the second image.

reflected appropriately. A general rule that will guide most clinicians properly is to always start with the bigger mirror and attempt to use it until proven that it is too large, and then only moving to a smaller mirror.

When working with mirrors, one should have a method to avoid fogging. There are many techniques to keep the mirror from fogging and they include heating pads and solutions that are applied to the glass. However, the easiest, quickest, and most sanitary way to keep mirrors from fogging is simply to run them under hot tap water for five seconds before drying and using them (Figure 7.21). Contrary to public perception, rhodium mirrors can be wiped down with paper towels for drying without causing damage. Lens cleaning paper and microfiber wipes are not necessary.

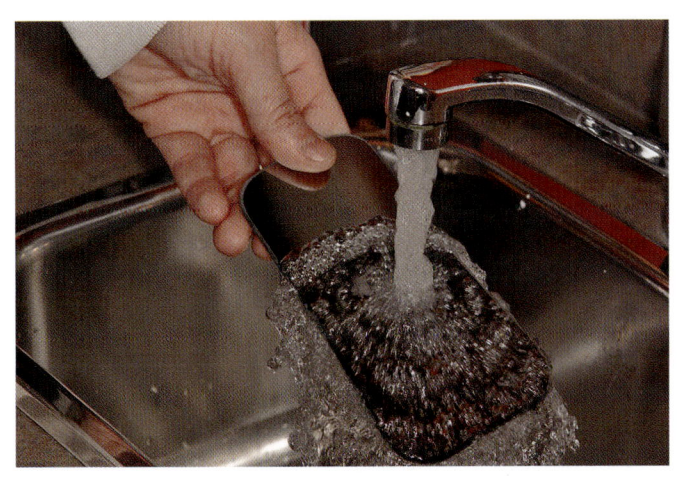

Figure 7.21 Warm running water is a great way not only to clean a mirror but also to keep it from fogging during use.

Retractors

To effectively use mirrors, retractors have been designed to keep the lips out of the way both in direct and nondirect mirrored images. Retractors can be made of either plastic or metal although it is the author's opinion that plastic offers a number of advantages. Because of the curved shape of plastic retractors, they do allow better retraction particularly in the anterior labial region. In addition, they can be shaped and cut down to match almost any clinical need which is something that metal simply cannot do. There are a variety of shapes and sizes that have been developed for retractors with each one providing advantages for certain clinical settings (Figure 7.22). Keep in mind that most retractors will become cloudy rather than clear over time with repeated autoclaving. As a result, many clinicians choose alternate disinfectant solutions like the ones used for X-ray holders. It is also important to remember that all retractors should be moistened before being placed inside the patient's mouth. It makes it easier to place a retractor and makes it a much more comfortable experience for the patient. Learning how to properly use mirrors and retractors in unison is of key importance for ideal outcomes. Although there is a learning curve associated with the clinical use of mirrors and retractors, the benefits of proper placement and angulation are immense.

Composition of images

There are dozens of standard images than one can capture depending on the proposed use of the pictures. Furthermore, many organizations mandate certain images as part of their documentation protocols. Regardless of the image needed, the following "basic set" of images, made up of 11 individual shots, will allow any clinician to develop the skills necessary to meet any future needs. This protocol includes the following images: full-face smile, full-face repose, full-face profile, close-up smile, close-up repose, retracted closed, retracted open, left lateral, right lateral, maxillary arch, and mandibular arch (Figure 7.23A–K).

Full-face smile

The purpose of this particular image is to view the entire face and to evaluate the soft and hard tissue and their harmony. The image should include everything from slightly below the chin to above the top of the head. The ears are an excellent guide for how far away one should stand (Figure 7.24). One should attempt to capture the width of the head by leaving a little bit of background space to the left and right of the ears. That will put one in a perfect position to better capture the face in the proper magnification. The patient should be standing for this image rather than seated as it makes it much easier for the dentist to capture what is necessary. If the patient is taller or shorter than the dentist, one should not use any step stool or ladder for either the patient or the dentist. Numerous accidents have been reported by patients standing on foot stools or doctors who have slipped off of them.

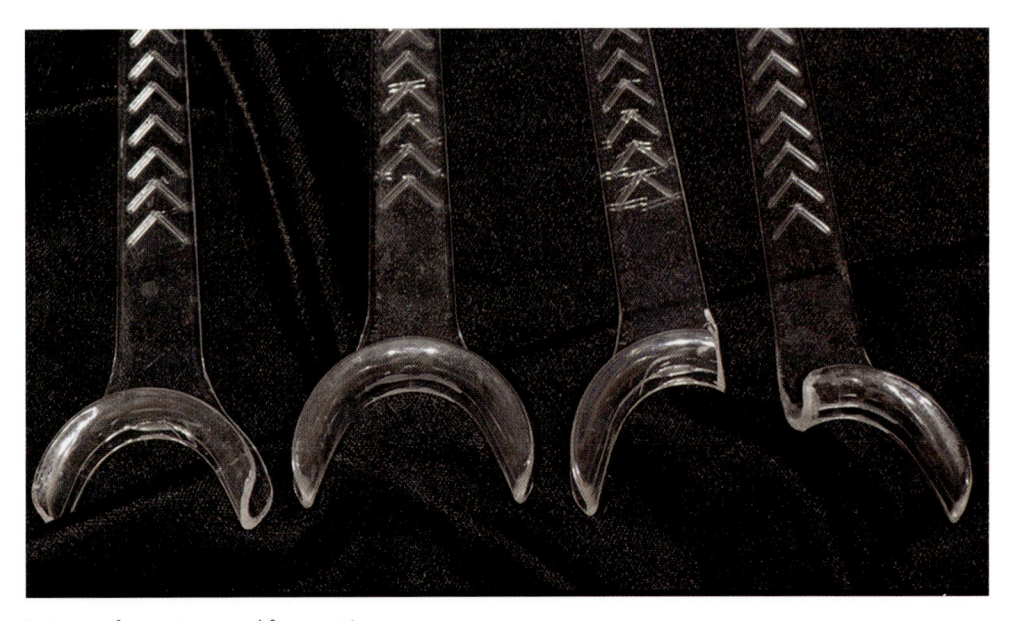

Figure 7.22 The basic types of retractors used for most images.

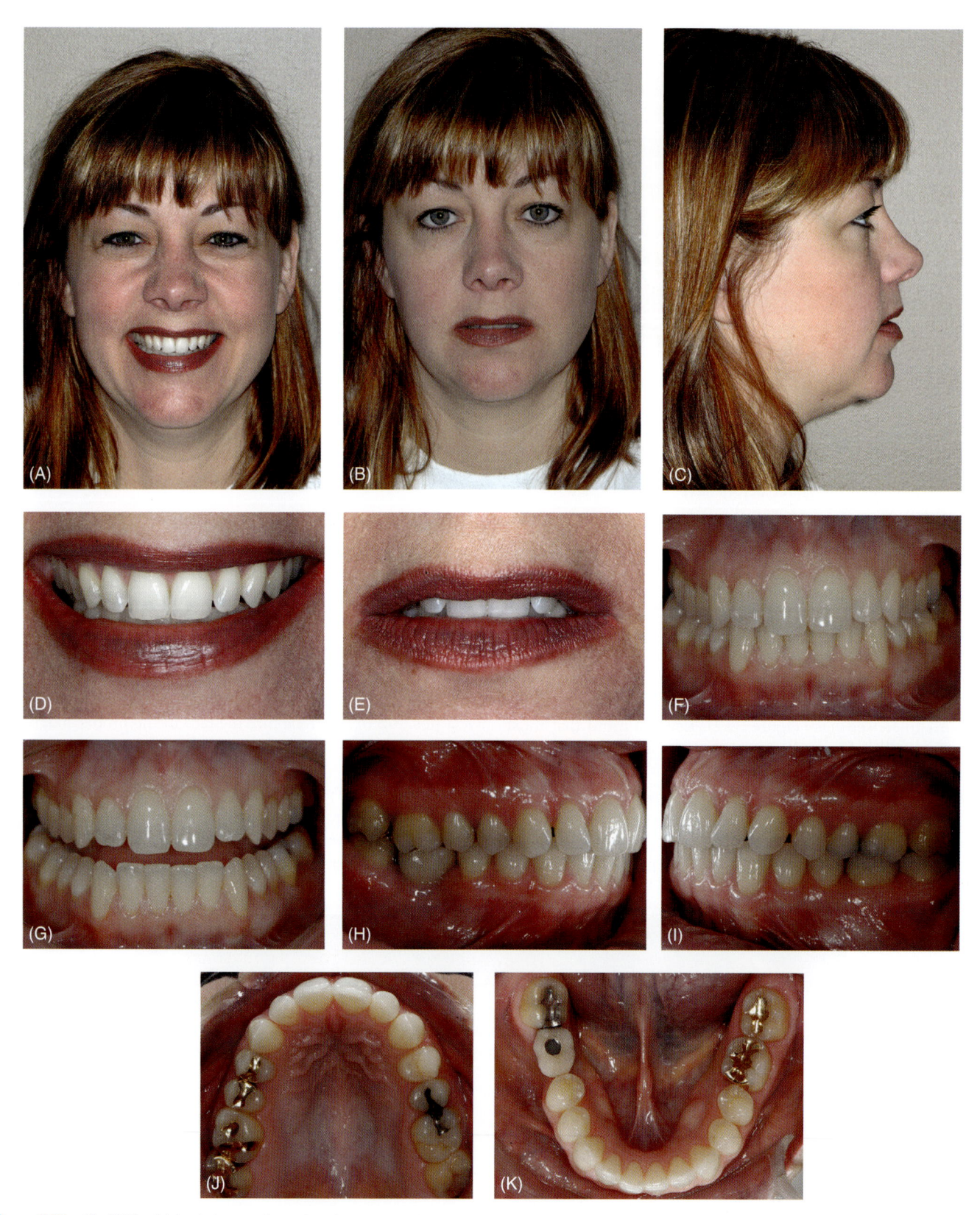

Figure 7.23 (A–K) The 11 basic images in composite.

It is far easier for both the patient and the doctor to be standing and one of them to adjust ever so slightly for a few seconds to capture the image. It is safe, effective, and consistent. The camera should be held vertically rather than horizontally because it will mimic the shape of most heads, which are elongated and not wide. Hair should be tucked behind the ears to view them as part of our landmarks. Glasses should be off, and distracting earrings should be removed. The patient should hold their head as

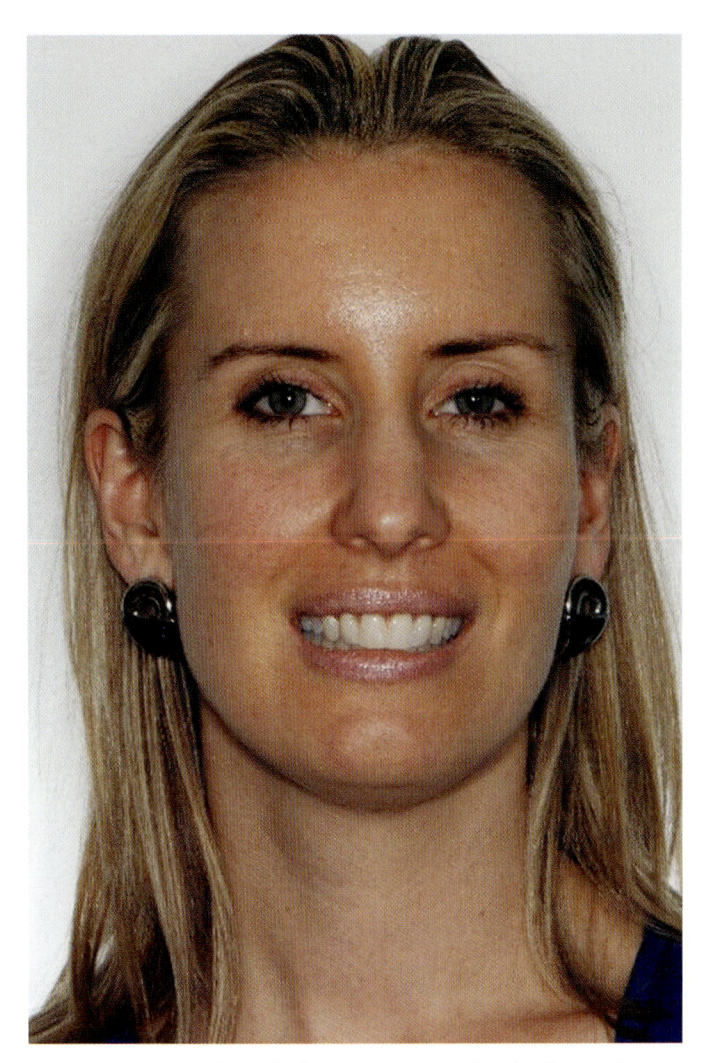

Figure 7.24 Notice how the face is not centered in the frame. The ears are an excellent way of judging how the patient should be positioned. This patient is also turned slightly to her left and this is also demonstrated very nicely by looking at the ear display. It is important to look at the patient, not through the camera, after capturing the image to determine whether the image accurately represents the patient or if there is some sort of misrepresentation caused by poor positioning.

straight as possible and should not smile until told to directly before capturing the image. Otherwise the smile may not come across as natural.

Full-face repose

The full-face repose image should be captured with exactly the same magnification as the full-face smiling image. Nothing should be changed in terms of settings, and both the dentist and patient should be standing exactly where they were for the full-face smile. The only difference between the full-face smile and full-face repose is that we need to see incisal edge at repose. To do so, have the patient say the name "Emma" and then relax. This will allow a very comfortable incisal edge repose. One can also simply have the patient lick the teeth to allow the teeth to fall into repose. Nonetheless, no matter what method is chosen, all settings and distances should be exactly the same as the full-face smile. It is for this reason that autofocus is never recommended. When one presses the shutter release button on a camera, the camera will automatically try to autofocus for a moment. If one has changed the distance slightly between the subject and photographer, the image will now reflect that, and the full-face images will not be taken from the same distances. For this reason autofocus should always be turned off.

Full-face profile

The goal of this image is to capture the profile on either smile or repose. It is completely at the discretion of the clinician depending on personal preference. The full-face profile image should be set up exactly like the first two images; however, the patient merely turns to his or her left or right side. This can be taken as a smile or as a repose depending upon the needs of the clinician. But once again, the distances in camera settings are identical as the first two full-face images.

Close-up smile

The next image is the close-up smile. The goal of this image is to view the teeth and lips and their relation to one another. There is no reason to include the nose or chin because they are already present in the full-face images. The patient should now be seated in a dental chair with the head against the headrest to minimize movement. Sunglasses should be placed on the patient to avoid over exposure to the eyes. Unlike the full-face images, the camera is now held horizontally. The shooting goal of this image is to capture a full smile from one corner of lip to the other corner of lip with a little bit of space on each side. The way to do this is to have the patient smile as big as they can while looking through the view finder. The dentist should move forward or back until the entire smile (but not much more) is seen to fit on the screen. The clinician should then adjust the lens to bring everything into focus. With the patient now relaxed, the dentist can tell the patient to smile again, being ready to capture the image shortly after the smile occurs. It is vital that if one is going to capture a smile image, let it truly be of a "natural" smile and not the one that has been held for 10 or 15 seconds (Figure 7.25A–C).

The incisal plane and lips should be captured as they are naturally. If the patient has a cant, do not correct it by adjusting the camera (Figure 7.26A and B). Remember that the goal of these images is to capture clinical information the way it is. To alter it by changing camera angles will misrepresent the patient's information and may lead the clinician down the path of incorrect diagnostic choices.

A common mistake is to have the patient's head tilted back or to have the chair reclined too far. As a result, the image will look as if it is being "shot up" at the patient and the diagnostic information will not be appropriate (Figure 7.27). Try to remain perpendicular to the patient's face thereby giving a natural view of their smile. If there is something in the image that doesn't look natural (i.e., asymmetry in the smile or buccal corridor), do not simply dismiss it as a poor shot. Evaluate the patient relative to the image to determine whether, in fact, it does accurately represent the subject.

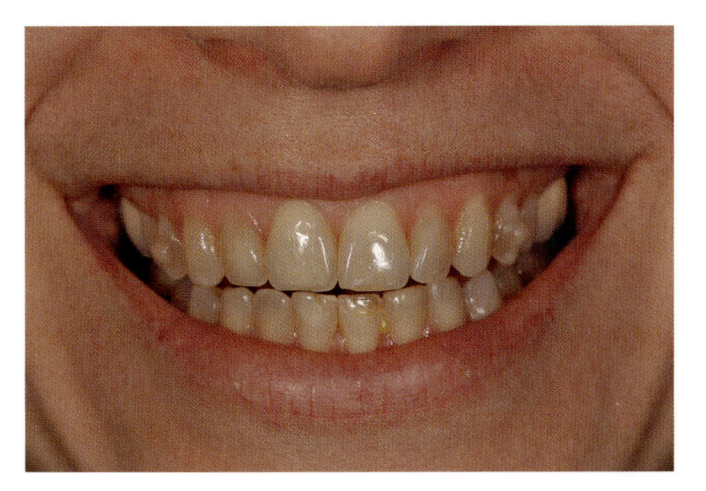

Figure 7.25 **(A)** Image of a laugh.

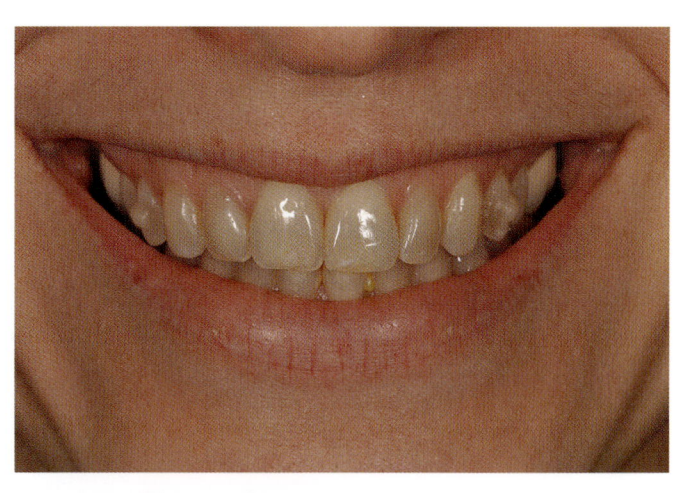

Figure 7.25 **(B)** Image of a smile.

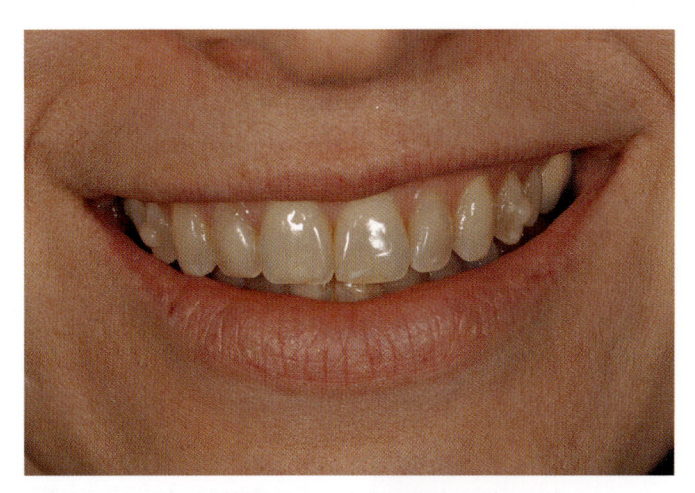

Figure 7.25 **(C)** Smile held for too long with same patient.

(A)

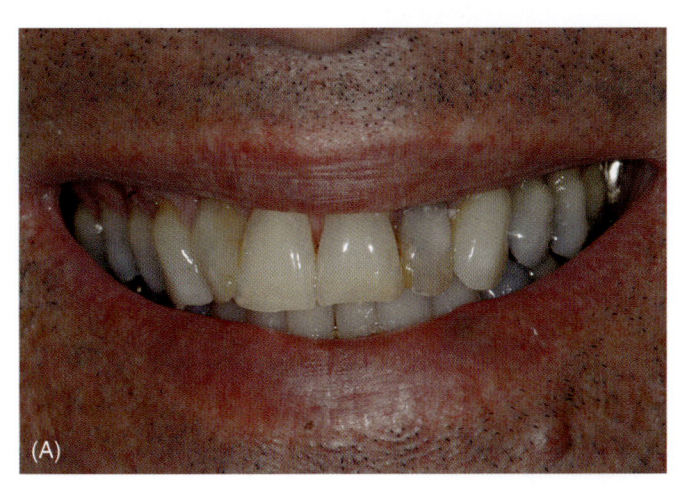

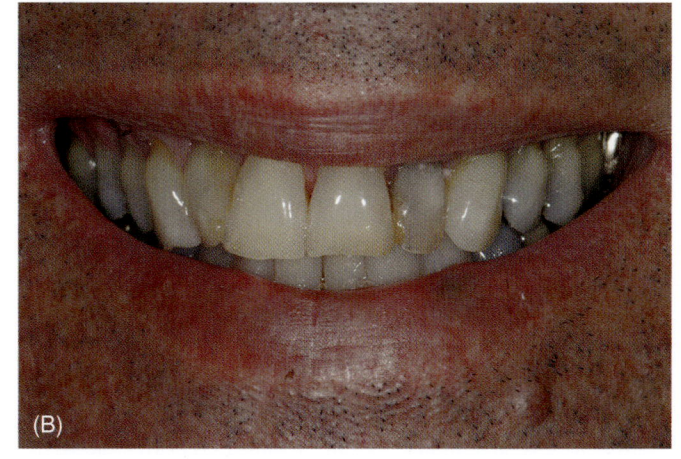

(B)

Figure 7.26 Images of a cant as found naturally **(A)** and an artificially corrected through camera rotation or software manipulation **(B)**.

Close-up repose

Just like the full-face repose image, the goal of the close-up repose image is to capture the incisal edge at rest. All settings of the previous close-up smile image are maintained for this shot. It is identical to the close-up smile with only the amount of tooth demonstrated altered. Simply have the patient go into repose exactly like the full-face repose and then capture the image. It is important to keep in mind that one must capture the close-up smile before the close-up repose for the following reason: if the close-up repose is captured first and fills the frame, when the

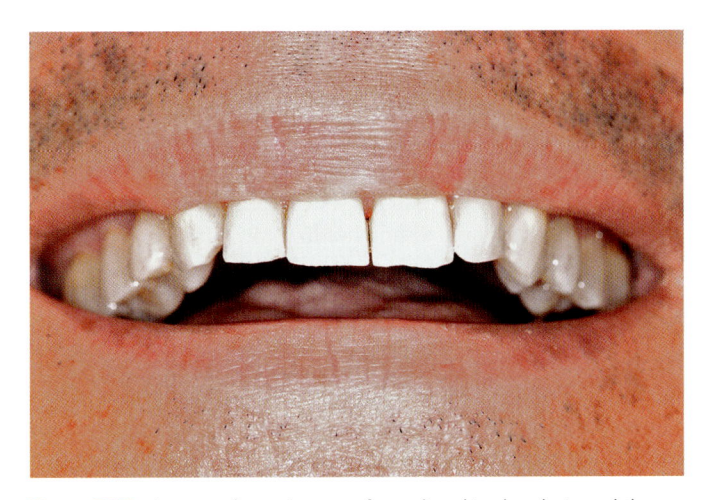

Figure 7.27 Image of a patient too far reclined in the chair and the resultant image. Notice how it looks as if one is looking up at the patient rather than straight on.

mucosa. The image should be taken straight on to the patient just like the close-up repose and smile images. Retractors should be placed in the patient's mouth and held outward and forward to move the lips out of the way. Retractor placement plays a huge role in capturing this image without the presence of lips or secondary structures.

With the patient turned slightly toward the operator and the occlusal planes seen as they present naturally, the image should be taken. The ideal image would allow second molar to second molar with everything in focus. This is where the understanding depth of field plays a vital role and why a higher f-stop really does make a difference. Traditional TTL images of this particular shot will have many teeth out of focus (Figure 7.29). Gone are the days of having to simply focus on the lateral incisors and hope that the bicuspids and molars are in focus. If the f-stop has been appropriately adjusted and lighting is correct, one can truly capture second molar to second molar in focus.

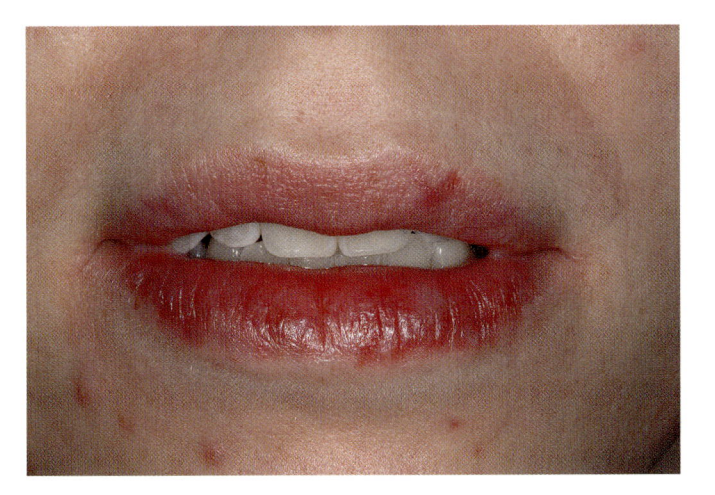

Figure 7.28 **(A)** Examples of a visible incisal edge at repose.

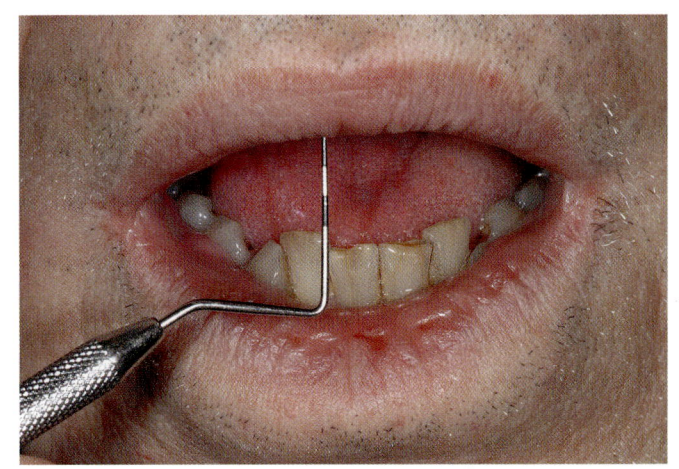

Figure 7.28 **(B)** The need to use a periodontal probe to demonstrate an incisal edge that is superior to the lip, and therefore not visible. Without a probe, one cannot determine whether the incisal edge is 1, 3, or even 8 mm above the lip at repose.

patient smiles the corners of the lips will be off of the field. Therefore, frame the full-face smile and then have the patient do the repose. There may be skin visible on the left and right of the lips in repose, but that is okay. It merely represents the difference in the facial features between smiling in repose for this particular patient.

A common issue with this image is the patient who demonstrates no visible incisal edge at repose; however, even that is relevant clinical information. One must capture this information for future evaluation. Simply have the patient in repose and place a periodontal probe on the nonvisible incisal edge. Capture the image as if it were any other close-up repose and one will be able to effectively evaluate how far above the lip the incisal edge truly rests (Figure 7.28A and B).

Retracted closed

The goal of the retracted closed image is to capture as much of the teeth, attached gingiva, and oral mucosa as possible, in focus without lips or retractors in the way. Think of capturing from second molar to second molar with all attached gingiva and oral

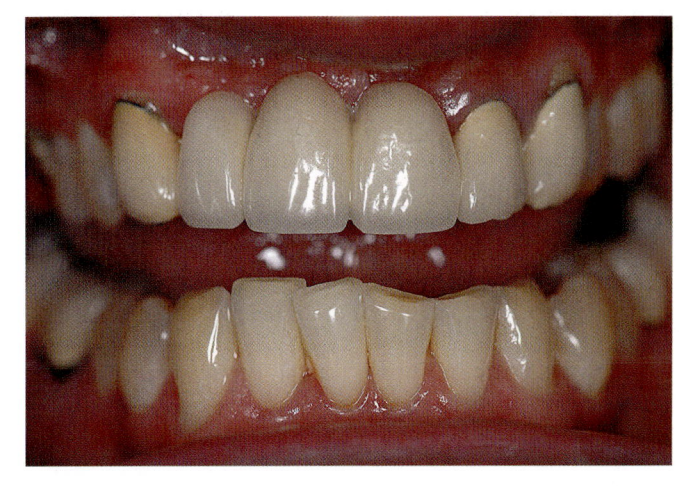

Figure 7.29 An image taken using TTL. Notice how the camera has arbitrarily chosen an f-stop that doesn't allow all of the teeth to remain in focus.

Retracted open

The retracted open is exactly the same as the retracted closed but with a goal of seeing the lower and upper incisal edges without overlap. Simply have the patient open, so that the anterior teeth clear one another by 4–6 mm and shoot the image. Looking at the lower incisal wear patterns is often the key to understanding a case (Figure 7.30A and B). The retracted open and retracted closed images should look almost identical with the exception of an open, rather than a closed mouth. One should be careful of accidentally shifting the camera either up or down to follow the opening of the jaw. It is a common mistake that can cause other vital information to be left out of the image. The easiest way to avoid this problem is to maintain the incisal edge of the maxillary teeth in the same position as in the retracted closed image (Figure 7.31A–C).

Left and right lateral

With the left lateral image, the introduction of mirrors now occurs. This is where altered retractors make a big difference. If one simply uses traditional retractors to capture an image, the tension on the lips is such that retracting the mirror for a full lateral arch view becomes very difficult. One should use a standard retractor with the tips cut off. This is placed in the contralateral side from the desired arch. A full-size retractor is placed on the side of the arch that one does want to capture. While holding both retractors, a lateral arch mirror can be placed on the side of the arch to be captured. While holding the mirror in place, the retractor on the same side is removed. The patient finds themselves holding the mirror on the side that will be captured and the smaller retractor on the side that will not be captured. This is where most doctors run into trouble. By keeping a full set of full-size retractors in the mouth, the tension is such that it is nearly impossible to capture a proper image. By removing one retractor and leaving a smaller retractor in the mouth, one will find that there is more elasticity to stretch the mirror. Furthermore, if one slides the cut-down retractor toward the midline, it will allow even more room for the mirror to be extended (Figure 7.32).

Another common mistake for novice photographers is to not stretch the patient enough (Figure 7.33). It is a valid concern that the patient is going to experience discomfort. However, most beginning photographers are amazed to find how far they can

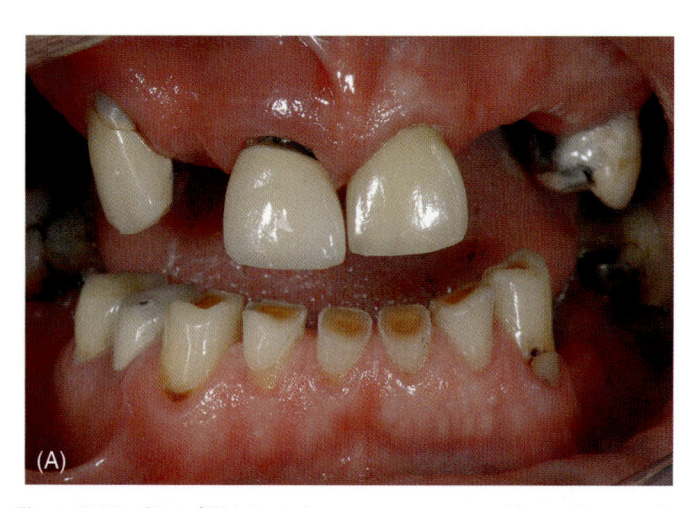

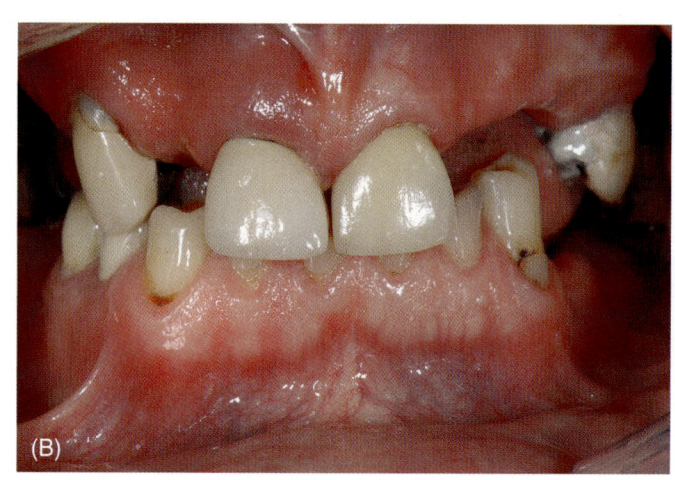

Figure 7.30 (A and B) It is vital to capture a retracted "open" image after the "closed" image. Often, vital information is not visible if only a closed image is captured.

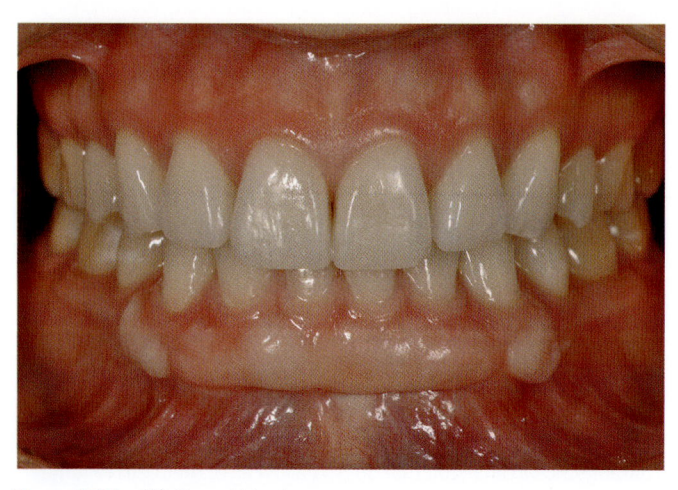

Figure 7.31 (A) Closed bite image.

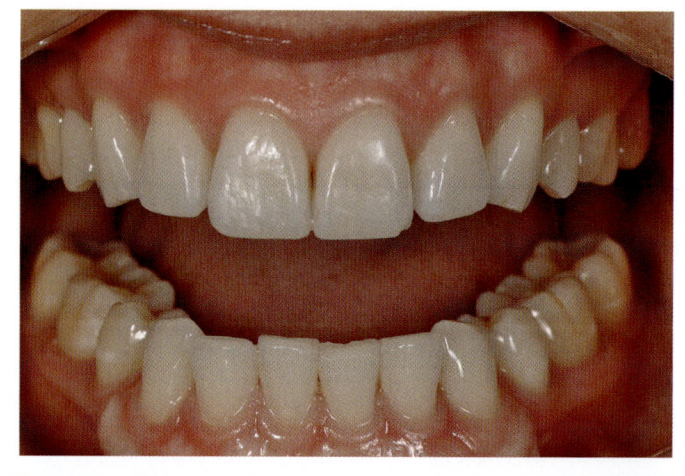

Figure 7.31 (B) Image with patient opening too wide and distorting image.

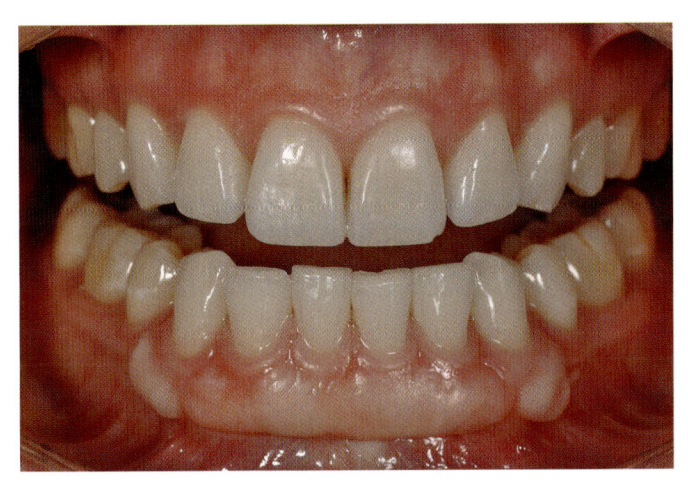

Figure 7.31 **(C)** Image captures important information below the lower central incisors missed in previous image.

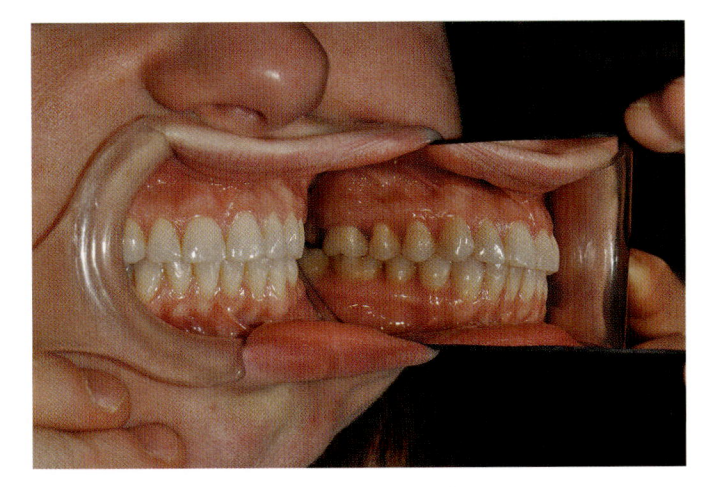

Figure 7.32 To properly capture a lateral arch image, one must not pull the contralateral retractor very far back. Ideally, one wants to move it as close to the midline as possible to reduce "pull" on the working side lips through tension. In this case, the height of concavity for the mirror is between the lateral and cuspid.

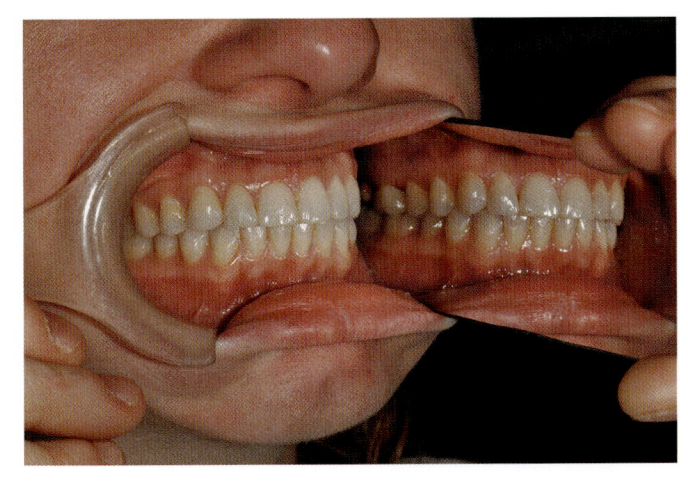

Figure 7.33 In contrast to Figure 7.32, notice how much more the contralateral retractor is being pulled, not allowing the mirror to be rotated and how misrepresented the angles classification has become.

stretch the lips with the mirror before any discomfort actually does occur. If one does not feel that they are capturing the entire image and also feels they have the proper size mirror in place, continue to stretch a little bit further and generally one will find that the patient does not feel any discomfort. As long as the distal end of the mirror is not resting on the attached gingiva, it is almost impossible to cause discomfort to the patient. Explain to the patient that they will feel tension, but not pain, and most patients will come through the process without trouble.

Of primary importance for the right and left lateral images is a proper representation of the angles/classification of the first molar and cuspids. Many dentists attempt to capture second molars with poor angulation and the images are simply useless (Figure 7.34). It is better to capture the arch from the first molar forward in the proper angles classification than it is to capture a second molar with an improper representation (Figure 7.35). Also worth noting is that after the mirror has been placed properly, one should use high-speed suction to dry the arch. Blowing air tends to create a lot of saliva over the mirror, whereas

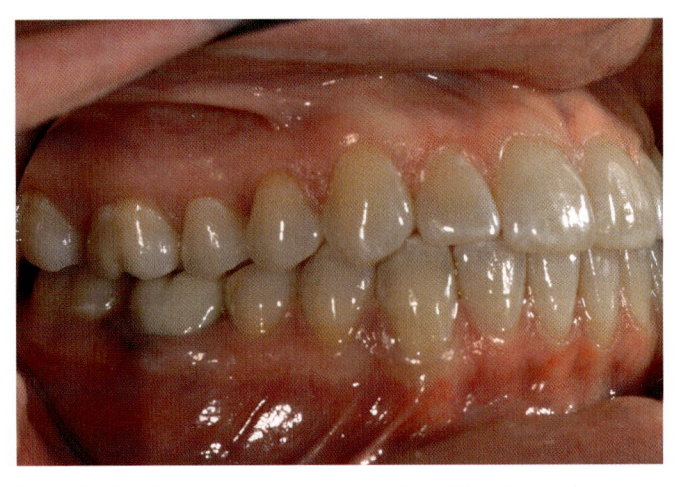

Figure 7.34 Although this image looks "clean," the clinician has captured the second molars at the expense of a misrepresented angles classification.

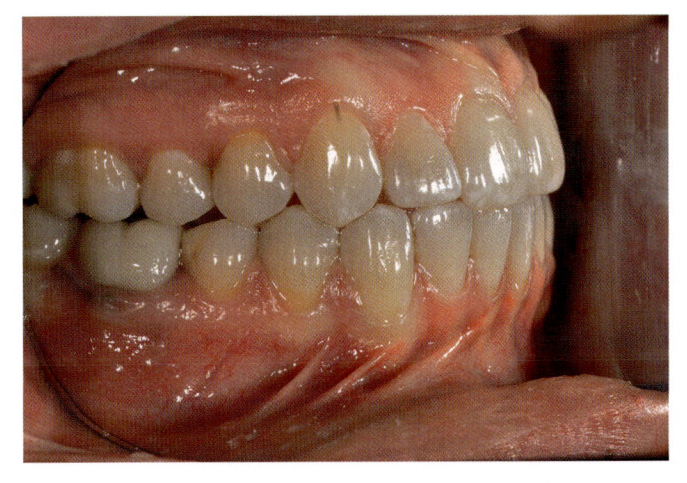

Figure 7.35 In contrast to Figure 7.34, this clinician has chosen to omit the second molar to properly position the mirror for an accurate representation of the angles relationship.

suctioning tends to dry things off. As mentioned earlier, to prevent fogging the best method is to run the mirror under hot water for a few seconds and then dry it. By doing so, the mirror will stay warm and will not fog for a period of 3–5 min, allowing the clinician to capture an ideal image without any fog.

Maxillary arch

For this image, the patient is seated flat in a chair with the dentist standing behind the patient (Figure 7.36A and B). Once again retractor and mirror use is the key for proper representation of maxillary arch. One should try to capture an image that shows all of the maxillary teeth straight on with the buccal surfaces of each tooth ever so slightly visible. The lip, nose, and retractor should be out of the way and one should only be looking at teeth and the palate. To achieve this consistently, a couple of steps should be followed: customized retractors should be used to hold only the upper lip out of the way. By using standard retractors and holding the lower lip at the same time, tension is put in places that do not allow mirrors to properly fit. By using specialized retractors, tension is released and the patient can actually open farther (Figure 7.37A and B). The patient should tip their head back after the mirror has been placed and the dentist's nose should be directly over the nose of the patient. All too often, clinicians attempt to capture this image from too far behind the patient. If this happens, the patient will appear as if they cannot open wide enough to capture an ideal image. Moving closer to the patient will assist in easier capture every time. Patients should not open fully until the operator is ready to capture the image. Having patients open for too long also makes capturing more difficult. By holding the mirror and angling it appropriately, a full arch image can be captured quickly and easily.

Mandibular arch

The final image in a standard set is the mandibular arch image. The goal is to capture all of the mandibular teeth without saliva or the tongue, or lips in the way. Unlike the maxillary arch, the clinician should be in front of the patient, not in back. By placing the split retractors on the lower lip only, tension is released from

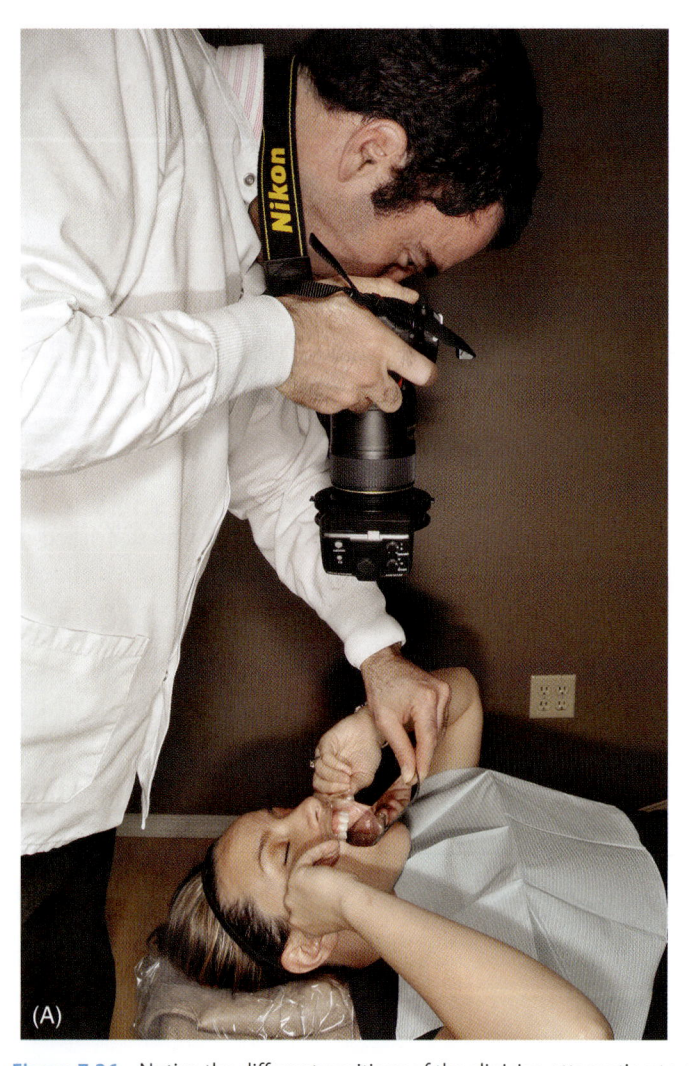

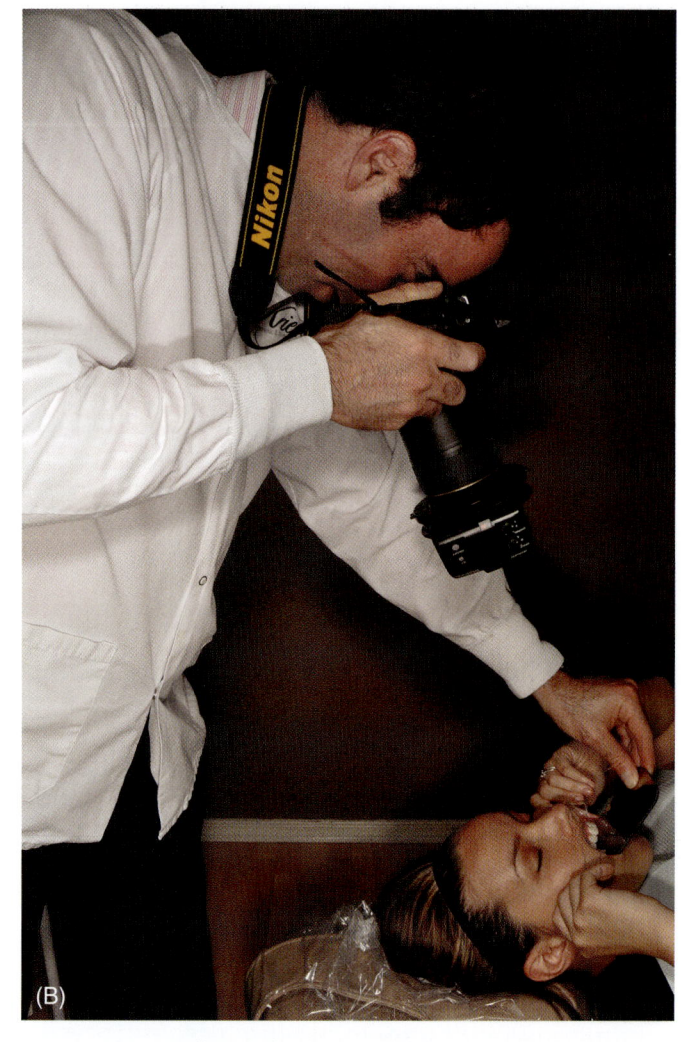

Figure 7.36 Notice the different positions of the clinician attempting to capture a proper maxillary occlusal image. **(A)** Demonstrates proper positioning where the patient's head is tilted back and the doctor's nose is directly over the patient's nose. **(B)** Very common example of improper patient positioning where the clinician's nose is behind the patient's head. It is nearly impossible to capture a proper occlusal image from this position. Most clinicians who are in this position generally feel that they cannot get the patient to open wide enough.

Figure 7.37 **(A)** The differences in using split retractors and full retractors for occlusal images are considerable.

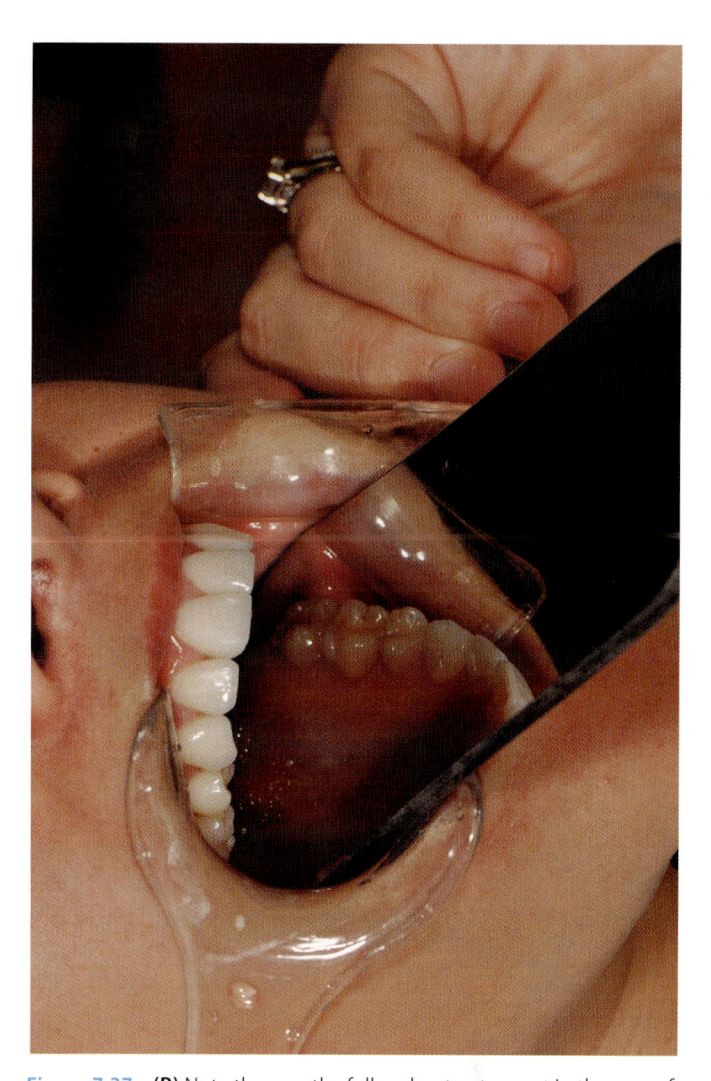

Figure 7.37 **(B)** Note the way the full-arch retractors get in the way of the mirror and stretch the lips in places not necessary to capture the image, thereby reducing opening.

the upper lip and the patient can open wider. The mirror should be placed in the mouth and the patient should be asked to place their tongue behind the mirror. The operator can then slowly and gently slide the mirror back in the mouth, keeping the tongue retracted behind it. With the head tilted back slightly and in a reclining flat position, the patient is asked to open as wide as they can and the image is captured. This will allow ideal capture every time of a mandibular arch. If one is "tongue tied," it is okay for the tongue to be in the image. However, wherever possible, having the tongue behind the mirror is preferable because it allows better visibility of the entire arch. Although there is as tongue to contend with, because the lower arch is generally smaller than the upper arch, the mandibular image is usually easier to capture than the maxillary image.

Image storage and presentation

Once images have been captured, there are many option regarding the importing, saving, and presentation of the images. This topic is a broad one which would require far more space than allotted here; however, there are a few key ideas to keep in mind when designing a digital image workflow.

Importing images

There are three basic ways in which an image can be imported to a computer. The camera can be connected to the computer via a cable and images are downloaded directly from the camera, the storage card is removed from the camera and the images are uploaded via a card reader (Figure 7.38A and B) or a wireless transmission of images can be accomplished using a variety of methods. The last method is brought with many potential technical glitches and in the author's opinion is not the most desireable way to bring images to an image server. Although it might seem easier to simply attach a wire to the camera, the correct choice is to use a card reader. Using a card reader reduces the wear on the camera, is faster, and allows the camera to be in use with another patient with an alternate card while the images are being uploaded from the first card.

Saving images

Regardless of the method used, one must give consideration to the software that will be used for editing and saving the images.

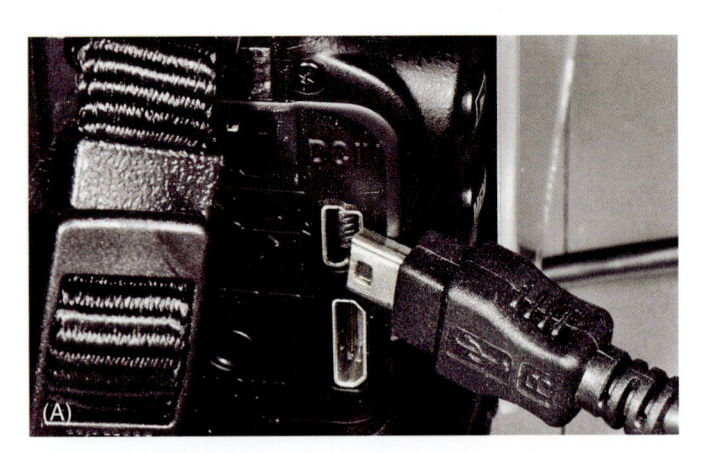

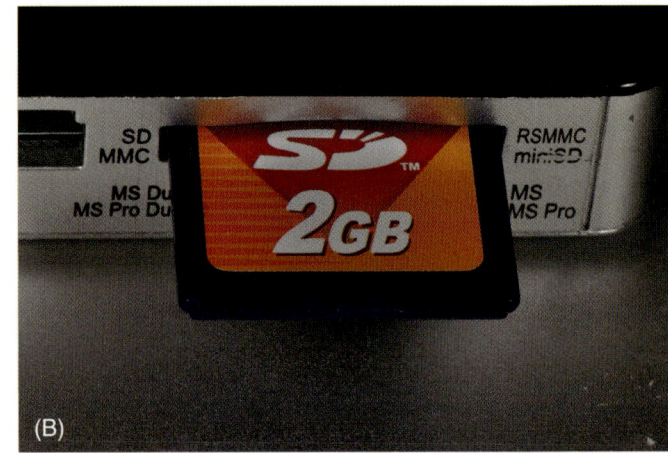

Figure 7.38 One can upload information either directly from the camera using a cable (**A**) or from the memory card using a reader (**B**).

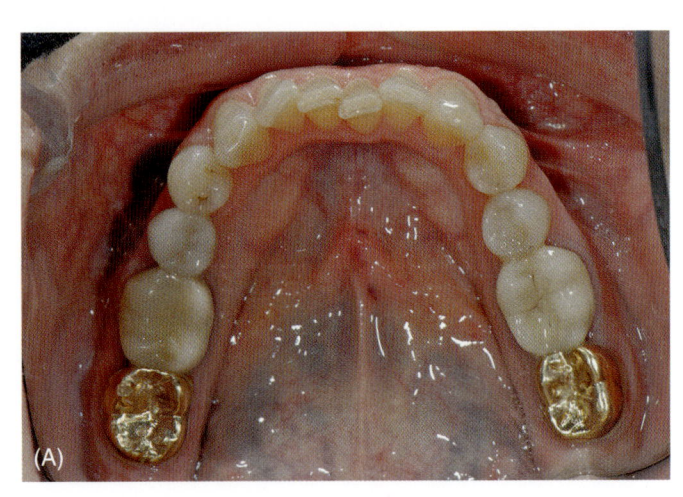

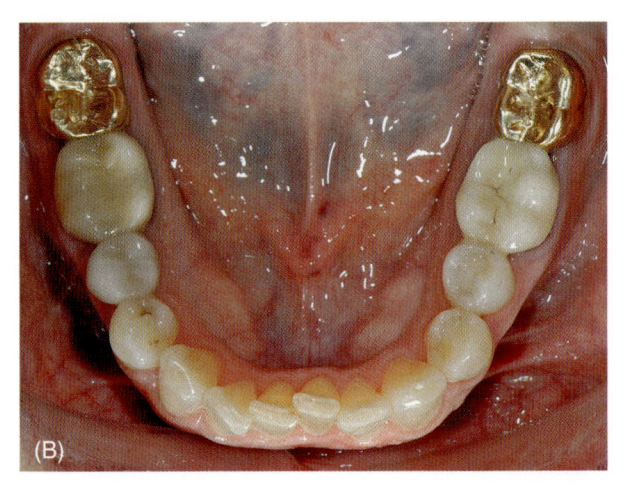

Figure 7.39 Notice the differences in the original (**A**) and edited (**B**) images. It's important to note that only "global" changes have been made (histogram adjustment, sharpening the entire image, rotating and flipping the arch) and not "regional" changes such as whitening a specific tooth or "morphing" proposed changes.

Just like an articulator needs to be cleaned before showing it to a patient, images should also be "cleaned up" before presentation (Figure 7.39A and B). There are a number of products available for this process, and clinicians need to determine which one is right for them. With programs ranging from free software that comes with a computer to programs that cost over $900 to dental software designed to work in conjunction with practice management programs, each has advantages and disadvantages. Dentists should evaluate each and every program and determine which one fits them best.

One must consider where to store images after editing. Many practice management programs allow images to become a part of the patient's chart; however, they might not allow the images to be transferred easily to another program should the office decide to change management software. Once should check with their software company to find out the limitations before making a decision.

Microsoft Windows Explorer comes free with every PC and is a built-in database management system. It allows one to easily and inexpensively (i.e., for free) store images in a format for quick access (Figure 7.40). The downside is that is doesn't integrate the images into the patient's chart, but every office needs to evaluate whether that is important.

Presenting images

There aren't many choices when it comes to presenting images. There are two main choices, and they simply depend on the operating system being used. If one is using a PC, then Microsoft PowerPoint is the proper presentation software. It is easy to learn, creates "shows" very quickly, and is very cost effective. If one is using a Mac, Keynote is the proper program. Although slightly more difficult to learn than PowerPoint, it allows more options, although most will never be used in dentistry. In the end, there is really little choice: PowerPoint for PCs, Keynote for Macs.

Video

There are many instances where video can be an excellent tool for the clinician. Unlike the static information presented by images, video allows a dynamic representation of the oral condition. Whether it's demonstration of lip dynamics while

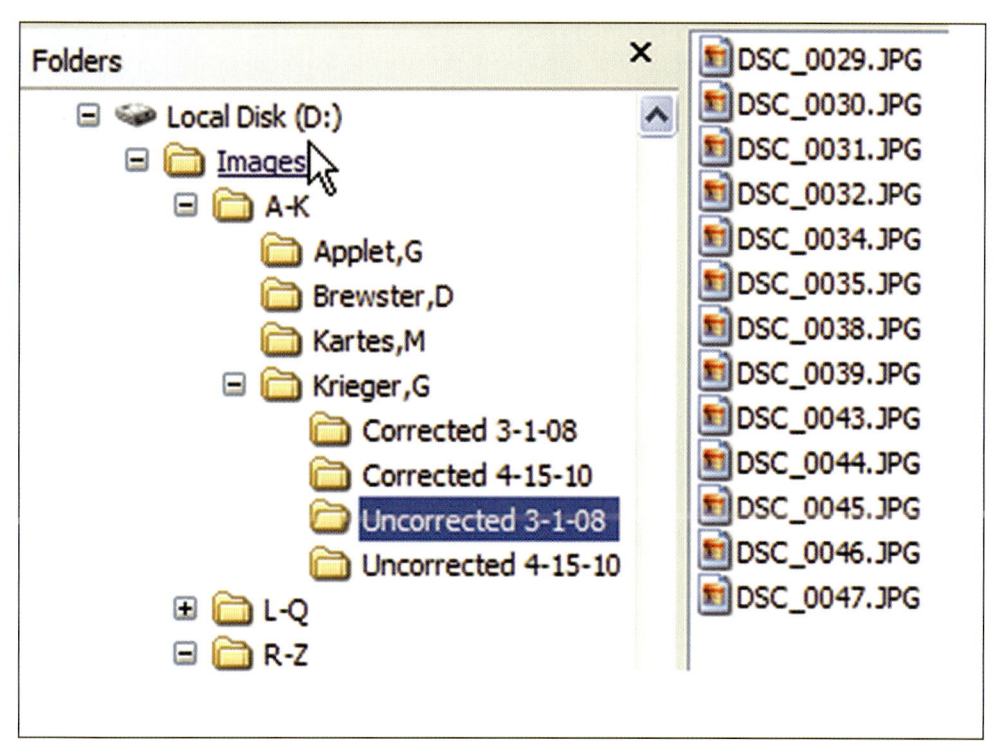

Figure 7.40 One example of database management using Windows Explorer.

speaking or smiling, or examining the facial form during function, video is an excellent way to communicate information to a laboratory or for collaboration among team members. Another excellent application for video is documentation. During the consultation, there is often so much information being exchanged between the dentist and patient that some points may be lost in the process. By capturing a video of the consultation, review of findings, and other pertinent doctor/patient discussions, one has the opportunity to archive and review the patient's exact words and gestures as they discuss goals, desires, or histories. Of course, having a video of patient discussions is always an excellent way of reviewing patient goals both during and after the treatment has been rendered. Once again, the goal is not to practice defensively, but video allows a level of protection that is not offered by any other medium, as the patient's exact words and gestures can be reviewed at any time. One does not need to spend thousands of dollars to start using video. There are many inexpensive options available today, and quality of video is not as important as photography because most video-capture devices that are in use today can offer more than enough resolution to capture what is necessary. Nonetheless, because regulations related to capture of video and audio can differ among regions, one should become familiar with their municipality's rules related to such use.

Video camera recorders (camcorders)

There are a variety of video camera recorders (camcorders) available today. They range from small, ultra-portable to large professional cameras, capable of producing exceptional-quality video. Prices can range from under $100 all the way to tens of thousands of dollars. For almost all clinicians, there is a camcorder that meets their price point. Unless a dentist is producing videos for professional purposes such as for creating DVDs or for educational use, almost any camcorder will serve; however, even for those looking for near-professional quality video, a camera to suit their needs can be purchased for far less than $1000. Advances in technology allow a $500 camcorder today to have more features and better quality than cameras 10 times their price just 5 years ago. The size of camcorders has also been significantly reduced in the past 5 years. Although helpful in terms of portability, their small size and light weight make these cameras somewhat difficult to hold still when being hand-held. It is for this reason, among others, that a tripod is always recommended when using a camcorder for clinical use. Of course, if the camera is going to be used to film a clinical procedure, having it mounted to a rigid, nonmoving system above the patient is generally the best idea. Another consideration is that many high end DSLR cameras have remarkable video capabilities. One need only switch the lens to the appropriate one for the desired effect and professional looking video can be captured. Not to be forgotten is the myriad of phones with HD video capability. Technology in the camera realm changes so frequently that it would be impossible to do justice to a review of systems, but the increase of web driven video for social media and advertising purposes means that one can quickly and easily capture simple video and post it immediately, without ever needing to use anything more than a phone.

Screen resolution and size should be taken into consideration when looking at a clinical camcorder. Like digital still cameras, most digital video cameras today have screens that are more than large enough for most users. However, screens do vary by size and the amount of pixels, and if one needs a larger screen or one with better resolution, solutions are readily available. Most camcorders being manufactured today record on microdrives or flash memory with the cost of storage being exceptionally low. Like a still camera, you need only to remove the storage media and replace it with a new one to keep recording when the card becomes full. As of right now, storage capacities are far greater than any dentist needs for clinical practice, and due to cost of storage clinicians can easily have many cards send to laboratories or collaborating clinicians. Best of all, uploading the video to a patient's digital chart is as simple as uploading a digital image. Simply connect the camera or storage device and upload.

The biggest issues facing most dentists when it comes to video capture are space and cost of good lighting systems. When it comes to lighting video, there are many more choices than simple camera-mounted lights. It is while thinking of lighting that clinicians must decide how far they are willing to go when it comes to their investment in a good lighting system. Unlike intraoral clinical photography, where the light source must be able to be directed into the mouth, limiting the choices to camera-mounted systems, videography is more like studio photography. One can set up multiple light sources around the room, each one serving a specific purpose. For instance, one could have one soft light to light the face, another to create shadows around the head and neck with a third to light up the background. For the clinician looking for this type of arrangement, it will create beautiful light once properly set up, but the cost can easily run to over $1000, and one needs a specific space with enough room to adequately position the lights, camera, and the subject. For dentists looking for simpler solutions with adequate, but reduced, quality, simple "clamp-style" lights can be used to capture all of the relevant details required for documentation and communication. These lights can generally be found for as little as $10 and are a good way to start. Don't fall into the trap of feeling that you must make this more complicated than it is. Some clinicians appreciate the "art" of video while one simply needs to remember that if the details can be visualized in the video, it is generally acceptable.

The last piece to the video puzzle is sound. Like lighting, one can make this as complicated as desired, but generally the choices fall into four basic categories: the camcorder's built-in microphone, a camcorder-mounted (shotgun) microphone, a wired microphone, or a wireless microphone. Because most clinical situations do not involve broad movement, a wireless microphone is generally not necessary and "on-board" camcorder microphones usually produce very good sound. Though generally a step up from the built-in microphone, camcorder-mounted microphones generally cost more and sound inferior to equally priced wired microphones. One can make the choice of wired microphone complicated; however, most electronic stores sell a relatively inexpensive wired microphone that will serve the needs of most clinicians quite nicely. Video is a great adjunct for the clinician who is looking for more complete documentation. However, no matter how good the quality of video, it serves as a supplement and not as a replacement for high-quality digital still photography.

Conclusion

There are many reasons why every dentist should be employing the use of clinical images on a regular basis. Using ever improving technology in today's digital cameras, capturing images has never been easier. Nonetheless, it takes time and energy to develop a system and protocol that allows the dental team to seamlessly move through the process from capture to presentation. If one approaches clinical photography like any other aspect of dental practice, with discipline and patience, it will offer a return on investment that is greater than any other tool in the office. There are many camera choices but, in the end, it is simply about picking up a camera, capturing images, and improving the patient care. Regardless of the system or program used, dentists will find that excellent images combined with good verbal skills will create a situation where patients will become partners in their care, leading to higher case acceptance and better relationships.

Additional resource

Ahmad I. Digital dental photography. Part 2: purposes and uses. *Br Dent J* 2009;206(9):459–464.

Bauer R. Using dental photography for predictable results from your dental lab. *Today's FDA* 2010;22(2):48–51.

Galdino GM, Vogel JE, Vander Kolk CA. Standardizing digital photography: it's not all in the eye of the beholder. *Plast Reconstr Surg* 2001;108(5):1334–1344.

Goldstein RE. Digital dental photography now? *Contemp Esthet Restor Pract* 2005;9(6):14.

McLaren EA, Chang YY. Photography and Photoshop®: simple tools and rules for effective and accurate communication. *Inside Dent* 2006;2(8):97–101.

McLaren EA, Figueira J, Goldstein RE. A technique using calibrated photography and Photoshop for accurate shade analysis and communication. *Compend Contin Educ Dent* 2017;38(2):106–113.

McLaren EA, Terry DA. Photography in dentistry. *J Calif Dent Assoc* 2001;29(10):735–742.

Terry DA, Snow SR, McLaren EA. Contemporary dental photography: selection and application. *Funct Esth Rest Dent* 2007;1(1):37–46.

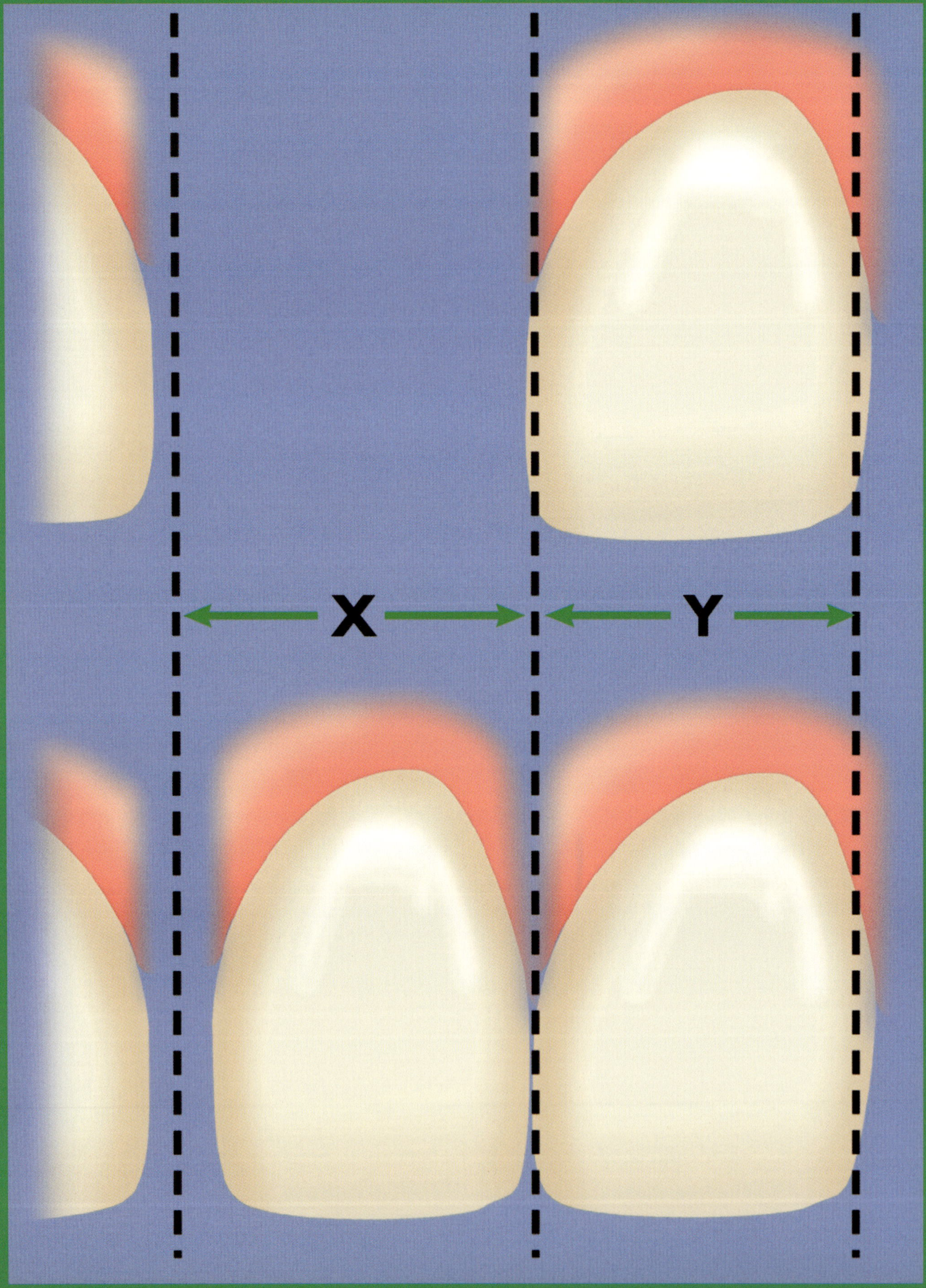
X
Y

Chapter 8 Creating Esthetic Restorations Through Special Effects

Ronald E. Goldstein, DDS, Jason J. Kim, CDT,
Pinhas Adar, MDT, CDT, and Adam Mieleszko, CDT

Chapter Outline

Seeing teeth in a different light	185
Positive and negative smile line	186
Lips and gums: the frame of our teeth	186
Illusions	188
Principles of illusion	188
Shaping and contouring	189
Arrangement of teeth creates illusion	190
Staining	193
Tips on technique	195
Techniques for resolving various problems	206
Space available is wider than the ideal replacement tooth	206
Space available is narrower than the ideal replacement tooth	209
The too-short tooth	214
The too-long tooth	215
Creating optical illusions with form and color	216
Insufficient differentiation between teeth	218
Influencing facial shape	218
Incorporating age characteristics	219
Incorporating sexual characteristics	223
Incorporating the personality of the patient	225
Loss of interdental tissue	225
Porcelain veneer alternate construction techniques	229

One cannot overestimate the magnificent contributions that dental laboratories and specifically dental ceramists have made in the advancement of esthetic dentistry. They are true partners in our quest for the best esthetic dentistry has to offer in all forms of dental prosthesis. They help us solve problems with dissimilar spaces, irregularities, and contour and shade problems, plus so many more situations that it would be difficult to practice prosthetic dentistry without them. This chapter will deal with both simple and complex problems that dentists and dental technicians face daily. It is our hope that you will better understand what it may take to better improve your restorations, since our overall goal is always to please our patients.

Special contribution was made to this chapter by Lukus Kahng, CDT, Nasser Shademan, and Guilherme Cabral, DDS, CDT.

Seeing teeth in a different light

When a technician fabricates teeth in a dental lab, he or she does so under the bright fluorescent lights typical of any modern dental laboratory. The individual restorations look great when bathed in direct light from all sides, and when placed on a typodont or stone model. Likewise, when a dentist receives the restoration from the lab and places it in the patient's mouth for the first time, it will be in a controlled situation: the dentist asks the patient for a big smile while shining the operatory light on those new pearly whites. They look just as great as they did in the dental lab, and both the dentist and patient are happy with the results. However, once the restorations are permanently seated in the patient's mouth, and the patient steps outside of the dental office, the teeth are no longer in a staged

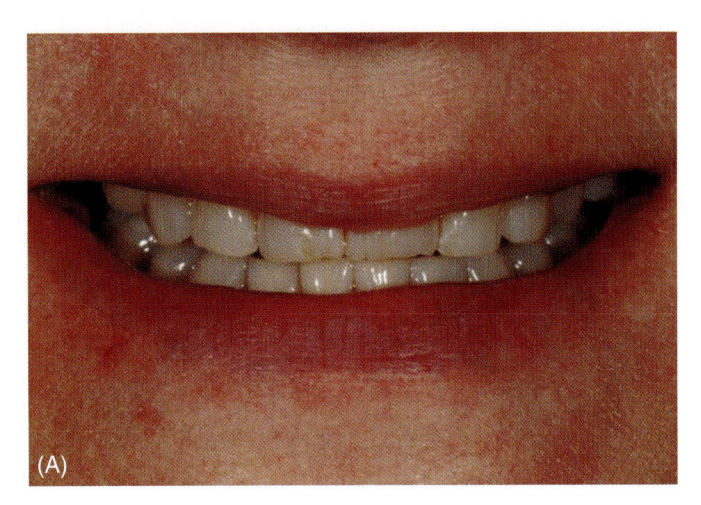

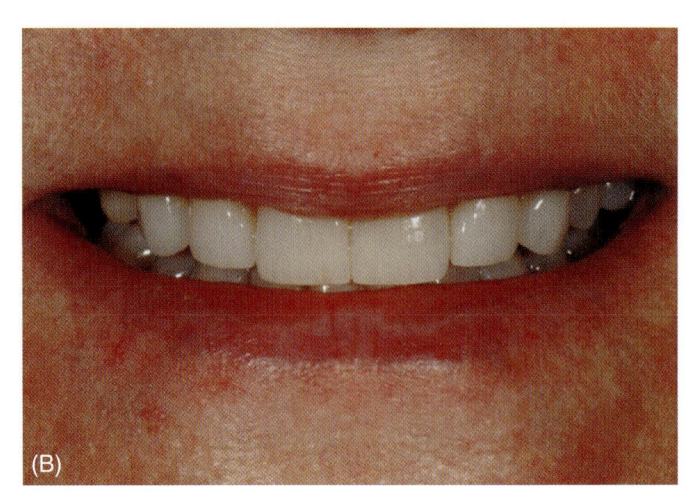

Figure 8.1 **(A and B)** Correction of negative smile line with porcelain veneers.

or controlled environment. The patient's teeth are now framed by the mouth, lips, and face. The mouth is not static but always changing as we smile, frown, laugh, and speak. The appearance of our teeth change as our facial features interact with available light that strikes our teeth. Various types of light affect the appearance of the teeth: daylight, incandescent, fluorescent, the strength and brightness, direct, indirect, light from above and below, and light that is diffused and shadowed by the shape and size of the lips. Our environment is filled with these various types of lighting that can affect the appearance of shape and color of teeth (Figure 8.1A and B).

Positive and negative smile line

Smile line refers to the line formed when going along the incisal edges of the upper front teeth. This line should roughly follow the contours of the lower lip line. Teeth should always be arranged or in alignment with the lips (Figure 8.1A). The more curved the lower lip, the more curved the incisal line of the upper teeth should be (Figure 8.1B). In most cases, the central incisors should be equal to or slightly longer than the cuspids.

Lips and gums: the frame of our teeth

Teeth are framed by lips and gingival tissue. Actually, the lips act more like the frame, and the gingival tissue acts as the backdrop, or the stage on which the teeth stand. Both the lips and gingival tissue affect the way we perceive the color and shape of teeth. The lips act like a curtain and can produce a shadowing effect on teeth. Gingival tissue is naturally light-reflective and light-transmitting; light will pass through it to varying degrees of intensity, depending on the tissue thickness. Because the gingiva transmits light, darker roots, implants, and metal posts will also affect gingival color. For example, if the root is darker, the restoration will look slightly darker near the gum line. It's that sensitive, and it is little nuances such as this that we must always be aware of, as even tiny details can have a big influence the way we perceive the color and shape of the restoration.

The importance of lip thickness on teeth appearance

The structure of the lips has much influence on the appearance of the restored teeth. Thicker lips can create a shadowing effect on teeth, which can make a white crown take on a gray cast once seated in the mouth. When the lips come down over the teeth, the area where the line angle begins to roll off becomes darker, and the tooth looks narrower. With the lips pulled back, such as when using a retractor, everything looks bigger because there is no shadowing effect.

Smile Midfacial Display	Lip Distance from Dental Arch	Customized Ceramic Value
High	Far	Increased Value
Medium	Average	Higher Value
Low	Close	Natural Translucency Level or Decreased Value

Thin lips = close lip distance from dental arch. No adjustment to translucency: teeth are virtually unobstructed and unaffected by thin lips. When designing restorations for a thin‑lipped person, there is no need to deviate from the natural translucent level.

Smile Midfacial Display	Lip Distance from Dental Arch	Customized Ceramic Value
High	Far	Increased Value
Medium	Average	Higher Value
Low	Close	Natural Translucency Level or Decreased Value

Medium lips = average lip distance from dental arch. Adjustment to translucency: with a medium smile line, the restorations need to be brighter. A modified value ranging between 10 and 20% greater than natural translucency would be sufficient..

Smile Midfacial Display	Lip Distance from Dental Arch	Customized Ceramic Value
High	Far	Increased Value
Medium	Average	Higher Value
Low	Close	Natural Translucency Level or Decreased Value

Thick lips = far lip distance from dental arch. Increased opacity: a person with thick, full lips will reveal a very small fraction of their teeth, which appear even less prominent due to shadowing. Although it may seem counterintuitive, creating restorations with increased opacity would help make the teeth appear brighter and more natural.

Illusions

Creating illusions is one of the most important objectives of esthetic dentistry. The ability to make a tooth look wider or thinner, smaller or larger, is an invaluable aid when solving difficult esthetic problems. Esthetic effects of dental restorations are controlled by factors such as form, size, alignment, contour, surface texture, and color of the original teeth. The patients' lip line and gingival tissue can also make a difference in the esthetic effect of dental restorations. When using restorative or prosthetic techniques on one or more teeth, duplicating the conditions and esthetics of the remaining natural dentition should be the ultimate goal. When patients request a "natural appearance," it does not necessarily mean that they want an exact copy of the adjacent or opposite tooth as the goal; the dentist frequently must alter tooth form by illusion to accomplish the desired esthetic results. The presence of space limitations—too much or too little—or other problems may make it impossible to duplicate the original tooth. Nevertheless, in many esthetic situations, the desired objective is to duplicate the natural teeth to attain symmetry in the smile. This chapter presents many of the problems encountered in esthetic restoration and offers techniques of illusion that help overcome these barriers to a desired appearance.

Principles of illusion

Several basic principles of illusion, such as those used to describe form, light, shadow, and line, may be applied specifically to dentistry. In the presence of excess light or in the absence of light, form cannot be distinguished since shadows are necessary to help the viewer perceive the contour or curvature of a surface. The edge of any form is described as a line; therefore, an object with many edges can be drawn "linearly" with little difficulty in visual interpretation (Figure 8.2A). If the object has smooth curved surfaces rather than edges, the form may not be easily comprehended (Figure 8.2B), unless one brings light and shadow into play (Figure 8.2C).

Light has the ability to change the appearance of a surface by its relation to that form. This ability relies on an observer's learned, intellectual approach to perception. For example, we learn that sunlight comes from above; therefore, when we view geometric designs drawn with another light source, an illusion is created. The classic example of this is where three cubes are seen when one side of a figure is up, but five appear when the figure is turned around (Figure 8.2D). This manipulation of light and perception is used in esthetic dentistry to create the ideal dentition: by staining to simulate shadow, creating appropriate shadows through the arrangement of teeth, and shaping or changing the contours of a tooth.

The relationship of lines plays an important role in creating illusion. To anyone who is not perceptually sophisticated, the vertical line seen in Figure 8.2E appears longer than the horizontal line because horizontal movements of the eyes are executed more easily than vertical movements. More time is spent "seeing" the vertical line, so the brain interprets the longer time spent as being due to a longer line. Figure 8.2F illustrates the effect of convergent and divergent lines. One's attention is directed outward on the right and inward on the left, altering perception, even though both lines are the same length.

The application of light, shadow, and linear elements to illusion and their relationship to each other is seen in Figure 8.2G1. The folded piece of paper in this line drawing may be interpreted as being folded forward or backward. When shade is applied to this linear image (Figure 8.2G2 and 3), form is more easily understood (arrows indicate direction of light). This illusion is aided by the fact that white "comes forward" while dark recedes.

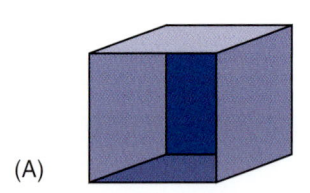

Figure 8.2 (A) Visual interpretation is relatively simple for a linear drawing with many edges.

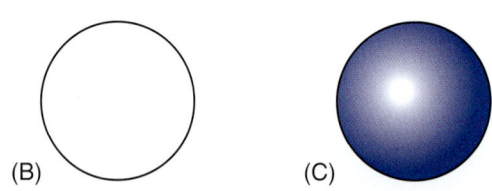

Figure 8.2 (B and C) (B) Form is not so easily understood in an object with smooth curved edges. (C) Added light and shadow help to clarify form interpretation.

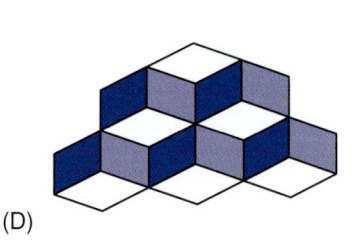

Figure 8.2 (D) Like the illusion created in this drawing, the perception and manipulation of light are used in cosmetic dentistry by staining, shaping, and contouring the dentition.

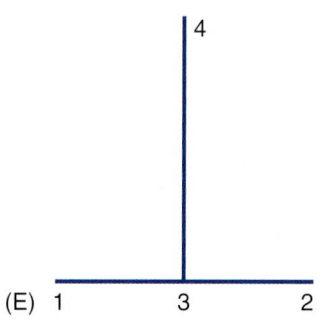

Figure 8.2 (E) Although the lines are of equal length, the vertical line appears longer because the brain spends more time "seeing" the vertical and interprets longer time as longer length.

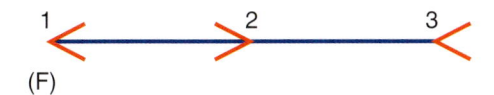

Figure 8.2 **(F)** Illusion is created by the angled direction of the arrows. The outward position of the arrows of line 1–2 gives the illusion that it is shorter in length than is line 2–3.

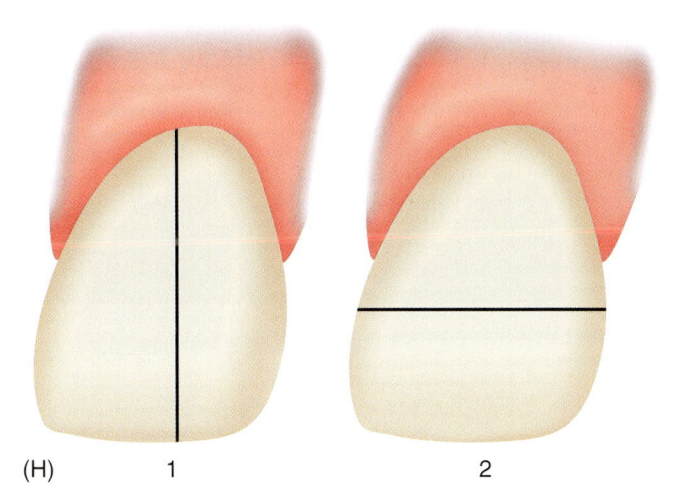

Figure 8.2 **(H)** Although teeth 1 and 2 are equal in size, the accent lines make tooth 1 appear longer and tooth 2 appear wider.

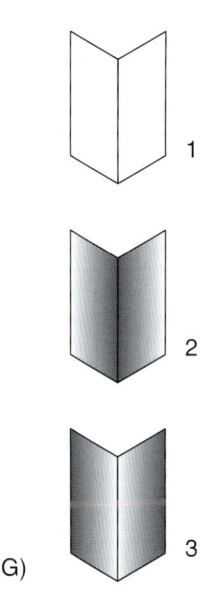

Figure 8.2 **(G)** The interpretation of whether this folded paper is outward or inward can be more accurate when shading is added.

We are accustomed to seeing distant objects as darker and receding objects as darker or shaded from light.

Given two teeth possessing identical shading, the presence of vertical and horizontal accent lines can create the illusion of length or width, respectively (Figure 8.2H). Although one figure may seem wider or longer than the other, both are identical in size, illustrating that combinations of light, shadow, and emphasizing lines are essential in creating effective illusions. Illusions in dentistry are created using three techniques, which are discussed in the following text:

1. shaping and contouring
2. arrangement of teeth
3. staining.

Shaping and contouring

The most frequent illusion is the creation of a different outline by shaping or carving the tooth. The eye is quite sensitive to silhouette form, so the incisal edges of a relatively white tooth will be easily seen silhouetted against the shadows of the oral cavity. The slight alteration of tooth structure done by shaping can alter this silhouette form to create a desired illusion.

Basic principles of illusion regarding shape and outline:

- Vertical lines accentuate height and de-emphasize width.
- Horizontal lines accentuate width and de-emphasize height.
- Shadows add depth.
- Angles influence the perception of intersecting lines.
- Curved lines and surfaces are softer, more pleasing, and perceived as more feminine than sharp angles.
- The relationship of objects helps determine appearances.

The creation of successful illusions is an art that requires advance planning. If the patient has a size, space, or arrangement problem that will need to be solved through illusion or other special effects, the following actions should be considered:

- Look for problems during the clinical examination and when reviewing the study casts.
- Consider whether repositioning through orthodontics, periodontics, preprosthetic surgery, or any other means will lessen or eliminate the problem. If so, the patient should be encouraged to undergo such treatment since the best illusion is none at all.
- If it is necessary to create illusions, begin planning by determining how much tooth reduction is necessary, allowing for any increase or decrease in the size of the intended restoration. Computer imaging will help you see which possibilities will have the best potential solution. Use the images, incorporating the illusion you have created, to show your patient all the possibilities and how his or her new smile can look.

Once this determination has been made, make detailed notes on the shade chart. The teeth are then prepared and the temporary restoration is fabricated. It is essential to make the temporary restoration after tooth preparation and before the final impression is made. The temporary restoration provides a preview of the illusions that are planned for the final restoration and also gives the dentist a working model on which any necessary alterations in the treatment plan may be made. Therefore, the temporary restoration acts as the blueprint for a successful esthetic illusion. Since the final impression will be made at a subsequent appointment, the patient has time to adjust to and voice any criticism of the temporary restoration. The dentist

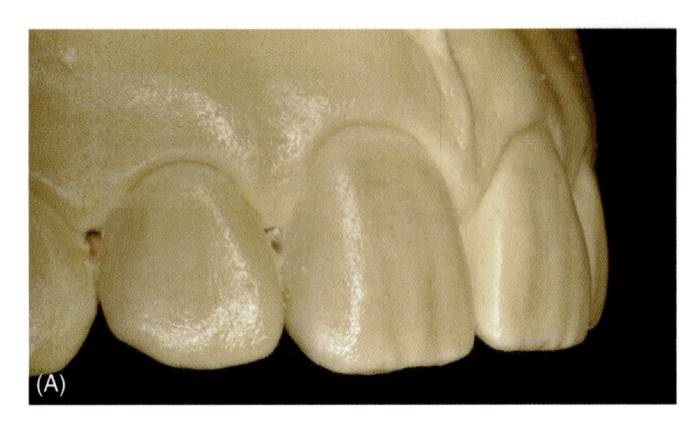

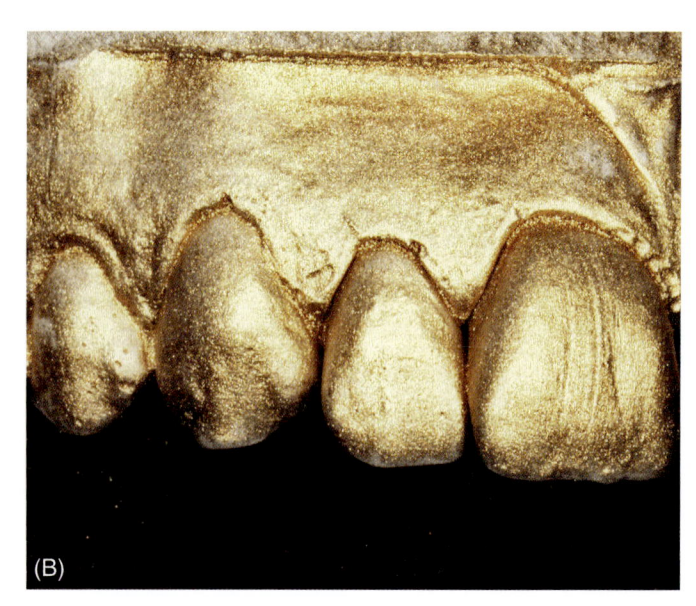

Figure 8.3 **(A and B)** A study cast in yellow or green stone is sprayed with model spray **(A)** or gold powder **(B)** to show texture and highlights.

also has the additional opportunity to alter the tooth preparation, the surrounding tissue, and the shape, size, or arrangement of the temporary restoration. During this appointment make an impression and study cast of the finished temporary restoration. (This can be done while waiting for the anesthetic to take effect for the final impression.) Send this impression, along with the final impression, to the laboratory. This will eliminate any guesswork by the laboratory technician as to the illusion desired.

The next step, shaping and contouring, is done at the try-in appointment. This is the time when any necessary correction through illusion is performed (see Chapter 43). After fitting the restoration to the teeth, examine it for size-of-space deformities. Before correcting with a disc or porcelain stone, outline the intended correction with a black alcohol marker to provide greater perspective. Then proceed with the necessary shaping and contouring. Although the eye is more sensitive to outline than to surface form, it is surface contour, a basic part of good illusion, which controls light reflection. Application of surface characterizations should be done with this in mind.

When planning surface characterizations, these procedures should be followed:

- Study the teeth being restored prior to tooth preparation.
- Study adjacent teeth before and during treatment.
- Make notes on the texture desired. Include convexities and concavities, grooves, fissures, stains, shadows, and highlights. Determine whether the lines are vertical, horizontal, or a mixture of both.
- Take an accurate study model and pour it in yellow or green stone to best show the texture (Figure 8.3). Use model spray (J.F. Jelenko and Co., Kuzler Lab Products) to bring out the highlights (Figure 8.3A). Gold powder can also be used to accomplish a similar effect (Figure 8.3B).
- Then take a digital photograph of the adjacent or opposite teeth. This can be helpful in observing texture and its influence on light reflection.
- Match the degree of smoothness or roughness of adjacent teeth.

When there are no guidelines and the anterior teeth have faulty or unesthetic restorations that must be replaced, it is important to remember that in older patients the enamel is usually worn on the incisal edges and is generally smoother in overall surface texture; younger patients have more textured teeth. If you observe the opposite arch, there may be indications of the type of texture required. Characterized or textured surfaces produce shadows, and shadow position can determine how the mind will interpret contour. A tooth with a shadow or shading on the incisal portion will cause the gingiva to appear more prominent. Shadows or shading can also cause a 2D object to appear 3D and can change the apparent length, width, or height.

Arrangement of teeth creates illusion

The second most frequently used technique for creating illusions involves the arrangement of the teeth being restored. The arrangement of teeth can be modified or changed to create a special esthetic effect. The position or arrangement of teeth can create the illusion of decreased or increased width. If a tooth is rotated distally, it will take on a thinner appearance (Figure 8.4A and B). Conversely, if it is rotated mesially, it will look wider (Figure 8.4C and D).

Alterations of the axial inclination of labial/lingual and mesial/distal surfaces can dramatically change appearance. This is accomplished by placing or building one tooth in front of, behind, overlapping, or rotated with respect to another. Planning must be done at the outset.

Lombardi[1] offers good, simple advice for those taking the first steps in altering tooth arrangement. His one, two, three guide

(A)

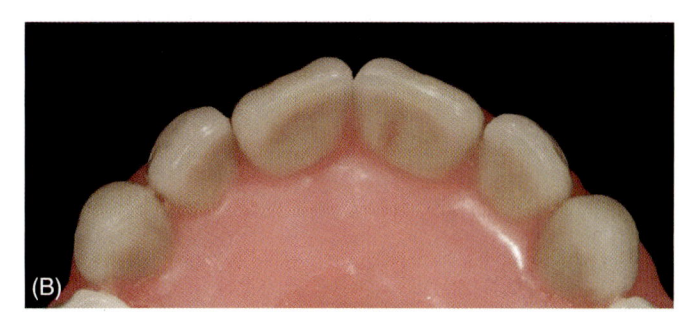

(B)

Figure 8.4 **(A and B)** Narrow, thinner look created with distal rotation of teeth.

(C)

(D)

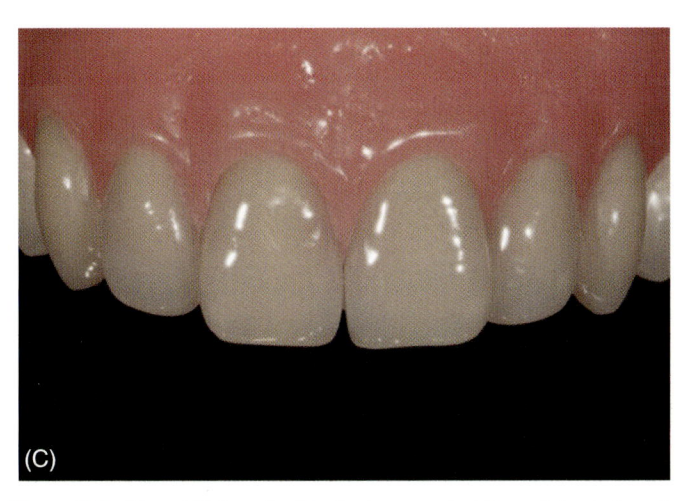

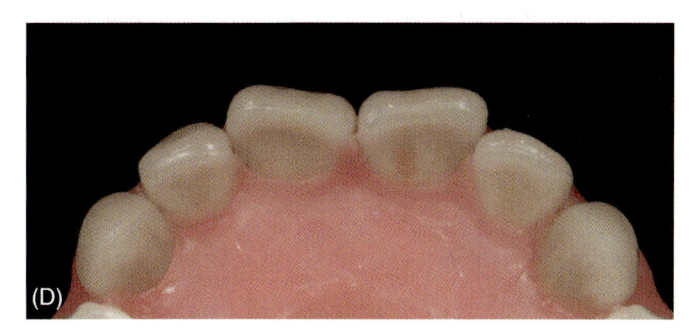

Figure 8.4 **(C and D)** Broad, wider look created with mesial rotation of teeth.

includes incisal modifications (Figure 8.5). One refers to the central incisor, which expresses age; two to the lateral incisor, which expresses sex characteristics; three to the cuspid, which denotes vigor. This guide shows how to use the "negative" or dark space behind the teeth. Alteration of incisal edges, which are then silhouetted against the dark intraoral background, helps to create a nearly limitless variety of illusions.[1]

To predict what type of arrangement will be necessary, construct the temporary restoration before taking the final impression. The effect can then be seen in the temporary restoration or fixed partial denture, and, if necessary, the preparation can be refined before taking the final impression. The patient is allowed time to live with the newly constructed restoration, evaluate acceptability, and express any desires for change. This is especially important in cases where a nonideal arrangement such as overlapping or crowding is to be included. Unless patients have a chance to visualize the arrangement conceived by the dentist, they may react unfavorably when the final restoration is inserted. This can be avoided by allowing the patient to try the restoration and to understand the

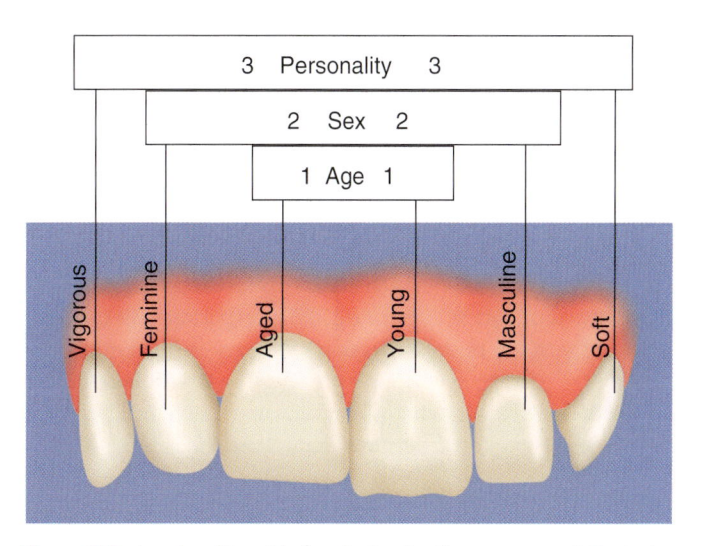

Figure 8.5 Lombardi's guide for altering tooth arrangement illustrates incisal edge modifications that affect personality, sex, and age characteristics.

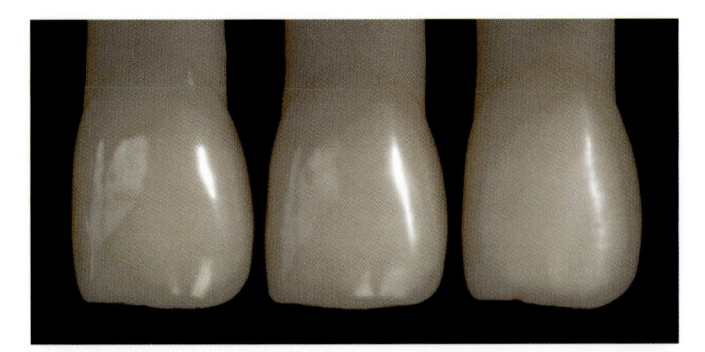

Figure 8.6 **(A)** A smoother surface results in greater light transmission through the tooth, which results in increased translucency and lower value.

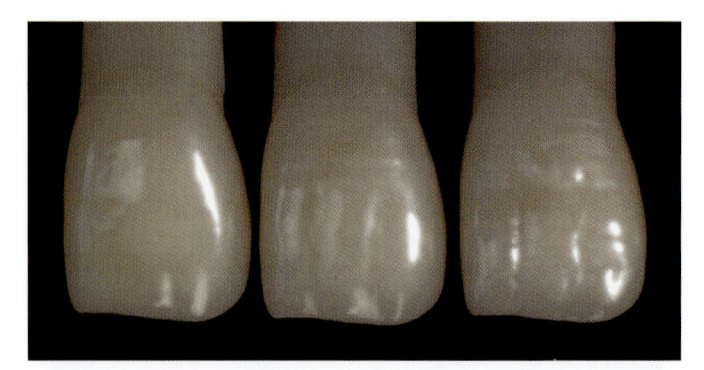

Figure 8.6 **(B)** Incorporating greater texture into the restoration will reflect more light, so the tooth can be designed with a slightly higher value while maintaining a natural appearance.

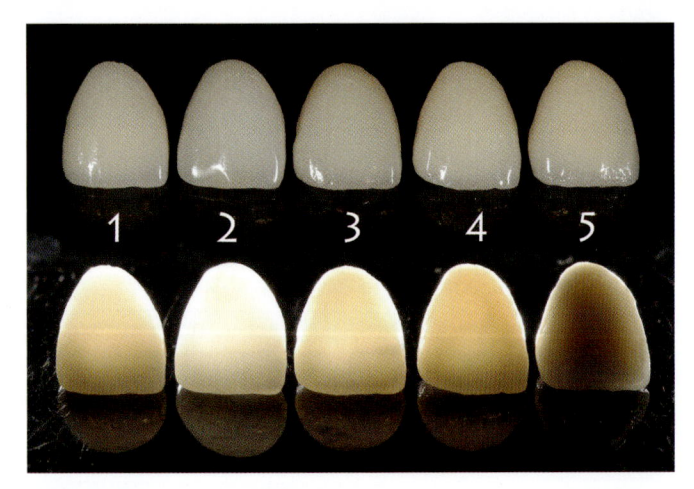

Figure 8.6 **(C)** Note the difference in light interaction of restorations depending on substructure. Top row: reflected light; bottom row: transmitted light. Figure courtesy of Adam J. Mieleszko.

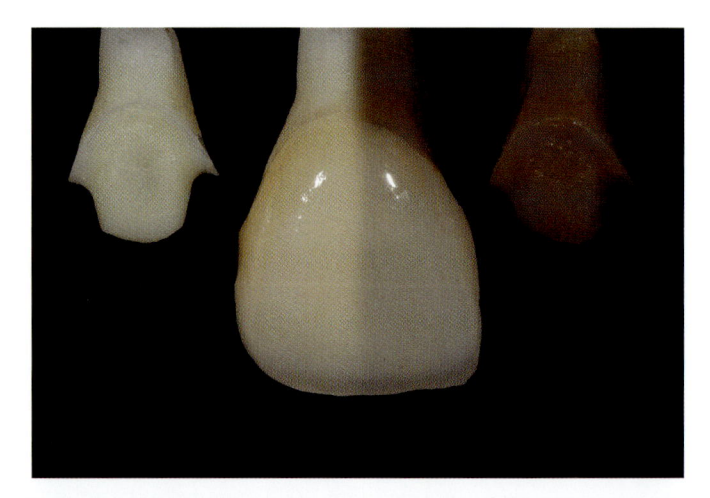

Figure 8.6 **(D)** Split view of the same restoration with different stump preparation color. Notice the value decrease with darker preparation. Figure courtesy of Adam J. Mieleszko.

reasons and space limitations that caused you to elect this type of illusion. For example, a patient who had overlapping centrals may not realize that overlapping laterals can be much more attractive when combined with straight centrals. By creating the new appearance in the temporary, the patient can gain the necessary confidence that will make the final restoration acceptable. It is difficult for most dentists to look at a particular patient and tell what type of tooth arrangement will be best suited for that type of face.

Although there is no convincing research to show that certain types of faces should have certain types of teeth, there are principles that can aid you in selecting the appropriate appearance. These include understanding the patient's personality, age, and esthetic wishes. It is only through trial and error that the delicate balance that creates harmony can be achieved. This takes time and the willingness on your part to experiment and re-experiment in the temporary stage. It is a mistake to wait until the try-in appointment to create or recreate arrangement possibilities. The try-in appointment already takes a great amount of your time and skill to make a properly chosen restoration appear as natural and esthetic as possible.

Special effects by manipulating teeth shape and arrangement

Modifying the surface texture of a tooth will affect its luster and brightness. A smoother restoration surface results in greater transmission of light through the tooth, which in turn results in increased translucency and lower value (Figure 8.6A). If we incorporate a lot of texture into the restoration, the tooth will reflect more light, so the tooth can be designed with a slightly higher value and still look natural (Figure 8.6B). In order for the translucency level, opalescence, coloring, and fluorescence of a tooth to "behave" correctly in the mouth, these characteristics need to be intrinsic—they need to be built in to the actual ceramic structure, rather than applied externally to the surface using stains and glazes.

Substructure material choices and their influence on tooth appearance

Choosing the correct substructure for a restoration is often overlooked, as we tend to pay more attention to the build-up or layering ceramics; however, substrate materials affect light in different ways, and it is important to know what those effects will be ahead of time. Additionally, the color (lightness or darkness) of the patient's tooth stump preparation may affect the final appearance of the restoration (Table 8.1, Figure 8.6C–E).

Staining

Previously, no dental material had the same ability as enamel to absorb or reflect light under all conditions. However, the development of a new generation of ceramic materials for both ceramic and ceramometal restorations makes it much easier to mimic the natural dentition. Staining is the final opportunity to enhance the original shade and to correct or improve restorations. Even though illusions through contouring may have been attempted, a combination of contouring and staining may be necessary to accomplish the desired results. Figure 8.7A illustrates a successful mandibular reconstruction made necessary by periodontal disease. The patient wished to maintain a natural appearance through crowning; effective shading, shaping, arrangement, and staining accomplished this goal (Figure 8.7B).

Staining may be used not only to duplicate the natural variations in tooth color (see Chapter 10 for a full discussion) but also to create and enhance illusions through manipulation of shape and surface characterization. There are two basic aspects of color that you can use to create and enhance illusion. First, by increasing the value of the color (increasing whiteness), you will make the area to which it is applied appear closer. Second, by decreasing the value of the color (increasing grayness), you will make the area to which it is applied appear less prominent and farther away.

Although most dentists leave staining to the laboratory technician, it is desirable to have a small porcelain oven in the office where this type of correction can be done. Staining in the office saves time, and it allows experimentation with different stains until the desired effect is achieved. To rely entirely on the laboratory technician to create the desired stain may require several visits by the patient before the effect is successfully achieved. Unfortunately, after a few visits, the patient or dentist may become impatient and insert a restoration that could have been further improved with additional staining. If the dentist does not employ a laboratory technician, an interested dental assistant who likes to paint is a good candidate to learn the art of staining porcelain or acrylic and may become quite proficient. An important consideration is to refer to a natural tooth while staining. A model constructed from extracted teeth is also an excellent aid when attempting to achieve a more natural result. Whenever possible, staining should be incorporated into the body of the restoration. The closer to the final shade the opaque and body layers are, the more lifelike will be the result. Opaquing material of various colors can influence the appearance of porcelain and add depth to the color. Basic modifying colors can be used for certain effects. Ideally, surface stains should be used only to add the final touch of realism and exactness to the restoration. Figure 8.8A shows

Table 8.1 Substructure Material Choices and Tooth Appearance

Type of Material	Light Reflected	Light Transmitted	Tooth Stump Effect
Feldspatic ceramic	Low	High	High
Lucite reinforced	Low	High	High
Lithium disilicate	High	High	Medium low
Zirconia	High	Low	Low
Metal	High	Low	No effect

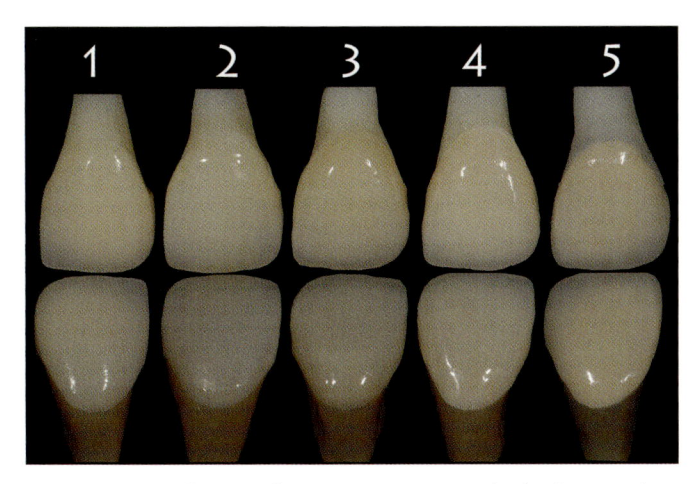

Figure 8.6 (E) Influence of stump preparation on final color is evident with all restorations except those with a metal substructure. Top row, light stump; bottom row: dark stump. Figure courtesy of Adam J. Mieleszko.

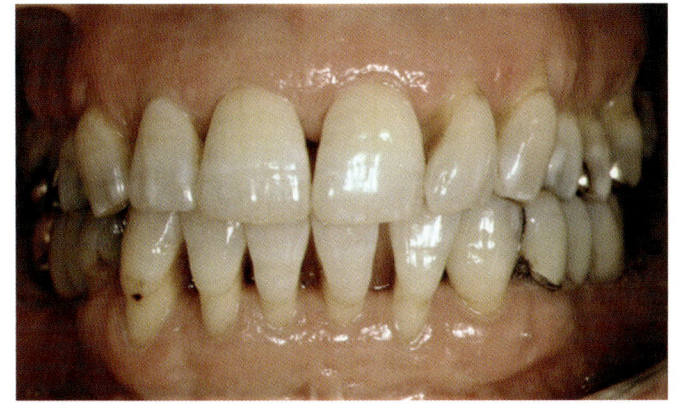

Figure 8.7 (A) This patient required anterior splinting to correct the effects of mandibular periodontal disease and therapy which left her with large interdental spaces.

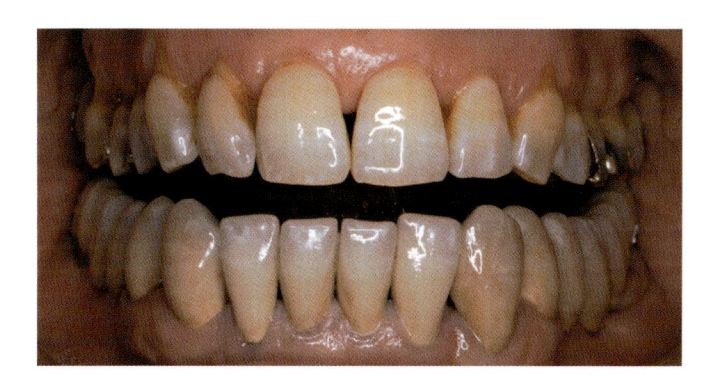

Figure 8.7 (B) A combination of staining, contouring, and effective arrangement of the mandibular anterior crowns gave this patient a natural-appearing result.

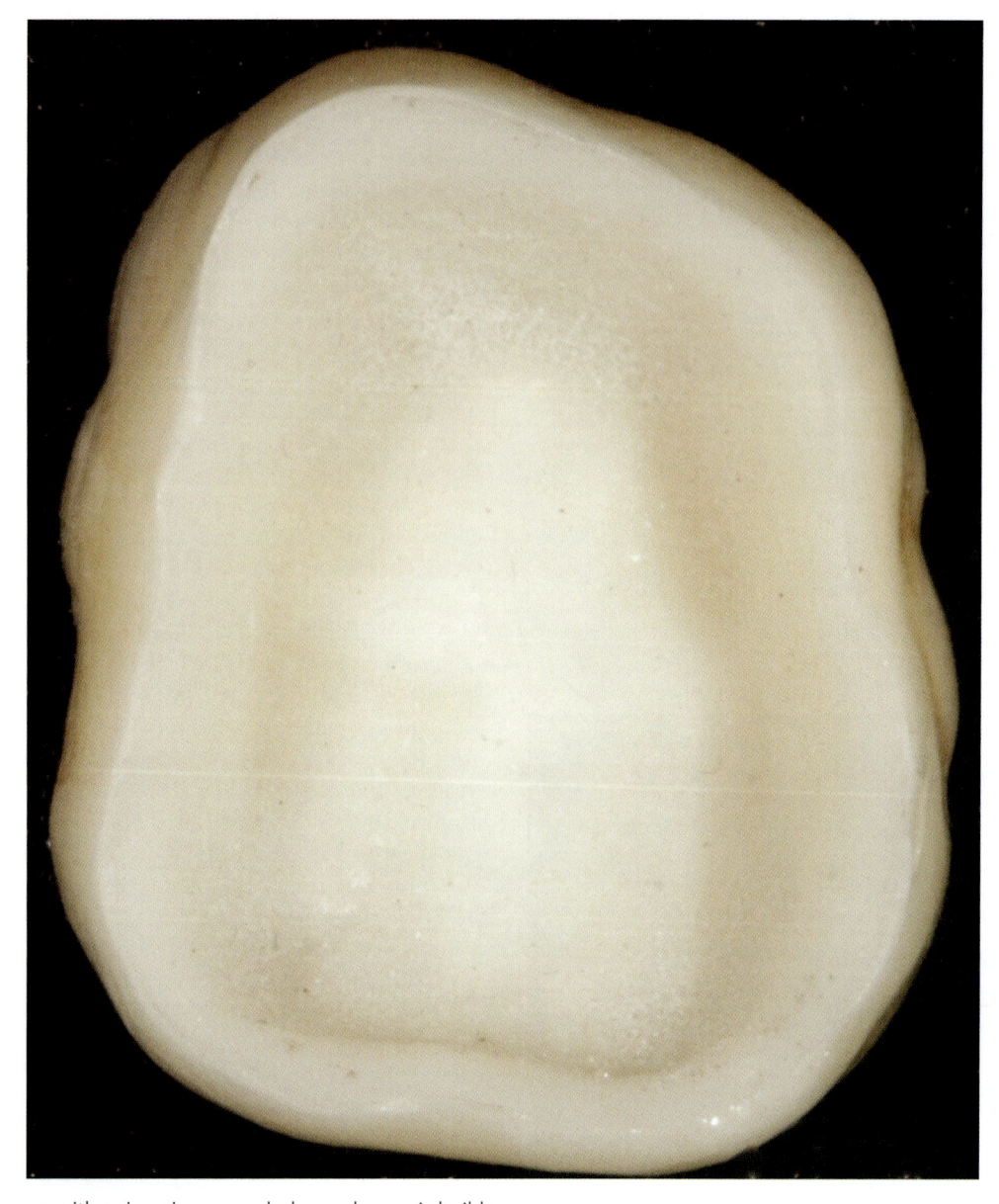

Figure 8.8 **(A)** A crown with a zirconia core and a layered ceramic buildup.

crown with a zirconia core and a layered ceramic buildup. Finally, Figure 8.8B shows the crown after glazing. Note the many colors used to create a more realistic and natural looking tooth.

Techniques used with surface stains

- **Glaze the crown first**. This allows surface stains to be applied over the glaze in a separate operation. However, Aker et al.[2] state that unless a second glaze is applied over the surface stain, the resultant wear will be accelerated approximately 50%, wearing through the stain in 10–12 years.
- **Cut into the porcelain**. The porcelain may be slightly cut back and fluorescence stains placed on the surface. An incisal or translucent opalescent porcelain is then added and the crown is reglazed (Figure 8.9A and B).
- **Combine glaze with stains**. Apply the glaze first, using the technique described here:

1. Mix the glaze to the consistency of thick cream.
2. Moisten a dry glaze brush in a small pool of liquid medium and squeeze any excess medium from the brush.
3. Load the brush with glaze mix.
4. Cover the surfaces to be glazed with a thin, even coat.
5. Vibrate the tooth using a serrated instrument to make the glaze flow evenly.
6. Rebrush only where necessary to assure a smooth, even coat with no pooling.
7. Stain as desired.

Figure 8.10A–D illustrates this technique at the try-in appointment. After the restoration has been thoroughly checked for fit, shape, and occlusion, it is removed and cleaned (Figure 8.10A). The preselected stain is mixed as instructed in step 1 (Figure 8.10B). The stain and glaze combination is applied to the

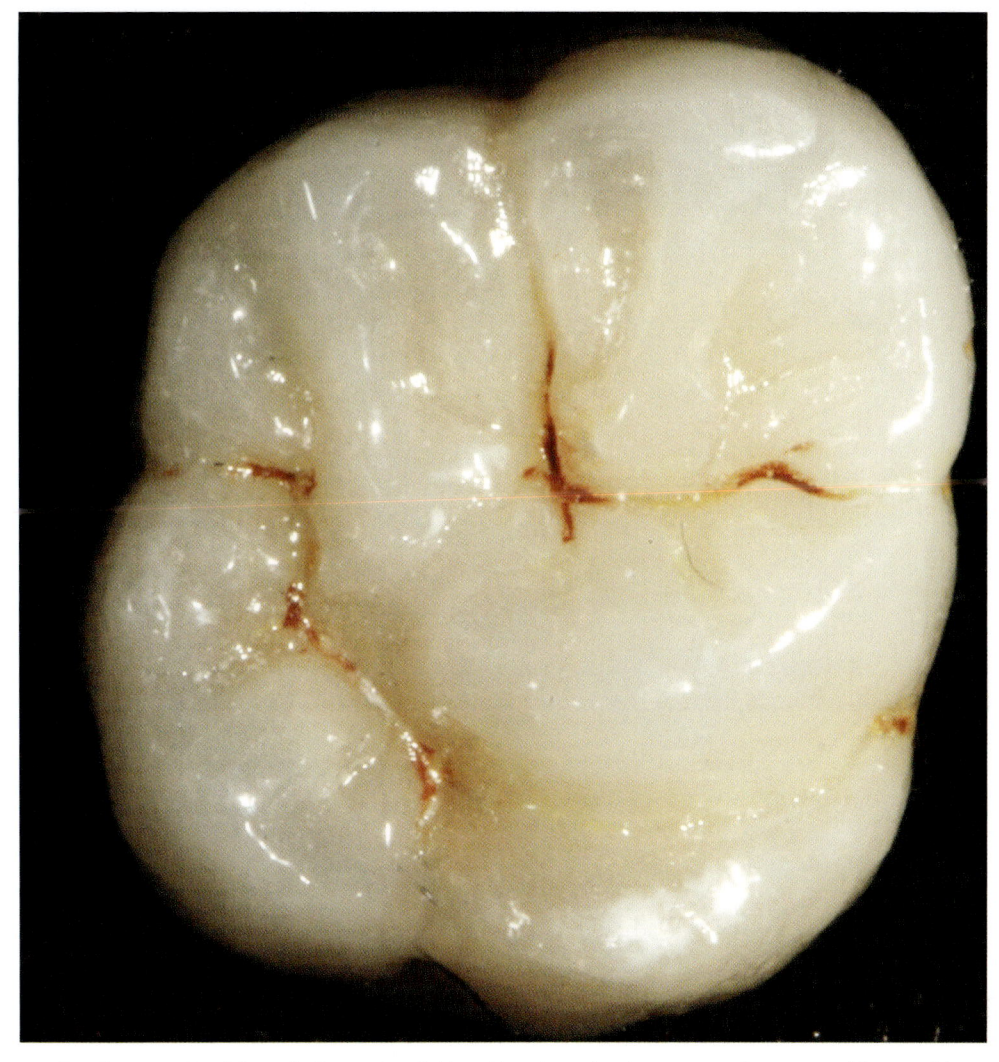

Figure 8.8 (B) The completed crown after firing, glazing and polishing. Note how the deep orange-brown modifier provides a more realistic crown.

restoration (Figure 8.10C) and fired at 960 °C (1760 F). The result after firing is seen in Figure 8.10D. When selecting a particular shade of stain, mix enough powder into the liquid medium to achieve a creamy mix. Refer to a color wheel to observe the effects of combining hues.

The decision of which type of stain to use will be based on the degree of shade alteration required and observation of the type of stains in the natural tooth under fluorescence (Figure 8.11A and B). Note that although the stains appear similar in conventional light, they change their behavior under black light (Figure 8.11B). Lack of fluorescence is evident in the conventional stains. The final crowns should look natural both in normal light (Figure 8.11A) and black light situations (Figure 8.11B and C).

When first building the porcelain, it is important to select the proper shade from the guide. If a guide tooth selection cannot be made, it becomes necessary to establish a basic shade with stains. Select a guide tooth that is lighter than the desired one and free from undesirable underlying hues.

Tips on technique

- Keep stain colors pure. Constantly check the porcelain for dirt specks. If you find any, cut back the porcelain and repair. Keep colors far apart to avoid contamination. Wearing magnifying loupes, lenses, or telescopes (Designs for Vision) is helpful.
- If your experience in the art of staining is limited, do not overstain.
- Staining should be done on a smooth surface. The tooth can be textured, but the surface should be free of pits and stone marks. Diamonds may scar the surface and puddles can form. An even, all-over texture is best. Avoid using any stones that could leave a residue that could be incorporated into the porcelain. (Use Dedeco [Dedeco International Inc.], Shofu [Shofu Dental, Lab Division], or Busch [Pfingst and Co.] chipless porcelain stones.)
- Opaque white can be applied better when a small amount of glaze is mixed with it.

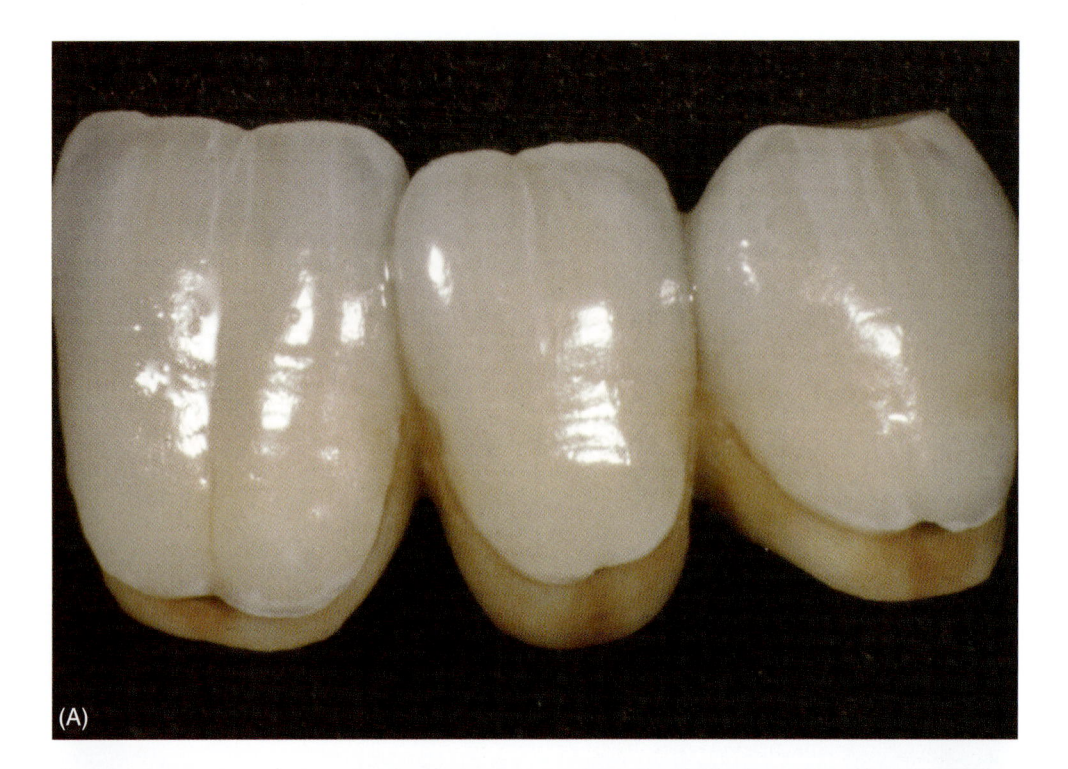

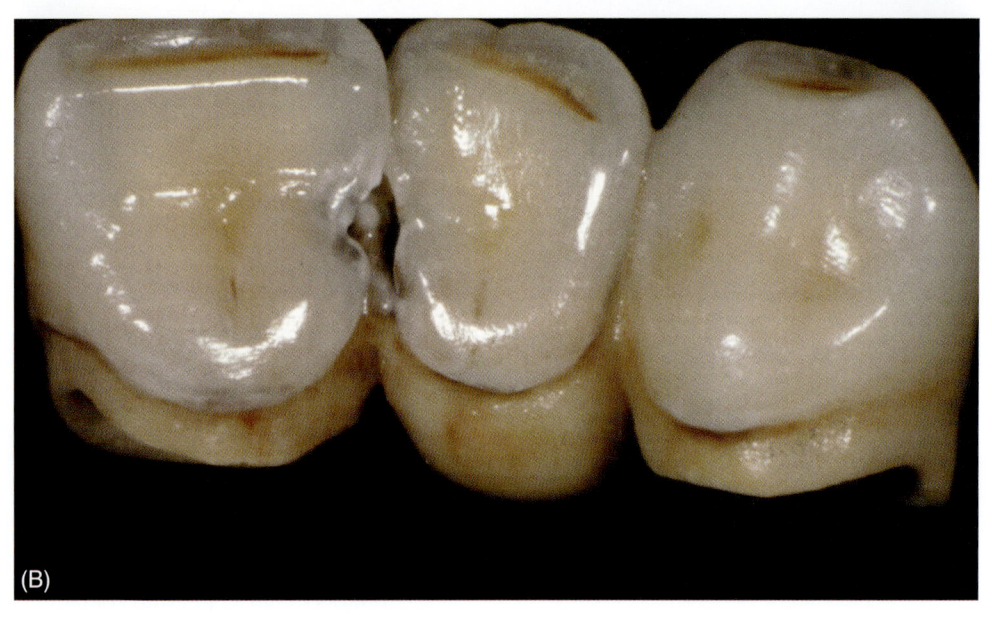

Figure 8.9 **(A and B)** This is a good example of internal characterization to mimic the natural effects sometimes seen in the naturally aged dentition.

- While wet, stains have essentially the same color value as when fixed.
- Stains should be dried carefully in front of the furnace door so they do not run or bleed.
- When simulating a "check line" or microcrack with surface stains, apply a broad line first with the chosen shade of stain (Figure 8.12A). Using a flat edge of the brush, carefully wipe away each side of the line until the desired thinness is achieved (Figure 8.12B). After inserting additional characterization as needed, fire the crown according to instructions (Figure 8.12C). Similar effects can be created with white microcracks instead of brown (Figure 8.12D). This can be helpful in younger patients.
- The guides for staining to alter shades and add characterization (Tables 8.2 and 8.3) should serve as a reference to help solve esthetic problems or to improve results. Some of the techniques can make the difference between unenthusiastic patient acceptance and complete satisfaction.

Too many firings may cause the restoration to lose its original vitality and alter shading. However, Barghi[3] states that repeated firings (up to nine) do not normally affect the porcelain shade but that repeated firings could cause reduction and loss of

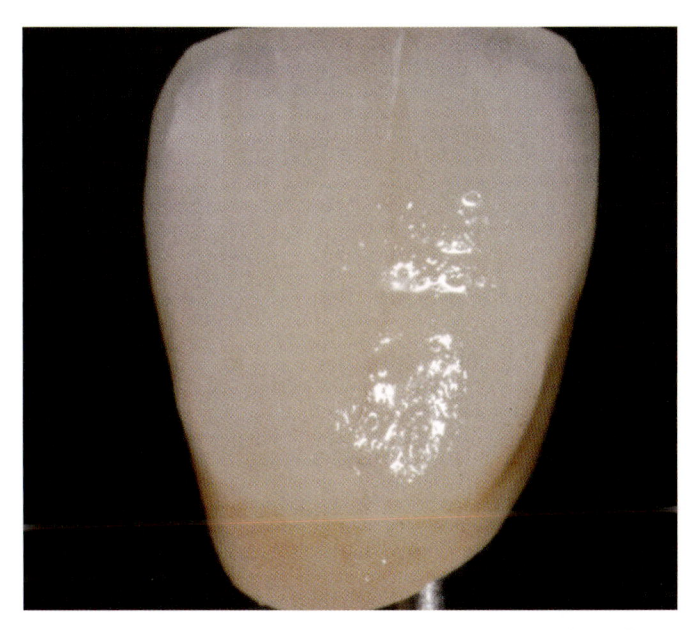

Figure 8.10 (A) A combined glaze and stain technique is shown here at the try-in appointment. The restoration has been checked for fit, shape, and occlusion.

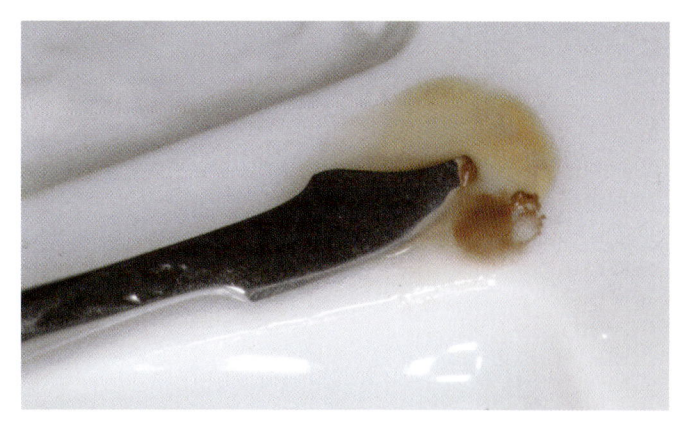

Figure 8.10 (B) The appropriate shade of stain is mixed to a thick, creamy consistency.

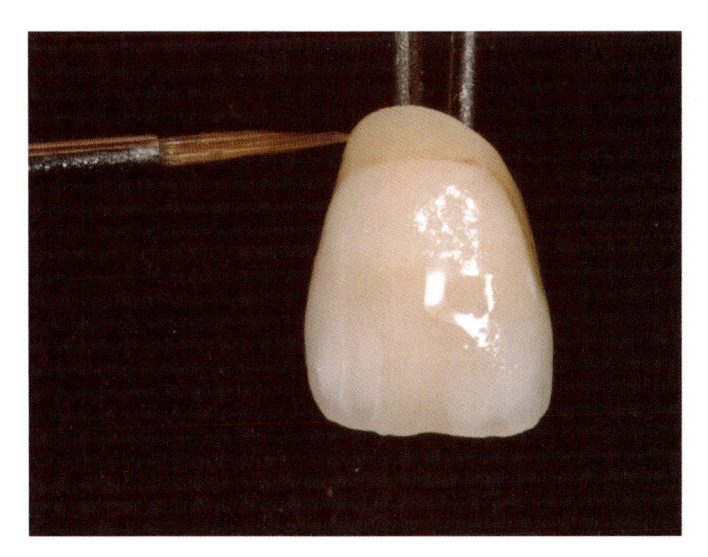

Figure 8.10 (C) The stain and glaze mixture is applied to the restoration.

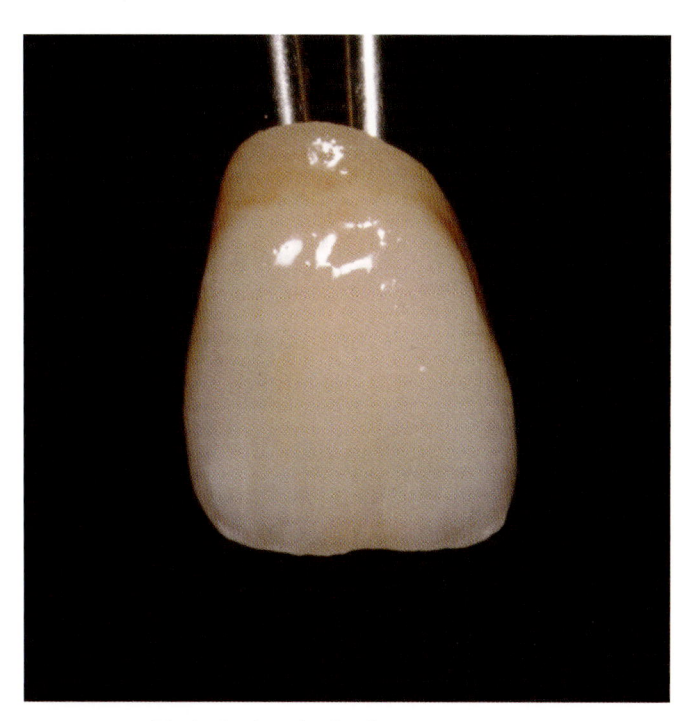

Figure 8.10 (D) The final result after firing. Note how the contrast between orange, brown, and blue can help create a more natural look.

autoglaze in porcelain. Nevertheless, try to incorporate as much staining as possible into the original bake and glaze. Place stains on the tooth and fire the restoration at a temperature slightly less than for glazing until all the desired effects are achieved. Then glaze at the proper temperature. Multiple staining effects are better achieved in this fashion.

Communication with the laboratory

Proper communication with your laboratory is essential if you expect to receive an accurate rendition of your esthetic concept. One of the most frequent complaints dentists have is that their laboratory did not return a finished product that had the anticipated esthetic qualities. There are five basic ways to achieve proper communication:

1. Computer imaging can provide a good idea of what the final result should look like. This is especially true if the images are taken by an intraoral camera, which allows occlusal and labial views to be included. Thus, the correction can be visualized on two or more planes. Eventually, computer-aided design/computer-aided manufacture (CAD/CAM) will provide the most useful information to the technician. If your technician does not have a direct link to your computer but has a similar system, you can arrange an email or file transfer with your intended results; otherwise, send a printout.
2. A waxed model may be sufficient to illustrate to you, your technician, and your patient the suggested changes.
3. Another effective way to let patients visualize just how their esthetic correction will appear is to apply ivory wax directly

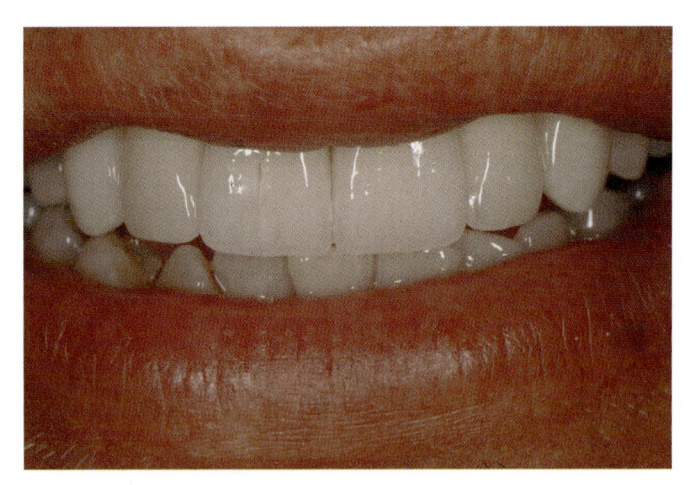

Figure 8.11 (A) The final close-up smile shows the two new ceramo-metal crowns combined with porcelain veneers.

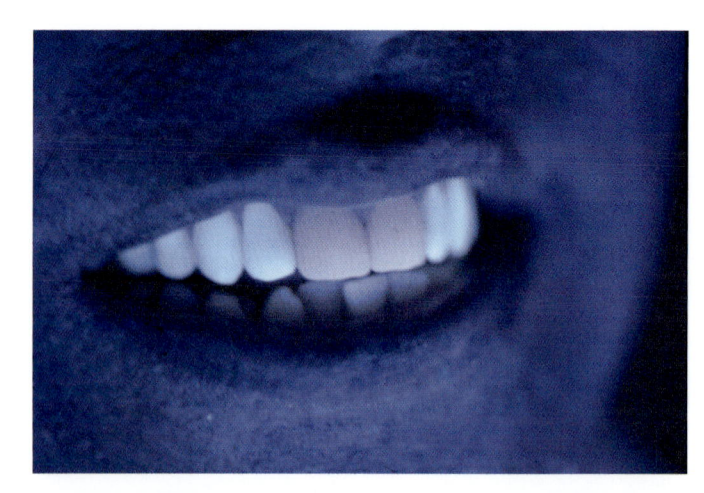

Figure 8.11 (B) This photograph of two central incisor crowns taken under black light demonstrates that they did not fluoresce like the adjacent natural enamel, causing the crowns to appear different under various light conditions.

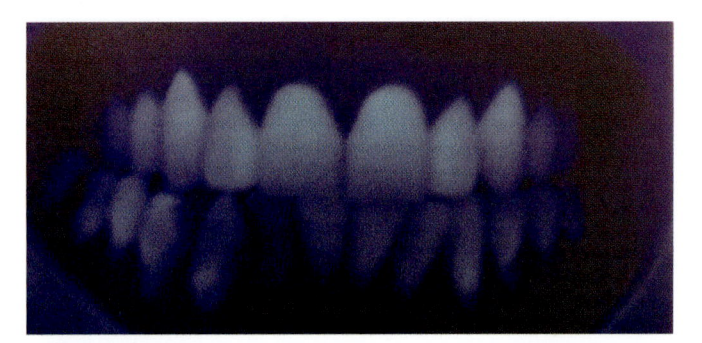

Figure 8.11 (C) Black light helps to show how naturally the new crowns and porcelain veneers fluoresce.

to the teeth. Use cotton rolls or plastic retractors to keep the teeth dry, and place a 2 × 2 gauze over the lower lip to protect it in case the hot wax accidentally drips. Flow tooth-colored or ivory-type wax onto the incisal edges of the teeth, shape with a wax carver, and then show your patient the anticipated result. Be sure to remind the patient to hold the mirror at arm's length to get the proper illusion.

4. The same effect can also be achieved by using the vacuform matrix/composite resin technique. Take a diagnostic cast and wax-up the intended correction. Make a plaster model of the corrected wax-up and then make a vacuform matrix of this. Fill the inside with old or outdated composite resin and place in the mouth without polymerizing. An alternative is to line the inside of the vacuform matrix and polymerize only after eliminating undercuts by trying in the matrix several times.

5. To assure that a restoration will have the desired shape, contour, and size when it is returned from the laboratory, detailed instructions must be written. Written communication may be the only source of information or may be a secondary

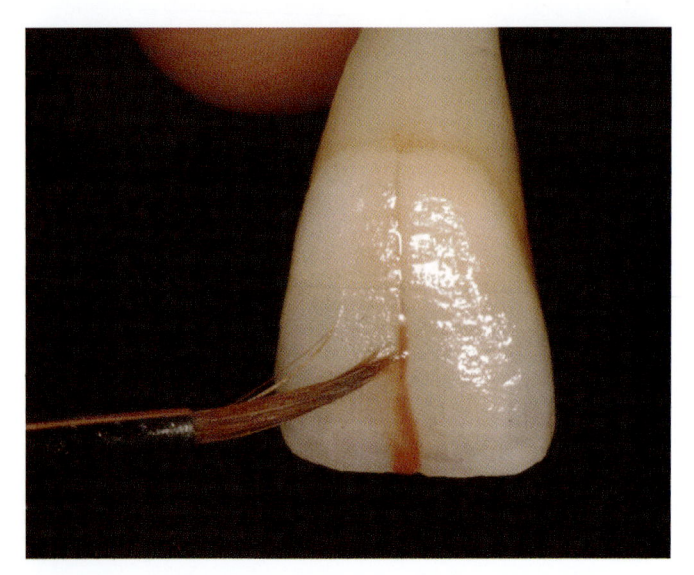

Figure 8.12 (A) A "natural-looking" microcrack is added by first applying a broad band of the selected shade of stain.

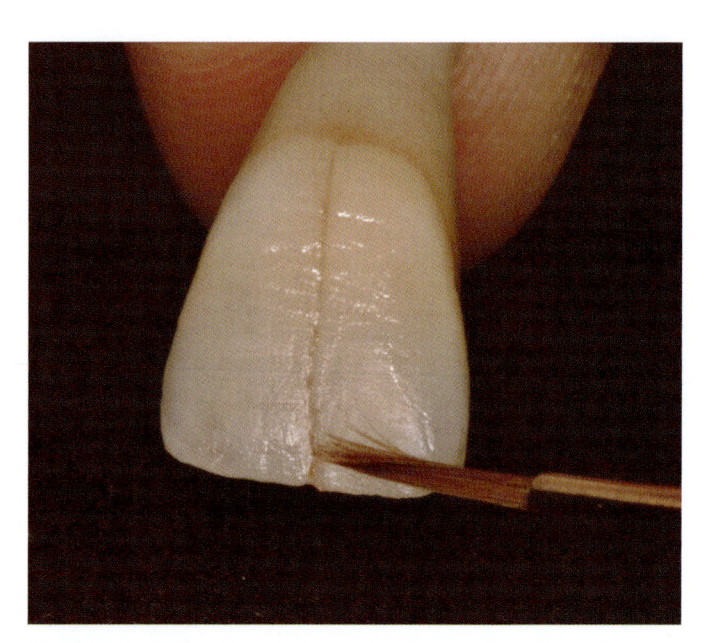

Figure 8.12 (B) The flat edge of the brush is used to achieve the desired thinness.

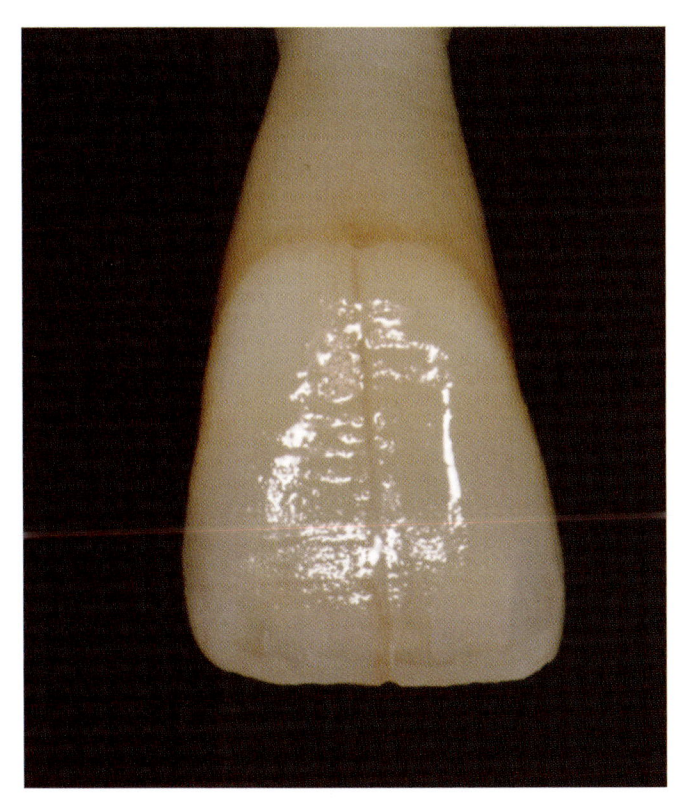

Figure 8.12 (C) The final result including additional "characterizations" after firing gives the appearance of realism.

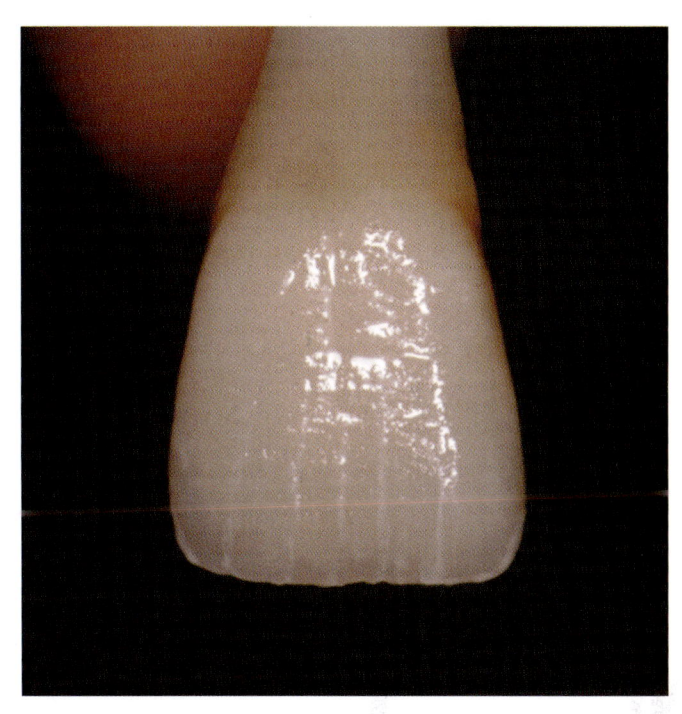

Figure 8.12 (D) These white "microcracks" may be more esthetically pleasing, especially for a younger patient.

source. Carefully written instructions are essential and leave no room for misinterpretation. For example, in the case of a diastema, the technician should be instructed to carve the contact areas to the lingual surface in order to diminish the apparent width of the crowns. This kind of communication makes it more likely that you can achieve the desired results before the restoration is even tried in the mouth.

In cases of illusion through arrangement, a diagram on the prescription blank is most helpful. If you want a tooth overlapped, rotated in labio- or linguoversion, or in any other position not commonly used by the laboratory, planning must be done at the outset. If you desire the ultimate in esthetics, then spend the necessary time to write a detailed, graphic laboratory prescription.

Providing your technician with digital photographs of whatever you need to communicate can help the technician better understand both your patient's esthetic problem and what you want to accomplish in the restoration. Try taking a close-up photograph holding the chosen shade tab against the area to be restored. Often, even slight differences in chroma and value can be seen. The more pictures you take, the better the technician will be able to visualize what he or she must do to help achieve the desired esthetic result.

Shade guide

One of the biggest frustrations for the ceramist is interpreting what both the dentist and patient visualize. Unfortunately, typical shade guides fail to show the range of special inlaid effects that natural teeth possess. One such system has been developed by Kahng (Chairside Shade Guide, LSK121) (Figure 8.13A).

Because of different translucencies, transparencies, dentin overlays with enamel, and enamel modifications, a traditional shade tab cannot match natural dentition. It is merely to be used as a guide. The Kahng shade system takes into consideration the theory behind these colors, looking at natural teeth but also the synthetic made colors we see when patients bleach their teeth. The Chairside Shade Guide ceramic shade tabs are divided into different categories, with 20 tabs in each grouping.

- Shade guide 3.0
  - Cosmetic (six colors)—historically, there has not been an extensive tool to guide dentists in the area of cosmetic color. Many patients want, specifically, bright color with translucency, light with warm tones. The tabs are created with that in mind.
  - Early Age (14 colors)—occlusal two-thirds area includes white calcification and opal blue, more dentin color and less translucency. For the incisal one-third bright color with deep translucency is provided (Figure 8.13B).
- Shade guide 4.0
  - Middle Years (20 colors)—includes variation of color in enamel, a 20–30% reduction compared to 3.0 in between the dentin and enamel. The tabs in this grouping consider outside enamel, translucency, and dentin. Expect to see 50% enamel and 50% translucency in these shade tabs. There are included three white calcification possibilities and a variety of translucency with mamelon (Figure 8.13C).
- Shade guide 5.0. Later Years (20 colors)—in the mouth, there is more intensive color saturation with deep dentin, translucency, and transparency, as well as a variety of

Table 8.2 Guide for Staining to Alter Shade

Objective	Color of Stain	Formula	Application	Rationale
Reduce real translucency				
Make coping invisible	Gray black or blue	Match value level with gray, black and blue	Match value level of incisal area	Method maintains value, chroma, hue, and blend
Masking small flaws and dirt specks	Orange	Gingival effect with orange		Complementary hue lowers value (grays) and reduces chroma (weakens)
Control apparent translucency				
Incisal edge				
To intensify translucency	Blue/ blue violet/blue-green	Use complementary color to neutralize orange, yellow, or pink	Brush lightly over labioincisal or linguoincisal area 0.5 mm from edge in an irregular pattern	Complementary hue lowers value (grays) and reduces chroma (weakens)
	Orange/orange-brown/ brown		Apply orange adjacent to incisal area and feather lightly into proximal contact areas. Applying thin area to incisal edge helps increase translucency and makes tooth appear more natural.	(Same as above) and complementary hues applied adjacent to one another enhance each other; also helps to create third dimension
To decrease translucency	Orange/red/yellow/ gray/white	Add complementary color to compensate for the increased value due to the white	Add white sparingly; adjust value with orange, red, yellow If necessary to lower value further, use gray	Complementary hue can alter value or chroma
Incisal-gingival blend				
To increase incisal translucency	Violet	If yellow body shade, use a violet stain	Add small increments brushing lightly	Use a hue that complements the body shade
	Blue	If brownish-orange body shade, use a blue stain (others hues similar procedure)		
To eliminate green	Pink		Add to body color as stain	A yellow body color with a gray opaquer results in a green cast. Red complements green
Control chroma (strength)				
Thin areas (gingival third)	Yellow or orange	Use opaquer of the same hue desired in thin areas		Color of thin area greatly influenced by the color of opaquer
Between abutment and pontic	Select desired hue		The final buildup and opaquer of the abutments and pontic should be of equal thickness	Thickness of area will influence chroma

Increase chroma (strength)	Red/yellow/blue	Add three primary colors in equal amounts; emphasis on hue to be strenghtened	Addition of the three primary colors will not change the shade (extremely difficult procedure)
Decrease chroma	Clear		Add clear material sparingly
Reduce value (brilliance)			Do not use white; it will increase the value (brilliance of the shade)
Match a too-light (too-bright) crown with the natural dentition	Complementary hue of desired shade	Add sparingly	Graying the shade by using a complementary hue reduces value
Example: yellow shade	Violet		
Increase value (This is practically impossible to do with stains.)			Choose a shade of higher value, if necessary

Table 8.3 Guide for Staining to Add Characterization

Effect Sought	Color of Stain	Formula	Application	Rationale
Random discoloration	White/orange/brown-blue/yellow	Combine small amount of white with body shade	Randomly intensify chroma over labial surface (adds dimension)	Cervical and interproximal discoloration can tolerate some opacity
Labial mottling	Same		Same as above	
Fissures and apertures				
Sulci and proximal apertures	Orange to brown	Use lighter yellow-orange in young people; deeper burnt orange as aging progresses	Apply thin lines asymmetrically	
Worn enamel and exposed dentin (incisal edge lower anteriors of the aged)	Orange to brown		May take two bakes	
Exposed dentin of smoker	Orange-brown or brown, blue		Vary shading, reduce incisal surface in center of teeth; increase incisal translucency at interproximals	
Incisal wear/erosion	Yellow-brown	One part yellow/one part brown/two parts diluent (medium)	Strain center area of incisal edge. Undiluted or slightly diluted brown may be placed centrally to depict exposed and heavily stained dentin. Mix with orange to radiate from center.	Adds depth and feeling of naturalness to incisal edge if worn
Enamel cracks (young patients)	Gray (distal)/white (mesial)/yellow/black	Use thick consistency	Strain runs 3–5mm (1/3 length of crown) (gray-white) to the incisal edge	Add depth to surface (third dimension)
			Place brush tip in the center of the crown, with a fast light stroke bring to incisal edge	
			Apply thicker line with correct shade	
			Wipe away mesially and distally until desired thickness is achieved. Create shadow effect by abutting the (gray/white) stain with black. Apply only a faint line.	
Check-lines	Brown/black/yellow/orange	Brown with a small amount of black or yellow/four parts stain/one part diluent (medium)	A wide strip of stain is applied, this is brushed until a very fine sometimes not continuous line remains. These lines can slant mesial or distally towards the embrasure terminating at the incisal edge.	
Grooves and pits (on the occlusal of posterior teeth and lingual surface of anteriors)	Brown/black/orange/blue	Brown with a small quantity of black or orange for a young person	Stain as fine lines, except in occlusal pitting.	Creates lifelike appearance to the tooth
			Combine pitting and grooves with bluish enamel staining of adjacent ridges.	

Decalcification/ hypocalcification	Opaque white yellow/brown/gray	Opaque white alone or with a trace of yellow, brown, gray	Use a thick layer of opaque applied irregularly in various areas. Effective if used on several teeth evenly in gingival area. Otherwise, vary	Used to match adjacent teeth. Note area and intensify
Cervical stain/gingival erosion	Brown/yellow/gray or lime-green	Three parts brown/one part yellow or gray/four parts diluent (medium) or lime-green	Blend with body shading where it begins. Occasionally dark brown spots may be placed using the feathered edge of a brush.	Ditching possible to actually create an eroded area
Existing silicate or composite				
Stained outline	Orange/brown/gray	Limit diluent added to stain	Paint the outline form using brown/gray/orange It should fade out irregularly	
		Opaque white with small amounts of any combination using gray, yellow or brown	Place the inside portion with opaque white	
Restoration itself	Opaque white Gray/yellow/brown			
Amalgam stain	Gray/black/blue	Match adjacent teeth	Gray or bluish stain on the proximal angle over a distance of 2 mm on the labial surface	
Gold inlay	Gold pottery stain		Superglaze surface to be stained. Paint a thin layer of gold stain over super glaze. Fire the layer and then coat with two thin layers of white glaze.	

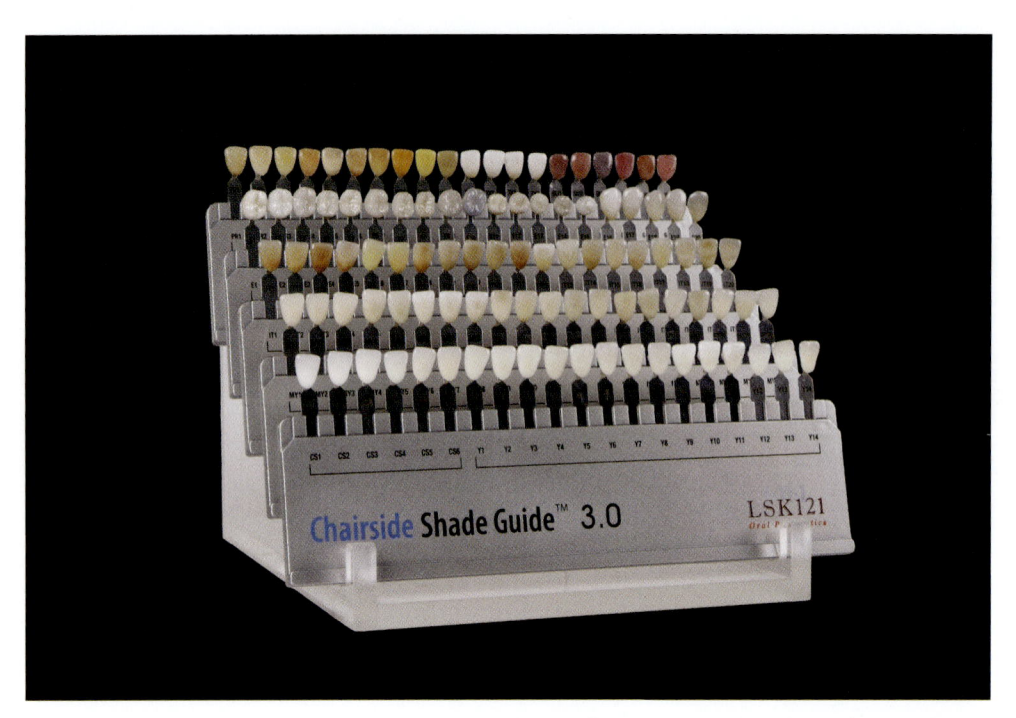

Figure 8.13 **(A)** The Chairside Shade Guide ceramic shade tabs are divided into different categories, with 20 tabs in each grouping. Figure courtesy of Lukus S. Kahng.

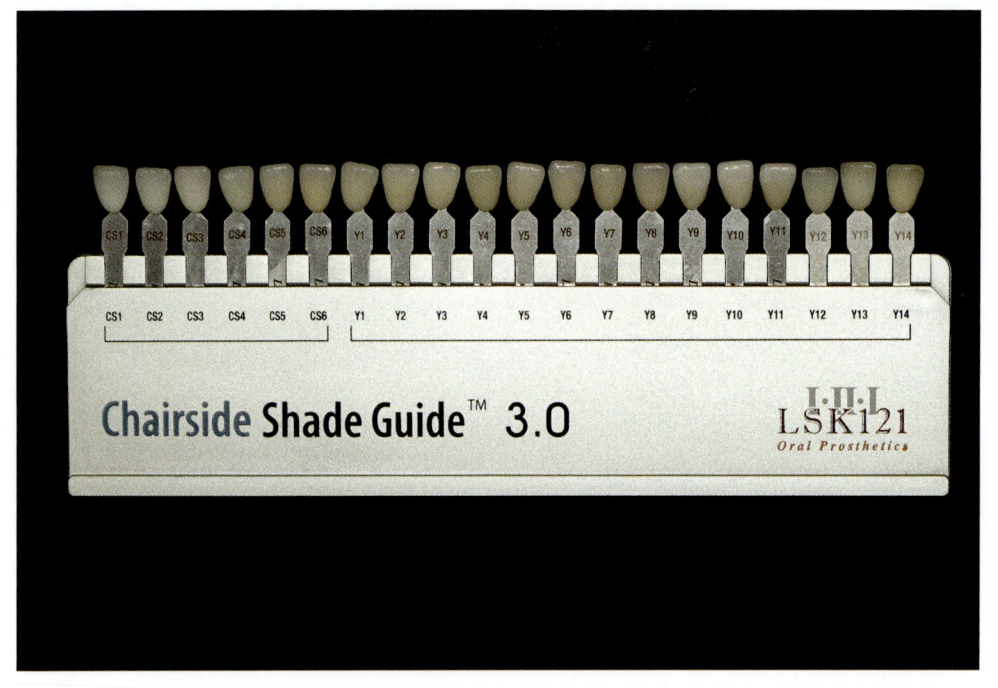

Figure 8.13 **(B)** Early Age (14 colors). Shade tabs range from bright to warm colors with different degrees of translucency. Figure courtesy of Lukus S. Kahng.

enamel translucencies. The shade tabs mimic those colors (Figure 8.13D).

- Shade guide 6.0: Pre-molar (five), Molar (10), and Canine (five) selections with two-thirds occlusal enamel along with occlusal stain, gray, tan, opal, and blue enamel and a variety of canine enamels, with consideration also given to the incisal one-third (Figure 8.13E).

- Shade guide 7.0: After Preparation Color (10) mimics natural teeth color and after preparation from implant to veneer cases and dark after-prep colors. Surface Texture (four) includes vertical, vertical horizontal, misty, and natural polish. Surface texture relates to anterior cases because without the proper texture application, the restoration will tend to have a fake appearance. Gingival Color (six) includes

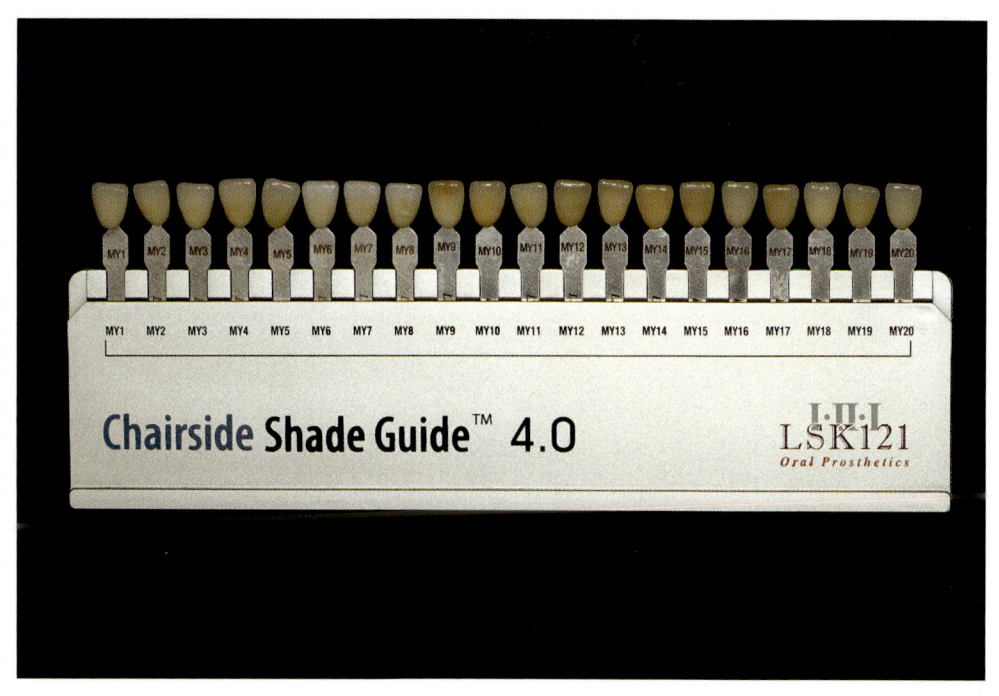

Figure 8.13 **(C)** Middle Years (20 colors) include variation of color in enamel in ratios of 50% enamel and 50% translucency with three white calcification possibilities. Figure courtesy of Lukus S. Kahng.

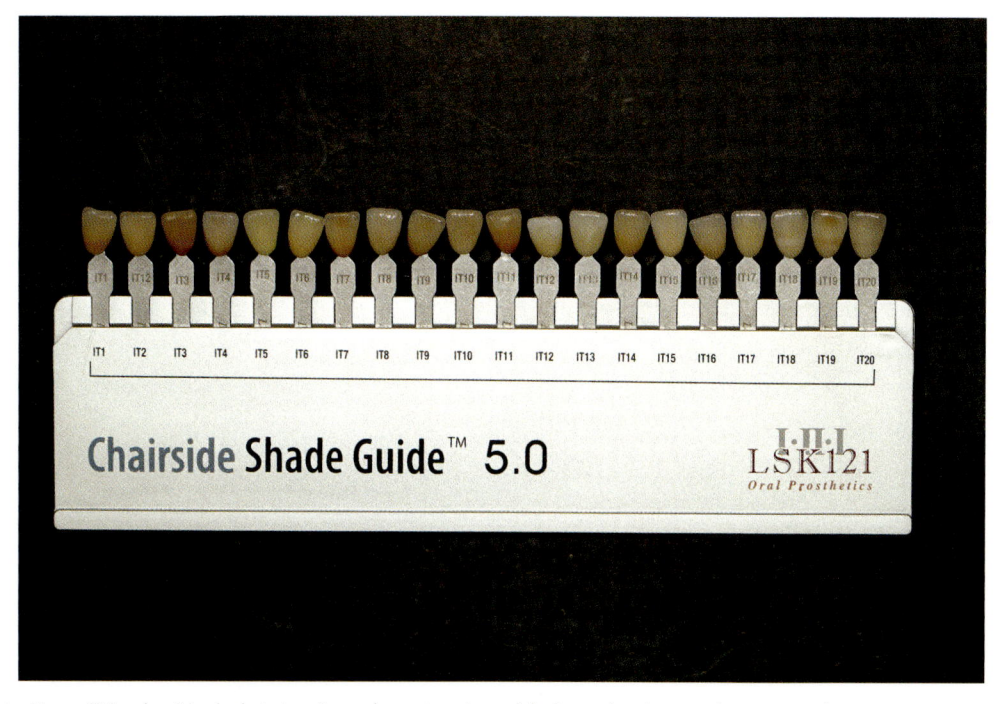

Figure 8.13 **(D)** Later Years (20 colors) include intensive color saturation with deep dentin, translucency, and transparency, as well as a variety of enamel translucencies. Figure courtesy of Lukus S. Kahng.

a variety of pinks with enamel overlay included in the color. This is especially important for implant and edentulous cases because the tissue color can create an unnatural appearance if it does not match the natural dentition (Figure 8.13 F).

These shade tabs are based on the theory behind custom shade matching and are each overlaid with different enamel colors so that they harmoniously match with natural teeth. A traditional 1–3 solid color shade tab opposes natural dentition and enamel, serving merely as a guide to color matching. It is also important to properly photograph the shade tabs with the teeth to be matched to show the ceramist any shade discrepancies (Figure 8.13G and H).

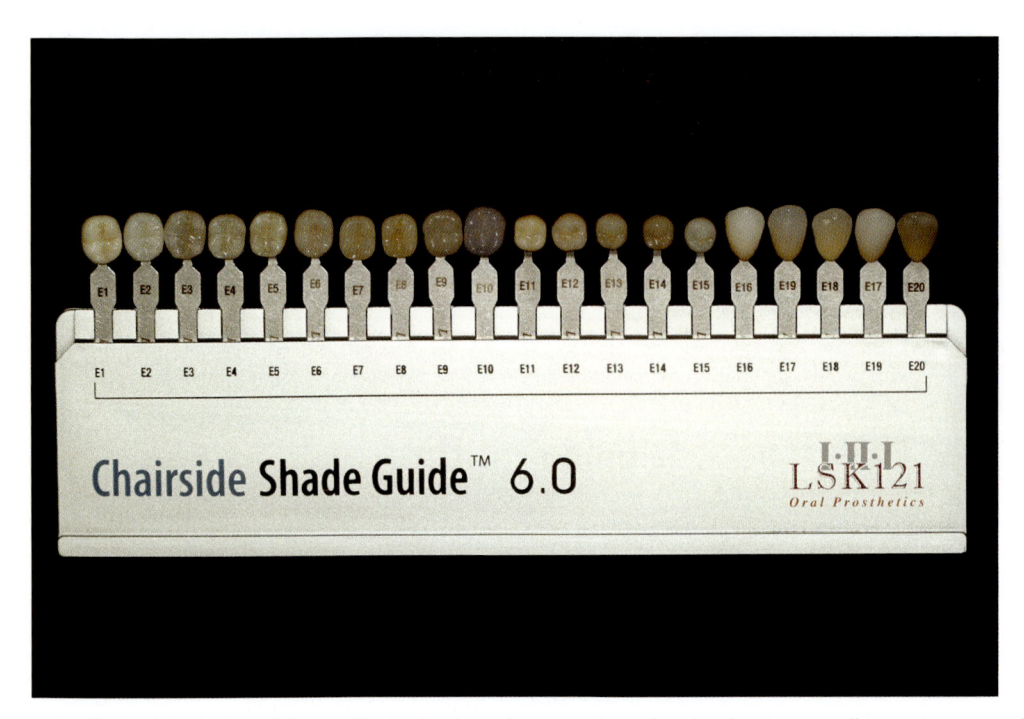

Figure 8.13 **(E)** Pre-molar (five), Molar (10), and Canine (five) selections show a variety of occlusal stains as well as canine enamel incisal variance. Figure courtesy of Lukus S. Kahng.

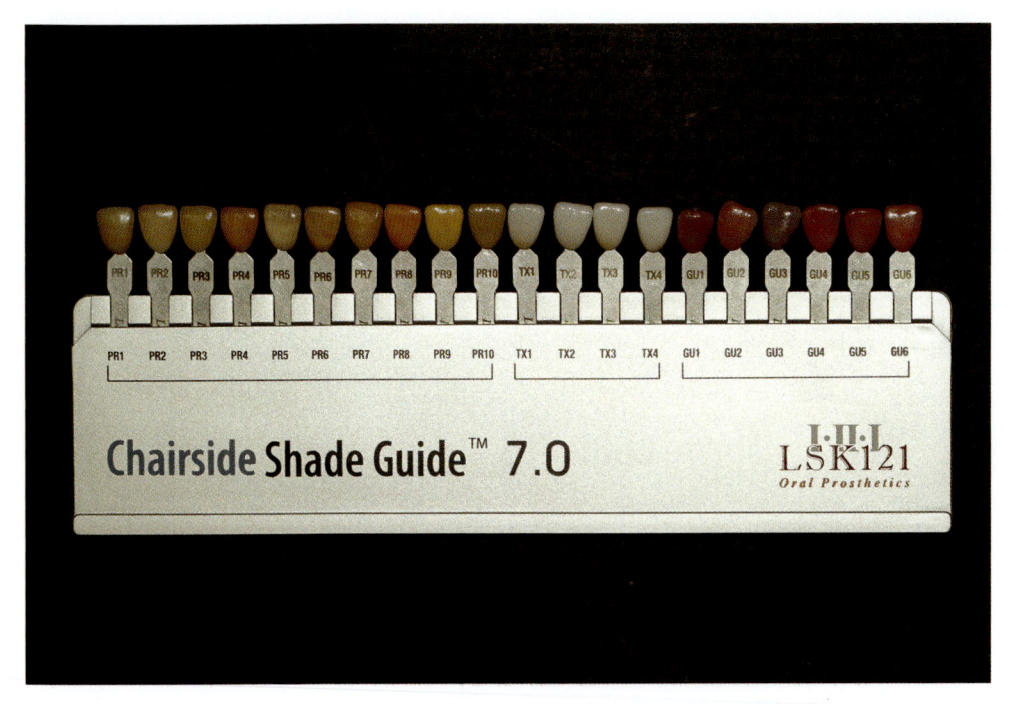

Figure 8.13 **(F)** After Preparation Color (10)—shows a variety of colors of prepared teeth. Surface texture (four) is also seen as well as a variety of pinks with enamel overlay. Figure courtesy of Lukus S. Kahng

Techniques for resolving various problems

The most commonly encountered problems that can be corrected through illusions are discussed below.

Space available is wider than the ideal replacement tooth

This problem is typically encountered either when space was present between the teeth prior to extraction or when drifting has occurred to widen the space. If the space is to be restored

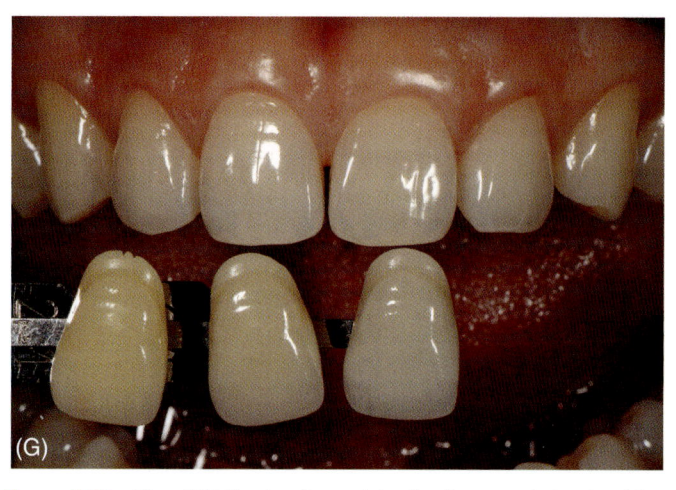

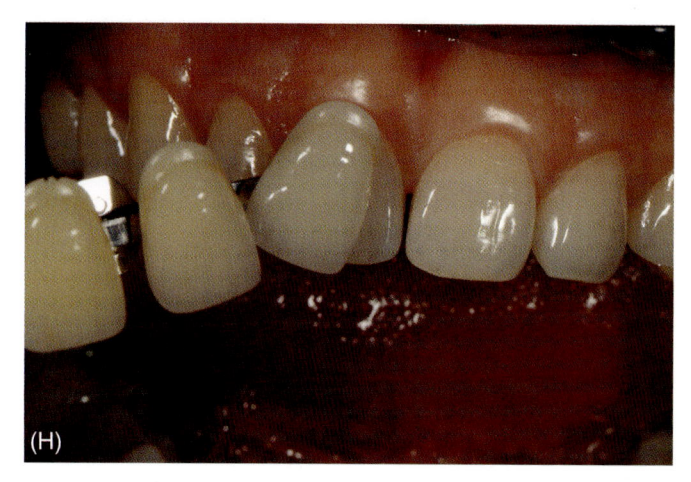

Figure 8.13 **(G and H)** Shade tabs position in photograph is critical for communicating color property. Shade tabs should be placed below and in the same plane as teeth.

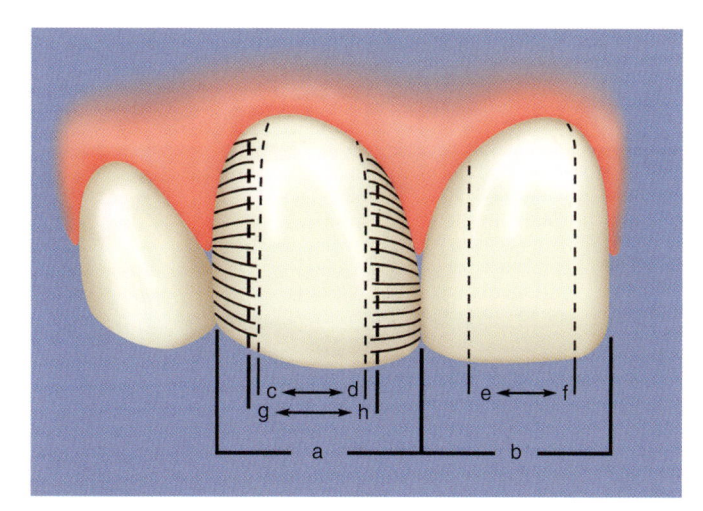

Figure 8.14 Tooth "a" is made to appear thinner than it actually is by carving the mesial and distal line angles to the lingual, thus presenting less labial surface.

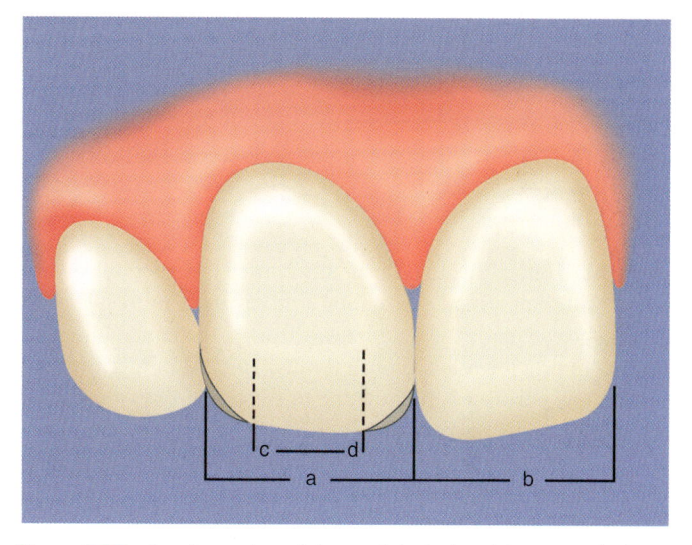

Figure 8.15 Gentle curving of the mesioincisal and distoincisal edges, as well as a slight indentation at the midincisal edge, alters visual perception.

with the correct number of teeth and tooth contact is to be re-established, avoid horizontal lines, edges, and characterizations, and incorporate as many vertical ones as possible into the restoration.

Shaping and contouring illusions

The width of the replacement tooth or teeth will have to be wider than ideal; therefore, various illusions achieved through shaping and contouring should be used. The width needed to close the space is gained in the areas of contact.

Illusions for incisors

The extra width can be disguised by placing the contact areas more lingually and cervically. In Figure 8.14, the diameter of tooth "a" is larger than that of tooth "b", but by carving the mesial and distal line angles to the lingual the tooth appears thinner. One reason for this illusion is the reflection created by shaping and contouring the tooth. Light usually reflects from the flat labial surface. Line angles "e" and "f" usually reflect light and give the appearance of width to the tooth. The corresponding lines on the right central would be "g" and "h". By moving the mesial and distal line angles slightly to the middle of the tooth, new line angles "c" and "d" are created and thus a less flat labial surface remains. This reduction in the reflective surface makes the tooth appear narrower than it really is. Although these should be subtle carvings, at times labial prominences can be created to actually catch light rays. In this manner, more precise distance can be interpreted by the observer.

In summary, the mesial and distal line angles in Figure 8.14 are moved toward the center of the labial surface (c and d). The mesial and distal surfaces are then made more convex, curving from the line angles into the areas of contact. The shape of the incisal edge can abet the illusion of decreased width. The mesioincisal corner is rounded, and a gentle curve is created from the middle third of the incisal edge to the distal contact (Figure 8.15). The incisal edge can be notched slightly to break

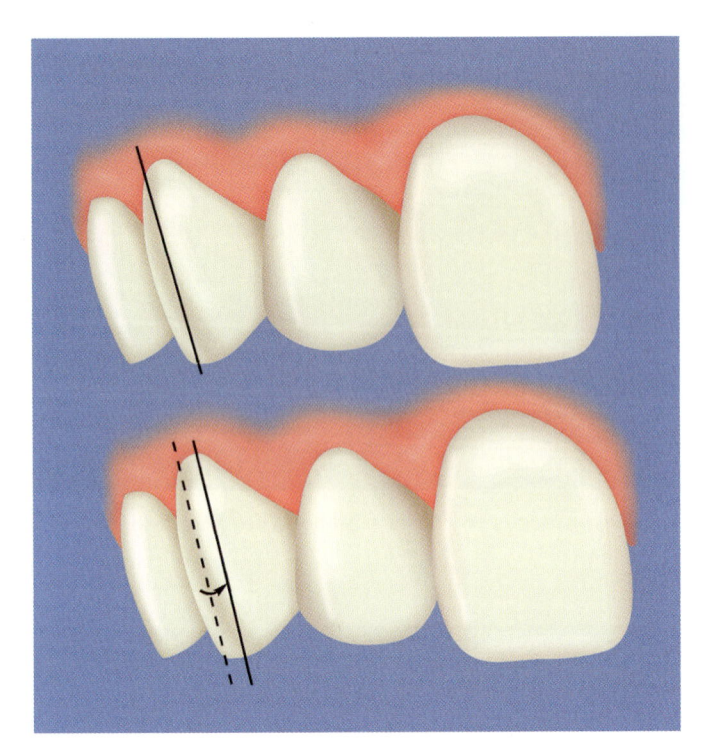

Figure 8.16 This figure illustrates a too - wide cuspid. The buccal ridge is carved to the mesial to disguise the excess width in the cuspid.

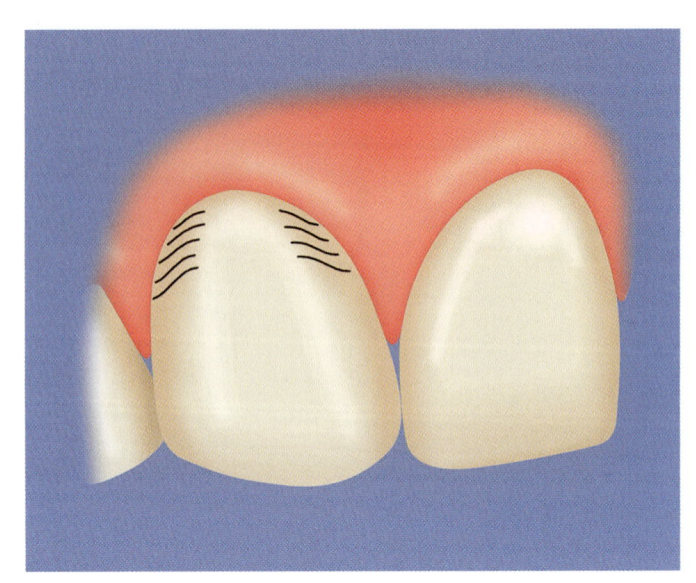

Figure 8.17 Shallow developmental grooves which break up the smooth labial reflecting surface make the tooth appear less wide.

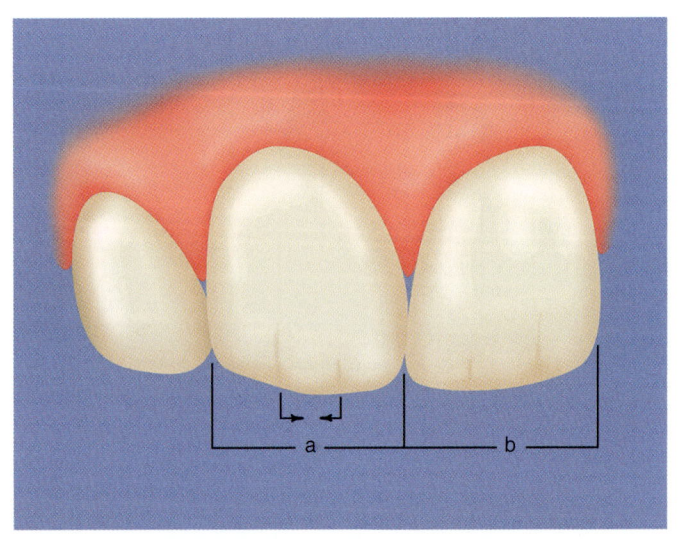

Figure 8.18 A more pronounced curve carved into the cemento-enamel junction which is in a more incisal or occlusal position is another technique used to make the tooth appear thinner.

up the horizontal line. Even a slightly curved indentation, a wave result, will alter visual perception and create a more pleasing effect. The eye tends to wander away from a horizontal line, and the curves provide relief. Only a limited amount of mesioincisal rounding is permitted, mainly due to the possibility of creating asymmetry in the restoration by overdoing it. It is possible, however, to create the illusion of a slight incisal diastema by moving the mesial contact of the larger tooth gingivally. This produces an entirely different effect than a complete diastema. The open incisal diastema can be natural in appearance and quite effective in balancing space variations. More incisal shaping is possible from the distal side. Since the observer sees the patient mainly from straight ahead, it is possible to achieve much of the space illusion by opening the distoincisal embrasure. The distance c and d is also re-emphasized by carving mainly from this point, both mesially and distally. At times, it may even appear as if a diastema is placed distally, depending on how much the contact is placed gingivally. This is still a much better esthetic choice than having an oversized contralateral central incisor.

Illusions for cuspids

Extra width can be disguised by moving the visual center of the labial or buccal surface more to the mesial by carving the buccal ridge to the mesial (Figure 8.16). The cusp tip should then be moved mesially if this is compatible with functional requirements. Contact areas should also be moved lingually and cervically.

Illusions for anterior or posterior teeth

The developmental grooves are moved closer together (Figure 8.17). These grooves do not have to be deep to be effective. Shallow grooves will give the desired shadows. To further this illusion, any characterizations ground into the labial or buccal surface should be vertically oriented. By breaking up the smooth unbroken labial or buccal reflecting surface with characterizations, you make the tooth appear less wide. The curve of the cementoenamel junction carved into the restoration can be made more pronounced and brought into a more incisal or occlusal position in the interproximal gingival embrasure areas (Figure 8.18). When shaping the restoration, the opposite tooth should be kept in mind as the ideal. Slight concavities in the gingival third also give the illusion of a narrower tooth. Special attention should be paid to duplicating ridges and depressions that reflect light (Figure 8.18). One should remember that it is the individual

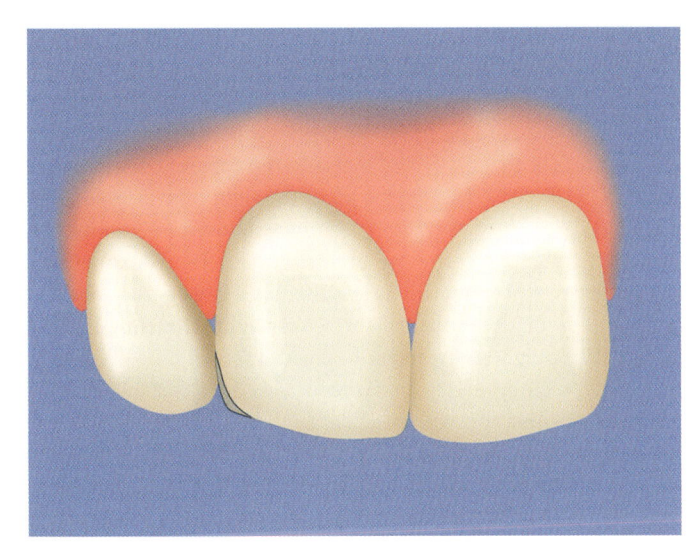

Figure 8.19 All three shaping special effects are combined on this restoration to produce the illusion of a thinner tooth.

pattern of light and color reflection that determines tooth character. Figure 8.19 shows all the shaping effects combined to produce the illusion of a thinner tooth.

Staining to mask tooth size

For masking a large tooth, color can be used to advantage in one of several ways. By selecting a body color barely darker than that of the approximating teeth, the larger tooth appears less prominent. The mesial and distal thirds of the labial or buccal surface can be stained grayer (Figure 8.20A and B) than the middle third. The gray color disappears in the mouth and the appearance of size is transmitted to the glancing eye by the normally colored area. Note how much thinner the teeth appear in Figure 8.20B after using the above technique. The developmental grooves and characterizations ground into the surface can also be emphasized with gray stain. Indefinite, barely perceptible, vertical lines can be incorporated to accent the vertical aspects of the tooth. This is done by using a stain slightly lighter than the body color and by running it from the tooth body to the incisal or occlusal edge. To further highlight the lighter lines suggested earlier, an opaque white, yellow, orange, or brown stain can be used to create vertical check or microcrack lines.

Arrangement of teeth can create the illusion of decreased width

The position or arrangement of the teeth can create the illusion of decreased width. When a tooth is placed in linguoversion, not only is its real width masked by the more prominent approximating teeth but also the effect of the increased shadowing masks its size (Figure 8.21). Rotation of a tooth from its normal labiolingual position will accomplish several illusions. Through rotation, the normal perception of the tooth is changed, and the tooth loses some of its identity. Depending upon the degree of rotation, the tooth can be made to appear less wide. In Figure 8.22A, the right central appears wider than the left central; actually the left central is rotated distally, so it looks thinner (Figure 8.22B). When the mouth is viewed from midway between the rotated and non-rotated teeth, the teeth look much the same width (Figure 8.22C). When two central incisors are replaced, the distal aspects of the wide crowns are rotated lingually, thereby narrowing the area that reflects light forward and decreasing the apparent width (Figure 8.23). You can create a diastema to avoid widening the replacement teeth. Position the teeth so that the space left on the distal aspect of the restoration is not prominent (Figure 8.24).

If the space to be filled is much wider than the replacement teeth, the only reasonably esthetic solution may ultimately be the addition of an extra tooth. This method of handling the extra space works especially well when replacing the lower anteriors. (See Chapter 26 on restorative treatment of diastema.)

Space available is narrower than the ideal replacement tooth

This problem is usually encountered when extraction was not immediately followed by replacement and the adjacent teeth drifted or tilted to encroach upon the space. If the space is to be

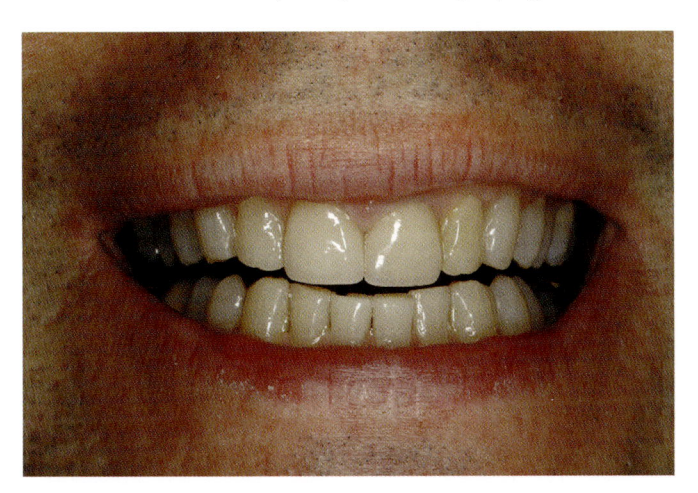

Figure 8.20 (A) These two central incisors appear too wide with respect to the other teeth in the patient's dentition.

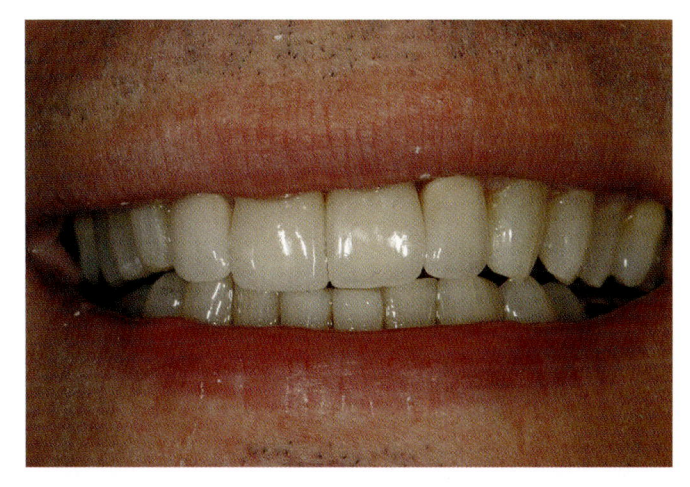

Figure 8.20 (B) To accomplish thinner looking central incisors the ceramic restorations were made slightly longer and more translucent stains were used in both mesial and distal proximal areas to give the appearance of thinner-looking teeth.

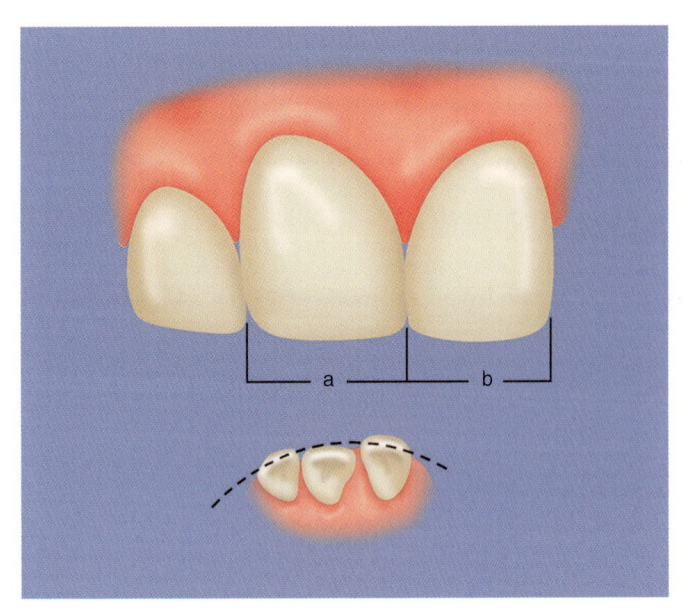

Figure 8.21 Placing the wider tooth in linguoversion masks its real width by diminishing its prominence with the adjacent teeth and adding shadowing.

restored with the correct number of narrower teeth, avoid vertical lines, edges, and characteristics, and incorporate as many horizontal lines as possible.

Shaping

Before the replacement crowns are shaped, the proximal surfaces of the adjacent teeth should be reduced slightly to increase as much as possible the space available. Most or all of the needed space can be obtained in this fashion. If this procedure is used, the reduced enamel surfaces must then be refinished (see Chapter 11). By altering the contour of the labial or buccal surface and the incisal or occlusal edge, an illusion of width can be achieved, even when the actual tooth is narrowed.

Illusion for incisors

The contact areas are moved labially and incisally, as illustrated in Figure 8.25. In this case, the right central is narrower than the left central and needs to be made to appear wider. By extending the contact areas both labially and incisally, the apparent width of line angle "X" is increased and helps make the right central look wider than it really is. If the previous technique is used in conjunction with flattening the entire labial surface and the proximal line angles, the overall effect will be lengthening of the incisal edge and development of a broad labial surface for light reflection. Both of these effects heighten the illusion of width (see Figure 8.25).

Another technique is to leave the incisal edge as flat and as horizontal as is compatible with adjacent teeth (see Figure 8.25). It may also help to reshape the incisal edge of the adjacent teeth slightly to help make the entire effect more esthetically harmonious. The adjacent central incisor can be shaped to look narrower by carving its distoincisal edge gingivally.

Illusions for cuspids

The narrowness of the crown can be disguised by moving the visual center of the labial or buccal surface (Figure 8.26) more distally. This is accomplished by carving the buccal ridge to the distal. The cusp tip should be moved distally if this is compatible with functional requirements, and the contact areas should be moved labially and incisally to accent the horizontal aspects of the narrow tooth.

Illusions for anterior or posterior teeth

The curve of the cementoenamel junction can be influential. It should be at the same level as the curve on the adjacent natural teeth but should have a flatter appearance (Figure 8.27A). To further accentuate the horizontal, additional grooves can be carved gingivally on the original one (see Figure 8.27A). However, if the adjacent natural teeth have strong vertical lines, this cannot be done effectively; therefore, the effort should be directed toward de-emphasizing as much as possible any vertical lines or edges. If there are only a few vertical lines on the adjacent natural tooth, it may be possible to cosmetically contour the labial surface on that tooth to diminish their effect.

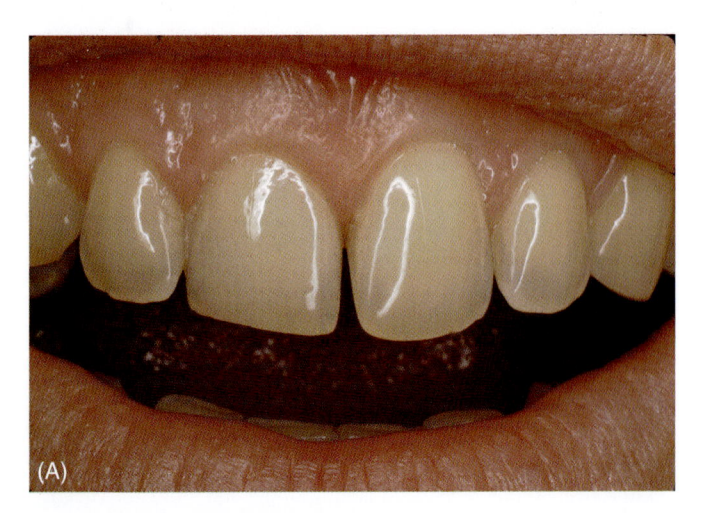

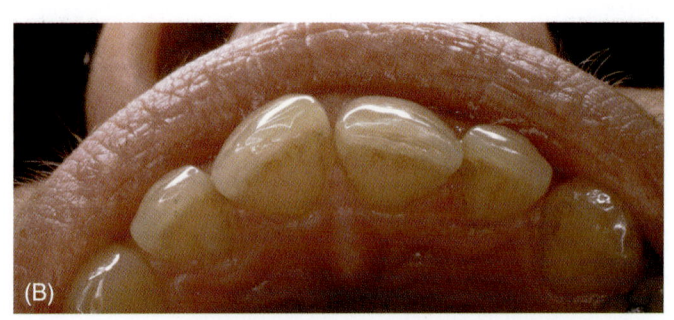

Figure 8.22 (A and B) Although the right central appears wider than the left central, the left central is actually rotated distally, which causes it to look thinner.

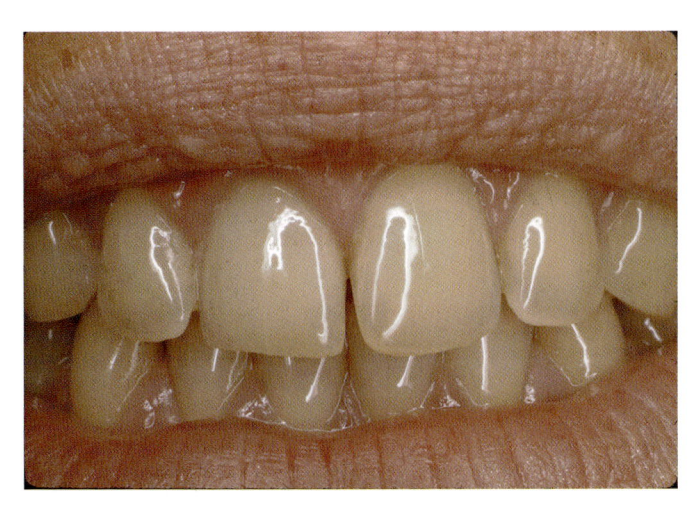

Figure 8.22 (C) When the patient is viewed from a different angle (halfway between the rotated and non-rotated teeth) the teeth look proportional.

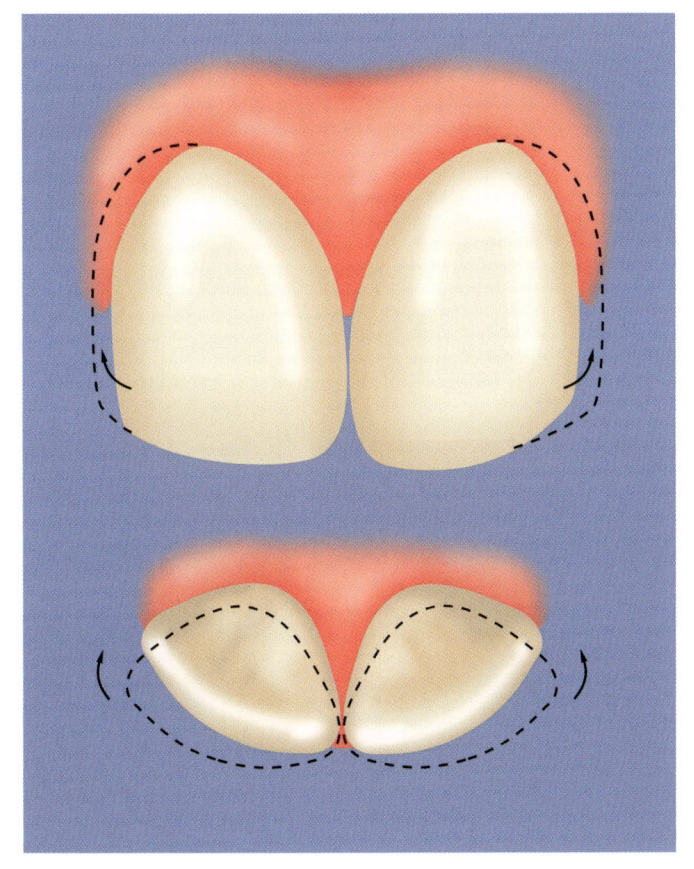

Figure 8.23 The distal aspects of both the replaced central incisors are rotated, which narrows the light - reflecting surface and decreases width perception.

By eliminating developmental grooves and lobes, the labial surface can be carved to develop a broad, flat surface to provide an area for unbroken light reflection. This area will appear broader than the same area that has the surface broken with grooves and characterizations that scatter the reflections (see Figure 8.27A).

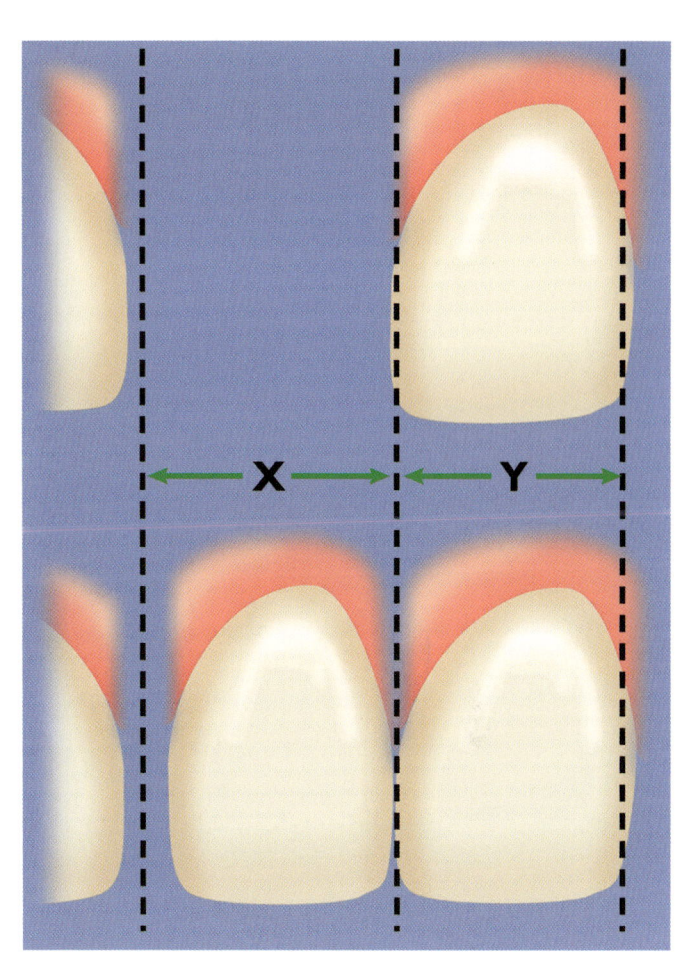

Figure 8.24 When a space is too wide (X) a distal diastema is preferable to making the replacement tooth too wide (Y).

Staining

Color can also be used to increase the illusion of width. For instance, when a body color is selected that is slightly lighter than that of the adjacent teeth, the narrow tooth will appear more prominent and therefore wider. The mesial and distal thirds can be stained a shade lighter than the middle third, to highlight the proximal aspects and the width of the tooth. Any horizontal grooves or lines that have been carved into the labial surface can be accentuated with a light stain. Definite, barely perceptible, horizontal lines can be created to accentuate width. This is done by choosing a stain slightly lighter than body color and running it from mesial to distal. To further accentuate these lines, a light, thin orange, yellow, brown, or white opaque line can be placed on the labial surface (Figure 8.27B).

Another way to accentuate width is to simulate multiple decalcification spots running horizontally across the middle third of the tooth (Figure 8.27C). Other horizontal lines can be created by using staining to indicate one or two anterior restorations that have been carried out onto the labial surface. If adjacent teeth show cervical erosion, this erosion should be either restored or reproduced in the replacement tooth (Figure 8.27C). Staining can also be used to create an illusion of incisal erosion (Figure 8.27D). Finally, shade modification can and should be done when patients want to have a more natural look (Figure 8.27E).

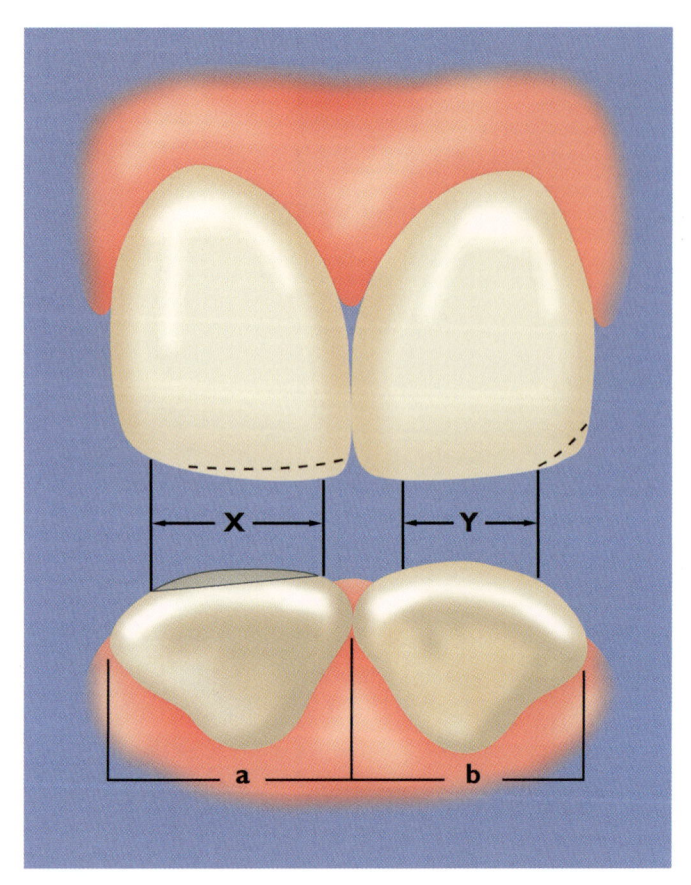

Figure 8.25 The narrow right central incisor needs to appear as wide as the left central incisor. The line angle "X" is extended labially and incisally, making the right central appear wider. If necessary, the distoincisal angle of the wide incisor can be reshaped, making it appear slightly narrower (Y).

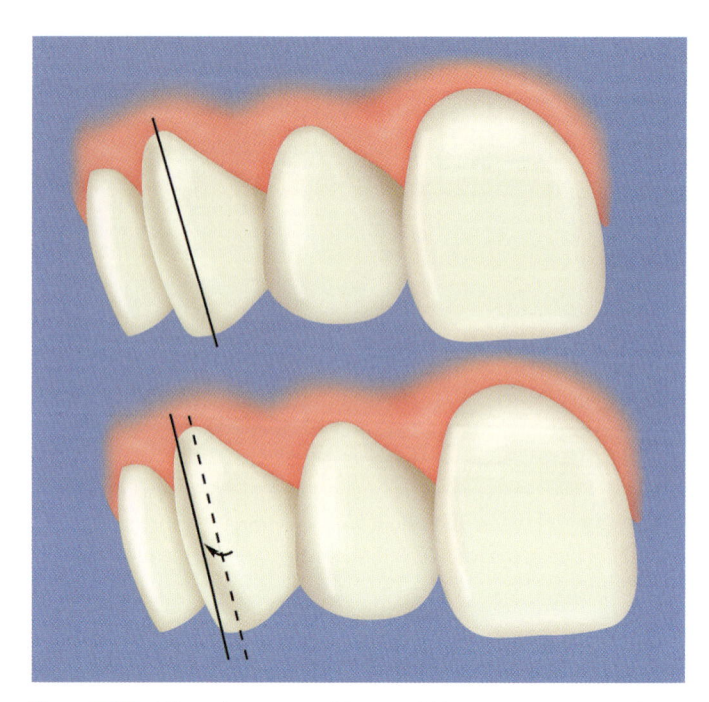

Figure 8.26 When the crown of the cuspid is too narrow, move the visual center of the labial surface distally by carving the buccal ridge distal to the usual position if this remains compatible with functional requirements.

Arrangement

The most simple and direct solution for inadequate space is to rotate and overlap the replacement crowns or teeth without reducing their ideal widths. If rotation and overlapping are unacceptable or impossible, and if the encroachment on the space has

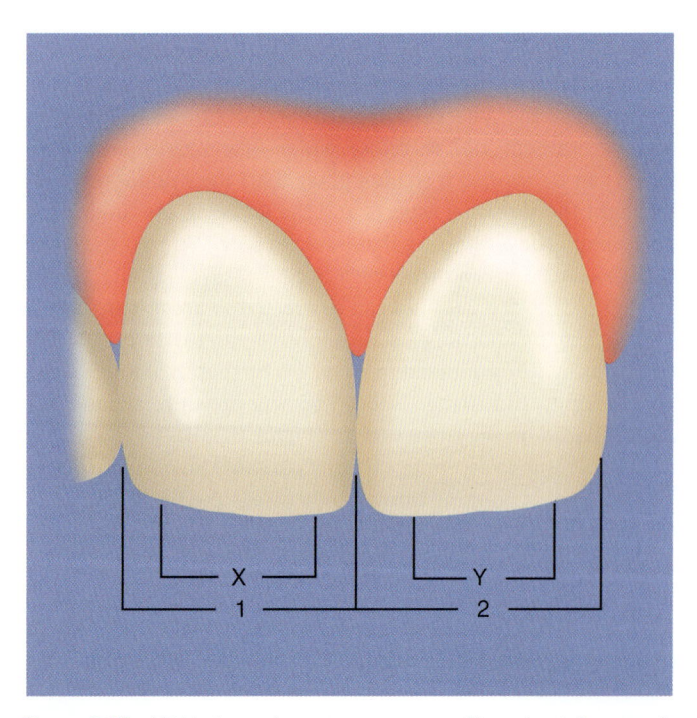

Figure 8.27 **(A)** Horizontal grooves were carved into the right central (1) to give it a wider appearance.

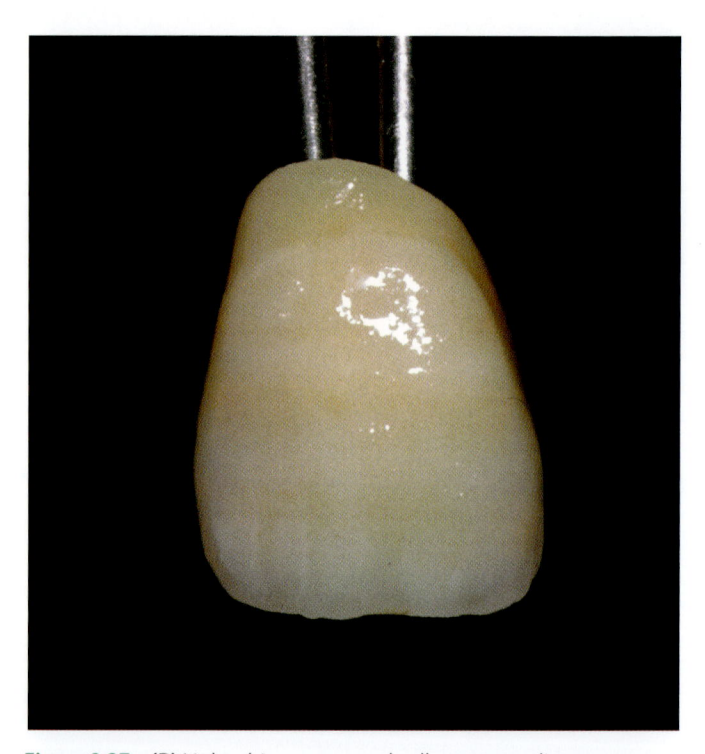

Figure 8.27 **(B)** Light, thin, orange and yellow opaque lines were placed on the surface to further enhance the carved horizontal lines.

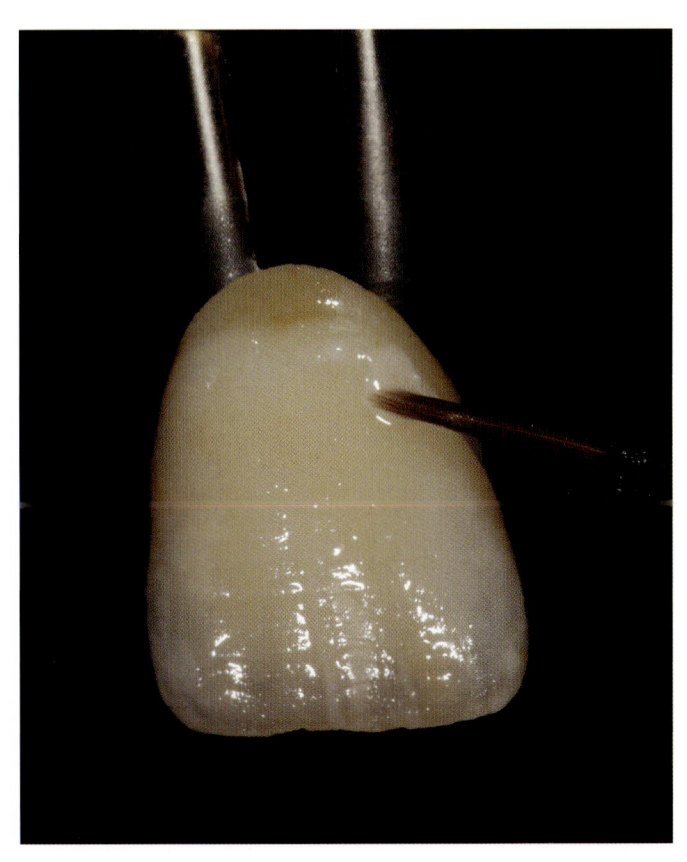

Figure 8.27 **(C)** White calcification spots running horizontally across the middle third of the tooth further accentuate width.

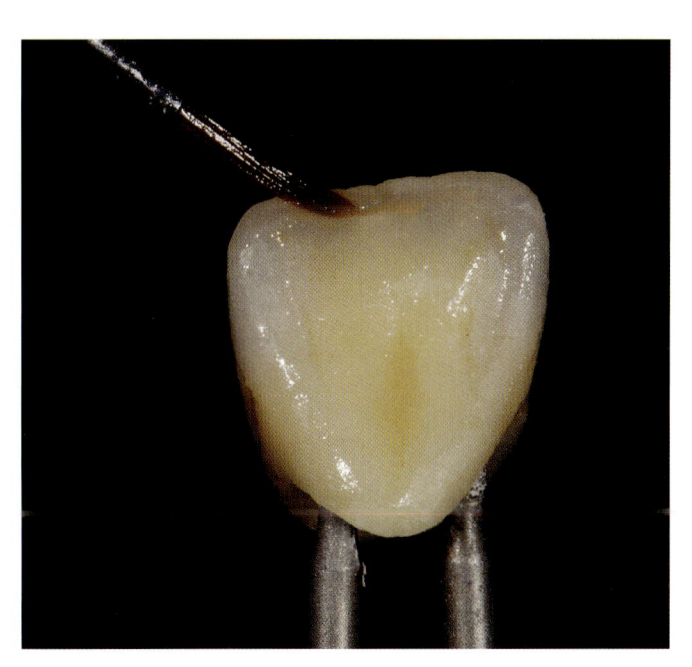

Figure 8.27 **(D)** Staining used to create the illusion of incisal erosion to match adjacent teeth also emphasizes width if the crown is horizontal and flat.

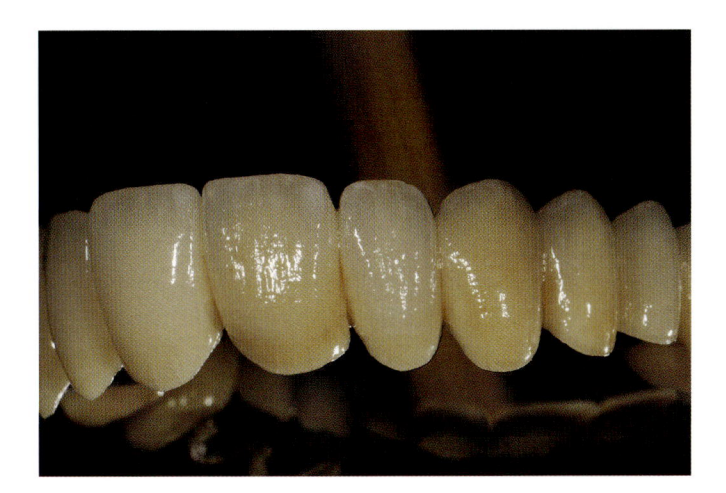

Figure 8.27 **(E)** This photo of a ceramometal splint shows the ability to modify shades to the patient's natural looking teeth.

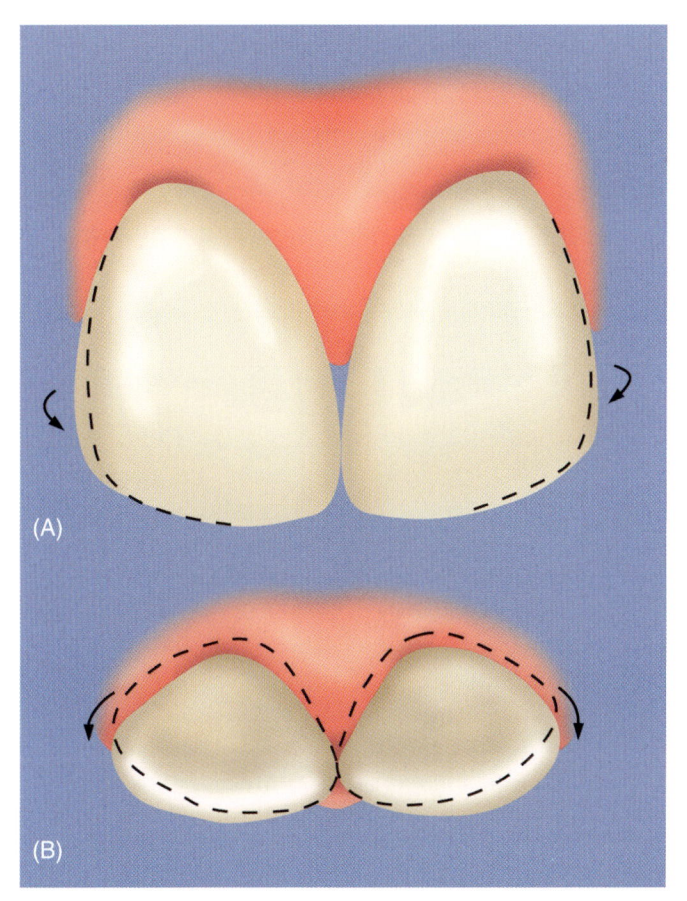

Figure 8.28 For an inadequate space involving central incisors, the teeth can be slightly rotated labially and lapped rather than reducing their ideal width, making them appear wider and more prominent.

been severe, it may be possible to eliminate one tooth entirely with good results, especially in cases involving lower anteriors. In cases where the maxillary central incisors are involved, the distal aspects can be rotated labially, making these teeth appear more prominent and wider (Figure 8.28). The principle involved here is to create prominent distolabial line angles to create more horizontal reflections.

When the problem involves both maxillary central and lateral incisors, the centrals can be placed normally and the laterals can

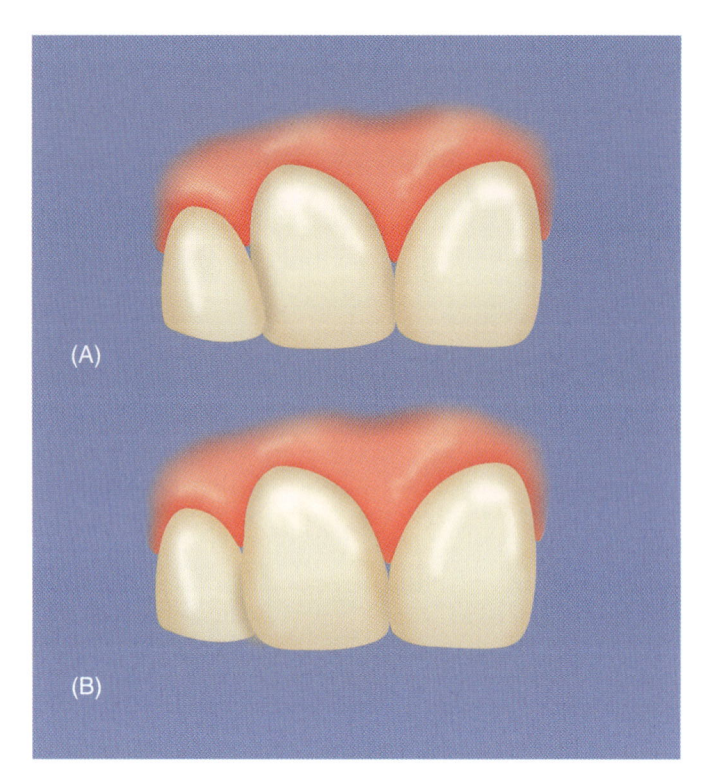

Figure 8.29 **(A)** For a female, the mesial aspect of the lateral incisor is rotated labially and lapped in front of the centrals to increase a soft, feminine appearance without increasing the space needed for the replacement teeth. **(B)** The mesial aspect of the lateral incisor of this male patient is rotated and lapped lingually behind the central to project width and boldness without requiring additional space.

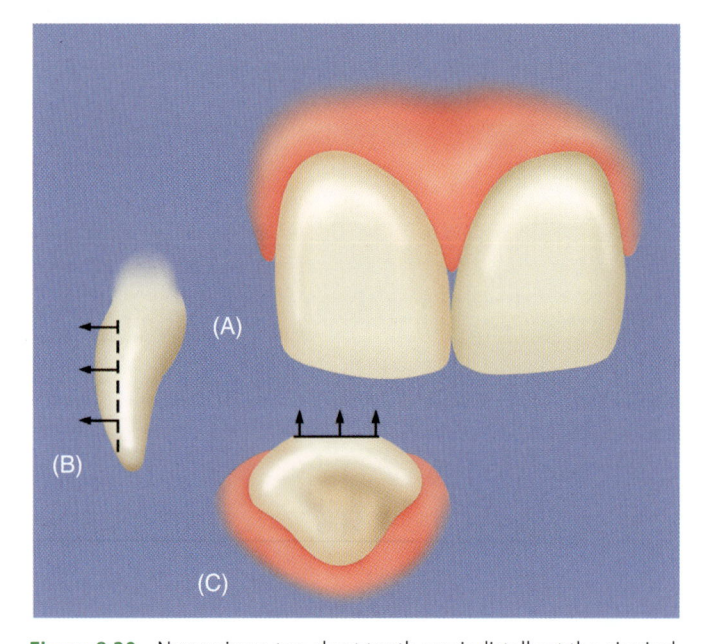

Figure 8.30 Narrowing a too-short tooth mesiodistally at the gingival one-third creates the illusion of length **(A)**. To further this illusion, vertically flatten the labial middle third (B, C).

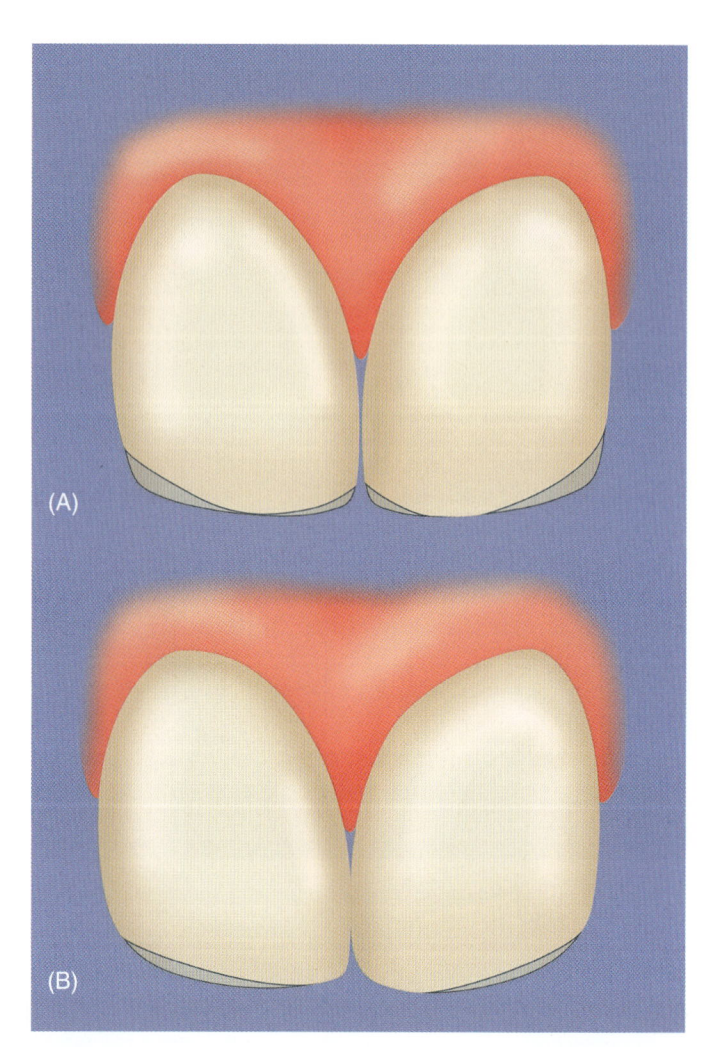

Figure 8.31 **(A)** An illusion of length can be created by gently sloping the mesial and distal halves of the incisal edge toward the gingiva from the midline to the contact areas. **(B)** If two adjacent anterior teeth need to appear longer, each incisal edge should be made to slope gingivally away from the approximating common incisal angles, lending the illusion of length.

be rotated. In the case of a male, the mesial aspects of the laterals are rotated and lapped lingually behind the centrals increasing the overall appearance of width and boldness and decreasing the amount of space needed (Figure 8.29A). In the case of a female, the mesial aspects of the laterals are rotated labially and lapped in front of the centrals, increasing the feminine appearance (Figure 8.29B).

The too-short tooth

If a tooth appears too short, as is likely if it is wider than normal, several techniques can be used to create the illusion of length.

Shaping

If the gingival third is narrowed mesiodistally, the tooth will appear more tapered and longer (Figure 8.30A). This illusion can be further enhanced by having a vertically flat labial middle third to increase the vertical reflecting surface (Figure 8.30B and C).

The shape of the incisal edge can be altered to create an illusion of greater length in the anterior region. For each involved tooth, the mesial and distal halves can be sloped gently toward the gingiva from the midline to the contacts (Figure 8.31A). In the specific case of the central incisors, each incisal edge can be

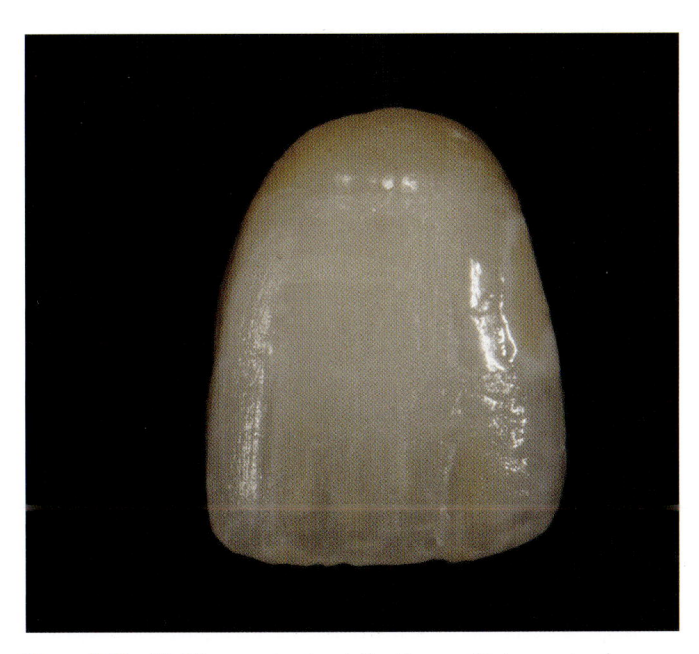

Figure 8.32 (A) Microcracks, decalcification, and interproximal restoration staining has produced the illusion of length.

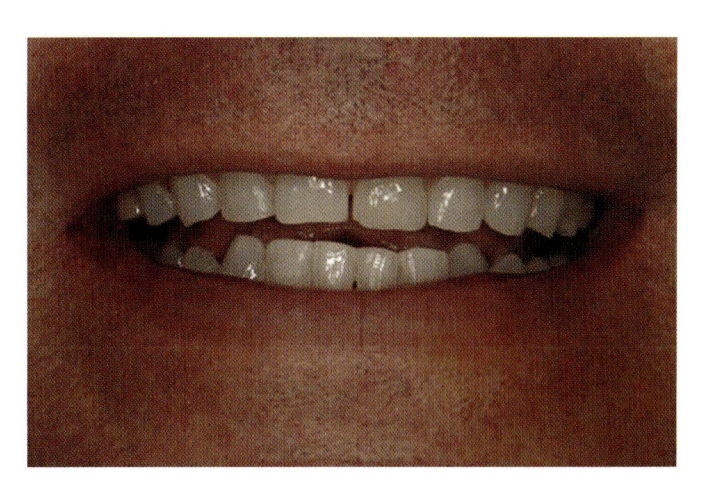

Figure 8.32 (B) This 49-year-old patient had an extreme case of bruxism resulting in an older-looking smile.

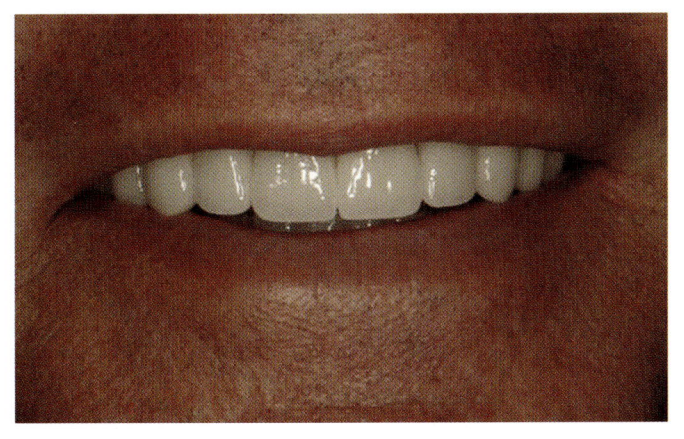

Figure 8.32 (C) A more youthful look was attained with all ceramic restorations consisting of slightly altering vertical dimension to be able to lengthen teeth. Interincisal distance was re-established and incisal embrasures restored.

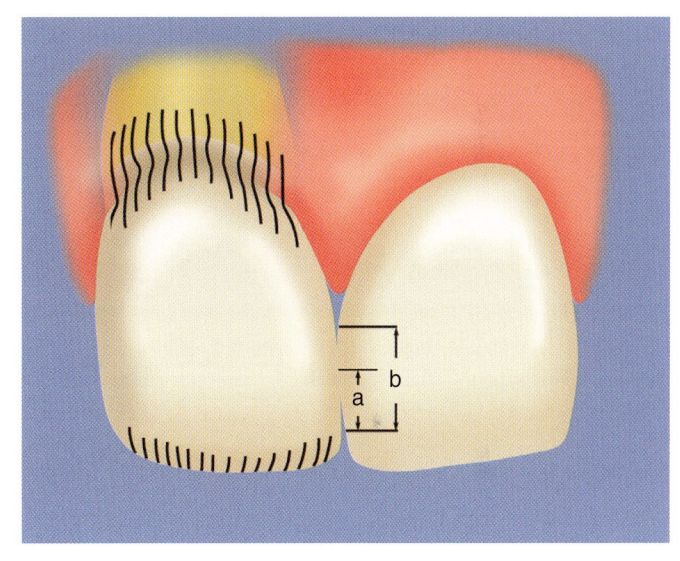

Figure 8.33 For the too-long tooth, increase the vertical contact area ("a" to a wider contact "b"), keep the embrasures as narrow as possible, and lingually incline the cervical and incisal one-fifth areas.

made to slope gingivally away from the approximating common incisal angles, lending the illusion of length (Figure 8.31B).

Staining

The main principle to remember when using staining to increase height is that stains of higher value (whiter) make the area to which they are applied more noticeable. A fine, opaque, white check line running from the body of the tooth to the incisal edge accentuates the height. A white decalcification spot placed close to the incisal edge also increases the height illusion. Staining can be used to duplicate the appearance of a long, vertical interproximal anterior restoration, which increases the illusion of length (Figure 8.32A).

Arrangement

If the maxillary six anterior teeth have worn unnaturally, producing noticeably shorter teeth, vertical dimension may need to be altered to be able to lengthen the teeth and reopen the incisal embrasures (Figure 8.32B and C). Be careful of using too much incisal staining, otherwise the teeth may still appear too short.

The too-long tooth

When alveolar or gingival recession has been severe, the length of the pontics or crowns must be made to appear shorter. Basically, vertical grooves or lines should be diminished and horizontal lines emphasized. This can be accomplished by several methods.

Shaping

The areas of contact can be lengthened as much as is physiologically acceptable while the gingival embrasures are kept as narrow as possible (Figure 8.33). The cervical portion and the incisal one-fifth of the pontic or crown should be inclined lingually (Figures 8.33 and 8.34). By changing the inclination of these

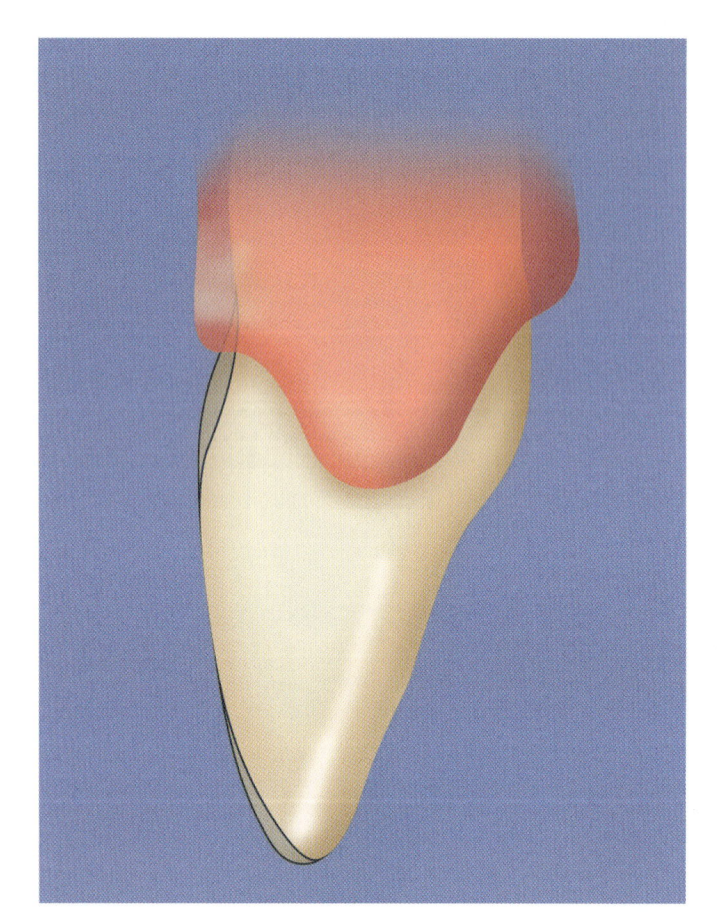

Figure 8.34 A lateral view demonstrating the lingual inclination of the cervical and incisal one-fifth areas which decreases the appearance of length.

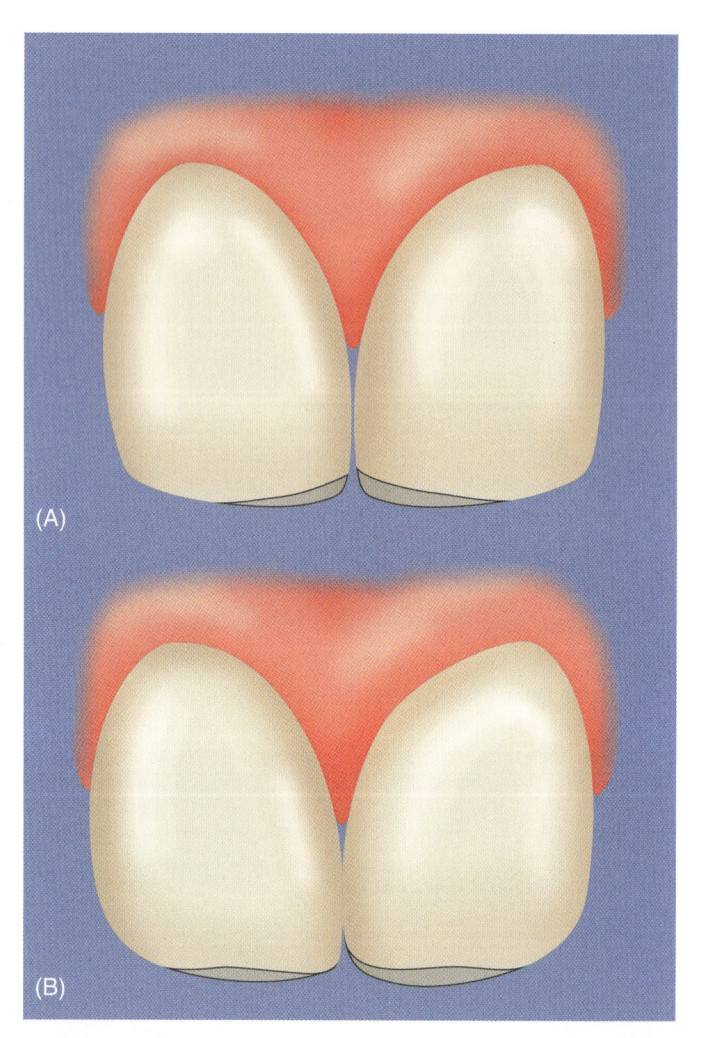

Figure 8.35 When two teeth are involved, reduce the incisal edges to converge gingivally at the proximal common contact (**A**). The length of the tooth will appear to decrease by the notching of the center of the incisal edge (**B**).

surfaces, the effective reflecting surface is shortened, decreasing the appearance of length. The incisal edge may be shaped to seemingly decrease length by notching the center (Figure 8.35B). If there are two adjacent teeth that need to appear shorter, grind the incisal edges to converge gingivally at the proximal contact (Figure 8.35A).

Staining

A definite demarcation at the cementoenamel junction decreases the apparent length, and this can be carved into the restoration and further accentuated with stain. The color of the cervical portion should be deepened by staining it either a deeper body or cervical shade.

To mask the height of extremely long teeth, either stain the gingival portion of the crown or pontic pink (to simulate gingival tissue) or use a combination of tissue-colored porcelain stains when baking the crown.

Creating optical illusions with form and color

Modifying shape and form, along with the color and shade of teeth can create a myriad of special effects or illusions (Figure 8.36A–L). Table 8.4 and accompanying photographs provide real-world examples of these special effects in action.

Need to disguise long-axis inclinations

When restoring a severely tipped tooth, it may be impossible to achieve correct alignment simply by altering the preparation. In these cases, the use of illusions can confer the appearance of good alignment.

Increasing mesial inclination

In an anterior tooth (Figure 8.37), the distal contact is moved cervically and the mesial contact is moved incisally. The distal line angle is carved toward the center of the incisal edge. To help complete this illusion, the incisal edge is pointed on the mesial and notched toward the distal. In a posterior tooth, the distal contact is moved cervically and the mesial contact is moved occlusally. The buccal ridge is carved to curve from the distogingival to the mesio-occlusal. The cusp tip can be moved mesially if this is compatible with functional requirements.

In both anterior and posterior teeth, the illusion of mesial inclination can be increased by incorporating light lines, by

(A)

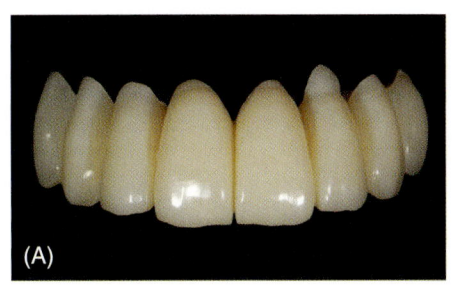

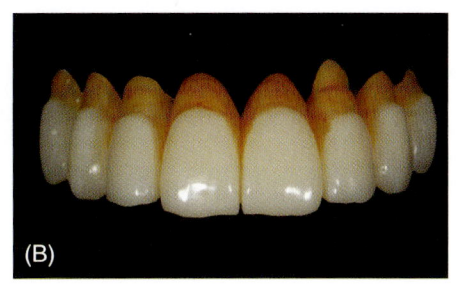

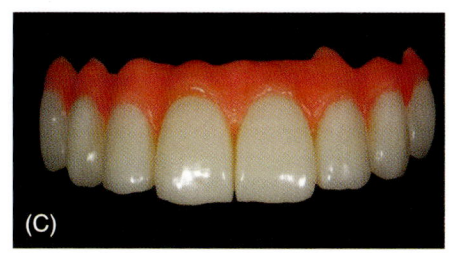

(B)

(C)

Figure 8.36 (A–C) Modifications of form and color can create illusion of better proportion of teeth.

(D)

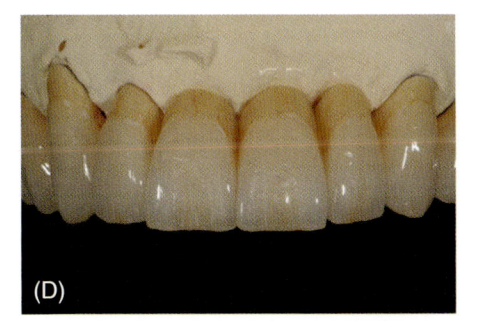

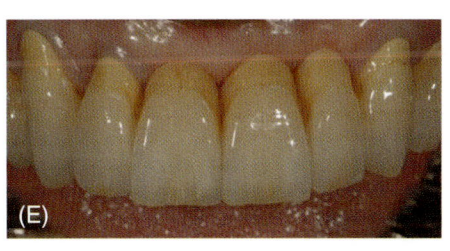

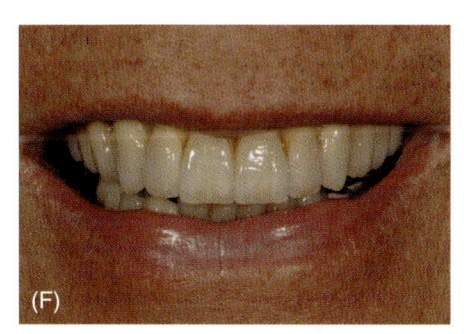

(E)

(F)

Figure 8.36 (D–F) Darker gingival color and root formations create shorter tooth appearance.

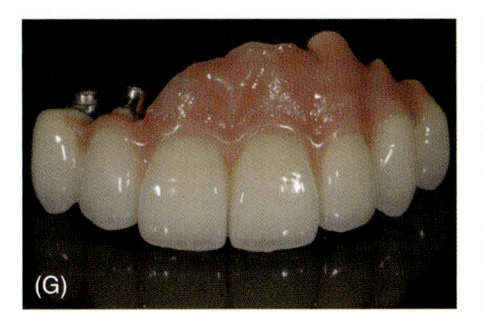

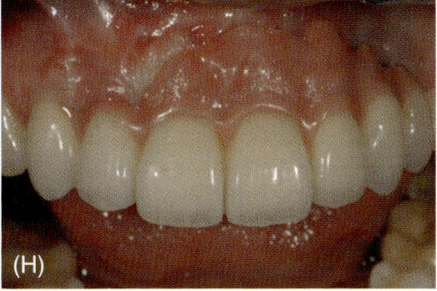

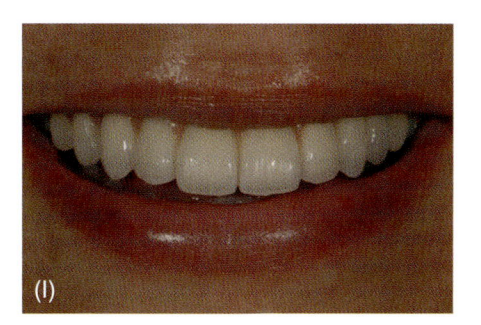

(G)

(H)

(I)

Figure 8.36 (G–I) Pink gingival ceramics used to re-establish correct proportions of teeth and gingival levels.

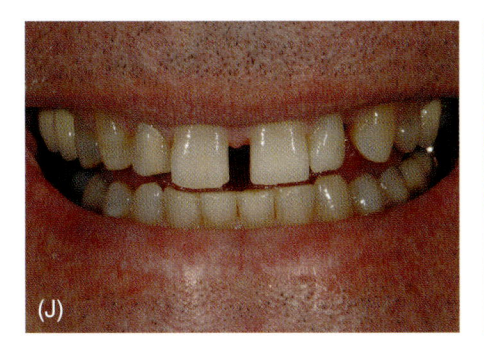

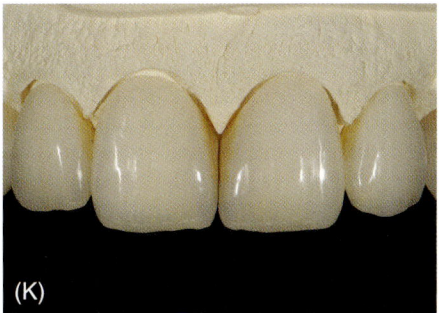

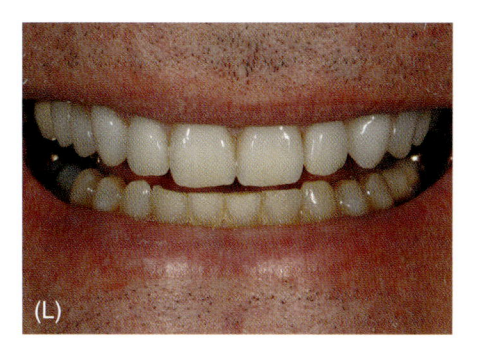

(J)

(K)

(L)

Figure 8.36 (J–L) Designing darker proximal wings and adjusting line angles gives a smaller/narrower appearance of the restoration. This is useful in diastema closure cases with excessive space to maintain the illusion of proper tooth proportion.

staining, that follow the distal line angle, or buccal ridge, or that run approximately parallel to them.

Increasing distal inclination

To increase the perception of a distal inclination, reverse the preceding instructions on mesial inclination. In an anterior tooth, the mesial contact is moved cervically and the distal contact is moved incisally. The mesial line angle is carved toward the center of the incisal edge. The incisal edge is pointed on the distal and notched toward the mesial. In a posterior tooth, the mesial contact is moved cervically, and the distal contact is moved occlusally. The buccal ridge is carved to curve from the mesio-gingival to the disto-occlusal. The cusp tip can be moved distally if this is compatible with functional requirements. In both

Table 8.4 Form and Color to Create Optical Illusions

Shape and Form	Desired Effect	Color and Shade
Pink ceramics (Figure 8.36A–C)	Long teeth	Darker root form
Vertical grooves and ridges (Figure 8.36D–F)	Make longer	Long vertical crack lines
Horizontal grooves and lines (Figure 8.36G–I)	Make shorter	Horizontal hypocalcification bands
Proximal wings (move in line angles) (Figure 8.36J–L)	Wide teeth	Darker, more chroma in proximal
Line angles out	Larger teeth	High value, bright, opacious
Line angles in	Smaller teeth	Low value, darker, translucent

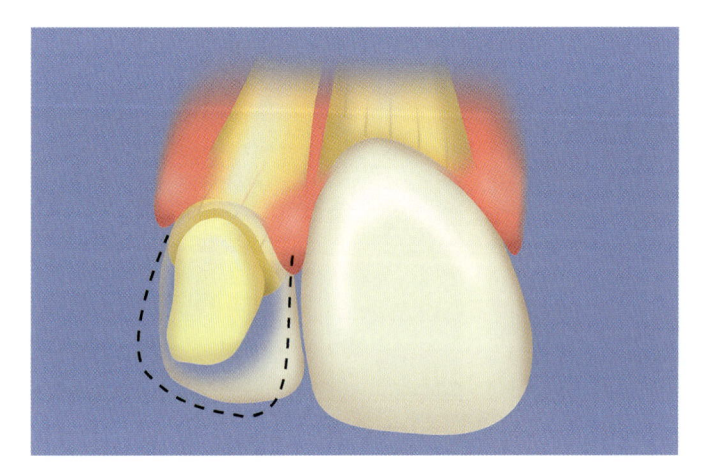

Figure 8.37 Increasing the mesial inclination on a severely tipped tooth is an illusion that increases the appearance of good alignment.

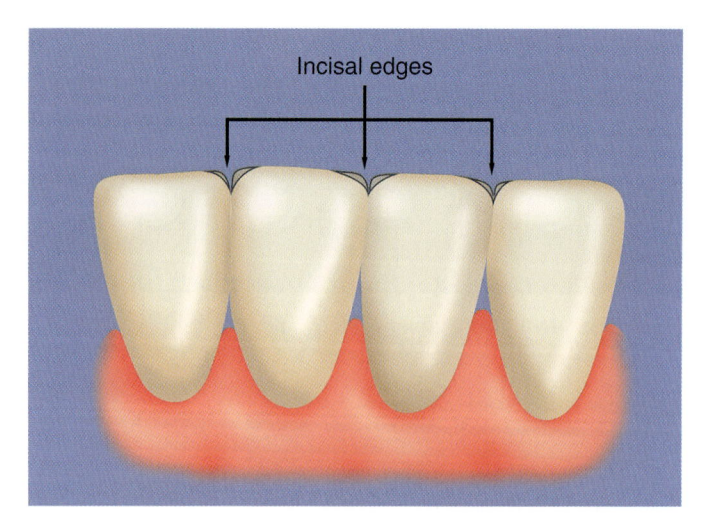

Figure 8.38 In addition to staining the interproximal areas where they curve into the embrasures, the incisal edges are slightly curved to create differentiation between teeth.

anterior and posterior teeth, the illusion of distal inclination can be increased by incorporating lightly stained lines that follow the mesial line angle or buccal ridge or that run approximately parallel to them.

Insufficient differentiation between teeth

Special problems occur in the attempt to achieve a natural appearance in the multiple unit anterior ceramometal restoration. The major objective is to give the illusion that the teeth are actually separate and not a connected series. This can be accomplished by placing the proximal connector as lingual as possible to allow for maximum interdental separation between the teeth. Staining should be used to give the teeth the appearance of individual units. Most restorations appear artificial because of stains that are too light or the absence of stains between the teeth. By the use of darker stains, the interproximal areas can be shaded where they curve into the embrasures. This will add an illusion of interproximal depth and separateness. Use an orange-brown or gray-green combination, whichever approximates the color of the adjacent or opposing teeth.

Sometimes, it is still difficult to obtain the desired illusion of separation in crowded lower anterior units. An alternative technique is postsoldering when multiple crowns are involved. The actual separation between the crowns, even though minimal, may create an individual, natural-looking restoration. Make certain not to create too much space between the crowns. Complete visualization of the result should occur before the final soldering. It is advisable to examine the framework and try to picture the degree of separation before the porcelain buildup. A slight depression in the framework strut in the contact area will also increase the illusion of separation by allowing a deeper depth-cut in the porcelain veneer. The incisal edge (ie) can also be curved into the interproximals, heightening the illusion (Figure 8.38).

Arch irregularity

On smiling, an arch irregularity can cause exposure of more crowns or more of the crowns on one side of the mouth than on the other (Figure 8.39A and 8.40A). You need to discuss this problem with the patient before treatment, explaining that the crowns will not be bilaterally symmetrical in the final restoration. All other unusual conditions should be noted at the second appointment during the esthetic diagnosis. Pre-restorative photographs should be taken to preserve a good record of both smiling and lip-retracted positions. It is a good idea to give a copy of these photographs to the laboratory as well.

Treatment for arch irregularity usually involves gingival raising, tooth shortening and/or lengthening, or a combination to help achieve the illusion of a more balanced arch (see Figure 8.39A–C). In addition, an artificial tissue insert can be made (Figure 8.40D–G) or tissue-colored ceramic composite be applied.

Influencing facial shape

In general, the oval is considered the ideal facial shape. If the face is too long, shortening long teeth will help to add width. Reduce the interincisal distance (the vertical height between the central

Figure 8.39 **(A)** This lady has a maxillary arch that drops down on the right side.

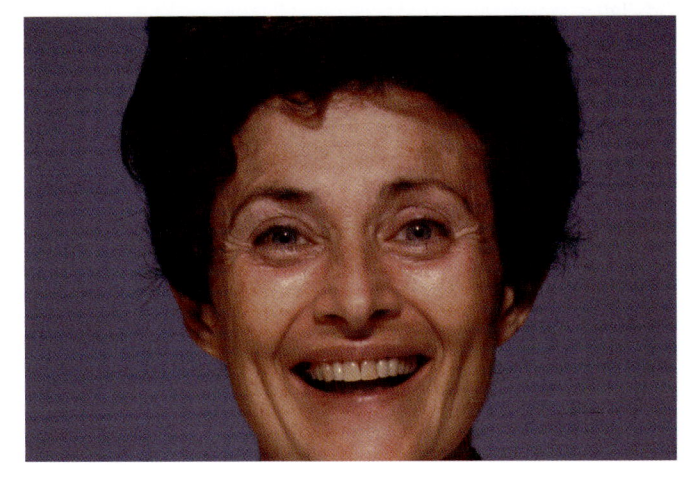

Figure 8.39 **(C)** After contouring, the patient's smile shows a balanced arch.

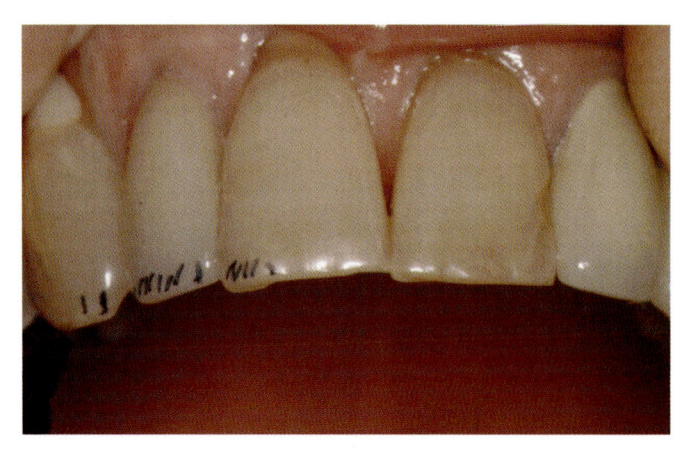

Figure 8.39 **(B)** The teeth are outlined with an alcohol marker to show where they will be contoured.

incisal edges and the lateral incisal edges) if the central incisors are extra long or extended. Also, horizontal lines and characterizations can be added or emphasized. The reverse procedure can be used on the round face by emphasizing tooth length, and using vertical lines and characterizations.

Incorporating age characteristics

Once the correct form and function have been achieved in a crown or pontic, the wear and stains that normally accumulate with age should be incorporated into the new restorations to blend with the appearance of the remaining natural teeth. Foods and various filling materials leave stains and discoloration. A clean, new, perfect tooth would be quite noticeable if set among others with worn incisal edges, multiple restorations, and tobacco stains. Overall, teeth are generally lighter in young people than in the aged, and rarely are all of the teeth uniform in shade in the older dentition.

Nature incorporates in each tooth many colors that usually become more pronounced with age; for example, the gray and yellow tones. A prosthesis prepared for an older individual should be stained to simulate the color variations found in the remaining natural teeth. For example, the presence of Class III restorations can be simulated with stains (see Figure 8.32A). If the patient desires, actual gold restorations may be placed in artificial replacement teeth to increase the illusion of age and realism.

Careful shaping and polishing can effectively mimic abrasion and imply advancing age. Wear on the incisal edge accumulates with increasing age, shortening the anatomic crown by abrading its translucent edge. This aging is simulated by carving the incisal edges and cusp tips to simulate accumulated abrasion. The grinding should not be a flat reduction in height but should simulate natural, angled wear facets produced by opposing teeth. Note in Figure 8.41A, how incisal wear can occur in natural teeth, and in Figure 8.41B and C, how cuspids can wear. To maintain harmony of appearance, if there is cemental erosion or erosion on the gingival one-third of the remaining teeth, carving and staining a similar pattern into the replacement tooth is indicated. Tooth migration, shifting, or rotation may also occur with aging. If the long axes of the remaining teeth are variable and if some of the teeth are rotated, a row of straight, perfectly aligned pontics or crowns will stand out. A slight rotation or shift of the long axis can mean the difference between an artificial appearance and a natural one (Figure 8.42). Although most patients request a younger look, never assume that this is what all patients prefer.

Reducing age effects on the smile

Many patients are motivated to seek esthetic dental treatment to make them look younger. They want to eliminate the aging effects just described. This is usually possible by the use of various restorative techniques. A too-light shade will look false, so avoid the temptation to follow the patient's wishes for "white teeth." When patients look at a single tooth tab from a shade guide, their inclination may be to choose the lightest color. What

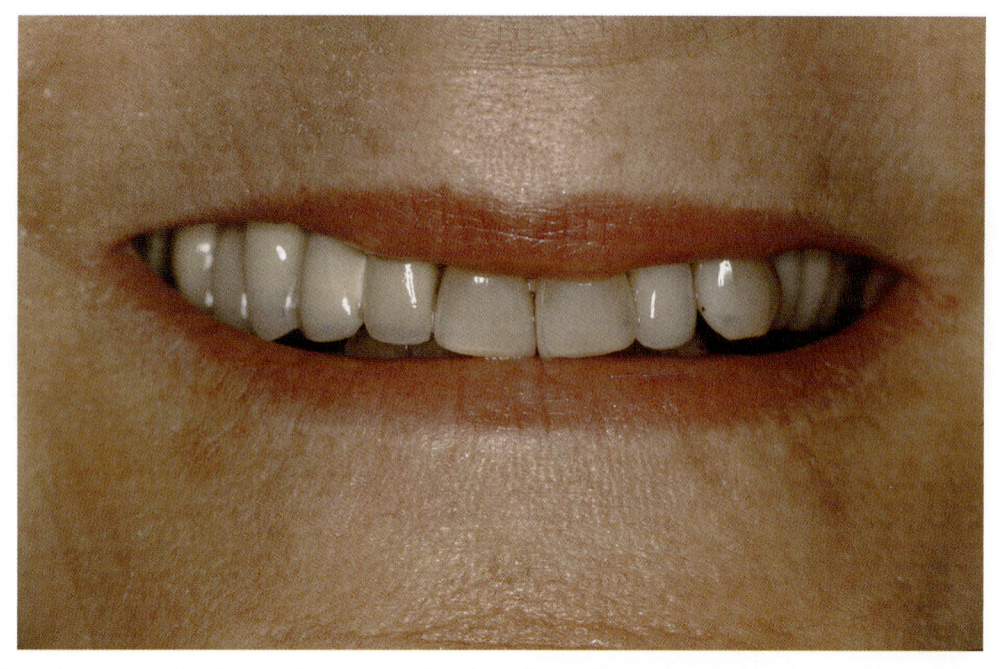

Figure 8.40 **(A)** When this patient smiles she reveals more tooth length on the maxillary right side than the remainder of the arch.

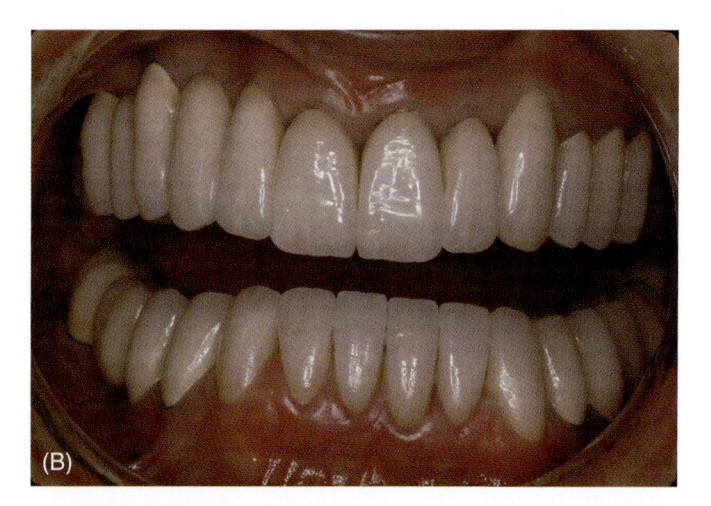

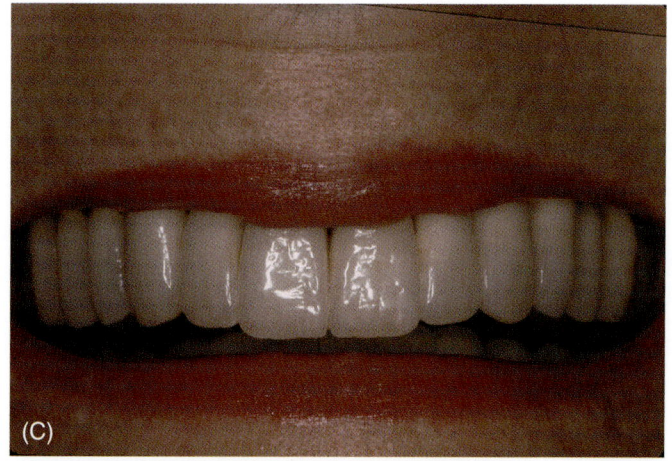

Figure 8.40 **(B and C)** After periodontal surgery and full ceramometal crown restoration, the maxillary crowns are extremely long.

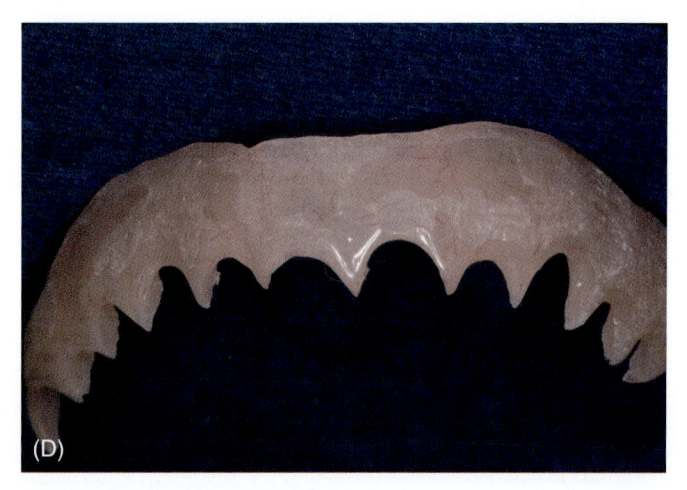

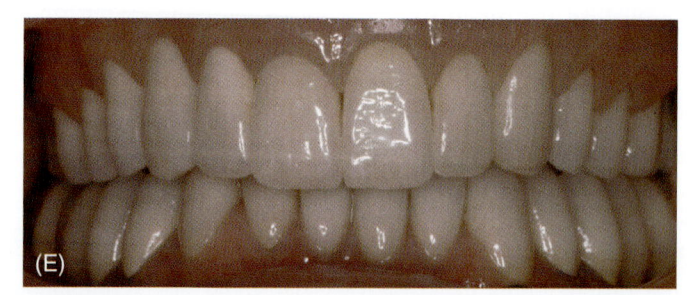

Figure 8.40 **(D and E)** An artificial tissue insert was made to mask the extra tooth length.

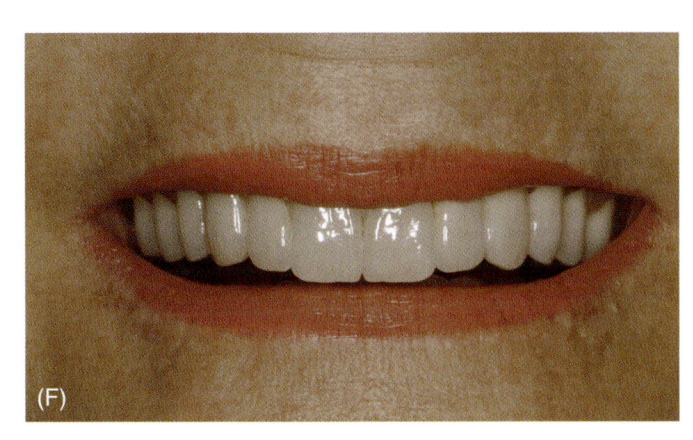

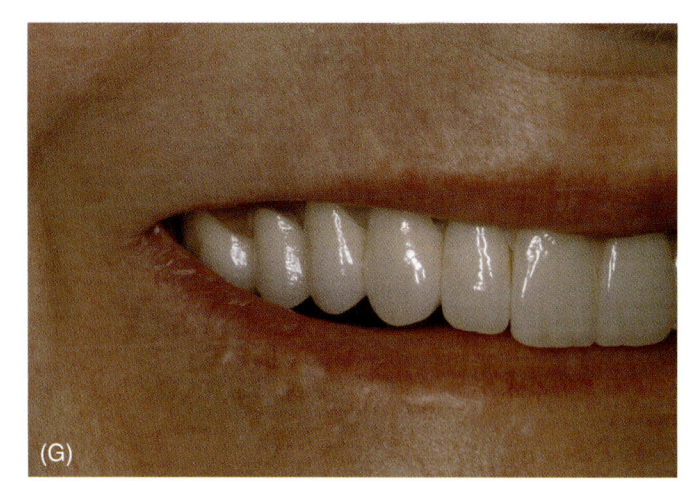

Figure 8.40 **(F and G)** The final result shows how wearing the artificial tissue insert enhances this woman's smile.

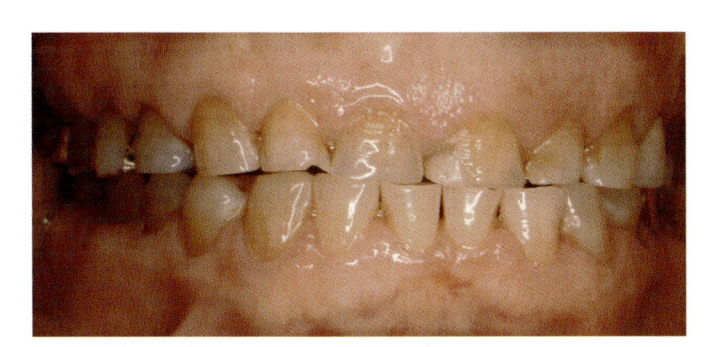

Figure 8.41 **(A)** This patient has uniform incisal and occlusal wear on all of the teeth due to bruxism (LSK121 Oral Prosthetics).

they usually fail to understand is that multiple teeth of a lighter shade will appear even whiter in the mouth when they are all together. The shade can be lighter, but vary the intensity of body color when staining the tooth. Use a deeper gingival shade that blends to the incisal edge. Avoid too much incisal shading. To make the tooth appear natural, the incisal edge should be mostly body colors, with bluish translucency appearing on the mesial and distal edges where the enamel may have worn thin. A bluish incisal surrounded by light opaque orange on the incisal edge intensifies the color, creating a halo effect, and helps give a much younger look (Figure 8.43A and B).

Aging wears down the incisal edges, usually drastically shortening the central incisors. Increasing the interincisal distance by making the centrals again longer than the laterals can help make the individual appear younger.

Most aged individuals show either too little tooth structure or none at all. If occlusion permits, make the entire anterior segment of teeth longer. Consider bevelling or cosmetic contouring on the lower anterior teeth to permit lengthening the upper incisors. In certain patients, it may even be possible to restore lost vertical dimension after which you can lengthen the upper anteriors. If this is attempted, begin with a removable or fixed interim appliance for several months to make sure your patient is comfortable with the new occlusal position. Then temporarily restore the teeth with veneers, crowns, or bonding that incorporate the new length. It is best to keep the patient in these temporary restorations for an additional 3 months before constructing the final restorations to allow for any occlusal adjustments, should your patient develop any temporomandibular joint (TMJ) discomfort.

Incisal embrasures

The incisal embrasure is the triangle formed between the edges of two adjacent anterior teeth. The incisal embrasures should display a natural, progressive increase in size or depth from the central incisor to the canine (Figure 8.44A and B). This is a function of the natural anatomy of the front teeth and, as a result, the contact point moves further toward the gum line as the teeth proceed from the centrals to the canines. This mimics the smile line and failure to provide adequate depth and variation to the incisal embrasures will make teeth appear too uniform and make contact areas too long, which will impart a box-like appearance to the teeth (Figure 8.44C and D). The individuality of the incisors will be lost if their incisal embrasures are not properly created. Also, if the incisal embrasures are too deep it will tend to make the teeth look unnaturally pointed. Incisal edge wear can eliminate the incisal embrasures, a characteristic identified with the elderly. Carving the embrasures into the restoration helps create a younger look (Figure 8.45A and B).

- **Problem**—This case shows the effect of discolored irregular teeth on a 67-year-old female (Figure 8.45E). Unfortunately, the teeth did nothing but create an even older appearance. No amount of makeup or any other cosmetic improvement could disguise the feeling of old age one got from her smile. Lipstick only helped to call attention to this.
- **Treatment**—Treatment consisted of full-mouth reconstruction with a fixed porcelain fused-to-metal prosthesis.
- **Result**—For purposes of this chapter, the patient illustrates the importance of the final esthetic result, particularly its effect on the lip line. With proper restoration, a more youthful look has been created by lengthening the central incisors and producing a more feminine (rounded) appearance in the anterior teeth. Note the overall improvement achieved by the use of a harmonious shade (Figure 8.45 F).

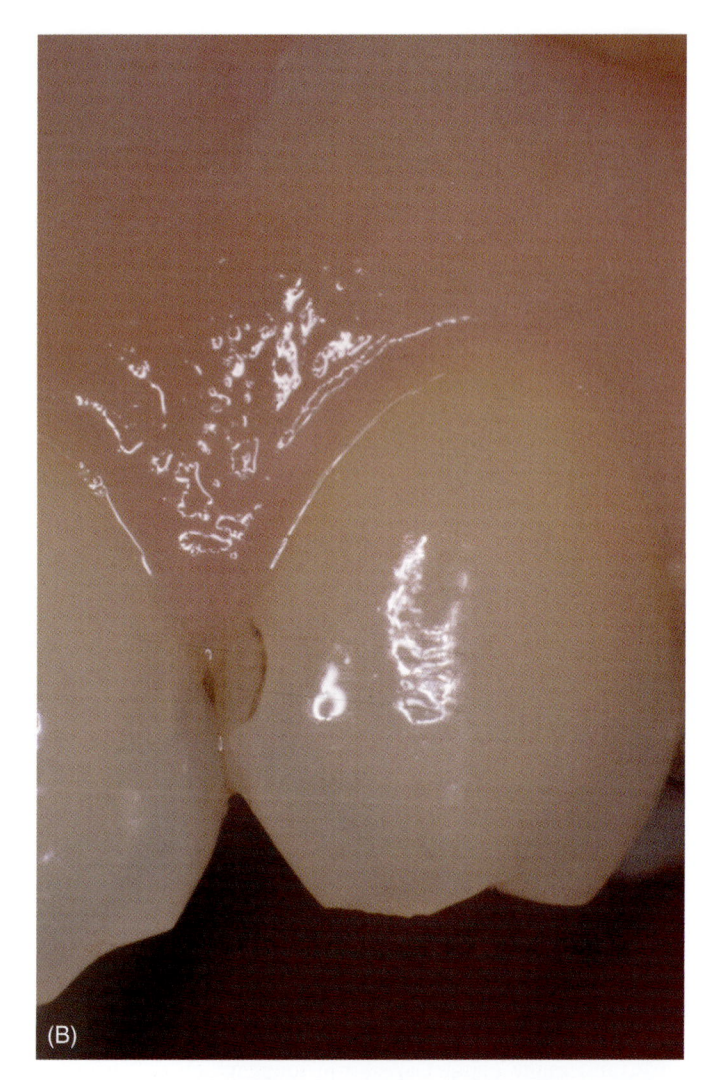

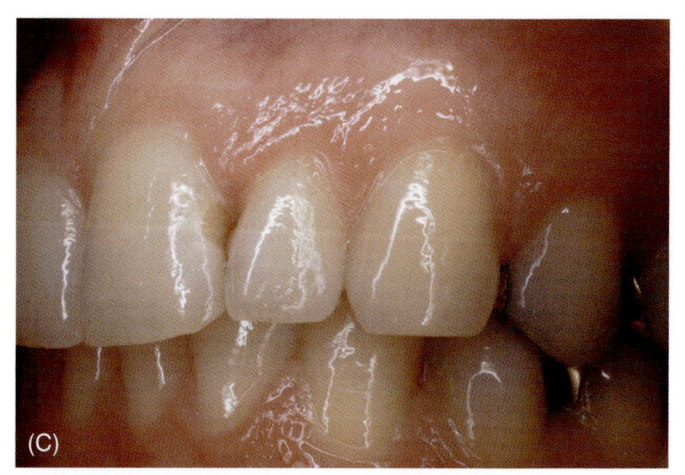

Figure 8.41 **(B and C)** These are examples of individual incisal tooth wear that often occurs in cuspids.

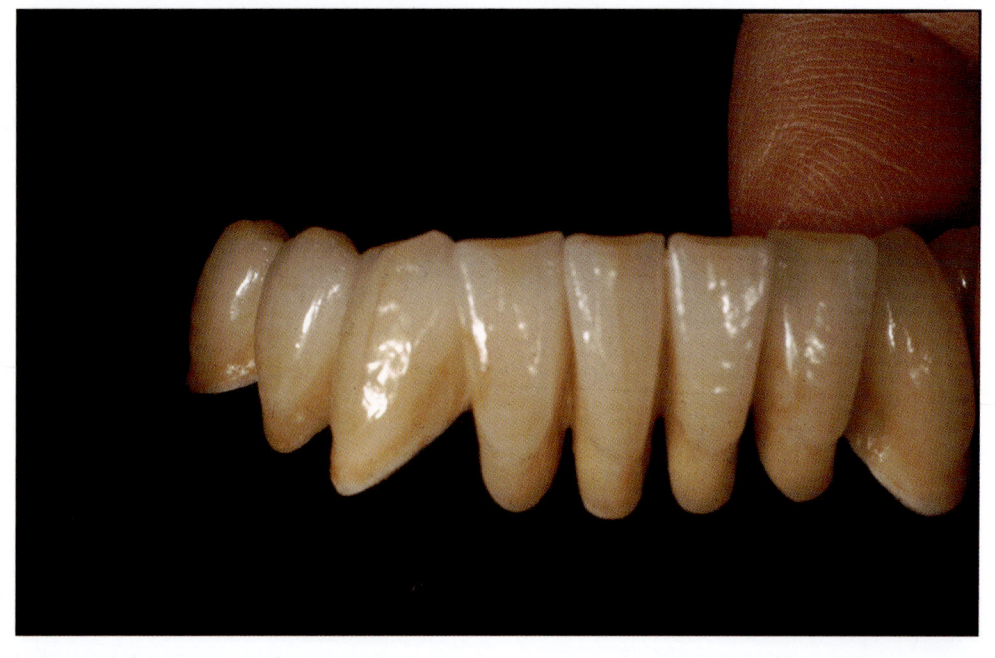

Figure 8.42 The slight rotation of the long axis of some teeth in a prosthesis can result in a more natural look. Figure courtesy of Magna Laboratories, Richard E. Resk.

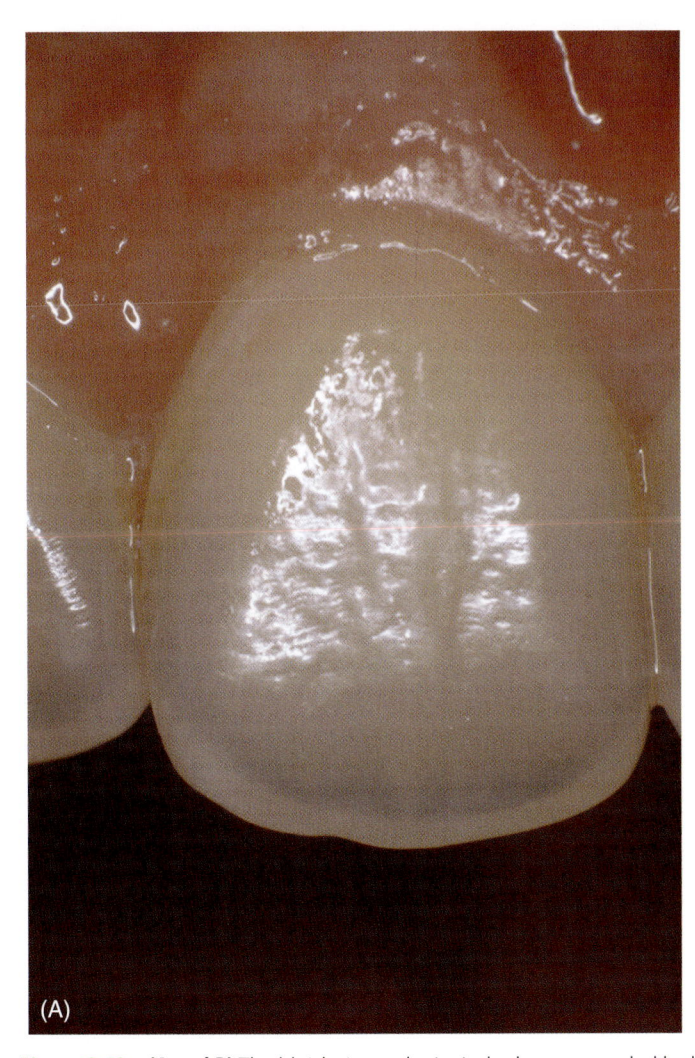

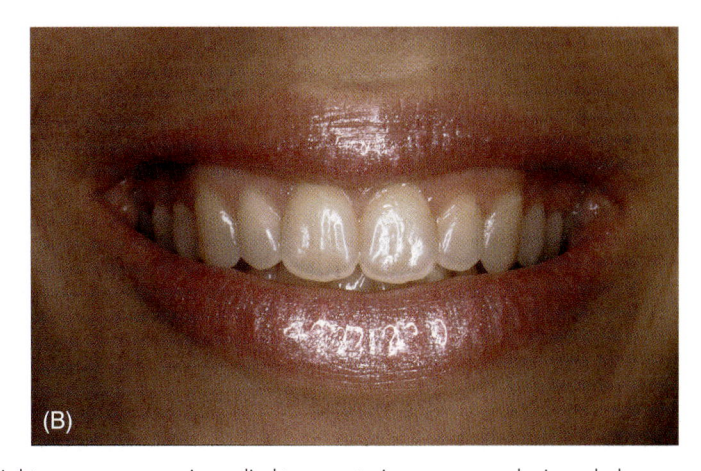

Figure 8.43 (A and B) The bluish tint at the incisal edge surrounded by light opaque orange is applied to an anterior crown, producing a halo effect and giving a younger-looking appearance to the teeth.

How color affects the way we perceive teeth

See Table 8.5 for examples of how color affects our perceptions of teeth and aging.

Incorporating sexual characteristics

Wear of incisal edges eliminates certain sex characteristics. When teeth are contoured or crowns carved, you may need to incorporate either feminine or masculine characteristics. The remaining teeth should be observed to see if the replacement tooth is in harmony. We tend to interpret a female mouth as one where the contours and lines are more rounded and curved than those in the male, which are usually flatter, sharper, and more angular. By rounding angles and edges, a more feminine appearance can be achieved (see Figure 8.45B). By squaring angles and edges, a more masculine feeling is created (Figure 8.46 and 8-47). The idea of masculinity can be further enhanced by slightly abrading the incisal surface. Staining the prosthesis to simulate tobacco, coffee, or tea stains can also aid this masculine illusion, as will the incorporation of light microcrack lines. Figure 8.48A and B show stained characteristics used to obtain a more masculine look, accomplished in Figure 8.45C and D. Note the simulated restorations and hypocalcified areas. Staining of women's teeth could consist of adding a touch of blue to the incisal edge (Figure 8.43A and B).

It is not always necessary to match adjacent, natural, untouched teeth. In fact, many times the opposite should be the case. During the planning stage, a decision should be made about the type of esthetic result desired by the patient. Since it is possible to alter the patient's masculine or feminine appearance through conservative procedures such as cosmetic contouring, bonding, or laminating on the adjacent teeth, determination should first be made about the extent of the masculine or feminine character that is desired before creating the final restorations. For example, for a female who has worn her incisal edges until they now appear angular and masculine, you may elect to recontour her natural dentition before carving the new restoration.

This is not to say every female should have a soft, curvaceous look to her mouth, or every male should look sharp and angular. The degree of femininity or masculinity is dependent on the patient's personality, habits, and (most of all) desire. Patients have an unquestionable right to help choose what type of appearance they will eventually have. The dentist must be sensitive enough to go beyond the patient's apprehensions about being considered vain and find out their true desires.

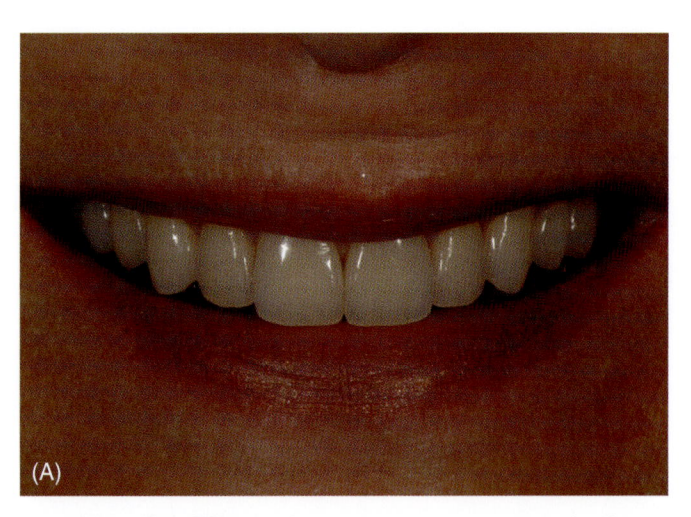

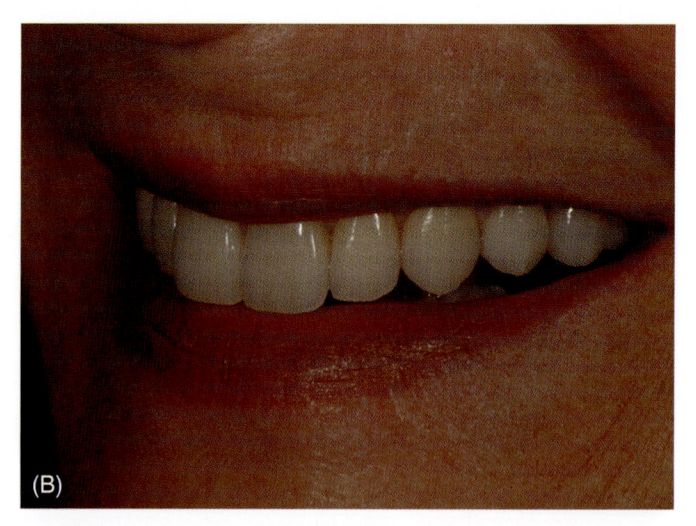

Figure 8.44 **(A and B)** Natural, progressive increase in incisal embrasures (Naperville).

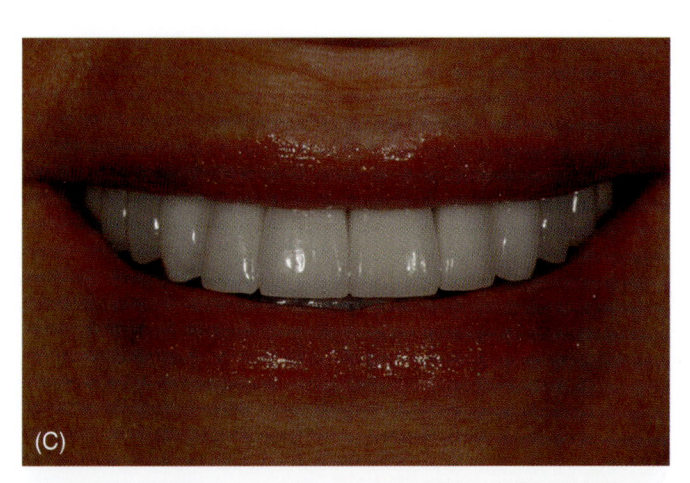

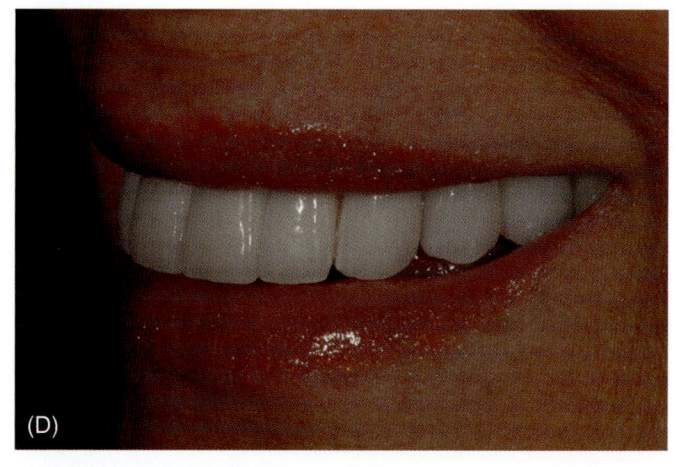

Figure 8.44 **(C and D)** Unnatural, too uniform incisal embrasures, described as "chicklets."

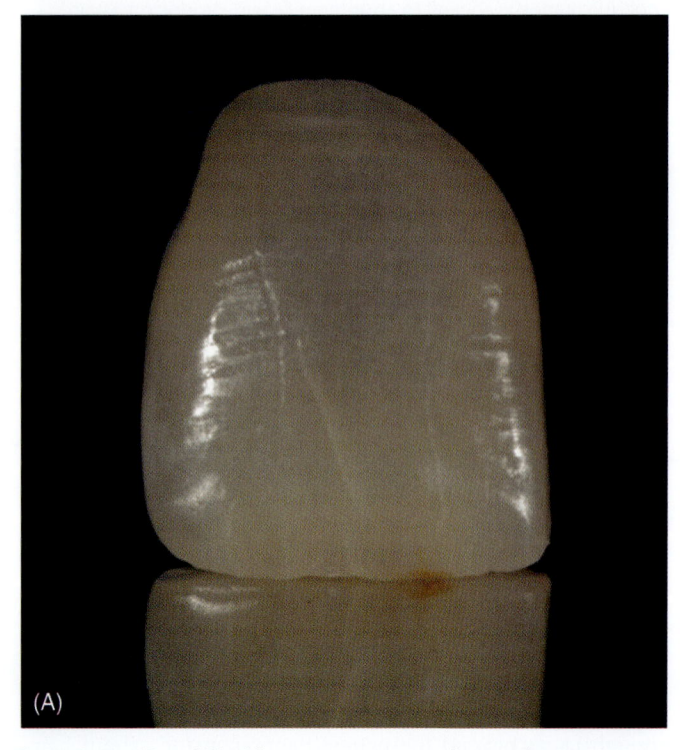

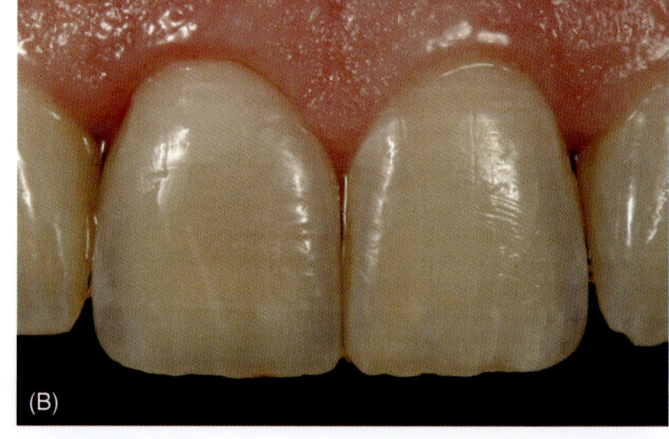

Figure 8.45 **(A and B)** Older, more mature tooth reproduction.

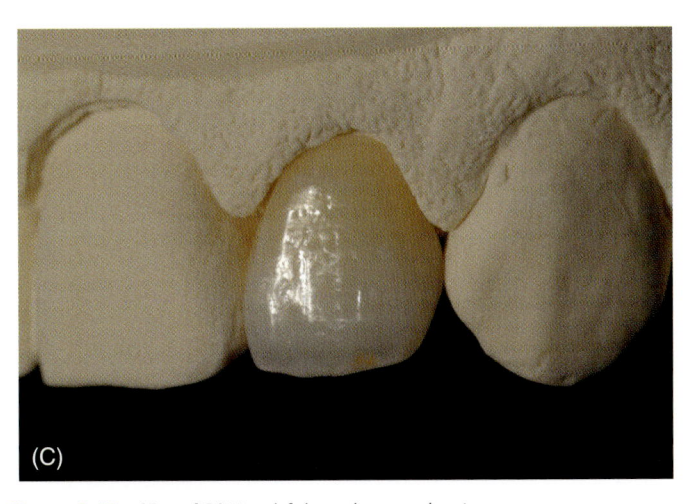

Figure 8.45 **(C and D)** Youthful tooth reproduction.

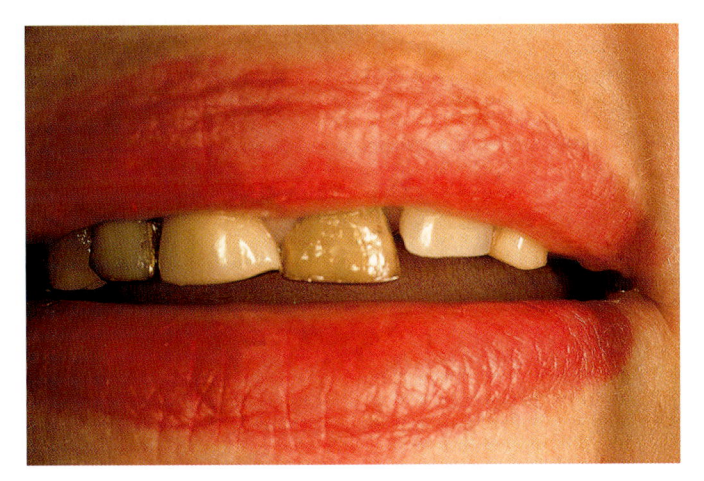

Figure 8.45 **(E)** Irregular and discolored teeth contribute to an older-appearing smile.

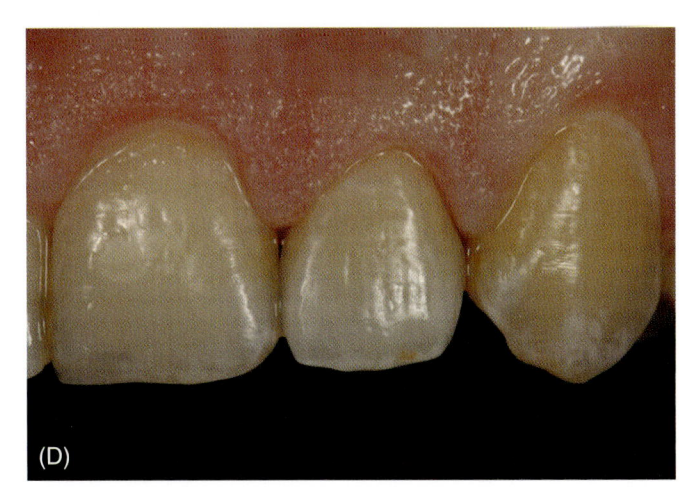

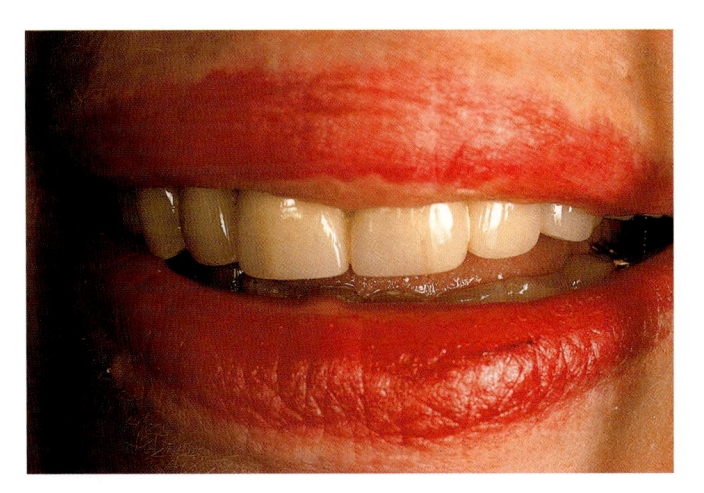

Figure 8.45 **(F)** A younger-looking appearance achieved by restoring the teeth with rounded, even, more feminine lines and a more uniform and harmonious shade.

Table 8.5 Color and Our Perception of Teeth

Younger-Looking Teeth	Older, More Mature-Looking Teeth
White hypocalcification	Yellow/orange staining
High texture	Low texture (surface polishing)
Include mammalons	Include signs of wear (flat edges)

* Some of these characteristics illustrated in Figure 8.43A and B.

Incorporating the personality of the patient

A delicate personality can be differentiated from the vigorous one by the degree of characterization, coloring, and arrangement of teeth. Overaccentuation of color, bold characterization, and nonuniform arrangement are compatible with an aggressive personality. The mild, demure personality is associated with less starkness and less color differentiation. The patient and his or her teeth should be evaluated carefully to achieve the desired final effect.

Many patients wish to improve the appearance of their teeth and want a very bright shade but fear a too-perfect look might alter their image. They want a natural appearance that retains their personality. An example was seen in a 47-year-old female patient (Figure 8.49A and B) who wanted a younger-looking, more feminine smile with a very bright shade. A combination of periodontal crown lengthening, full crowns, porcelain veneers, and even composite resin bonding created the final result. Figure 8.49B shows the patient's choice for a natural, youthful appearance.

Loss of interdental tissue

Minimizing the loss of interdental tissue and concealing the fact that it is missing are problems that intrigue both the periodontist and the general practitioner, as well as the prosthodontist. Patients who have had periodontal surgery resulting in the loss of interdental tissue that then created holes or spaces between the teeth can be miserable about their appearance. Occasionally, surgical techniques can be altered to include either a lingual approach or other procedure that does not expose as much root surface.

Both the restorative dentist and the periodontist should always examine the patient's smile line to see exactly how much

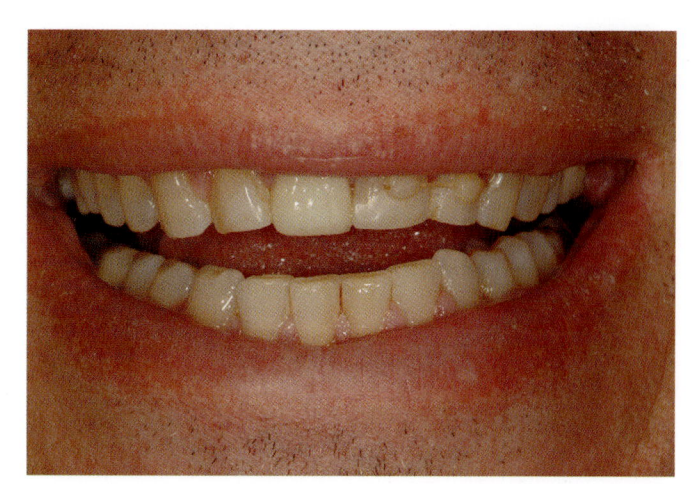

Figure 8.46 (A) Worn, irregular and discolored teeth contribute to an older-appearing smile in this 52-year-old man.

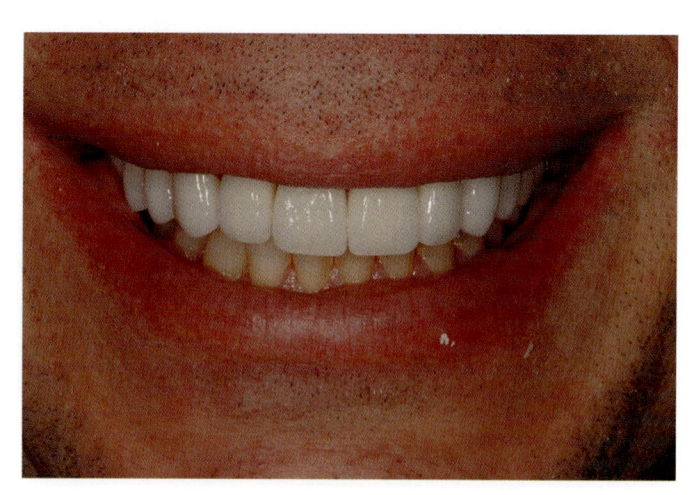

Figure 8.46 (B) An improved appearance was achieved by restoring the teeth with more masculine-shaped, lighter-colored ceramic crowns. Note the central incisors are a little longer than the lateral incisors, creating a greater interincisal distance and resulting in a younger-looking smile.

tissue would be exposed by each of several different procedures. If no compromise is possible, then a special effect may have to be created after the tissue has healed. There are generally four solutions to this problem: (1) a removable artificial interdental tissue appliance, (2) composite resin bonding or porcelain veneers, (3) full crowning, or (4) fixed porcelain interdental addition (Figure 8.40A–G).

Composite resin bonding or porcelain veneers

It is possible, by use of an acid-etch composite resin technique, to proportionally bond composite resins to each tooth so that the space is closed. This method is perhaps the easiest, and certainly the quickest, to perform. When doing so, it is important to add the material mainly from the linguoproximal surface, so that the size of the tooth is not changed appreciably (Figure 8.50A). The lingual, proximal, and mesiolabial surfaces of both central incisors were etched, and the composite resin was placed. The final attractive result was achieved by not overbuilding the tooth and yet hiding the unsightly spaces left by the missing interdental tissue (Figure 8.50B). When using this technique, it is important to take as much time as necessary for shaping and forming the composite resin. For this reason, a light-polymerized composite

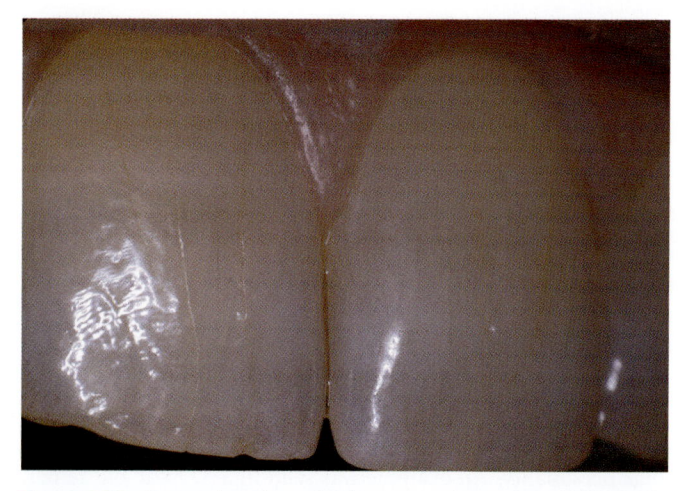

Figure 8.47 Squared angles and edges create a more masculine look.

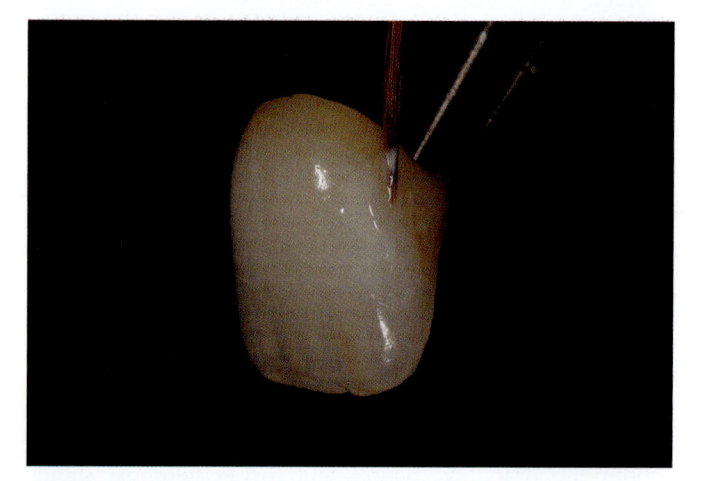

Figure 8.48 (A) Light microcracks, simulated restorations, and hypocalcified areas can help create a more natural and youthful look.

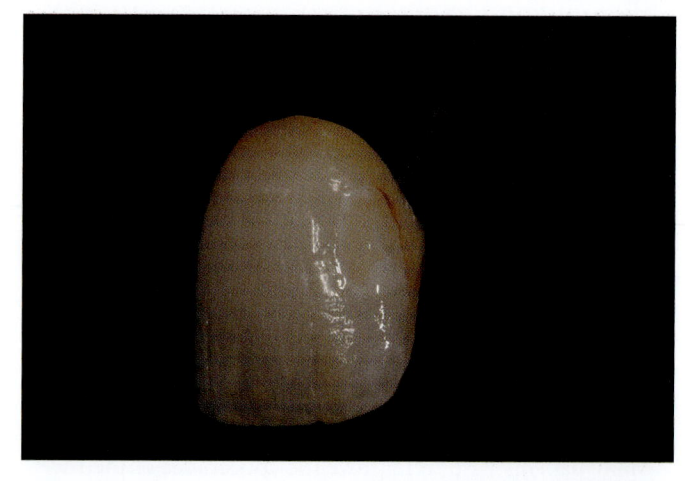

Figure 8.48 (B) Yellow/orange staining is a natural characteristic of the older dentition.

Chapter 8 Creating Esthetic Restorations Through Special Effects

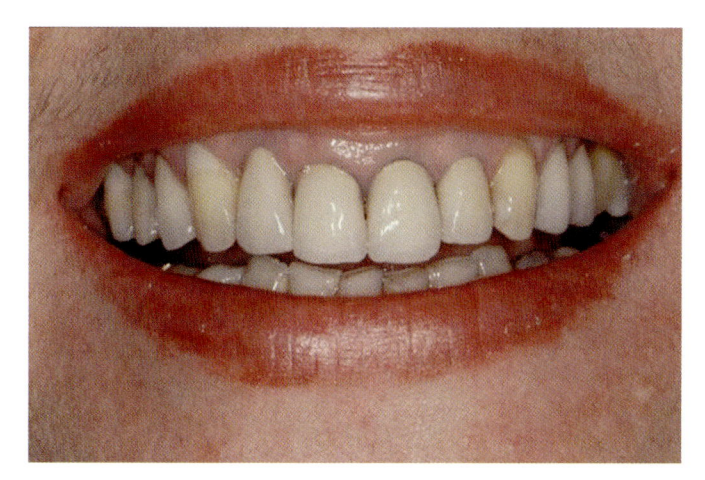

Figure 8.49 **(A)** This 47-year-old female wanted to restore her teeth and have a more attractive smile.

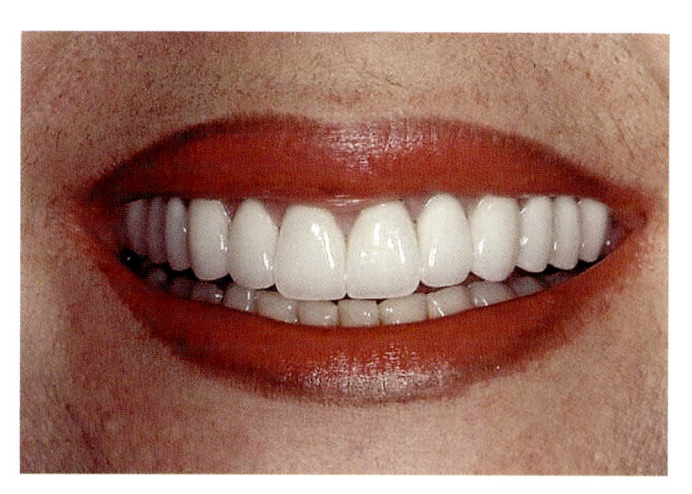

Figure 8.49 **(B)** A combination of crown lengthening, full crowns, porcelain veneers and composite resin bonding were done to create the final result.

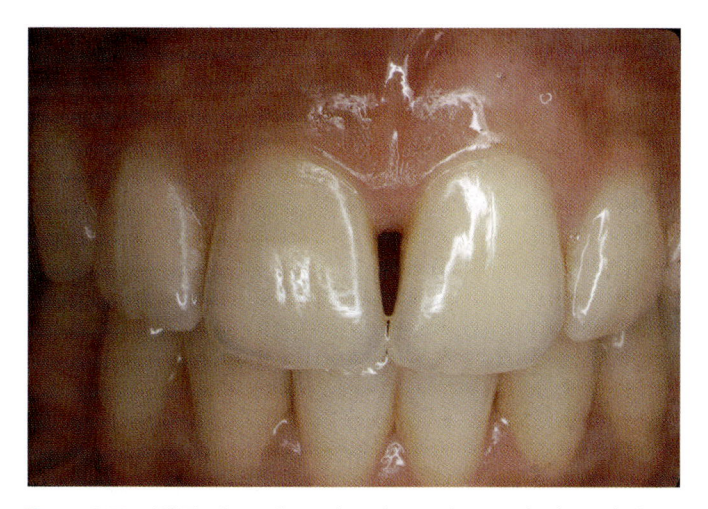

Figure 8.50 **(A)** The loss of interdental tissue has resulted in a dark, unattractive space between the two central incisors.

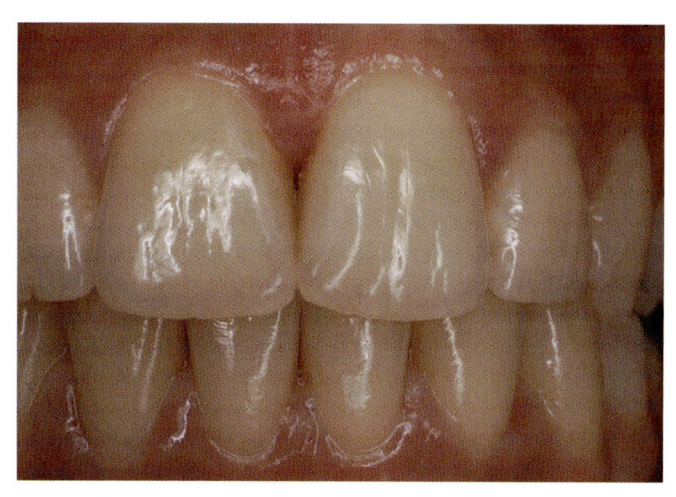

Figure 8.50 **(B)** Conservative composite resin bonding of the lingual, mesial, and labial surfaces of both central incisors hides the space while not overbuilding the teeth.

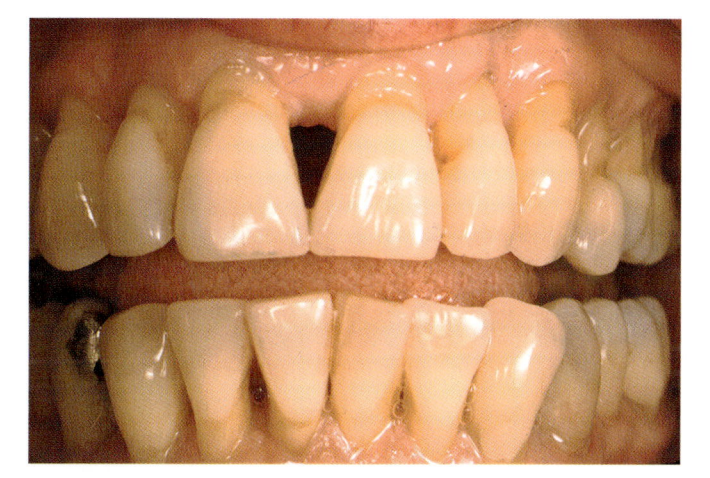

Figure 8.51 **(A)** Interdental spaces from periodontal surgery plus severe cervical erosion may require more than the usual conservative treatments of bonding or laminating.

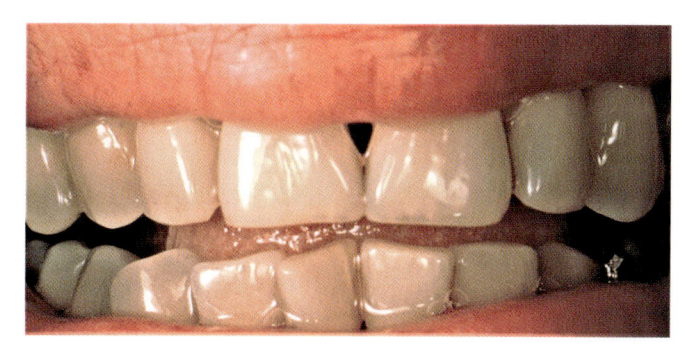

Figure 8.51 **(B)** An unsightly dark space was clearly visible between the central incisors in the before-treatment smile.

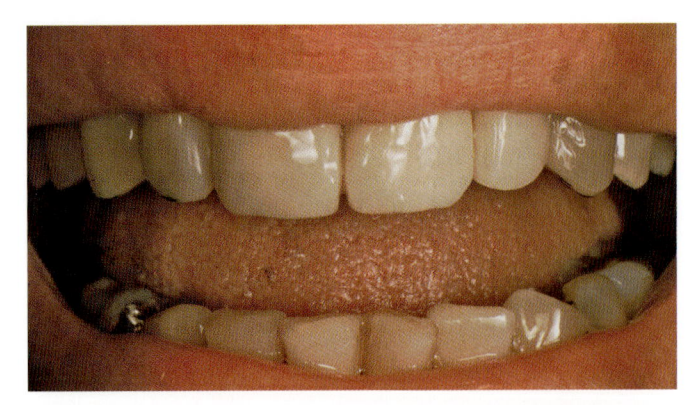

Figure 8.51 **(C)** Full-arch splinting with a telescopic prosthesis allowed for both raising the contact area gingivally and the addition of material lingually to lessen the space. After treatment, the interdental space is not evident, and the patient now has a more attractive smile line.

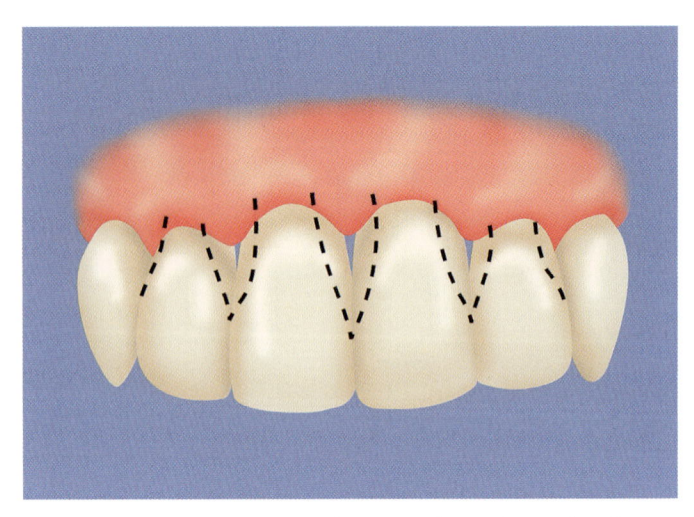

Figure 8.51 **(D)** This illustrates where to add porcelain so that the spaces are masked and the restorations do not appear too bulky.

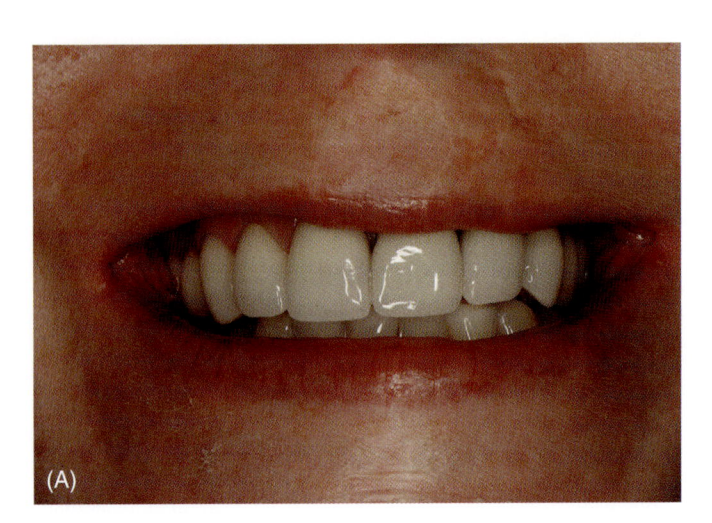

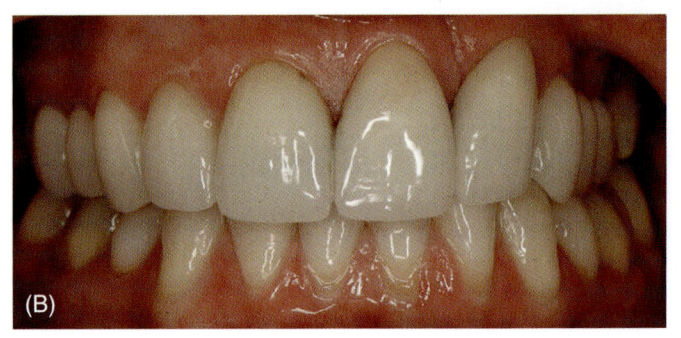

Figure 8.52 **(A and B)** This 45-year-old female presented with older, discolored porcelain veneers with slight loss of interdental papilla.

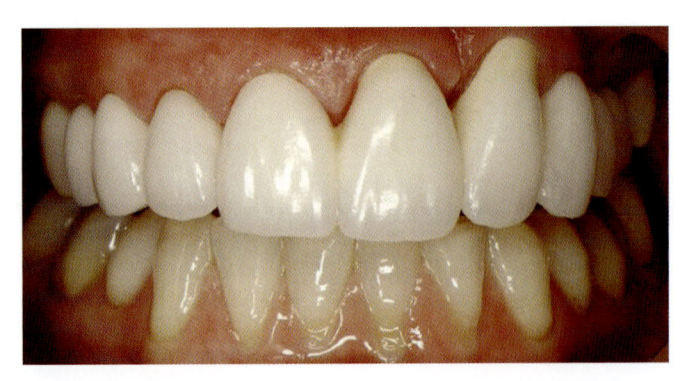

Figure 8.52 **(C)** New all-ceramic crowns were made and splinted together due to her cleft palate. However, a fixed pink ceramic insert was chosen to replace the missing interdental papilla.

resin is best. Adequate time is then available to fully carve each tooth to obtain a good esthetic result. An alternative to this technique is to use porcelain veneers to mask the spaces. If this is done, make sure the proximal surfaces of the teeth are prepared deeply into the embrasure space.

Full crowning

Full crowning can also be used to mask the loss of interdental tissue; however, it is generally not advised unless the teeth also need to be restored. In Figure 8.51A and B, we see a patient after periodontal surgery left him with unsightly interdental spaces. Since individual gold telescopes plus full-arch splinting were necessary, closure of these spaces could be adequately handled with the fixed prosthesis. By raising the contact areas gingivally

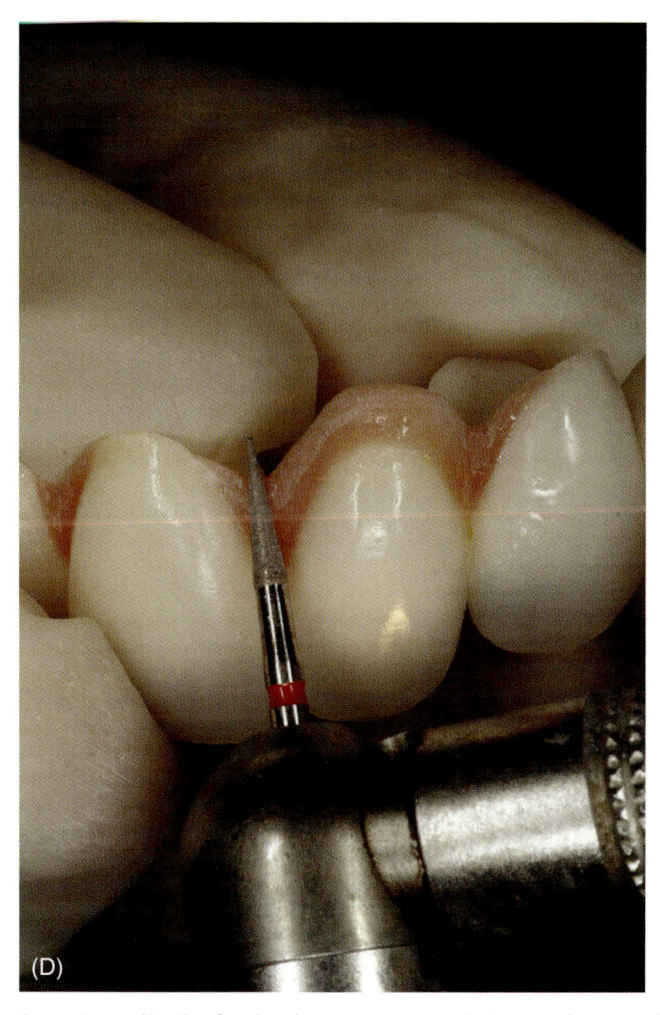

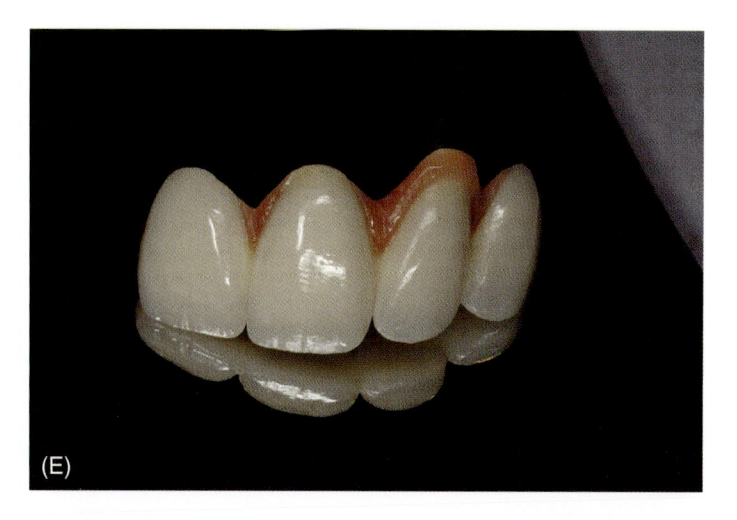

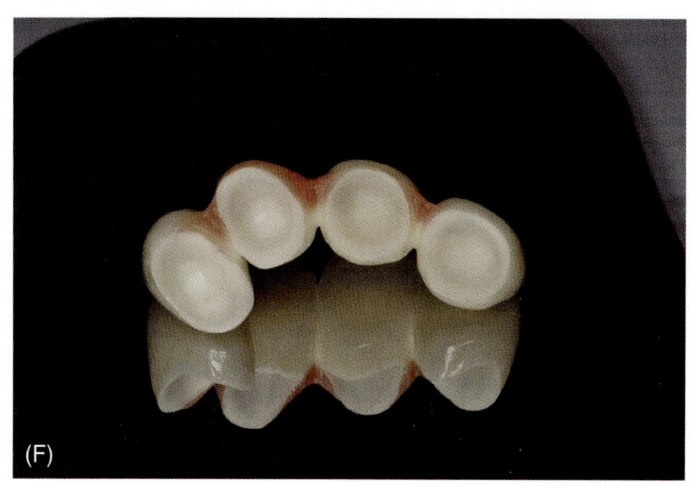

Figure 8.52 (D–F) A fixed pink ceramic was applied to the four-unit fixed bridge to replace the missing interdental papilla.

and by adding additional porcelain lingually to close the interdental spaces, an improved smile line is created (Figure 8.51C). Figure 8.51D shows graphically where the porcelain is added to hide the spaces and keep the crowns from looking too bulky. Note that the visible gold bands at the gingival margins are concealed by the patient's medium lip line.

Fixed porcelain interdental addition

An alternative solution to the interdental space problem is adding a gingiva-colored porcelain insert attached to the fixed partial denture. This method works well when there are missing anterior or posterior teeth and extreme ridge resorption. The following case illustrates the technique for construction. A female patient, aged 45, presented with an older, discolored anterior restoration (Figure 8.52A and B). The patient was conscious of her unattractive smile and tried to hide it by keeping her upper lip as far down as possible. Her main problem was loss of interdental tissue. The treatment included a fixed splint with a fixed pink ceramic interdental insert (Figure 8.52C–H).

Lost interdental tissue can be effectively and esthetically treated with the above techniques. However, another type of porcelain addition has been suggested by Cronin and Wardle.[4] They describe a cantilevered porcelain papilla that features a convex gingival form, which can be easily cleaned with dental floss. Treatment could also consist of a combined therapy including orthodontics to erupt the central and cuspid, bringing the tissue level down to balance the opposite side, followed by ridge augmentation as necessary, and completed with a single-tooth implant replacement or a conventional three-unit bridge.

Another alternative to the fixed porcelain interdental tissue is to use a fixed composite resin addition. A major advantage to composite resin is the ease of masking the add-on and the ability to repair it in the mouth (Figure 8.53A–N).

Porcelain veneer alternate construction techniques

There are times when preparation for a porcelain veneer might result in insertion problems with too much bonding cement in undercut areas. Therefore, master ceramist and artist Nasser Shademan has developed a two-tier quattro veneer construction that can be seen in Figure 8.54A–V.

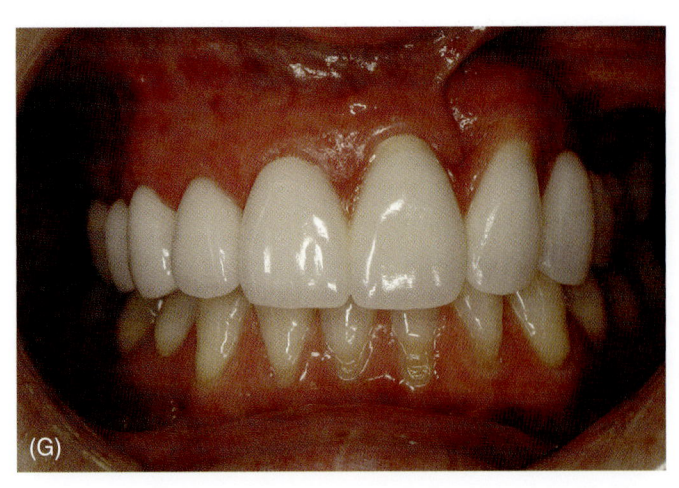

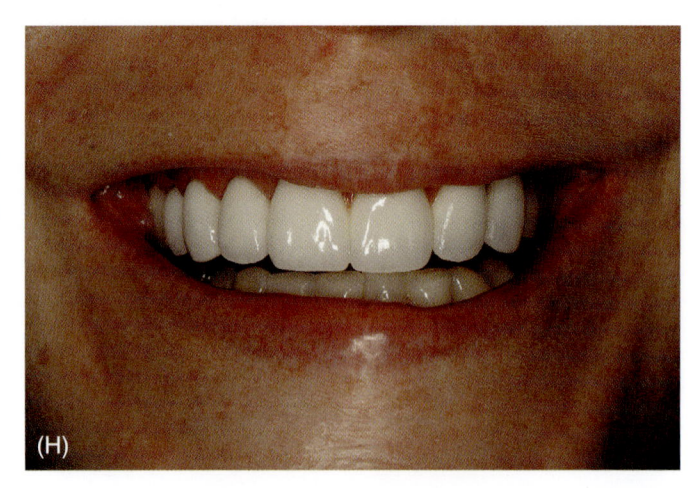

Figure 8.52 (G and H) Note a more attractive smile line was created by full crown restorations and using the pink porcelain addition to replace her missing papilla.

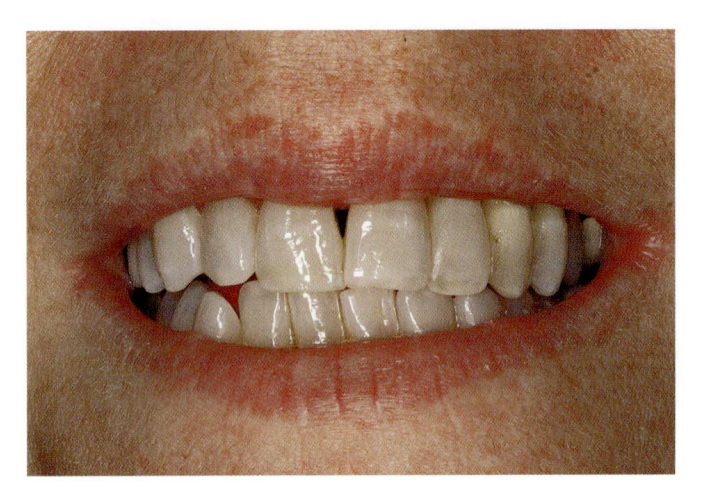

Figure 8.53 (A) This patient was concerned about the interdental space between her centrals.

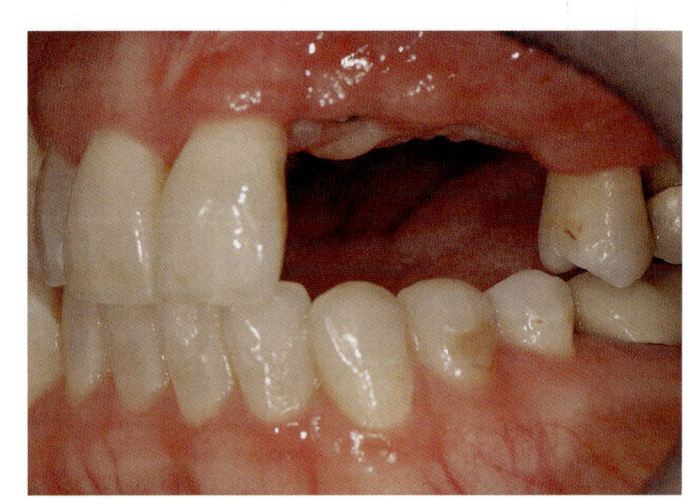

Figure 8.53 (B) After implant placements make spaces where interdental papilla will be missing.

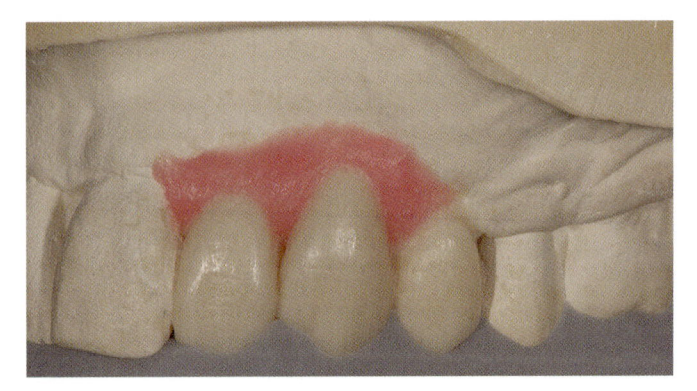

Figure 8.53 (C) Wax-up of the proposed implant bridge and gingival papilla. Note how Siltek matrix will be used in the design.

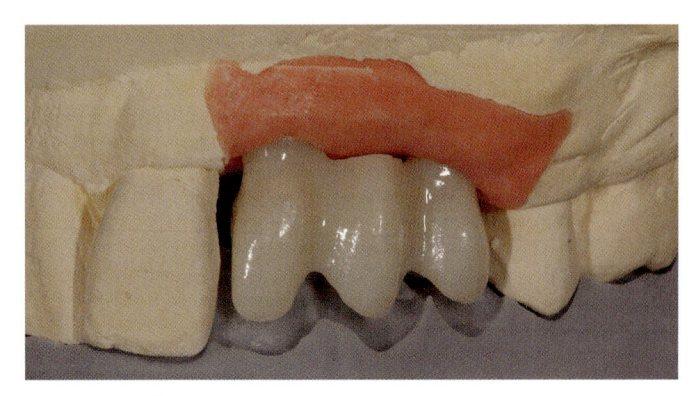

Figure 8.53 (D) Zirconia framework.

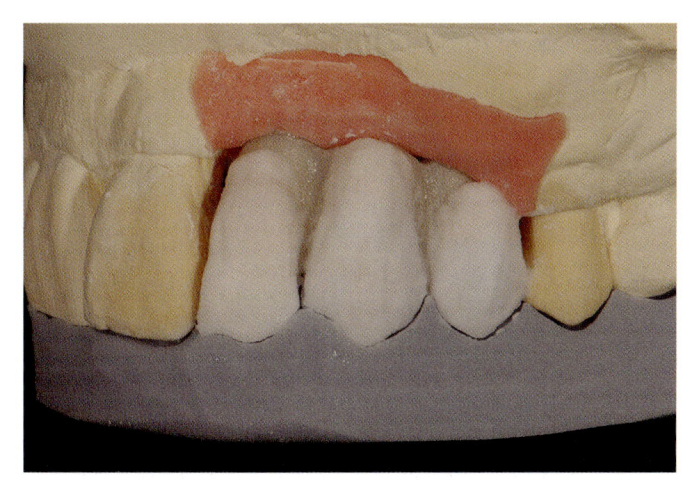

Chapter 8 Creating Esthetic Restorations Through Special Effects

Figure 8.53 (E) Porcelain buildup following the Siltek design.

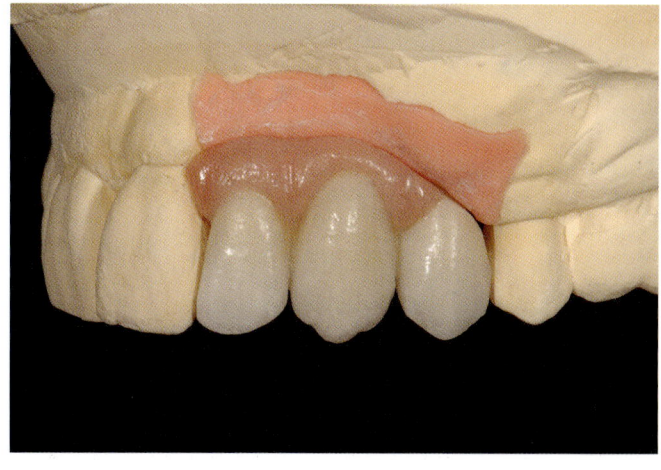

Figure 8.53 (F) Final restorations in place on the model.

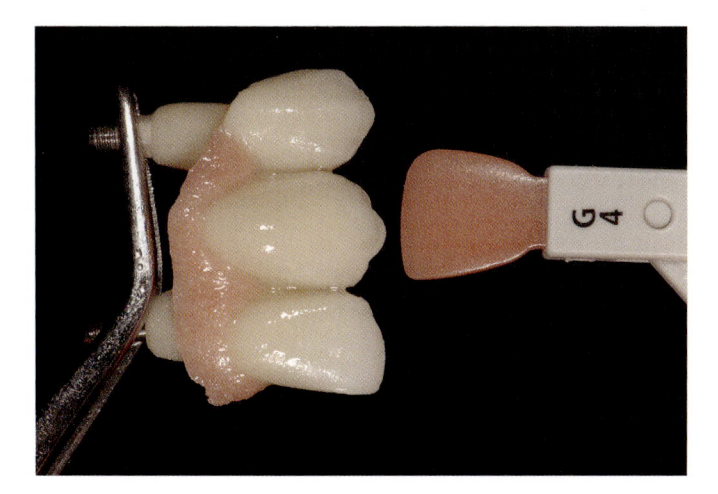

Figure 8.53 (G) Checking the pink shade.

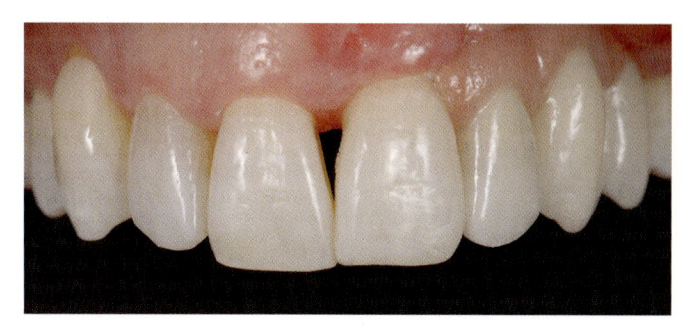

Figure 8.53 (H) After the implant was seated the patient's concern turned to the missing gingival papilla between her natural central incisors.

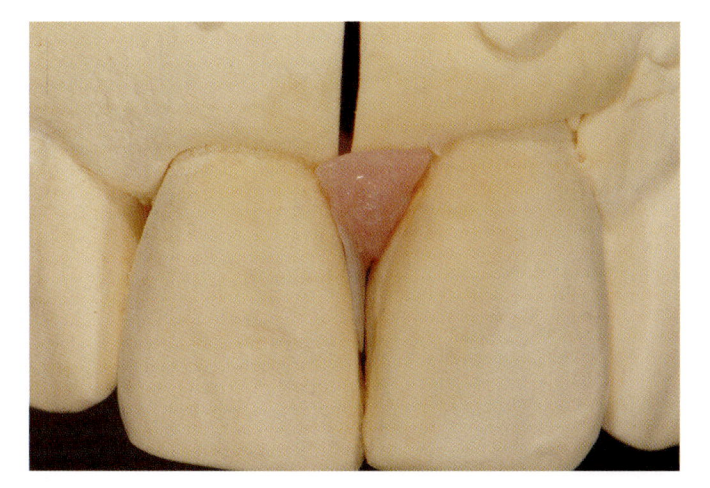

Figure 8.53 (I) An EMAX white tooth fragment was constructed with a pink composite resign gingival papilla bonded to the porcelain.

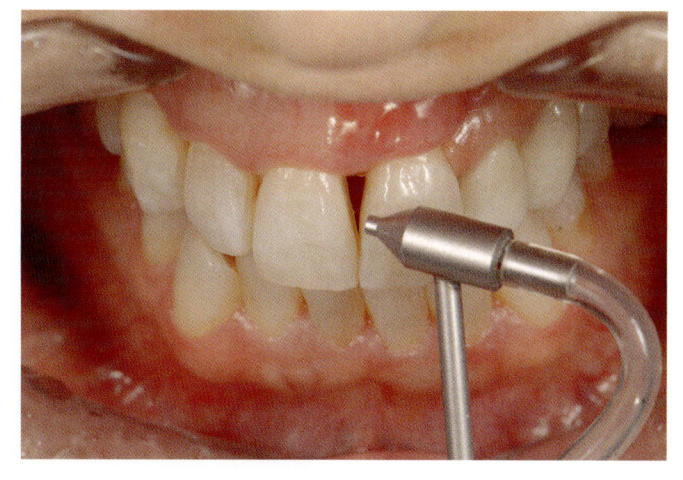

Figure 8.53 (J) Air abrasion was used to help clean and etch the enamel. This procedure also corrected the provisional defect.

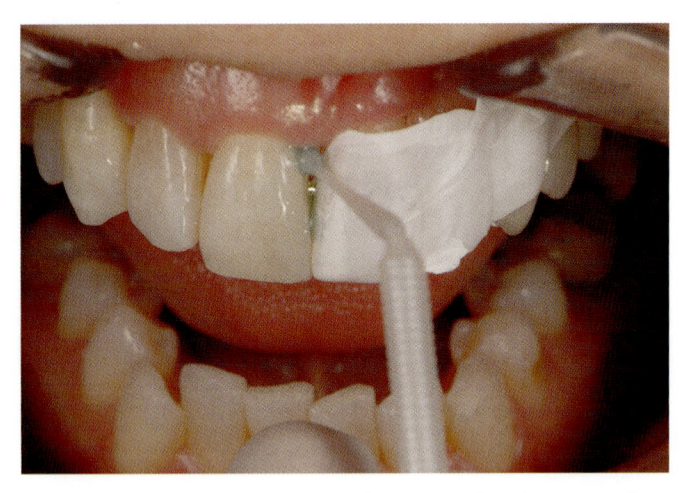

Figure 8.53 **(K)** Teflon tape was used to protect the adjacent tooth as etch is applied to the other central incisor.

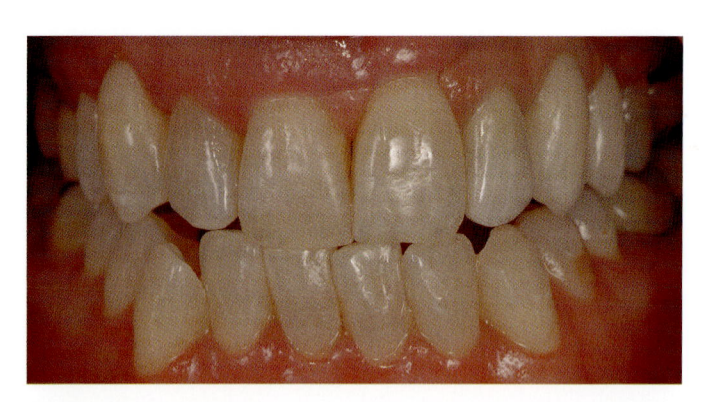

Figure 8.53 **(L)** The final central incisor tissue insert and the implant bridge are in good health.

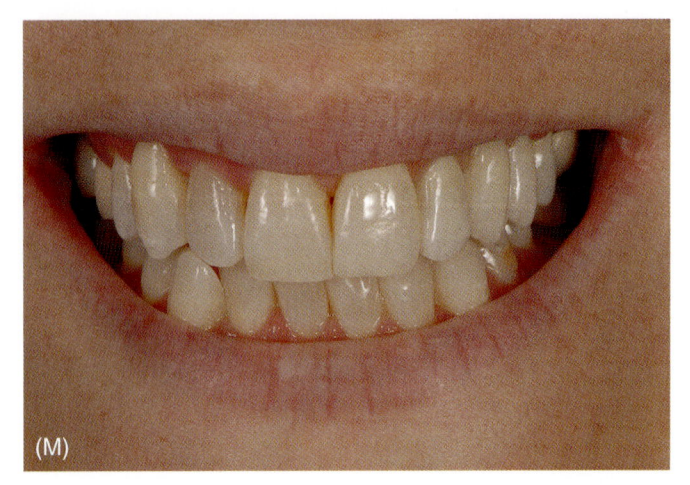

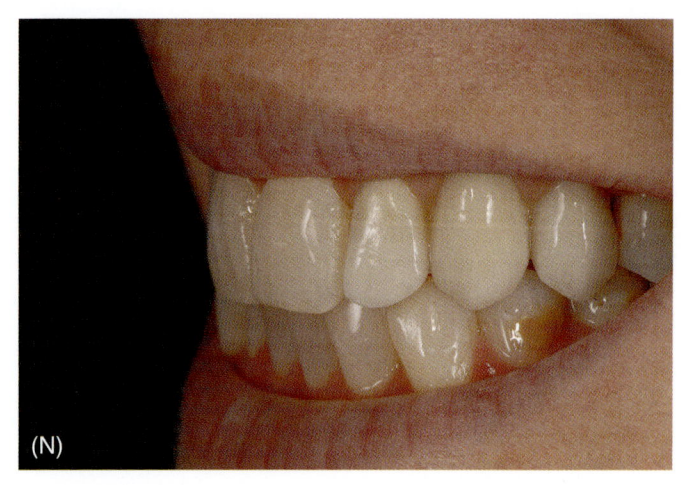

Figure 8.53 **(M and N)** Extraoral close-up photos show how esthetics look 2 years postoperatively. Figure courtesy of Guilherme Cabral.

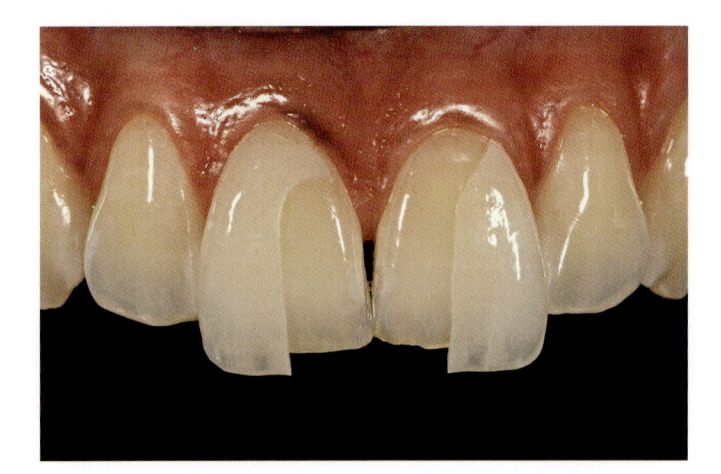

Figure 8.54 **(A)** All-ceramic quattro veneers on the maxillary central incisors are a new solution to allow intimate marginal adaptation and a perfect fit. This may eliminate excessive tooth reduction especially with triangular tooth shapes. Figure courtesy of Nasser Shademan.

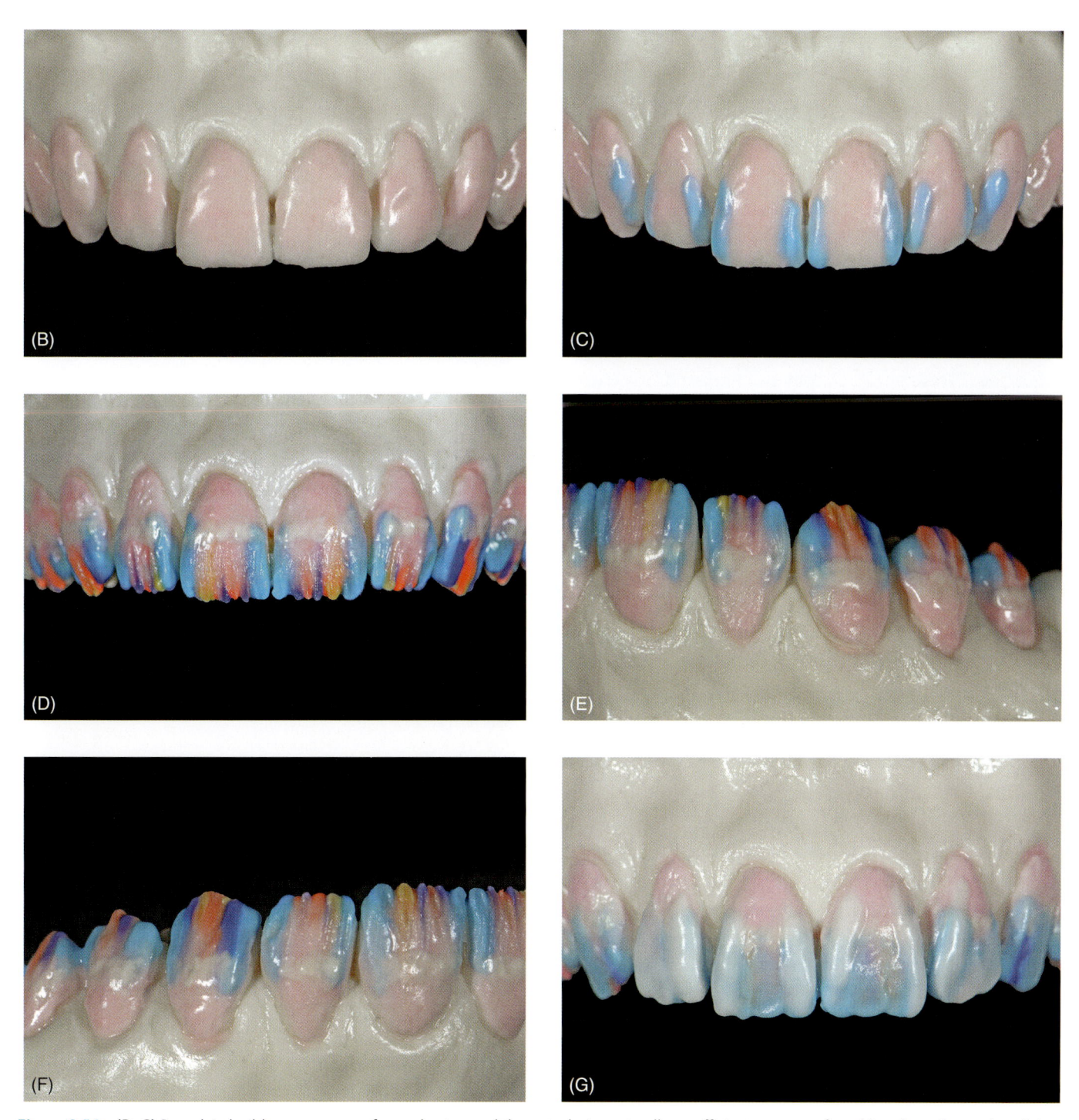

Figure 8.54 **(B–G)** Porcelain buildup process performed using multilayer technique, to allow sufficient amount of masking the yellow color of the tooth beneath, while at the same time displaying natural translucency on layers closer to the labial surface on refractory dyes. Figures courtesy of Nasser Shademan.

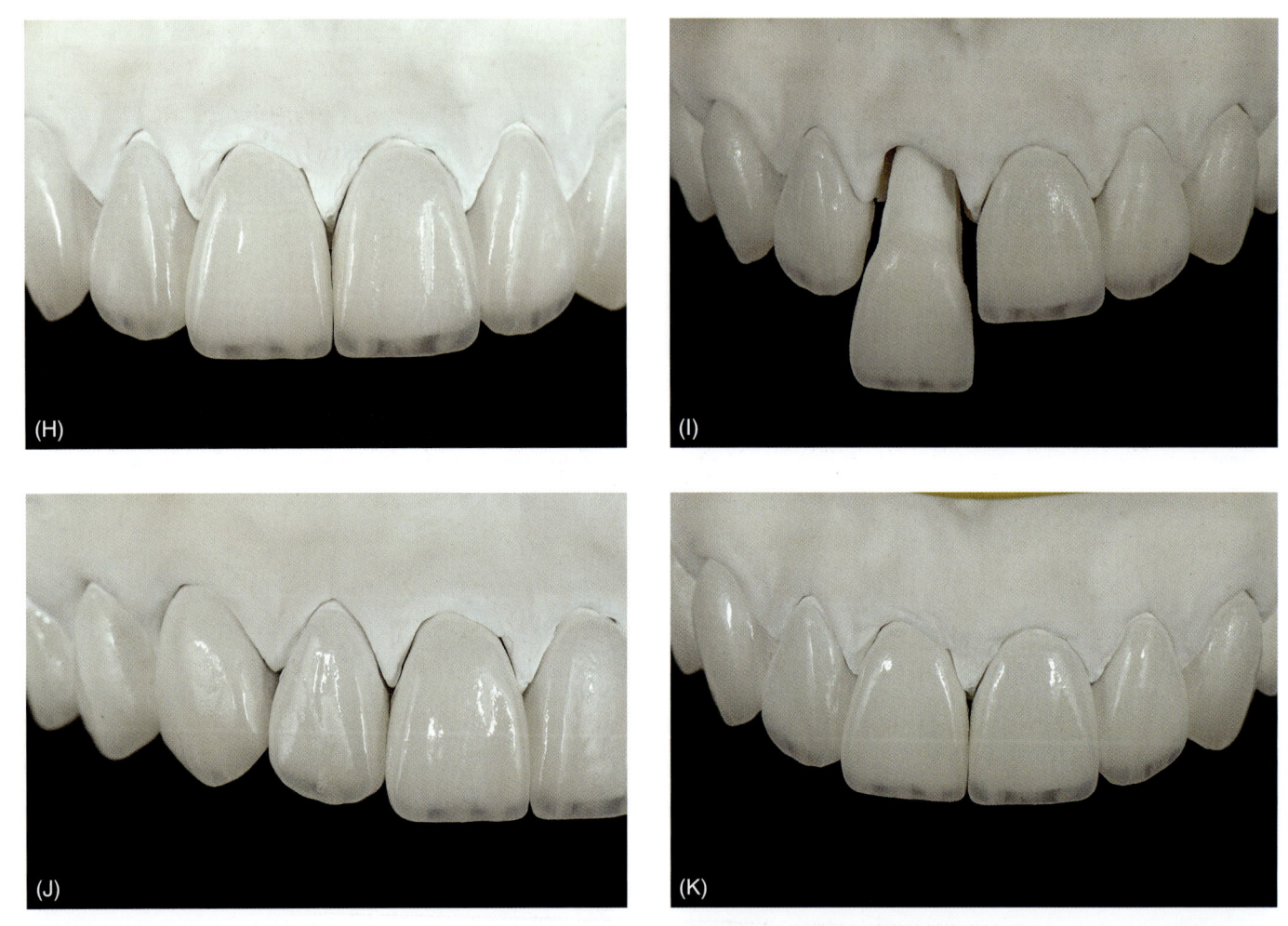

Figure 8.54 (H–K) The porcelain buildup is completed and the ceramic surface is glazed and manually polished under the microscope. Figures courtesy of Nasser Shademan.

Summary

This chapter has presented a variety of methods to help make artificial teeth look more realistic. Selecting material with optical properties closest to the natural dentition in all light conditions is a good start. The ceramometal crown can be just as realistic as the all-ceramic crown. Splinted teeth can look just as individual as single units. However, in the final analysis, the quality of the result is directly proportional to good communication and the ability and artistry of the dental ceramist (Figure 8.55A and B).

Natural tooth positions, contours, surface characterizations, and blemishes can be quite esthetic. Asymmetry is a normal occurrence. Neither dentist nor patient may wish to reproduce that which is grotesque, but the classic ideal may be just as unesthetic. All or some of these factors must be analyzed and resolved before an esthetic result can be achieved. There is an obligation to the patient to restore not merely healthy function but the esthetics that are so important to a healthy personality. Through the use of illusion, this end can often be achieved, despite seemingly impossible esthetic problems.

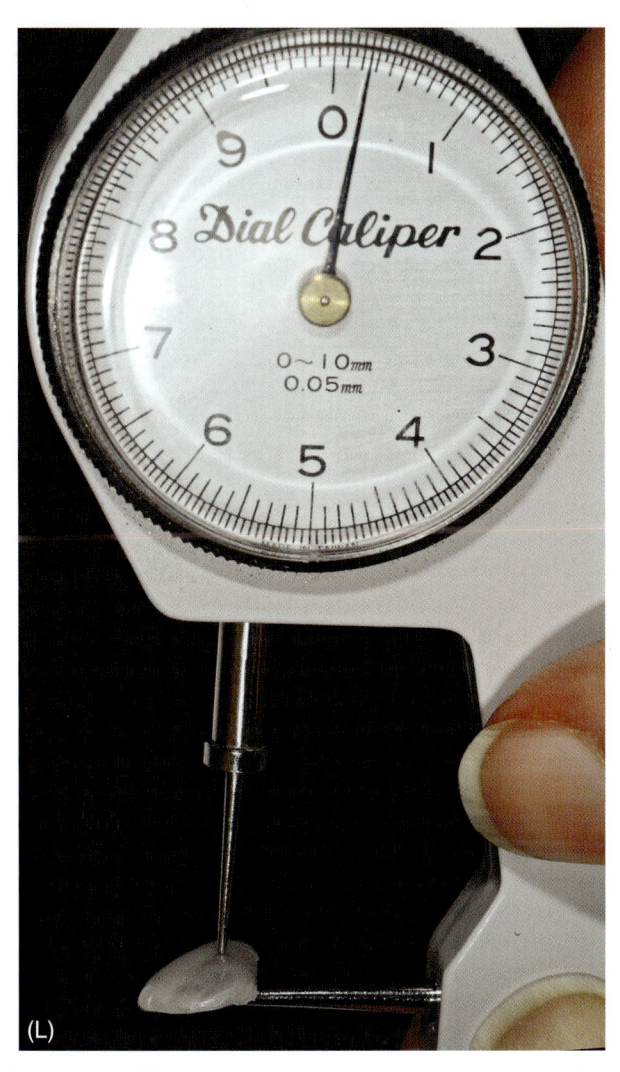

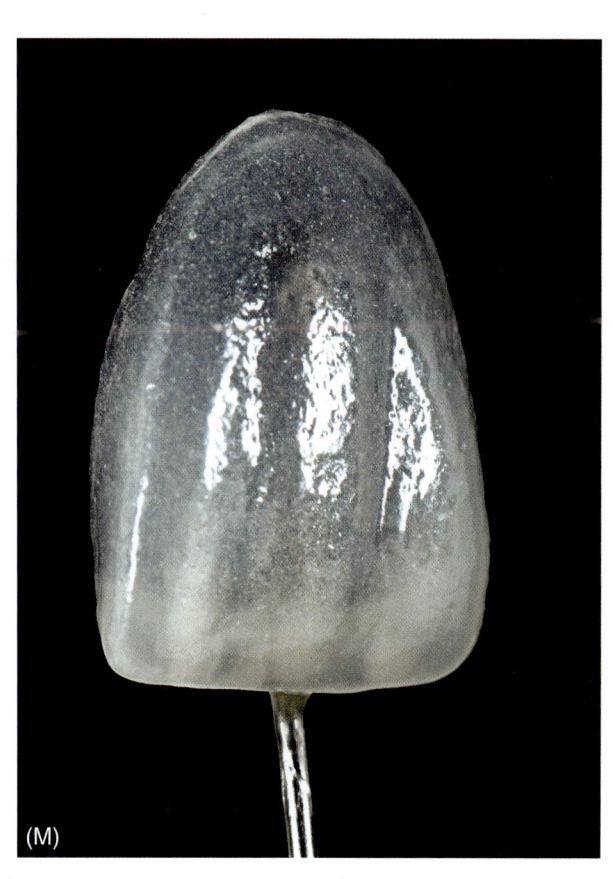

Figure 8.54 **(L and M)** The maxillary central incisor after removal of the refractory dye material that was sand blasted earlier shows a thickness of less than 0.5 mm. Figures courtesy of Nasser Shademan.

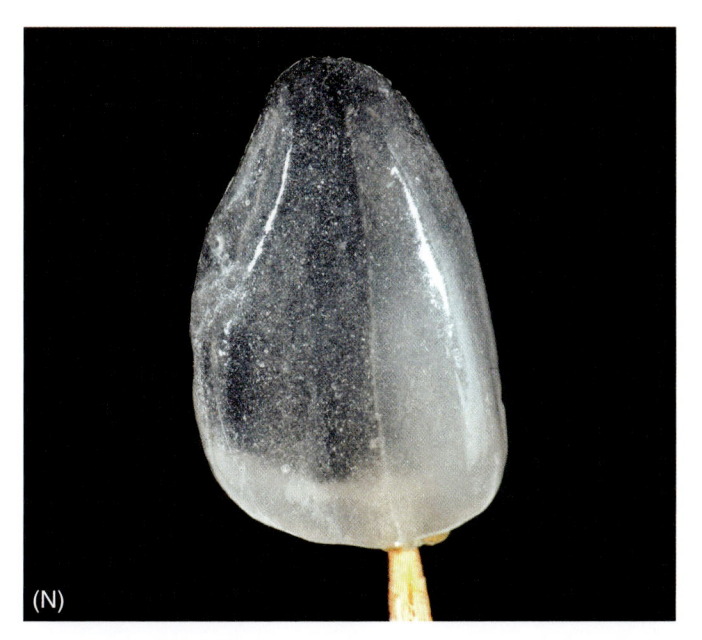

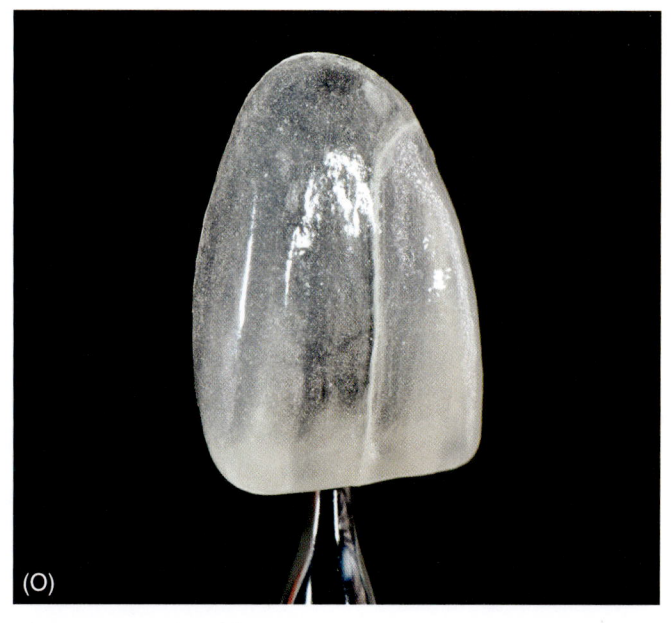

Figure 8.54 **(N and O)** Using a well-sharpened ceramic cutting bur the vertical groove was created from inside the veneer under the microscope, outlining the design of a dual-section veneer. Figures courtesy of Nasser Shademan.

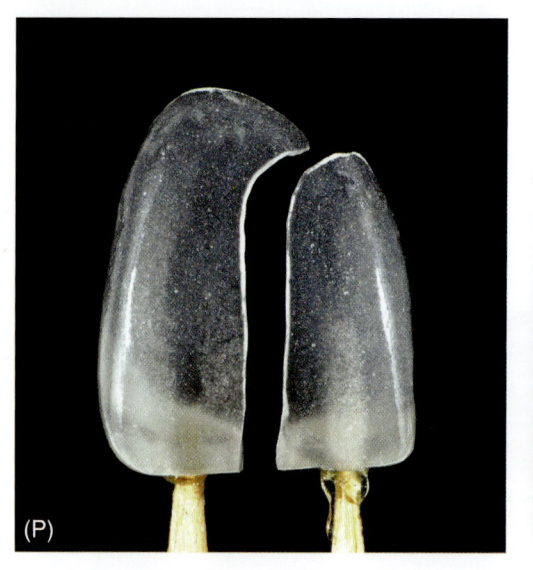

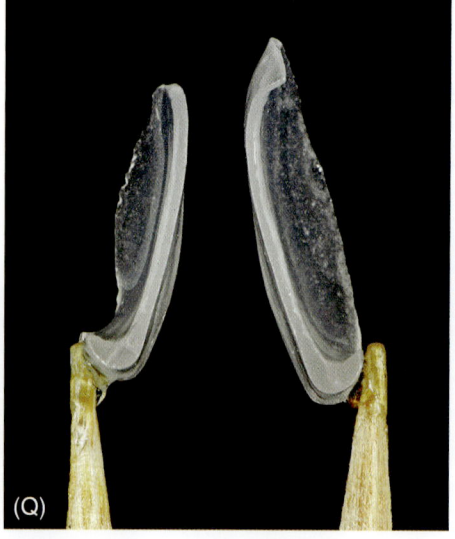

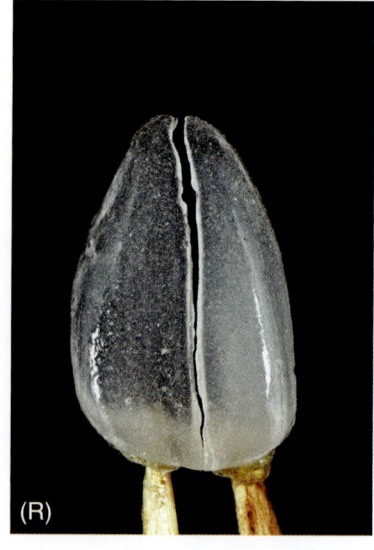

Figure 8.54 **(P–R)** With a little pressure the single porcelain veneer is now separated into two sections, just as planned. Figures courtesy of Nasser Shademan.

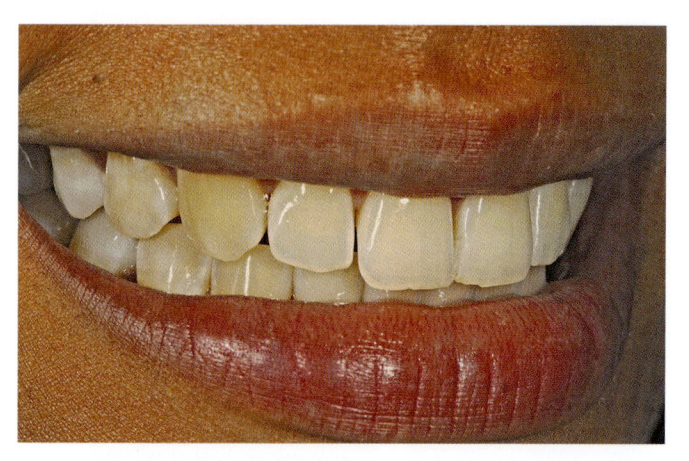

Figure 8.54 **(S)** The preoperative close-up image shows the triangular interproximal shape as well as excessive yellow staining on the canine. Figure courtesy of Nasser Shademan.

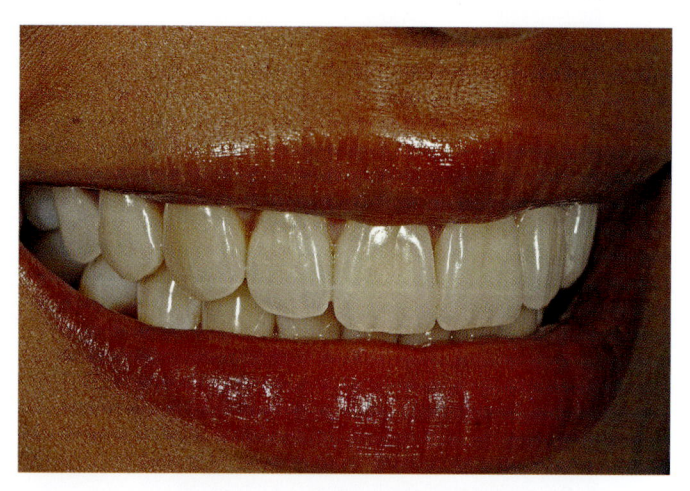

Figure 8.54 **(T)** Postoperative close-up image from the same patient after insertion of all-quattro veneers. Figure courtesy of Nasser Shademan.

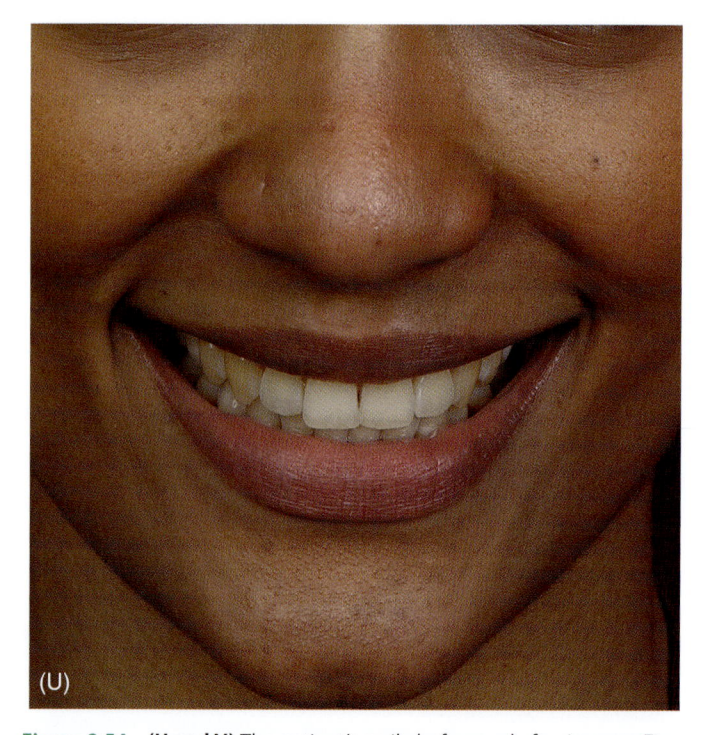

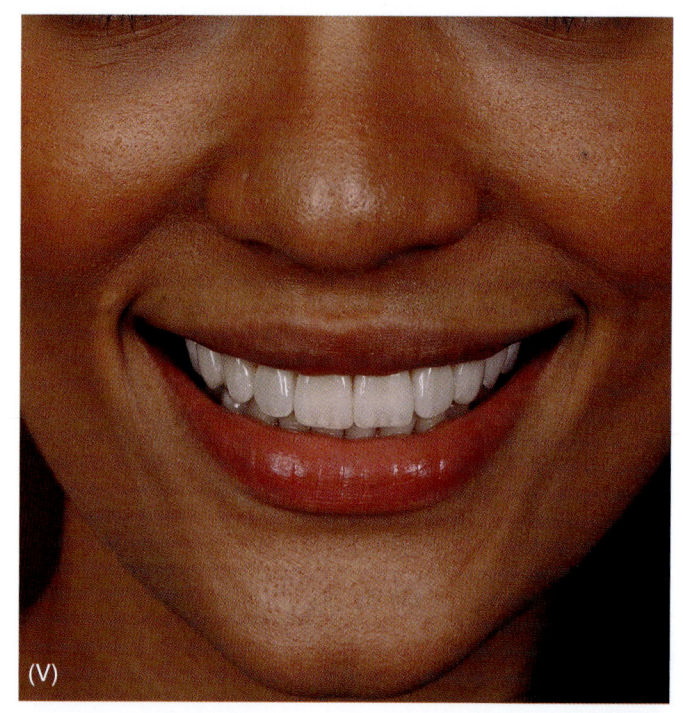

Figure 8.54 **(U and V)** The patient's smile before and after images. Figures courtesy of Nasser Shademan.

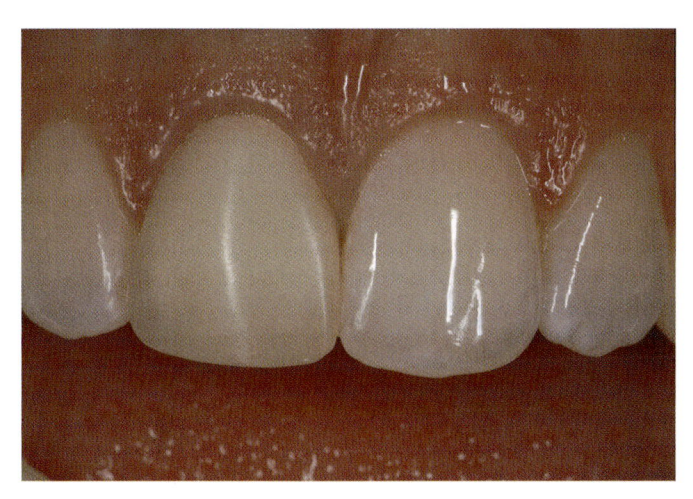

Figure 8.55 **(A)** A preoperative view of the patient's existing left central incisor crown shows a lack of (1) color match, (2) proper tooth form, (3) luster, and (4) texture. Figure courtesy of Guilherme Cabral.

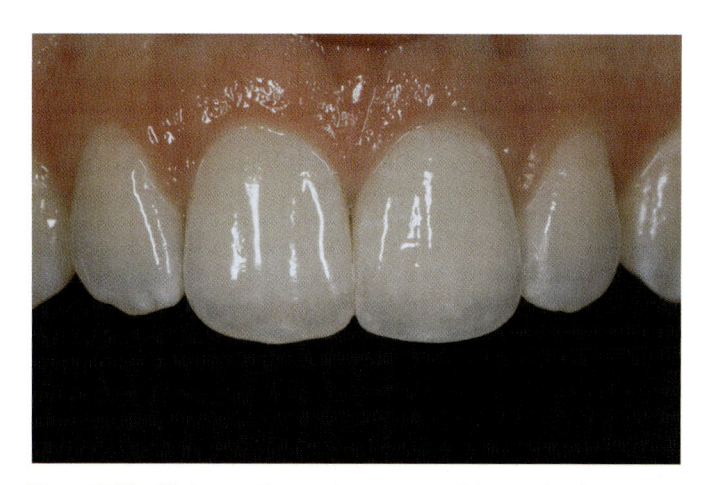

Figure 8.55 **(B)** A new all-ceramic crown was fabricated to better mimic the natural dentition. Note the type of shade characterization, the density of calcified spots, and the finishing texture and luster which give the illusion of a natural tooth. Figure courtesy of Guilherme Cabral.

References

1. Lombardi RE. The principles of visual perception and their clinical application to denture esthetics. *J Prosthet Dent* 1973;9:358.
2. Aker DA, Aker JR, Sorensen SE. Toothbrush abrasion of color-corrected porcelain stains applied to porcelain fused-to-metal restorations. *J Prosthet Dent* 1980;44(2):161–163.
3. Barghi N. A study of various factors influencing shade of bonded porcelain. *J Prosthet Dent* 1978;39(3):282–284.
4. Cronin RJ, Wardle WL. Loss of anterior inter-dental tissue: periodontal and prosthodontic solutions. *J Prosthet Dent* 1983;50:505–509.

Additional resources

Adisman IK. Management of esthetic problems in unconventional denture prosthesis. *Dent Clin North Am* 1967;March:101–114.

Aeziman HT. Use of surface stains for ceramic restorations. *Northwest Dent* 1971;50:215.

Anusavice KJ. Stress distribution in atypical crown designs. In: Preston J, ed. *Perspectives in Dental Ceramics*. Chicago, IL: Quintessence; 1988:175.

Aoshima H. *A Collection of Ceramic Works: A Communication Tool for the Dental Office and Laboratory*. Tokyo: Quintessence; 1992.

Arnheim R. *Visual Art and Perception*. Berkeley, CA: University of California Press; 1966.

Baumhammers A. Prosthetic gingiva for restoring esthetics following periodontal surgery. *Dent Digest* 1969;75:58.

Baumhammers A. *Temporary and Semipermanent Splinting*. Springfield, IL: Charles C. Thomas; 1971.

Bazola FN, Maldne WF. A customized shade guide for vacuum-fired porcelain-gold combination crown. *J Am Dent Assoc* 1967;74:114.

Bazos P, Magne P. Bio-emulation: biomimetically emulating nature utilizing a histo-anatomic approach; visual synthesis. *Int J Esthet Dent* 2014;9(3):330–352.

Beagle JR. Surgical reconstruction of the interdental papilla: case report. *Int J Periodontics Restorative Dent* 1992;12(2):145–151.

Beder OE. Esthetics and enigma. *J Prosthet Dent* 1971;25:588.

Berger RP. Esthetic considerations in framework design. In: Preston J, ed. *Perspectives in Dental Ceramics*. Chicago, IL: Quintessence; 1988:237.

Blancheri RL. Optical illusions. *J S Calif Dent Assoc* 1950;17:24.

Blancheri RL. Optical illusions and cosmetic grinding. *Rev Assoc Dent Mex* 1950;8:103.

Borenstein S. Effects of the age factor on the layering technique. In: Preston J, ed. *Perspectives in Dental Ceramics*. Chicago, IL: Quintessence; 1988:257.

Boucher CO, ed. *Swenson's Complete Dentures*, 6th edn. St. Louis, MO: C.V. Mosby; 1970.

Boucher CO. Esthetics and occlusion. In: *Esthetics*. New York: Medcom; 1973.

Bourelly G, Pruden JN. Influence of firing parameters on the optical properties of dental porcelains (FRE). *Rev Fr Prothes Dent* 1991;27:33–40.

Brecker SC. *The Porcelain Jacket Crown*. St. Louis, MO: C.V. Mosby; 1951.

Brecker SC. *Clinical Procedures in Occlusal Rehabilitation*. Philadelphia, PA: W.B. Saunders; 1966.

Bronstein BR. Problems in porcelain rehabilitation. *J Prosthet Dent* 1967;17:79.

Buckner RC. Cosmetics in denture prostheses. *J Am Dent Assoc* 1963;66:787.

Bulanov VI, Strelnikov VN. The planning of the design of combined crowns with regard to tooth display during conversation and smiling (RUS). *Stomatologiia* 1991;4:60–62.

Calamia JR. Dental restorations of firmly bonded porcelain in anterior and posterior regions. *Quintessenz Zahntech* 1991;17:821–838 [in German].

Cappello N, Bazzano F, Ferrero A. Anthropometric assessments in dental esthetics (ITA). *Minerva Stomatol* 1991;40:613–617.

Carlson C, Krueger KR. Full coverage cosmetic dentistry and gingival health. *J Esthet Dent* 1991;3:43–45.

Celenza FV. Occlusal management of metal ceramic restorations. In: Preston J, ed. *Perspectives in Dental Ceramics*. Chicago, IL: Quintessence; 1988:457.

Ceramco Color System. *Long Island City*. New York: Ceramco Equipment Corporation; 1956.

Chase RF. Sex and the upper central incisor. *Tex Dent J* 1972;90:39.

Chiche GJ, Aoshima H. *Smile Design*. Japan: Quintessence; 2004.

Chiche G, Pinault A. *Esthetics of Anterior Fixed Prosthodontics*. Chicago, IL: Quintessence; 1993.

Chu SJ. A biometric approach to predicatble treatment of clinical crown discrepancies. *Pract Proced Aesthet Dent* 2007;19:401–409.

Chu SJ, Tan JH, Stappert CF, Tarnow DP. Gingival zenith positions and levels of the maxillary anterior dentition. *J Esthet Restor Dent* 2009;21:113–120.

Coachman C, Salama M, Garber D, et al. Prosthetic gingival reconstruction in the fixed partial restoration. Part 3: laboratory procedures and maintenance. *Int J Periodontics Restorative Dent* 2010;30:19–29.

Coachman C, Salama M, Garber D, et al. Prosthetic gingival reconstruction in the fixed partial restoration. Part 1: introduction to artificial gingiva as an alternative therapy. *Int J Periodontics Restorative Dent* 2009;29:471–477.

Crispin B. *Contemporary Esthetic Dentistry: Practice Fundamentals*. Tokyo: Quintessence; 1994.

Crispin BJ, Hewlett E, Seghi R. Relative color stability of ceramic stains subjected to glazing temperatures. *J Prosthet Dent* 1991;66:20–23.

Cross TP. Creating the appearance of white enamel dysmineralization with bonded resins. *J Esthet Dent* 1991;3:30–33.

Culpepper WD. Esthetic factors in anterior tooth restoration. *J Prosthet Dent* 1973;30:576.

DeFabianis E, Preti G. The esthetic factor in total prosthesis. *Minerva Stomatol* 1968;17:51.

de Kloet JJ, Steneker C. Cosmetic aspects of dental treatment. *Ned Tijdschr Tandheelk* 1991;98(6):198–202 [in Dutch].

Dickerman MJ. Esthetics and optical illusions. *Certified Dent Technol* 1964;2:4.

Dunn W. Staining artificial teeth to match exceptional natural ones. *Am J Dent Sci* 1983;17:302–307.

Dwork HR. The godfather takes his family to the dentist. *Dent Survey* 1972;48:26.

Fabelis N. The four harmonies of esthetics. *J Ky Dent Assoc* 1964;16:71.

Feigenbaum NL. Aspects of aesthetic smile design. *Pract Periodontics Asthet Dent* 1991;3(3):9–13.

Feigenbaum NL. Reshaping tooth contours with direct resins. *J Esthet Dent* 1991;3:57–61.

Feinberg E. *Full Mouth Restoration in Daily Practice*. Philadelphia, PA: J.B. Lippincott; 1971.

Ferreia D, Monard LA. Measurement of spectral reflectance and colorimetric properties of Vita shade guides. *J Dent Assoc S Afr* 1991;46(2):63–65.

Frisch J, Jones RA, Bhaskar SN. Conservation of maxillary anterior esthetics: a modified approach. *J Periodontol* 1967;33:11.

Frush JP, Fisher RD. Introduction to dentogenic restorations. *J Prosthet Dent* 1955;5:586.

Frush JP, Fisher RD. How dentogenic restorations interpret the sex factor. *J Prosthet Dent* 1956;6:160.

Frush JP, Fisher RD. How dentogenics interprets the personality factor. *J Prosthet Dent* 1956;6:441.

Frush JP, Fisher RD. The age factor in dentogenics. *J Prosthet Dent* 1957;7:5.

Frush JP, Fisher RD. The dynesthetic interpretation of the dentogenic concept. *J Prosthet Dent* 1958;8:558.

Frush JP. Dentogenics: its practical application. *J Prosthet Dent* 1959;9:914.

Glickman I. *Clinical Periodontology*, 4th edn. Philadelphia, PA: W.B. Saunders; 1972.

Gmur O. News about the metal porcelain technique. *Zahntechnik* 1970;28:450.

Goldstein CE, Goldstein RE, Garber DA. Computer imaging: an aid to treatment planning. *J Calif Dent Assoc* 1991;19(3):47–51.

Goldstein RE. Diagnostic dilemma: to bond, laminate, or crown? *Int J Periodontics Restorative Dent* 1987;87(5):9–30.

Goldstein RE. Esthetics in dentistry. *J Am Dent Assoc* 1982;104:301–302.

Goldstein RE. Solving tooth color problems in esthetic dentistry. Presented at Hinman Dental Meeting. *Clinical Topics in Dentistry*. University of Nebraska Medical Center; #81, 1992.

Goldstein RE. Study of need for esthetics in dentistry. *J Prosthet Dent* 1969;21:589.

Goldstein RE, Adar P. Special effects and internal characterization. *J Dent Technol* 1989;17(11):48–49.

Goldstein RE, Feinman RA, Garber DA. Esthetic considerations in the selection and use of restorative materials. *Dent Clin North Am* 1983;27(4):723–731.

Goldstein RE, Adar P. Immediate conservative corrections of esthetic problems. *J Dent Technol (Jpn)* 1990;75(3):50–59.

Goodsir L. *Creating Illusions of Tooth Size by Varying Tooth Form. The Thermotrol Technician, vol. 25*. New Rochelle, NY: JF Jelenko and Co; March–April 1971.

Goodsir L. *Creating Illusions of Tooth Size by Shading and Characterizing. The Thermotrol Technician, vol. 25*. New Rochelle, NY: JF Jelenko and Co; September–October 1971.

Grant D, Stern IB, Everett FG. *Organ's Periodontics*, 2nd edn. St. Louis, MO: C.V. Mosby; 1963.

Hallarman E. *A Statistical Survey of the Shape and Arrangement of Human Male and Female Teeth [master's thesis]*. NY University College of Dentistry; 1971.

Hawkins CH, Sterrett JD, Murphy HJ, Thomas JC. Ridge contour related to esthetics and function. *J Prosthet Dent* 1991;66:165–168.

Henderson D. The dentist, the technician, and work authorizations. In: *Esthetics*. New York: Medcom; 1973.

Henderson D, Frazier Q. Communicating with dental laboratory technicians. *Dent Clin North Am* 1970;14:603.

Hickey JC. The esthetics of anatomy. In: *Esthetics*. New York: Medcom; 1973.

Hickey JC, Boucher C, Woelfel J. Responsibility of the dentist in complete dentures. *J Prosthet Dent* 1962;12:637.

House MM. *Form and Color Harmony in Denture Art*. Whittier, CA: House & Loop; 1939.

Hubbard JR. Natural texture and lustre in ceramics. In: Preston J, ed. *Perspectives in Dental Ceramics*. Chicago, IL: Quintessence; 1988:263.

Hulten P, Dudek RP. The importance of translucency and fluorescence in dental ceramics. In: Preston J, ed. *Perspectives in Dental Ceramics*. Chicago, IL: Quintessence; 1988:273.

Jinoian B. The importance of proper light sources in metal ceramics. In: Preston J, ed. *Perspectives in Dental Ceramics*. Chicago, IL: Quintessence; 1988:229.

Johnston JF, Dykema RW, Mumford G, Phillips R. Construction and assembly of porcelain veneer gold crowns and pontics. *J Prosthet Dent* 1962;12:1125.

Johnston JF, Phillips RW, Dykema RW. *Modern Practice in Crown and Bridge Prosthodontics*, 3rd edn. Philadelphia, PA: W.B. Saunders; 1971.

Jones D. Ceramics in dentistry. *Dent Technol* 1971;24:64.

Kataoka S, Shoji T, Okubo Y. Layering technique with opal ceramic for natural color in front teeth. *Quintessence Int* 1991;17(2):189–200 [in German].

Katz SR. Aesthetics in ceramics. *J Can Dent Assoc* 1966;32:224.

Kina S. *Equilibrium*. Sao Paulo: Artes Medicas Ltd; 2009.

Klaffenbach AO. Dental porcelains, glazes, stains and their application to dental restorations. *Dent Cosmos* 1928;19:1185.

Kohler FD. Personalizing the teeth. In: *Esthetics*. New York: Medcom; 1973.

Kornfeld M. *Mouth Rehabilitation: Clinical and Laboratory Procedures*. St. Louis, MO: C.V. Mosby; 1967.

Korson D. *Aesthetic Design for Ceramic Restorations*. London: Quintessence; 1994.

Krajicek DD. Dental art in prosthodontics. *J Prosthet Dent* 1969;21:122.

Krajicek DD. Anatomy of esthetics. In: *Esthetics*. New York: Medcom; 1973.

Kurzeja R. Translucency and esthetics. In: Preston J, ed. *Perspectives in Dental Ceramics*. Chicago, IL: Quintessence; 1988:267.

Landa LS. Anterior tooth selection. In: *Esthetics*. New York: Medcom; 1973.

LaVere AM, Marcroft KR, Smith RC, Sarka RJ. Denture tooth selection: an analysis of the natural maxillary central incisor compared to the length and width of the face: Part 1. *J Prosthet Dent* 1992;67:661–663.

Lee JH. Immediate full upper denture. *Dent Pract* 1952;2:336.

Lee JH. *Dental Aesthetics: The Pleasing Appearance of Artificial Dentures*. Bristol, CT: John Wright and Sons; 1962.

L'Estrange PR, Strahan JD. The wearing of acrylic periodontal veneers. *Br Dent J* 1970;128:193.

Levin EI. Dental esthetics and the gold proportion. *J Prosthet Dent* 1978;40:244.

Lombardi RE. A method for the classification of errors in dental esthetics. *J Prosthet Dent* 1974;32:501.

Luckiesh M. *Visual Illusions*. New York: Dover Publications; 1965.

Magne P, Magne M, Belser U. The diagnostic template: a key element to the comprehensive esthetic treatment concept. *Int J Periodontic Restorative Dent* 1996;16:560–569.

Marcushamer E, Tsukiyama T, Griffen TJ, et al. Anatomic crown width/length ratio of unworn maxillary teeth in asian subjects. *Int J Periodontics Restorative Dent* 2011;31:495–503.

Marquis PM. Optimizing the strength of all-ceramic jacket crowns. In: Preston J, ed. *Perspectives in Dental Ceramics*. Chicago, IL: Quintessence; 1988:15.

Martinelli N. *Dental Laboratory Technology*. St. Louis, MO: C.V. Mosby; 1970.

Martone AL. Complete denture esthetics and its relation to facial esthetics. *Dent Clin North Am* 1967;March:89–100.

Mclaren EA. *The Art of Passion: A Photographic Journey*. Tustin, CA: Edward A. McLaren, 2007.

McLean JW. The alumina reinforced porcelain jacket crown. *J Am Dent Assoc* 1967;65:621.

McLean JW. *The Science and Art of Dental Ceramics*, vol. 2. London: Quintessence; 1980.

McLean JW, Kedge M. High-strength ceramics. In: Preston J, ed. *Perspectives in Dental Ceramics*. Chicago, IL: Quintessence; 1988:153.

Miller CJ. *Inlays, Crowns and Bridges*. Philadelphia, PA: W.B. Saunders; 1962.

Miller IF. Complete restorative dentistry. *J Prosthet Dent* 1973;30:675.

Miller L. A clinician's interpretation of tooth preparation and the design of metal substructures for metal-ceramic restorations. In: McLean JW, ed. *Dental Ceramics*. Chicago, IL: Quintessence; 1983:153.

Mitchell RG. Method used to obtain optimum esthetics in the porcelain gold crown. *Tex Dent J* 1968;85:7.

Morali M. Esthetics. *Rev Belge Med Dent* 1970;25:421.

Morley J. Smile designer's workshop. *Dent Today* 1991;10(1):42.

Morrison K, Warnick M. Staining porcelain-bonded-to-metal restorations. *J Prosthet Dent* 1967;15:713.

Muia P. *Esthetic Restorations: Improved Dentist-Laboratory Communication*. Chicago, IL: Quintessence; 1993.

Myers GE. *Textbook of Crown and Bridge Prosthodontics*. St. Louis, MO: C.V. Mosby; 1969.

Nelson AA. The aesthetic triangle in the arrangement of teeth: face form, tooth form, alignment form, harmonious or grotesque. *Natl Dent Assoc J* 1922;9:392.

Newman A. Dental porcelains and furnaces. *Dent Technol* 1968;2:14.

Nixon RL. Smile showcase—redesigning the narrow smile. *Pract Periodontics Aesthet Dent* 1991;3(4):45–50.

Owall B, Kayser AF, Carlsson GE. *Prosthodontics: Principles and Management Strategies*. St. Louis, MO: Mosby; 1996.

Owen EB. A study of the human complexion and a means of determining hues and shades in edentulous cases. *J Am Dent Assoc* 1925;12:944.

Palmieri CJ, Platzer KM. Orthodontic-plastic surgical collaboration in aesthetic facial remodeling. *N Y State Dent J* 1991;57(4):32–33.

Patur B, Glickman I. Gingival pedicle flaps for covering root surfaces denuded by chronic destructive periodontal disease: a clinical experiment. *J Periodontol* 1968;29:50.

Payne AGL. Factors influencing the position of artificial upper anterior teeth. *J Prosthet Dent* 1971;26:26.

Payne SH. Contouring and positioning. In: *Esthetics*. New York: Medcom; 1973.

Pensler AV. Shade selection: problems and solutions. *Compendium Cont Educ Dent* 1998;19:387–396.

Philippe J. Esthetics of the face and teeth. *Orthod Fr* 1991;62:423–432 [in French].

Pilkington EL. Esthetics and optical illusions in dentistry. *J Am Dent Assoc* 1936;23:641.

Pincus CL. Building mouth personality. *J Calif Dent Assoc* 1938;14:125.

Pincus CL. New concepts in model techniques and high temperature processing of acrylic resins for maximum esthetics. *J S Calif Dent Assoc* 1956;24:26.

Pincus CL. The role of jacket crown and fixed bridge restorations in the prevention and treatment of periodontal lesions. *J S Calif Dent Assoc* 1956;24:19.

Pincus CL. Light reflections. In: *Esthetics*. New York: Medcom; 1973.

Potter RB. Impressionism in denture esthetics. *J Tenn Dent Assoc* 1970;50:16.

Potter RB. Dentoesthetics through visual aids. *J Tenn Dent Assoc* 1970;50:19.

Pound E. Esthetics and phonetics in full denture construction. *J Calif Dent Assoc* 1950;26:179.

Pound E. Recapturing esthetic tooth position in the edentulous patient. *J Am Dent Assoc* 1957;55:181.

Pound E. Modern American concepts in esthetics. *Int Dent J* 1960;10:154–172.

Pound E. Applying harmony in selecting and arranging teeth. *Dent Clin North Am* 1962;3:241.

Pound E. Lost—fine arts in the fallacy of the ridges. *J Prosthet Dent* 1964;4:6.

Preston J. The elements of esthetics—application of color science. In: McLean JW, ed. *Dental Ceramics*. Chicago, IL: Quintessence; 1983:491.

Prichard JF. *Advanced Periodontal Disease*, 2nd edn. Philadelphia, PA: W.B. Saunders; 1972.

Prinz R. An error and its correction. *Quintessence Int* 1971;2:47.

Renner RP. *An Introduction to Dental Anatomy and Esthetics*. Chicago, IL: Quintessence; 1985:241–273.

Risch JR, White JG, Swanson HM. The esthetic labial gingival prosthesis. *J Indiana Dent Assoc* 1977;56:15.

Roach RR, Mujia PJ. Communication between dentist and technician: an esthetic checklist. In: Preston J, ed. *Perspectives in Dental Ceramics*. Chicago, IL: Quintessence; 1988:445.

Rosenstiel SF, Land MF, Fujimoto J. *Contemporary Fixed Prosthodontics*, 2nd edn. St. Louis, MO: Mosby; 1994.

Rufenacht CR. *Fundamentals of Esthetics*. Chicago, IL: Quintessence; 1990.

Saklad MJ. Achieving esthetics with the porcelain jacket. *Dent Clin North Am* 1967;March:41–55.

Salama M, Coachman C, Garber D, et al. Prosthetic gingival reconstruction in the fixed partial restoration. Part 2: diagnosis and treatment planning. *Int J Periodontics Restorative Dent* 2009;29:573–581.

Saleski CG. Color, light shade matching. *J Prosthet Dent* 1972;25:589.

Scharer P. A clinician's view of porcelain reconstructions. In: McLean JW, ed. *Dental Ceramics*. Chicago, IL: Quintessence; 1983:293.

Schweitzer JM. Esthetics and hygiene after extensive periodontal treatment. *J Prosthet Dent* 1960;10:284.

Sharry JJ. *Complete Denture Prosthodontics*. New York: McGraw-Hill; 1968.

Shavell HM. Dentist-laboratory relationships in fixed prosthodontics. In: Preston J, ed. *Perspectives in Dental Ceramics*. Chicago, IL: Quintessence; 1988:429.

Shelby DS. Practical considerations and design of porcelain fused to metal. *J Prosthet Dent* 1962;12:542.

Shelby DS. Cosmetic restorative problems: initial study with television. *J Prosthet Dent* 1964;14:107.

Shelby DS. Esthetic needs in anterior tooth restoration. *N Y J Dent* 1967;37:108.

Shelby DS. Esthetics and fixed restorations. *Dent Clin North Am* 1967;March:57–70.

Shelby DS. *Anterior Restoration, Fixed Bridgework, and Esthetics*. Springfield, IL: Charles C Thomas, 1976.

Sieber C. *Voyage: Visions in Color and Form*. Chicago, IL: Quintessence; 1995.

Silver M, Howard M, Klein G. Porcelain bonded to a cost metal understructure. *J Prosthet Dent* 1961;11:132.

Silverman HN, Wolf ROL. Posterior restorations. *Dent Manage* 1991;31(8):41–43.

Spear FM, Kokich VG, Mathews dP. Interdisciplinary management of anterior dental esthetics. *J Am Dent Assoc* 2006;137:160–169.

Staffileno H. Management of gingival recession and root exposure problems associated with periodontal disease. *Dent Clin North Am* 1964:11.

Stappert CF, Tarnow DP, Tan JH, Chu SJ. Proximal contact areas of the maxillary anterior dentition. *Int J Periodontics Restorative Dent* 2010;30:471–7.

Stoloff CI. The fashionable tooth. *J Oreg Dent Assoc* 1972;42:6.

Sturdevant CM, Roberson TM, Heymann HO, Sturdevant JR. *The Art and Science of Operative Dentistry*, 3rd edn. St. Louis, MO: Mosby; 1994.

Sulikowski AV, Yoshida A. Three dimensional management of dental proportions: a new aesthetic principle: "the frame of reference". *Quintessence Dent Technol* 2002;25:8–20.

Swenson HM, Hanson NM. The periodontist and cosmetic dentistry. *J Periodontol* 1961;32:82.

Tanaka A. Successful technologist-dentist teamwork. In: Preston J, ed. *Perspectives in Dental Ceramics*. Chicago, IL: Quintessence; 1988:439.

Tarnow D, Chu S, Kim J. *Aesthetic Restorative Dentistry*. Mahwah, IL: Montage Media Corporation, 2008.

Tashma J. Coloring somatoprostheses. *J Prosthet Dent* 1967;17:303.

Tillman EJ. Modeling and staining acrylic-resin anterior teeth. *J Prosthet Dent* 1955;5:497.

Touati B, Miara P, Nathanson D. *Esthetic Dentistry & Ceramic Restorations*. New York City: Martin Dunitz, 1999.

Tsukiyama T, Marcushamer E, Griffin T, et al. Comparison of the anatomic crown width/length ratios of unworn and worn maxillary teeth in Asian White subjects. *J Prosthet Dent* 2012;107:11–14.

Tylman SD. *Theory and Practice of Crown and Fixed Partial Prosthodontics (Bridge)*. St. Louis, MO: C.V. Mosby; 1970.

Valderhaug J. A 15-year clinical evaluation of fixed prosthodontics. *Acta Odontol Scand* 1991;49(1):35–40.

Viana PC, Correia A, Neves M, et al. Soft tissue waxup and mock-up as key factors in treatment plan: case presentation. *Eur J Esthet Dent* 2012;7:310–323.

Vig RG. The denture look. *J Prosthet Dent* 1961;11:9.

Vryonis P. Aesthetics in ceramics: perceiving the problem. In: Preston J, ed. *Perspectives in Dental Ceramics*. Chicago, IL: Quintessence; 1988:209.

Wehner PJ, Hickey JC, Boucher CO. Selection of artificial teeth. *J Prosthet Dent* 1967;18:222.

Williams DL. Prosthesis for a lost gingival papilla. *Dent Surv* 1977; November:36.

Williams Gold Refining Co. *Basic Colormanship*. Buffalo, NY: H.D. Justi Co.; 1968.

Woon KC, Thong YL. A multidisciplinary approach in achieving aesthetics and function. *J Ir Dent Assoc* 1991;37(1):15–17.

Zarb GA, Bolender CL, Carlsson GE. *Boucher's Prosthodontic Treatment for Edentulous Patients*, 11th edn. St. Louis, MO: Mosby; 1997.

Zena RB, Abbott LJ. Light harmony of crowns and roots: understanding and managing the black line phenomenon. *Pract Periodontics Aesthet Dent* 1991;3:27–31.

House 1:16 Rule

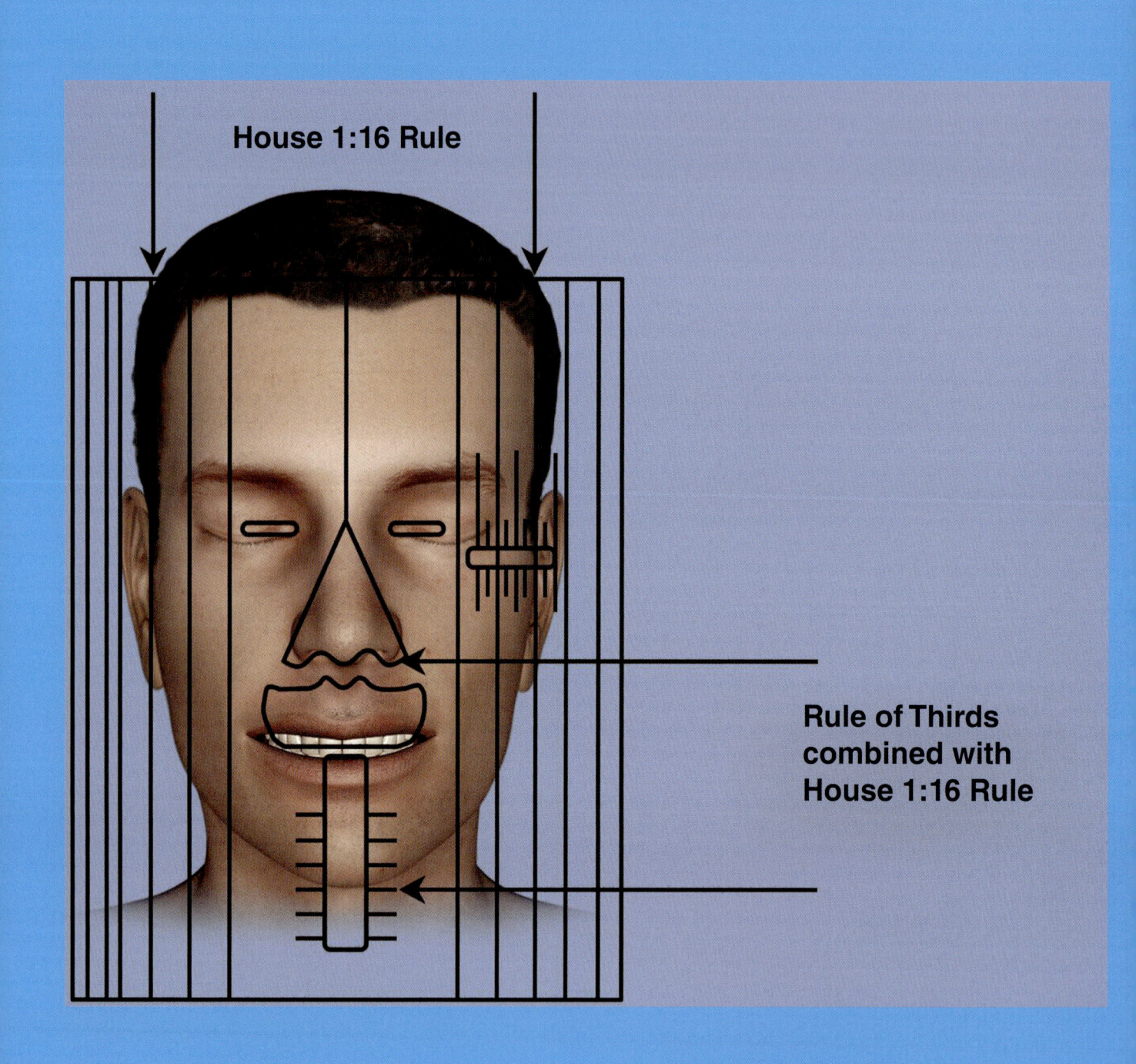

Rule of Thirds combined with House 1:16 Rule

Chapter 9 Proportional Smile Design

Daniel H. Ward, DDS, Stephen J. Chu, DMD, MSD, CDT, and Christian F.J. Stappert, DDS, MS, PhD

Chapter Outline

The golden proportion	243	Proportional dental/facial analysis	253
Proportions of the esthetic face	245	Width/length ratio of maxillary central incisor	253
Smile design principles	245	Tooth-to-tooth width proportion theories	254
Determinants of incisal edge position	246	Recurring esthetic dental (RED) proportion	257
Embrasures	247	Dentist proportion preferences	258
Size and shape of individual teeth	248	Using the RED proportion to calculate ideal tooth widths	260
Apical tooth forms	248	Clinical use of the RED proportion	261
Proportion of tooth size to face size	249	Simplified use of the RED proportion	263
Digital dental photography	251	Use of computer simulation	265
Facial image view evaluation (FIVE)	253	Patient preferences and individuality	268

The modern paradigm of dentistry merges an esthetic element with a functional restorative component. An analytical approach in conjunction with a stylistic expression of smile design is essential to balance the artistic and scientific aspects of the discipline. A few gifted operators have the ability to internally visualize the potential outcome of a smile without formal analysis. This subjective approach may be effective for the most experienced and talented professionals, but a more objective method for evaluating and predetermining the final outcome is essential for the majority of dentists. Some professionals may feel this diminishes the creativity of their efforts, but in today's consumer-oriented environment, patients often demand a clear visualization of the end results. On closer evaluation and study, specific characteristics and patterns of what is considered esthetic become evident. Certain key proportions emerge as being present in smiles considered to be pleasing to the eye.

The golden proportion

Balance, symmetry, and proportion are essential to create the perception of beauty and harmony in objects viewed as esthetic (Figure 9.1). The concept of beauty and its correlation with nature and mathematics was a central theme in the development of the "golden proportion." Attributed to Phidias in ancient Greece over 2000 years ago, it has been believed by many to possess mystical powers.[1] Leonardo da Vinci denoted the presence of the golden proportion in his book of illustrations depicting the human body (Figure 9.2). The golden proportion occurs when the length of two objects have a special relationship in which the proportion between the shorter to the longer is the same as the proportion of the longer to the sum of the shorter plus the longer (Figure 9.3). The proportion in which this occurs is 0.618:1 or 62%. The golden proportion has been observed to

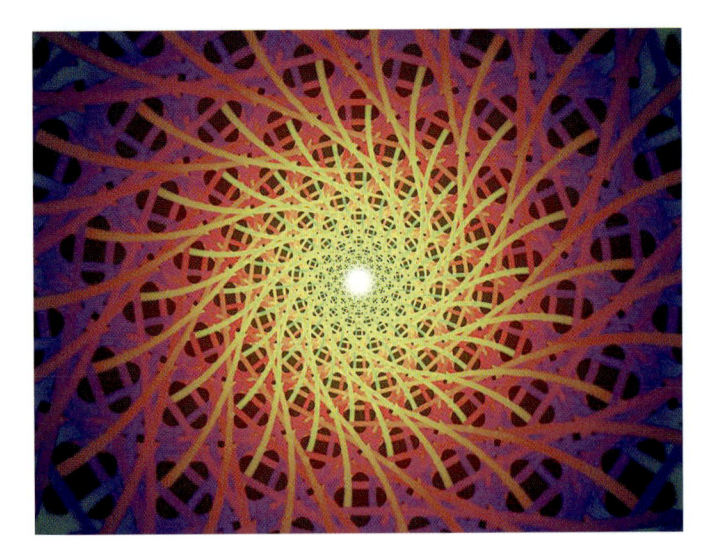

Figure 9.1 Esthetic balance and symmetry.

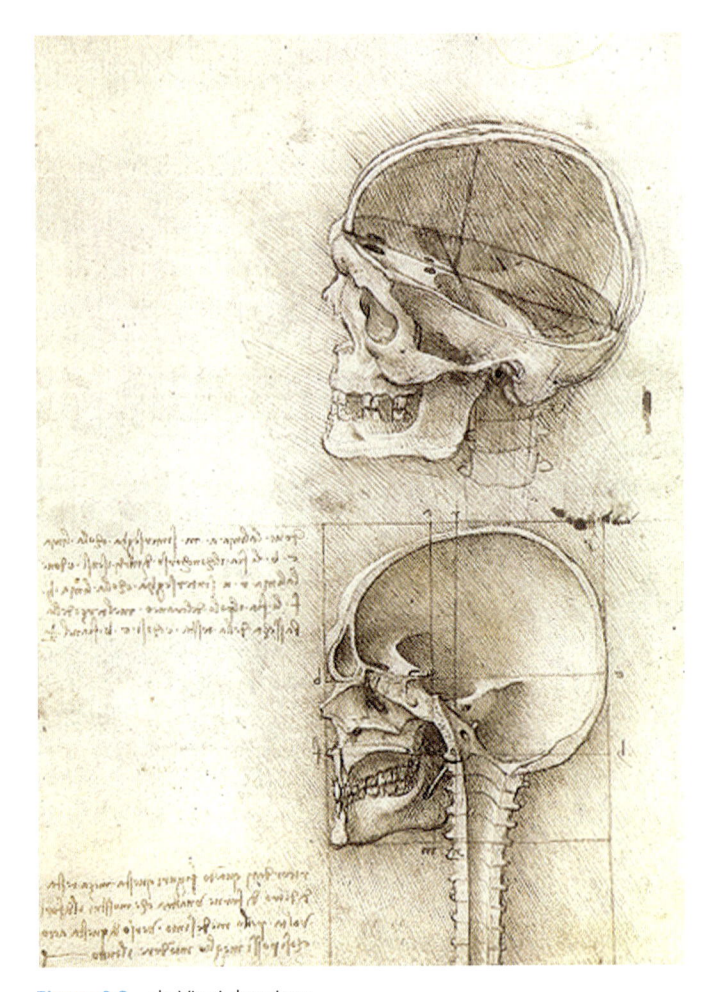

Figure 9.2 da Vinci drawings.

Golden Proportion

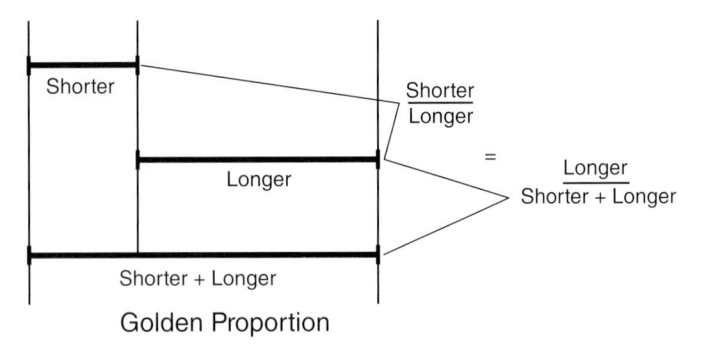

Figure 9.3 Lines in golden proportion.

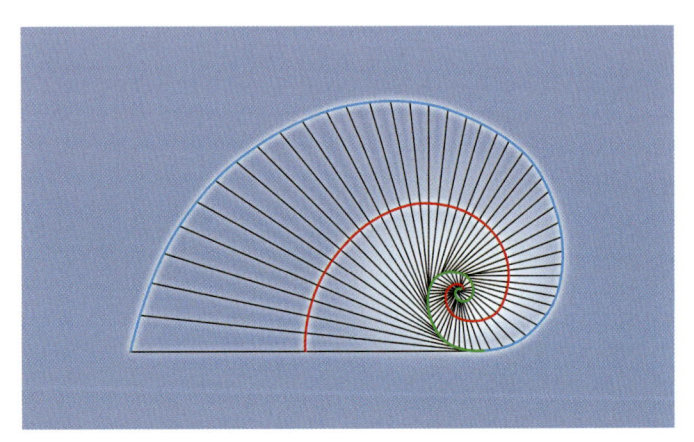

Figure 9.4 The golden proportion is observed in many organisms, such as a snail's shell.

$$\frac{\text{Golden}}{\text{Proportion}} = \frac{\text{Shorter}}{\text{Longer}} = \frac{\text{Longer}}{\text{Shorter + Longer}} = 0.62 = \left(\frac{\text{Shorter + Longer}}{\text{Longer}} - 1\right)$$

Figure 9.5 Unique golden proportion mathematical properties.

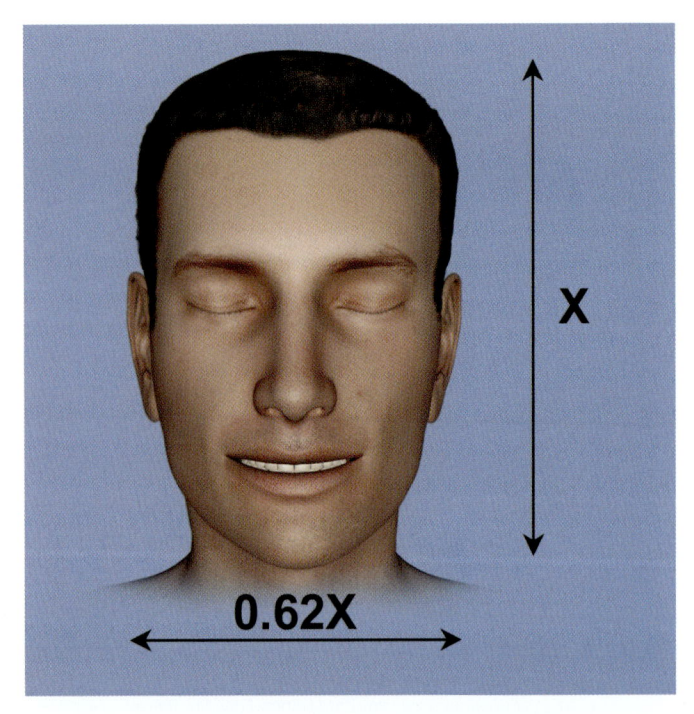

Figure 9.6 Width and length of face in golden proportion.

be present in nature in the growth of many organisms (Figure 9.4). It is interesting to note that the reciprocal of the golden proportion is equal to the sum of 1 plus the golden proportion (Figure 9.5). Authors have described various proportions of body parts as being golden (Figure 9.6).[2] Ricketts suggests that the golden proportion registers in the mind at the subconscious level and provides beauty, comfort, and pleasure to the senses.[3]

Proportions of the esthetic face

Other proportions have been reported to be present in humans. Modeling agencies often have measured their models in search of esthetic proportions deemed to be desirable for employment. A common lay observation has been that models are often tall. The average head is one-seventh of the total body height, yet the desired ratio by some modeling agencies is one-eighth (Figure 9.7) (L. Guthrie, personal communication, 1992). Artists have defined the facial rule of sevenths: the hair comprises the top seventh, the forehead the next two-sevenths, the nose two-sevenths, the space between the nose and mouth one-seventh, and the chin the final seventh (Figure 9.8).[4] Plastic surgeons speak of the rule of facial thirds and the rule of facial fifths.[5] Vertically, the esthetic face can be subdivided into approximately equal thirds. The superior third is from trichion to glabella, the middle third from glabella to subnasale and the inferior third from subnasale to menton. Of further interest to dentists is if the inferior third is equally divided into thirds, the incisal plane is generally located at the junction of the superior and middle thirds (Figure 9.9). It is interesting to note that these facial proportions may change as a patient ages, suggesting that certain proportions may be age-specific or age-appropriate (Figure 9.10). Similarly, plastic surgeons have noted the esthetic face can be divided into approximately equal fifths horizontally with one-fifth being the width of an eye (Figure 9.11).

Smile design principles

Every culture has its own esthetic preferences. The definitions reported are generally accepted standards for North America and may not be applicable worldwide. The original definitions of an esthetic smile were relative to the fabrication of

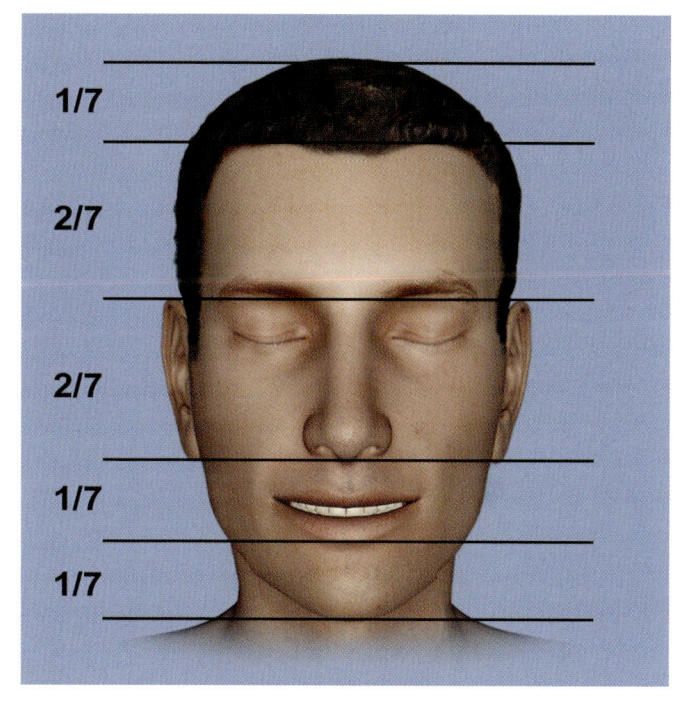

Figure 9.8 Facial rule of sevenths.

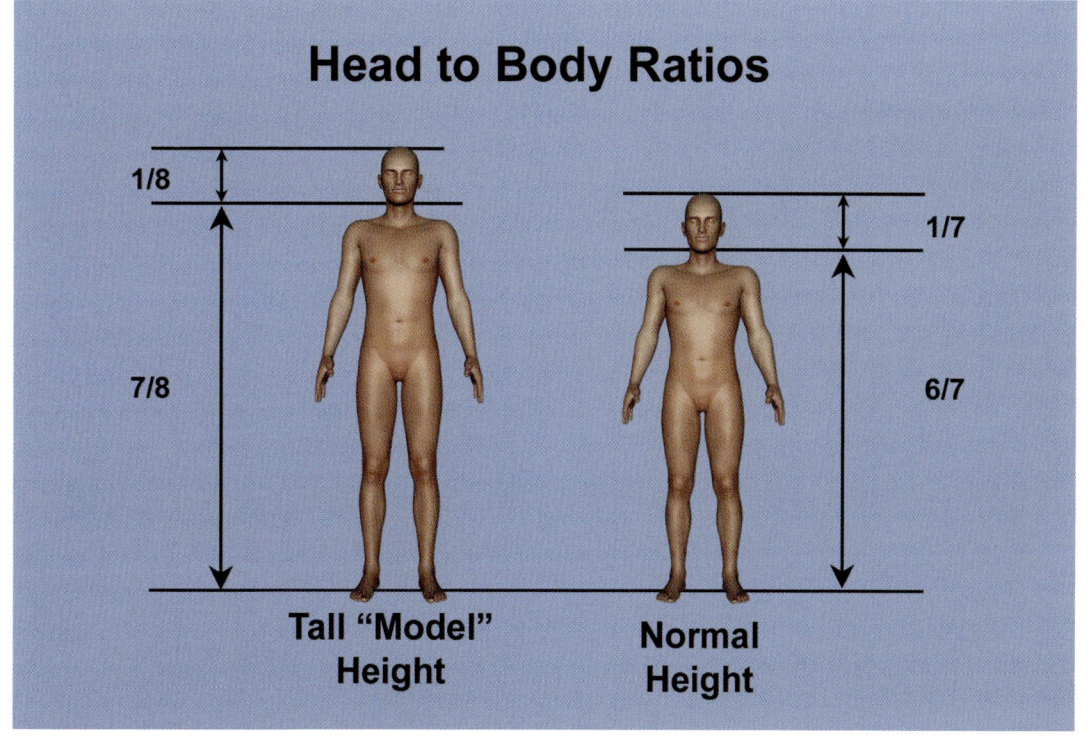

Figure 9.7 Head to body ratios.

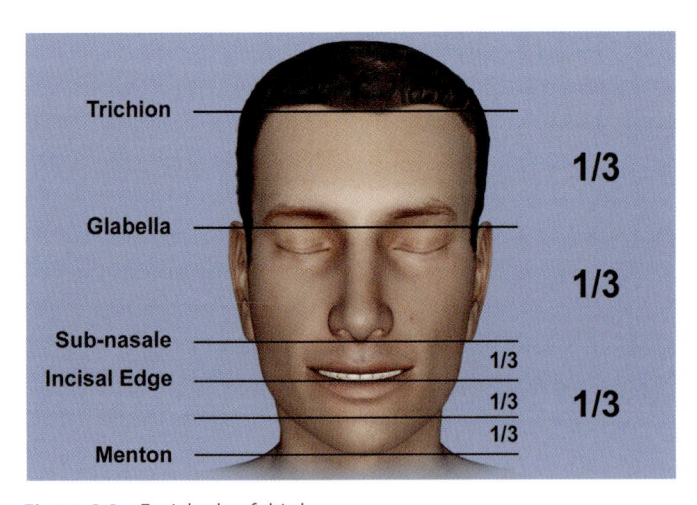

Figure 9.9 Facial rule of thirds.

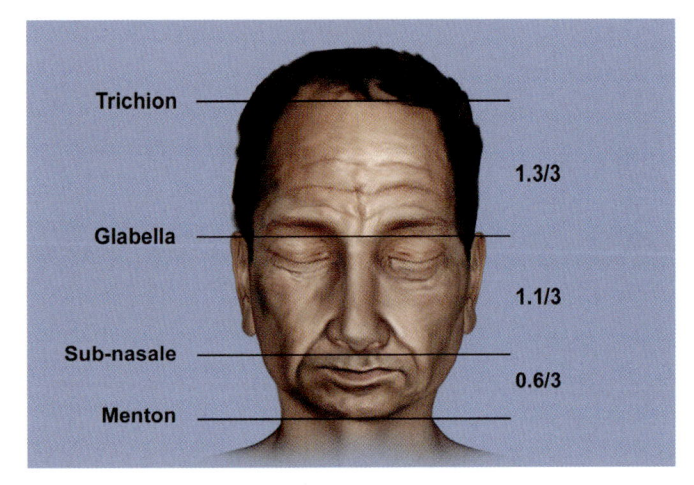

Figure 9.10 Aging facial proportions.

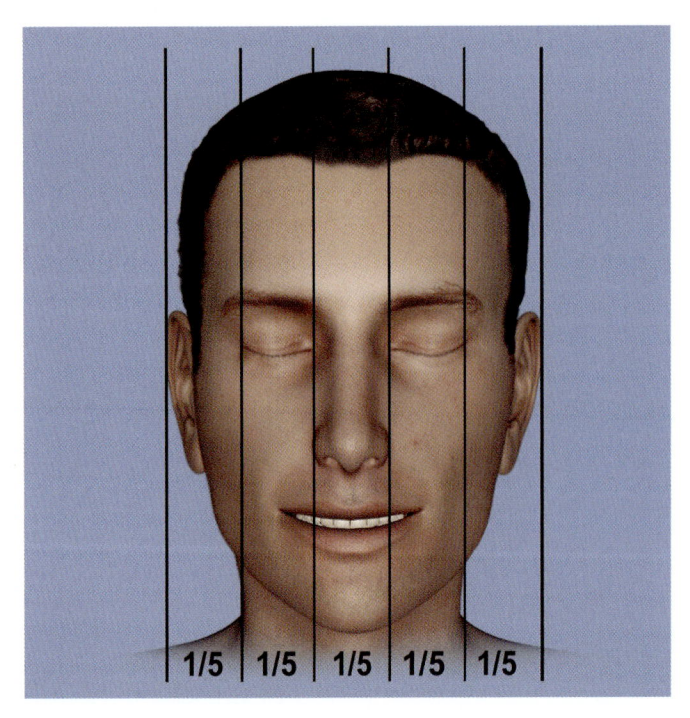

Figure 9.11 Facial rule of fifths.

complete dentures. Many classic and still often cited papers helped to define much of smile design as we know it today. "Dentogenics" was defined over 60 years ago as the art, practice, and techniques used to achieve esthetic results in dentistry.[6] No individual smile ever follows all these rules, nor would it look natural if all were followed, but a basic definition of an ideal smile is an important reference.

Determinants of incisal edge position

The starting point for smile evaluation is the position of the incisal plane. It should be parallel to the interpupillary line and the midline centered with the philtrum (Figure 9.12).[7] The superior/inferior position of the incisal plane can be selected by the use of four determinants.[8] The first determinant of incisal plane placement is esthetics. The incisal edges should follow the curvature of the lower lip (Figure 9.13).[9] The position of the buccal cusp tips of the teeth should progressively move apically

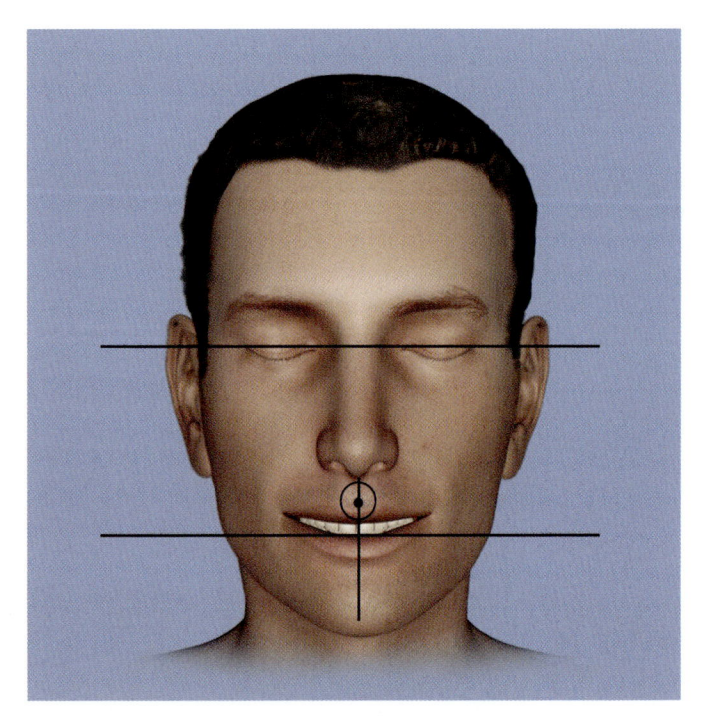

Figure 9.12 Incisal plane parallel to interpupillary line and the midline centered with the philtrum.

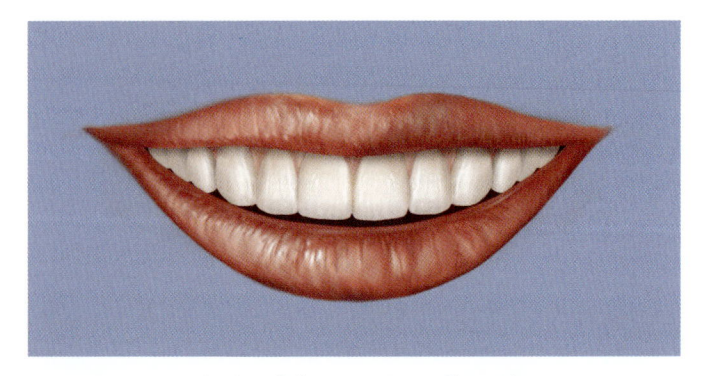

Figure 9.13 Incisal edges follow curvature of lower lip.

as you move distally. This curvature has been referred to as the curve of Spee (Figure 9.14).[10] The opposite of this curvature is referred to as a "reverse smile curve" and is considered to detract from the overall appearance of the smile (Figure 9.15).[11] The clinical crown should be outlined by the upper and lower lip and the marginal gingival display should be confined to the interdental papilla (Figure 9.16).[12] The second determinant of incisal edge position is phonetics. The incisal edges of the incisors should meet at the junction of the wet and dry zone when the fricative ("f" and "v") sounds are pronounced (Figure 9.17).[13] Words that begin with "th" can be pronounced by the patient and the relative ease and sound of the enunciation can help to evaluate the superior/inferior position of incisal edge placement. The third determinant of incisal placement is occlusion and anterior guidance. Anterior guidance is the key to protecting the posterior teeth while developing the esthetics of the smile. The lingual surfaces of the maxillary anterior teeth should disclude the posterior teeth immediately on forward movement of the mandible.[14] The fourth determinant is condylar border movements. The maxillary anterior teeth should meet the mandibular anterior teeth in full protrusive movements. The angle the lingual surfaces of the maxillary teeth disclude the mandibular teeth should be slightly greater than the angle of the eminentia.[15] The requirements of esthetics, phonetics, and adequate anterior guidance greater than the angle of the eminentia must be satisfied for long-term success.

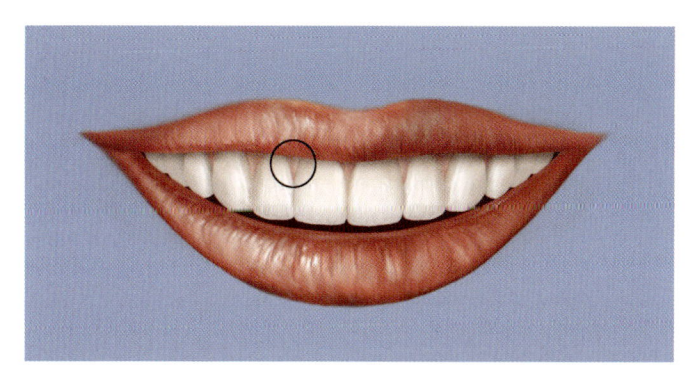

Figure 9.16 Marginal gingival display should be confined to the interdental papilla.

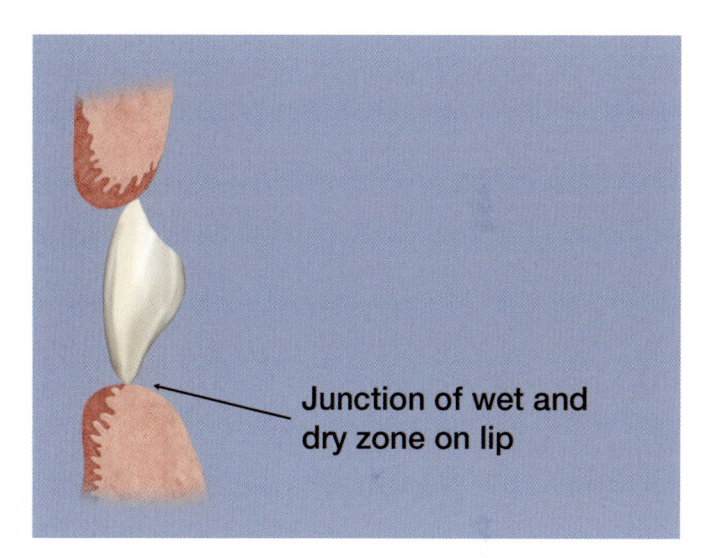

Figure 9.17 The incisal edges should meet at the junction of the wet and dry zone when the fricative ("f" and "v") sounds are pronounced.

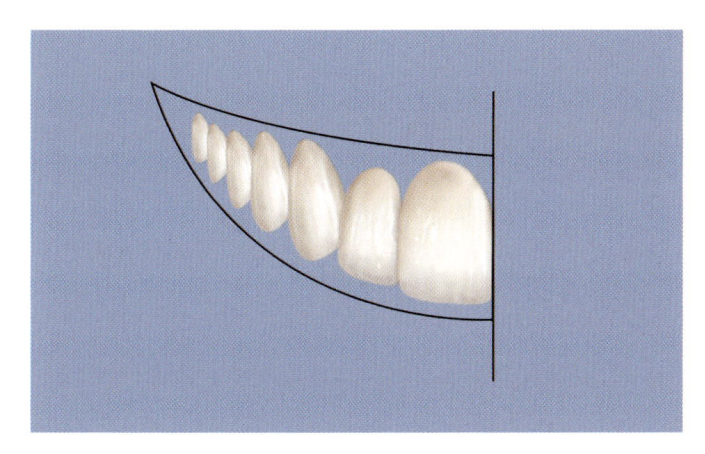

Figure 9.14 Curve of Spee.

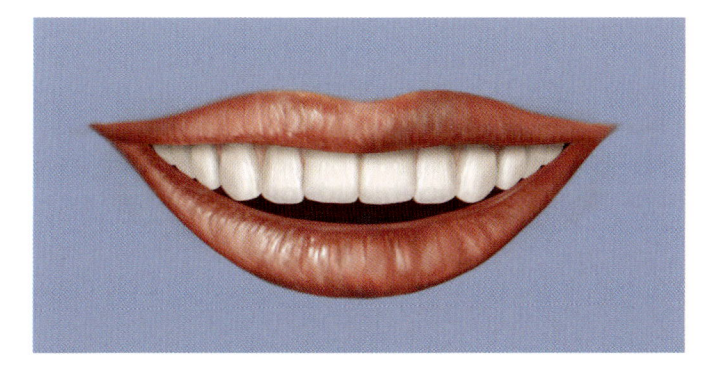

Figure 9.15 Reverse smile curve.

Embrasures

The shape of the incisal edges as they blend into the interproximal area at the incisal embrasures is important to the overall smile and may change due to aging, trauma, or biting patterns.[16] The incisal embrasures should become larger as you move distally (Figure 9.18). The mesial-incisal line angle of the maxillary incisors should be more of a right angle whereas the distal-incisal line angle should be more acute and rounded.[17] The location of the contact points between adjacent teeth should move apically as you move distally.[18] The amount of perceived contact between adjacent teeth has been referred to as the "connector area" and decreases as you move distally in the anterior area. The connector area between the maxillary central incisors should be 50% of the incisal length of the teeth. The connector area should be 40% between the central and lateral incisor and 30% between the lateral incisor and canine (Figure 9.19).[19] The incisal edges and embrasures are an important factor in the visual age perception of a patient.[20] As a patient ages and the incisal edges become worn, the incisal embrasures become smaller.

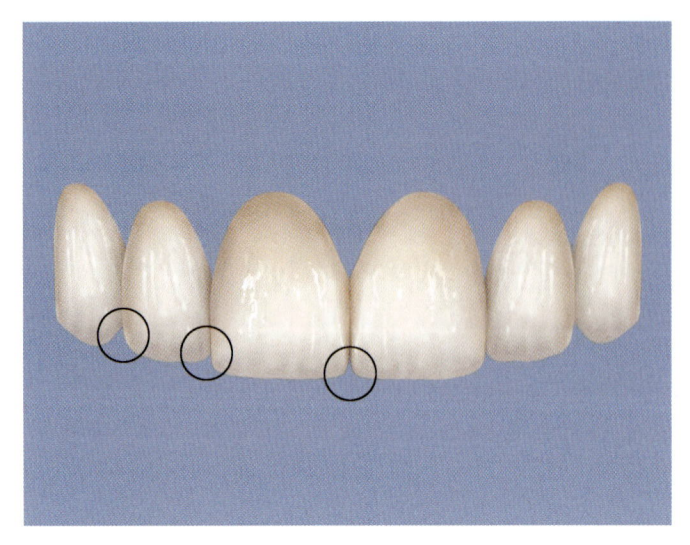

Figure 9.18 The incisal embrasures should become larger as you move distally.

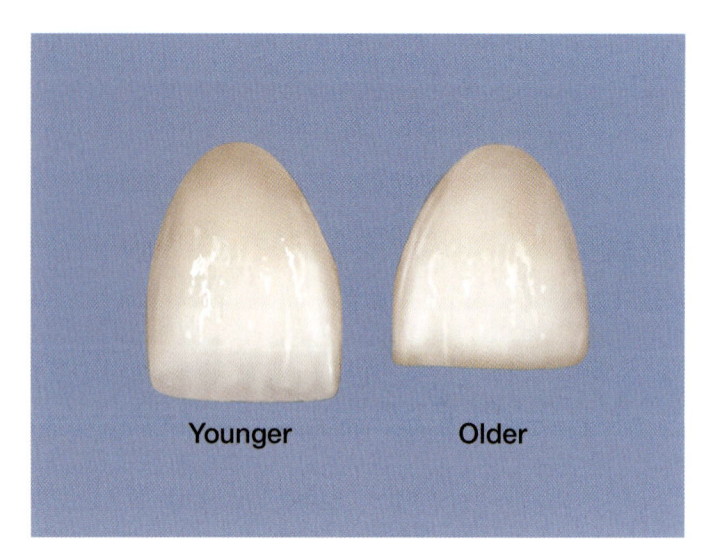

Figure 9.20 Central incisor SPA factor reflects age.

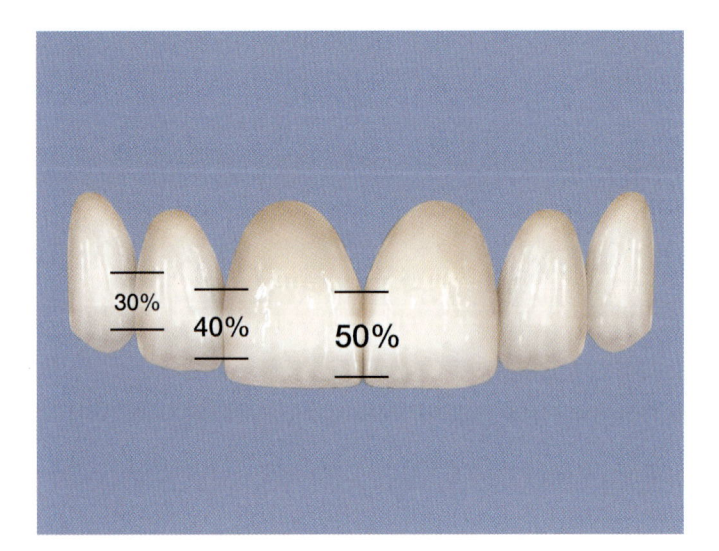

Figure 9.19 Connector area should be 50% between the central incisors, 40% between the central and lateral incisor, and 30% between lateral incisor and canines.

Size and shape of individual teeth

The individual teeth have certain characteristics associated with their form. The shapes of the maxillary anterior teeth have been associated with the "SPA" (sex, personality, age) factor.[6] The incisal edge wear of the maxillary central incisor may coincide with the age of the patient since it may shorten and flatten as a patient ages (Figure 9.20).[21] There is a gradual reduction of maxillary central incisor exposure with an increase in age accompanied by a gradual increase in mandibular tooth exposure.[22] To impart a younger appearance to a smile, distinct angular embrasures may be created along with incisal indentations coinciding with the developmental lobes. The outline form of the central incisor has been recommended to be the inverted facial form of the patient.[23] A person with a square jaw would exhibit a square central incisor and a person with a tapered jaw would have a tapered central incisor (Figure 9.21). The shape of the maxillary lateral incisor may be associated with the sex of a patient.[24] A female lateral incisor exhibits more rounded line angles and curved facial surfaces. The length of the lateral incisor may be less in the feminine form (Figure 9.22). The masculine lateral incisor has sharper line angles, is more similar in length to the central incisor, and has a flatter facial profile. The maxillary canine may coincide with the personality of the patient.[25] A more aggressive personality is projected by a prominent and pointed canine whereas a more passive feel is imparted by a rounded cusp tip (Figure 9.23). The SPA factors should be considered as a guide when designing a smile to satisfy the desired persona projected by the patient.

Apical tooth forms

The shapes and angles of the apical portions of the tooth may be a factor in the esthetic appearance of a smile. In situations where the lip is lifted above the clinical crowns of the teeth upon smiling, the form of the free marginal gingival becomes visibly important. The free gingival margin outlines of the respective contralateral maxillary central incisors and canines should be mirror images of each other and symmetrical. Slight variations of the maxillary lateral incisors are permissible and often desired to give variation. The free gingival margins of the lateral incisors should be located slightly coronal to lines connecting the free gingival margins of the central incisors and canines.[26] A more feminine appearance is portrayed when the free marginal gingivas of the lateral incisors are positioned 0.5–1.0 mm coronal to this line. A more masculine appearance is present when it is more in line (Figure 9.24). The apical zeniths of the maxillary central incisors should be located approximately 1 mm distal and the lateral incisors 0.4 mm distal to the midline of the long axis of the teeth. The apical zeniths of the canine teeth should be nearly in line with the long axis of the tooth (Figure 9.25).[27] The apical angulations of the long axes of the maxillary anterior teeth should become more inclined toward the distal as you move distally (Figure 9.26).

Chapter 9 Proportional Smile Design

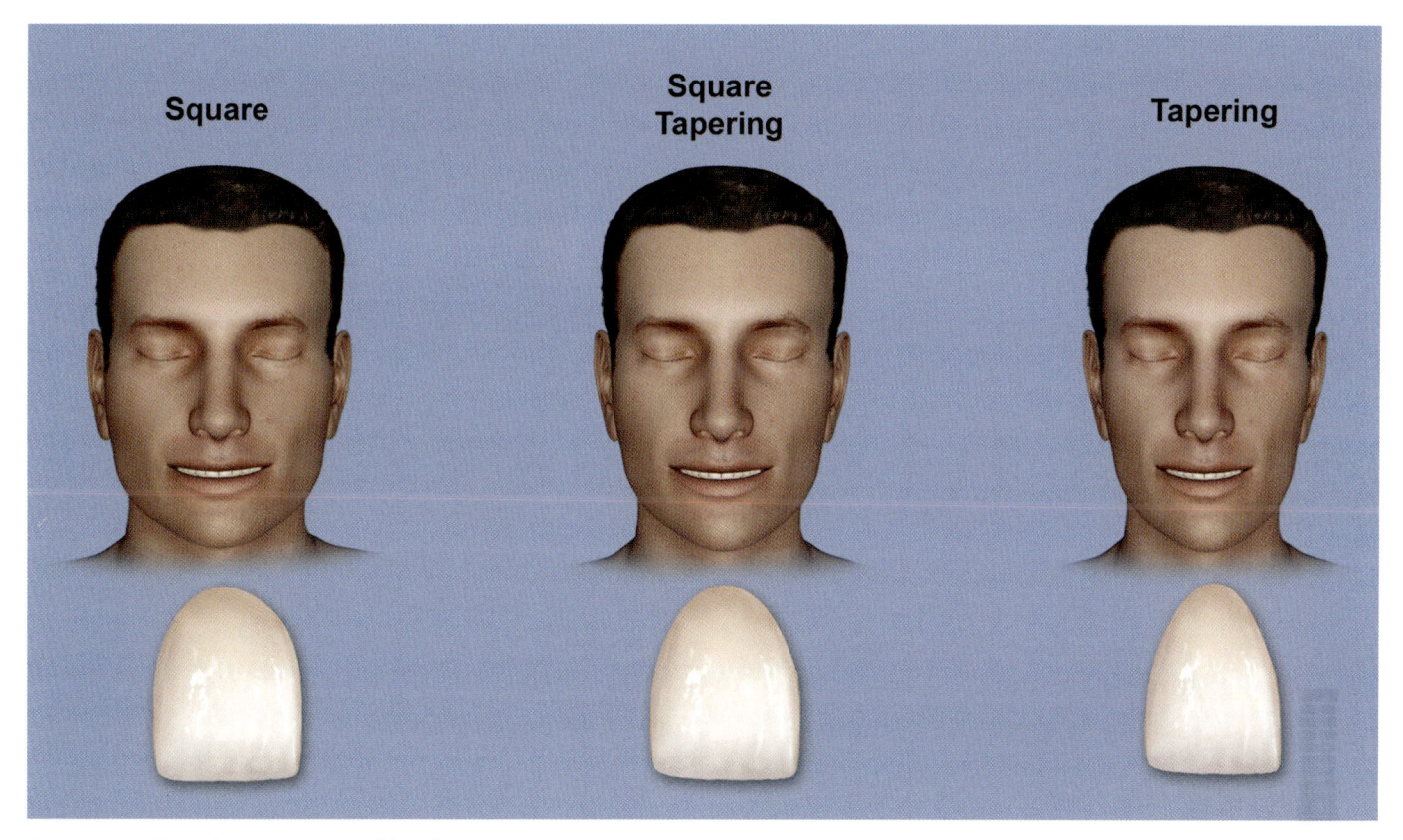

Figure 9.21 Central incisor is inverted face form.

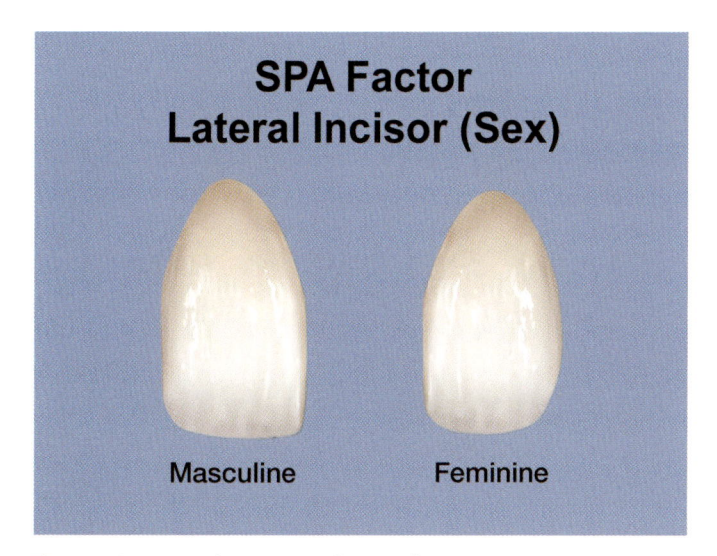

Figure 9.22 Lateral incisor SPA factor reflects sex.

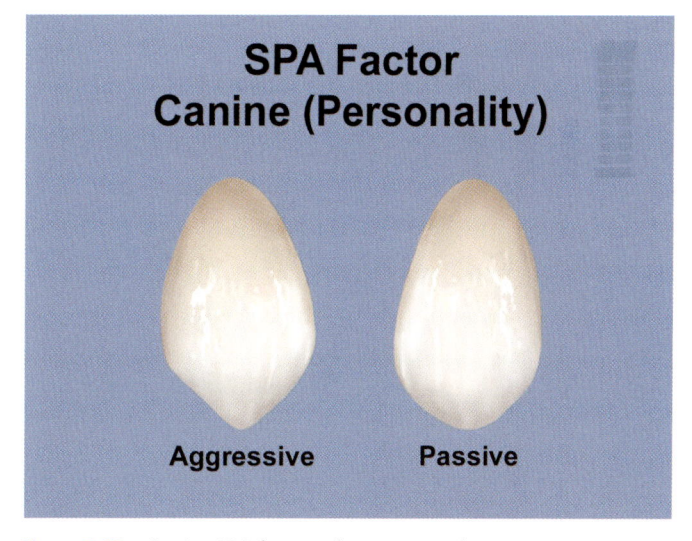

Figure 9.23 Canine SPA factor reflects personality.

Proportion of tooth size to face size

One of the earliest references correlating the proportion of tooth size to face size states the ideal length of the central incisor should be 1/16 the length from trichion to menton (Figure 9.27).[28] Similarly, the ideal width of the central incisor should be 1/16 the interzygomatic width (Figure 9.28). A manufacturer of denture teeth combined the concepts of the rule of thirds with the 1/16 proportion to produce a clear plastic guide which can be placed over the face to determine the appropriate dimensions of the central incisor relative to the size of the face. Position the guide over the face by lining up the nose and eyes in the slots. The recommended length and width can be read by recording the corresponding numbers aligned with the lowest aspect of the chin and the widest part of the zygoma on the guide (Figure 9.29). House and Loop[28] also reported that the interzygomatic width divided by 3.3 gave the approximate width of the maxillary anterior six teeth as viewed from the frontal (Figure 9.30). Others have recommended that the width of the maxillary anterior six teeth (the intercanine width, ICW) as viewed from the frontal

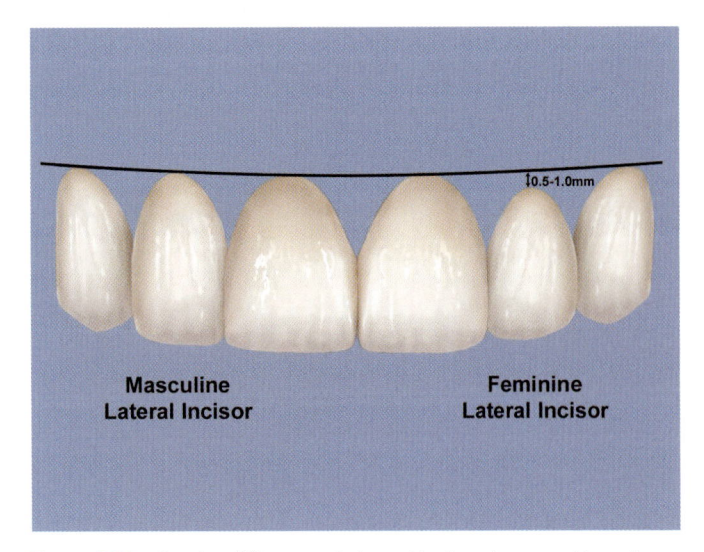

Figure 9.24 Gender differences in lateral incisor shape and length.

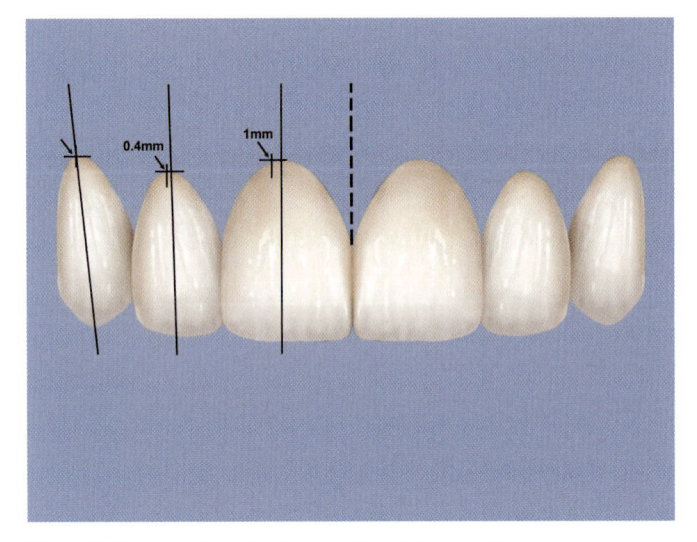

Figure 9.25 Location of apical zeniths of the maxillary anterior teeth.

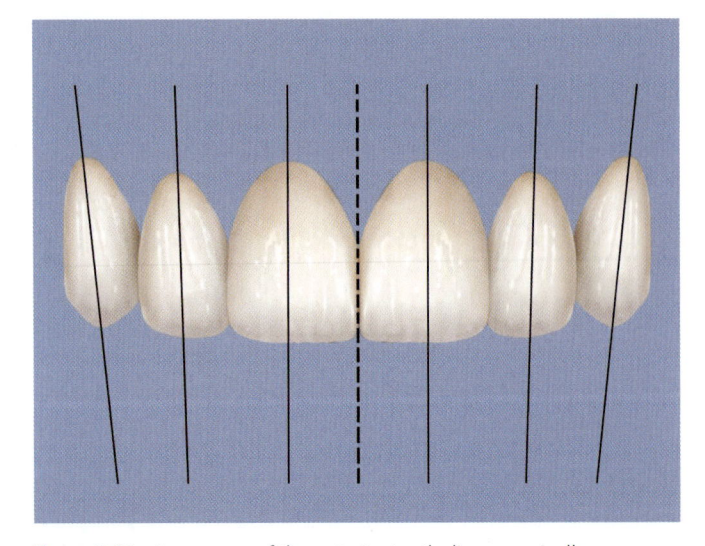

Figure 9.26 Long axes of the anterior teeth diverge apically as you move distally.

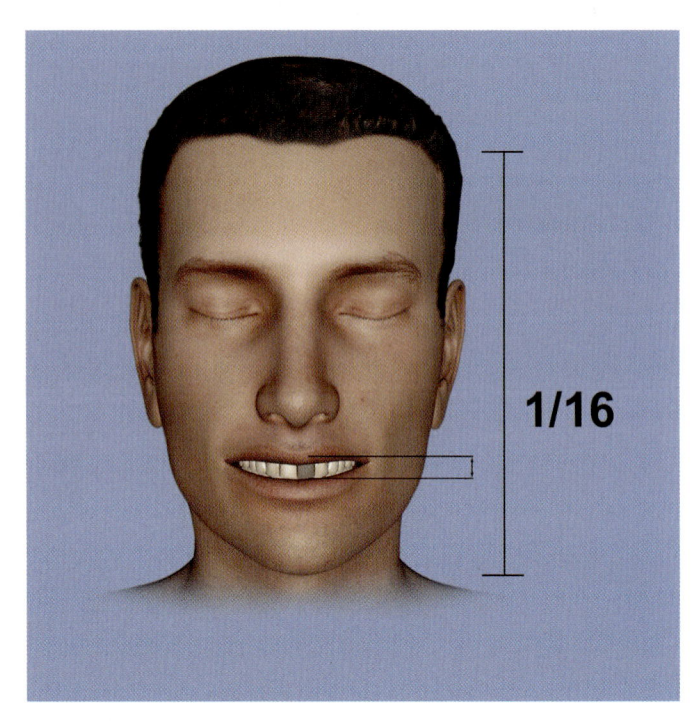

Figure 9.27 The vertical 1/16 rule.

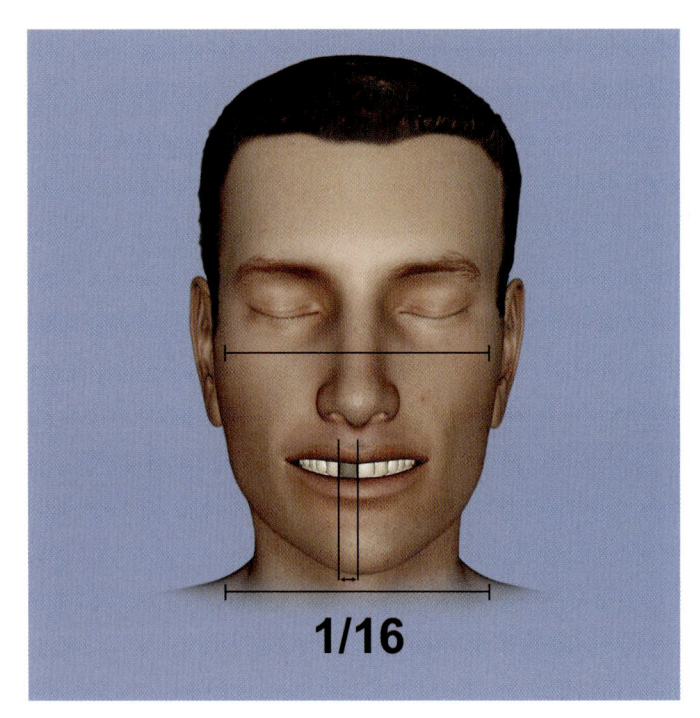

Figure 9.28 The horizontal 1/16 rule.

should be in golden proportion to the intercommisural width when smiling[29] (Figure 9.31).

Recent studies have reported that the average width of each maxillary anterior tooth as measured parallel to the facial surface of each tooth to be 8.5 mm for the central incisor, 6.5 mm for the lateral incisor, and 7.5 mm for the canine (Figure 9.32).[30] It is interesting to note that in this study 80–84% of all teeth measured ranged within ±0.5 mm of the average size. A majority of males exhibited tooth measurements between the average

Chapter 9 Proportional Smile Design

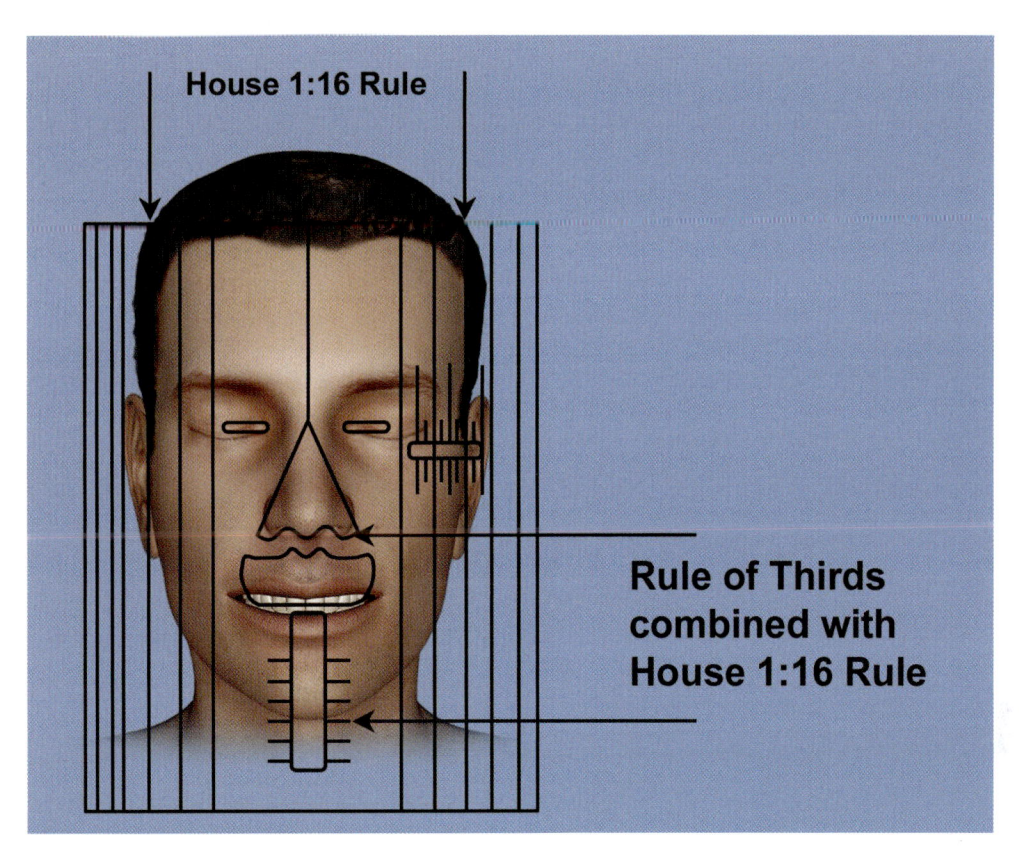

Figure 9.29 The Dentsply tooth size facial guide.

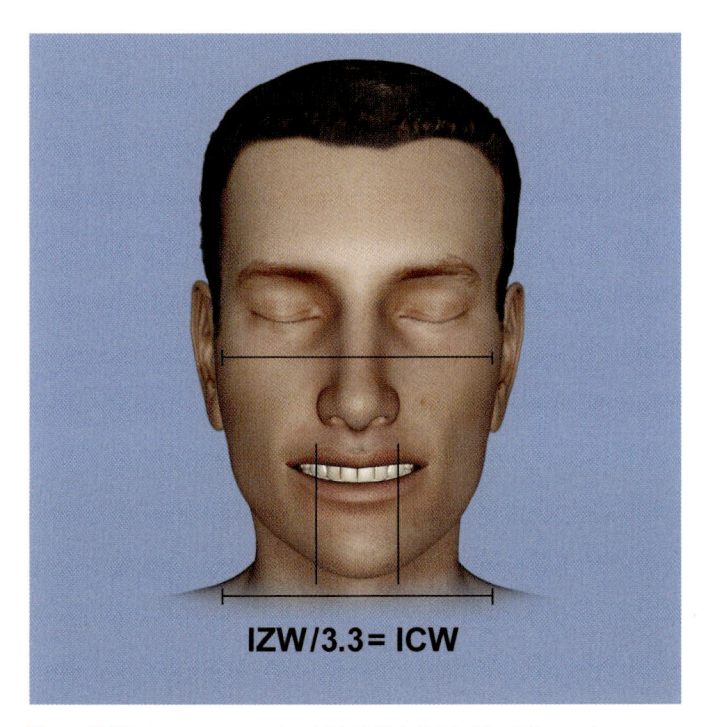

Figure 9.30 Interzygomatic width (IZW) divided by 3.3 equals intercanine width (ICW).

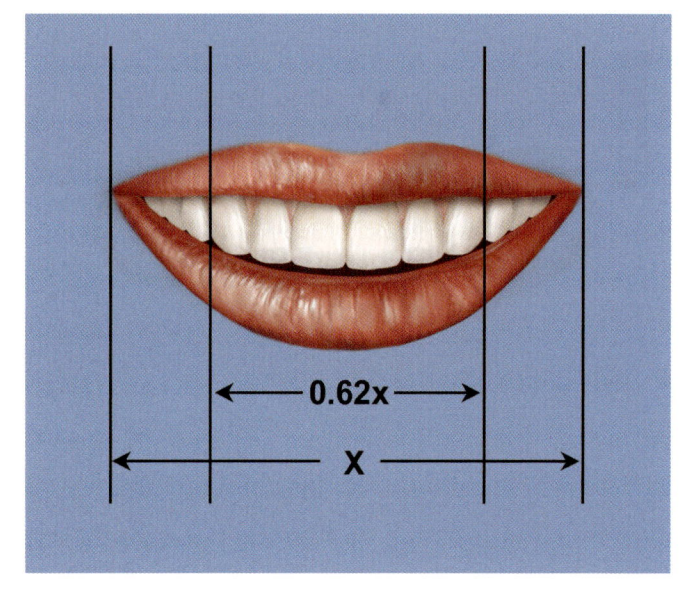

Figure 9.31 Intercanine width in golden proportion to intercommissural width.

width and 0.5 mm wider while a majority of females exhibited tooth measurements between the average width and 0.5 mm narrower (Figure 9.33). However; only 35% of patients showed all three average tooth widths concurrently.

Digital dental photography

The use of dental photography is essential for the evaluation of a smile. Facial images allow for the diagnostic analysis of the smile and are invaluable in treatment planning. Photos give the dentist and adjunct personnel an unlimited time to evaluate the smile. Photos allow the patient to more readily view their own smiles

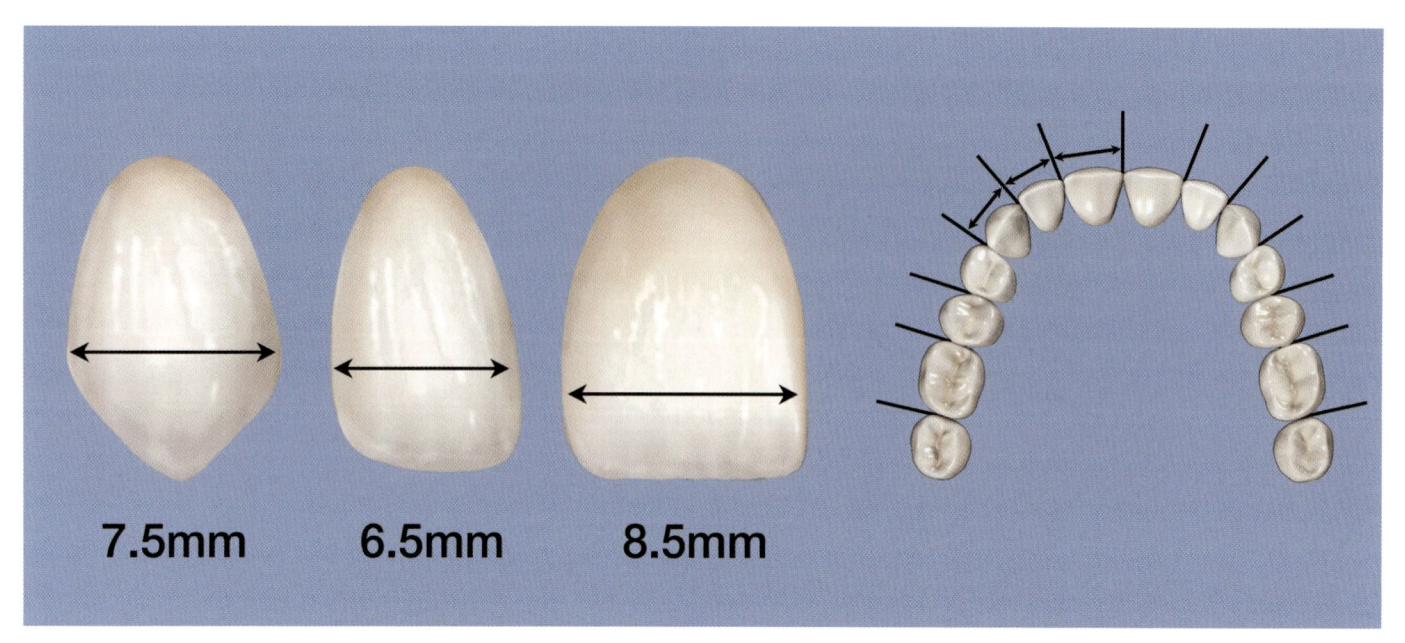

Figure 9.32 Average cast view widths of maxillary anterior teeth.

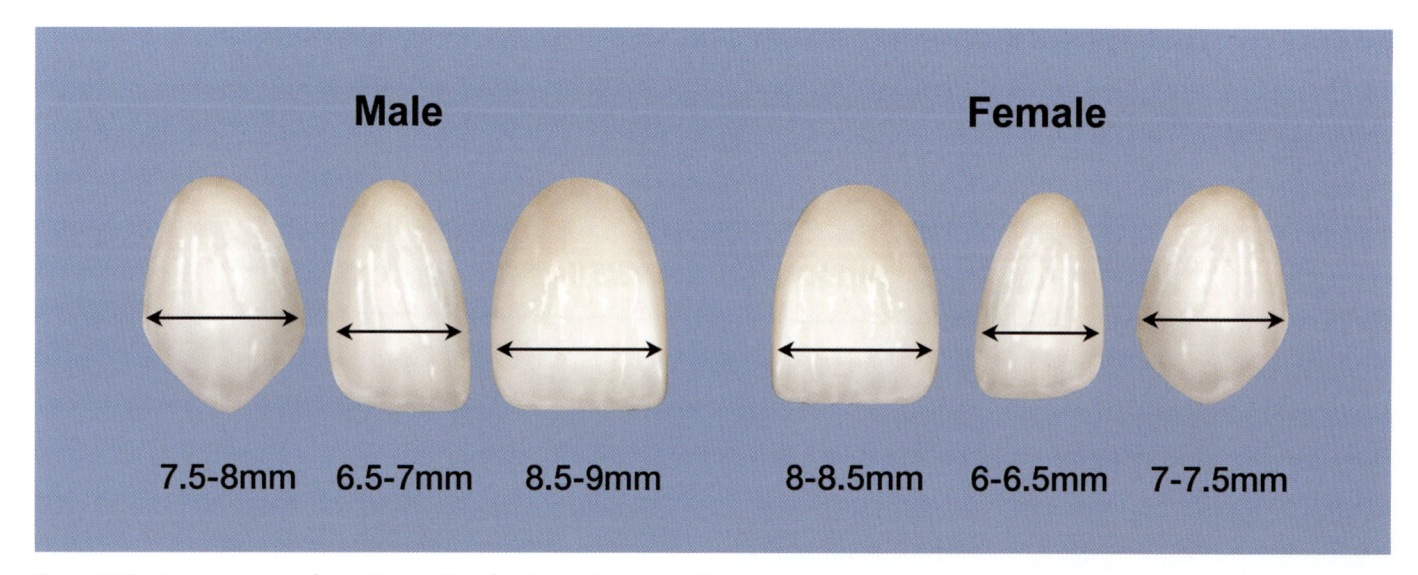

Figure 9.33 Average range of cast view widths of male and female maxillary anterior teeth.

and afford effective communication regarding treatment rationale and potential desired outcomes. Photos are useful when communicating with specialists and the dental laboratory and are easily emailed. Outward personality, appearance, and the role of the smile in the face, can be better understood by the ceramist. Archived pretreatment photos are important should questions arise after treatment begins or is completed.

Digital photography offers many advantages to print or slide film formats. Images can be instantly previewed to evaluate the exposure (Figure 9.34). Alignment and focusing can be viewed. Multiple views can be exposed since there is no additional expense incurred for external processing. A single-lens reflex (SLR) camera is recommended for better exposure control, precise focusing, and standardized image magnifications (see also Chapter 7). The SLR should be fitted with a telephoto/macro lens to allow the production of distortion-free images for accurate 2D

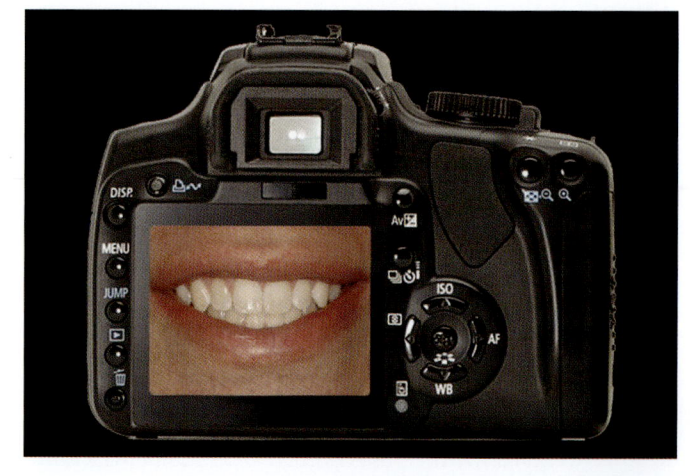

Figure 9.34 Digital single-lens reflex (SLR) instant image preview.

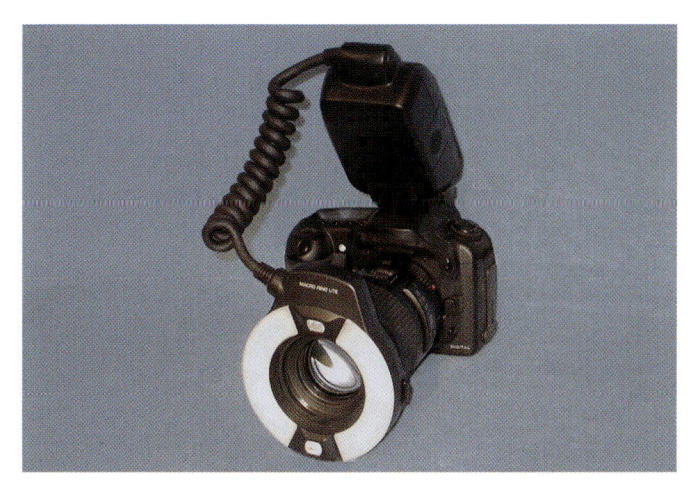

Figure 9.35 Digital SLR camera setup for dental photography.

proportional measurements (Figure 9.35). Standardized views at a consistent magnification produce useful before and after pictures and insure all cases can be analyzed in the same manner. The lens should be set on manual focus and the desired magnification selected. The photographer moves closer to or further away from the subject until the image is in focus. This results in all pictures of each magnification and view being exposed from the same distance away. The photographer should carefully preview the image in the viewfinder to properly center the view parallel to the incisal plane and properly align the angles and borders before taking the picture. Using a protocol of standardized views is important for review and documentation of all esthetic treatment (Figure 9.36).

Facial image view evaluation (FIVE)

The reference for any smile assessment is the view by an observer directly in front of the patient. This view gives a 2D representation of a 3D smile. The use of properly exposed photographic views to evaluate a smile is termed facial image view evaluation (FIVE). Aligned photographic views exposed parallel to the facial plane are essential to allow proper analysis of the smile and accurate relative tooth dimensions. It is important to understand the relative measurements of teeth when using FIVE may be significantly different than the sizes of teeth measured from varying angles (Figure 9.37). The teeth located further distal from the midline will be significantly smaller with FIVE than when measured parallel to each tooth's facial or buccal surface. Changes in tooth positions will change the FIVE. A maxillary canine extruded out buccally will have a larger FIVE width than one intruded palatally.

To use the FIVE method, a correlation must be established between the size of the teeth in the photo and the size of the teeth in the mouth. A common measurement should be made of a readily viewable dimension of a central incisor. Typically the length of the maxillary central incisor is used if the entire tooth can be viewed when the patient smiles. Otherwise the width can be used. The measurement in the mouth is divided by the size of the same measurement in the photograph, giving a fraction.

The photograph is measured and the dimensions multiplied by this fraction to yield the FIVE widths and lengths. This produces the perceived sizes of the individual teeth in the smile by a viewer located directly in front of the patient (Figure 9.38).

Studies of Asian patients report the frontal view width of the maxillary anterior six teeth (intercanine width or ICW) is typically 5–6 mm less than the individual widths of the anterior teeth if the teeth were extracted and laid on a flat surface similar to the manner in which denture teeth are measured (Figure 9.39).[31] These same studies report the mesial/distal 2D angulations of the maxillary anterior teeth from parallel to the facial plane are 8° for the average maxillary central incisor, 26° for the average lateral incisor, and 56° for the average canine.

Proportional dental/facial analysis

Proportional and angular analysis is often employed by the dental specialties. Facial esthetic treatment planning must be directed toward balanced proportions and a harmonious arrangement of facial parts.[32] The measurement of frontonasal, nasal tip, nasolabial, interlabial, labiomental, and lip-chin-throat angles may be useful in evaluating the face as a whole.[33] Orthodontists routinely employ cephalometric analysis of facial bony components to predict clinical success (Figure 9.40).[34] Periodontists may measure papilla proportions to evaluate esthetic norms.[35] The measurement of proportions is equally important to the restorative dentist during treatment planning.

Width/length ratio of maxillary central incisor

One of the most important proportions for the esthetic success of a smile is the width/length ratio of the maxillary central incisor.[36] Studies have reported a wide range of naturally occurring width/length ratios. According to one often quoted study, the average width/length ratio of the North American central incisor is reported to be 85–86%.[37]

Another North American study cites the average as 90%.[38] A North American study of extracted teeth reveals that worn central incisors had an average width/length ratio of 87% but that unworn incisors had an average width/length ratio of 78%.[39] Several European studies reported an average width/length ratio of 81–84% for the central incisor.[40,41] However, several studies have recommended the use of maxillary central incisor width/length ratios in the range of 75–80%, which are smaller than those observed in nature (Figure 9.41).[42,43] Studies have revealed the width/length ratio to be a major determinant in smiles preferred by dentists with different tooth-to-tooth width ratios. In these studies, the majority of dentists chose the smiles with central incisors that were as close to the 75–78% width/length ratio as possible.[44] A useful plastic guide has been created which allows for easy reproduction of the 78% width/length ratio when held up in front of a maxillary central incisor in the mouth (Figure 9.42). The similarly colored vertical and horizontal lines are consistent with a 78% width/length ratio.

Photographic Protocol

Full Face View 1:10

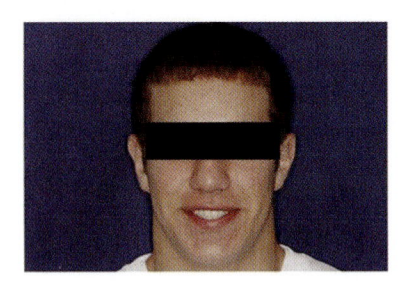

Frontal Retracted View 1:2

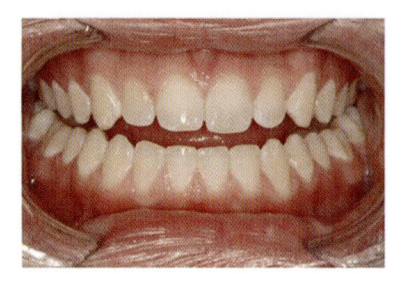

Maxillary Anterior Lateral View 1:1

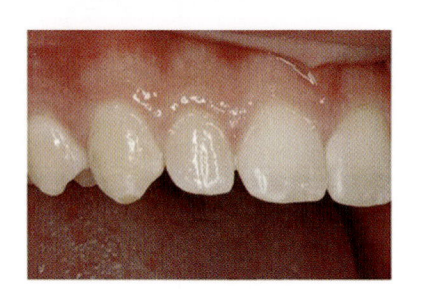

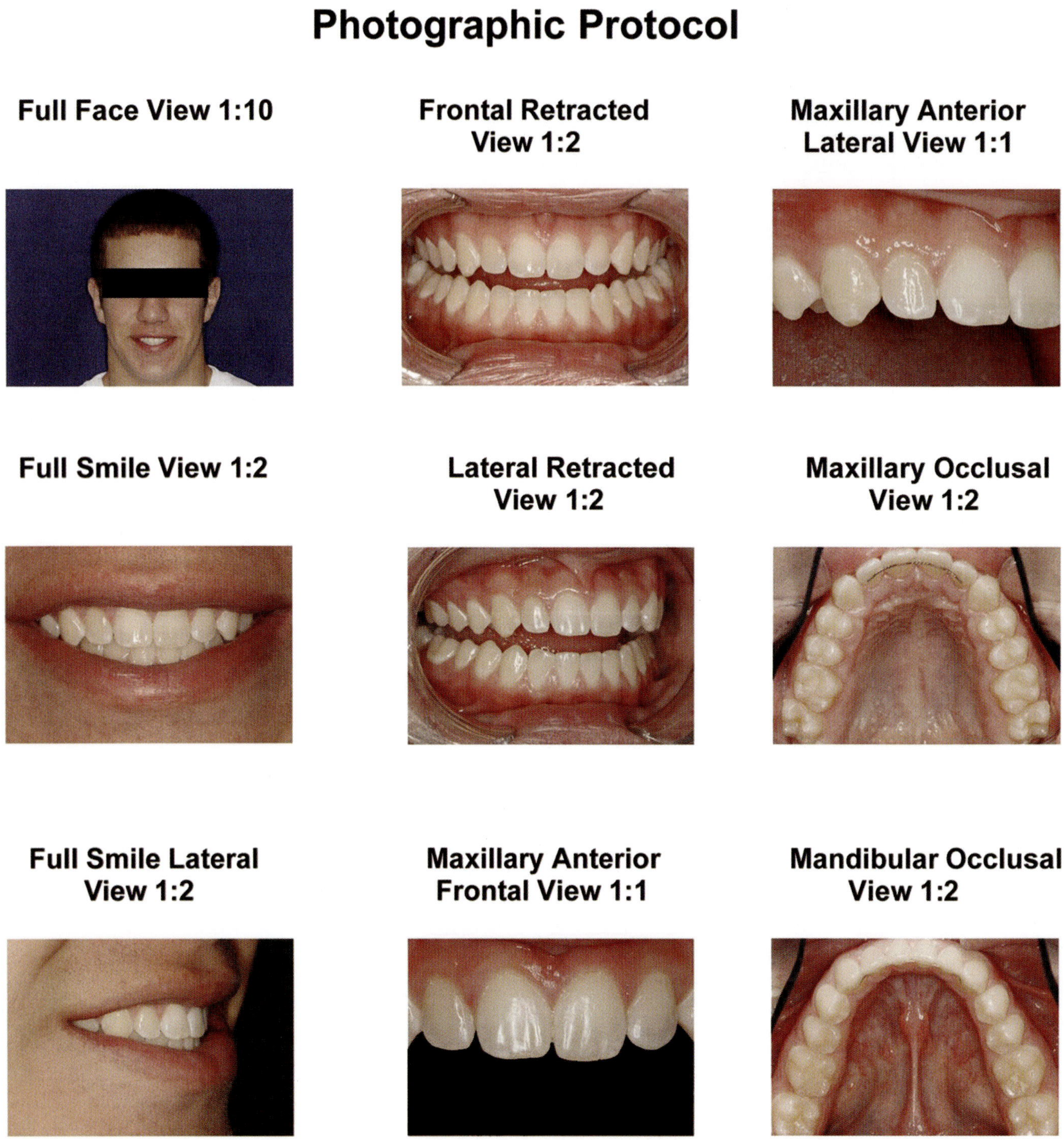

Full Smile View 1:2

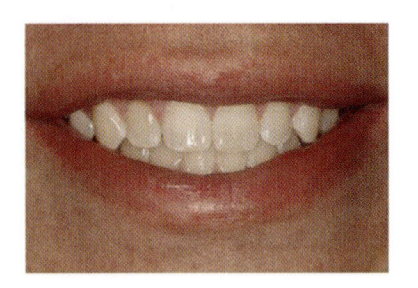

Lateral Retracted View 1:2

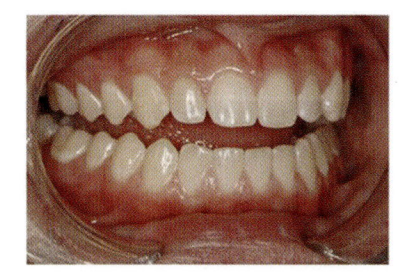

Maxillary Occlusal View 1:2

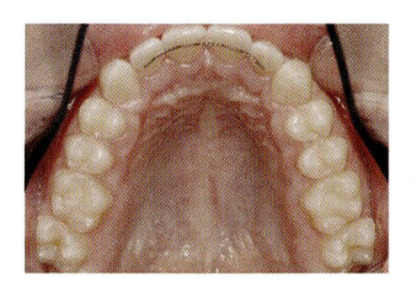

Full Smile Lateral View 1:2

Maxillary Anterior Frontal View 1:1

Mandibular Occlusal View 1:2

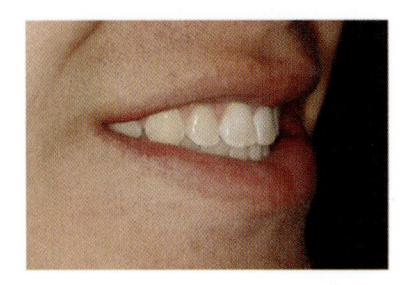

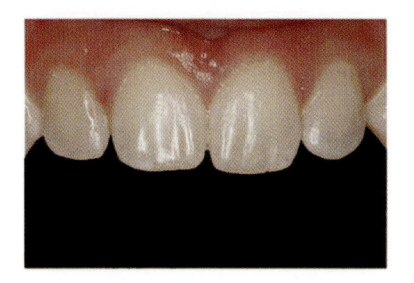

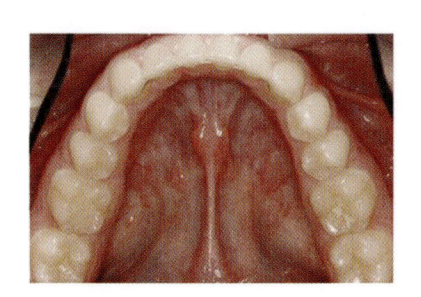

Figure 9.36 Standardized dental photographic series.

Tooth-to-tooth width proportion theories

One of the earliest to discuss the tooth-to-tooth width proportions of the maxillary anterior teeth was Lombardi.[45] He spoke of the need for a "repeated ratio" in which the facial view width proportion which existed between the maxillary lateral incisor and central incisor was repeated between the teeth progressing distally. He felt it gave the teeth unity and order. Beaudreau[46] proposed a "proportionate ratio" in which the actual width of each tooth was measured separately, parallel to the facial surface of each tooth. He suggested a ratio in which an 8 mm-wide maxillary central incisor should have a 6 mm-wide lateral incisor and 7 mm-wide canine. This would result in the cast view width of the lateral incisor being 75% the width of the maxillary central incisor and the canine being 87.5% the cast view width of the lateral incisor.[46] Levin used the concept of the repeated ratio but preset the ideal repeated ratio as the golden proportion or 62% (Figure 9.43).[47] Using the golden proportion, the facial view

Chapter 9 Proportional Smile Design

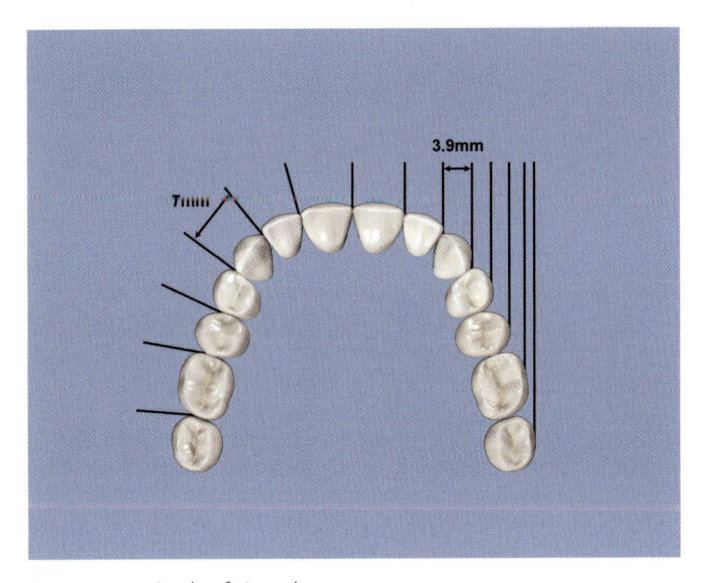

Figure 9.37 Angle of view changes measurements.

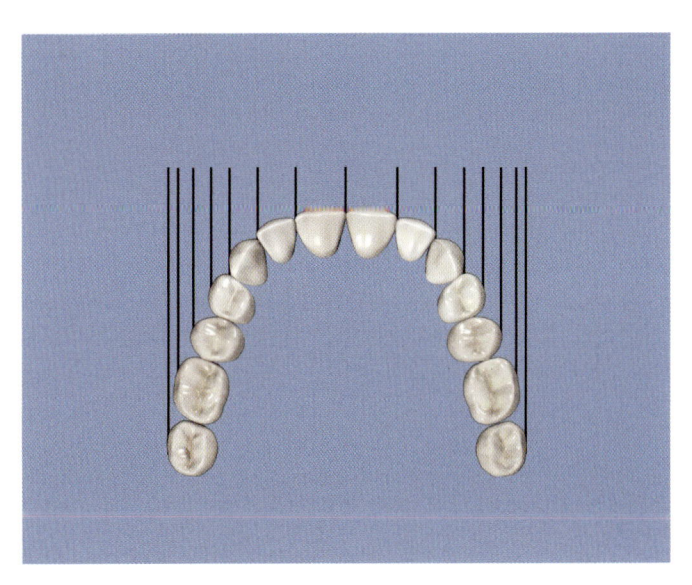

Figure 9.38 FIVE widths of maxillary teeth.

Cast View Widths

ICW + 5-6mm

(2-dimensional measurement)

"FIVE" View Widths

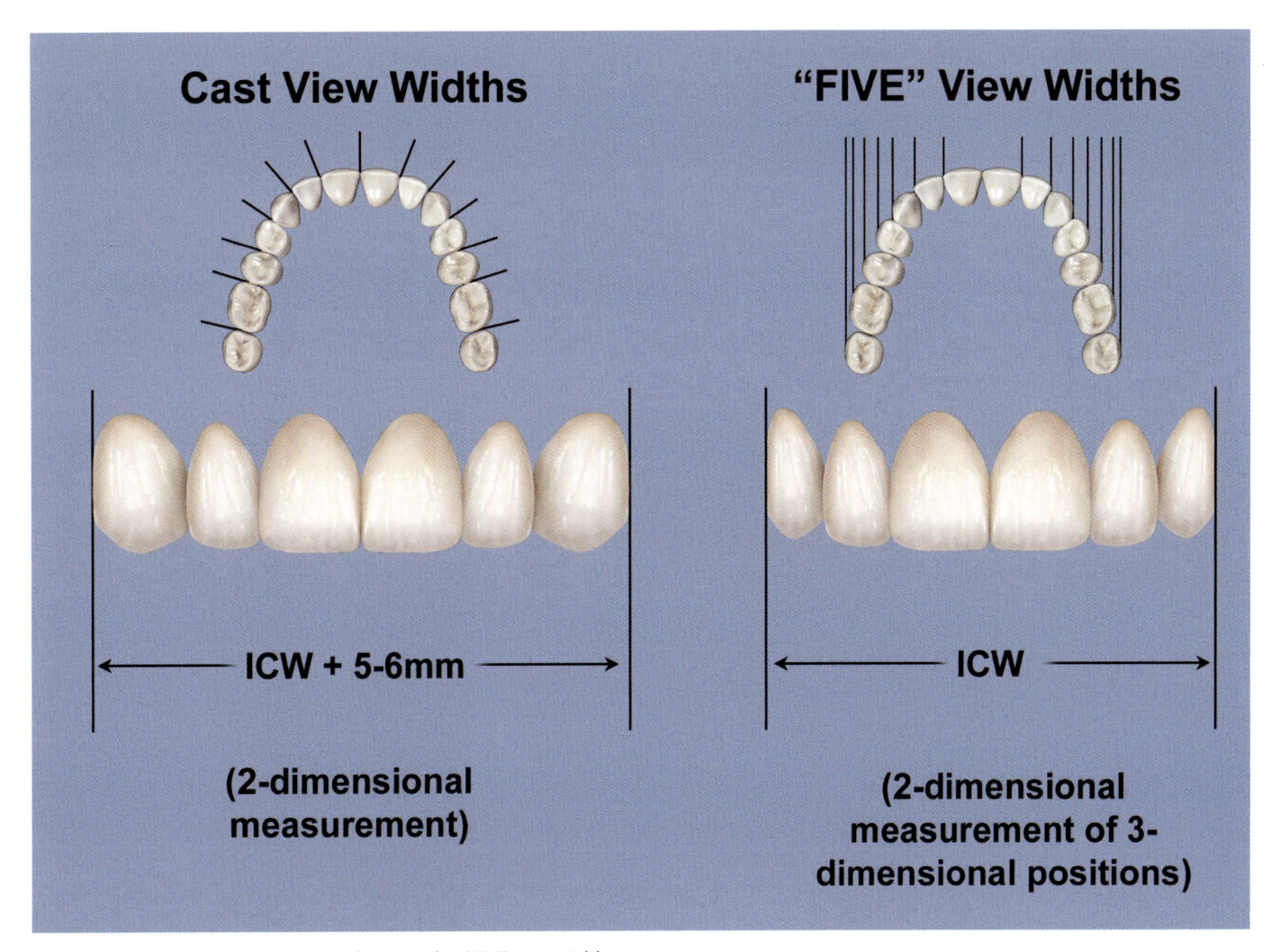

ICW

(2-dimensional measurement of 3-dimensional positions)

Figure 9.39 Cast view widths versus photographic (FIVE) view widths.

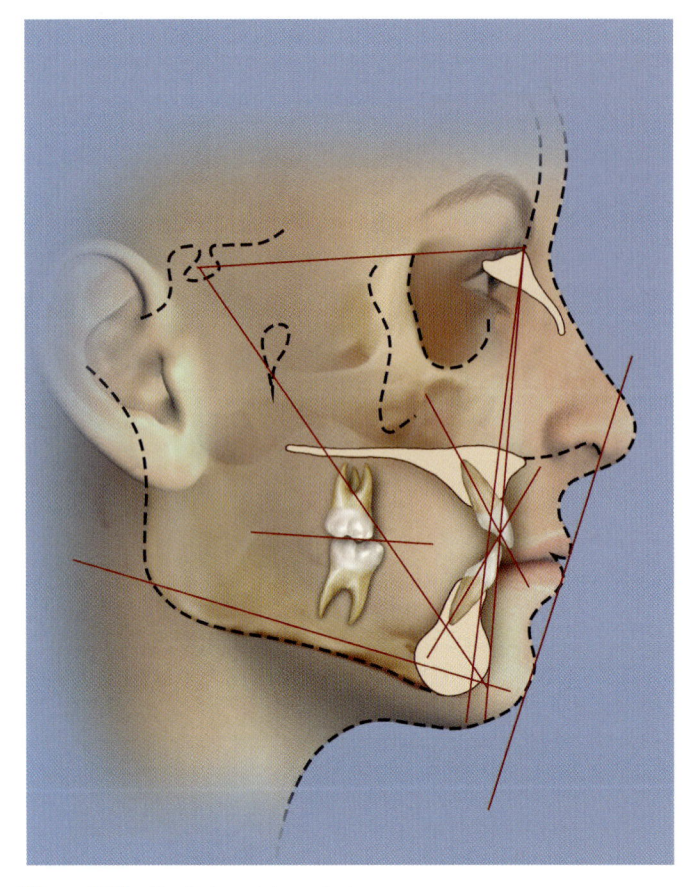

Figure 9.40 Cephalometric analysis.

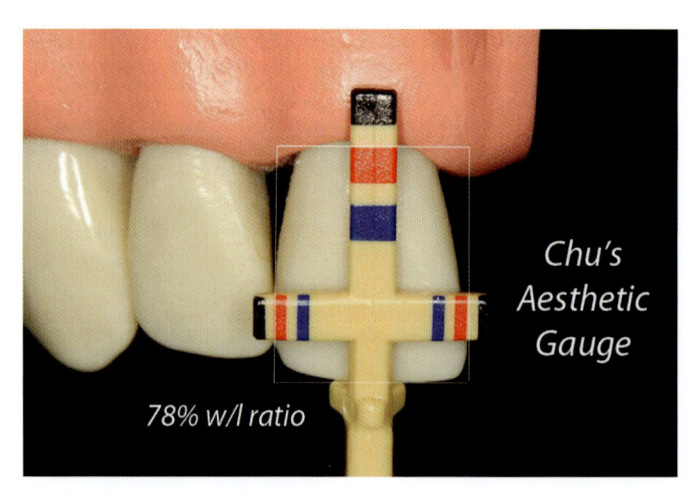

Figure 9.42 Chu aesthetic gauge.

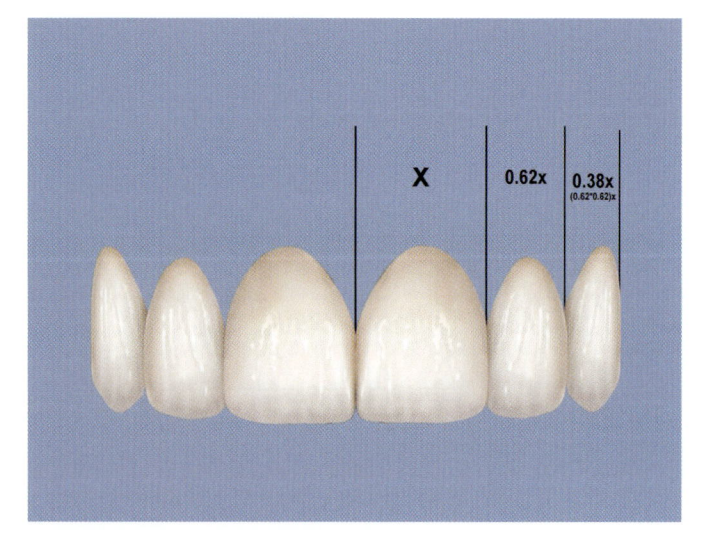

Figure 9.43 Golden proportion.

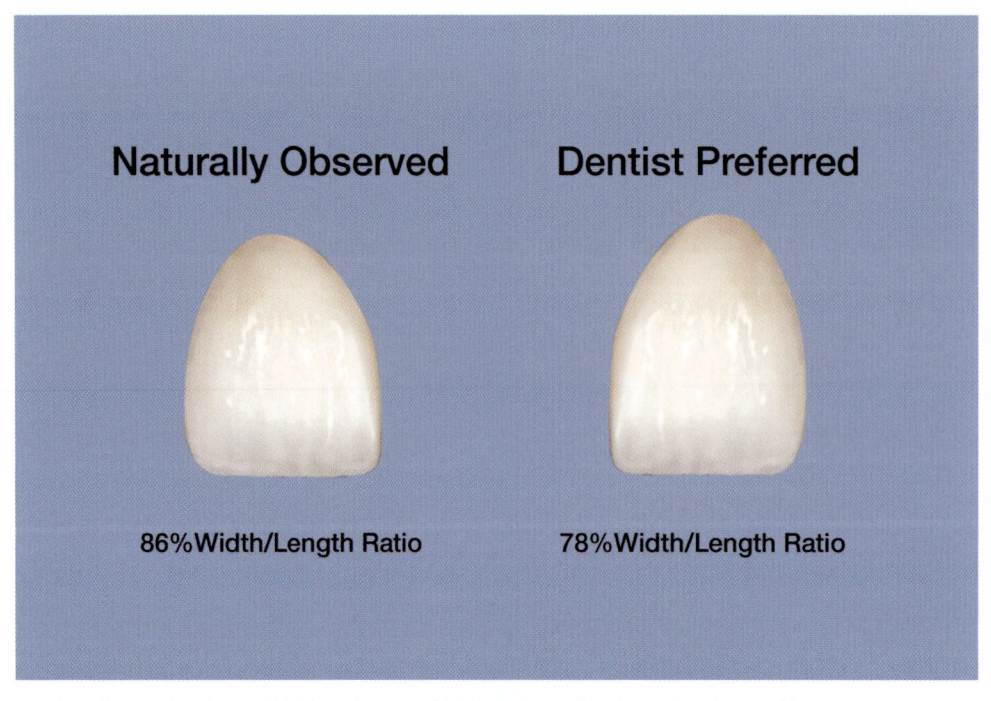

Figure 9.41 Dentist-preferred central incisor width/length ratio of 75–80% is smaller than that observed in nature.

FIVE width of the maxillary lateral incisor is 62% the FIVE width of the central incisor, and the FIVE width of the canine is 62% the width of the maxillary lateral incisor. Snow defined a "golden mean" in which each of the central incisors occupied 25% of the facial view width of the maxillary anterior six teeth (ICW), the laterals each 15% of ICW, and the canines 10% of ICW (Figure 9.44).[48] Albers discussed a number of fixed tooth-to-tooth width proportions including the 57% Plato beauty proportion, the 75% quarter 3:4 proportion, and the 80% human norm 5:6 proportion.[49]

Studies have evaluated tooth proportions observed in nature. Preston observed in a North American dental student population that the average maxillary lateral incisor was 66% the frontal view (FIVE) width of the central incisor and the average maxillary canine was 84% the FIVE width of the lateral incisor (Figure 9.45).[50] Gillen reported that the golden proportion (62%) was rarely observed in the casts evaluated.[38] Other studies have observed similar results, although the findings vary according to the ethnic population evaluated.[40,51]

Studies have attempted to correlate different factors to the size of the teeth.[52,53] In spite of many proposals for determining the ideal size of the teeth, they are not consistently found to exist in patients. The golden proportion was not routinely found in patients determined as possessing an esthetically pleasing smile.[54] Selecting one static tooth-to-tooth width proportion may not be suitable for universal use.

Recurring esthetic dental (RED) proportion

Fixed tooth-to-tooth width proportions or tooth sizes do not take into consideration the relationship between the teeth, the bony support, and the face. Considerations for the length of the teeth, the gingival architecture, and the facial view width of the anterior teeth should be factors for making decisions about the desired size of the teeth in a smile. The recurring esthetic dental (RED) proportion incorporates the existing or desired length of the maxillary central incisors with the ICW to calculate the sizes of the maxillary teeth. It allows the dentist to select the desired tooth-to-tooth width proportions, rather than accepting the existing width relationships, using the the repeated ratio or being confined to the 62% golden proportion or golden mean. The RED proportion states that the proportion between the successive frontal view widths of the teeth should remain constant as you move distally (Figure 9.46).[55] It allows for the selection of a successive width proportion which remains consistent throughout the designed smile. The proportion between the FIVE widths of the maxillary lateral incisor and the central incisor should be the same as the FIVE width proportion between the maxillary canine and the lateral incisor and continues as you proceed distally. RED proportions are in the range of 62–80% with 70% considered the standard for average or normal length teeth (Figure 9.47). The 70% RED proportion results in a maxillary central incisor identical in width to the central incisor identified by Preston's "naturally occurring" proportion.

Research has shown that dentists prefer using a RED proportion that will yield a width/length ratio of the maxillary central incisor between 75 and 78%.[44] Given a specific ICW, a number of RED proportions may be used dependent upon the relative length of the teeth, the size of the face, and the wishes of the patient. The ICW may be allocated to the anterior six teeth in a number of ways. The percentage of the ICW for each of the maxillary anterior teeth has been calculated according to the RED proportion selected (Figure 9.48). A patient with tall teeth requires wider maxillary central incisors in order to maintain the preferred 75–78% width/length ratio (Figure 9.49). Less space remains for the lateral incisors and canines, necessitating the use of a smaller RED proportion. A smaller RED proportion results in each successive distal tooth being a smaller percentage of the width of the preceding tooth. When using a smaller RED proportion the central incisor is wider or more dominant since the lateral incisor and canine diminish their widths at a greater rate. In fact, when using the 62% RED proportion (i.e. the golden proportion), 50% of the ICW is occupied by the two central incisors. It is understandable why fashion models who are usually tall look best when restored with tall teeth, dominant central incisors, and the golden proportion tooth-to-tooth width proportions.

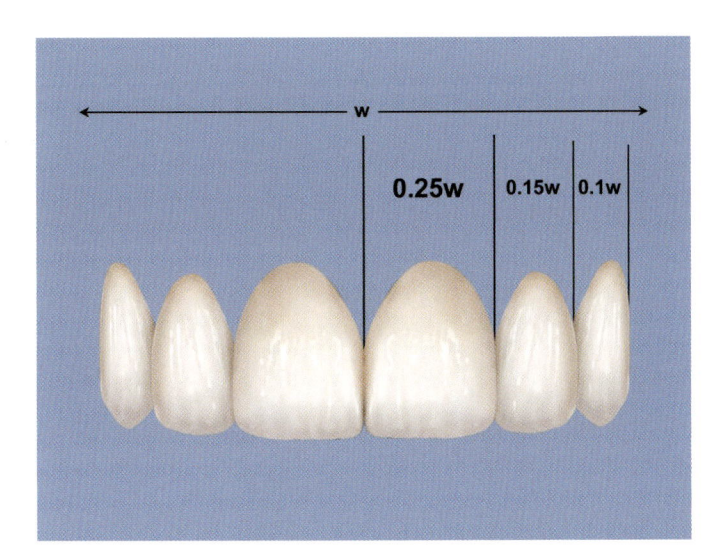

Figure 9.44 Golden mean.

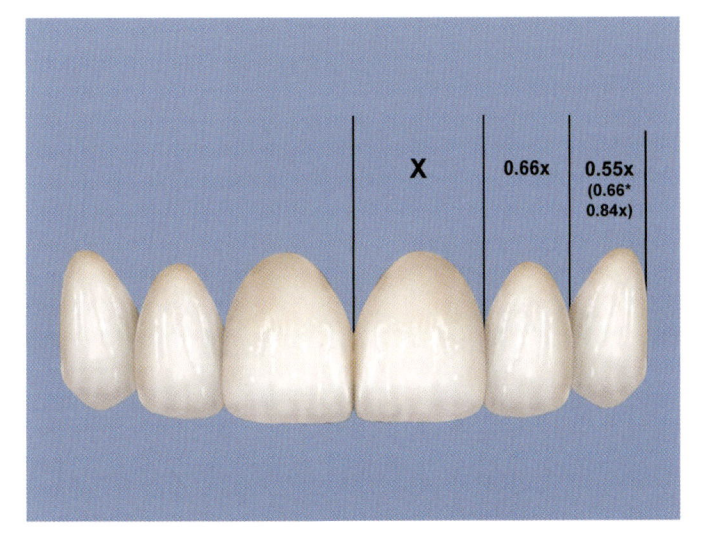

Figure 9.45 Preston proportion (naturally occurring).

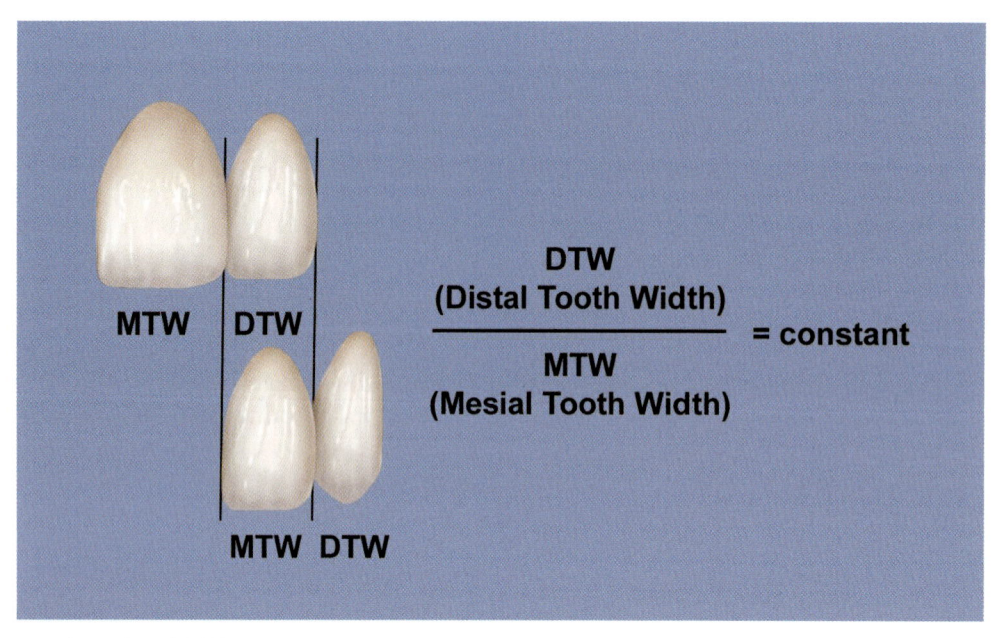

Figure 9.46 Recurring esthetic dental (RED) proportion.

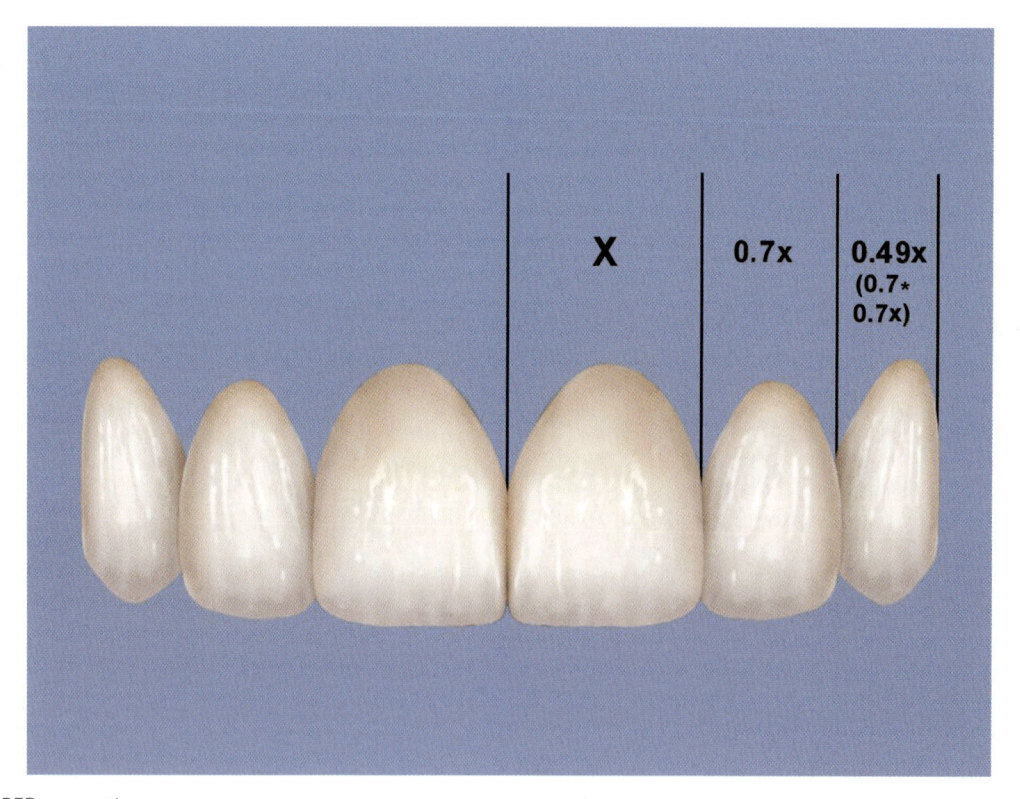

$$\frac{\text{DTW (Distal Tooth Width)}}{\text{MTW (Mesial Tooth Width)}} = \text{constant}$$

Figure 9.47 70% RED proportion.

Dentist proportion preferences

Studies have been conducted to evaluate preferred successive tooth-to-tooth width ratios of teeth by dentists in conjunction with the relative tooth lengths.[44] The golden proportion was clearly not preferred for normal length teeth by dentists surveyed. With normal length teeth dentists preferred the size of the maxillary central incisor recommended by the 70% RED proportion (Figure 9.50). With very short teeth, dentists preferred the 80% RED proportion, which results in successive teeth more similar in width (Figure 9.51). With very tall teeth, the 62% RED proportion (golden proportion) was preferred (Figure 9.52).

In another study, dentists surveyed overwhelmingly preferred the 70% RED proportion and the Preston (naturally occurring) proportion to the golden proportion for normal-length teeth (Figure 9.53).[56] The golden proportion was preferred only in very tall teeth. They preferred the 70% RED proportion to the

Figure 9.48 Individual tooth width percentage of ICW for different RED proportions.

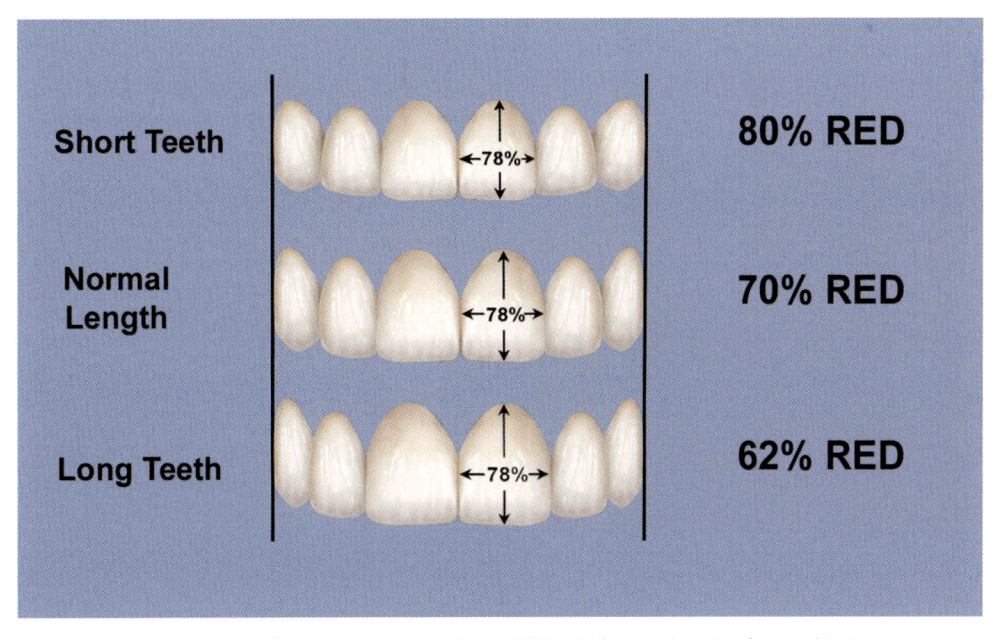

Figure 9.49 RED proportions incorporating tooth lengths which maintain 78% width/length ratio of central incisors.

Preston (naturally occurring) proportion (Figure 9.54). Both the 70% RED proportion and the Preston proportion have the same-size central incisor, the difference being that the lateral incisor is slightly larger and the canine slightly smaller in the 70% RED proportion.

Even though the RED proportion has not been readily observed in nature, dentists surveyed preferred it to natural proportions. Patients desiring a change in their smile likewise may not always find naturally occurring proportions to be the most desirable. In other areas of elective esthetic treatment, the final

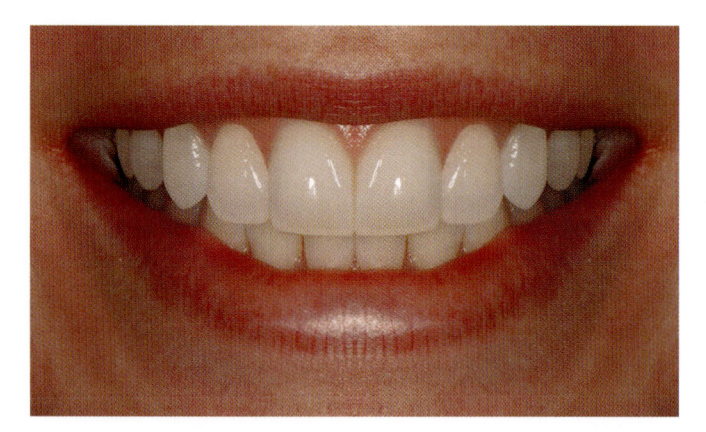

Figure 9.50 Preferred 70% RED proportion for normal-length teeth. Reproduced from reference 56 with permission.

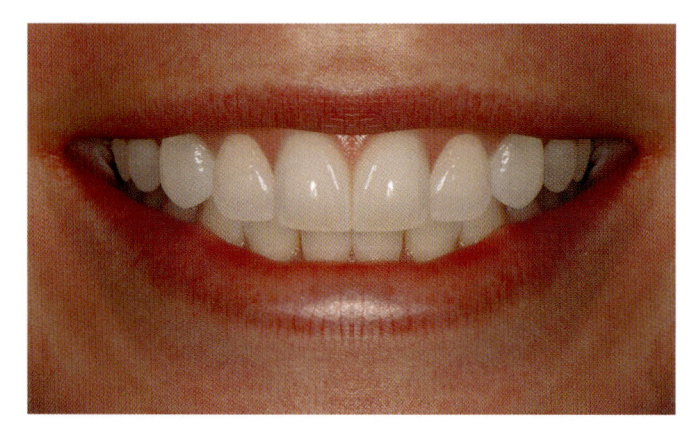

Figure 9.51 Preferred 80% RED proportion for very short teeth. Reproduced from reference 56 with permission.

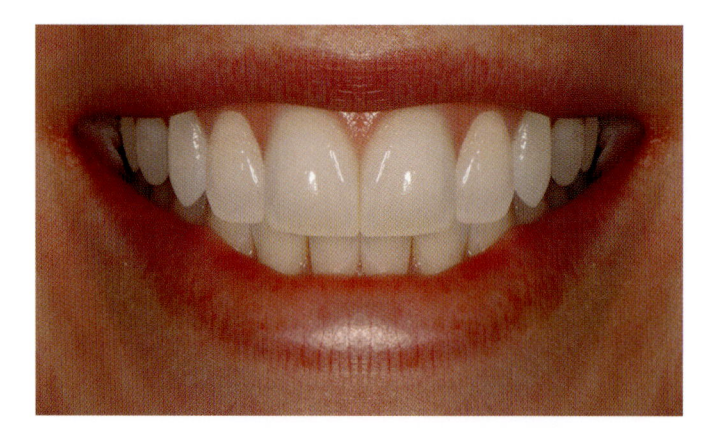

Figure 9.52 Preferred 62% RED proportion for very tall teeth. Reproduced from reference 56 with permission.

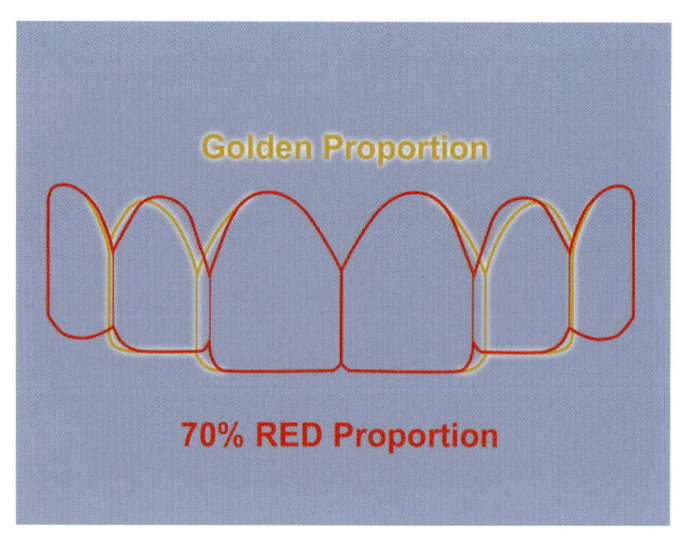

Figure 9.53 Comparing golden proportion to 70% RED proportion (normal-length teeth). Reproduced from reference 56 with permission.

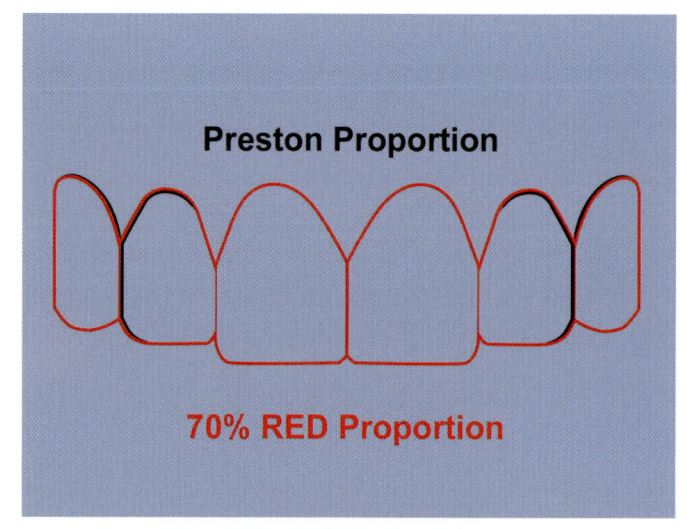

Figure 9.54 Comparing Preston (naturally occuring) to 70% RED proportion. Reproduced from reference 56 with permission.

Using the RED proportion to calculate ideal tooth widths

Understanding the relationships among the overall length of the teeth, the width/length ratio of the central incisor, and the recommended RED proportion allows the dentist to propose different tooth-to-tooth width proportions for different length teeth. For any given maxillary ICW, there are a number of different tooth lengths and tooth-to-tooth width proportions that may be utilized. It is dependent upon the desired length of the teeth (Figure 9.55). Patients who elect to have the clinical crowns of their teeth lengthened should have wider, more dominant central incisors fabricated (Figure 9.56). Longer clinical crowns can be achieved by placing the incisal edges more coronally, by crown lengthening, or a combination of the two (Figure 9.57).

results often do not mimic what is present in nature. Tooth whitening and orthodontic treatment are popular but often result in smiles different than the norms observed in nature. Likewise smile design concepts using proportions preferred by dentists but not readily observed in a patient population may be successfully employed.

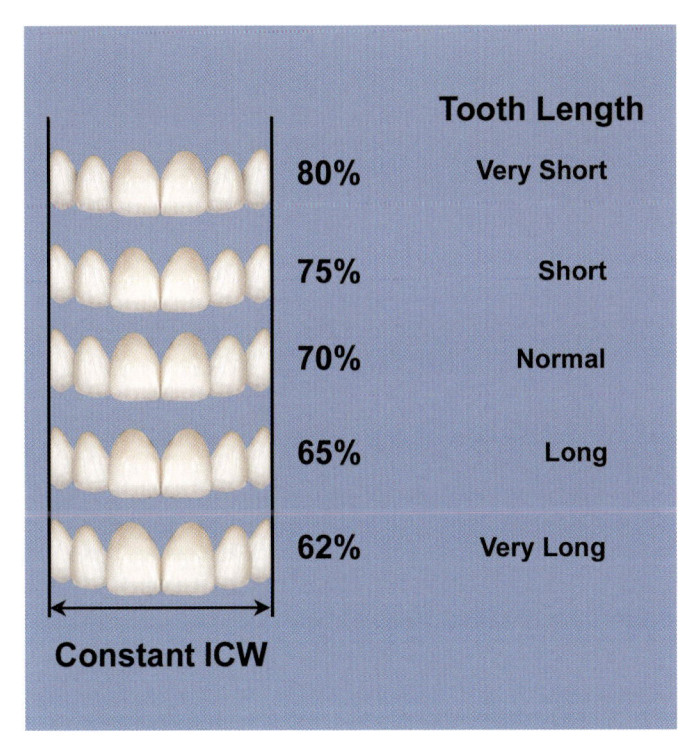

Figure 9.55 Different RED proportions (central incisor 78% width/length ratio) for the same ICW.

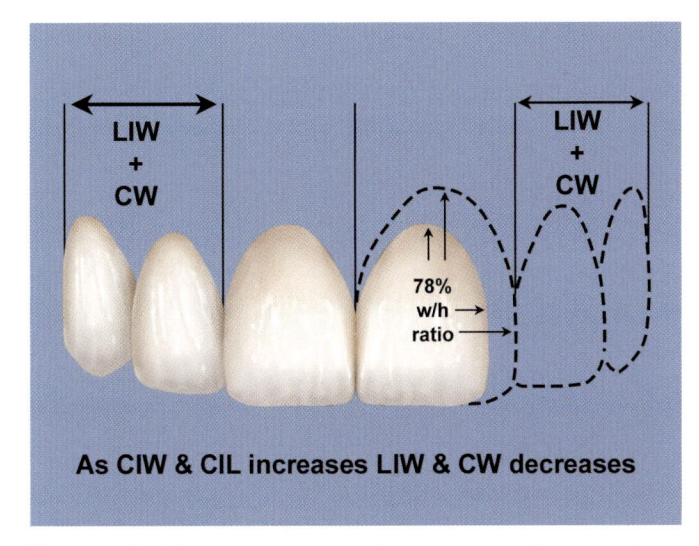

Figure 9.56 Taller tooth gives more dominant central incisor and narrower lateral incisor and canine. CIL, central incisor length; CIW, central incisor width; CW, canine width; LIW, lateral incisor width.

The incisal edge determinants, periodontal considerations, and desires of the patient will ultimately determine the final length of the clinical crowns.

Clinical use of the RED proportion

Correlating the preferred RED proportions of different length teeth with the preferred 78% width/length ratio of the central incisor provides a powerful tool for determining the ideal sizes of the maxillary teeth. The central incisor width (CIW) relative to any RED proportion can be calculated by the equation:

$$\text{Central incisor width} = \frac{\text{FIVE ICW of anterior six teeth}}{2(1+\text{RED}+\text{RED}^2)}$$

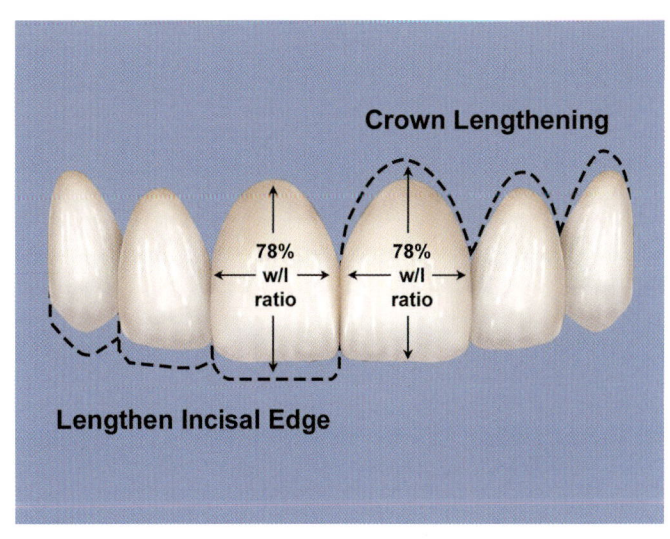

Figure 9.57 Methods to gain favorable width/length ratio in short teeth.

If you substitute into the equation the values of RED for the very tall (62% or 0.62), tall (66% or 0.66), normal (70% or 0.7), short (75% or 0.75), and very short (80% or 0.8) teeth you can calculate the divisor for the intercanine width (ICW) appropriate to calculate the central incisor width (ICW). This equation was used to solve for the divisor of the 70% RED proportion:

$$\text{Central incisor width} = \frac{\text{FIVE ICW of anterior six teeth}}{2(1+(0.7)+(0.7)^2)}$$
$$= \frac{(\text{ICW})}{4.38}$$

Table 9.1 shows the RED proportions associated with relative tooth lengths and how to calculate the maxillary anterior tooth widths. To use this table first determine if the general lengths of the teeth are very tall, tall, normal, short, or very short. Measure the same dimension (usually the length of a central incisor) on the cast and on the photograph and divide the cast dimension by the photographic dimension to calculate a conversion factor. This relates the actual size of the tooth to the size of the tooth on the photograph. Next, measure the width between the distal aspects of the maxillary canine teeth on the photograph and multiply by the conversion factor to determine the facial view (FIVE) ICW (Figure 9.58). Determine the RED proportion recommended width of the maxillary central incisor (CIW) by dividing the facial view ICW of the maxillary anterior six teeth (ICW) by the divisor listed in the table for the relative tooth

Table 9.1 Calculating Anterior Tooth Widths using Relative Tooth Lengths and the RED proportion

Relative Tooth Length	RED Proportion	Central Incisor Width (CIW) (rounded)	Lateral Incisor Width (LIW)	Canine Width (CW)
Very tall	62% RED	ICW/4.0	CIW*0.62	LIW*0.62
Tall	66% RED	ICW/4.2	CIW*0.66	LIW*0.66
Normal	70% RED	ICW/4.4	CIW*0.70	LIW*0.70
Short	75% RED	ICW/4.6	CIW*0.75	LIW*0.75
Very short	80% RED	ICW/4.8	CIW*0.8	LIW*0.80

Using a conversion Factor to determine FIVE (Facial Image View) ICW (Inter-canine Width)

Step 1

$$\frac{\text{Cast length of Central Incisor}}{\text{Photographic length of Central Incisor}} = \text{Conversion factor (Decimal less than 1)}$$

Step 2

Photographic width between distal aspects of canines × Conversion factor = FIVE ICW (*Facial Image View inter-canine width*)

Figure 9.58 Using the conversion factor to calculate the facial image view ICW.

Table 9.2 Using RED Proportions to Determine Anterior Tooth Widths and Central Incisor Length

Step 1. Determine relative tooth length	Select very tall, tall, normal, short, or very short relative tooth length
Step 2. Determine conversion factor	Measure same dimension on cast and photo, divide cast dimension/photo dimension to calculate conversion factor
Step 3. Determine facial image view ICW	Measure distance between distal aspects of both maxillary canines on photo and multiply by conversion factor to determine ICW
Step 4. Determine central incisor width (CIW)	Divide ICW/divisor of desired relative tooth length (4.0, 4.2, 4.4, 4.6, 4.8) to determine CIW
Step 5. Determine lateral incisor width (LIW)	Multiply CIW × RED (0.62, 0.66, 0.7, 0.75, 0.8) of desired relative tooth length
Step 6. Determine canine width (CW)	Multiply LIW × RED (0.62, 0.66, 0.7, 0.75, 0.8) of desired relative tooth length
Step 7. Determine central incisor length (CIL)	Divide CIW/0.78

length. Multiply the resulting central incisor width (CIW) by the RED proportion decimal equivalent listed in the table for the determined relative tooth length to produce the lateral incisor width (LIW). Finally, multiply the calculated LIW by the same decimal listed in the table to calculate the facial view canine width (CW). To determine the central incisor length (CIL) divide the CIW by 0.78. Table 9.2 is a review of the steps to use the RED proportion to determine the anterior tooth widths for appropriate relative tooth lengths.

To determine the tooth widths for normal-length teeth using the RED proportion first determine the ICW. Look up in the chart the divisor for normal length teeth, which is 4.4. Divide the ICW by 4.4 to determine the width of the maxillary central incisor. Look up in the chart the RED proportion to be used for normal-length teeth which is 70%. Multiply the CIW by 0.7 (70% RED) to determine the LIW. Multiply the lateral incisor width by 0.7 (70% RED) to calculate the CW (Figure 9.59).

A patient being orthodontically treated with congenitally missing maxillary lateral incisors was referred for space evaluation (Figure 9.60). No alterations were planned to the width of the central incisor and the width/length ratio approximated 78%. The patient was determined to have very short teeth. The width of the central incisor was measured as 6.4 mm and the length was 8.3 mm (yielding a 77% width/length ratio). Looking at the chart and considering the very short 8.3 mm long maxillary central incisor, a RED proportion of 80% needed to be used. With an 80% RED proportion, the LIW should have been 80% of

CIW=ICW/4.4 (from chart)
LIW=CIW*0.7 (RED Proportion normal length teeth)
CW=LIW*0.7 (RED Proportion normal length teeth)

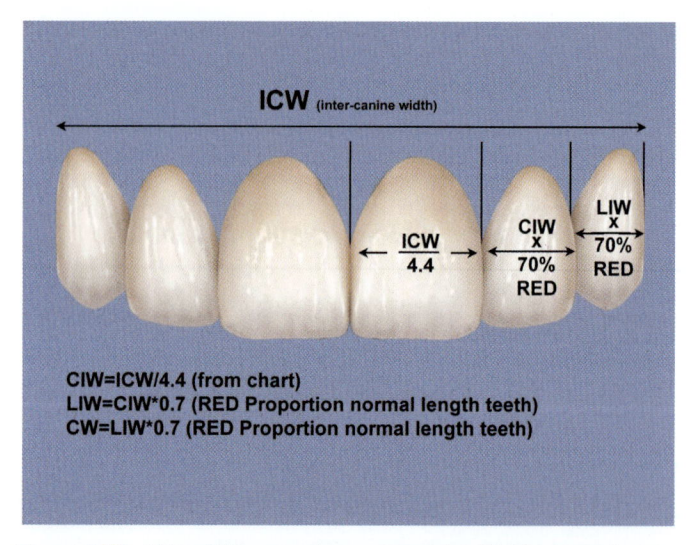

Figure 9.59 Using RED proportion to determine ICW for normal-length teeth. For definitions see text and Figure 9.56 legend.

Chapter 9   Proportional Smile Design

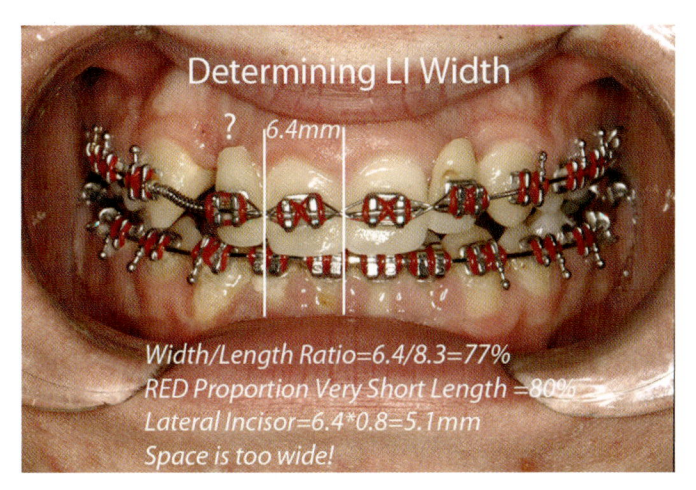

Figure 9.60 Figuring LIW using RED proportion.

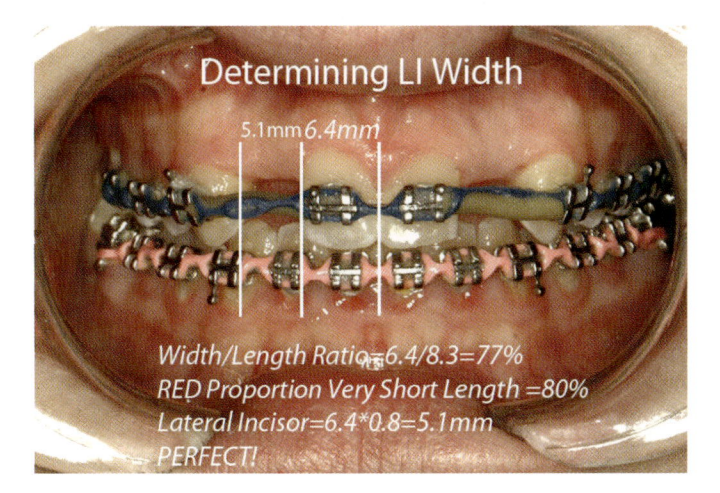

Figure 9.61 Verifying LIW width using RED proportion.

the width of the central incisor or 5.1 mm. The space was measured and deemed to be too wide. The patient arranged with the orthodontist to have their teeth moved to close the space to the desired 5.1 mm. The patient returned and the space was re-measured and determined to be correct (Figure 9.61).

Simplified use of the RED proportion

To further simplify the use of the RED proportion, a chart has been developed with the 78% width/length ratio substituted as a constant within the equation, the RED proportion tooth widths solved, and the quotient of the ICW divided by the CIL as the variable (Table 9.3). The facial view ICW is calculated and divided by the CIL (CIL) to produce a quotient (Figure 9.62). The quotient is looked up in the chart and the associated relative tooth lengths, RED proportion, and ICW divisors for each tooth are recorded. The ICW is divided by the divisors listed in the chart to determine the widths of the maxillary central incisor, lateral incisor, and canine. The length of a maxillary central incisor can be calculated by dividing the width of the maxillary central incisor by 0.78.

If the ICW/CIW quotient in the chart does not coincide with the desired relative tooth length, look up the quotient appropriate to the relative body height. Simple substitution gives:

$$\frac{ICW}{\text{Desired quotient}} = CIL$$

Divide the ICW by the quotient in the chart of the desired relative tooth length to calculate the CIL. Determine if the resulting length seems applicable. This is especially helpful when the incisal edges of the teeth are worn and can be lengthened and/or apical repositioning of the free gingival margin is possible. Using a longer central incisor often allows it to be proportioned to a 78% width/length ratio without making significant changes to the original widths of the teeth (Figure 9.63). Using the chart, repeat the calculations for the widths of the incisors and canines. Table 9.4 is a review of the above steps.

A patient presented requesting an improvement to her smile (Figure 9.64). Photos were taken and study models made. The left CIL measured 9 mm on the cast (Figure 9.65). The CIL on the photograph measured 25 mm (Figure 9.66). The measurements made on the photograph were multiplied by 9/25 or 0.36 to convert the photographic view measurements to the FIVE measurements (Figure 9.67). The width between the distal aspects of the two maxillary canine teeth measured on the photograph was 92.8 mm. Multiplying 92.8 mm by 0.36 gave a

Table 9.3 Chart using ICW/CIW Quotient to Determine Relative Tooth Lengths, RED Proportion, and Anterior Tooth Widths

ICW/CIL Quotient	RED Proportion	Relative Tooth Length	CIW	LIW	CW
3.1	62% RED	Very tall	ICW/4.00	ICW/6.47	ICW/10.43
3.2	65% RED	Tall	ICW/4.15	ICW/6.38	ICW/9.81
3.3	67% RED	Slightly tall	ICW/4.24	ICW/6.33	ICW/9.44
3.4	70% RED	Normal	ICW/4.38	ICW/6.26	ICW/8.94
3.5	73% RED	Slightly short	ICW/4.53	ICW/6.20	ICW/8.49
3.6	75% RED	Short	ICW/4.63	ICW/6.17	ICW/8.22
3.7	78% RED	Shorter	ICW/4.78	ICW/6.12	ICW/7.85
3.8	80% RED	Very short	ICW/4.88	ICW/6.10	ICW/7.63

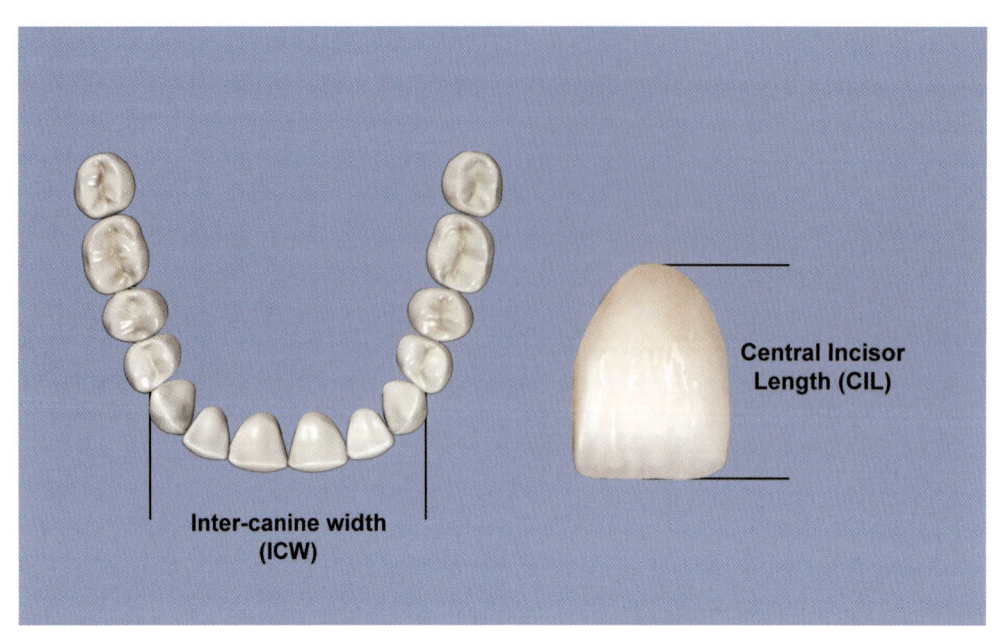

Figure 9.62 ICW is divided by the CIL to determine quotient.

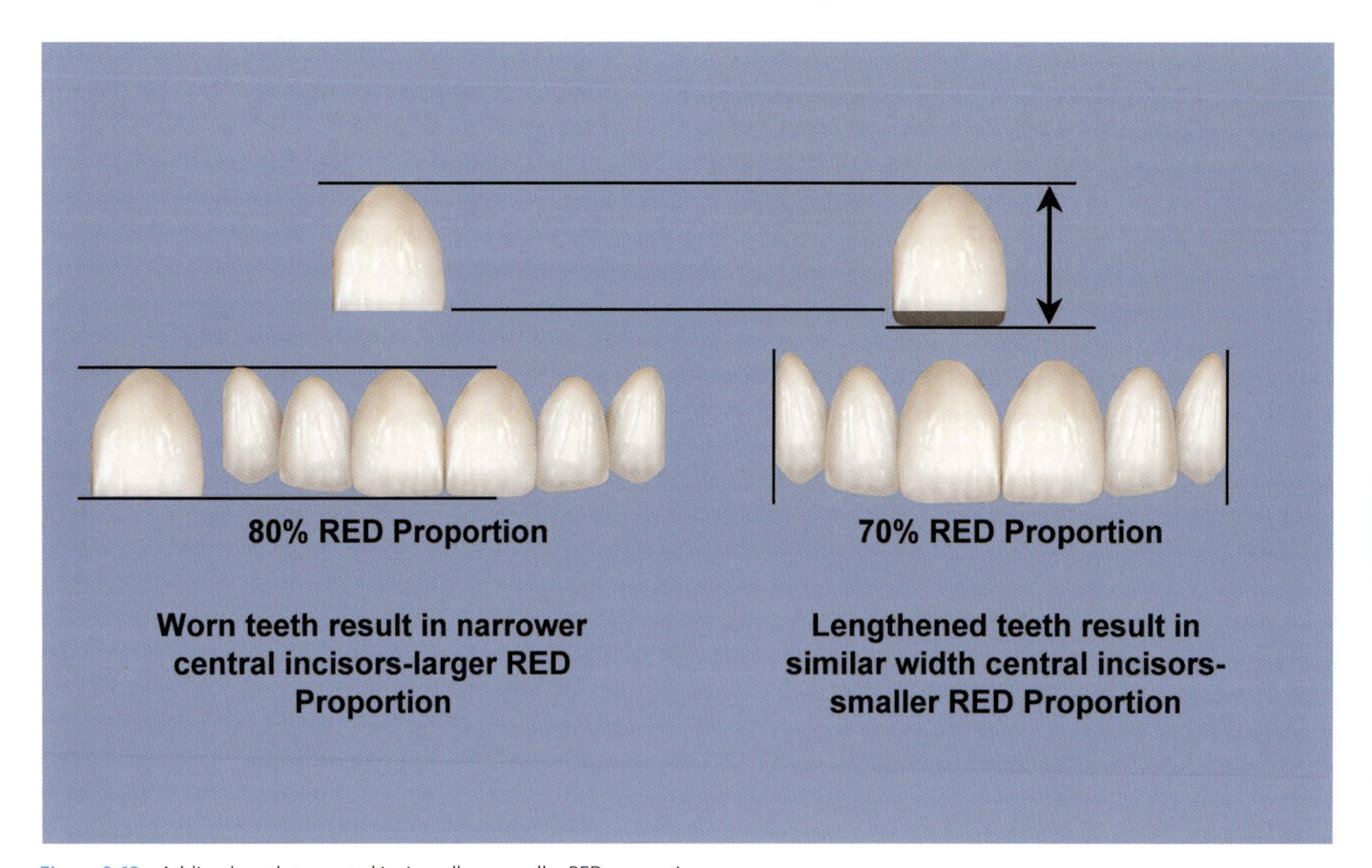

Figure 9.63 Adding length to central incisor allows smaller RED proportion.

FIVE ICW of 33.4 mm. Dividing 33.4 by the CIL of 9 gave a quotient of 3.7 (Figure 9.68). Looking at the chart shows that a quotient of 3.7 is appropriate for shorter teeth. The patient was a person of average height who preferred normal-length teeth. Looking at the chart, normal-length teeth have a quotient of 3.4 and RED proportion of 70%. Dividing 33.4 (FIVE ICW) by 4.38 (the divisor from Table 9.3 for the 70% RED central incisor) gave a 7.6 mm-wide central incisor. Dividing 33.4 by 6.26 (the divisor

Chapter 9 Proportional Smile Design

Table 9.4 Simplified Method using ICW/CIL Quotient Chart to Determine Anterior Tooth Widths and Central Incisor Length

Step 1. Determine conversion factor	Measure same dimension on cast and photo and divide cast dimension/photo dimension to calculate conversion factor
Step 2. Determine facial image view ICW	Measure distance between distal aspects of maxillary canines on photo and multiply by conversion factor to determine ICW
Step 3. Measure central incisor length	Measure CIL on cast
Step 4. Determine ICW/CIL quotient	Divide ICW/CIL and look up quotient on chart
Step 5. Evaluate relative tooth length of quotient	If quotient matches desired relative tooth length proceed to step 7
Step 6. Select a different quotient	If quotient does not match, look up the quotient appropriate to the relative body height; divide the ICW by desired relative tooth length quotient in chart to calculate CIL; if appropriate proceed to step 7; if not choose a different quotient and retry
Step 7. Determine central incisor width (CIW)	Divide ICW/divisor of selected relative tooth length for CIW
Step 8. Determine lateral incisor width (LIW)	Divide ICW/divisor of selected relative tooth length for LIW
Step 9. Determine canine width (CW)	Divide ICW/divisor of selected relative tooth length for CW
Step 10. Determine central incisor length (CIL)	Divide CIW by 0.78 for CIL

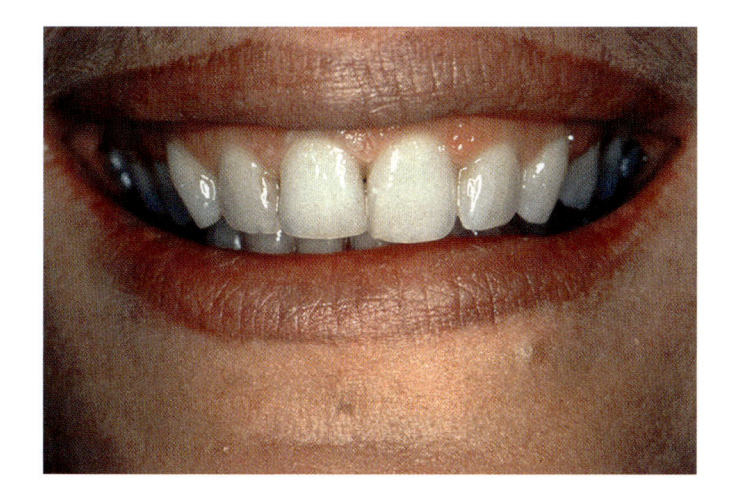

Figure 9.64 Preoperative smile to be analyzed using simplified RED proportion method.

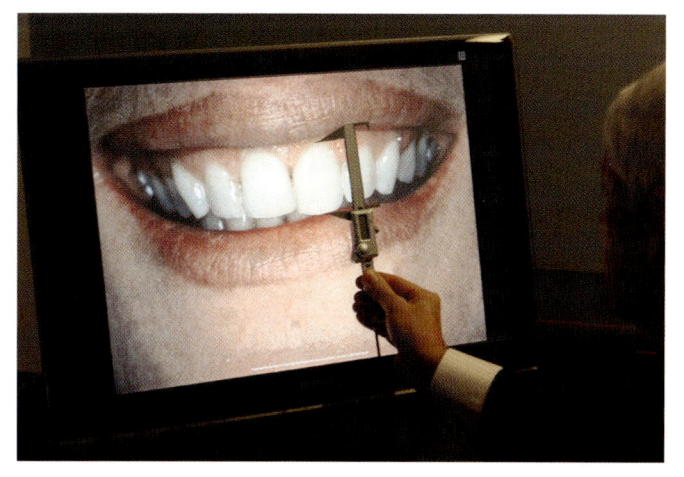

Figure 9.66 Measuring photographic view lengths and widths.

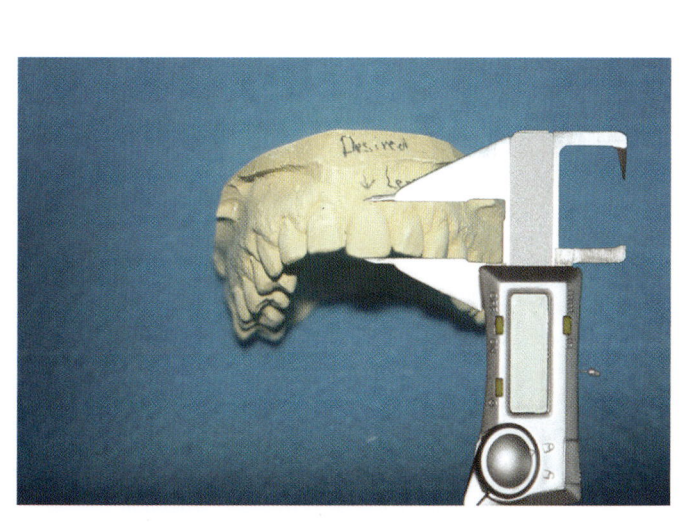

Figure 9.65 Measuring cast view length.

from Table 9.3 for the 70% RED lateral incisor) yielded a 5.3 mm-wide lateral incisor. Finally, dividing 33.4 by 8.94 (the divisor for the canine) gave a 3.7 mm-wide canine (Figure 9.69). The CIL was determined by dividing the CIW of 7.6 by 0.78 (desired width/length ratio) to yield a 9.8 mm-long central incisor. (Figure 9.70). The final dimensions of the maxillary anterior six teeth were calculated and inserted into a chart (Figure 9.71).

Use of computer simulation

Effective communication between the patient, dentist, and laboratory is important to satisfy the esthetic requirements of the patient. With the advent of the computer, smile analysis has become more objective. Tooth and smile proportions can be evaluated and the widths and lengths of the maxillary anterior teeth calculated according to RED proportion principles. A grid can be placed over the photograph with the appropriate RED proportion

Cast central incisor length	9 mm								
Photo central incisor length	25 mm								
Cast/photo proportion	0.36								

	Photographic Widths								Widths
	5	6	7	8	9	10	11	12	#6-11
Width	2.7	12.4	13.8	20.6	20.6	13.8	11.6	4.7	92.8
Length	14.0	20.0	19.8	22.6	25.0	19.8	19.7	15.4	

Calculated Cast Widths (FIVE widths)
(Photo widths X Calculated Cast/Photo Proportion)

	5	6	7	8	9	10	11	12	ICW
Width	1.0	4.5	5.0	7.4	7.4	5.0	4.2	1.7	33.4 mm
Length	5.0	7.2	7.1	8.1	9.0	7.1	7.1	5.5	

Figure 9.67 Correlating cast lengths with photo lengths to calculate FIVE widths.

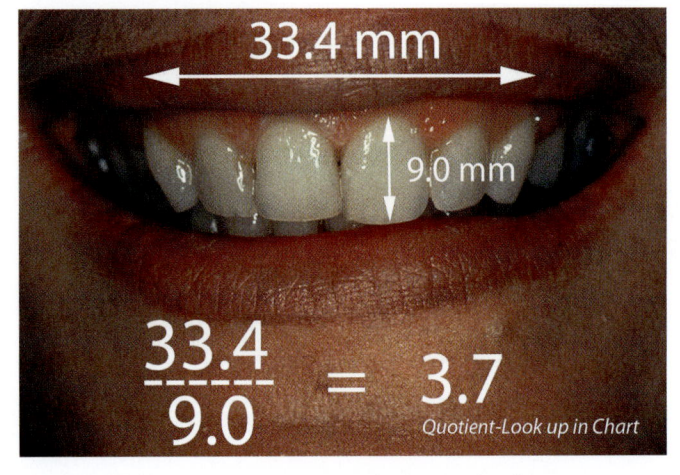

$$\frac{33.4}{9.0} = 3.7 \text{ Quotient-Look up in Chart}$$

Figure 9.68 Calculating a quotient to look up in the chart.

Using CIW & W/L Ratio

CIW/0.78 = CIL
7.62/0.78 = 9.8 mm *long central incisor*

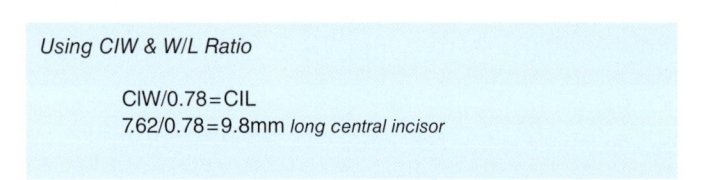

Figure 9.70 Calculating central incisor tooth length.

Normal Length (ICW = 33.4 mm)

ICW/CIH quotient	RED Proportion	Relative tooth length	Central incisor width (CIW)	Lateral incisor width (LIW)	Canine width (CW)
3.4	70% RED	Normal	ICW/4.38	ICW/6.26	ICW/8.94

CIW = 33.4/4.38 = 7.6 mm (wide lateral incisor)
LIW = 33.4/6.26 = 5.3 mm (wide lateral incisor)
CW = 33.4/8.94 = 3.7 mm (wide canine)

Figure 9.69 Using ICW, calculating a CIL (shown as CIH, or central incisor height on the figure) quotient to calculate anterior tooth widths for patient.

(ICW = 33.4 mm)

RED Proportion Measurements (in mm)

	6	7	8	9	10	11
Width	3.7	5.3	7.6	7.6	5.3	3.7
Length	9.8	8.8	9.8	9.8	8.8	9.8

70% RED proportion   78% W/L Ratio

Figure 9.71 Completed chart using RED proportion.

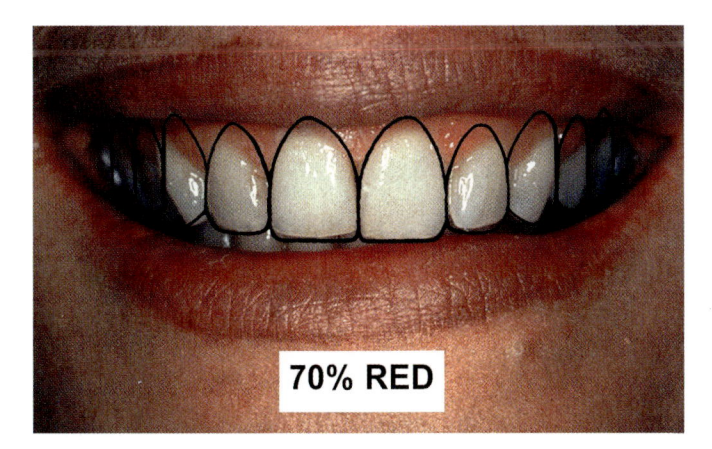

Figure 9.72 RED proportion template overlay.

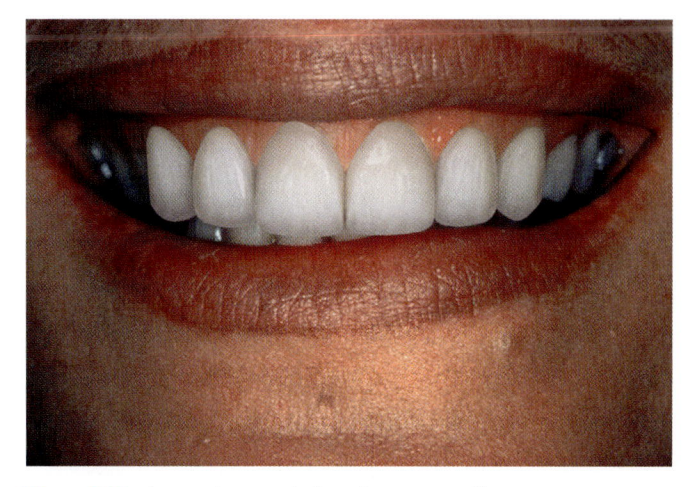

Figure 9.73 Imaged nonperiodontal surgery smile.

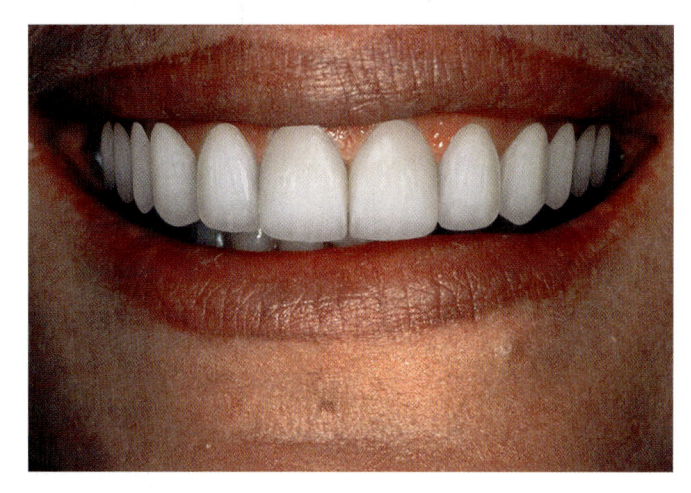

Figure 9.74 Imaged periodontal surgery smile.

outlines of the desired teeth (Figure 9.72). Using computer imaging software, an image of the final desired sizes of the teeth can be produced. It is important to create simulations with the patient's own gingiva to show results that can knowingly be accomplished. The use of a smile library to insert other patients' teeth and gums within the lips of a patient may not accurately portray what is possible. A computer image of the final desired obtainable result allows open discussion before operative treatment begins.

The patient was originally interested in only six porcelain laminate veneers but wanted them to be lighter. After evaluating the display of her buccal corridor when smiling, it was determined there would be a sharp contrast between the veneers and the darker maxillary posterior teeth. A computer simulation of the probable final appearance without crown lengthening was prepared (Figure 9.73). Elective crown lengthening would allow for a more desirable width/length ratio of the central incisor. A RED proportion could be selected that coincided with the overall height of the patient. Using the calculations derived above, a simulation was produced for the likely outcome of crown lengthening and placement of eight porcelain laminate veneers. Extending treatment distally to the first premolar helps to visually fill the buccal corridor, give better unity to the anterior teeth, and allow for lighter final restorations. The RED proportion was used to determine the appropriate facial view width of the first bicuspids (Figure 9.74). The patient viewed both simulations and was able to make an informed decision. She elected to have crown lengthening performed and eight porcelain laminate veneers placed.

The patient was referred to the periodontist to have crown lengthening and gingival recontouring performed (Figure 9.75). It is important to inform the specialist the desired lengths of the final restorations, so that the free gingival margin can be placed in the proper position. The teeth that will be restored must be communicated as well. The tissue was allowed to heal and final

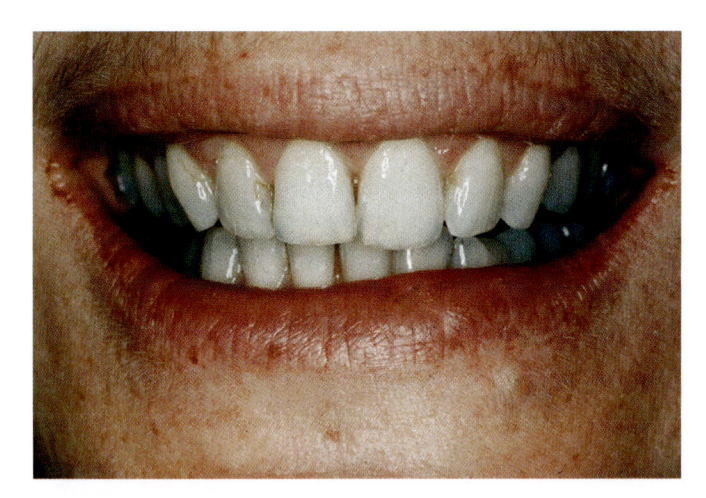

Figure 9.75 Postperiodontal surgery.

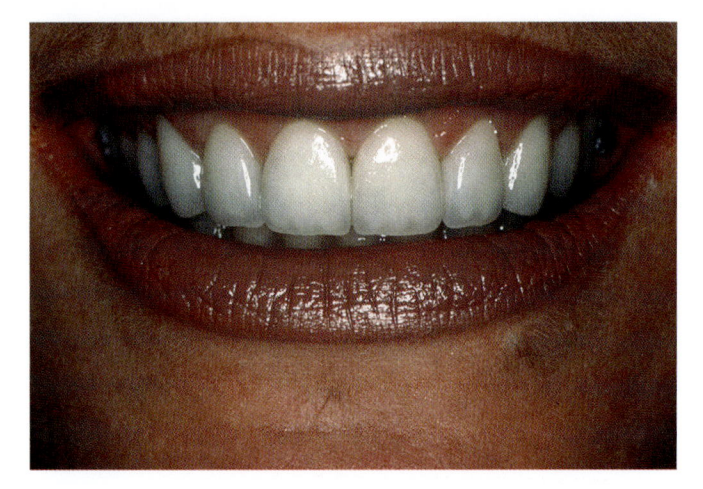

Figure 9.76 Postoperative smile designed using the 70% RED proportion.

gingival sculpting was performed. The anterior eight teeth were prepared for porcelain laminate veneers and the case completed (Figure 9.76).

Patient preferences and individuality

Studies have evaluated the smile preferences of patients. Their general likes and dislikes compared to dentists are similar but their acceptable variance is much broader. Patients accept greater deviance from defined norms.[57,58] Laypersons are not as discerning about likes and dislikes.[59,60] Patients often have a different order of criteria for what is considered esthetic.[61,62] In one study, patients were willing to accept variations of width/length ratio of the maxillary central incisor between 75 and 85% compared to dentists, who preferred 75–80%.[63] However, patients surveyed, like their professional counterparts, did not prefer the golden proportion to other suggested tooth-to-tooth width proportions with normal-length teeth.[64] Another aspect which has only briefly been investigated is variation in preference by gender. Members of each group may place different emphasis and regard for factors that comprise an esthetic smile. The bias of a dentist of one gender treating the other gender could result in minor differences of opinion.[56]

It is important to understand the characteristics which comprise an esthetic smile and then incorporate variations for the individual. A natural smile rarely exhibits all the ideal components of a smile. Learning how and when to break these rules allows for an expressive smile. As stated over 60 years ago by Frush and Fisher, our goal should be to create eminently suited, fully expressive smiles that convey the person's charm, character, dignity, and beauty.[6] By incorporating the design principles of an esthetic smile, we can provide our patients the ability to display on the outside their inner feelings via a pleasing smile.

References

1. Huntley HE. *The Divine Proportion: a Study in Mathematical Beauty*. New York: Dover Publications Inc.; 1970.
2. Ghyka M. *The Geometry of Art and Life*. New York: Dover Publications Inc.; 1977.
3. Goldstein RE. *Esthetics in Dentistry*, 2nd edn. Hamilton, ON: B C Decker Inc.; 1998.
4. Bates B, Cleese J. *The Human Face*. New York: Dorling Kindersley Publishing Inc.; 2001.
5. Powell N, Humphreys B. *Proportions of the Aesthetic Face*. New York: Thieme-Stratton; 1984.
6. Frush JP, Fisher RD. Introduction to dentogenic restorations. *J Prosthet Dent* 1955;5:586–595.
7. Morley J, Eubank J. Macroesthetic elements of smile design. *J Am Dent Assoc* 2001;132:39–45.
8. Broderson SP. Anterior guidance-the key to successful occlusal treatment. *J Prosthet Dent* 1978;39:396–399.
9. Ahmad I. Geometric considerations in anterior dental aesthetics: restorative principles. *Pract Periodontic Aesthetic Dent* 1998;10:813–822.
10. Boucher CO. *Swenson's Complete Dentures*, 6th edn. St Louis, MO: C.V. Mosby; 1970.
11. Lombardi RE. A method for the classification of errors in dental esthetics. *J Prosthet Dent* 1974;32:501–513.
12. Frush JP, Fisher RD. The dynesthetic interpretation of the dentogenic concept. *J Prosthet Dent* 1958;8:558–581.
13. Pound E. Utilizing speech to simplify denture service. *J Prosthet Dent* 1970;24:595.
14. McIntyre F. Restoring esthetics and anterior guidance in worn anterior teeth: a conservative multidisciplinary approach. *J Am Dent Assoc* 2000;131:279–283.
15. McHorris WH. The importance of anterior teeth. *J Gnathol* 1982;1:19–36.
16. McIntyre FM, Jureyda O. Occlusal function. Beyond centric relation. *Dent Clin North Am* 2001;45:173–180.
17. Wheeler RC. *Dental Anatomy and Physiology*. Philadelphia, PA: WB Saunders; 1940.
18. Gürel G. *The Science and Art of Porcelain Laminate Veneers*. Berlin: Quintessence; 2003.
19. Morley J. The role of cosmetic dentistry in restoring a youthful appearance. *J Am Dent Assoc* 1999;130:1166–1172.
20. Morley J. The esthetic of anterior tooth aging. *Curr Opin Cosmetic Dent* 1997;4:35–39.
21. Frush JP, Fisher RD. The age factor in dentogenics. *J Prosthet Dent* 1957;7:5–13.
22. Vig RG, Brundo GC. The kinetics of anterior tooth display. *J Prosthet Dent* 1978;39:502–504.

23. Williams JL. A new classification of human tooth forms with special reference to a new system of artificial teeth. *Cosmos* 1941;56:627–628.
24. Frush JP, Fisher RD. How dentogenic restorations interpret the sex factor. *J Prosthet Dent* 1956;6:160–172.
25. Frush JP, Fisher RD. How dentogenic restorations interpret the personality factor. *J Prosthet Dent* 1956;6:441–449.
26. Weisgold A. Contours of the full crown restoration. *Alpha Omega* 1977;70:77–89.
27. Chu SJ, Tan JH, Stappert CF, Tarnow DP. Gingival zenith positions and levels of the maxillary anterior dentition. *J Esthet Restor Dent* 2009;21(2):113–120.
28. House MM, Loop JL. *Form and Color Harmony in the Dental Art*. Whittier, CA: Monograph; 1937:3–33.
29. Rufenacht CR. *Fundamentals of Esthetics*. Chicago, IL: Quintessence; 1990:67–134.
30. Chu SJ. Range and mean distribution frequency of individual tooth width of the maxillary anterior dentition. *Pract Proced Aesthet Dent* 2007;19(4):209–215.
31. Lee SP, Lee SJ, Hayaski K, Park YS. A three-dimensional analysis of the perceived proportions of maxillary anterior teeth. *Acta Odontol Scand* 2012;70(5):432–440.
32. Diamond O. Facial esthetics and orthodontics. *J Esthetic Dent* 1995;8:136–143.
33. Morris W. An orthodontic view of dentofacial esthetics. *Compendium* 1994;15:378–390.
34. Al-Balkhi KM. Orthodontic treatment planning: do orthodontists treat to cephalomatric norms? *J Contemp Pract* 2003;4(4):12–27.
35. Chu SJ, Tarnow DP, Tan JH, Stappert CF. Papilla proportions in the maxillary anterior dentition. *Int J Perodontics Restorative Dent* 2009;29(4):385–393.
36. Chiche GJ, Pinault A. *Esthetics of Anterior Fixed Prosthodontics*. Chicago, IL: Quintessence; 1994.
37. Sterrett JD, Oliver T, Robinson F, et al. Width/length ratios of normal clinical crowns of the maxillary anterior dentition in man. *J Clin Periodontol* 1999;26:153–157.
38. Gillen RJ, Schwartz RS, Hilton TJ, Evans DB. An analysis of selected normative tooth proportions. *Int J Prosthodont* 1994;7:410–417.
39. Magne P, Gallucci GO, Belser UC. Anatomical crown width/length ratios of unworn and worn maxillary teeth in white subjects. *J Prosthet Dent* 2003;89:453–461.
40. Wolfart S, Quaas AC, Freitag S, et al. Subjective and objective perception of upper incisors. *J Oral Rehabil* 2006;33:489–495.
41. Zlataric DK, Kristek E, Celebic A. Analysis of width/length ratios of normal clinical crowns of the maxillary anterior dentition: correlation between dental proportions and facial measurements. *Int J Prosthodont* 2007;20:313–315.
42. Naylor CK. Esthetic treatment planning: the grid analysis system. *J Esthet Restor Dent* 2002;14:76–84.
43. Wolfart S, Thormann H, Freitag S, Kern M. Assessment of dental appearance following changes in incisor proportions. *Eur J Oral Sci* 2005;113(2):159–165.
44. Rosenstiel SF, Ward DH, Rashid RG. Dentists' preferences of anterior tooth proportion-a web-based study. *J Prosthodont* 2000;9:123–136.
45. Lombardi RE. The principles of visual perception and their clinical application to denture esthetics. *J Prosthet Dent* 1973;29:358–382.
46. Beaudreau DE. *Atlas of Fixed Partial Prosthesis*. Springfield, IL: Charles C. Thomas; 1975.
47. Levin EI. Dental esthetics and the golden proportion. *J Prosthet Dent* 1978;40:244–252.
48. Snow SR. Esthetic smile analysis of anterior tooth width: the golden percentage. *J Esthet Dent* 1999;11:177–184.
49. Albers HA. Esthetic treatment planning. *Adept Report* 1992;3:45–52.
50. Preston JD. The golden proportion revisited. *J Esthetic Dent* 1993;5:247–251.
51. Fayyad MA, Jamani KD, Aqrabawi J. Geometric and mathematical proportions and their relations to maxillary anterior teeth. *J Contemp Dent Pract* 2006;7(5):62–70.
52. Al Wazan KA. The relationship between intercanthal dimension and the width of maxillary anterior teeth. *J Prosthet Dent* 2001;86:608–612.
53. Basting RT, Trindale RS, Flório FM. Comparative study of smile analysis by subjective and computerized methods. *Oper Dent* 2006;31:652–659.
54. Mahsid M, Khoshvaghti A, Varshosaz M, Vallaei N. Evaluation of "golden proportion" in individuals with an esthetic smile. *J Esthet Restor Dent* 2004;16:185–192.
55. Ward DH. Proportional smile design using the RED proportion. *Dent Clin North Am* 2001;45:143–154.
56. Ward DH. A study of dentists' preferred maxillary anterior tooth width proportions: comparing the recurring esthetic dental proportion to other mathematical and naturally occurring proportions. *J Esthet Restor Dent* 2007;19:323–336.
57. Brisman AS. Esthetics: a comparison of dentists' and patients' concepts. *J Am Dent Assoc* 1980;100:345–352.
58. Kokich VO, Kiyak HA, Shapiro PA. Comparing the perception of dentists and lay people to altered dental esthetics. *J Esthet Dent* 1999;11:311–324.
59. Carlssan GE, Wagner IV, Odman P, et al. An international comparative multicenter study of assessment of dental appearance using computer-aided image manipulation. *Int J Prosthodont* 1998;11:246–254.
60. Witt W, Flores-Mir C. Laypeople's preferences regarding frontal dentofacial esthetics. *J Am Dent Assoc* 2011;142(6):635–645.
61. Wagner IV, Carlsson GE, Ekstrand K, et al. A comparative study of assessment of dental appearance by dentists, dental technicians, and laymen using computer-aided image manipulation. *J Esthet Restor Dent* 1995;8:199–203.
62. Jørnung J, Fardel Ø. Perceptions of patients' smiles: a comparison of patients' and dentists' opinions. *J Am Dent Assoc* 2007;138:1544–1553.
63. Ker AJ, Chan R, Fields HW, et al. Esthetics and smile characteristics from the layperson's perspective: a computer-based survey study. *J Am Dent Assoc* 2008;139(10):1318–1327.
64. Rosenstiel SF, Rashid RG. Public preferences for anterior tooth variations. *J Esthet Restor Dent* 2002;14:97–106.

Additional references

Conniff R. What's behind a smile? *Smithsonian* 2007;38(5):46–53.
Sorokowski P, Pawlowski B. Adaptive preferences for leg length in a potential partner. *Evol Hum Behav* 2008;29(2):86–91.
Trumble A. *A Brief History of the Smile*. New York: Basic Books; 2004.
Ward DH. Using the RED proportion to engineer the perfect smile. *Dent Today* 2008;27(5):112–117.

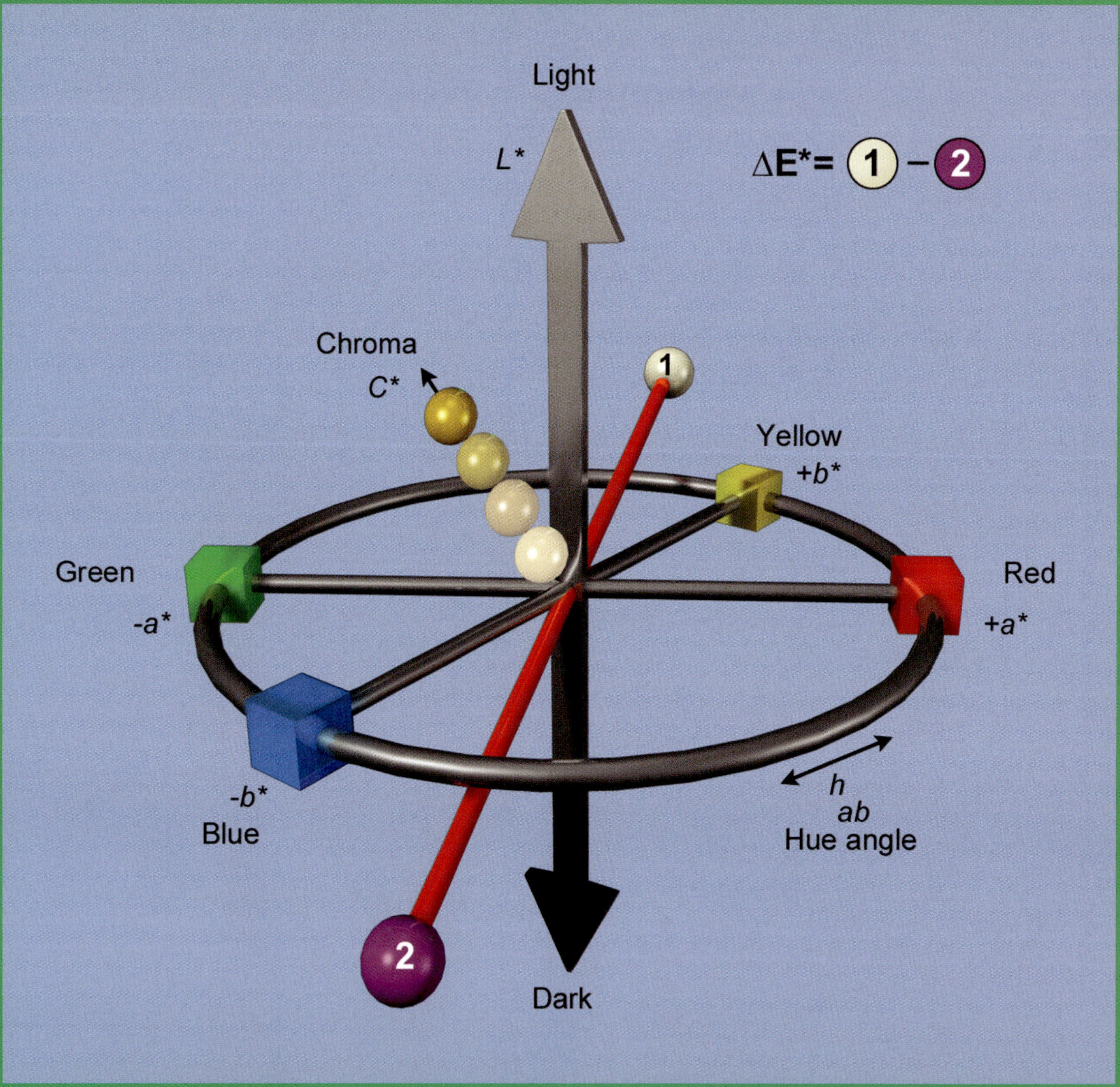
Light
L*
ΔE*= 1 − 2
Chroma
C*
1
Yellow
+b*
Green
-a*
Red
+a*
-b*
Blue
h
ab
Hue angle
2
Dark

Chapter 10 Understanding Color

Rade D. Paravina, DDS, MS, PhD

Chapter Outline

Basics of color	272	Color matching method	282
Color triplet: light, object and observer	272	Myths and facts about visual color matching	284
Color dimensions	272	Color matching instruments	284
Color notation systems	273	Communicating color	285
Color in dentistry	273	Verbal and written instructions and sketches	285
Tooth color	274	Modified and custom-made shade guides	285
Gingival color	274	Color modification	286
Skin color	274	Color-related properties of dental materials	286
Visual color matching	274	Color education and training	287
Color matching conditions	274	A look to the future	292
Color matching tools—shade guides	276		

This book amply documents the many areas that must be coordinated to achieve the intangible result called "esthetic." Color must take its place as merely another building stone, a part of the total perceptual impression. However, just as the disharmony is created by a discordant note in a symphony, the wrong color can destroy a result so painstakingly sought.

To the untrained eye, all teeth are white. To the dentist, who must match the natural teeth using a restorative material, the wide and subtle gamut of color is a real, perceptual challenge. Although the need to know accepted color matching procedures is a basic requirement, it is often ignored in dental education. It is also usually poorly understood by the dentist, the technician, and manufacturers of dental materials. The science of color matching involves physics, psychophysics, psychology, and even philosophy. Knowledge of advanced algebra and calculus is helpful. The nature of light, color vision theories, spectrophotometric studies, color dimensions, color order systems, and other equally confusing matters are all part of the color scientist's world.[1,2] These advanced concepts are not required for perceiving and equating colors, but if one is to truly understand what is occurring in color perception and matching, they are essential.

This chapter is intended to provide practical guidelines for color matching. In a text that emphasizes the clinical approach to esthetics, the reader has the right to expect clinical guidelines on color matching instead of a technical discourse. Only that technical information essential to accomplish these goals is presented. Clinical color matching involves more than picking a tab from a shade guide and having a restoration of the same color processed. One often wishes it were that simple; unfortunately, that is the extent of understanding that usually accompanies the shade selection procedure. To develop an ability to select a shade that will ultimately result in a restoration matching the adjacent natural dentition, it is essential to have an appreciation of the role of the three-dimensional nature of color. There must also be a realization of the benefits and limitations of existing guides and materials.

Basics of color

E. Bruce Clark, an early leader in color matching in dentistry, succinctly stated the need for learning the three-dimensional nature of color: "In the study of color not only is an intimate acquaintance with its three dimensions the first requisite that should be acquired, but it is, without exception, the most important."[3] Familiarity with the three-dimensional nature of color is the key to successful clinical color matching. A mental image of an object such as a box can be conveyed to another person by describing its length, width, and depth. It is easy to give instructions on modifying its dimensions, or to make comparisons of its size and shape with those of another box. This is possible because other people know what a "box" is, they understand the concept of three dimensions, and the scales, such as meters, centimeters, and millimeters, by which those dimensions can be expressed. The dimensions of color—hue, value, and chroma—enable similar type of communication regarding color. The mechanism of visual color perception—a light-object-observer triplet, color dimensions, and color notation systems—will be described in this section.

Color triplet: light, object and observer

Color is a psychophysical sensation produced in the eye by visible light reflected from an object and interpreted by the brain.[4-6] The color triplet consists of light source, object, and observer.

Light

There is no color without light. Visible light is merely one small portion (lies in a narrow band from 380 to 760 nm) of the electromagnetic spectrum (Figure 10.1). More detail about desirable light characteristics for work with color in dentistry will be provided in the section on color matching conditions.

Object

The light can be reflected, transmitted, and absorbed by the object (we seldom look at the light source). We see the reflected light, either from the surface (surface reflection), or from the body of the translucent material or tissue (volume reflection). Tooth color matching is closely related to volume reflection. Depending on the angle, reflection can be specular (mirror angle compared to incident light), diffuse (light reflected in any other angle), or total.

Observer

Light rays reflected from an object have the ability to stimulate the rods and cones, cells of the retina that enable color perception. Rods enable an achromatic component, while cones (red-, green-, and blue-sensitive) enable color perception. The information is then conveyed to the brain, which interprets it and allows the sense of sight.

Color dimensions

Colors differ in many ways: they may be red, orange, yellow, blue, and so on, or they may be light or dark, weak or strong. The description of these differences is the basis for the clinical approach to color matching in dentistry. The description of color dimension, similar to one provided by Munsell for his color notation system and later adapted in other systems, will be presented here.

Hue

The dimension of hue is most easily understood. It is "that quality by which we distinguish one color family from another, as red from yellow from blue or purple."[7] All hues are placed in a closed hue circle in Figure 10.2 (only green, red, blue, and yellow are shown). The order of hues in the visible spectrum is violet, blue, green, yellow, orange, and red. It is important to understand that these hue names are descriptive of a family of sensations and there is no clear distinction between where one hue terminates and another begins. The spectrum is a continuum of sensations to which we have given convenient (although sometimes meaningless) names.

Value

This is an achromatic dimension, ranging from black to white, with all the grays in between, as represented by a vertical value axis in Figure 10.2. Value relates to the quality (not quantity) of a color's grayness. A black and white image of a colored object would be a one-dimensional (value) rendition of a three-dimensional (colored) object.

Chroma

This color dimension enables discrimination between a strong color and a weak one. Chroma is represented by the distance of certain color from the point of the same value on an achromatic

Gamma rays	X rays	Ultraviolet	Infrared	Microwave	Radio
<0.02 nm	0.01–10 nm	10–400 nm	750–1 nm	1mm–1 meter	1 m–100,000 km

Visible spectrum 400–700 nanometers

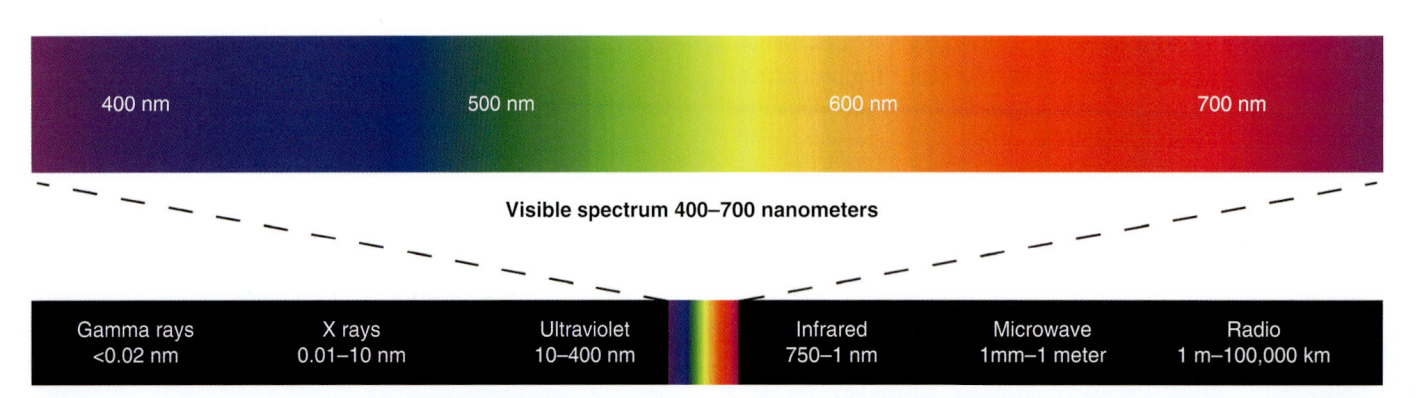

Figure 10.1 Electromagnetic spectrum with relative wavelengths and frequencies, and expanded visible light.

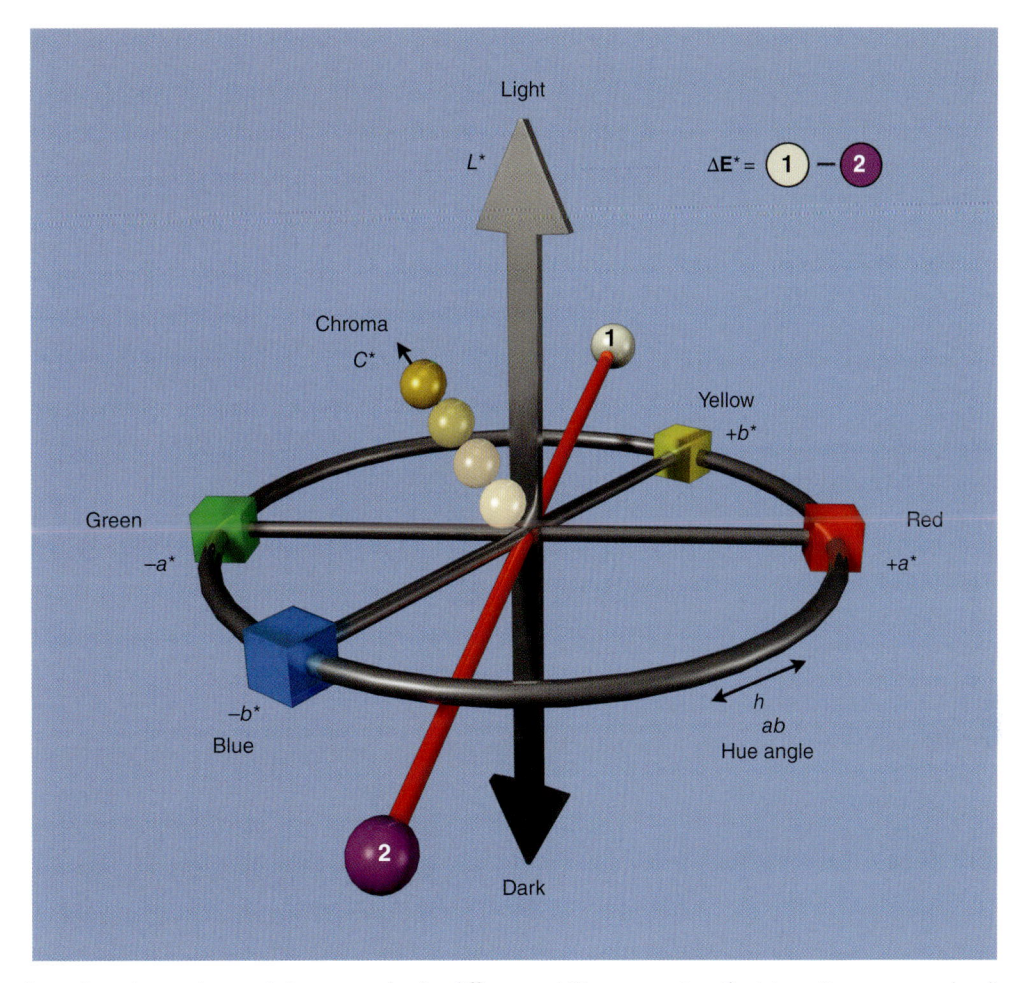

Figure 10.2 Color dimensions: hue, value, and chroma, and color difference, ΔE*, representing the interaction among color dimensions.

axis—it increases with the increase of this distance (Figure 10.2). Therefore, hue differences are associated with different colors, while chroma differences are related to different strength of the same color.

A large portion of this chapter has been devoted to understanding color dimensions because it is basic to comprehending a logical basis for color matching in dentistry. This will become more apparent when shade guides and their use are discussed. However, before familiarity with the three-dimensional nature of color can be a practical aid, one must know how to identify color differences and attribute them to hue, value, or chroma.

Color notation systems

Color dimensions—hue, value, and chroma—are used in different color notation systems and formulae. Familiarity with color dimensions can contribute to the traditional means of color matching, communication (for indirect restorations), reproduction, and verification. In addition, these systems are of the great benefit for color research in dentistry. The Munsell hue-value-chroma color notation system is probably mostly important historically, while different formulae of the Commission Internationale de l'Éclairage (CIE; International Commission on Illumination) system are presently most frequently used and will be more thoroughly described.

Commission Internationale de L'Éclairage (CIE) System

Similarly to the Munsell system, CIE system has achromatic (value) and chromatic component (hue and chroma). The CIELAB formula was developed in 1976 and it utilizes the following color coordinates: L* (lightness; synonym for Munsell Value), a* (−a* green, +a* red), b* (−b* blue, +b yellow), H* (hue), and C* (chroma), where H* and C* are calculated from a* and b* coordinates. Color difference in the CIELAB formula is denoted ΔE* (Figure 10.2); it represents the difference in sensation (the symbol delta, Δ, means the difference, while E is the first letter of the German word *Empfindung*, which means sensation), and represents the interaction of L*a*b* or L*C*H* differences.[1] A more recent and more advanced CIE formula, CIEDE2000,[8] has been subsequently introduced and it is increasingly used in dental color research.[9,10]

Color in dentistry

One of the best descriptions of the importance of color was offered by Bergen. He said "Color is unimportant to the physiologic success of a dental restoration, yet it could be the controlling factor in the overall acceptance by the patient."[11]

Dental professionals are routinely performing matching, replication, and/or creation of color of hard and soft oral tissues, while maxillofacial prosthodontists are dealing with color in the entire maxillofacial area. Therefore, this section is related to color of teeth, gingiva, and skin.

Familiarity with the basics of color is essential to the understanding of color-related clinical and dental technology applications, and the remainder of this chapter. What is the practical meaning of ΔE^* values? What ΔE^* corresponds to perfect match, *perceptibility*, and *acceptability thresholds* (wait, what is color threshold)? A ΔE^* of 0 corresponds to perfect match—it is rarely seen and not really necessary. Visual thresholds are also known as industry tolerances, and these differ from one industry to another. A 50:50 perceptibility threshold is the difference in color that can be detected by 50% of observers. The other 50% of observers will notice no difference in color between the compared objects. A nearly perfect color match in dentistry is a color difference at or below the 50:50 perceptibility threshold. A 50:50 acceptability threshold is the difference in color that is considered acceptable by 50% of observers. The other 50% of observers would replace the restoration or correct its color. An acceptable color match in dentistry is a color difference at or below the 50:50 acceptability threshold.[12]

Tooth color

Color of human teeth differs by dentition: permanent teeth are darker and less chromatic than primary teeth. It differs by individual and by tooth type for the same person: incisors are in general the lightest while the canines are the darkest and most chromatic. It also differs for the same tooth, by the tooth area: from gingival to incisal, mesial to distal and buccal to lingual, and throughout the lifetime; "older" teeth are in general darker and more chromatic.[13,14]

The following color coordinate ranges of permanent teeth were reported: L* ranged from 56 to 90, a* ranged from –4 to 7, b* ranged from 4 to 39, C* ranged from –4 to 39, while H* ranged from 73 to 119.[15] When color of permanent teeth was compared by gender: female teeth were lighter, less red, and less chromatic, and the overall color difference (ΔE^*) was 3.0. The same was found for comparisons between bleached and nonbleached teeth, and teeth of smokers and nonsmokers: bleached and nonsmoker teeth were lighter, less red, and less chromatic, with $\Delta E^* = 4.6$ and 3.4, compared to nonbleached and smoker teeth, respectively.[16] In general, lighter teeth are less chromatic and less red, regardless of all variables mentioned above. Based on the literature, the 50:50 perceptibility threshold for teeth ranges from ΔE^* of 1 to 2,[17,18] while the 50:50 acceptability threshold ranges from ΔE^* of 2.7 to 3.5.[5,18,19]

Gingival color

Color range of healthy human gingiva is far beyond the "ideal" light pink. A lightness range from 27 to 81, a* range from 4 to 38, and b* range from 5 to 27 were reported.[20] Wide ranges of color coordinates make restoring color of the gingiva more challenging whether dental materials (ceramics, acrylic, or composite resins) or human tissues are used.[21] Restorations that do not primarily involve gingiva can also affect its color: partial dentures, implants, crowns, and veneers. Inflammation and tooth whitening can also cause reversible color changes of gingival tissue.

Skin color

There are numerous reports of dissatisfaction with the longevity, function, esthetics, or color stability of facial prostheses.[22–24] When perceptibility and acceptability thresholds for human skin replications were evaluated, significant differences were found by primary specimen color and type of threshold. CIELAB perceptibility thresholds for light and dark skin replications were 1.1 and 1.6, respectively. Corresponding values for acceptability thresholds were 3.0 and 4.4, respectively.[25]

Visual color matching

Tooth color is most frequently matched through visual comparison with dental shade guides. Visual comparison is subjective and to a certain extent inconsistent, and also includes variables such as color matching conditions, tools, and method. Several traditional myths persist: (a) dental professionals are gifted for shade matching; (b) females are better in shade matching than males; and (c) experienced practitioners are better than novices.

The truth is that ability to see and differentiate color for dental professionals varies from individual to individual, comparable to the general population. According to the results of the Farnsworth–Munsell 100 Hue Test, humans have 16% superior, 68% average, and 16% low color-discrimination abilities.[26] There is no professional vision research or dental research that supports female "supremacy" in color matching ability for color-normal individuals.[27,28] However, color deficiency is far more frequent in males (1 in 12, or 8%) than females (1 in 200, or 0.5%).

There is no sufficient evidence to show that those with more years of experience have superior skills. If experience has been with inadequate color matching conditions, inappropriate shade guides and color matching methods, this could hardly be considered good color training experience. Experience is important, but so is the status and age of the eyes. Typically a healthy 25 year old has better vision than a 50 year old. It would be beneficial to test color vision of all dental students and professionals using both conventional (nondental) and customized (dental) tests. Testing *color discrimination competency* (CDC) in dentistry has been described in the technical report by the International Organization for Standardization (ISO TR 28642).[12] The dental test includes matching pairs of tabs from two shade guides under controlled conditions and method. Superior, average, and low CDCs correspond to a score of 85, 75, and 60%, respectively.

Color matching conditions

Appropriate lighting and environment are of critical importance for work with color in dentistry. Poor color matching conditions can reduce chances for successful color matching before one even starts.

Lighting

When a wavelength of light is lacking in the light source, it cannot be reflected from the object being viewed. Full-spectrum color-corrected lighting is needed to elicit all the color a tooth is capable of reflecting. For example, teeth fluoresce a blue color when seen in a light source that includes ultraviolet energy (such as daylight). This blue fluorescence acts as a whitening agent, through the principles of additive color. Without getting into the technicalities, the blue light emitted by fluorescence neutralizes some of the yellow light and makes the tooth appear whiter. Therefore, the light source should have a near-ultraviolet component.

Daylight varies from morning to evening, with the cloud cover, the air pollution, and from any colored object from which it is reflected. Therefore, it is not recommended to use natural daylight for dental color matching; furthermore, the solution is just a "click away"—there is a huge selection of appropriate ceiling, portable (floor and table lamps), and hand-held lights (Figures 10.3 and 10.4).

There are several parameters that describe an ideal light for shade matching in dentistry. The first one is called *correlated color temperature* (CCT). Color-corrected lights resembling standard daylight at 5500 and 6500 K (D55 and D65) are recommended. Another key factor is termed the *color rendering index* (CRI)—a light source that has CRI of 90 or greater is appropriate. Lighting of these characteristics would have a *spectral power distribution* (SPD) that is similar to standard daylight. Finally, the light needs to be of adequate intensity, which is termed the *illuminance*, and measured in lux (abbreviated to lx). The level of illuminance at the color matching area should be 1000 lx.[1] More intense light, up to 1500 lx, might be used to overcome other ambient lighting. The importance of proper light intensity cannot be overemphasized: low intensity reduces our color matching ability, while the outcome of very intense light is similar: it can "wash out" color differences between the tooth and shade tab or restorative material. Light meters (lux meters, flash meters, exposure meters), like the ones used by photographers, should be used to control the illuminance.

High-quality lights are widely available in specialized stores and online. Sales people or customer support can provide invaluable help—one just needs to ask for color-corrected light of appropriate CCT, CRI, and light intensity.

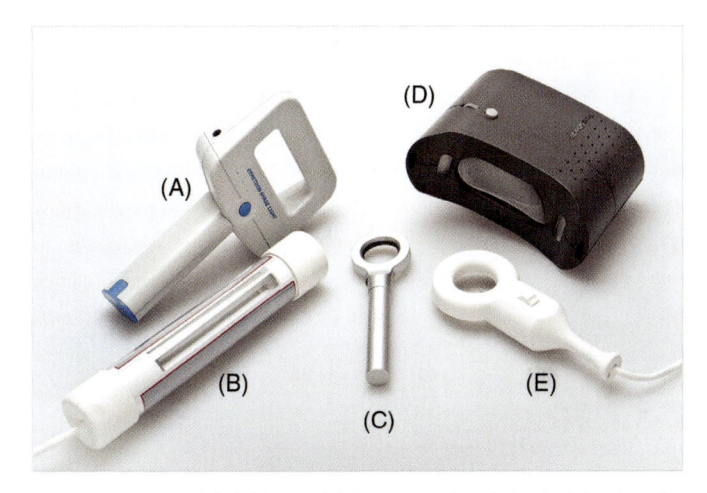

Figure 10.3 Hand-held lights. **(A)** Demetron Shade Light (KerrHawe); **(B)** Shade Wand (Authentic Dental Lab); **(C)** Ritelite (AdDent); **(D)** Optilume Trueshade (Optident); **(E)** Esthelite Shade Matching Light (EFOS).

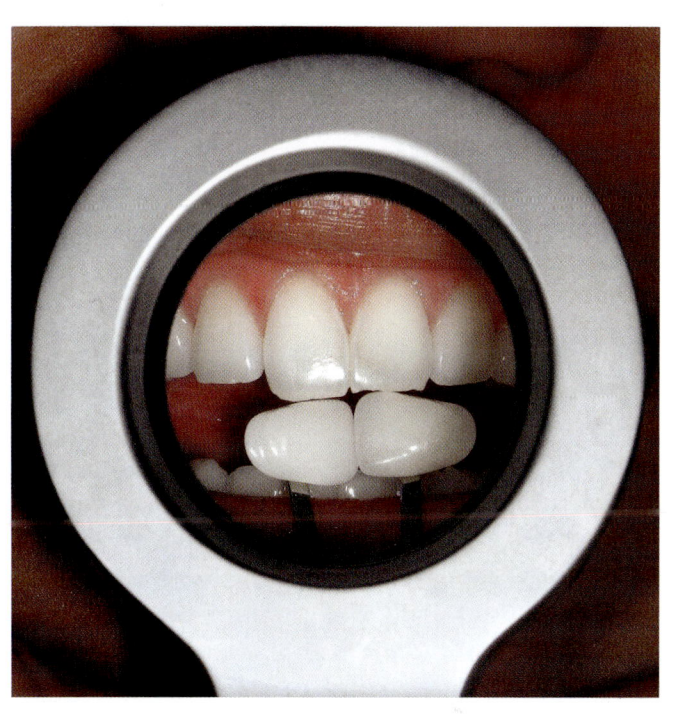

Figure 10.4 Color matching with a Ritelite hand-held light.

Metamerism

Teeth, shade tabs, and restorative materials are composed of different materials, and have different spectral curves. When the color of a pair of specimens having different spectral reflectance functions matches under one set of illuminant and observer conditions, but mismatches under another set of conditions, this phenomenon is called metamerism, conditional match, or non-spectral match, while these specimens are called metamers.[5] Inversely, specimens with identical spectral reflectance functions (spectral or unconditional match) are called isomers. There are several types of metamerism: *illuminant* (different lighting conditions), *observer* (different persons), *geometric* (different viewing angles), and *field size* (different viewing distances) *metamerism*. Ideally, dental restorations would match color of natural teeth under any of mentioned conditions. Because of the different nature and composition of hard dental tissues and dental materials this is not always achievable.

Environment

Shade matching environment encompasses the *background* and the *surround*. These two terms are closely related to *visual angle of subtense*, which is calculated from the size of the observed object and viewing distance. The background is defined as the surface upon which specimens are placed; the environment of the stimulus extending for about 10° from the edge of the stimulus in all, or most, directions. For tooth color matching, this would correspond to up to a 100 mm circular area around the tooth, and include adjacent teeth, soft oral tissues, lips, and skin. The surround is defined as the field outside the background.[12] In practical situations, the surround can be considered to be the entire environment in which the stimulus is viewed.[2] The surround should be matte and neutral light gray. Hand-held lights are very useful for overcoming the influence of the surround on color matching, especially when overhead lights are turned off.

Color matching tools—shade guides

Shade matching tools for visual shade matching are called dental color standards or shade guides.[5] Depending on their purpose, basic division encompasses shade guides for teeth (ceramic and resin-made shade guides), oral soft tissues, and facial skin. The latter two types are not routinely used in dentistry.

Tooth shade guides

Shade guides designed by Clark and Hayashi are among the most important shade guides historically. Clark created the Tooth Colour Indicator, a ceramic shade guide consisting of 60 ceramic tabs (Figure 10.5),[11] while the Hayashi shade guide consisted of all the combinations of five lightness, five chroma, and five hue levels, for a total of 125 printed chips. The Spectratone shade guide, consisting of 256 three-dimensionally arranged ceramic tabs, was also a noteworthy attempt to create a systematic dental color standard.[5] Logical order and adequate color distribution have been emphasized as two primary requirements for dental shade guides for a long time.[29-31] Current shade guides fulfill these criteria to different extents and they are divided into three main groups as follows:

1. VITA classical A1–D4
2. VITA System 3D-Master
3. others: proprietary or classical-proprietary shade guides.

The VITA classical A1–D4 (VITA classical, VITA Zahnfabrik, Bad Säckingen, Germany) was a gold standard for shade matching in dentistry for decades and to a large extent it still is. The vast majority of resin composites, dental ceramics, and denture teeth are keyed to this shade guide. VITA classical contains 16 shade tabs. The original tab division is known as the "A to D" arrangement (Figure 10.6a). The four groups are created based on hue: A is reddish-brown (A1, A2, A3, A3.5, A4), B is reddish-yellow (B1, B2, B3, B4), C is gray (C1, C2, C3, C4), and D is reddish-gray (D2, D3, D4). Within the groups, tab arrangement is based on increasing chroma and decreasing value—the higher the number, the higher chroma and the lower the value.[5]

An alternative tab arrangement, known as the "value scale," has been established according to the "degree of brightness," with no group division (Figure 10.6b). The value scale tab order

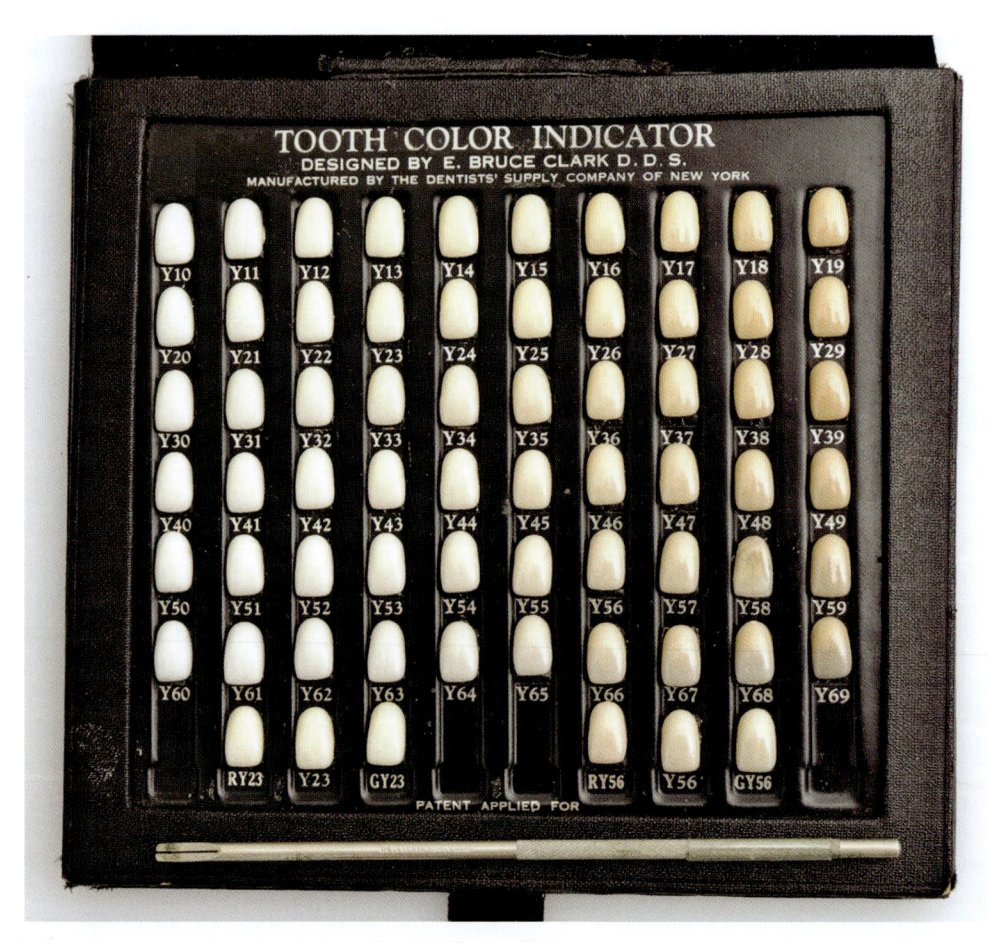

Figure 10.5 Tooth Color Indicator, a shade guide designed by E.B. Clark in 1931.

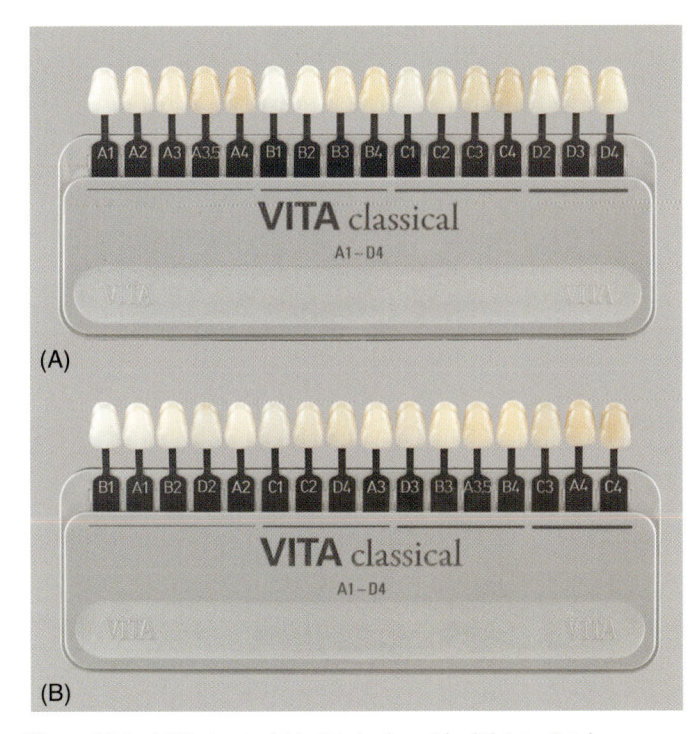

Figure 10.6 VITA classical A1–D4 shade guide: **(A)** A-to-D tab arrangement; **(B)** value scale.

is B1, A1, B2, D2, A2, C1, C2, D4, A3, D3, B3, A3.5, B4, C3, A4, and C4. The value scale is a gold standard for monitoring tooth whitening, expressed in *shade guide units* (sgu)—tab number (from B1, tab 1 to C4, tab 16) before bleaching minus the tab number after bleaching. Visual and instrumental change of 3, 4, and 5 *color change units* (ccu) of the value scale are the American Dental Association thresholds of clinical success for over-the-counter home-use tooth whitening products, dentist-dispensed home-use products, and professional in-office bleaching products, respectively.[32–34] The value scale is more logical and preferred by many over the A-to-D arrangement when it comes to color matching for dental restorations. However, several significant shortcomings of the value scale have been emphasized when it comes to monitoring whitening: (a) it does not correspond to visual light-to-dark order; (b) it has narrow range and inconsistent color distribution; (c) it is poorly correlated with the increase in chroma; and (d) it lacks very light tabs, which dictates exclusion of huge percentage of the population from whitening studies.[35,36] These concerns compromise findings on tooth whitening efficacy to a certain extent. Given its empiric nature and concept, and the fact that the classical was not originally designed for monitoring tooth whitening, the above-mentioned shortcomings are not surprising.

VITA System 3D-Master Shade Guides have been developed based on research on color of natural teeth. There are three 3D-Master shade guides: Toothguide, Linearguide, and Bleachedguide. 3D-Master tabs are marked using a number-letter-number combination. The first number designates the group and represents value, from 0 (the lightest) to 5 (the darkest). The letters L, M, and R represent hue: L corresponds to yellowish (or less red), M to medium, and R to reddish.

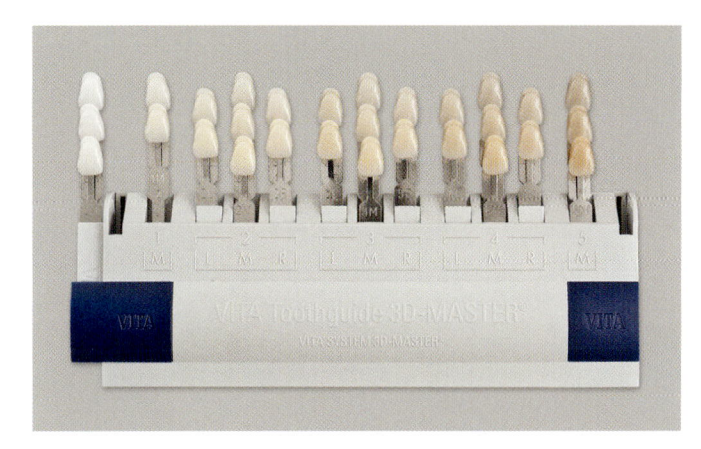

Figure 10.7 VITA Toothguide 3D-Master.

The number after the letter represents chroma, which increases from 1 to 3, with designations 1.5, 2, and 2.5 in between.

The VITA Toothguide 3D-Master (Figure 10.7) consists of 29 tabs divided into six groups according to lightness. Within the groups, tabs are arranged according to chroma (vertically) and hue (horizontally). Groups 0 and 5 have three tabs each; group 1 has two tabs, while groups 2, 3, and 4 have seven tabs each.[5] Shade matching with the Toothguide is basically a three-step procedure. In the first step, the value (group 0–5) is determined using the entire shade guide, thus reducing the number of possible shades. The second step is to determine chroma, while hue is determined in step three. Given that hue variations are present only in groups 2, 3, and 4, there are only two steps for groups 0, 1, and 5. This method can be challenging for those with little experience in tooth shade matching. The same is true for users with little knowledge about the physical background of the system.[6]

The VITA Linearguide 3D-Master (Figure 10.8) has the same shade tabs as the Toothguide. The differences are in its design and shade-matching method. Similarly to the Toothguide, the group selection occurs in step one, but using only a single linear scale that contains the middle tabs from each group (0 M2 to 5 M2, dark gray tab holder; Figure 10.9). The initial selection is simplified by a small number of tabs with huge color differences and the familiar linear tab arrangement. The second step is "fine tuning" by selecting the best match within the group selected in step one. The tabs from groups 0–1, 2, 3, 4, or 5 are placed into five separate light gray holders (Figure 10.10). The Linearguide 3D-Master was viewed as superior compared to the Toothguide and many users described the shade-matching method with Linearguide as self-explanatory and user-friendly.[37]

The VITA Bleachedguide 3D-Master (Figure 10.11) has been developed specifically for visual monitoring of tooth whitening. It has 15 shade tabs, marked in the same letter-number-letter style as the Toothguide and Linearguide tabs. The Bleachedguide tabs are also marked with odd numbers 1 to 29 sgu, representing 29 original 3D-Master tabs, from 0 M1 to 5 M3. Even numbers have been added as interpolated sgus, to comply with the American Dental Association recommendation that 1 ccu = 1 sgu = $1\Delta E^*$, and to increase its precision (when a tooth shade is in between two shade tabs) and sensitivity. Tooth whitening causes a decrease in chroma and hue, and an increase in lightness

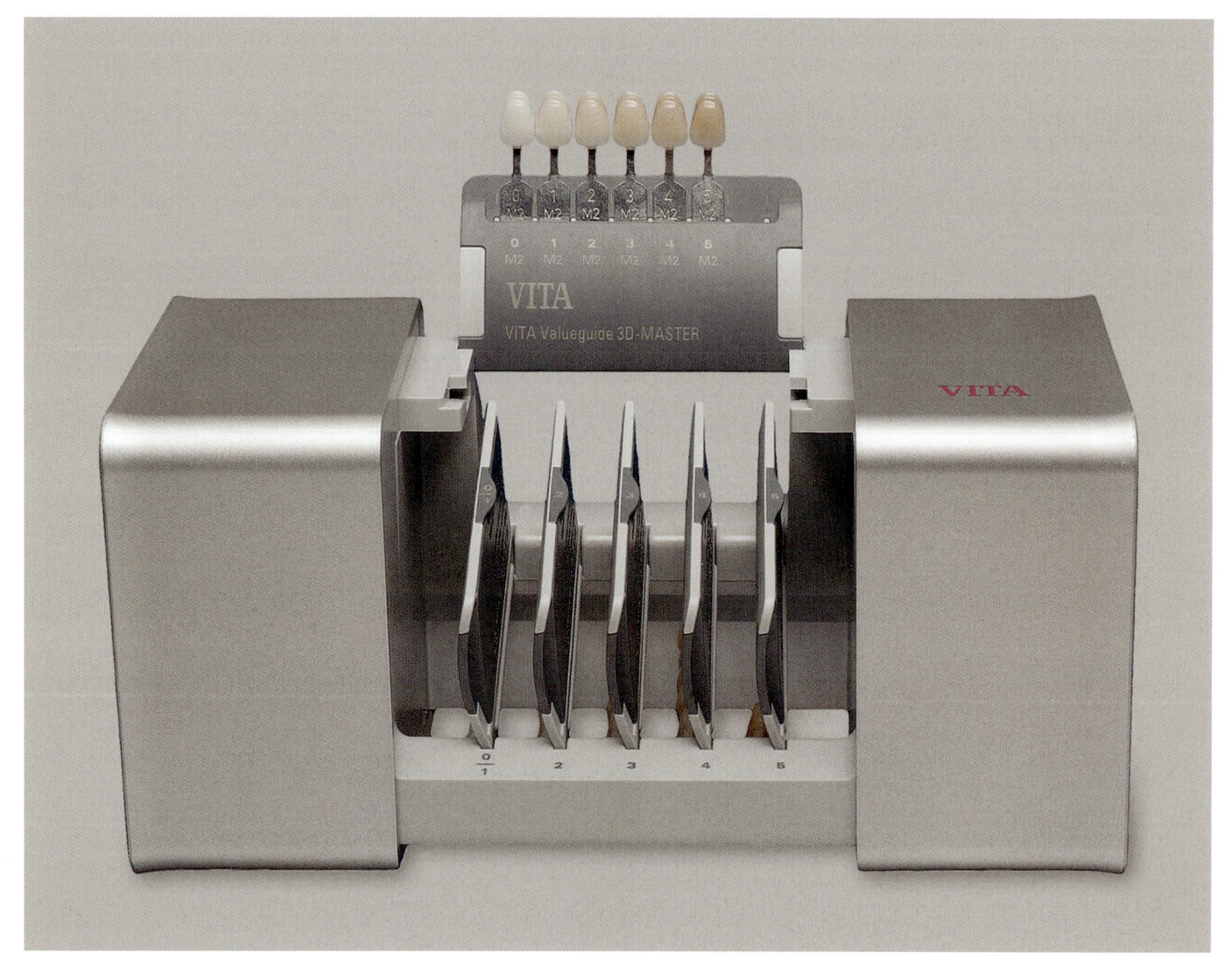

Figure 10.8 VITA Linearguide 3D-Master.

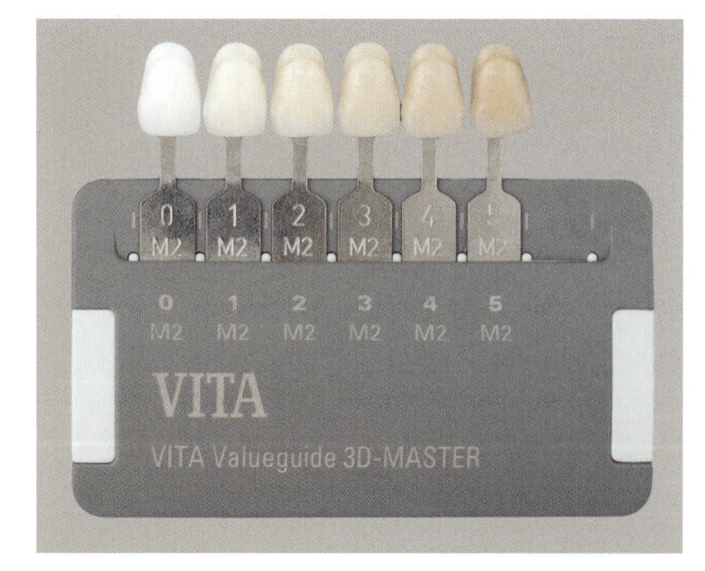

Figure 10.9 VITA Linearguide 3D-Master: dark gray holder for initial shade matching (step 1, select the group).

of natural teeth: changes in chroma are the most pronounced, followed by changes in lightness and hue. Chroma over lightness is called saturation, and it decreases upon bleaching (teeth are becoming less saturated). The Bleachedguide is a color scale (not a value, chroma, or hue scale), with lighter tabs being less chromatic and less red than the darker tabs.

Given the number of people who bleach their teeth and mentioned shortcomings of the classical value scale when it comes to monitoring whitening, the development of an advanced shade guide for this purpose was greatly needed. The Bleachedguide exhibits a wider color range and a more consistent color distribution than the classical value scale and some other products. Inclusion of very light shades and interpolated shade guide units further complement contemporary esthetic dentistry, starting from the fact that no patient inclusion/exclusion needs to be done based on their tooth shade before bleaching. Even a patient with the classical B1 shade before whitening can be included—this would correspond to number 6 on the Bleachedguide. This is a huge advantage compared to the classical value scale. In order

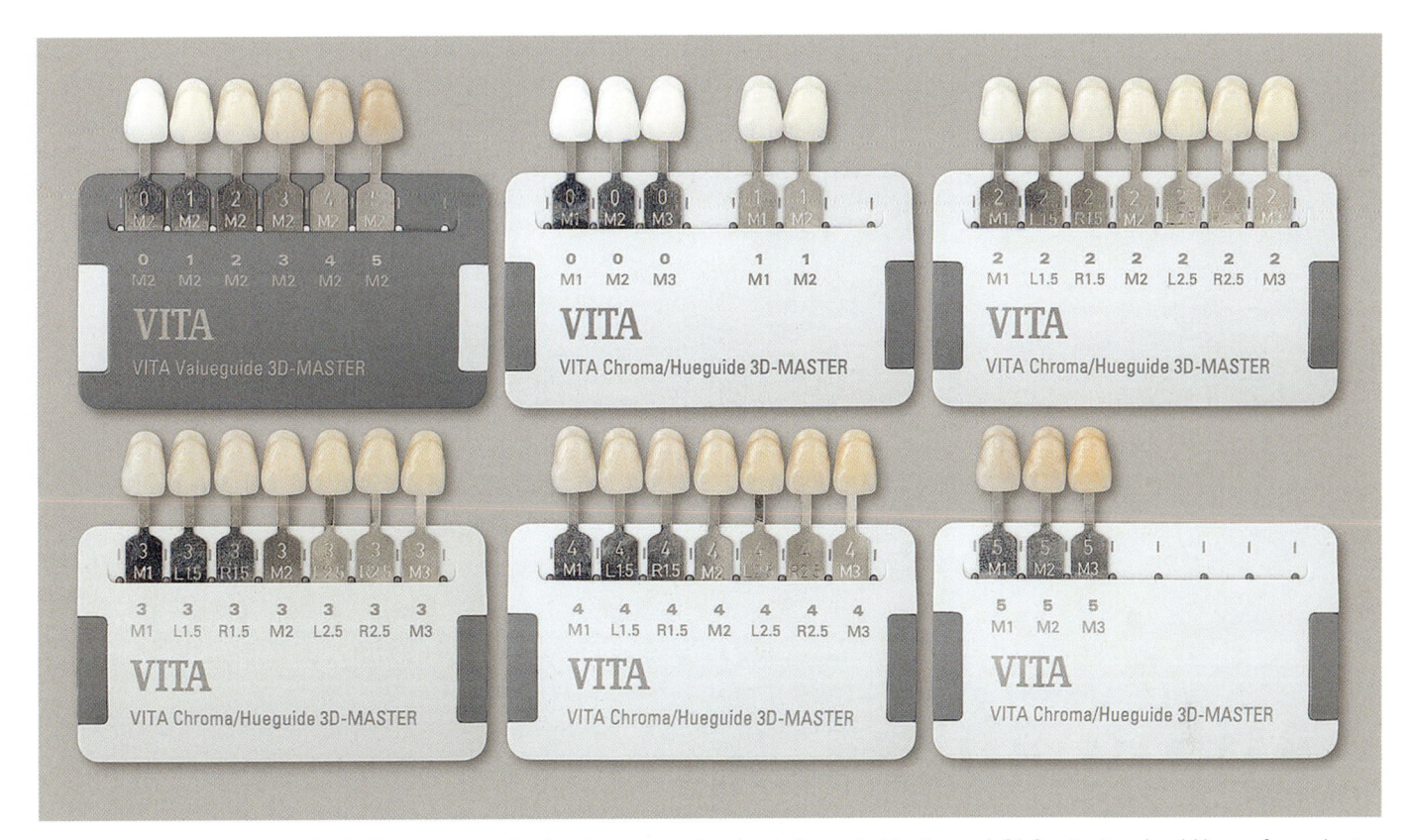

Figure 10.10 VITA Linearguide 3D-Master: upon selecting the group using the dark gray holder (upper left), fine tuning should be performed using the corresponding light gray holder (step 2, select within the group).

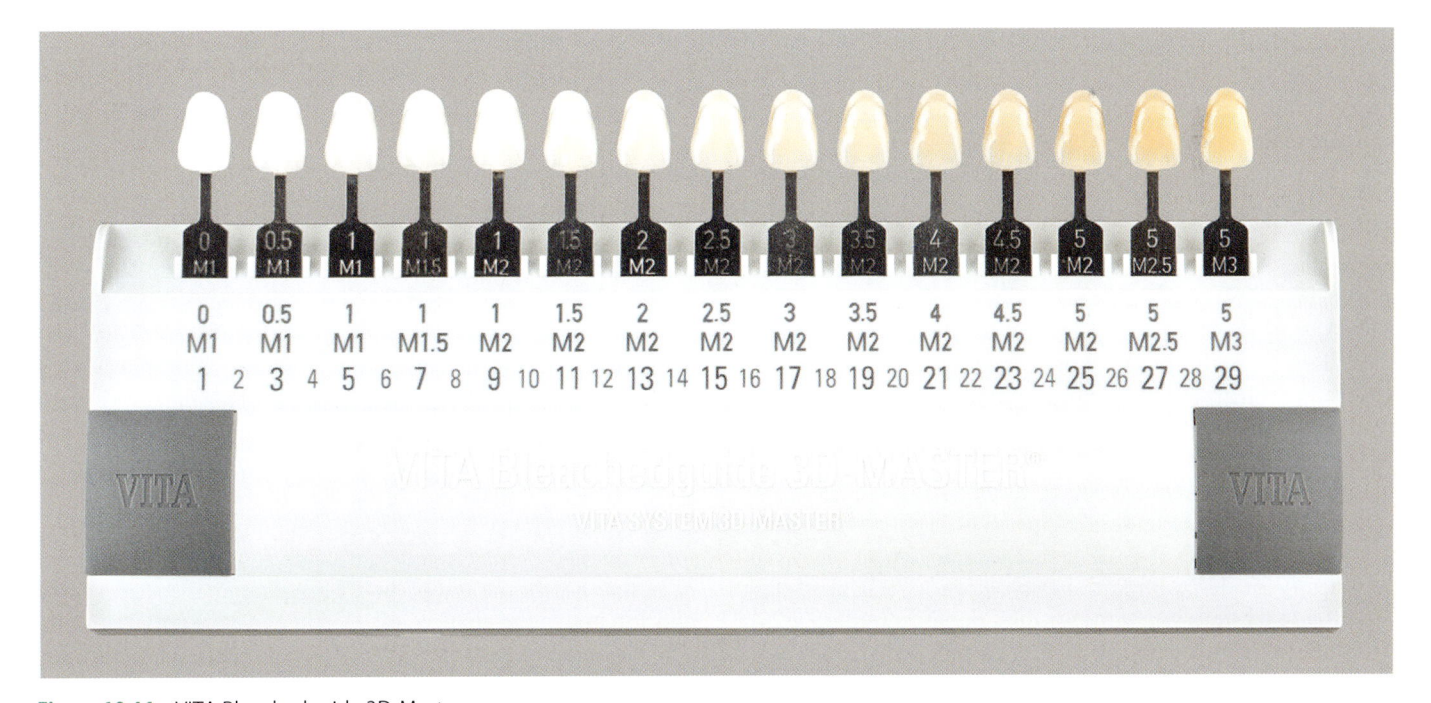

Figure 10.11 VITA Bleachedguide 3D-Master.

to compensate for a lack of lighter shades (lighter than B1), many studies included only patients whose teeth were A3 or darker before bleaching, thus excluding more than 52% of population.[13]

Proprietary or classical-proprietary shade guides: there are many shade guides made of dental ceramics, or single-layer or multilayer resins, with proprietary shades, or partly keyed to VITA classical (Figures 10.12–10.15).

The Ivoclar Chromascop (Ivoclar Vivadent, Schaan, Liechtenstein; Figure 10.12, top) is a proprietary shade guide with the same group division principle as VITA classical. It is

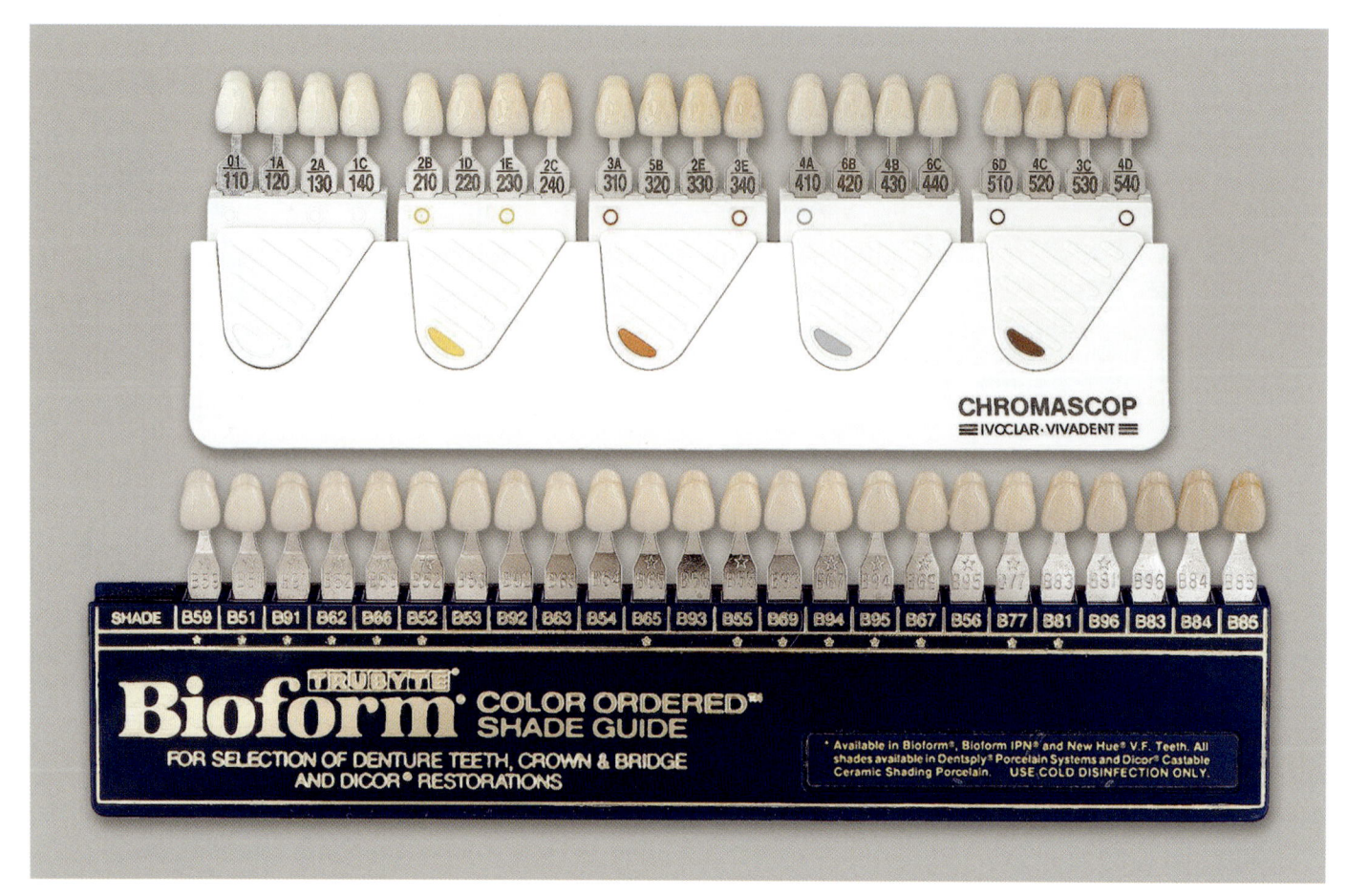

Figure 10.12 Proprietary or classical-proprietary shade guides: (top) Ivoclar Chromascop; (bottom) Trubyte Bioform.

divided into five groups according to the hue: group 1, white; group 2, yellow; group 3, light-brown; group 4, gray; and group 5, dark-brown. Each group consists of four tabs, marked by adding the numbers 10, 20, 30, or 40 after the group number (e.g., 310, 320, 30, and 340 for group 3). As in VITA classical, the tabs with higher number within each of the group are darker and more chromatic. A group 0, consisting of four extra light shades (010, 020, 030, 040), was later added to the original shade guide. In addition to the three-digit number marking, each Chromascop tab is additionally marked with a number-letter combination, without explanation on the meaning of these markings.

Trubyte Bioform (Dentsply International; Figure 10.12, bottom) is a classical/proprietary ceramics/resin shade guide arranged according to hue and as the VITA classical value scale. The former includes A-to-D classical arrangement and eight proprietary shades, while the latter represents a light-to-dark order of 24 tabs marked with two-digit numbers (order: 59, 51, 91, 62, 66, 52, 53, 92, 63, 54, 65, 93, 55, 69, 94, 95, 67, 56, 77, 81, 96, 83, 84, 85). As in many other shade guides, the additional bleached tabs are also available.

Pros and cons of tooth shade guides

Dental color standards are the only tools available for visual shade matching and should be used to their best advantage. Familiarity with these products, including the awareness of their good and bad sides, is probably the most logical starting point.

As mentioned previously, dental shade guides have different characteristics and indications. A single shade guide should not be used for all purposes. For example, VITA classical is the most frequently used shade guide in the dental profession, and it is appropriate for color matching for composites and ceramics, but much less appropriate for monitoring whitening. VITA 3D-Master shade guides enable the best color match to human teeth (see next paragraph) and have the most uniform color distribution. However, the Linearguide was found to be more user-friendly than its "peer," the Toothguide, and the biggest concern about this shade guide appears to be the absence of resin composites keyed to it. The Bleachedguide has been designed specifically for visual monitoring of tooth whitening.

Coverage error (CE) is a very convenient and simple method for evaluation of how well dental shade guides match the color of human teeth: the lower the CE, the better the shade guide and the better the chances of selecting an appropriate match. The CE actually quantifies the mean color difference between each evaluated natural tooth and the best matching tab from a particular shade guide. As shade guides are schematic representation of tooth color space, they have to have some CE. Although the reported CE values vary due to differences among color measurement instruments and techniques, it is evident that VITA classical and Trubyte Bioform have the highest CE, while VITA 3D-Master has the smallest CE. Other shade guides are in between these boundaries: Chromascop

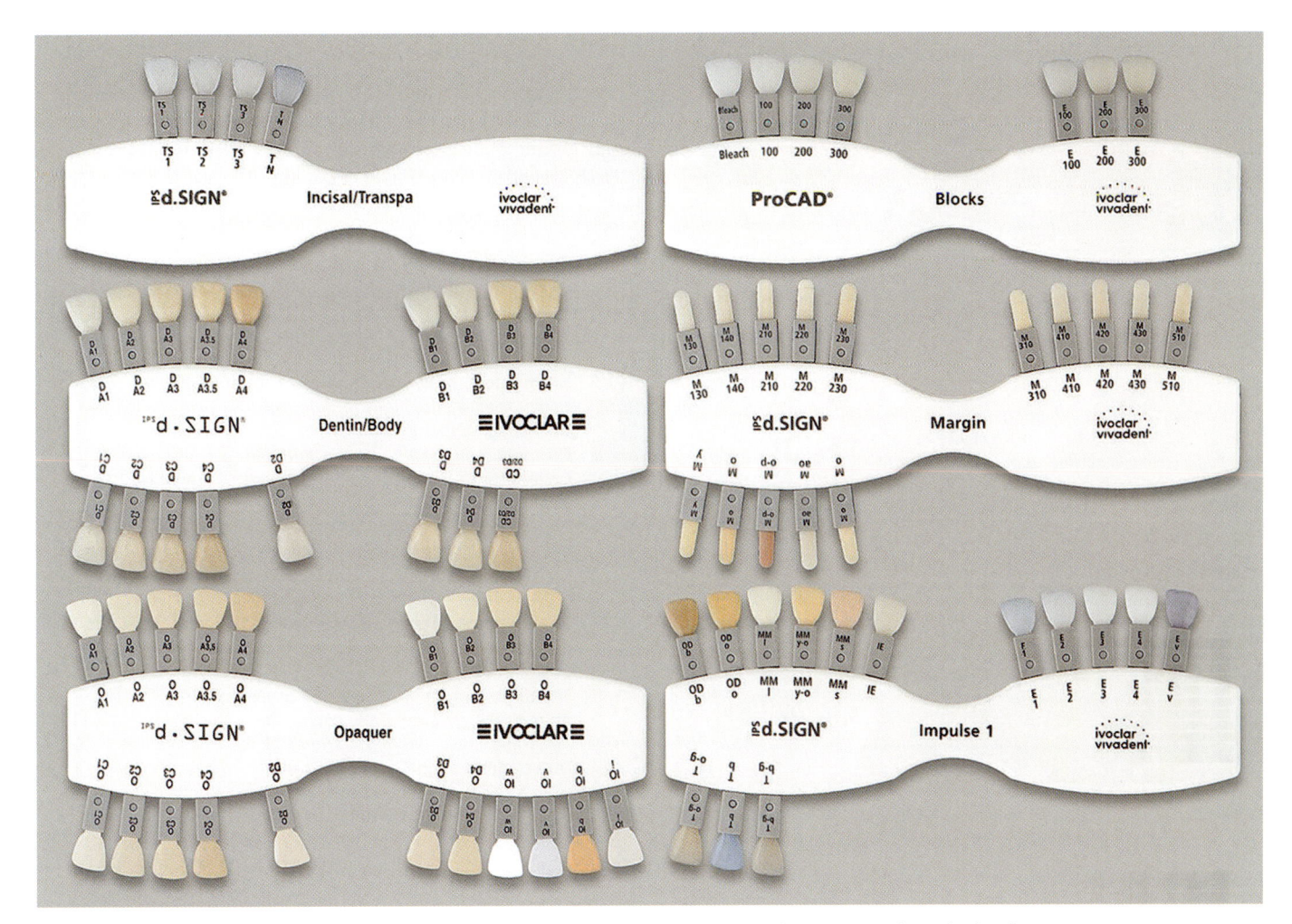

Figure 10.13 Proprietary or classical-proprietary shade guides for different layers and different materials, and color characterization (Ivoclar Vivadent).

and Vintage Halo are closer to classical, whereas Vintage Halo NCC is closer to the 3D-Master.[38]

Inadequacies of various dental shade guides have been reported many times in the literature and throughout this section. These concerns, summarized in Table 10.1, apply to some shade guides more than to others.

Shade Guides for Oral Soft Tissues

Color reproduction of the wide variety of shades of human gingiva and the other oral soft tissues requires the full attention of the dental profession. An esthetically pleasing result can be achieved by using adequate basic shades (custom or commercially made), by custom intrinsic and extrinsic characterization, or both. Ethnic differences and shade tab size, shape, and thickness should be taken into consideration when designing respective shade guides.

The Lucitone 199 shade guide (Dentsply Trubyte) consists of four glossy shade tabs of the same shape: original, light, light reddish pink, and dark. The IPS Gingiva (Ivoclar Vivadent) is a shade guide available in 10 shades: five "regular shades" (G1, G2, G3, G4, G5), four gingival modifier shades (GM1, GM2, GM3, GM4), and one gingival opaquer shade (GO). The Gummy gingival indicator (Shofu Dental) is available in three gingival shades (light, medium, and dark) and enables color matching combined with tooth shade tabs.[5]

Shade guides for facial prostheses

There is no gold standard for color matching of maxillofacial prosthetics—color matching and reproduction of a wide range of human skin are commonly performed using the trial-and-error method. Esthetic, social, and cultural demands suggest development of shade guides for facial prostheses for growing numbers of patients. Physical specimens that represent color of available maxillofacial materials and pigments cannot be considered skin shade guides. In addition, they are frequently limited to white skin shades, which is not adequate to serve the full ethnical diversity of our patients.[5]

Development of facial skin shade guides and color formulations for facial prosthetic materials can help clinicians achieve better and more predictable shade-matching results, thereby saving time and money. Furthermore, improving the quality of facial prostheses through the development of reliable facial skin shade guides will enhance quality of life for prosthetic patients. Another significant concern is poor color stability of some maxillofacial elastomers, and this issue has to be addressed simultaneously with the development of facial shade guides.

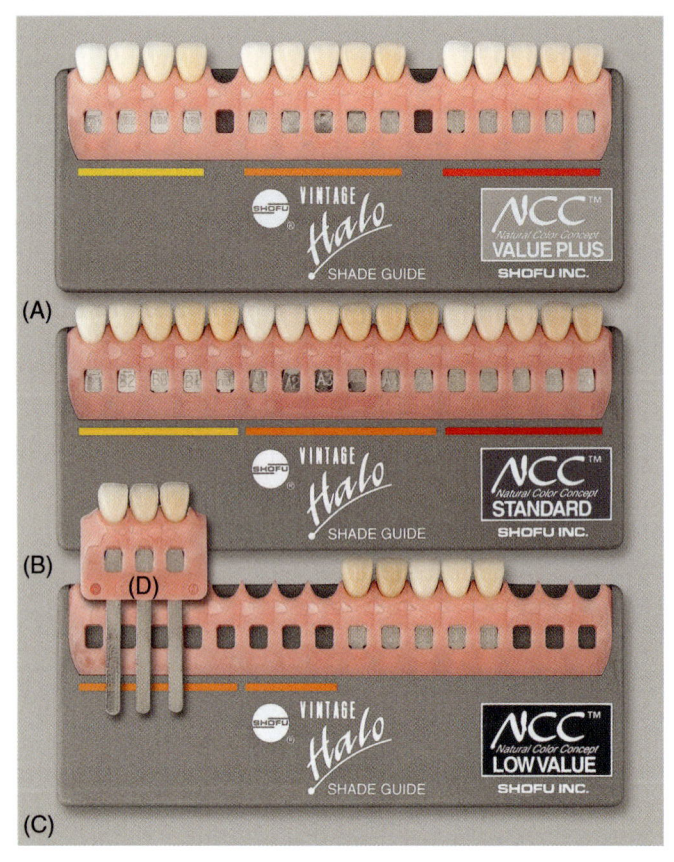

Figure 10.14 Proprietary or classical-proprietary shade guides, Vintage Halo NCC (Shofu): **(A)** Value Plus; **(B)** Standard; and **(C)** Low Value.

Color matching method

An adequate color matching method should complement the appropriate color matching conditions and the selection of the appropriate shade guide. This phase is of critical importance and "from the patient's point of view, the selection of a shade for the conservative anterior esthetic restoration that will match the

Table 10.1 Top 10 Concerns Regarding Some Dental Shade Guides

	Concerns Regarding Dental Shade Guides
1	Narrow color range compared to natural teeth; lack of darker and redder shades[7,31,39]
2	Uneven color distribution[30,40,41]
3	Different reflection curves compared to natural teeth[42]
4	Color differences among shade guides of the same manufacturer[43,44]
5	Shade guides keyed to VITA classical match color of original classical tabs with various success[5]
6	Lack of color stability of some resin-made shade guides due to factors such as disinfecting solutions, heat, and age[5]
7	Anatomy and optical characteristics of upper central incisors are not ideal for color matching of all teeth, especially posteriors[45]
8	Tab arrangement is sometimes confusing[46]
9	Shade tabs are frequently considerably thicker than the final restoration[40]
10	Other appearance attributes of shade tabs do not fully match natural and denture teeth, and restorative materials[5]

Adapted from reference 5.

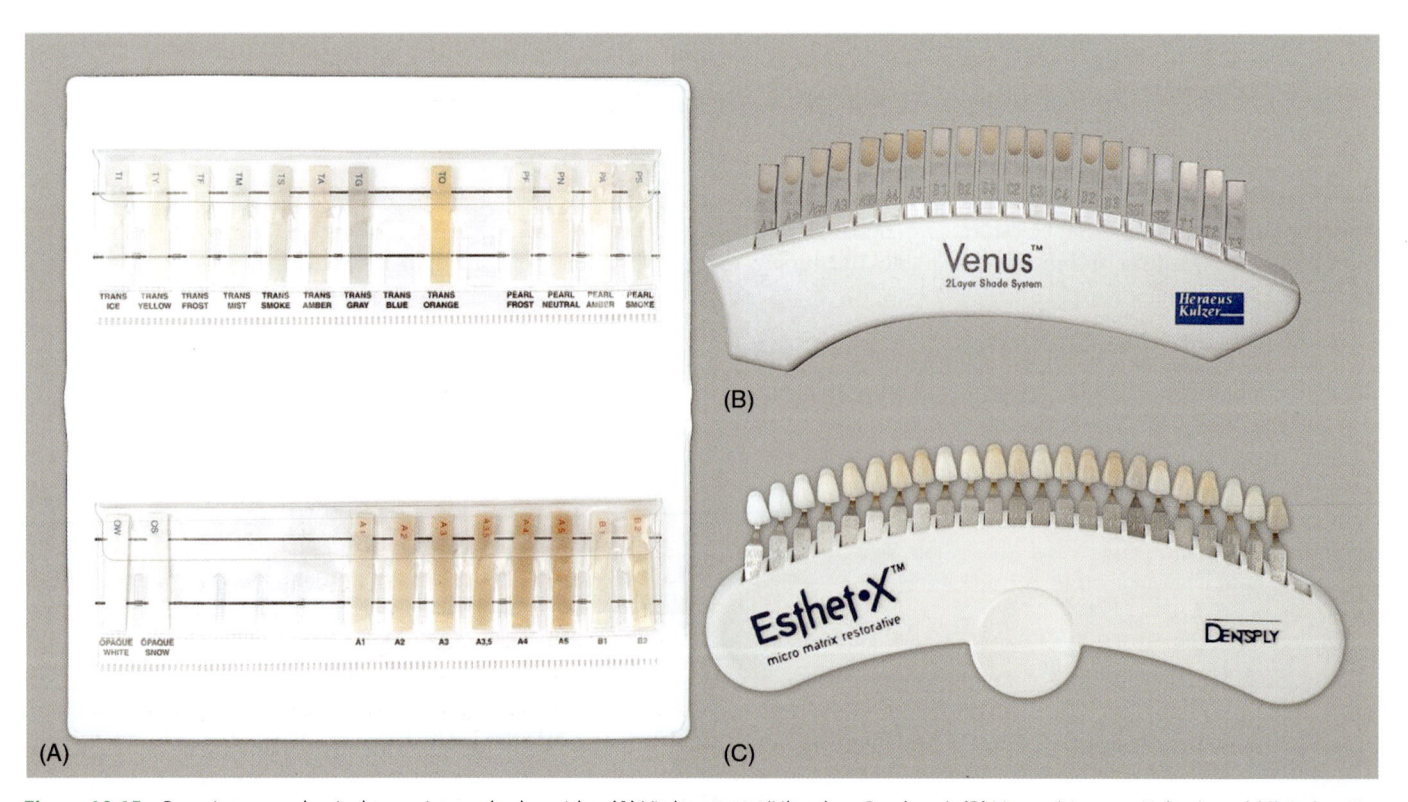

Figure 10.15 Proprietary or classical-proprietary shade guides: **(A)** Vit-l-ecsence (Ultradent Products); **(B)** Venus (Heraeus Kulzer); and **(C)** Esthet-X (Densply Caulk).

color and translucency of the tooth to be restored is probably the most important part of the appointment period."[47] Before the shade matching, patients need be asked to remove any lipstick and anything that could distract our attention or influence our judgment (large jewelry, eyeglasses, and similar). Teeth need to be cleaned and traces of prophy paste should be removed.[48]

Dental professional should not wear tinted eyeglasses or contact lenses while working with color as they can affect color perception. Shade matching should be performed at the beginning of the appointment as dentist eye fatigue and tooth dehydration could occur during the appointment—when teeth are allowed to dry out, they appear whiter and more opaque. The traditional belief that shade matching should be performed at arms' length is incorrect since that distance would create too small a *visual angle of subtense* (which, depending on the object size and viewing distance, should not be smaller than 2°).[1] Therefore, the arms' length distance would cause a decrease of visual precision. Color matching distance should be 25–35 cm.

The *optical geometry* is defined by the angle of illumination and the angle of viewing relative to the surface of the object. Several types of optical geometries are recommended for visual shade matching in dentistry. A 45°/0° optical geometry (45° illumination geometry/0° viewing geometry; Figure 10.16a) or a diffuse/0° optical geometry are more frequently seen in clinical shade matching. A 0° illumination geometry and 45° viewing geometry (Figure 10.16b) or 0°/diffuse geometry are more frequently seen in the dental laboratory setting. It is recommended to perform color matching using different lights because of the potential existence of illuminant metamerism. The dentist's eyes should be on the patient's tooth level. Whenever possible, shade tabs should be placed in the same plane and with the same relative edge position as the tooth. When the adjacent tooth is present, tabs can be placed horizontally or vertically in between the upper and lower teeth (Figure 10.4). The tab carrier should be along the tab's normal axis.[6]

The first impression of tooth color is frequently the most accurate. Since the vision pigment is used up quickly and to prevent the eye fatigue, an individual shade-matching trial should last 5–7 seconds, and the number of potentially adequate tabs should be reduced as quickly as possible. The traditional belief that it is good to gaze at a blue card between two shade-matching trials because this will increase the eye sensitivity to yellow is questionable. Staring at blue card will increase sensitivity to yellow, but it also provokes the chromatic induction effect, where a neutral field may appear slightly yellow. Therefore, one should observe a gray card between trials.

There is a huge difference between color dimensions and physical dimensions of an object (height, width, and length)—individual color dimensions cannot be distinguished when a single object is observed. What we see is the interaction of all three color dimensions. When we compare two objects, like in dental color matching, the eye cannot distinguish individual color dimensions of either tooth or shade tab, but can pretty accurately detect subtle color differences between them. However, our ability to detect the magnitude and direction of this difference (hue, value, and/or chroma) is much lower. Hue differences are, perhaps, the only dimensional differences that most individuals have been accustomed to judging with any degree of accuracy. Differences of value and chroma are often vaguely lumped together and used interchangeably. The danger in confusing a value difference (rod function) with chroma difference (cone function) is clear. It is evident that even with a correct level of one color dimension, differences in the other two may still prevent a color match.

It appears that "select the best match" is the best and most appropriate color matching method in dentistry (and in the best accordance with physiology of color vision). There is no standard combination or rule for the origin of color differences between tooth and shade tab or restoration.[5] The "dimension by dimension" method can be a subsequent, fine-tuning supplement once color matching using the former method is completed. This includes squinting for orientation about the value. Indeed, color vision can be excluded at scotopic (very low) levels of light, which is hard to achieve without sacrificing other useful visual information. However, a digital image converted to grayscale is a good alternative and can be beneficial for color communication and reproduction. The use of several shade

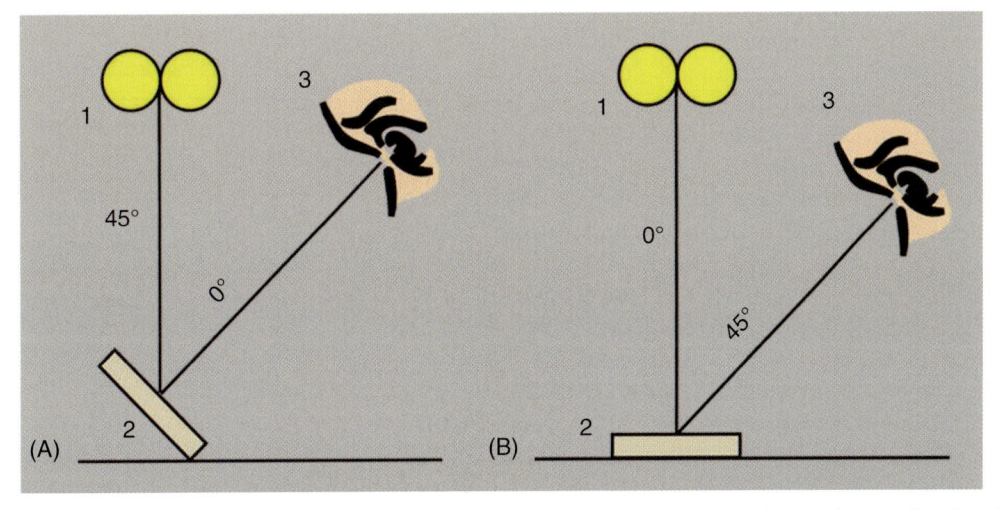

Figure 10.16 Illumination/viewing geometries for work with color in clinical and laboratory: **(A)** 45°/0°, more frequently utilized in clinical shade matching; **(B)** 0°/45°, more frequently utilized in dental laboratory (in both cases 1 = illuminant, 2 = tooth/specimen, and 3 = observer).

guides (and corresponding materials) would expand the choice of shades thereby increasing the likelihood of identifying a good match. The same is true for the use of extended shade guides, with the tabs representing different layers of the restoration.

Color transitions and local color characteristics of a single tooth sometimes dictate selection of more than one shade tab. The success of shade selection can also be enhanced by noting the color of dentin after enamel is removed. Color differences among different teeth of the same patient dictate selection of more than one shade tab for restorations of multiple teeth. Magnification is helpful to discern nuances of shading as well as the presence of any local color characteristics. Such custom color matching and reproduction requires more time, is more demanding of both the ceramist and the dentist, and yields greater satisfaction for everyone.

Other appearance attributes should also be visualized and matched. Translucency, denoting the state between total opacity and transparency, is probably the most important one. Translucency is the opposite of opacity—the higher the former, the lower the latter, and vice versa. Surface roughness and gloss are also of importance and could influence the tooth's appearance. The tab and the tooth should be wet with water in order to neutralize the influence of surface texture differences during color matching. Patients must also be made to understand that although a restoration, a single central incisor in particular, may look good in one lighting environment, it may not in another (metamerism). For this reason, the dentist may wish to select a shade in a specific critical environment.

Myths and facts about visual color matching

The myths related to visual color matching in dentistry and corresponding facts have already been elaborated throughout this section. In order to emphasize them, a summary is given in Table 10.2.

Color matching instruments

Dental color matching instruments and systems have potential advantage over visual shade matching due to their objectivity and ability to quantify differences in color and its dimensions compared to the closest match from different shade guides. Although hand-held color matching instruments are accurate and user-friendly, the role of dental professionals is still a decisive one—the more we know about instrument's features and limitations, the more useful they are for color matching, communication, reproduction, and verification. Instrumental and visual color matching methods complement each other and their combined use can lead toward predictable esthetic outcome.[49,50]

Spectrophotometers measure reflectance throughout the visible spectrum.[51] Two such devices will be described here: SpectroShade Micro (MHT Optic Research; Figure 10.17a) and VITA Easyshade V (VITA; Figure 10.17b). Both instruments consist of a cordless handpiece and a base unit.

The SpectroShade Micro is an imaging spectrophotometer that measures the complete tooth surface providing a tooth

Table 10.2 Top 10 Myths and Facts About Visual Color Matching

	Myth	Fact
1	Dentists are gifted for shade matching because of their ability to differentiate color.	There is no sufficient evidence that dental professionals can differentiate color better than others, but there is evidence that education and training can improve one's color matching skills.
2	Gender and experience influence shade-matching quality.	There is no sufficient evidence of this as far as color-normal individuals are concerned.
3	Northern daylight and huge windows are ideal for color matching.	Daylight is highly variable in color temperature and intensity, while tinted windows further limit this option. A plethora of excellent office/lab lighting is available.
4	One shade guide fits all (our needs).	No. Shade guide should be selected based on the purpose, restoration type, and selection of restorative material.
5	VITA classical value scale should be used for monitoring whitening.	VITA classical is an inferior product for monitoring whitening compared to a new VITA Bleachedguide 3D-Master (highly recommended).
6	"Tooth whitening" accurately describes the effects of bleaching.	Not really. All three color dimensions change upon bleaching: teeth become less chromatic (most pronounced), lighter, and less red (least pronounced). Overall, teeth are becoming less saturated (chroma over lightness ratio).
7	Arms' length is the best shade-matching distance.	Color matching distance should be 25–35 cm.
8	Observe a blue card in between shade-matching trials.	A gray card should be observed in between two color matching trials.
9	Matching one color dimension at a time is the best color matching strategy.	We cannot see color dimensions separately—we see only their interaction. Therefore, we should start by identifying the best color match and then potentially detect and describe differences in individual color dimension.
10	Squint to match value.	Very low levels of light can hardly be achieved without sacrificing other useful visual information. A digital image converted to grayscale may be a good alternative.

"color map." It uses a digital camera connected to an LED spectrophotometer, and an internal computer with storage capacity. Its software matches and calculates color differences between the tooth and selected shade tab, providing laboratory

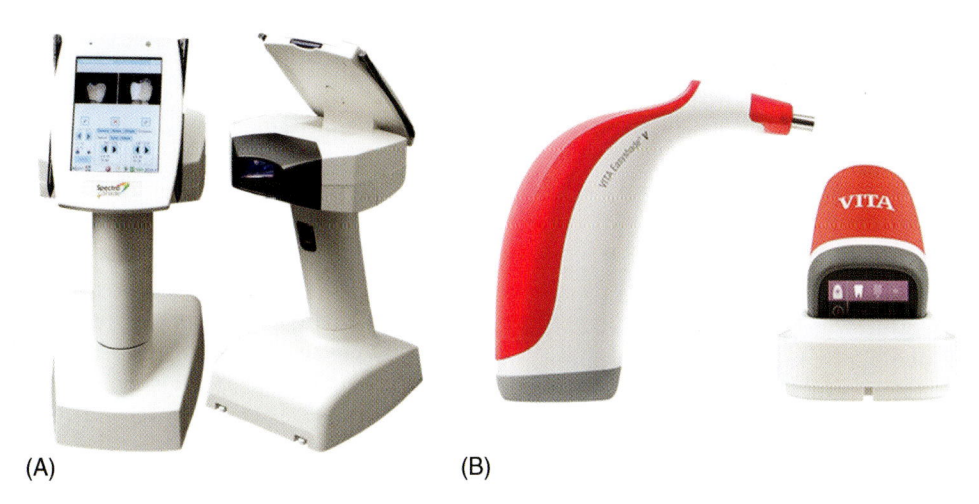

Figure 10.17 Dental color measuring instruments: **(A)** SpectroShade Micro; and **(B)** VITA Easyshade V. Figure courtesy of VITA Zahnfabrik.

information about lightness, chroma, and hue. Tooth positioning guidance system, shown on the LCD screen, enables controlled measurements.[52]

The VITA Easyshade V is the newest-generation spectrophotometer for tooth color matching, communication, reproduction, and verification. The device enables quality measurement through different mechanisms including neural network. Basic tooth shade or color by area, from cervical to incisal/occlusal third, is displayed in VITA classical A1–D4 and VITA System 3D-Master shades. The instrument also indicates adequate shades for computer-aided design/ computer-aided manufacture (CAD/CAM) materials, layered crowns, denture teeth, materials for direct fillings, and veneers. Calculation of bleach shades is an additional unique feature of this device. The Windows-based software VITA Assist and the smartphone application VITA mobileAssist enable Bluetooth communication between office and dental lab and communication with patients. According to some calculations, the savings in color matching costs using the Easyshade exceed $9000 per year compared to visual color matching, which is more than four times the price of the instrument.

Color matching instruments and systems have also generated significant interest from dental researchers. The topics investigated include evaluation of color of natural teeth, gingiva, skin, and various dental materials,[13,53] tooth whitening,[54,55] comparison with visual findings,[56,57] and performance assessment.[58–60] In addition to dental spectrophotometers, colorimeters, digital cameras, and scanners can be used to record color information and provide a detailed image of the tooth surface and useful color mapping.

Communicating color

Color matching and reproduction are complex procedures that can only be simplified by an understanding of the factors involved, and better controls at each step. The dentist and technician need to work together on effective communication, and invoke the controls needed to optimize results. The rewards outweigh the efforts, and the patient benefits as a result. Verbal and written instructions and sketches, modified and custom-made shade guides, and digital images as tools for communication on color and appearance will be described in this section. Traditional photography and slide films have been valuable methods to communicate color and appearance in dentistry in the past. They have been progressively replaced with digital imaging, and presently have only historical importance.

Verbal and written instructions and sketches

Verbal and written communication are the basic methods to communicate information on color and appearance. A detailed diagram or chart of the tooth is a valuable addition to verbal and written instructions and so are sketches of the color zones and variations in translucency. Such sketches do not have to be artistic renderings but should adequately define areas of transition between shades, relative translucency and transparency, and characterizing colors. They should include not only the facial view, but a labiolingual cross-section to indicate the relative thickness of each layer. Such sketches require a narrative describing the meaning of each part of the drawing. Often just making oneself look closely enough at tooth color to attempt to minutely describe it in sketches improves perception of the actual color components.

Modified and custom-made shade guides

When a tooth closely approximates a specific shade tab, but has characterizations or deviations, those variations may be defined and communicated using a shade guide with the glaze removed and a set of dental surface colorants ("stains"). Airborne particle abrasion using aluminum oxide is recommended to remove the glaze although this may also be done using emery discs. The colorant may be applied, and removed or modified until the proper effect is achieved. Once the shade tab closely resembles the tooth to be matched, it should be placed in a vial to avoid smearing, and sent to the laboratory along with a description of the colorants used and the effects desired.

Custom shade guides made of the actual restorative material, especially the ones having an expanded shade range, are another advanced communication tool. Although fabrication of such a guide is time consuming, it provides a more realistic representation of what is achievable. Fabrication of a custom guide for metal ceramic restorations should include a metal backing. In all cases, custom shade guides should be of realistic thickness, achievable with clinical restorations. Guides having varying textures and gloss may also be helpful.

Digital images

Digital imaging is a rapidly evolving field and permits the easy transfer of images from the clinician to the technician through electronic and storage media. Accordingly, the reference digital photography is highly recommended for communication on tooth color.[49] The photos should be taken with selected shade tabs in proper orientation in reference to the tooth. For consistent color communication, camera and light settings and image format must be kept constant. It is beneficial to have photo of the three basic shade tabs representing the respective color in gingival, middle, and incisal third, next to the tooth in question. Photos of two additional reference shade tabs should be included to graduate and calibrate shifts in hue, chroma, and value between physical tabs visually in the laboratory. One of these tabs should be lighter in shade and one darker in shade in respect to the selected basic shades.

The digital image gives a vivid description of the relative translucency, opacity, color zones, and incisal variation. Although the technique requires photographic equipment, the cost of improved shade selection is rapidly offset by avoiding remakes and disappointment. Accurate information on color and appearance obtained through visual and instrumental shade matching combined with standardized reference shade communication photography can ensure a predictable esthetic outcome.[49]

Color modification

Color modifications may be either intrinsic (at the time of fabrication) or extrinsic (surface coloration). Without unnecessarily complicating this explanation, suffice it to say that the principles of modifying a restoration, either intrinsically or extrinsically, involves subtractive color mixing (as one adds color, the resulting color gets darker), and the use of complementary colors (colors of the "opposite" hue). For example, when modifying a completed restoration using surface colorants, the surface color blocks some bands of the spectrum (hues) and the resulting appearance is usually lower in value (less bright).

If the ceramist fabricating the restoration is familiar with the dimensions of color, some of the modifications may be accomplished during fabrication. If not, choosing a shade that is higher in value and lower in chroma will keep the restoration in the proper volume of color space that permits successful modification at the chair side. Of course, the dentist must have the proper materials and equipment to make such modifications, as well as the time and desire to do so. A few simple and relatively inexpensive supplies and pieces of equipment are needed including a selection of colorants for porcelain (usually termed "stains"), high-quality sable brushes, a ceramic or glass mixing surface, and a glazing oven in which to fire the restorations. Any porcelain furnace will suffice. Vacuum or sophisticated circuitry is not needed for glazing, but the unit should have automatic (and accurate) temperature control that will signal to the operator when the desired temperature has been reached.

Porcelain fusing is a result of time and temperature, so a restoration can be taken more rapidly to a higher temperature, or to a lower temperature and held at that temperature longer. Since porcelain is also a product of its thermal history, the type of porcelain and the number of times it has been fired as well as the temperatures used in fabrication will determine the temperature at which the desired maturation will occur. The smoothness and surface gloss must be visually inspected to evaluate the proper glazing temperature.

The choice of materials is optional, but it should evolve through a cooperative effort of the technician and dentist. "Stains" are metallic oxides in a modified porcelain base. Even though most stain kits use the same color names, the actual colors vary widely. Colorants from a number of kits may be used to supply the desired colors. The most useful colors are orange, yellow, violet, gray, and browns of different hues and concentrations, and whites of different translucencies. Violet is useful for neutralizing the basic hue, reducing chroma, and giving the appearance of a more gray (lower value) and translucent appearance of the incisal one-third. Brown plus the dominant hue will lower value, and increase chroma in the cervical portion. Yellow and orange are helpful in hue changes. White, gray, orange, and brown may all be used in characterizing.

There is no question that intrinsically building color in a tooth produces a superior restoration and is the preferred technique. Surface modifications should be reserved for minor changes to improve the initial results. This section is not intended as an extensive treatise on the technique of surface coloring but rather to point out the principles involved.

Color-related properties of dental materials

Esthetic dental materials have undergone amazing improvements related to optical properties during the last decade. Materials are now available that exhibit satisfactory color compatibility, good color stability, and color interactions that could reduce color mismatch, such as blending and layering (Table 10.3).[6]

Table 10.3 Color-Related Properties of Dental Materials

Property	Subdivision
Color compatibility	With natural teeth;[13] among restorative materials[61,62]
Color stability	During fabrication/at placement: firing/polymerization/other types of setting[63,64]; after placement: aging, staining[65]
Color interactions	Layering[66–68]; blending (chameleon effect)[69,70]

The material selection is an important component for the esthetic outcome. The "same hand, different outcome" results based solely on material selection is common in dentistry. Frequent updates from professional publications and other sources listed in the following section on color education and training can reduce this problem.

Color education and training

A clear conclusion on the importance of color education and training in dentistry can be drawn based on the statement of Sproull: "The technology of color is not a simple matter that can be learned without study neither is it a complicated matter beyond the comprehension of dentists."[7] Research on this topics and current publications and programs will be presented in this section.

Surveys

The first survey on education on color in dentistry was performed in 1967. Only three out of 115 institutions that responded had a color science course, with an average of 2.3 classes.[7] The results of the second survey were published in 1990. A total of 69 dental schools responded: courses on color were taught at 26% schools in core curriculum and at 17% as an elective course.[48] A survey from 1992 reported on 138 responses with an average of 6.6 hours on color-related topics.[71] Finally, the most recent survey, published in 2010, reported on teaching of color at 130 institutions. A course on "color" or "color in dentistry" was included in 80% of predoctoral and 82% of postdoctoral programs, with an average of 4.0 and 5.5 hours, respectively.[15]

The substantial increase of interest in color in dentistry is followed by the increase in number and variety of publications and programs. A Medline search using the keywords "color" and "dentistry" and limited to the time of the first survey (1967) returned fewer than 50 papers. On the other hand, more than 6500 papers were listed when the search was performed without the time limitation (at the time this chapter was prepared).

Current publications and programs

It has already been noted that many changes have occurred since the times of the first survey on color in dentistry. This includes the changes in color research, education, and training resources compared to the times and pioneer work of Sproull, Bergen, Preston, and Miller.[7,11,19,29–31,40,72] Currently available specialized resources are listed in Table 10.4.

The specialized publications and programs should be combined with nonspecialized resources such as Medline, clinical and research journals, meeting proceedings, and independent evaluation sources (US Air Force Dental Evaluation & Consultation Service, Dental Advisor, Clinicians Report, Reality Publishing, and similar).

Dental Color Matcher (DCM) is a free online color education and training program for esthetic dentistry, hosted through the SCAD website (www.scadent.org). This program is also available as a CD (Figure 10.18). The DCM is in essence a computer game and it consists of several different interactive color matching exercises: there are closest match (there in no exact match), exact

Table 10.4 Currently Available Specialized Resources for Color Education and Training

Resource (Publisher)	Format and Features
Color in Dentistry – A Clinical Guide to Predictable Esthetics (Quintessence Publishing)[73]	Clinically oriented textbook, appropriate for students, general practitioners, and specialists. Content: basics of color theory, followed by chapters on conventional and technology-based shade matching, digital photography, material selection, predictable color reproduction, and clinical cases
Esthetic Color Training in Dentistry (Elsevier)[5]	Research-oriented textbook with color training program on CD-ROM
Society for Color and Appearance in Dentistry, SCAD (www.scadent.org)	Professional group that promotes interdisciplinary collaboration and discovery among researchers, clinicians, and laboratory technicians, and relevant educational and training programs for dental professionals and students
Special Issues on Color and Appearance in Dentistry (Wiley Blackwell)	Peer reviewed journal, a permanent semi-annual issue of *Journal of Esthetic and Restorative Dentistry*
Dental Color Matcher, DCM (SCAD; VITA Zahnfabrik)[6]	Free online educational and training program for esthetic dentistry, www.scadent.org
Dentistry – Guidance on Color Measurement (ISO/TR 28642)[12]	Terms and definitions, visual and instrumental color assessment, qualification of observers, testing and interpretation of acceptability and perceptibility thresholds, reporting of color and color difference measurements
Color and Shade Selection for Prosthodontics (American College of Prosthodontists)[4]	Educational DVD; figures and instructional videos complement the text
Toothguide Trainer, TT and Toothguide Training Box, TTB (VITA Zahnfabrik)[74]	Color training program, software (TT), and physical shade tabs (TTB)

Adapted from reference 73.

match, and match the pairs exercises (Figures 10.19 and 10.20). VITA Linearguide 3D-Master is used in all exercises in the fashion described in the section on tooth shade guides (step 1: select the group from the dark gray holder; step 2: select the best match using corresponding light gray holder/s). Six different achromatic backgrounds are available for shade matching. In the exact and best match exercises, tabs are placed over the image of the upper edentulous jaw. Users can place up to two tabs next to the target tab (one on each side), and hide everything except

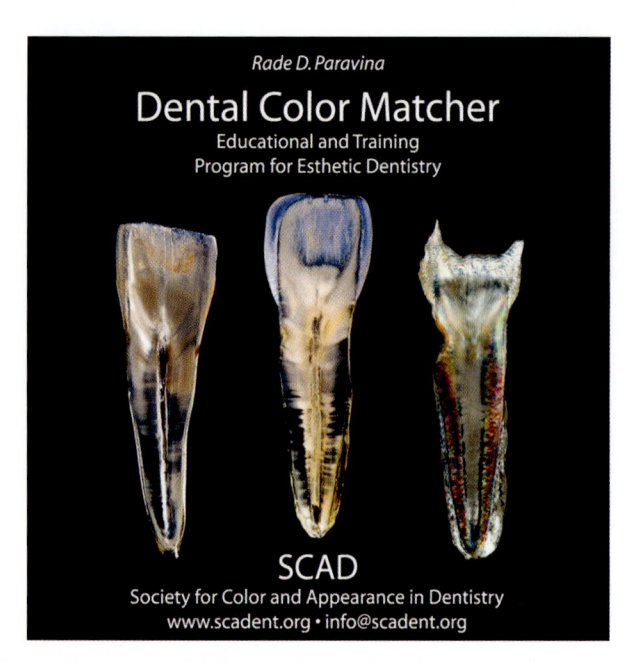

Figure 10.18 Dental Color Matcher, a color education and training program for esthetic dentistry: CD cover (also available online at www.scadent.org).

the immediate working area if distracted. In the "matching pairs" exercises, users are asked to separately match 15 lighter pairs and 14 darker pairs of Linearguide tabs. Breaks (light gray screen) are available during and in between all color matching exercises. A 20-minute didactic video addresses color matching conditions, tools, and techniques, while a 12-question quiz brings additional competitiveness. A diploma and two continuing education hours are available upon the program completion. DCM has had thousands of registered users from more than 100 countries since its September 2010 release.

Bottom line: education and training

Perceiving and analyzing color is a skill that can be taught, and one that can be improved with practice. Significant advances have occurred in color education and training resources in dentistry. Regardless of the differences, all mentioned resources have the same intention—to educate dental students and professionals on color and appearance in dentistry. Resources are available, now it is up to us to implement the philosophy of Thomas Jefferson, third president of the United States: "I'm a great believer in luck, and I find the harder I work the more I have of it". Indeed, we can't afford to have an undeveloped potential.

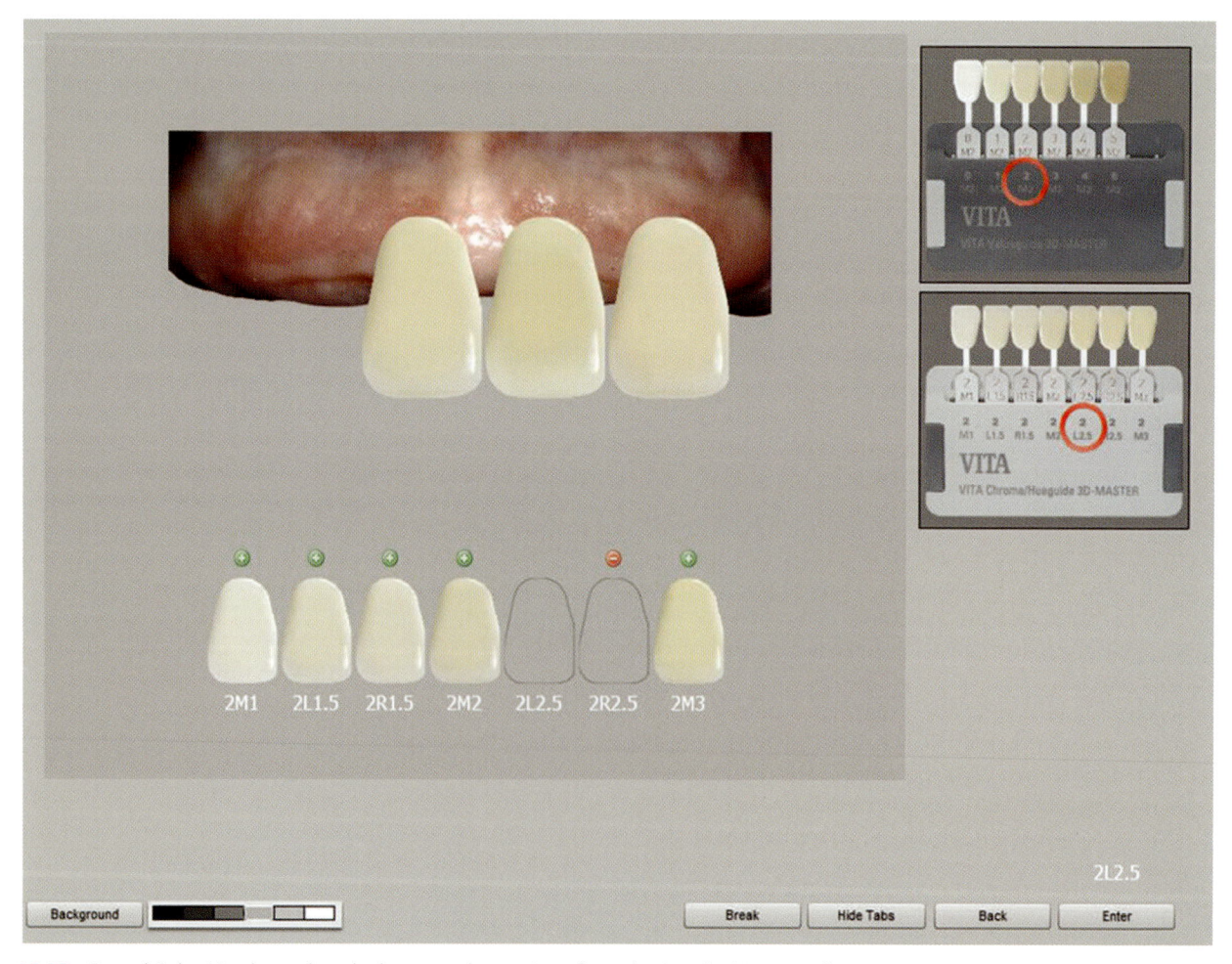

Figure 10.19 Dental Color Matcher, select the best match exercise: after selecting the Linearguide group in step 1 (group 2 tab is circled in red in a dark gray holder, upper right corner), optional matches have been selected in step 2 (select within the corresponding group); the first choice (2L2.5) is on the left (circled in red in a light gray holder underneath the dark gray holder), the target tab is in the middle, while the second choice (2R2.5) is on the right; a variety of achromatic backgrounds is shown.

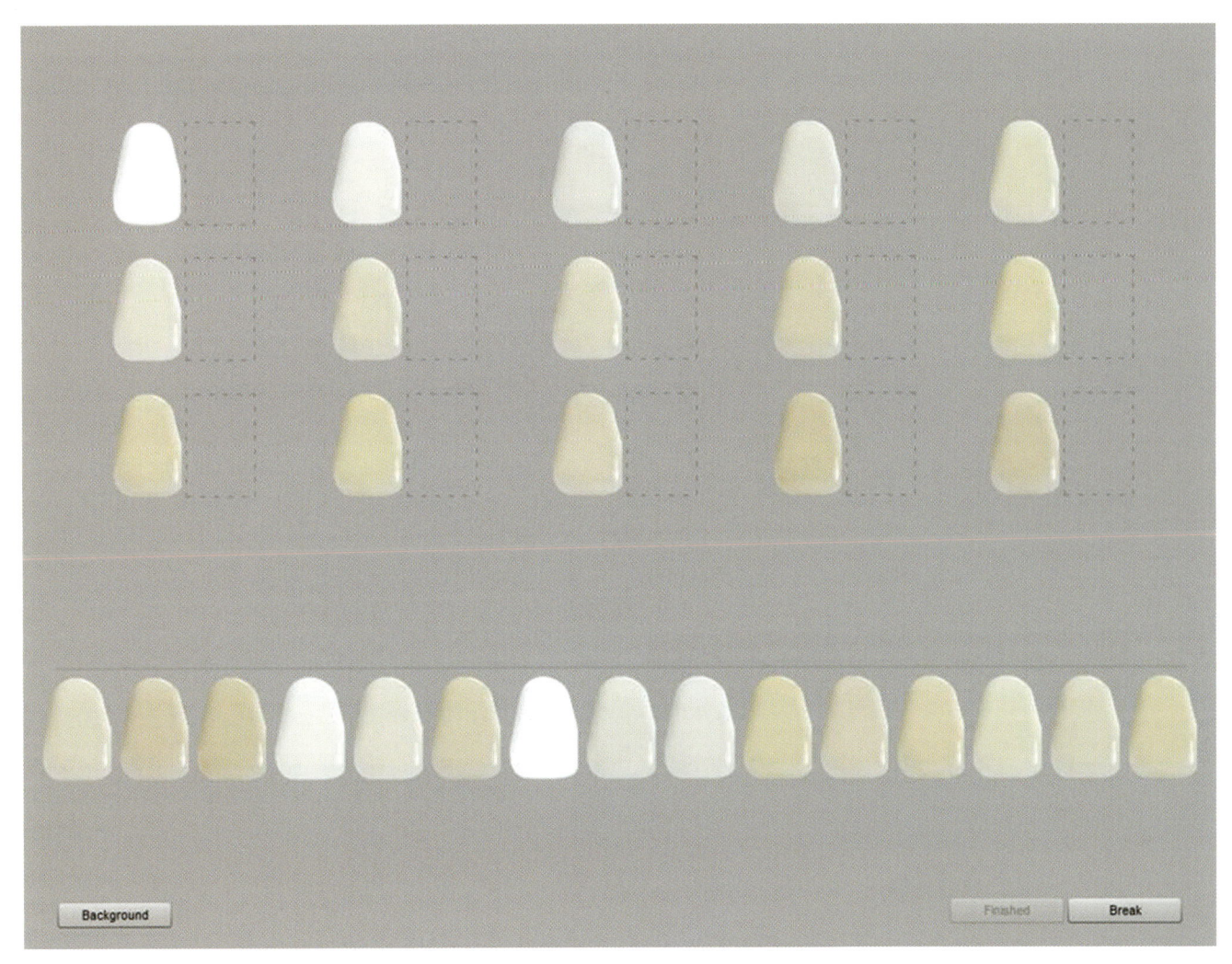

Figure 10.20 Dental Color Matcher, match the pairs exercise (light pairs): each of 15 tabs from the bottom row need to be arranged (using the drag-and-drop technique) next to the corresponding tab in the upper three rows.

Case study: Class IV restoration by Newton Fahl, Jr, DDS

This book details various aspects of esthetics dentistry and elaborates the most advanced materials and techniques for achieving the predictable success. The following case study demonstrates the ultimate synergy between art and science in reproduction of color and appearance. The technique used and thinking outside the box added an additional flavor and resulted in a superb esthetics.

Figure 10.A1 A defective Class IV restoration is present on the left central incisor and needs replacement.

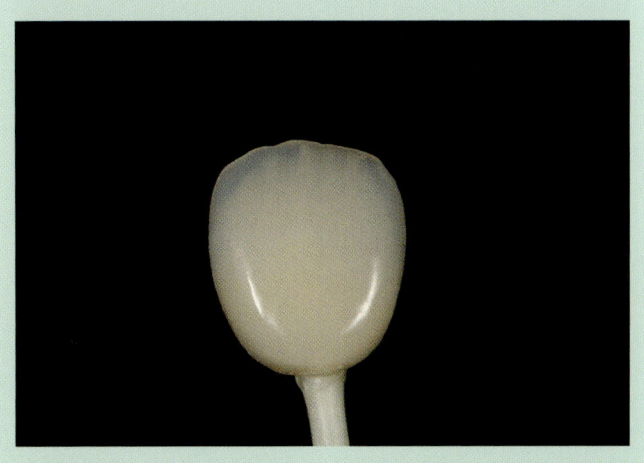

Figure 10.A2 Shades are selected for the composite resins to be used and are layered to form a color mock-up tab according to the precise thickness and contour of each layer.

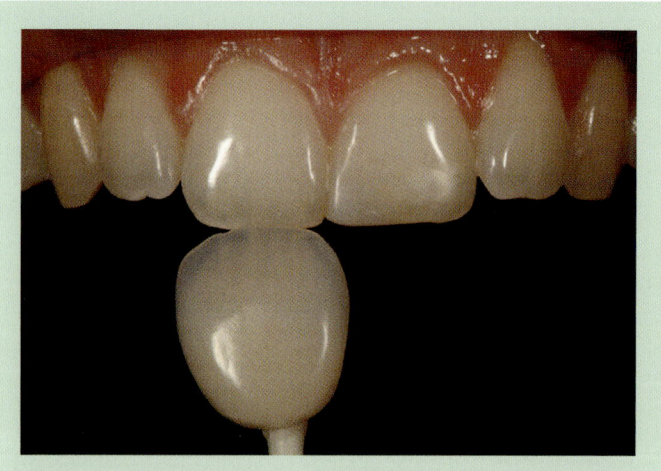

Figure 10.A3 The associated shades are compared to the natural tooth used as a color reference and aspects such as opacity, chroma, hue, value, and opalescence are ascertained. At this stage, the operator decides on changes in material selection and thickness of each layer to be implemented during the final restorative steps.

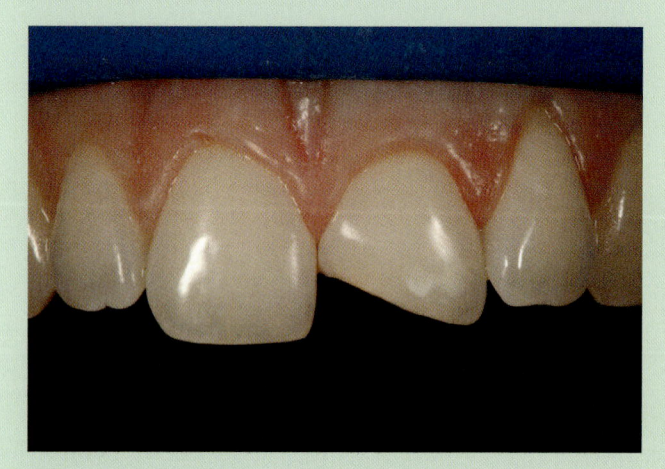

Figure 10.A4 Tooth preparation is carried out by placement of a 2.5 mm long bevel on the facial aspect and a small chamfer on the palatal aspect. The long, thick, and infinity-line bevel provides for generating a smooth optical gradient from tooth to synthetic materials after completion of the restoration.

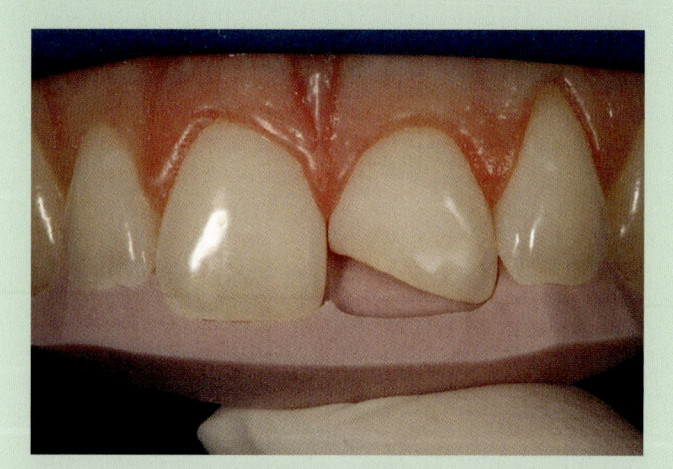

Figure 10.A5 From a wax-up model or an intra-oral mock-up, a silicone matrix is made to be used as a three-dimensional reference for the establishment of palatal contours and, most importantly, the incisal edge position.

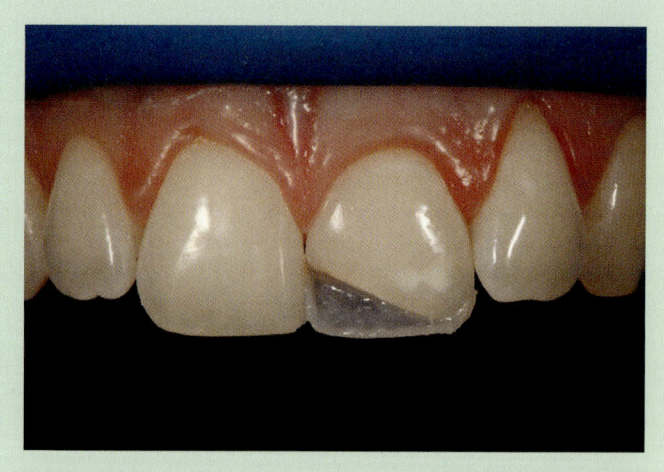

Figure 10.A6 A milky-white semi-translucent layer of composite is applied to the silicone matrix and sculpted to conform to the shape of a "lingual shelf." This layer should be approximately 0.3 mm in thickness but the incisal halo can be made slightly thicker to impart a more marked opalescent amberish-white appearance. Light curing is carried out and the silicone matrix is removed. For the application of the subsequent layers, there is no need for the use of the matrix because the three-dimensional landmarks are already established with this layer.

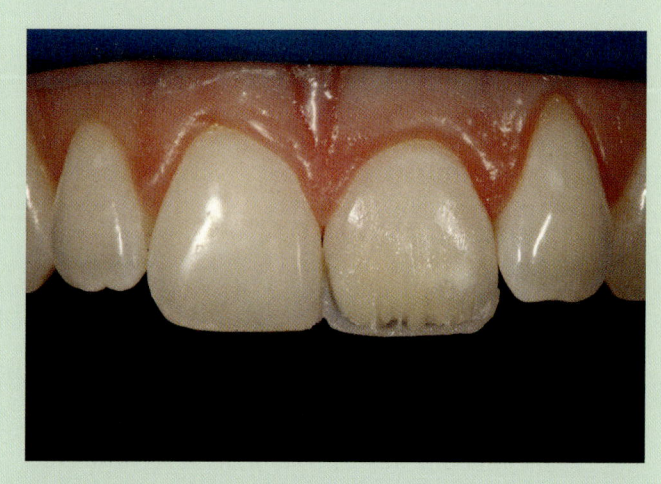

Figure 10.A7 A dentin composite resin of a chroma one tone higher than the intended final chroma is applied and contoured to mimic the histological boundaries of a natural tooth. The exception to this is present at the bevel area, where the artificial dentin should cover the beveled enamel about half of its width. The key element at this stage is to be able to fully conceal the fracture line with the dentin composite, which aids in determining a seamless transition between tooth and composite. At this stage, dentin mamelons are sculpted with a fine-tipped instrument to replicate the morphology of those of the contralateral tooth. This layer is light cured.

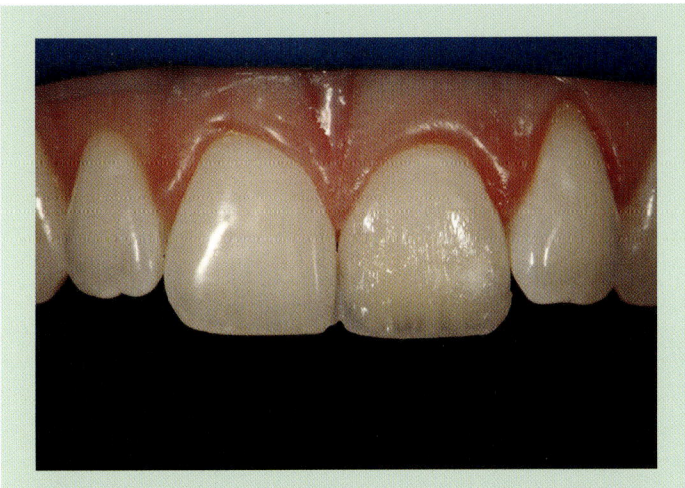

Figure 10.A8 An effect translucent enamel bearing opalescent properties is applied in between and around the mamelons, slightly covering them. By virtue of its chemical composition, the composite resin selected for this layer should reflect bluish wavelengths and transmit amber wavelengths of light. The amount of inner opalescent effect achieved is directly related to the thickness of this layer, which should be used sparingly so as not to overemphasize the bluishness nuance.

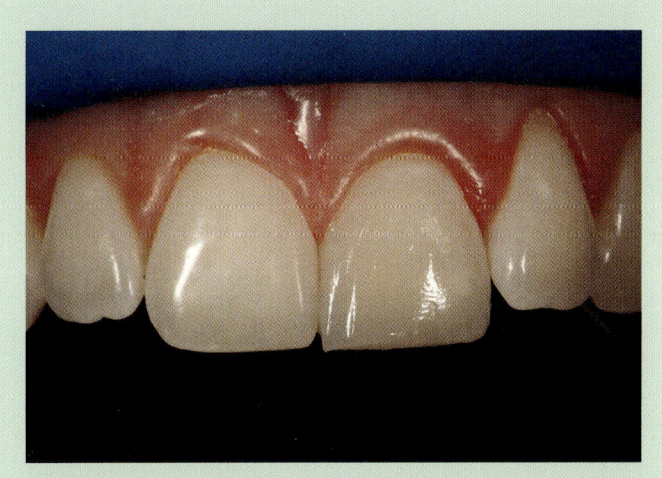

Figure 10.A10 A final layer of a non-VITA classical-based (achromatic) enamel is applied over the incisal one-third and thinly feathered over the VITA classical-based enamel. This enamel is also called value enamel, as it can corroborate or modulate the tooth value to the higher or to the lower, depending on the effect that is intended. A more translucent enamel of lower value allows more light transmission and thus a more obvious halo, opalescent, and dentin mamelon effect is perceived. If it is more opacious and, therefore, higher in value, a whitish appearance is achieved over the incisal one-third and less of the underlying effects are observed. As with any layer of composite, the modulating properties of this layer are directly dependent on thickness and opacity.

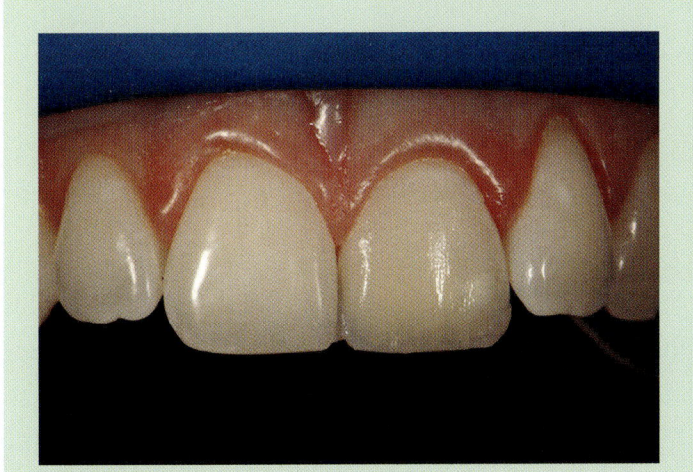

Figure 10.A9 A VITA classical-based (chromatic) enamel composite resin of the final intended hue, chroma, and value is applied beyond the bevel finish line and brought to almost final facial contour. A cut-back is realized along the incisal one-third to permit a greater degree of light transmission and to capture the details of the underlying dentin and enamel layers. This chromatic enamel layer brings both tooth and restoration into perfect color harmony. As the thickness of this enamel layer is thin and varies according to the areas over which it is applied based on the amount of chroma that is desired, a correct assessment of its blending properties is mandatory to ensure an ideal optical and color integration.

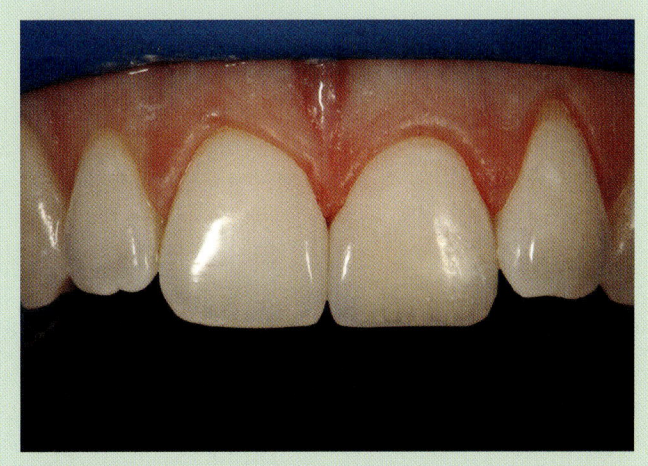

Figure 10.A11 The restoration is finished to primary anatomy, followed by sequential steps leading to secondary and tertiary anatomy placement. After final polishing with rotary instruments and polishing pastes, the surface gloss mimics that of the natural enamel.

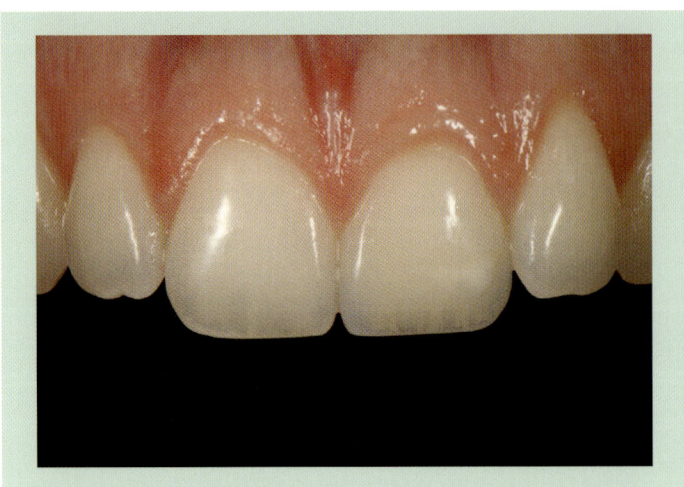

Figure 10.A12 Following complete rehydration, a few days later, the restoration depicts a harmonious form and color integration with the natural tooth tissues.

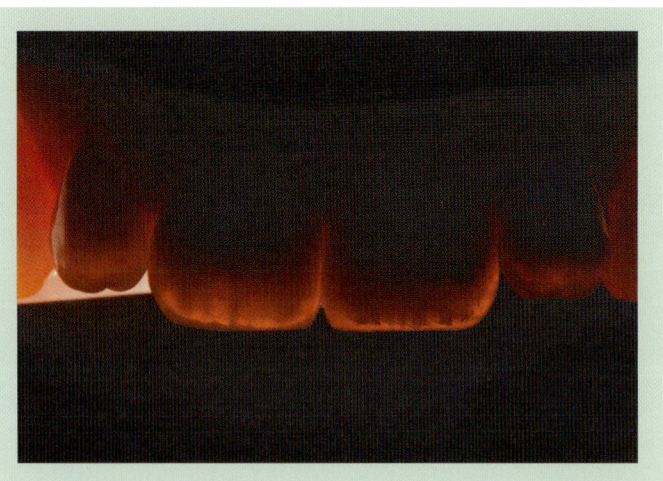

Figure 10.A13 Transmitted light shows the inner histological morphology and optical differences between artificial dentin and enamel. Composite resins with optical properties similar to the natural enamel show identical properties when compared to the natural dentition.

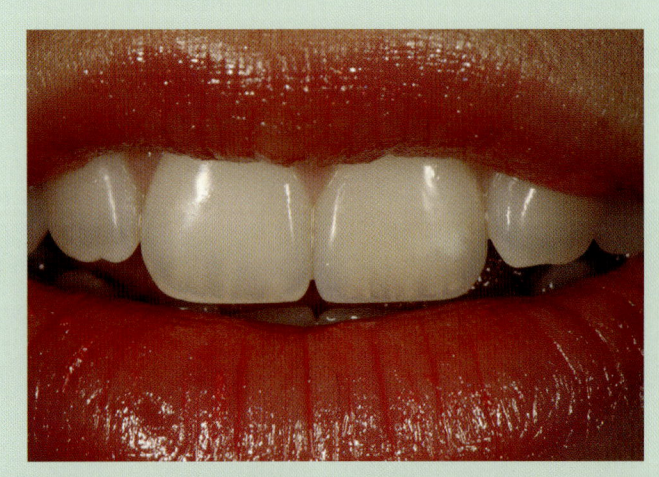

Figure 10.A14 The greatest challenge of the direct restorative dentist is to achieve seamless restorations. When selected according to a strict protocol, composite resins can emulate the natural dentition in all of its morphological, physical, color, and optical properties.

A look to the future

It is always risky to predict the future. However, chances are good that progress will occur in undergraduate and graduate education and training of dental students and professionals on color and appearance. This will likely be complemented by new technologies including the affordable, high-quality color matching instruments. Further improvements are expected from dental materials: new, improved shade guides and color-stable materials that correspond to the color of human teeth and exhibit pronounced blending will be a step in the same direction.

Cooperation between educators, practitioners, technicians, and manufacturers can lead to solutions to the color problem in dentistry. The combination of science, education, and training will allow objective color matching, communication, reproduction, and verification to become a routine part of dental education and practice. The acquired knowledge and skills should facilitate not only improved results but the enjoyment of accomplishing the difficult task of replicating natural beauty, with patients being the ultimate benefactors.

References

1. Berns RS. *Billmeyer and Saltzman's Principles of Color Technology*, 3rd edn. Hoboken, NJ: John Wiley & Sons; 2000.
2. Fairchild MD. *Color Appearance Models*, 2nd edn. Hoboken, NJ: John Wiley & Sons; 2005.

3. Clark EB. The color problem in dentistry. *Dent Digest* 1931;37: 499–509, 571–583, 646–659.
4. Goodacre CJ, Paravina RD, Bergen SF, Preston JD. *A Contemporary Guide to Color and Shade Selection for Prosthodontics* [DVD]. American College of Prosthdontists; 2009.
5. Paravina RD, Powers JM. *Esthetic Color Training in Dentistry*. St. Louis, MO: Elsevier-Mosby; 2004.
6. Paravina RD. *Dental Color Matcher*. http://www.scadent.org/dcm. Society for Color and Appearance in Dentistry; VITA Zahnfabrik, 2010; CD, 2011.
7. Sproull RC. Color matching in dentistry. Part I: the three-dimensional nature of color. *J Prosthet Dent* 1973;29:416–424.
8. Luo MR, Cui G, Rigg B. The development of the CIE 2000 colour difference formula: CIEDE2000. *Color Res Appl* 2001; 26:340–350.
9. Hu X, Johnston WM, Seghi RR. Measuring the color of maxillofacial prosthetic material. *J Dent Res* 2010;89:1522–1527.
10. Perez MM, Ghinea R, Herrera LJ, et al. Dental ceramics: a CIEDE2000 acceptability thresholds for lightness, chroma and hue differences. *J Dent* 2011;39 s:e37–e44.
11. Bergen SF. Color in esthetics. *NY State Dent J* 1985;51:470.
12. International Organization for Standardization. *Dentistry – Guidance on Colour Measurement, ISO/TR 28642*. Geneva: International Organization for Standardization; 2016.
13. Paravina RD, Majkic G, Imai FH, Powers JM. Optimization of tooth color and shade guide design. *J Prosthodont* 2007;16:269–276.
14. Paravina RD, Majkic G, Stalker JR, et al. Development of a model shade guide for primary teeth. *Eur Arch Paediatr Dent* 2008;9:74–78.
15. Paravina RD, O'Neill PN, Swift EJ, et al. Teaching of color on predoctoral and postdoctoral dental education in 2009. *J Dent* 2010;38 s:e34–e40.
16. Paravina RD, O'Keefe KL, Kuljic BL. Color of permanent teeth: A prospective clinical study. *Balkan J Stomatol* 2006;10:93–97.
17. Ishikawa-Nagai S, Yoshida A, Sakai M, et al. Clinical evaluation of perceptibility of color differences between natural teeth and all-ceramic crowns. *J Dent* 2009;37(suppl 1):e57–63.
18. Ghinea R, Pérez MM, Herrera LJ, et al. Color difference thresholds in dental ceramics. *J Dent* 2010;38(suppl 2):e57–e64.
19. Paravina RD, Ghinea R, Herrera LJ, et al. Color difference thresholds in dentistry. *J Esthet Restor Dent* 2015;27:S1–S9.
20. Bayindir F, Bayindir YZ, Gozalo-Diaz DJ, Wee AG. Coverage error of gingival shade guide systems in measuring color of attached anterior gingiva. *J Prosthet Dent* 2009;101:46–53.
21. Huang JW, Chen WC, Huang TK, et al. Using a spectrophotometric study of human gingival colour distribution to develop a shade guide. *J Dent* 2011;39(suppl 3):e11–e16.
22. Beatty MW, Mahanna GK, Jia W. Ultraviolet radiation-induced color shifts occurring in oil-pigmented maxillofacial elastomers. *J Prosthet Dent* 1999;82:441–446.
23. Haug SP, Andres CJ, Moore BK. Color stability and colorant effect on maxillofacial elastomers: Part III. Weathering effect on color. *J Prosthet Dent* 1999;81:431–438.
24. Kiat-amnuay S, Mekayarajjananonth T, Powers JM, et al. Interactions of pigments and opacifiers on color stability of MDX4-4210/type A maxillofacial elastomers subjected to artificial aging. *J Prosthet Dent* 2006;95:249–257.
25. Paravina RD, Majkic G, Perez MM, Kiat-Amnuay S. Color difference thresholds of maxillofacial skin replications. *J Prosthodont* 2009;18:618–625.
26. Munsell Color. *Farnsworth-Munsell 100 Hue Test*. http://munsell.com/color-products/color-vision-tests/ (assessed January 5, 2012).
27. Jasinevicius TR, Curd FM, Schilling L, Sadan A. Shade-matching abilities of dental laboratory technicians using a commercial light source. *J Prosthodont* 2009;18:60–63.
28. Poljak-Guberina R, Celebic A, Powers JM, Paravina RD. Colour discrimination of dental professionals and colour deficient laypersons. *J Dent* 2011;39 s:e17–e22.
29. Miller LL. Organizing color in dentistry. *J Am Dent Assoc* 1987;Special issue:26E–40E.
30. Preston JD. Current status of shade selection and color matching. *Quintessence Int* 1985;16:47.
31. Sproull RC. Color matching in dentistry. Part II: practical applications for the organization of color. *J Prosthet Dent* 1973;29:556.
32. American Dental Association Council of Scientific Affairs. *Acceptance Program Guidelines: Over the Counter Home-Use Tooth Bleaching Products*. Chicago, IL: ADA; 2006.
33. American Dental Association Council of Scientific Affairs. *Acceptance Program Guidelines: Dentist-Dispensed Home-Use Tooth Bleaching Products*. Chicago, IL: ADA; 2006.
34. American Dental Association Council of Scientific Affairs. *Acceptance Program Guidelines: Professional In-Office Tooth Bleaching Products*. Chicago, IL: ADA; 2006.
35. Paravina RD, Johnston WM, Powers JM. New shade guide for evaluation of tooth whitening – colorimetric study. *J Esthet Restor Dent* 2007;19:276–283.
36. Paravina RD. New shade guide for tooth whitening monitoring: Visual assessment. *J Prosthet Dent* 2008;99:178–184.
37. Paravina RD. Performance assessment of dental shade guides. *J Dent* 2009;37(suppl 1):e15–e20.
38. Paravina RD. Color in dentistry: improving the odds for correct shade selection. *J Esthet Restor Dent* 2009;21:202–208.
39. Paravina RD, Powers JM, Fay RM. Color comparison of two shade guides. *Int J Prosthodont* 2002;15:73.
40. Preston JD, Bergen SF. *Color Science and Dental Art: A Self-teaching Program*. St. Louis, MO: Mosby; 1980:42.
41. Sorensen JA, Torres TJ. Improved color matching of metal-ceramic restorations. Part I: a systematic method for shade determination. *J Prosthet Dent* 1987;58:133–139.
42. Grajower R, Revah A, Sorin S. Reflectance spectra of natural and acrylic resin teeth. *J Prosthet Dent* 1976;36:570.
43. Bell AM, Kurzeja R, Gamberg MG. Ceramometal crowns and bridges: focus on failures. *Dent Clin North Am* 1985;29:763.
44. O'Brien WJ, Boenke KM, Groh CL. Coverage errors of two shade guides. *Int J Prosthodont* 1991;4:45–50.
45. Sykora O. Fabrication of a posterior shade guide for removable partial dentures. *J Prosthet Dent* 1983;50:287.
46. Paravina RD, Powers JM, Fay RM. Dental color standards: shade tab arrangement. *J Esthet Restor Dent* 2001;13:254.
47. Charbeneau GT. Direct esthetic restorations. In: Charbeneau GT, ed. *Principles and Practice of Operative Dentistry*, 3rd edn. Philadelphia, PA: Lea & Febiger; 1988.
48. O'Keefe KL, Strickler ER, Kerrin HK. Color and shade matching: the weak link in esthetic dentistry. *Compendium* 1990;11: 116–120.
49. Chu SJ, Trushkowsky RD, Paravina RD. Dental color matching instruments and systems. Review of clinical and research aspects. *J Dent* 2010;38 s:e2–e16.
50. McLaren EA, Schoenbaum T. Combine conventional and digital methods to maximize shade matching. *Compend Contin Educ Dent* 2011;32(4):30–33.
51. Lehmann KM, Igiel C, Schmidtmann I, Scheller H. Four color-measuring devices compared with a spectrophotometric reference system. *J Dent* 2010;38(suppl 2):e65–e70.

52. Ristic I, Paravina RD. Color measuring instruments. *Acta Stomatol Naissi* 2009;25:925–932.
53. Yuan JC, Brewer JD, Monaco EA, Davis EL. Defining a natural tooth color space based on a 3-dimensional shade system. *J Prosthet Dent* 2007;98:110–119.
54. Chu SJ. Use of a reflectance spectrophotometer in evaluating shade change resulting from tooth-whitening products. *J Esthet Restor Dent* 2003;15(suppl 1):S42–S48.
55. Ontiveros JC, Paravina RD. Color change of vital teeth exposed to bleaching performed with and without supplementary light. *J Dent* 2009;37:840–847.
56. Li Q, Wang YN. Comparison of shade matching by visual observation and an intraoral dental colorimeter. *J Oral Rehabil* 2007;34:848–854.
57. Paul S, Peter A, Pietrobon N, Hämmerle CH. Visual and spectrophotometric shade analysis of human teeth. *J Dent Res* 2002;81:578–582.
58. Da Silva JD, Park SE, Weber HP, Ishikawa-Nagai S. Clinical performance of a newly developed spectrophotometric system on tooth color reproduction. *J Prosthet Dent* 2008;99:361–368.
59. Dozic A, Kleverlaan CJ, El-Zohairy A, et al. Performance of five commercially available tooth color-measuring devices. *J Prosthodont* 2007;16:93–100.
60. Kim-Pusateri S, Brewer JD, Davis EL, Wee AG. Reliability and accuracy of four dental shade-matching devices. *J Prosthet Dent* 2009;101:193–199.
61. Paravina RD, Kimura M, Powers JM. Color compatibility of resin composites of identical shade designation. *Quintessence Int* 2006;37:713–719.
62. Wee AG, Kang EY, Johnston WM, Seghi RR. Evaluating porcelain color match of different porcelain shade-matching systems. *J Esthet Dent* 2000;12:271–280.
63. Paravina RD, Kimura M, Powers JM. Evaluation of polymerization-dependent changes in color and translucency of resin composites using two formulae. *Odontology* 2005;93:46–51.
64. Sailer I, Holderegger C, Jung RE, et al. Clinical study of the color stability of veneering ceramics for zirconia frameworks. *Int J Prosthodont* 2007;20:263–269.
65. Paravina RD, Ontiveros JC, Powers JM. Accelerated aging effects on color of composite bleaching shades. *J Esthet Restor Dent* 2004;16:117–127.
66. Braun A, Glockmann A, Krause F. Spectrophotometric evaluation of a novel aesthetic composite resin with respect to different backgrounds in vitro. *Odontology* 2012;100.
67. Charisis D, Koutayas SO, Kamposiora P, Doukoudakis A. Spectrophotometric evaluation of the influence of different backgrounds on the color of glass-infiltrated ceramic veneers. *Eur J Esthet Dent* 2006;1:142–156.
68. Da Costa J, Fox P, Ferracane J. Comparison of various resin composite shades and layering technique with a shade guide. *J Esthet Restor Dent* 2010;22:114–126.
69. Paravina RD, Westland S, Imai FH, et al. Evaluation of blending effect of composites related to restoration size. *Dent Mater* 2006;22:299–307.
70. Paravina RD, Westland S, Johnston WM, Powers JM. Color adjustment potential of resin composites. *J Dent Res* 2008;87:499–503.
71. Goodkind RJ, Loupe MJ. Teaching of color in predoctoral and postdoctoral dental education in 1988. *J Prosthet Dent* 1992;67:713–717.
72. Bergen SF. *Color Education for the Dental Profession [master's thesis]*. New York: University of New York, College of Dentistry; 1975.
73. Chu SJ, Paravina RD, Sailer I, Meleszko AJ. *Color in Dentistry – A Clinical Guide to Predictable Esthetics*. Hanover Park, IL: Quintessence Publishing, 2017.
74. Haddad HJ, Jakstat HA, Arnetzl G, et al. Does gender and experience influence shade matching quality? *J Dent* 2009;37(suppl 1):e40–e44.

PART 2
ESTHETIC TREATMENTS

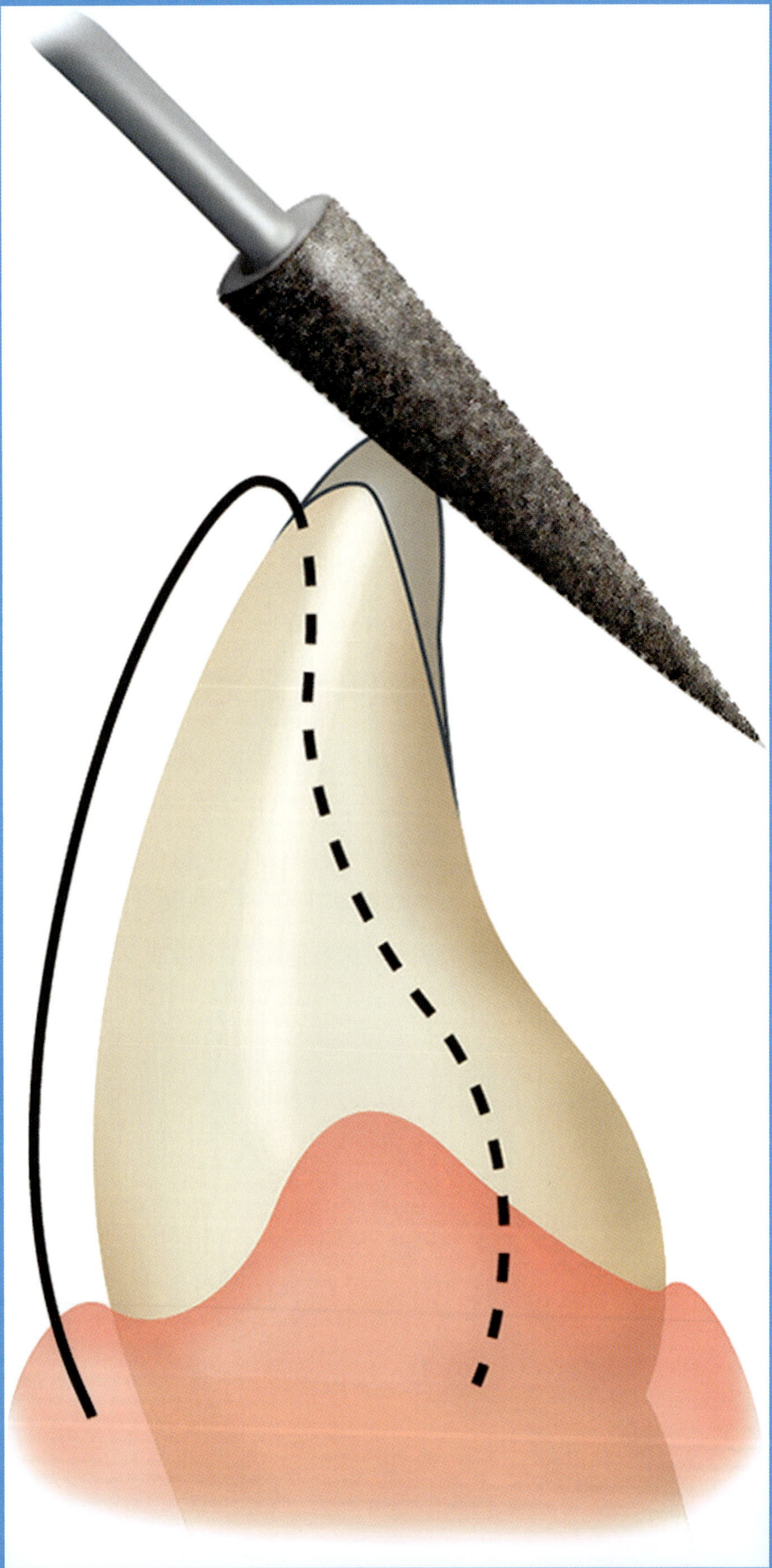

Chapter 11 Cosmetic Contouring

Ronald E. Goldstein, DDS

Chapter Outline

Early techniques	297	Large anterior restorations	303
Indications	298	Extensive anterior crowding or occlusal disharmony	303
Alterations of tooth structure	298	Principles of cosmetic contouring	303
Correction of developmental abnormalities	298	Proportion	303
Substitute for crowning	298	Gender differences	303
Minor orthodontic problems	300	Occlusion	303
Removal of stains and other discolorations	300	Treatment planning	304
Periodontal problems	300	Esthetic imaging	304
Bruxism	300	Diagnostic study casts	304
Contraindications	301	Intraoral marking	304
Hypersensitive teeth	301	Radiographs	304
Large pulp canals	301	Techniques of cosmetic contouring	305
Thin enamel	302	Achievement of illusions	305
Deeply pigmented stains	302	Angle of correction	305
Occlusal interferences	302	Reduction	306
Periodontal involvement	302	Altering tooth form	313
Susceptibility to caries	302	Arch irregularity	319
Negative psychological reactions	302		

Cosmetic contouring is the reshaping of the natural teeth to create an illusion of straightness for esthetic purposes. Such reshaping does not merely consist of filing and leveling the incisal edges—it involves shaping the mesial, distal, labial, and lingual surfaces as well. It is necessary to have a good concept of the original tooth anatomy and how that structure can be recarved into the teeth—only improved.

Early techniques

Cosmetic contouring is one of the oldest of all the esthetic procedures known, because as long as humans have had teeth, we have had tooth fractures. Since the file was an instrument known to early humans, it is easy to understand that the sharp edges on fractured teeth would be filed to a smoother surface

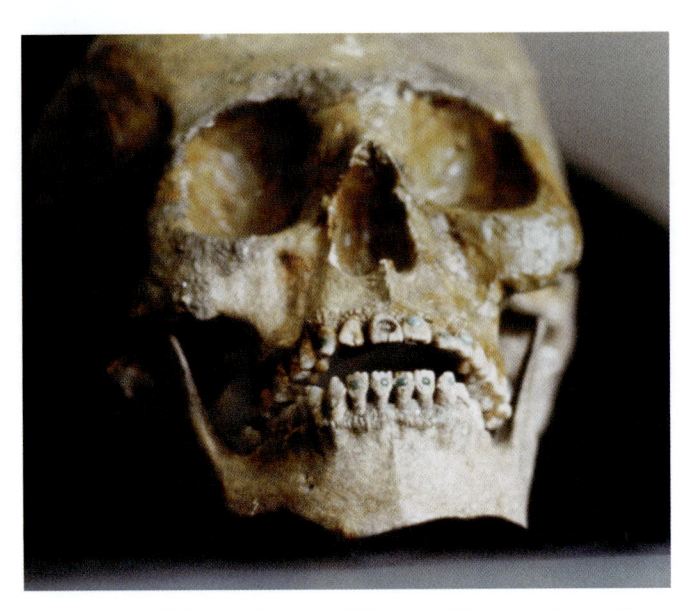

Figure 11.1 (A) This 2000-year-old Mayan skull bears evidence of how early civilizations used cosmetic contouring for cosmetic and possibly functional purposes.

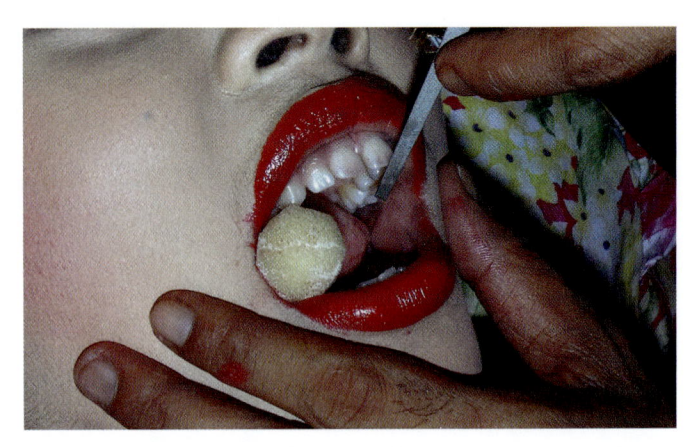

Figure 11.1 (B) In Bali, it is the custom for young women to undergo filing of their labioincisal enamel at puberty to make the edges appear even.

and that people in some cultures filed teeth merely to beautify them. A 2000-year-old Mayan skull shows teeth contoured into points for cosmetic purposes (Figure 11.1A). In fact, the ornamental use of jadeite inlays in anterior teeth and other decorative treatments is further evidence of ancient cosmetic tooth contouring. In Bali, it has been a custom for young women to undergo filing of the labioincisal enamel at puberty to make the edges of the teeth appear even (Figure 11.1B). This shortening of the anterior teeth is said to be necessary for eventual cremation and was thought to be a factor in assuring the normal growth and development of the child. Central African Wawira men point their teeth for esthetic reasons only. A man who does not do so may be unable to find a woman in the tribe who would want to marry him.

In our society, cosmetic contouring has become one of the major esthetic treatments and happens to be one of the most economical as well. Nevertheless, the public at large still is not aware of just how much the technique can help improve almost everyone's smile. For instance, in a landmark 2-year study performed on 60 beauty contestants, cosmetic contouring was strongly indicated in 40% of cases and almost all the rest of the contestants could have been helped through contouring as a compromise to more extensive treatment.[1] Cosmetic reshaping provides an excellent compromise in many situations when other procedures are prohibitively expensive. It is always better to offer a suggested treatment for less-than-ideal esthetic improvement than to tell the patient nothing can be done except veneers, crowning, or treatment that is considered ideal. If crowning is the ultimate answer but cosmetic reshaping could improve the appearance somewhat, there is no reason why crowning cannot be done later if the patient so decides. Finally, cosmetic contouring is one of the most valuable of all esthetic procedures because, in addition to esthetic benefits, function frequently is improved. Reshaping and polishing malposed teeth can make them more self-cleansing and even reduce the likelihood of chipping or fracture, especially in lower incisors.

Perhaps most importantly, cosmetic contouring is one of the dental treatments most appreciated by patients. As Pincus declared, "One must always keep in mind that one is dealing with organs which can change an individual's entire visual personality. Few things will cause a patient to enthuse as much as the results which may be obtained by a little rounding of very long sharp cusps, creating a 'softer' more rounded effect instead of the harsh angular appearance."[2] And as Shelby said, "In every restoration, contouring the teeth may lend that esthetic extra that creates life and character."[3]

Indications

Cosmetic contouring has a number of other advantages over other more involved esthetic procedures. Other than bleaching, it is perhaps the most inexpensive cosmetic treatment. It is a rapid procedure that gives immediate and long-lasting results. It is painless and therefore requires no anesthetic. Cosmetic contouring is indicated for the following purposes.

Alterations of tooth structure

The most frequent use of cosmetic contouring is in the reshaping of fractured, chipped, extruded (Figure 11.2A), or overlapped teeth to give them a more pleasing appearance. Reshaping and repolishing chipped incisal edges also decreases the chance of additional fracturing (Figure 11.2B).

Correction of developmental abnormalities

Often teeth that are malformed can be reshaped to correct unattractive areas at the incisal edges, such as nonfused mamelons (Figure 11.3A–C).

Substitute for crowning

Cosmetic contouring can sometimes be a substitute for bonding, veneering, or crowning anterior teeth. Too often the dentist,

Chapter 11 Cosmetic Contouring   299

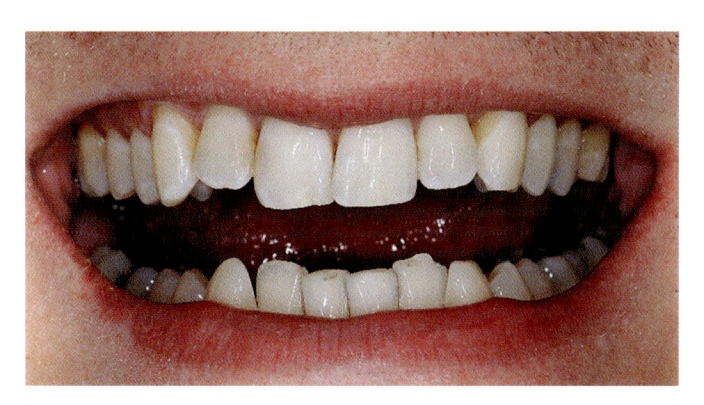

Figure 11.2 **(A)** This 35-year-old night club manager wanted a better-looking smile.

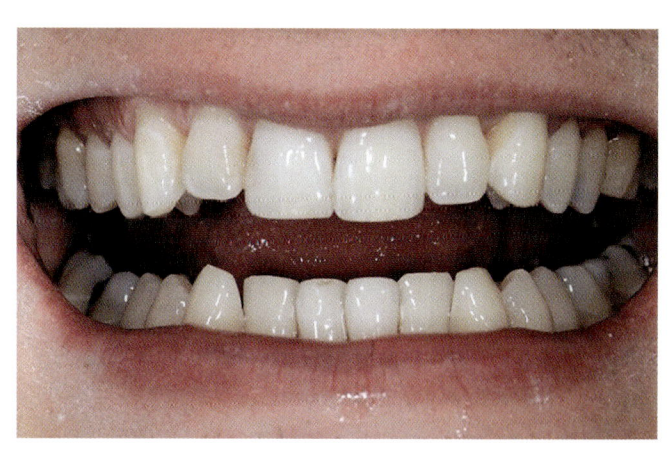

Figure 11.2 **(B)** It only required one cosmetic contouring procedure to produce a more pleasing smile.

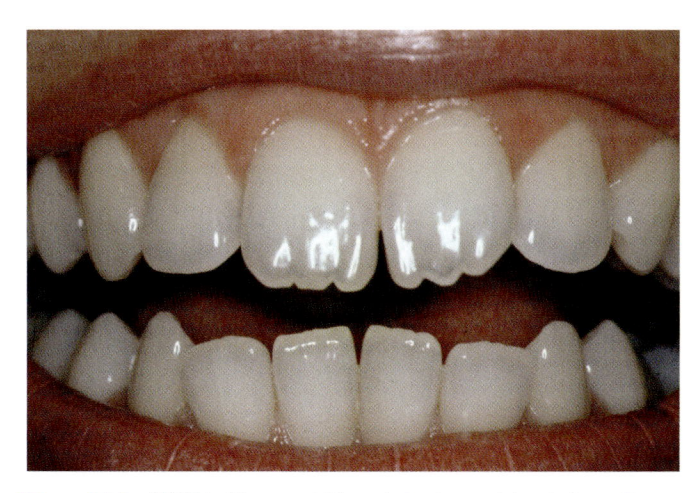

Figure 11.3 **(A)** This 33-year-old female had complained about the jagged appearance of her front teeth. Clinical examination revealed maxillary central incisors with nonfused mamelons. The mandibular incisors were slightly overlapped and distolingually inclined.

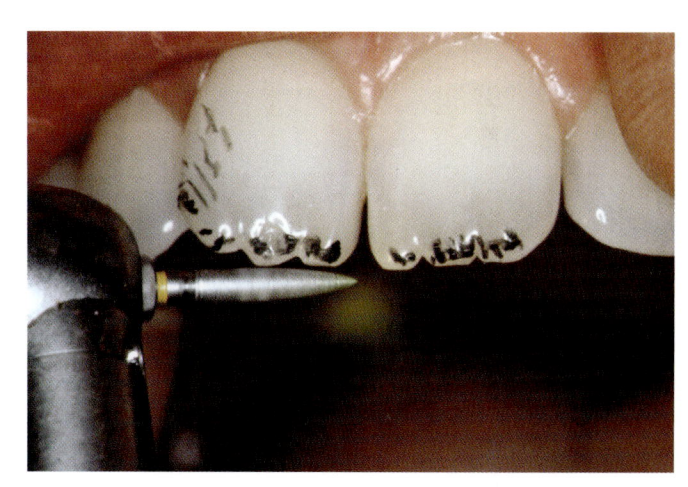

Figure 11.3 **(B)** The maxillary central incisors were cosmetically contoured to eliminate the spaces caused by the prominent mamelons and to reduce the amount of distolabial overlap of the mandibular central incisors.

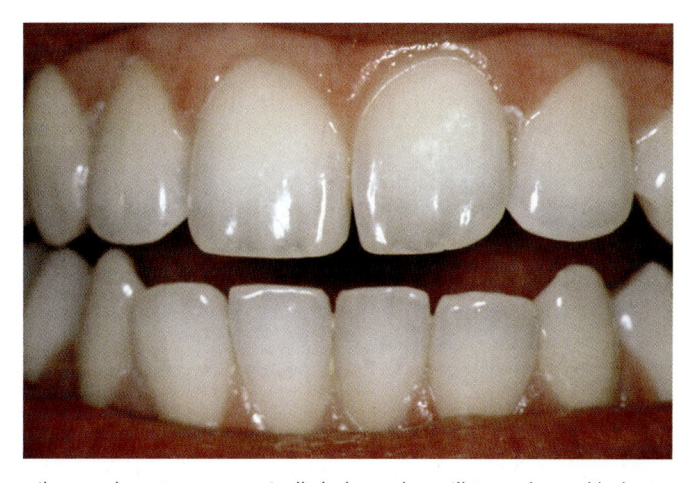

Figure 11.3 **(C)** The post-treatment smile reveals more symmetrically balanced maxillary and mandibular incisal edges. Note the right central incisor could be made to look more esthetic by bonding the distoincisal corner. However, the patient was completely satisfied with the esthetic result of contouring.

in an attempt to improve the patient's appearance, will think only of more invasive procedures, sacrificing tooth structure that might have been merely recontoured.

Minor orthodontic problems

Cosmetic contouring is a recommended treatment in patients with slightly crowded anterior teeth that are not sufficiently maloccluded to warrant orthodontic intervention. These teeth usually can be reshaped to create an illusion of straightness. Extruded teeth in Class II cases can be reshaped to appear more esthetic. Cosmetic contouring may be used after orthodontic treatment to obtain an even better esthetic result.

Removal of stains and other discolorations

Reshaping can cause light to be deflected at different angles and effectively "remove" a superficial hypocalcified area or make a stain appear lighter in certain cases (Figure 11.4A–C). If contouring and polishing are not successful, microabrasion may remove the stain, or a bonded restoration can effectively mask the stain.

Periodontal problems

Coronal recontouring is definitely indicated in cases where destructive occlusal forces have injured the periodontium. If significant evidence of injury such as tooth mobility, migration, or bone loss exists, the specific interferences should be found and eliminated. The usual specific problems that can be addressed by contouring include uneven incisal levels, overlapping, rotation, supraeruption, and insufficient horizontal overlap.

Bruxism

Bruxism can make the anterior teeth wear evenly across the front, producing sharp angular edges, which may be considered masculine. The teeth can be reshaped by rounding the corners to make the lateral and central incisors look more feminine, especially where the incisal embrasures have been obliterated by wear. Excessive grinding can also wear the incisal edges of the central incisors creating interincisal distance but wearing central and laterals. This wear can age the smile especially when the cuspid tips are worn flat as well. The following case illustrates how cosmetic contouring can improve the appearance of a patient with excessively uniform teeth caused by bruxism.

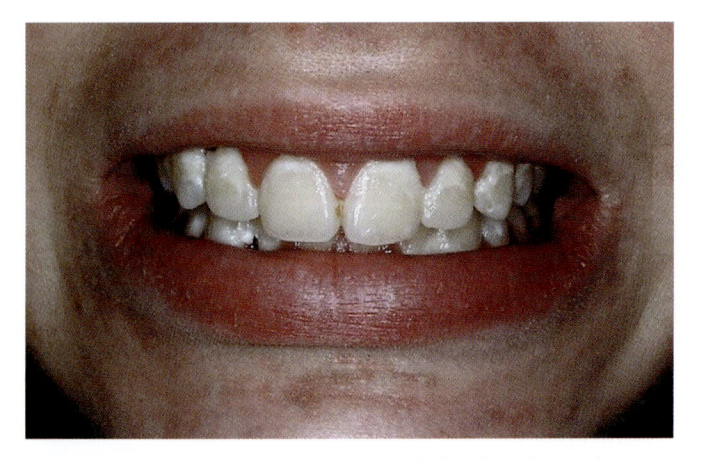

Figure 11.4 **(A)** This 13-year-old girl avoided smiling due to the hypocalcified areas on her teeth.

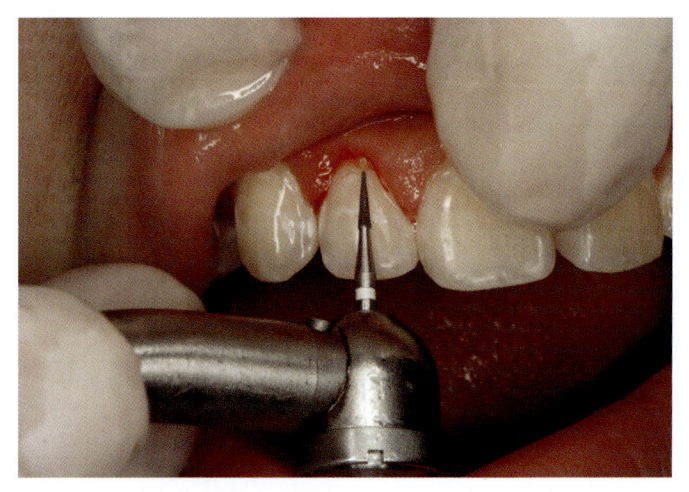

Figure 11.4 **(B)** A 6 mm 30-blade carbide bur (ET6UF Brasseler USA) was used to gently but effectively remove most of the hypocalcified areas.

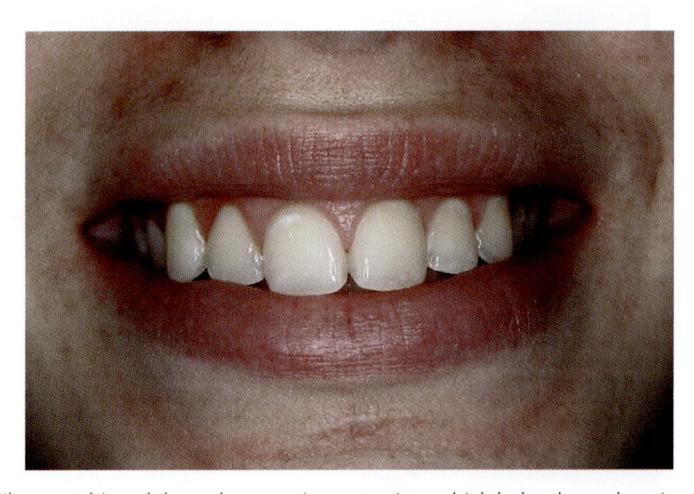

Figure 11.4 **(C)** A much improved smile was achieved through cosmetic contouring, which helped greatly to improve not only this young lady's smile but also her self-image and confidence.

Clinical case: Excessive uniformity of the maxillary incisors caused by bruxism

There are few habits that can cause so much tooth damage as unconscious grinding of the teeth. Bruxism is a major culprit that can ruin a beautiful smile. The shapes of both cuspid tips and incisal embrasures contribute to nature of the smile. It is unfortunate that more hygienists and dentists who constantly examine the same patient multiple times during each year fail to diagnose the obvious signs of grinding before severe wear occurs. Hygienists need to be trained to alert the dentist and patient about cuspal and incisal wear, so appropriate action can be taken to prevent further tooth loss. However, cosmetic contouring can many times help to restore tooth shapes and improve the smile.

A female model presented with excessive uniformity of the maxillary incisors and extrusion and crowding of the left lower anterior, which caused the lip to be shifted slightly to the right (Figure 11.5A). Cosmetic contouring of the maxillary and mandibular incisors was performed by reopening the incisal embrasures and varying the length of the incisal edges. The importance of feminine or masculine reshaping of the anterior teeth should be remembered when contouring in these cases. The result was a more attractive smile created with minimal effort (Figure 11.5B). To prevent additional, future damage, it is often necessary to correct the underlying problem of bruxism, and a night guard may well be indicated.

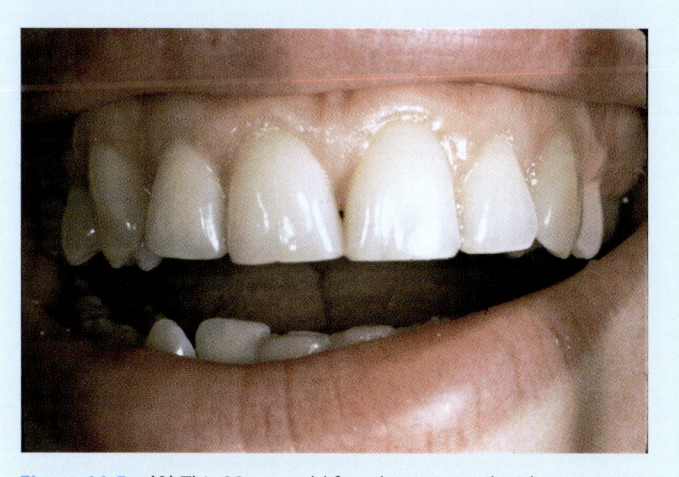

Figure 11.5 **(A)** This 23-year-old female presented with anterior edges worn flat due to bruxism which gave her a more masculine smile.

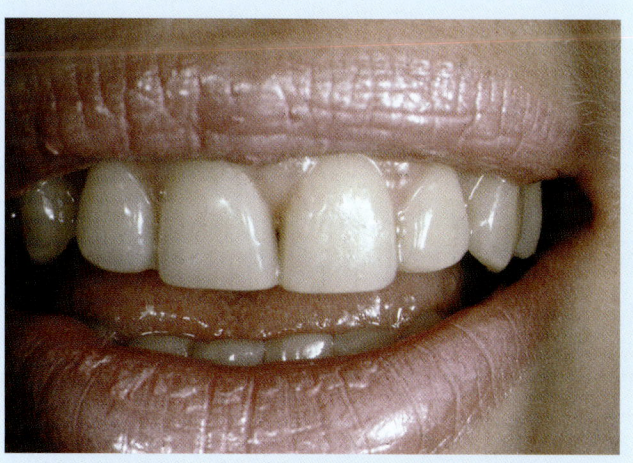

Figure 11.5 **(B)** A younger, more feminine, and attractive smile was accomplished with cosmetic contouring of the maxillary and mandibular incisors.

Contraindications

Cosmetic contouring cannot change the position of the teeth, and the position of the teeth may limit the amount of tooth structure that can be removed. Furthermore, the patient's occlusion may limit the amount of cosmetic treatment achievable. The following sections include the contraindications to cosmetic contouring.

Hypersensitive teeth

If a patient, usually a child or adolescent, complains that the tooth is sensitive, it is better to defer cosmetic contouring until the tooth becomes or can be made less sensitive. The patient should be encouraged to have orthodontic treatment to correct even minor crowding since there is a chance the tooth may remain sensitive for most of the patient's life. If you must contour a sensitive incisal edge, use a coarse diamond (AC2, Brasseler USA), which tends to create less heat as it cuts.

Large pulp canals

Young people with extremely large pulp chambers and pulp canals may be poor candidates for cosmetic contouring (Figure 11.6) because of possible discomfort during the

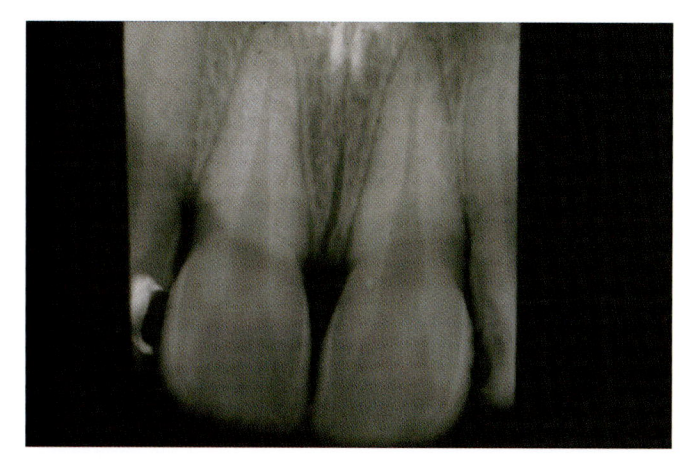

Figure 11.6 Due to the large pulp canals, sensitivity could be a problem for this 24-year-old student if extensive cosmetic contouring were performed.

procedure and sensitivity afterward. If contouring is absolutely necessary, the teeth can be desensitized but it is advisable to do as little contouring as possible in such cases. It may even be necessary to administer a local anesthetic. If crowding is the problem, orthodontic treatment may be the best option.

Thin enamel

Cosmetic contouring should be avoided in patients with overlapping incisors where proximal reduction might create translucency or expose dentin. Excessive removal of enamel from the labial surface of the incisors may result in the darker yellow dentin beneath showing through, creating an unesthetic problem. Excessive thinning at the mesio- and distoincisal corners of teeth that already have thin enamel may lead to future fracture. Teeth with thin enamel on the mesiolabial, distolabial, or incisolabial surfaces as the result of erosion, attrition, or abrasion should not usually be considered for cosmetic contouring. If, however, these teeth are in bucco- or linguoversion, it is sometimes possible to contour the linguoincisal or labioincisal to make them blend in and look straighter. It is important to preserve all possible enamel on the labioincisal and linguoincisal so that the tooth can resist further wear. In the final analysis, it is a value judgment based on experience of the dentist and the patient's goals for the esthetic treatment. A combination of conservative cosmetic contouring and bonding or veneering may be indicated.

Deeply pigmented stains

Hypocalcifications or stains that would require extensive reduction to eliminate or lighten should be treated by restorative procedures. Otherwise, the enamel may be too thin and the dentin may become more visible. In this situation, minor cosmetic contouring may be tried and, if it is unsatisfactory, microabrasion, bonding, or veneering should be considered. If there are doubts as to the thickness of the stain, be sure to let your patient know in advance that additional treatment may be necessary to completely eliminate the stain.

Occlusal interferences

Centric occlusion and lateral and protrusive excursions should always be checked before the treatment. Cosmetic contouring is contraindicated if it might create an occlusal disharmony, for example eliminating a cuspid rise, thus changing the occlusal relationships.

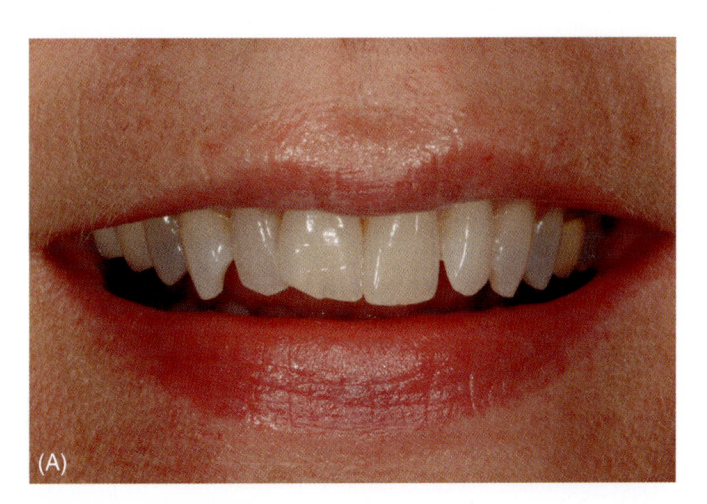

Periodontal involvement

In many cases the teeth may need to be orthodontically repositioned to make them easier to clean. There should never be any doubt that orthodontics would be the ideal treatment to achieve the best functional and esthetic result. In fact, by reshaping the incisal edges, cosmetic contouring might only postpone ideal treatment. For the most part, cosmetic contouring is usually a compromise treatment and should be explained as such to the patient and documented in the chart. Nevertheless, for the patient who will not consider orthodontic treatment, there may be considerable benefit to a compromise treatment of cosmetic contouring. Certainly, by making the teeth easier to clean and eliminating some food traps, the teeth will look better and the patient will feel better about his or her appearance. Thus, the patient will be more apt to take better care of the teeth and gums (Figure 11.7A–D).

Susceptibility to caries

As the enamel is made thinner a tooth could be more susceptible to caries. In situations of crowded teeth, however, this is partially offset because the now less-crowded teeth are easier to clean. In all cases the tooth must be repolished and treated with fluoride postoperatively.

Negative psychological reactions

Certain patients may be subconsciously afraid to look better. Cosmetic contouring can alter a person's smile, so the patient should be forewarned of the change in appearance. Occasionally, the spouse may be the concerned individual. Therefore, show the patient and spouse, if necessary, how the appearance will change by first doing esthetic imaging, or use a black alcohol marker to show your patient exactly where and how much reshaping you are intending to do. This step will help to create an illusion of how the final result will appear. When you give your patients a full-face mirror to visualize the result, make sure the mirror is held at arm's length. Also consider taking a full-face digital smile photo to compare the before smile with the intended treatment smile.

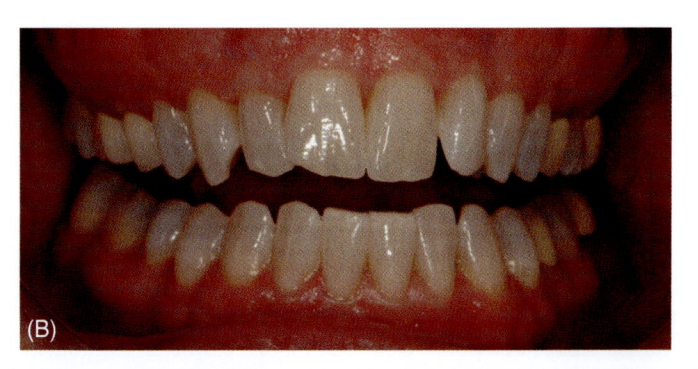

Figure 11.7 (A and B) This executive assistant was unhappy with her crooked, worn, and chipped teeth.

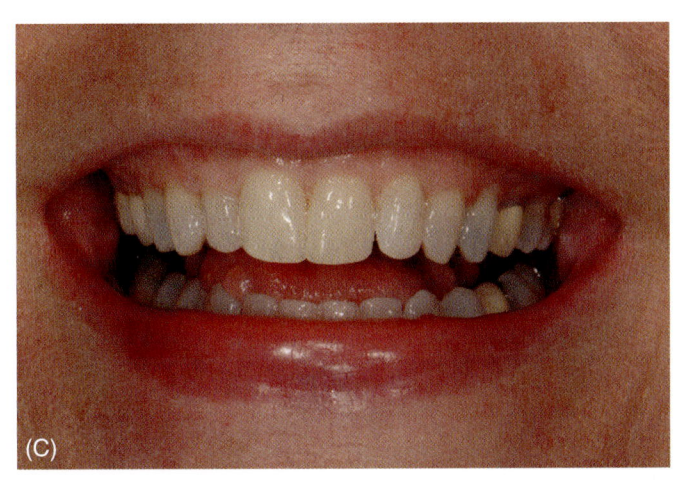

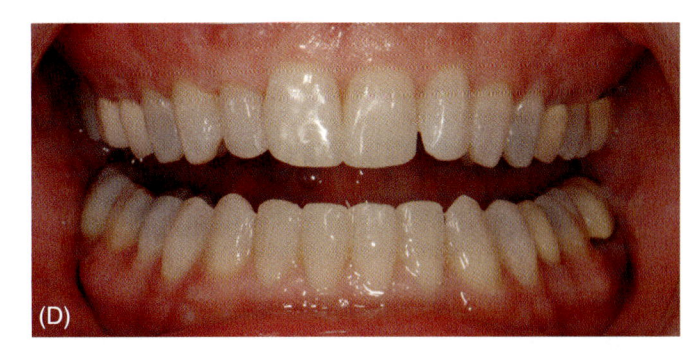

Figure 11.7 (C and D) Although orthodontic treatment would have been an ideal option, she chose cosmetic contouring.

Large anterior restorations

Large composite or other anterior restorations may limit the amount of contouring that can be done. When too much enamel is reduced, the remaining tooth structure may be weakened and eventually fracture.

Extensive anterior crowding or occlusal disharmony

Although cosmetic contouring can usually help improve the appearance of crowded anterior teeth, if there is severe crowding it may accomplish so little that it should not be attempted. In these situations, the patient should be strongly advised to undergo corrective orthodontic treatment. This also applies to those instances when there is extreme functional impairment in the dentition. Cosmetic contouring is never a substitute for definitive or complete occlusal adjustment or functional repositioning of misaligned teeth.

Principles of cosmetic contouring

Proportion

Dentists who perform cosmetic contouring must give foremost attention to the tooth proportion (see Chapter 9). Whether or not a tooth or other structure conforms to the golden proportion is best evaluated by visualizing the silhouette form of a tooth or an arch. The silhouette form is the shape of a tooth as defined by the outline of the tooth, and this, even more than color, governs what most people perceive as either attractive or unattractive. The outline of the tooth is usually determined by the portion of the tooth within the mesiolabial and distolabial line angles. This area defines the perception of how big, long, or short a tooth is. Total perception is gained not only by looking at the tooth but also by looking at the smile and at the entire face. It involves first focusing on the tooth and how the teeth relate to each other and then stepping back and visualizing the smile and its relation to the face and seeing what, if anything, can be done to improve the overall appearance. Opening or closing an incisal embrasure may make a difference. The silhouette form of a tooth that is out of proportion can be altered by adjusting the location and curvature of the mesiolabial or distolabial line angles. But a distoincisal line angle that is needed to preserve the proportion should not be curved. Care must be taken to also understand the effect on the illusion created by light reflection (see Chapter 8).

Gender differences

The assumption of gender differences in tooth form was introduced in the 1950s by Frush and Fisher in their series on full denture esthetics.[4-9] They said that the feminine tooth has more curves whereas the masculine tooth is more angular and boldly textured. However, according to Abrams there is no anthropologic basis for this claim. In 1981, Abrams conducted a survey at the American Academy of Esthetic Dentistry's annual meeting. He showed images of teeth from 60 patients from right, left, and center views with the lips blocked out so that the audience could not see whether the person was male or female. The 150 dentists who participated in the test were given 5 s to determine whether each person was a male or female and their degree of certainty. Only one participant guessed correctly more than 50% of the time. This study showed that dentists have prejudices about what is masculine and feminine, but according to Abrams these prejudices are not substantiated by the facts. In your clinical practice, however, you should be aware that rounding teeth can soften the appearance and making the mesioincisal and distoincisal line angles more angular can give a harder, more aggressive look. You should consider these appearances as descriptive rather than gender-specific.

Occlusion

Cosmetic contouring must always be done with the principles of proper occlusion in mind. Nothing should be added or eliminated that will produce occlusal disharmonies. Occasionally, the factors that produce poor esthetics are also responsible for the malocclusion, and an esthetic improvement may correct both. Simring et al. reviewed a series of occlusal considerations for anterior teeth.[10,11] Ideally, in mandibular anterior teeth a series of thin, symmetrical incisal edge contacts exist that produce vertical forces that are contained within the area of periodontal support.

When establishing a new incisal level for mandibular anterior teeth through contouring, consideration should be given to the following.

- Establish an incisal level that permits optimum contact without producing occlusal trauma. An uneven incisal level and a labiolingual curve produced by crowded teeth not only create problems in esthetics but also create occlusal trauma.
- Establish symmetrical incisal edge contacts, and when that is not possible, labial contacts should be created that are positioned as far incisally as possible.

In maxillary anterior teeth, the objectives for centric and protrusive positions and excursions are as follows.

- To reduce destructive forces occurring in these positions.
- To produce optimum contact and to eliminate deflecting contacts. Optimum contact is contact of the greatest possible number of teeth without poor esthetics or undesirable occlusion. Since the optimum mandibular incisal level should be established first, all additional grinding to obtain these objectives should be done on the maxillary teeth. Sometimes there will be a conflict between the amount of reduction that gives optimal function and the amount that gives optimal esthetics. The decision will have to be based on the degree of occlusal dysfunction that will remain, the esthetic importance, and the ultimate health of the dental organ.

Treatment planning

Cosmetic contouring is one treatment that should be considered in almost every patient's overall treatment plan. When deciding whether to bond, veneer, or crown, ask yourself the question: "Can cosmetic contouring help me to achieve a more successful esthetic result?" Four methods are useful in answering this question:

1. esthetic imaging
2. diagnostic study casts
3. intraoral marking
4. radiographs.

Esthetic imaging

One of the best ways to show your patient how cosmetic contouring can improve his or her smile is with esthetic imaging (Figure 11.8). The technique accomplishes two purposes: first, it serves as a good method for patient communication and, second, it can be invaluable in letting you know exactly how much tooth alteration is necessary to achieve the best result. Even if patients can appreciate basic principles of tooth alteration, it is almost impossible for the average patient to visualize the tooth changes you plan through cosmetic contouring, or how the new tooth shapes will affect the smile and the face. This can also be the

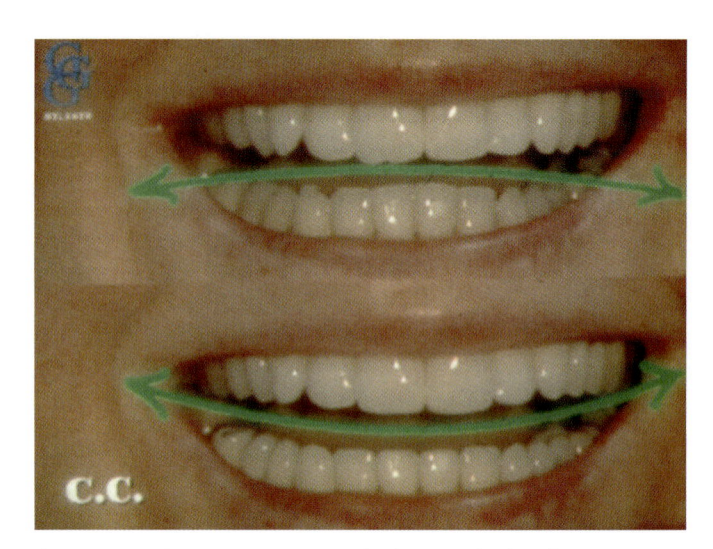

Figure 11.8 Computer imaging is the best method to show your patients how cosmetic contouring can improve their smiles. It can also show you just how much tooth alteration you will need to do to achieve the best result.

quickest method of determining if cosmetic contouring will suffice or if an alternative treatment should be chosen (Figure 11.9A–C).

Diagnostic study casts

Take impressions of both arches and pour a duplicate set of models. Analyze where and how tooth structure will have to be altered and perform the proposed treatment on the patient's duplicate study models (Figure 11.10). By practicing this way, the end result will be more predictable. In addition, the patient also can more easily visualize what the final result will be, and it gives you an exact record of what the teeth were like before they were reshaped. Finally, it will give you a good idea of where and just how much tooth structure you will have to contour to achieve the result you envision.

Intraoral marking

A third method of predetermining the effect of cosmetic contouring, which was previously mentioned, is to block out the tooth surfaces that will be contoured with a black alcohol marker. Dry the teeth with your air syringe and mark the visible overlapping tooth surfaces. Have your patient hold a mirror at arm's length or have the patient stand before a large mirror to see the effect of the new silhouette form. If the patient wears glasses, ask him or her to remove them for a more realistic view of the proposed silhouette form.

Radiographs

Radiographs, particularly of the anterior teeth, should be examined for thickness of the enamel as well as for the size and shape of the pulp. This is the best way to predict potential sensitivity and to give an indication of how much enamel you will safely be able to remove.

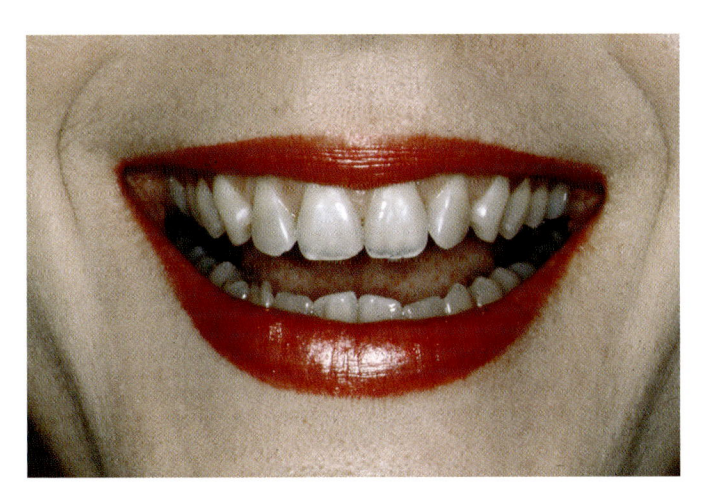

Figure 11.9 (A) This 30-year-old woman wanted straighter teeth without orthodontic treatment. Note the uneven appearance of the mandibular incisors.

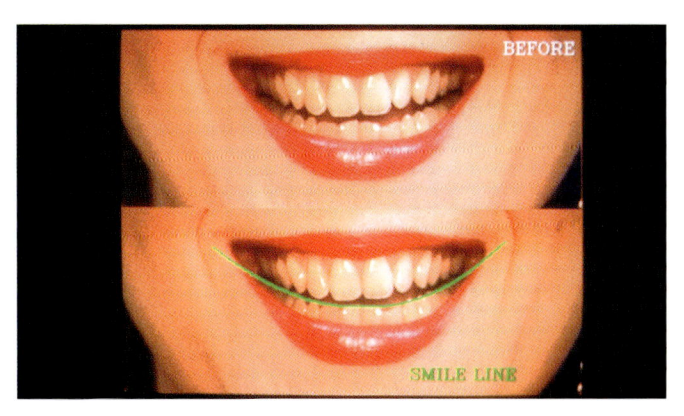

Figure 11.9 (B) By selecting an imaginary lower arc which mimics the lower lipline, it is possible to create an illusion of straightness, especially in the lower anterior area.

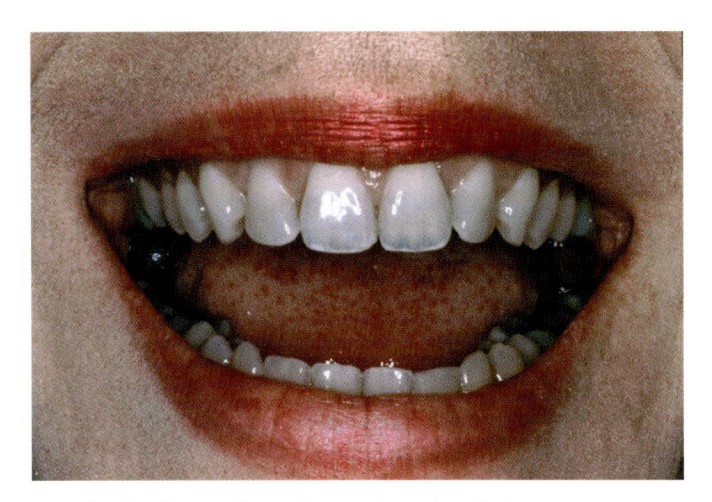

Figure 11.9 (C) Cosmetic contouring provides the illusion of straightness the patient desires.

Techniques of cosmetic contouring

Achievement of illusions

The purpose of planning is to determine how to achieve an illusion of straightness. This process must include different views and perspectives (Figure 11.11A–C). An optical illusion should work most effectively in the position from which most people will be viewing the patient, and you need to view the illusion from that standpoint first (see Figure 11.11C). The easiest way to determine if cosmetic contouring can obtain the result you want is to use computer imaging to record the way more people will view your patient. Draw an imaginary line to simulate the arc you wish to create by contouring (see Figure 11.11C). Most contour planning should be done by marking the teeth with a black marker when the patient is sitting. However, the patient should also stand with you sitting, and then both the patient and you should stand. Each time, the areas to be contoured should be dried and marked with a black alcohol marker. Areas to avoid cutting, such as a holding cusp in the cuspid areas, may be distinguished with a red alcohol marker. The patient should have an opportunity to visualize the planned reshaping or contouring with a mirror. Many times the patient will see something that you may not have observed.

Angle of correction

A lower incisor that actually or apparently extends above the lower incisal plane can be quite noticeable. The angle of view is important, especially in shaping a lower tooth. Owing to the relative positions of the eyes and mouth, most people look down at the lower arch. This is why, because of the angle of view, an anterior tooth that is in linguoversion appears to be much more prominent than the one in labioversion. To contour the tooth in linguoversion, its incisal edge should be beveled lingually (Figure 11.11D). Figure 11.11E shows the position of the diamond stone used to reduce the unsightly tooth. Correction must be done with this lingual aspect in mind. Using these principles helped create a much more attractive smile with straighter-looking teeth when this patient smiled or spoke (Figure 11.11 F).

Reduction

Before doing even preliminary contouring, you need to be aware of the fact that reshaping of the natural dentition must always be in relationship to the lip positions in both speaking and smiling. Failure to do this may lead to over-reduction in areas not actually needed for esthetics. In addition, the lips should be retracted as little as possible during the recontouring procedure so that their influence and natural relationship toward the dentition will always be apparent.

The entire process of contouring should usually be scheduled in two appointments instead of a single appointment simply because, after prolonged observation, the teeth tend to be seen as you want them to be, rather than as they actually are. In rare cases it may be necessary to desensitize the teeth. The teeth can be desensitized using one of the topical agents you routinely prescribe. These patients should also be advised to use a desensitizing toothpaste as necessary after treatment.

It is important during all cutting operations to use a water spray as a coolant. Furthermore, with the use of water, it is often possible to see a slight color shift before the enamel is completely penetrated. The last few layers of enamel are more translucent, so that the yellow dentin becomes more visible. Enamel removal should be stopped as soon as a color shift is observed and hopefully before. When such a tooth is dried and polished, it should look fine. As the teeth are contoured, it is important to move from one tooth to another frequently. Not only will this minimize frictional heat buildup but it helps maintain a proper perspective toward the overall goal.

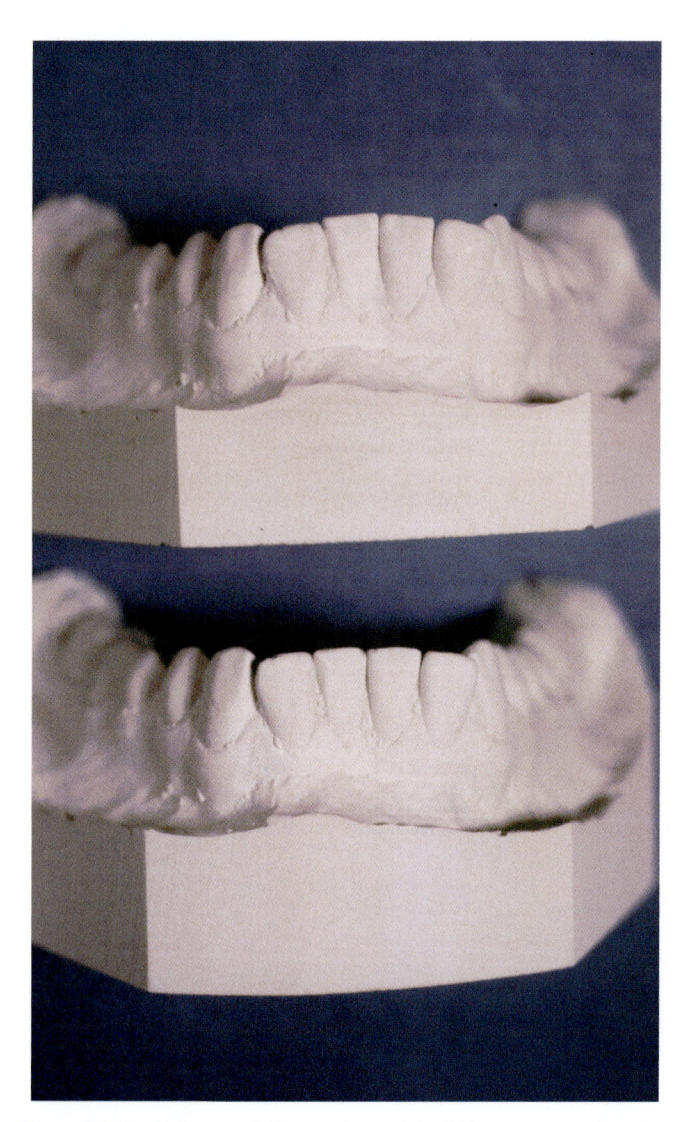

Figure 11.10 Before and after study models aid in treatment planning of cosmetic contouring. This helps both the dentist and the patient to better visualize the anticipated result.

> If a tooth is being shortened, it will need to be reduced labiolingually as well. If this is not done, the patient may be able to feel the difference in the widths of the incisal edges and the difference may also be visible.

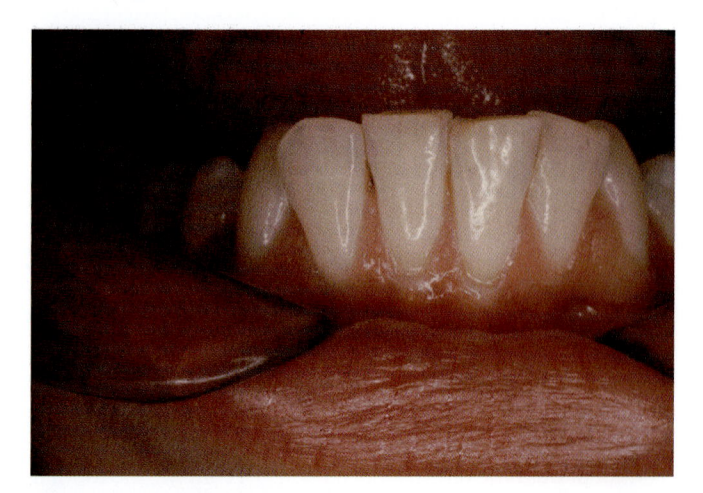

Figure 11.11 **(A)** This patient desired straighter-looking lower teeth. Although the teeth appeared to be even from a horizontal aspect, a more normal speaking position revealed lingually locked right central and left lateral incisors.

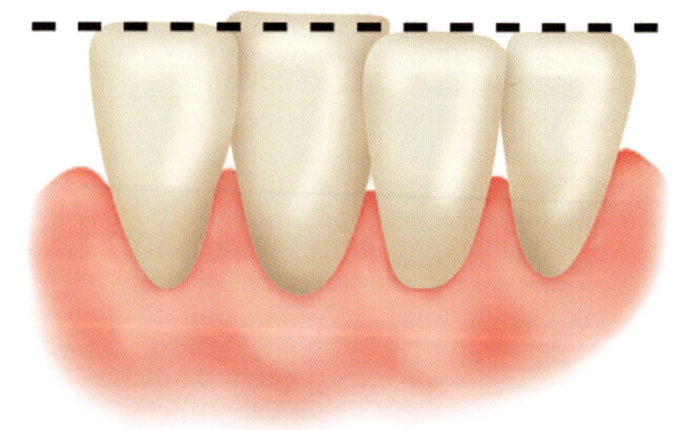

Figure 11.11 **(B)** This is the view of the lower arch as seen by a person at eye level.

Chapter 11 Cosmetic Contouring   307

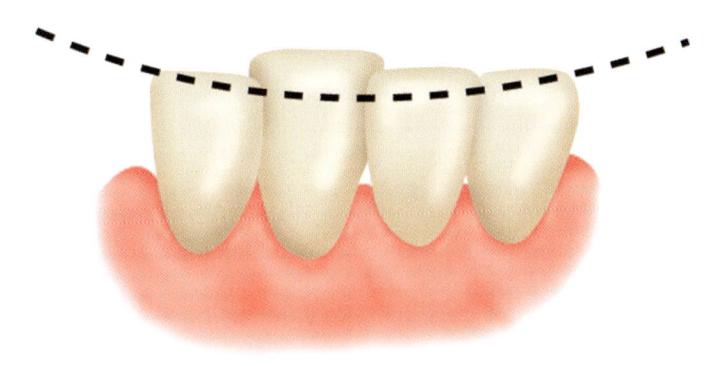

Figure 11.11 **(C)** Shows the same individual as viewed when speaking. A line is drawn to simulate the desired arc.

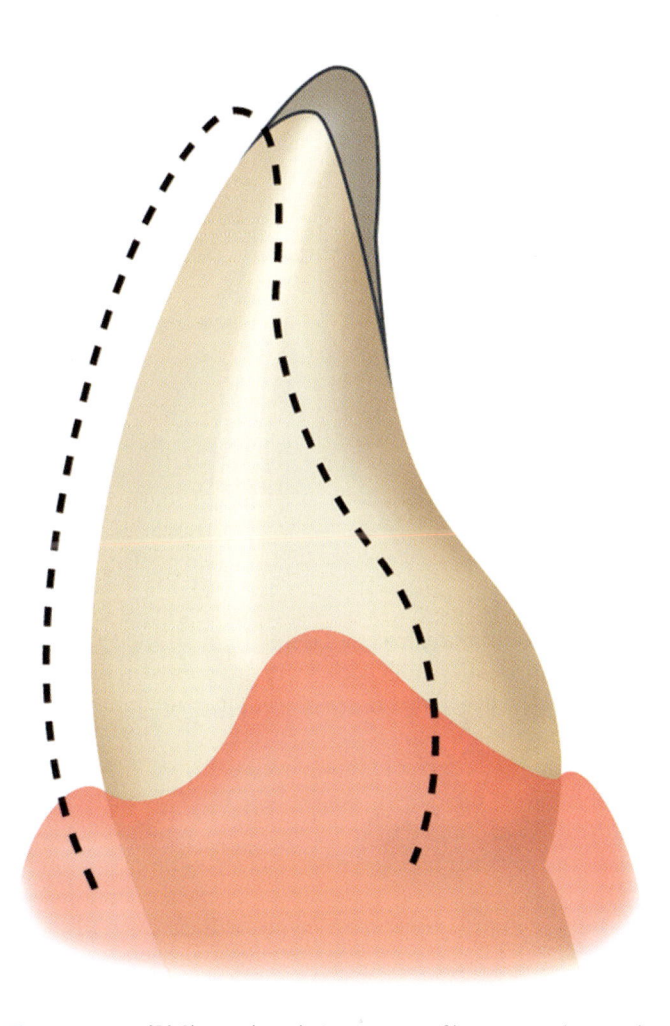

Figure 11.11 **(D)** Shows the relative amount of linguoincisal enamel necessary to alter to achieve a straighter look.

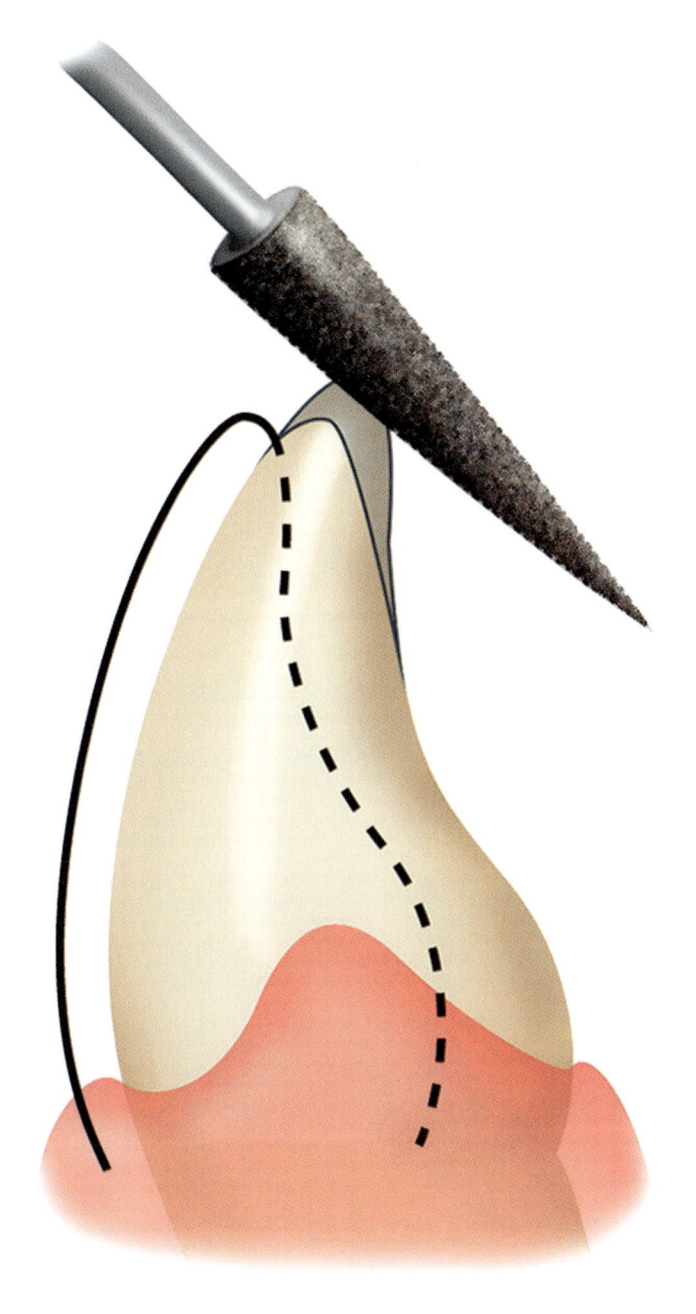

Figure 11.11 **(E)** Notice the correct angle to hold the bur.

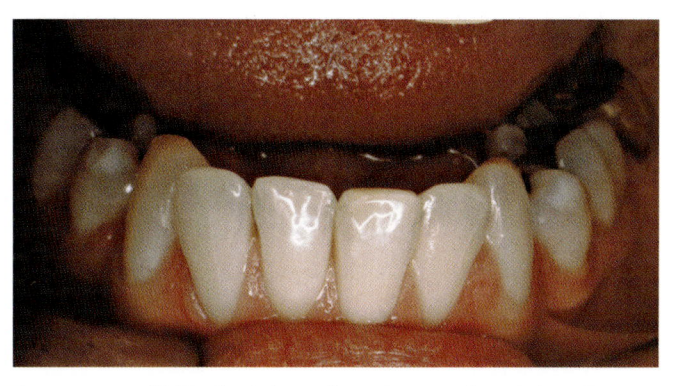

Figure 11.11 **(F)** The final photo shows how much straighter the lower teeth appear following cosmetic contouring. Both mesial and distal aspects of the adjacent labial surfaces were also contoured.

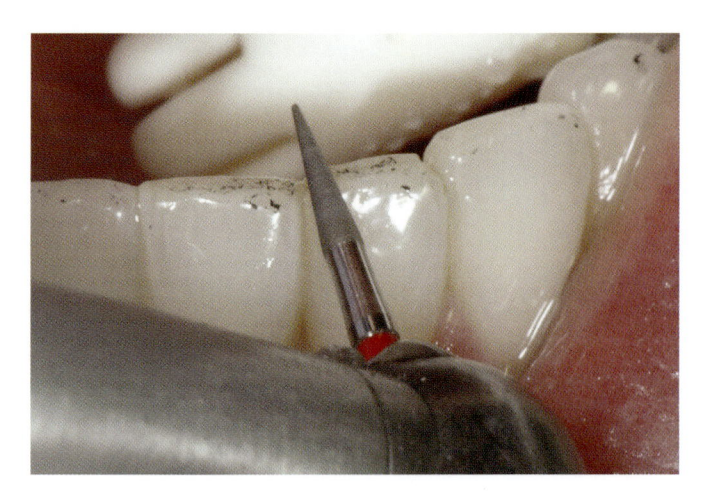

Figure 11.12 The 6 mm 30 μm diamond (DET-6, Brasseler USA) is the perfect shape and grit size to perform cosmetic contouring.

Anterior teeth in the lower arch should be shortened only to the level where they still occlude in protrusive movements. Simring et al. state, "Lower anterior teeth that are ground out of occlusal contact in the intercuspal position will not overerupt if they have occlusal contact in protrusive excursion."[11] Wear facets can detract from the esthetic shape of the teeth. These teeth can be esthetically contoured by rounding away from the flat planes of wear, thereby distributing the occlusal forces more evenly and creating a more pleasing appearance. There are times when initial shaping of the teeth is performed with fine and ultrafine diamonds on a high-speed handpiece with water spray. Excellent diamond shapes are the needle-shaped DET-6 (F and UF) and the DET-4 (F and UF) (Brasseler USA). Reduction is accomplished by carefully shaping the marked areas with a bulk reduction diamond, AC-2 (Brasseler USA), except for the lower anterior teeth. Bulk-reduction in these teeth should be done first with a fine (a 30 μm diamond DET-6) finishing diamond at high speed rather than with the bulk-reduction diamond (Figure 11.12). Because of the thinness of the enamel on these small teeth, if enamel is cut with a fine grit, little will be lost at one time. Therefore, there is less danger of cutting away too much tooth structure. After the initial reduction, the patient should be viewed again in all relevant positions and the teeth remarked.

Final shaping on the mesial, distal, incisal, and embrasure is done with the thin and extra-thin diamond points, because their shapes allow for better access to these areas. After facial shaping is complete, finishing is begun by using an extra-coarse sandpaper disc (Sof Flex, 3M or EP200, Brasseler USA). Finishing is continued by using the impregnated polishing wheels of varying grits in the following order: plain shank, single yellow band, and double yellow band. This will restore the enamel to its original luster; this procedure can also be used to refinish porcelain.

The following figures are a good step-by-step example of a patient who chose cosmetic contouring as an esthetic treatment. A female graphic illustrator, aged 40, presented with malposed, supererupted, and chipped anterior teeth for cosmetic analysis (Figure 11.13A). Orthodontics was ruled out because the patient wanted an immediate esthetic result. She also was reluctant to have her teeth reduced for crowning or veneering.

Treatment

Cosmetic contouring was the treatment of choice for an economical and quick esthetic solution. The first step in the procedure is to analyze the occlusion. The patient is asked to chew on articulating paper in various directions to determine existing centric holding cusps and lateral inclined planes (Figure 11.13B and C). It is necessary to determine how much the tooth structure can be altered without sacrificing functional occlusion. The angle from which most people see the patient determines the angle of view for which an illusion of straightness will be created. The areas where the initial reduction will be done are drawn on the teeth with a black alcohol marker, which creates marks that are removed by cutting with the diamonds and carbides (Figure 11.13D and E). Looking in a mirror, the patient can get some idea of how the teeth will look. The vertical correction was made first by reducing the incisal edges slightly to achieve an esthetic balance (Figure 11.13F). The distal edges of the overlapping laterals (Figure 11.13G) were then recontoured. The incisal symmetry is refined with a Soflex disc (Figure 11.13H). The incisal embrasure is then reopened for a more natural esthetic appearance (Figure 11.13I).

Figure 11.13 (A) Malposed, supererupted, and chipped anterior teeth are evident in this before photograph.

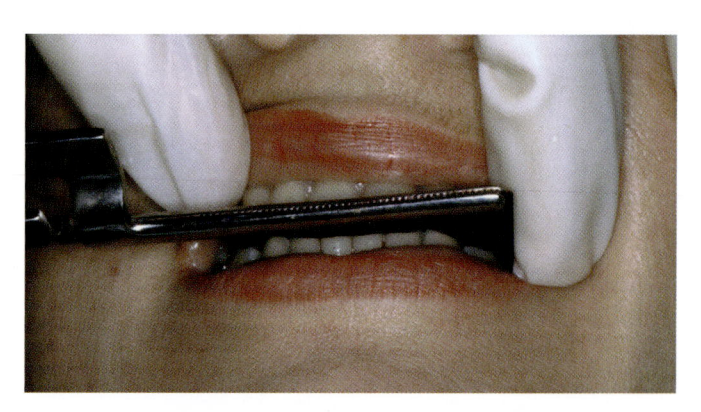

Figure 11.13 (B) Articulating paper is used to record the existing centric holding cusps and lateral inclined planes.

Chapter 11 Cosmetic Contouring

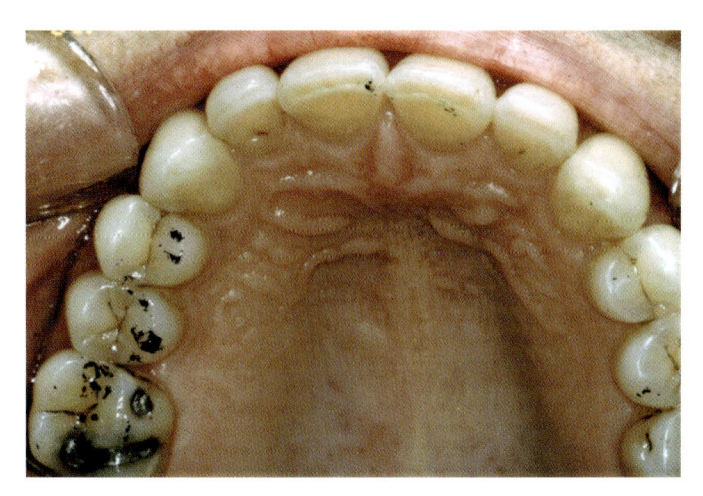

Figure 11.13 (C) Articulating paper is used to record the existing centric holding cusps and lateral inclined planes. Note the articulating paper marks on the patient's right side.

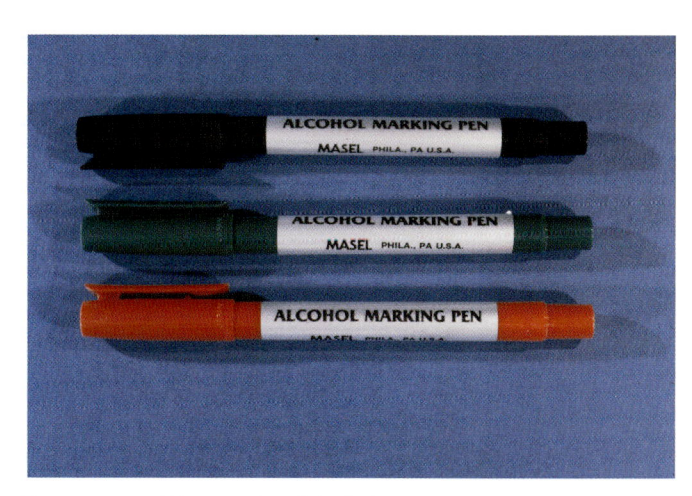

Figure 11.13 (D) Examples of alcohol marking pens (Masel, Inc., Bristol, PA, USA).

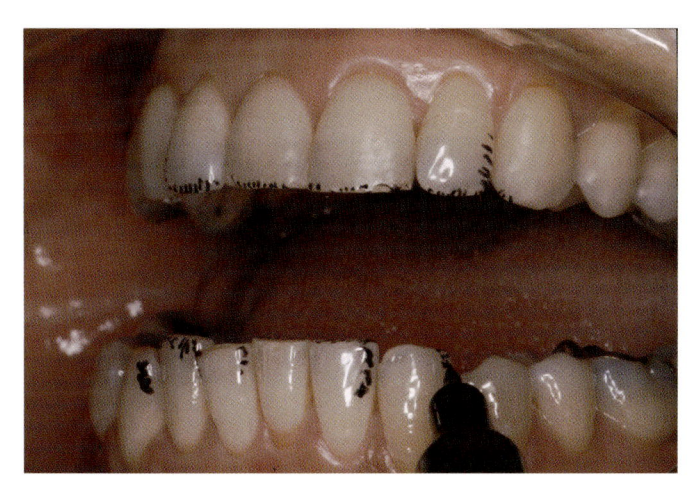

Figure 11.13 (E) After thoroughly drying the teeth, a black alcohol marker is used to outline the areas to be contoured.

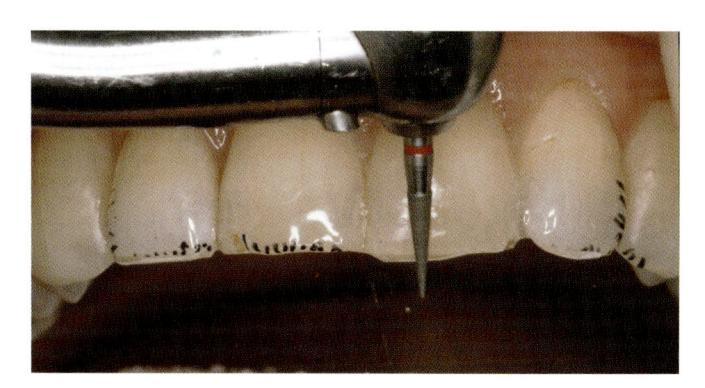

Figure 11.13 (F) Vertical correction was accomplished by leveling the incisal edges of the central incisors and slightly shortening the incisal edges of the laterals.

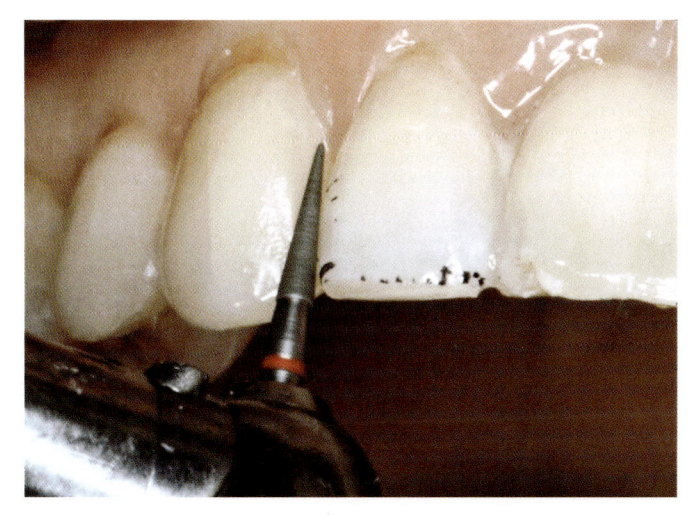

Figure 11.13 (G) Recontouring of the distolabial edges and line angles of the overlapping laterals helps to create better distolabial proportion and exposes more of the mesial surface of adjacent cuspids.

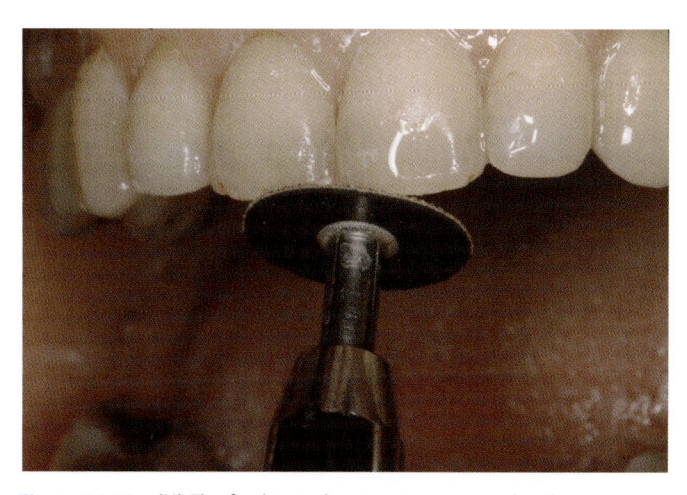

Figure 11.13 (H) The final incisal symmetry is created with an extra-coarse Soflex sandpaper disc (3 M, St. Paul, MN, USA).

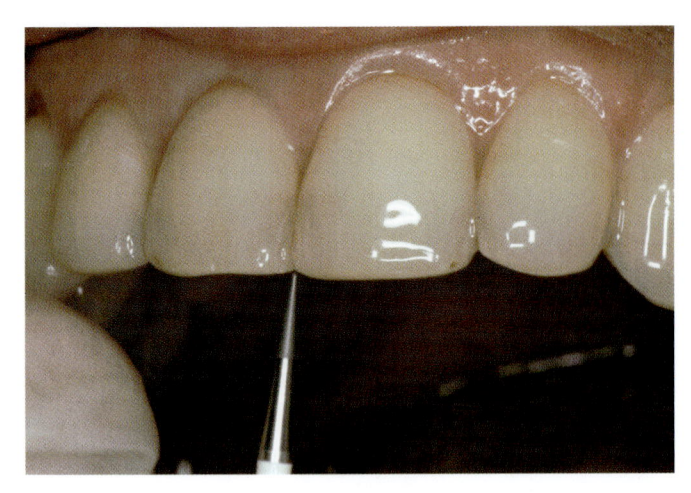

Figure 11.13 **(I)** An ET-3UF 8 μm grit diamond (Brasseler USA) is used to reopen and carve the incisal embrasure for a more natural esthetic appearance.

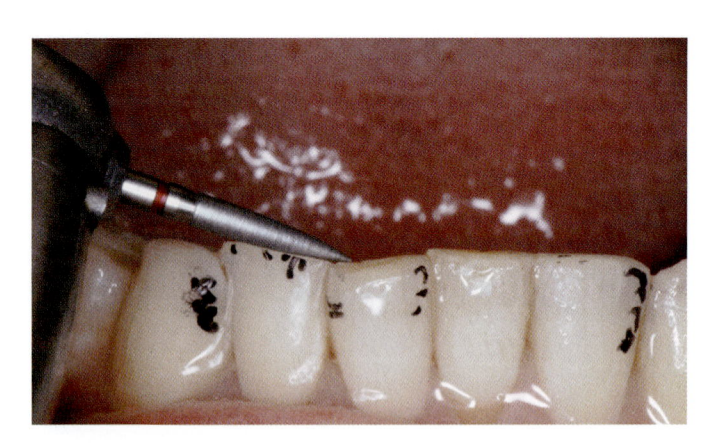

Figure 11.13 **(J)** Lingual shaping is done using an approximate 45° angle. This helps achieve a more natural look when the patient is speaking.

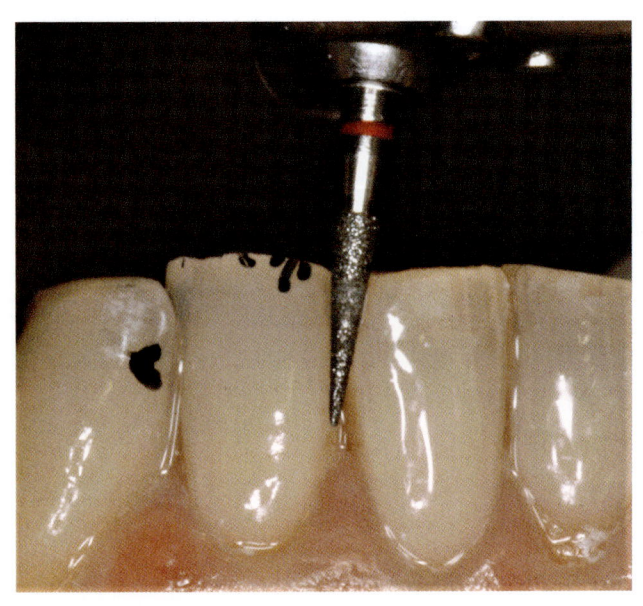

Figure 11.13 **(K)** Horizontal overlap, which is created by too-wide or poorly aligned incisors, is narrowed.

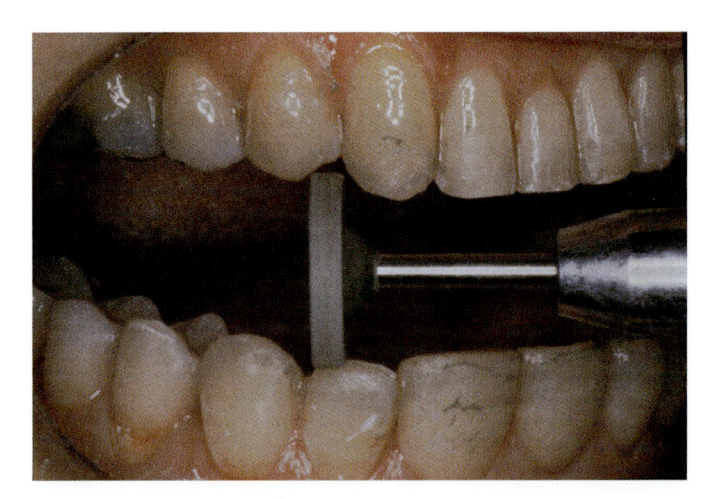

Figure 11.13 **(L)** The no-band wheel shape is used to finish the incisal edges of the maxillary incisors.

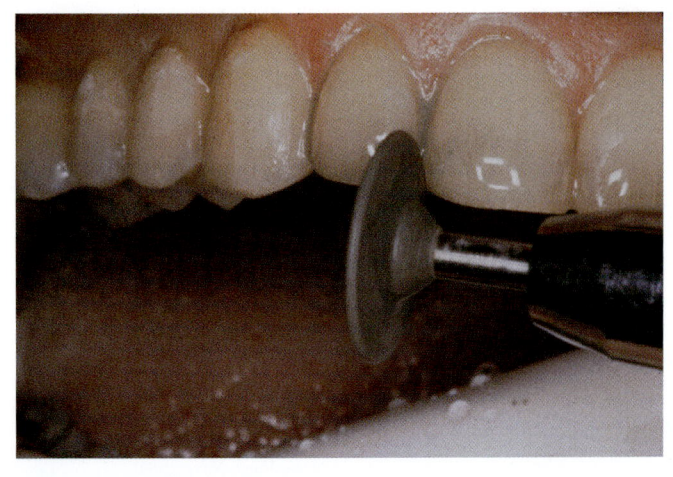

Figure 11.13 **(M)** Interproximal surfaces and incisal embrasures of maxillary central and lateral incisors are polished using the disc shape.

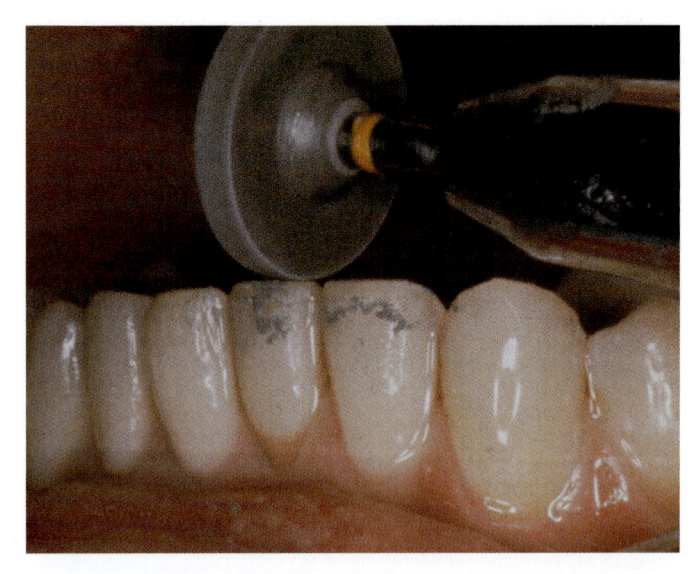

Figure 11.13 **(N)** Switch to the one yellow-banded wheel for further incisal edge and labial finishing.

Chapter 11 Cosmetic Contouring

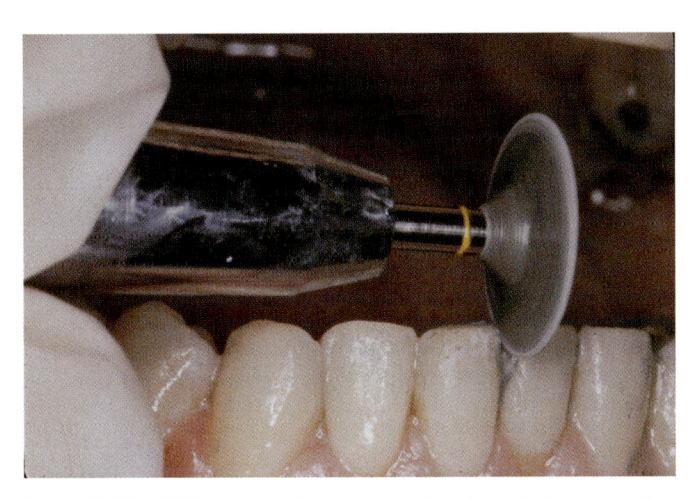

Figure 11.13 **(O)** The one yellow-banded disc shape further smooths the incisal embrasures and proximal surfaces.

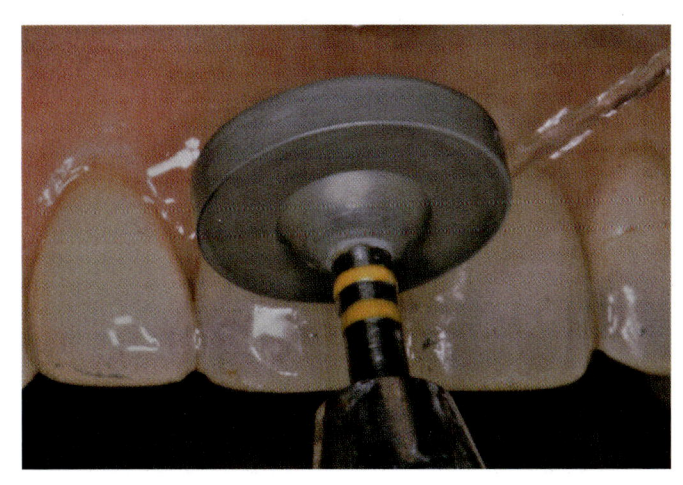

Figure 11.13 **(P)** The final finishing is done with the two yellow-banded wheel. Note how water is used to cleanse the tooth surface while reducing heat.

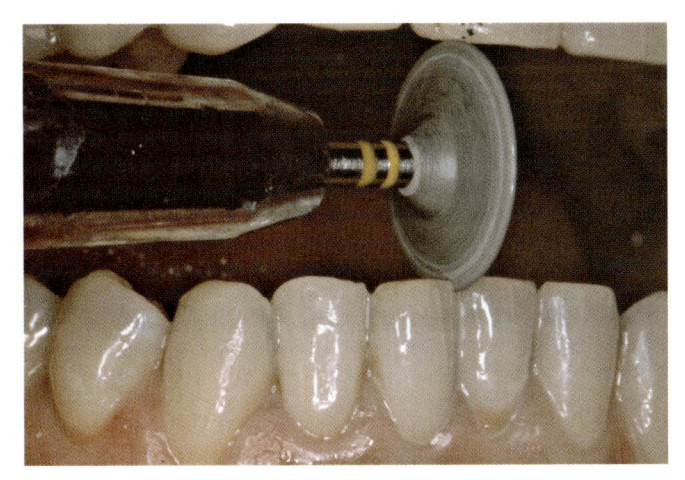

Figure 11.13 **(Q)** The two yellow-banded disc shape places the final finish on incisal embrasures.

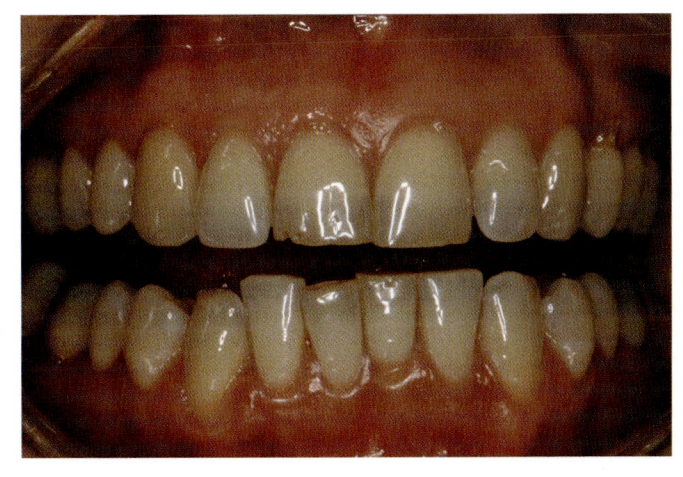

Figure 11.13 **(R)** Retracted view before cosmetic contouring.

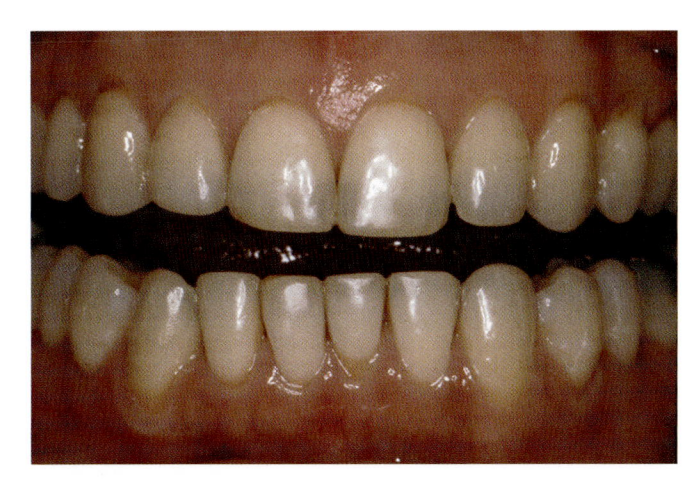

Figure 11.13 **(S)** Retracted view after cosmetic contouring shows the improved lower and upper incisal planes.

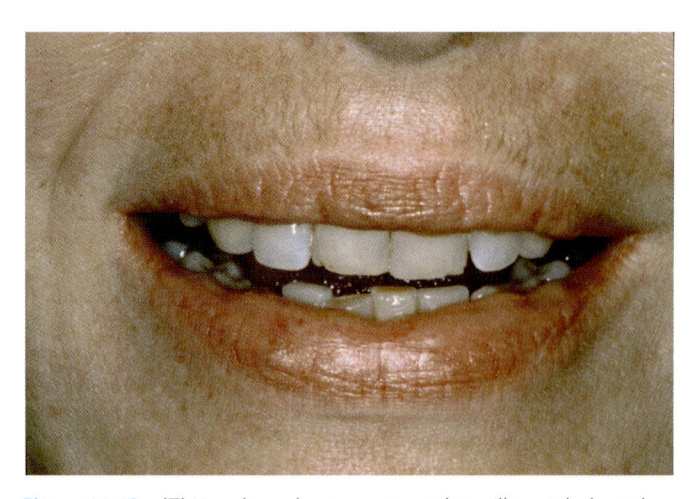

Figure 11.13 **(T)** Note how the supererupted maxillary right lateral and the lower crowding called unfavorable attention to the smile.

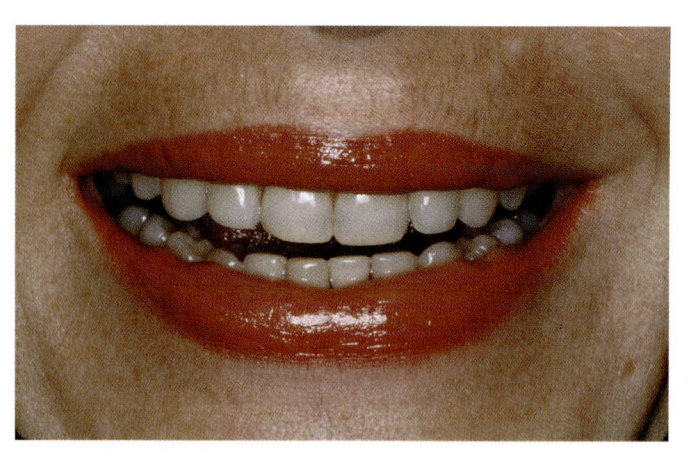

Figure 11.13 **(U)** This after smile shows how the lower incisal plane was improved. Shortening of the lateral incisors also helped to create a younger-appearing smile line.

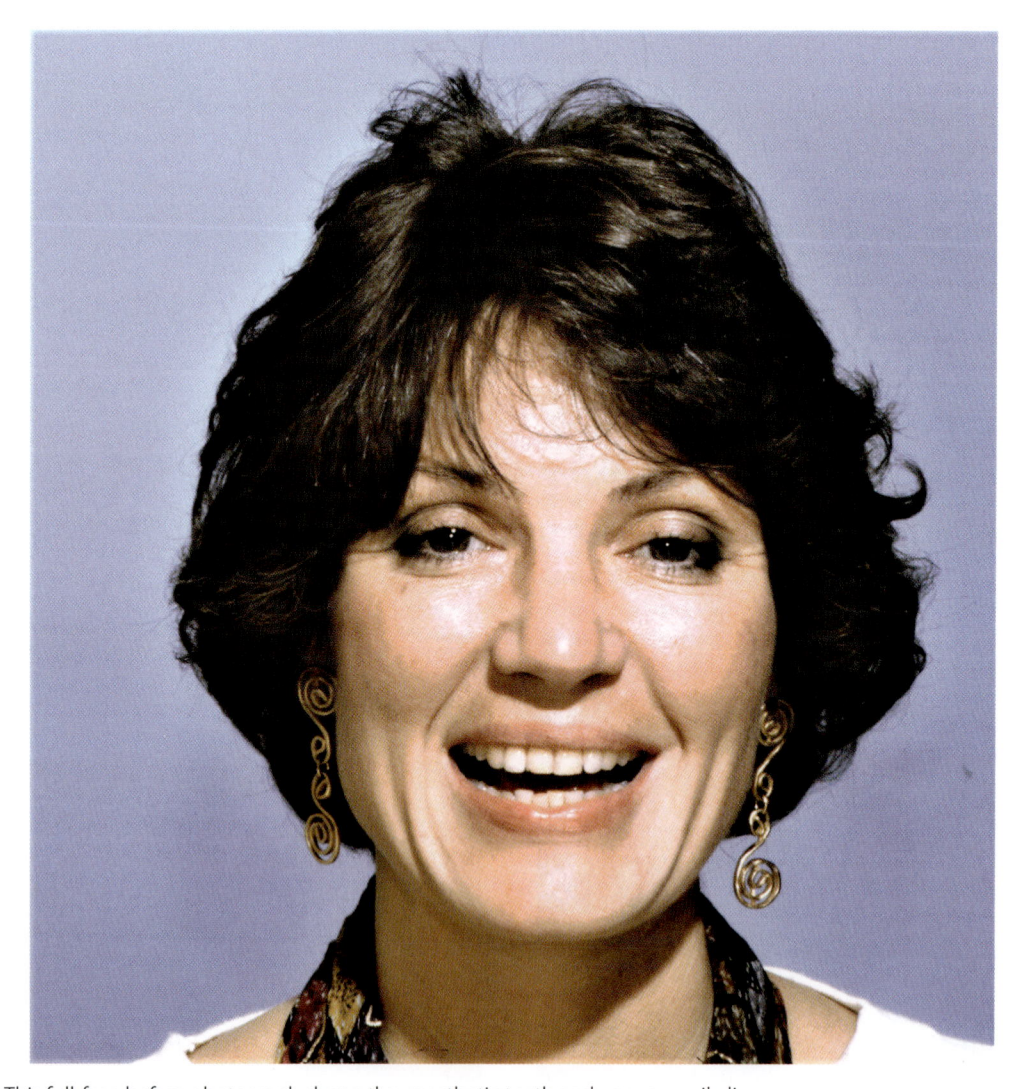

Figure 11.13 **(V)** This full-face before photograph shows the unesthetic teeth and uneven smile line.

The patient's chin drops down during normal conversation, and this, combined with the typical labial angulation of the lower incisors, presents an oblique view of these teeth to most viewers. So, in order to achieve a more natural look when the patient is speaking, an approximate 45° correction angle is used for lingual shaping (Figure 11.13 J). Next, any horizontal overlap created by overly wide or poorly aligned incisors is reduced (Figure 11.13 K). The mandibular teeth are then finished from

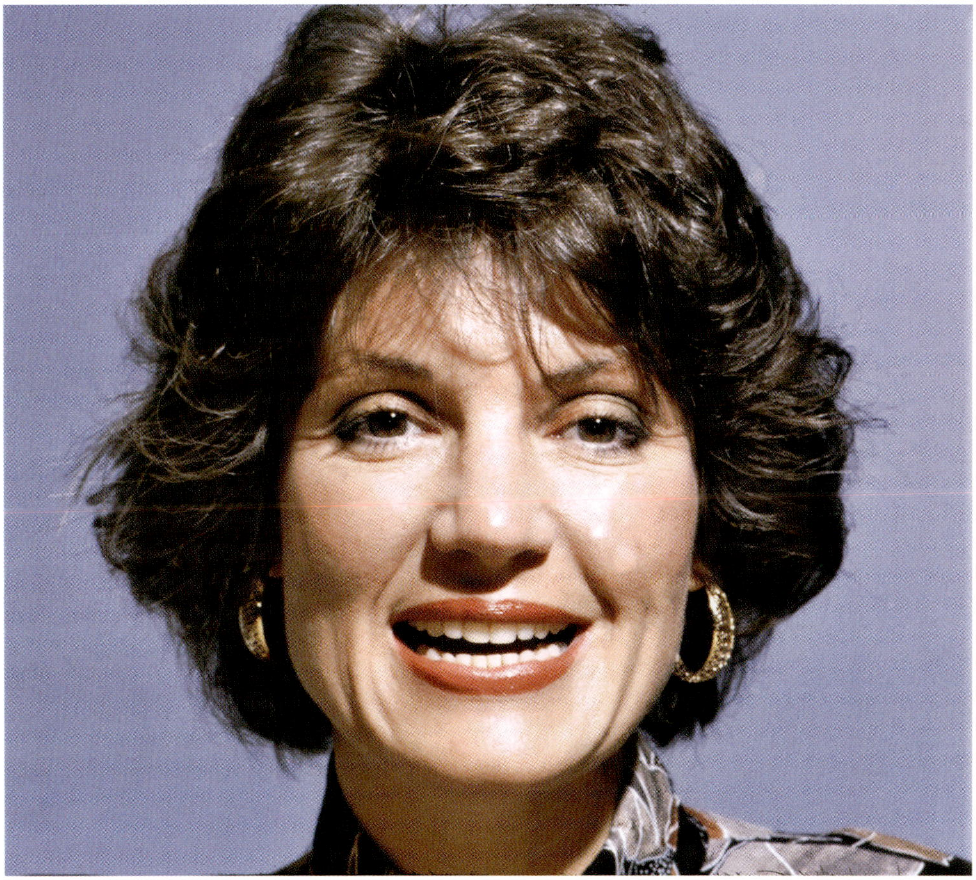

Figure 11.13 **(W)** The full-face after photograph shows the dramatic effect cosmetic contouring had on facial appearance by helping to achieve an illusion of straighter-looking teeth.

the lingual surface to make them appear even. After the original reshaping, the patient is viewed again in the given position to see if there is any further contouring required. It is a good idea to vary both your and the patient's position, for example sit up, stand up, and lean back, and don't forget lateral views. All of these views are helpful to make sure the illusion of straightness is as complete as possible. If necessary, remark and repeat the above steps.

Enamel finishing can be done with gray mounted points found in the Cosmetic Contouring Kit. The Shofu, wheel shape, with no yellow band (Figure 11.13 L) is used to polish incisal edges and labial and lingual surfaces. The disc shape is well suited for interproximal and incisal surfaces (Figure 11.13 M). Remember to always use these in sequence: no band, then one yellow band, then two yellow bands or one white band (Figure 11.13 N–Q).

Before and after views can be seen in Figure 11.13R and S. In studying the before and after retracted views, you can see how the lower incisal plane was improved by cosmetic contouring. Also, note how shortening the lateral incisors make the central incisors appear longer, thereby creating a younger-appearing smile line. If occlusion is a limiting factor, then consider restoring the opposing teeth to allow for your esthetic contouring. For instance, if you feel it is necessary to shorten a mandibular cuspid, it may be possible to bond or veneer the opposing maxillary cuspid to close the resulting interocclusal space so that your occlusion will not be altered.

When looking at the before smile (Figure 11.13 T) one's attention is subconsciously drawn to the super-erupted maxillary lateral incisor which has a fang-like appearance. This preoccupation with the mouth tends to compete with the eye-to-eye contact that most individuals strive for in speaking with others. The dramatic effect that cosmetic contouring can have on the facial appearance is shown in Figure 11.13 U–W. An illusion of straightness has been created.

Altering tooth form

Often the anatomic form of one tooth is altered to resemble another. A canine that has drifted or been repositioned into the space of an extracted or congenitally missing lateral incisor can sometimes be reshaped to resemble the missing tooth. Another example is the removal of part of the lingual cusp and reshaping of the labial surface of a first bicuspid so that it resembles a cuspid. Frequently, however, attempts to alter anatomic form do not produce the results that were hoped for. Nevertheless, in these cases, cosmetic contouring is still the most economical and least time-consuming method available, and the appearance may be quite acceptable. The next two cases are examples of how alteration of tooth form can create improved esthetics.

Clinical case: Esthetic shaping of incisal edges

Problem: A female, aged 24, presented with a worn cuspid (Figure 11.14A). She expressed a desire to have her anterior teeth "capped" to produce a more attractive smile but was willing to try cosmetic contouring first.

Treatment: Cosmetic contouring of the maxillary right cuspid is done by contouring the mesioincisal and distoincisal surfaces to open the incisal embrasures. New contours are created which give a softer look (Figure 11.14B).

Result: The patient was so pleased with the result that she no longer desired to have her teeth crowned. Most patients who want anterior esthetic improvement will usually ask to have their teeth crowned, or bonded. However, cosmetic contouring should always be considered as an alternative ideal or compromise solution.

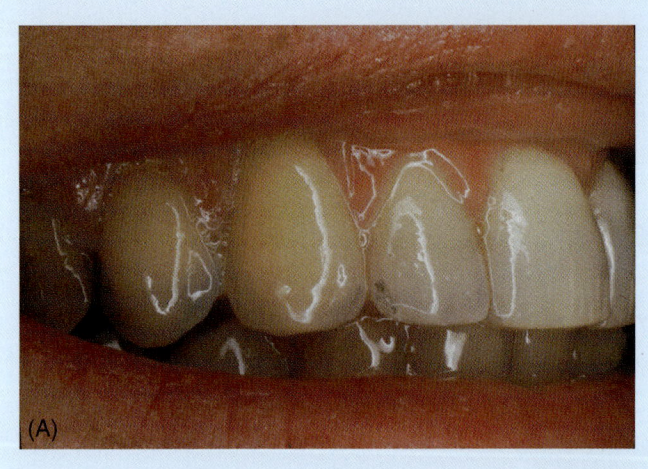

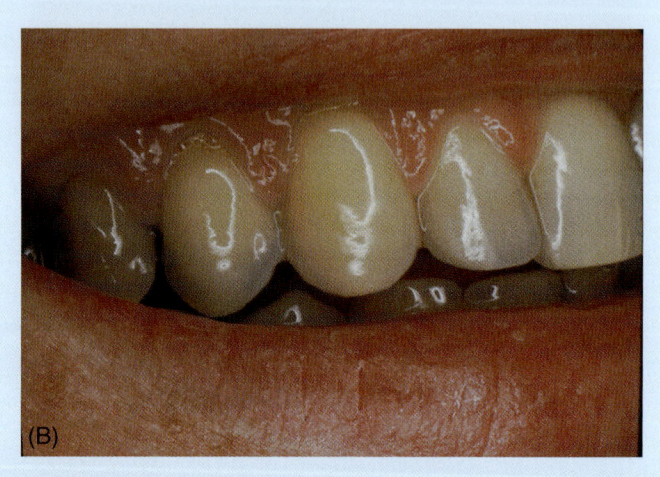

Figure 11.14 (A) This patient requested anterior crowns to produce a more attractive smile. (B) The mesioincisal and distoincisal surfaces of the maxillary right cuspid were contoured instead.

Clinical case: Changing cuspid anatomy

Problem: A female, age 31, presented with extremely long maxillary cuspids which gave her a "vampire" look. She stated that when she smiled her cuspids were so prominent that they detracted from her appearance (Figure 11.15A and B).

Treatment: The patient was told that a conservative procedure could be performed that could improve her smile. Cosmetic contouring of the labial surface of the cuspids was then done without exposing sensitive dentin (Figure 11.15C and D).

Result: The patient was extremely pleased at the dramatic improvement of her appearance that was accomplished in one appointment.

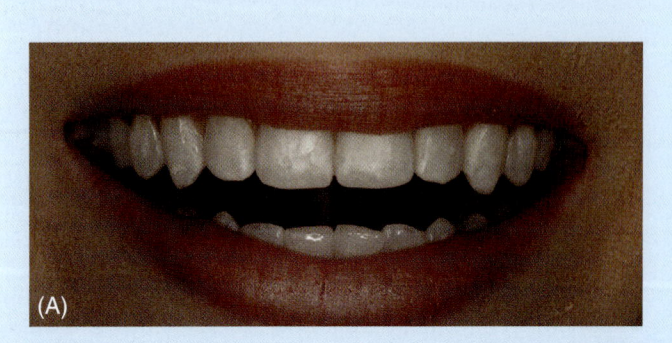

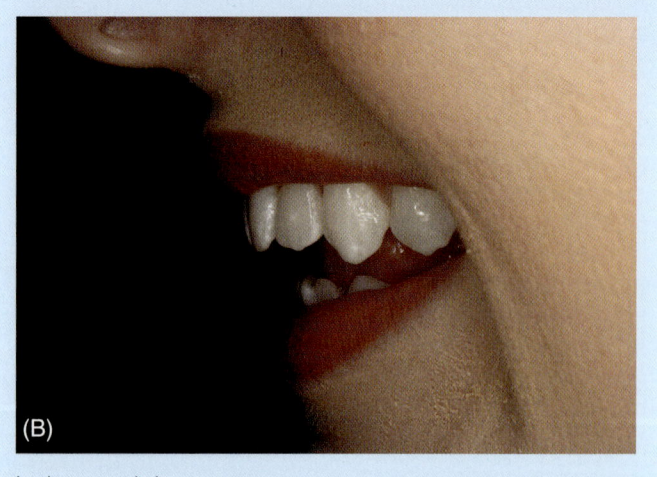

Figure 11.15 (A and B) This 31-year-old state beauty contestant winner had extremely long canines.

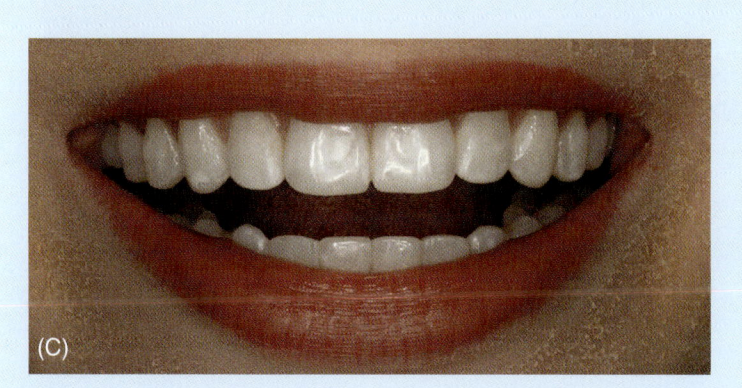

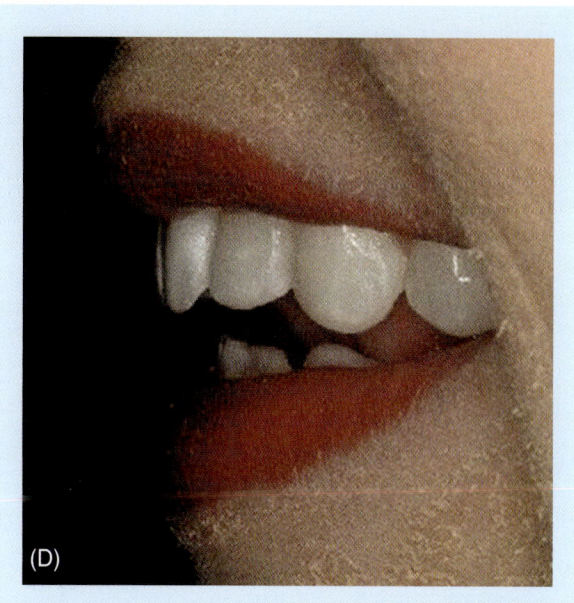

Figure 11.15 (C and D) After a 1 hour cosmetic contouring appointment, in which the canines were reshaped, the patient's smile line was improved.

Clinical case: Overlapping central incisors

The main objective in correcting overlapping incisors is to remove as much as possible of the tooth structure that overlaps the adjacent tooth by contouring the labial aspect of the labially malposed tooth and the lingual aspect of a lingually malposed tooth. This straightens the portion that overlaps the adjacent tooth and makes the long axis of the teeth more parallel to each other (Figure 11.16A–E).

An important consideration is the amount of tooth structure that will show when the patient speaks and smiles. This can be determined by having the patient repeat words that emphasize different lip positions. Also ask the patient to smile slightly and then to smile as widely as possible. If a compromise has to be reached, then make that determination during conversation so that the incisal one-third of the dentition—the part that shows

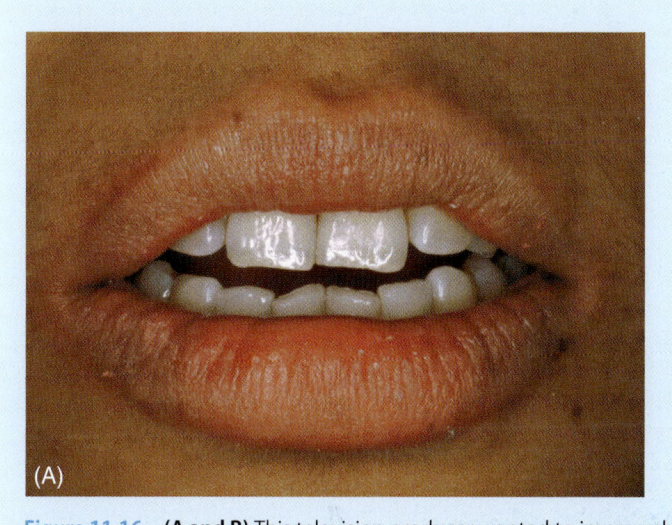

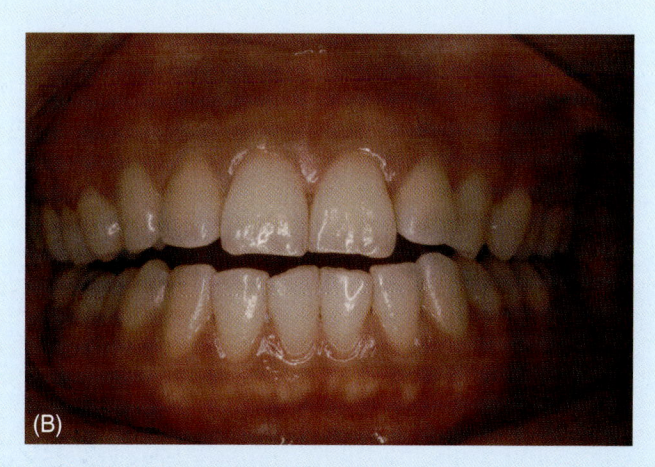

Figure 11.16 (A and B) This television producer wanted to improve her smile without wearing braces if possible.

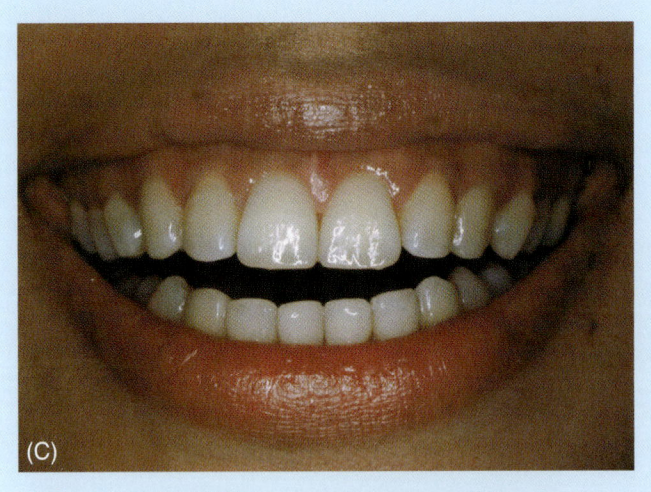

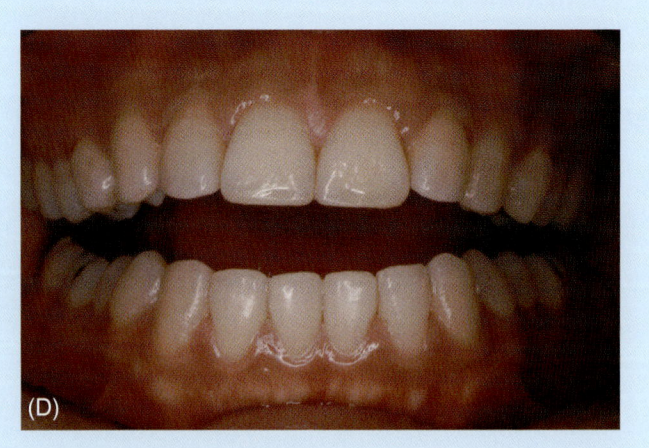

Figure 11.16 (C and D) A 1 h appointment was all it took to help create an illusion of straight teeth and a new smile.

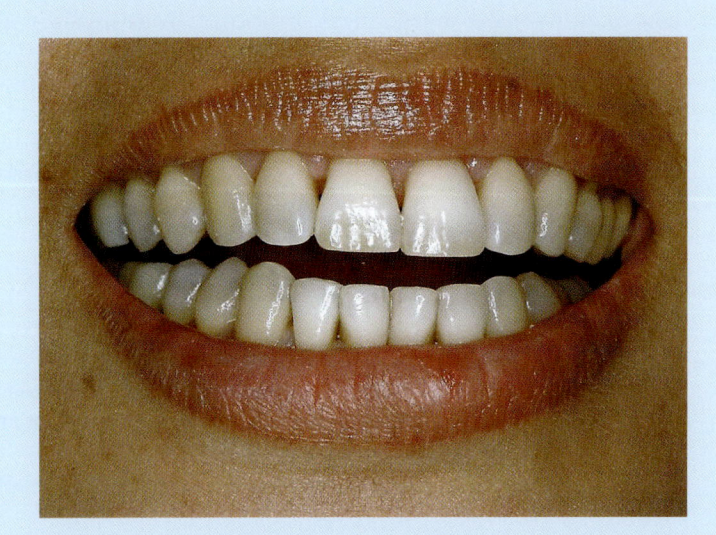

Figure 11.16 (E) The same patient 35 years later, with very little change despite presence of some bone loss. It has been the author's experience that if you maintain either centric or protrusive relations, the result will remain consistent.

most of the time—can be contoured to achieve the desired illusion of straightness.

One important point in reshaping is to make sure that the incisal embrasure between the teeth is reopened to at least 0.25–0.50 mm length. This is accomplished by using an extra-thin needle-shaped diamond (DET-3 or -4, Brasseler USA) (Figure 11.17A–C). This helps achieve an illusion of straightness. In the labiogingival area, the extension of an overlapping tooth is de-emphasized by blending the shape into the newly created contour.

Care must be taken in reducing the extended portion (circle) of an overlapping tooth (Figure 11.17A). One of the most common pitfalls in reshaping is to thin the tooth so much that the dentin shows through. If that happens, the tooth may appear discolored. The long axis of each of the teeth must be determined, as it will be used to correct the overlapping tooth. Usually the long axes of the teeth (lines a in Figure 11.17C) will vary from tooth to tooth when the lower anterior teeth are crowded (Figure 11.17C). Therefore, choose a parallel line (line b in Figure 11.17C) and do all of the mesial and distal reshaping with this line as the guide. Then reopen the incisal embrasure (Figure 11.17C). The following two cases are examples of two solutions to this problem—the first is solved with cosmetic contouring by itself and the second with cosmetic contouring and bonding.

Chapter 11 Cosmetic Contouring

Figure 11.17 (A) These are the areas to contour to reduce the horizontal overlap and make the teeth appear straight.

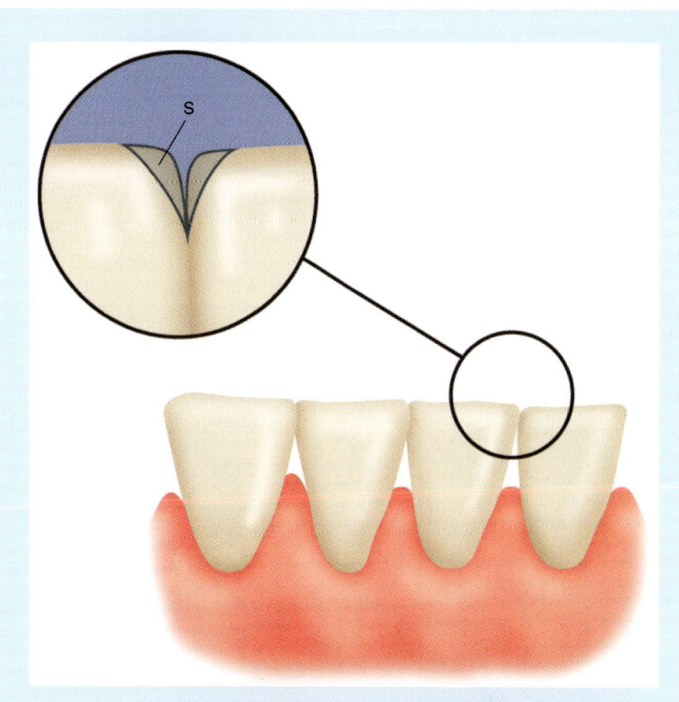

Figure 11.17 (B) An incisal embrasure(s) can break up a too-even, worn look at the incisal edge.

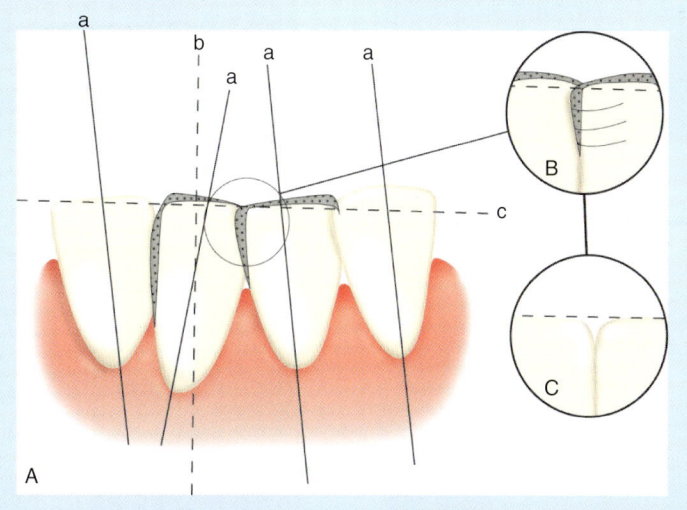

Figure 11.17 (C) The gingivoincisal angle of straightness between all the teeth must be determined as it will be used to correct the overlapping tooth. The long axes of overlapping teeth will usually vary when the lower anterior teeth are crowded; therefore, choose a parallel line (b) when doing your mesial and distal correction.

Clinical case: Reducing large teeth

Problem: A female, age 25, presented with extremely large, overlapping, and flaring central incisors (Figure 11.18A–F). Because of the arch alignment, the labioversion of the centrals called attention to their size. The patient's high lip line made it impossible to conceal the unesthetic appearance.

Treatment: Cosmetic contouring was selected as a compromise to orthodontics or crowns. The teeth on the diagnostic study casts were reshaped with a sandpaper disc, so that the patient could then visualize the anticipated result (Figure 11.18C). The areas to be reduced were marked in the mouth (Figure 11.18D). The procedure for reduction and polishing was followed, and the results can be seen in Figure 11.18E and F.

Result: A definite improvement is seen in the patient's smile, since the teeth are now in better proportion (Figure 11.18E and F).

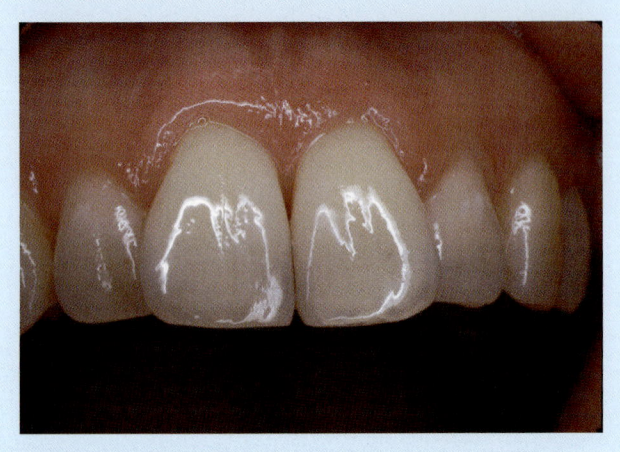

Figure 11.18 (A) Unesthetic central incisors can benefit from cosmetic contouring.

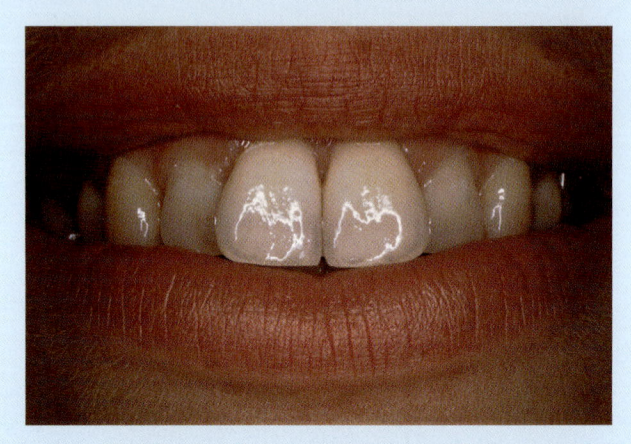

Figure 11.18 (B) A high lipline made it impossible to conceal the unesthetic appearance.

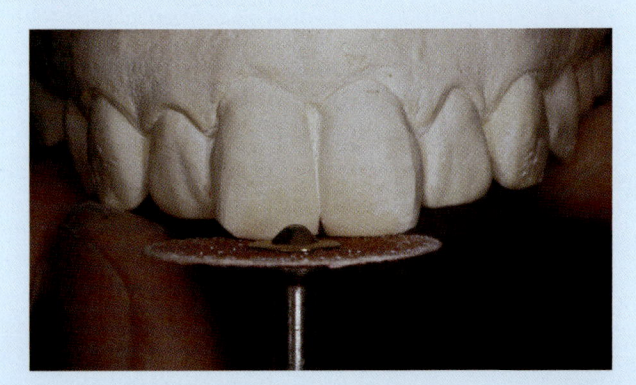

Figure 11.18 (C) The diagnostic study casts were shaped with a sandpaper disc, so that the patient could visualize the final result.

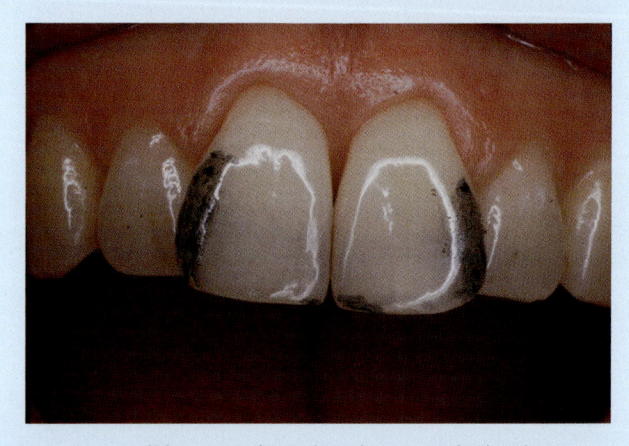

Figure 11.18 (D) Areas to be reduced were marked with an alcohol marking pen.

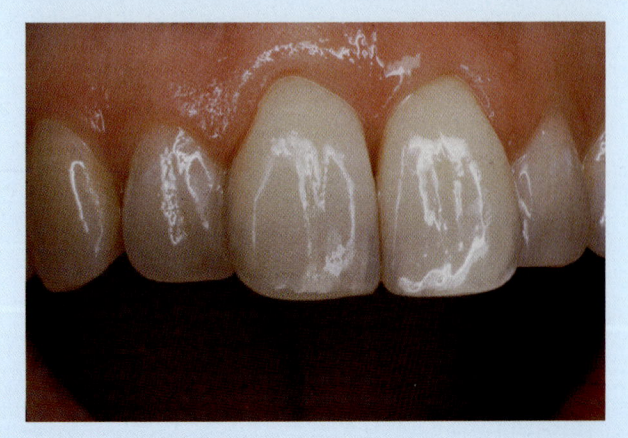

Figure 11.18 (E) Note the more proportional appearance created by cosmetic contouring and polishing the central incisors.

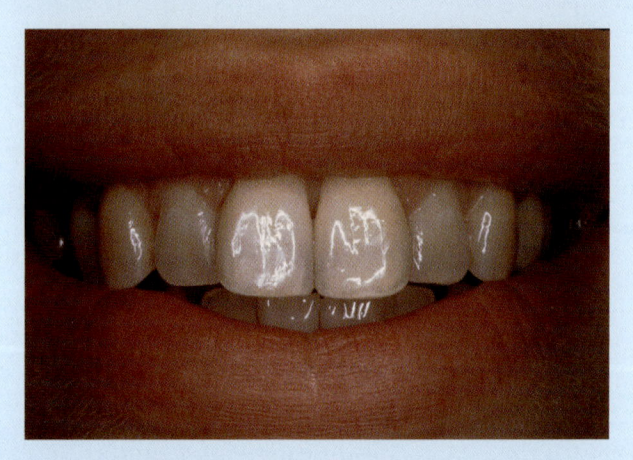

Figure 11.18 (F) Cosmetic contouring improved this patient's smile. The teeth are now in better proportion.

Clinical case: Combination cosmetic contouring and direct composite bonding

Cosmetic contouring is an important adjunct to bleaching, bonding, veneering, crowning, or any other treatment designed to make the teeth look better. In fact, the procedure is indicated to some degree in almost every patient who wants to achieve the best smile possible. This is a case that illustrates the combined therapy of cosmetic contouring and composite resin bonding.

Problem: This female wanted to improve her smile which was marred by two protruding, wide central incisors (Figure 11.19A and C).

Solution: Cosmetic contouring narrowed the central incisors and composite resin was added to the labial surfaces of the lateral incisors. Figure 11.19D shows the occlusal view of this newly improved arch relationship.

Result: Better tooth alignment and a balanced light reflection produced a more symmetrical smile (Figure 11.19B and D). Anterior teeth that are in linguoversion typically can benefit from bonding or veneering to improve the alignment and arch form.

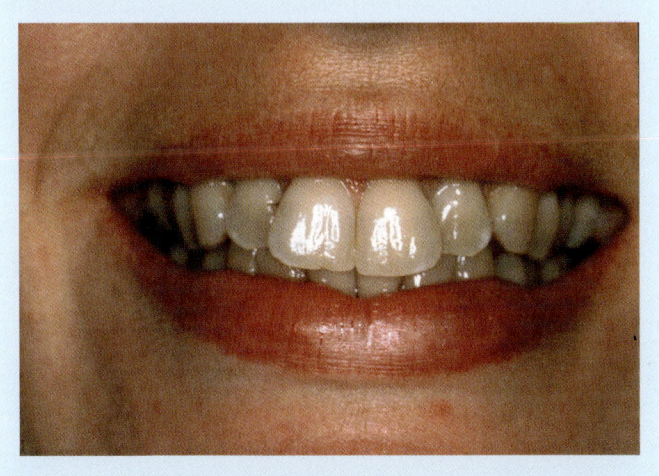

Figure 11.19 (A) This 35-year-old female's smile was marred by two extremely wide protruding central incisors.

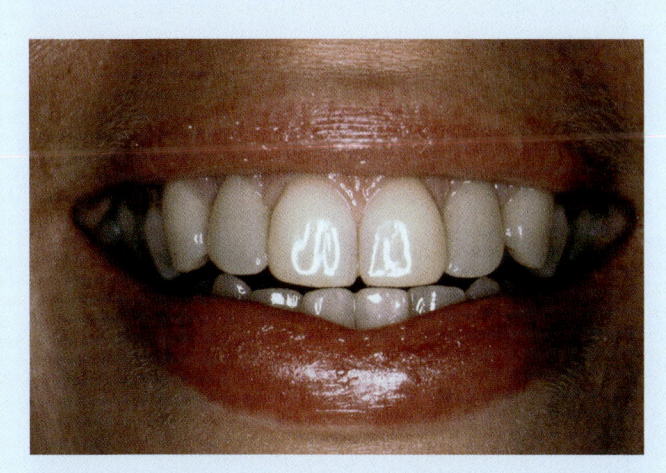

Figure 11.19 (B) The after smile photo reveals a more symmetrical smile produced in part by the balanced light reflection made possible by building out the lateral incisors with direct composite resin bonding.

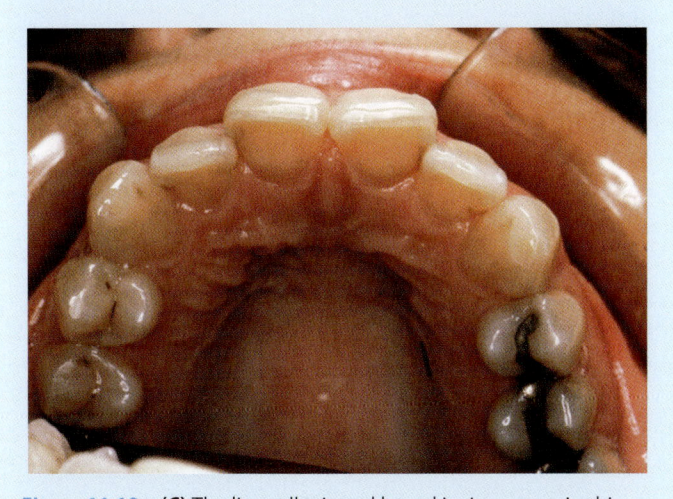

Figure 11.19 (C) The lingually tipped lateral incisors seen in this occlusal view needed to be built out labially with direct composite resin bonding.

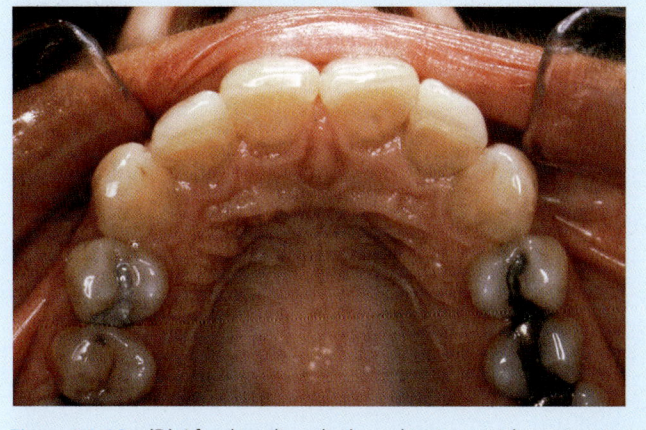

Figure 11.19 (D) After bonding the lateral incisors with composite resin, there is an improved arch relationship.

Arch irregularity

Few of us are born with perfectly symmetrical arches. But most of us rarely notice minor deviations. However, a serious discrepancy is usually noticeable to the patient but less to the viewer. This is especially true of a canted arch as in Figure 11.20A–F. Treatment to correct arch irregularity ranges from orthodontics, including orthognathic surgery at times, to restorative methods such as crowns, veneers, bonding, and especially cosmetic contouring. Treatment of choice can sometimes be conservative if the cant is not too severe. Cosmetic contouring alone or combined with restorative dentistry can be a viable option as seen in Figure 11.20C and D.

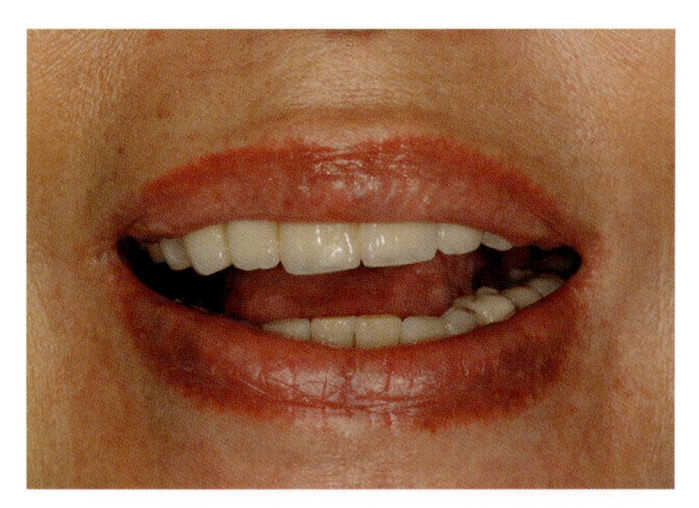

Figure 11.20 (A) This patient was unhappy with her canted smile.

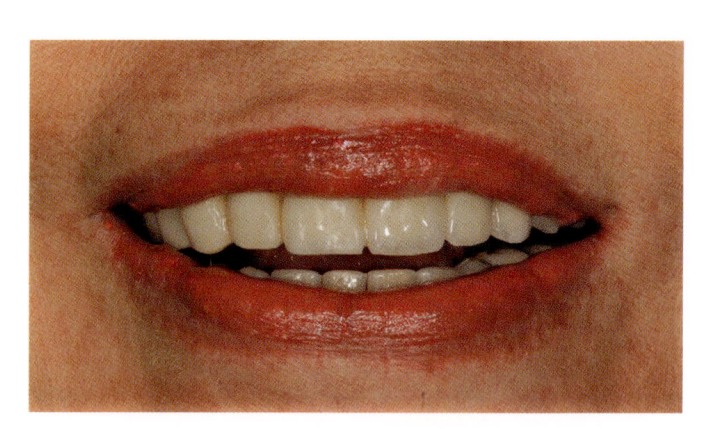

Figure 11.20 (C) The patient now has a more improved and symmetrical smile.

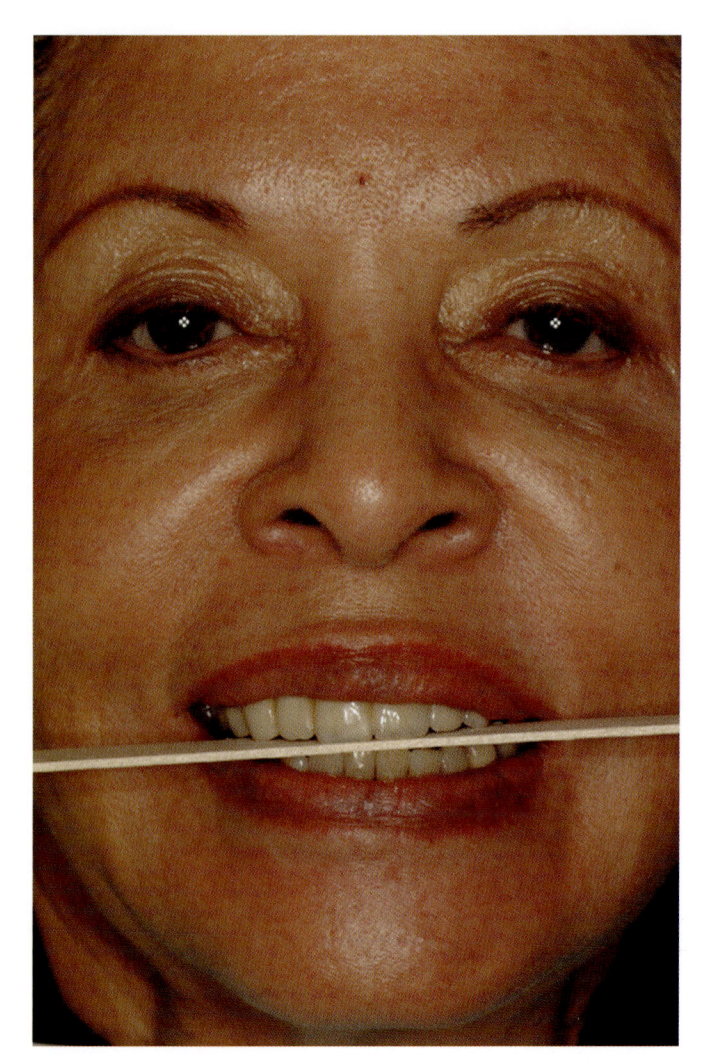

Figure 11.20 (B) By having the patient bite with a tongue depressor in place, you can easily see the amount of cant that needs to be corrected.

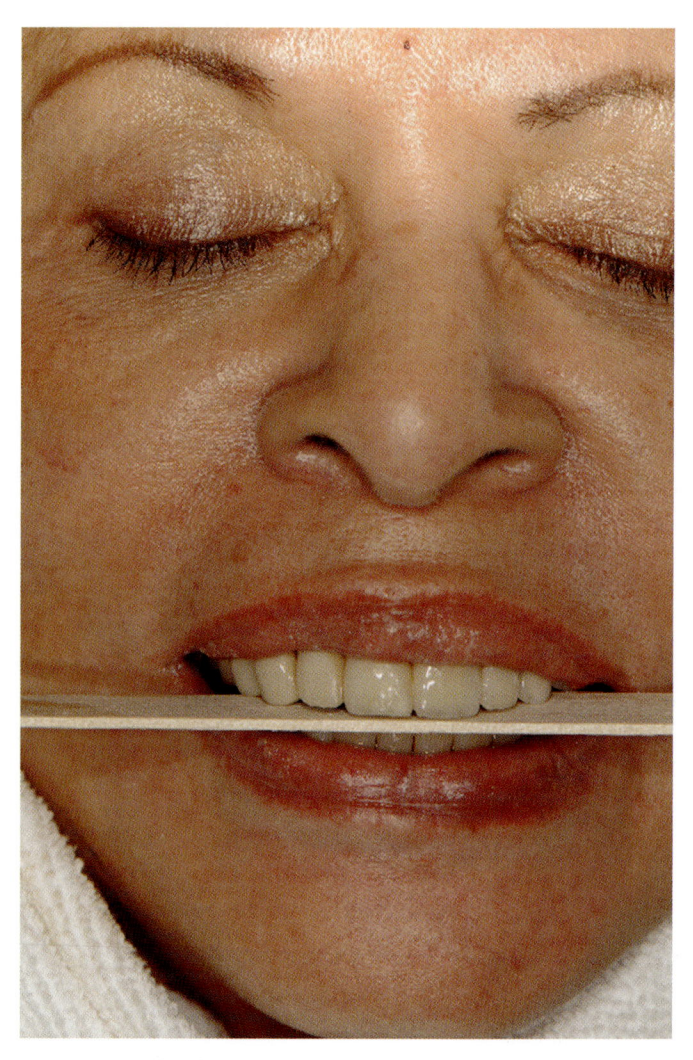

Figure 11.20 (D) The tongue depressor helps illustrate a more symmetrical arch, which was accomplished with cosmetic contouring alone, creating a straight illusion.

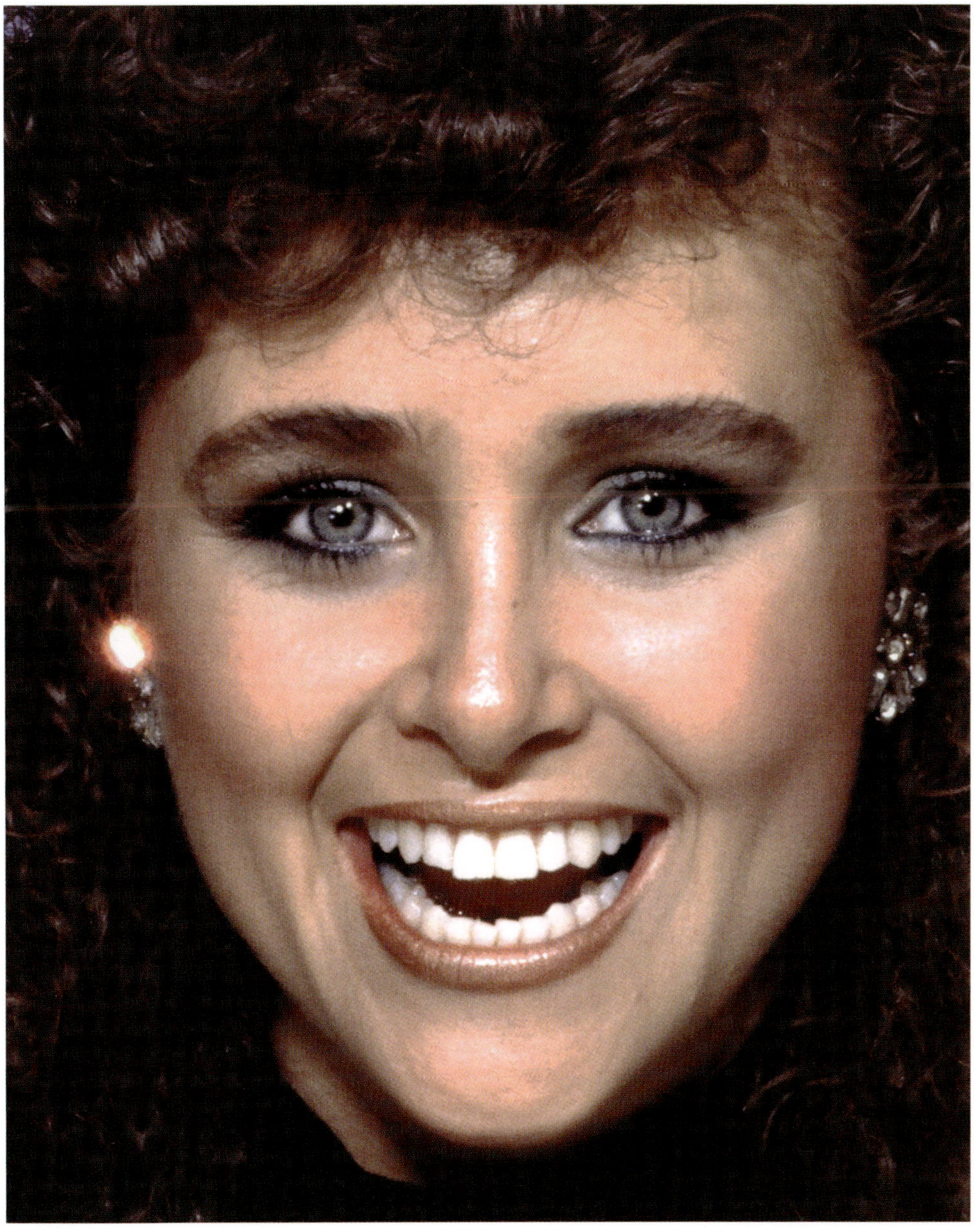

Figure 11.20 **(E)** This patient's lower and upper arch were affected by overlapping maxillary centrals plus lower crowding.

Summary

When I look at before and after smile results both in lectures and dental magazine publications I periodically see how the smile could have been improved through cosmetic contouring. The procedure takes an hour or less in most cases and it is a fee-based procedure. So what is lacking is remembering to examine each patient to see how much more you can improve his or her smile. I even ask my treatment coordinator or lead dental assistant to remind me if I fail to include cosmetic contouring in the treatment plan. In fact, there is a separate line devoted to the procedure in one of my treatment planning worksheets (Figure 3.17).

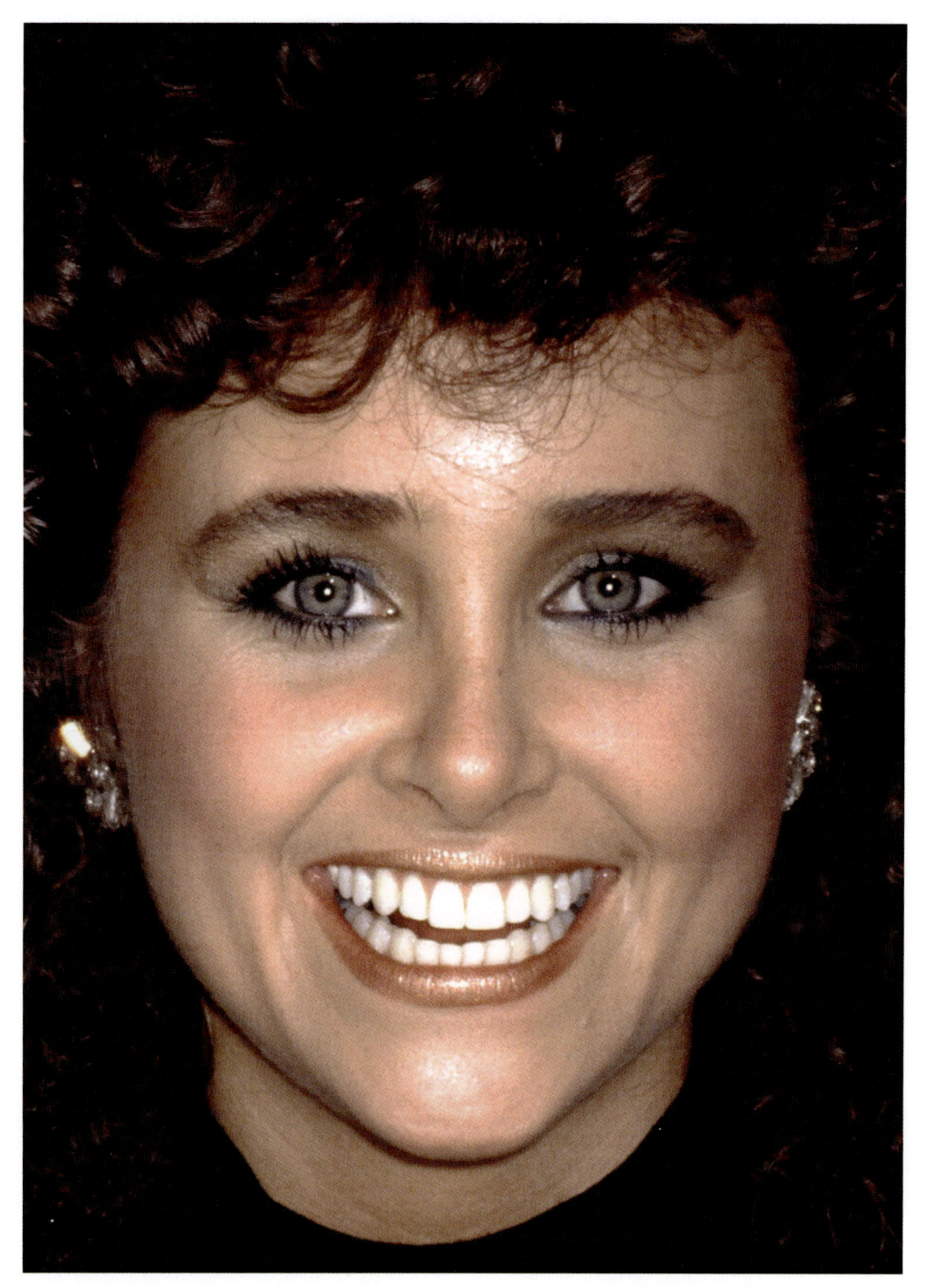

Figure 11.20 **(F)** Cosmetic contouring of both arches helped to hide the irregularities enhancing the smile of this young lady.

References

1. Goldstein RE. Study of need for esthetics in dentistry. *J Prosthet Dent* 1969;21:589.
2. Pincus CL. Cosmetics—the psychologic fourth dimension in full mouth rehabilitation. *Dent Clin North Am* 1967;March:71.
3. Shelby DS. *Anterior Restoration, Fixed Bridgework, and Esthetics* [postgraduate course]. First District Dent Soc. of NY; October 1967.
4. Frush JP, Fisher RD. Dentogenics: its practical application. *J Prosthet Dent* 1959;9:914.
5. Frush JP, Fisher RD. How dentogenic restorations interpret the sex factor. *J Prosthet Dent* 1956;6:160.
6. Frush JP, Fisher RD. How dentogenics interprets the personality factor. *J Prosthet Dent* 1956;6:441.
7. Frush JP, Fisher RD. Introduction to dentogenic restorations. *J Prosthet Dent* 1955;5:586.
8. Frush JP, Fisher RD. The age factor in dentogenics. *J Prosthet Dent* 1957;7:5.

9. Frush JP, Fisher RD. The dynesthetic interpretation of the dentogenic concept. *J Prosthet Dent* 1958;8:558.
10. Simring M. *Practical Periodontal Techniques for Esthetics* [postgraduate course]. First District Dent. Soc. of NY; November 1966.
11. Simring M, Koteen SM, Simon SL. Occlusal equilibration. In: Ward HL, Simring M, eds. *Manual of Clinical Periodontics*. St. Louis, MO: CV Mosby; 1973.

Additional resources

Adolfi D. Functional, esthetic and morphologic adjustment procedures for anterior teeth. *Quintessence Dent Technol* 2009;32:153–168.

Goldstein R. *Change Your Smile*, 4th edn. Hanover Park, IL: Quintessence Publishing Co.; 2009.

Guyana Chronicle Online. Enameloplasty. http://guyanachronicle.com/2013/03/24/enameloplasty (accessed January 10, 2014).

IEnhance. *Tooth Contouring and Reshaping*. http://www.ienhance.com/procedures/tooth-contouring (accessed July 23, 2014).

National Center for Aesthetic Facial and Oral Surgery. *Dental Contouring and Reshaping*. http://www.maxfac.com/dentistry/reshaping.html (accessed October 12, 2014).

Paliwal M, Thoma A, Azad A., Balani R, Ekka S. Application of cosmetic contouring in orthodontic esthetic dentistry-a case report. *Int J Adv Dent Sci Technol* 2013;1:10–13.

Sarver D. Principles of cosmetic dentistry in orthodontics: Part 1. Shape and proportionality in anterior teeth. *Am J Ortho Dentofac Orthoped* 2004;126:749–753.

Sarver D. Enameloplasty and esthetic finishing in orthodontics—differential diagnosis of incisor proclination—the importance of appropriate visualization and records Part 2. *J Esthet Restor Dent* 2011;23:303–313.

Sheehan J, Haynes C. Tooth reshaping and dental contouring. http://www.everydayhealth.com/dental-health/cosmetic-dentistry/tooth-reshaping.aspx (accessed November 3, 2014).

WebMD. *Dental Health and Recontouring Teeth*. http://www.webmd.com/oral-health/guide/recontouring-teeth (accessed November 1, 2014).

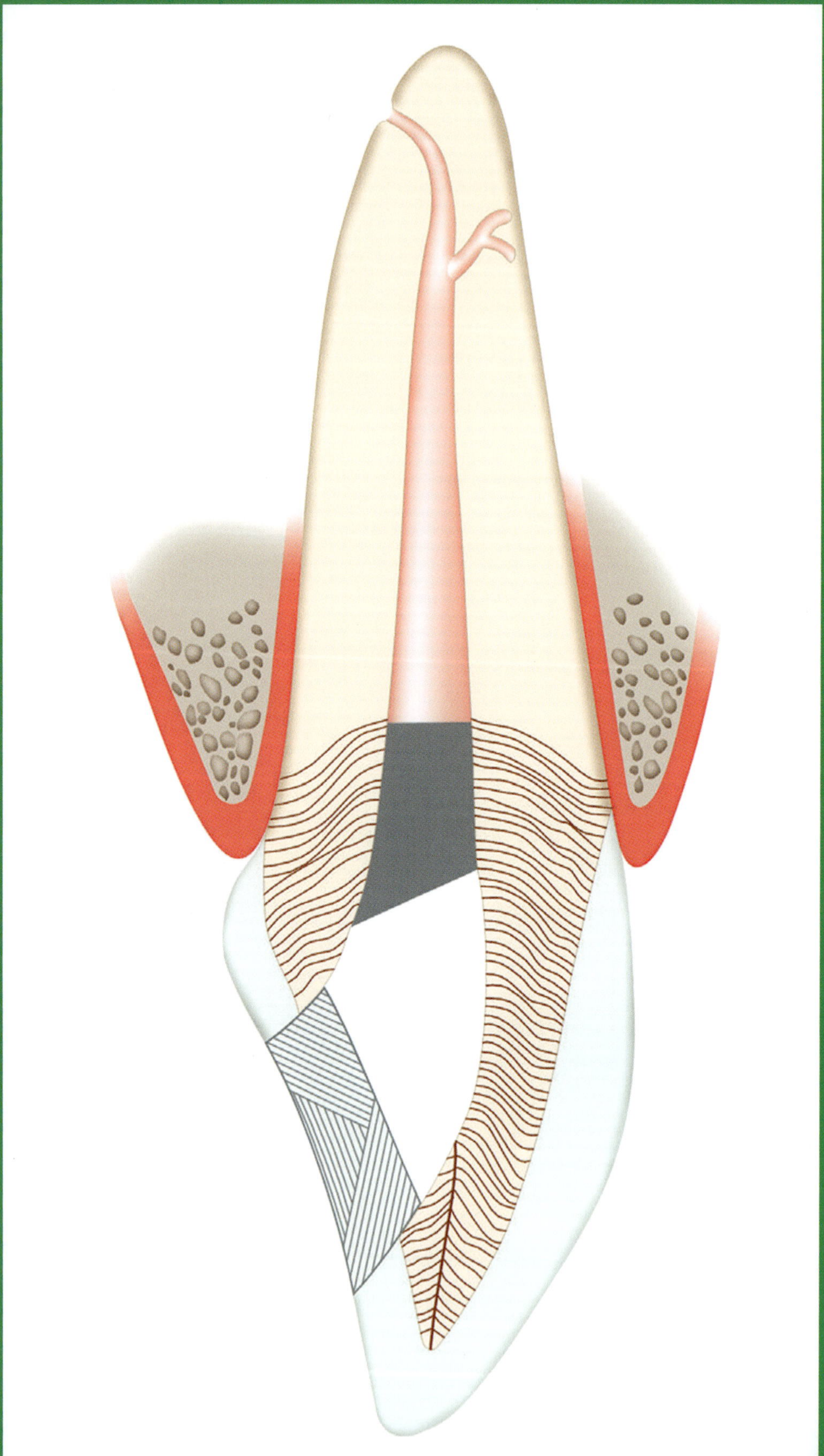

Chapter 12 Bleaching Discolored Teeth

So Ran Kwon, DDS, MS, PhD, MS and
Ronald E. Goldstein, DDS

Chapter Outline

Bleaching vital teeth	326
Etiology of discoloration	328
Extrinsic stains	328
Intrinsic stains	328
Tetracycline stain	328
Minocycline stain	329
Stain from dental conditions or treatments	330
Stain from systemic conditions	330
Discoloration due to aging	331
Contraindications to bleaching of vital teeth using in-office techniques	331
Level of expectation	332
Sequence of treatment	333
Combined bleaching and restorative dentistry	333
Bleaching combined with minor restorative treatment	334
Bleaching combined with orthodontics	334
Bleaching in patients with multiple caries, abrasion, and erosion	335
Bleaching combined with periodontics	335
Bleaching for children	335
Bleaching for elderly patients	335
Recording the baseline color	336
Techniques for in-office bleaching of vital teeth	336
Preparation and application of bleaching material	336
Microabrasion	341
Matrix bleaching (nightguard vital bleaching)	341
Power and monitored matrix bleaching: a combined approach	341
Preparing the patient for matrix-monitored bleaching	343
Home bleaching without dental supervision (over-the-counter systems)	345
Tooth sensitivity during vital bleaching	345
Maintaining bleaching results	346
In-office bleaching of nonvital teeth	346
Etiology of discoloration	346
Contraindications to bleaching of pulpless teeth with concentrated hydrogen peroxide (35%)	346
Techniques for bleaching pulpless teeth	346
Preparation	347
Inside-outside tray bleaching technique	348
Out-of-office bleaching technique (or walking bleach)	348
Finishing	349
Planning for continued treatment	349
Complications and risks	350
Cervical root resorption	350
Color relapse	350
The future of bleaching	350

Ask the average person how they would most like to improve their smile and the answer would often be "with whiter and brighter teeth." It is commonly known that people are responded to in a more positive manner when they have a dazzling, healthy smile. This chapter is about how we in dentistry can fulfill our patients' requests for a brighter smile through bleaching.

Most newly formed teeth have thick, even enamel. This enamel layer modifies the base color of the underlying dentin, creating a milky white appearance.[1] For many of your patients, that bright, white look can typify youth, health, and physical attractiveness. It is the look against which they measure the appearance of their own teeth.

For some, unfortunately, their teeth will seem dingy and discolored in comparison. Teeth become stained and discolored, sometimes before they even erupt, almost always as they age, for one or more genetic, environmental, medical, or dental reasons. The most common problems are the superficial color changes that result from tobacco, coffee or tea, or highly colored foods. Teeth that contain microcracks are particularly susceptible to these stains. Discoloration also occurs through the penetration of the tooth structure by a discoloring agent, such as a medication given systemically, excessive fluoride ingested during the development of tooth enamel, byproducts of the body such as bilirubin released into the dentinal tubules during illness, trauma (primarily the breakdown of hemoglobin), or pigmentation from the medicaments and materials used in dental repair. Wear and thinning of the enamel caused by aging, too abrasive cleaning materials, aggressive brushing, and acidic food and drink also can diminish the covering power of the white enamel, letting more of the darker-hued dentin show through.[1]

Severe discoloration of a tooth or teeth can be a major esthetic problem. If left untreated, this discoloration may produce social and psychological difficulties. Other chapters have described some of the ways in which dentistry has responded to patients' desire for whiter teeth, from full crowns to bonding and laminating with various veneers and inlays and onlays. For the appropriate patient, with careful diagnosis, case selection, treatment planning, and attention to technique, bleaching can be the simplest, least invasive, and least expensive approach to brighter teeth. Sometimes one office session is sufficient to change a patient's appearance dramatically. If considered as an adjunct to other procedures for correcting discoloration and other esthetic problems, bleaching extends promise to an even larger group of patients who seek more attractive teeth. This chapter will provide current concepts and the latest scientific evidence in tooth bleaching that can fulfill our patient's desire for a whiter and brighter smile.

Bleaching vital teeth

The earliest efforts to bleach teeth go back more than a century and focused on the search for an effective bleaching agent to paint on discolored teeth. As described in a detailed history by Zaragoza,[2] Abbot had introduced by 1918 the forerunner of the combination used to bleach vital teeth today: hydrogen peroxide and an accelerated reaction caused by devices delivering heat to the teeth.

In the early 1960s, Goldstein developed the first commercial bleaching light for in-office bleaching of vital teeth (Figure 12.1A–F).

The recent history of this procedure comprises the bleaching of stained vital teeth that became increasingly popular in the 1970s when a growing number of dentists saw how well it worked on the stains caused by tetracycline ingestion at critical developmental stages of the teeth.

Although many of the mechanisms by which bleaching removes discoloration may not be fully understood, the basic process almost certainly involves oxidation, during which the molecules causing the discoloration are released. The use of heat and light devices appears to accelerate the oxidation reaction.[3,4]

For the next 20 years, in-office bleaching or power bleaching by dentists proved helpful for this and other problems. More recently, dentists began combining in-office bleaching with further treatments that the patient continues at home. This combination is increasingly popular among dentists and patients alike, particularly because of the ease and lower costs of nightguard vital bleaching.

In the early 1990s, bleaching gained a new prominence in the public eye with the introduction and aggressive marketing of bleaching materials intended to be used without dental evaluation and monitoring.[5] The widespread acceptance of these products can also be seen as a disturbing trend due to the potential for misdiagnosis, use of bleaching for inappropriate conditions, poorly fitting mouthguards, and unesthetic or painful results. Bleaching materials applied inappropriately may make the existing situation worse, creating uneven color change or deleteriously affecting restorations. The availability of such products places additional responsibility on the dental profession to make people aware how well professionally applied bleaching works, or whether it works at all, depends on the discoloration itself, its cause, the length of time the discoloring agent has permeated the structure of the tooth, and other factors about which a dentist's advice and monitoring is critical.

A good visual examination usually will suggest the etiology of discoloration and consequently the appropriateness of bleaching as a treatment. The diagnostic workup should include pretreatment photographs, X-ray films, and an intensive prophylaxis to remove superficial staining that may be compounding more intrinsic discoloration. The presence and condition of all restorations must be noted, and special attention paid to the materials of which these are made. The medical history should focus on diagnosis of any systemic problems or medications that might have affected or be affecting tooth coloration. A behavior inventory should determine the possible contributions of tobacco, beverage, and foods. The workup should establish color baselines, note the condition of the teeth and mouth in general, and note the patient's tooth sensitivity in particular.

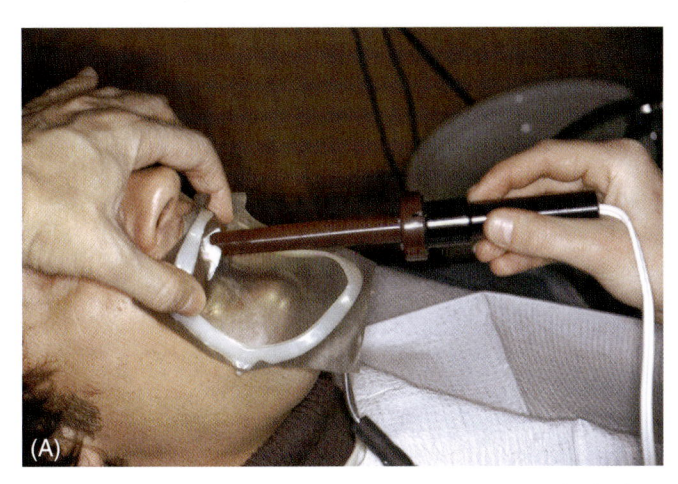

Figure 12.1 **(A)** In the early 1960s, Christensen showed individual teeth bleaching using a modified soldering iron.

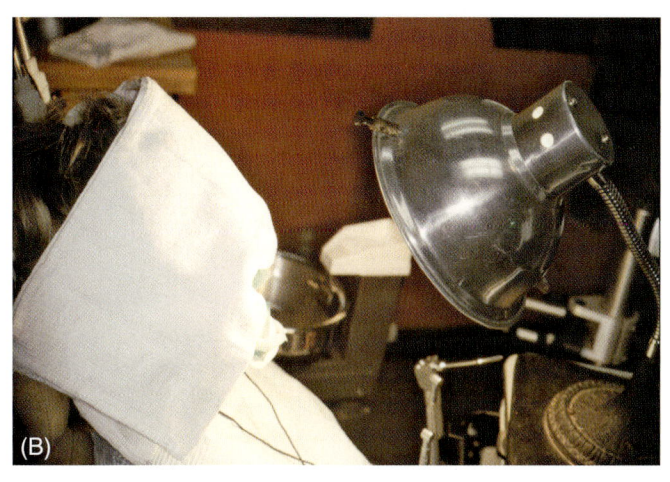

Figure 12.1 **(B)** Also in the 1960s, Goldstein showed in-office bleaching using a modified photoflood lamp in order to bleach multiple teeth.

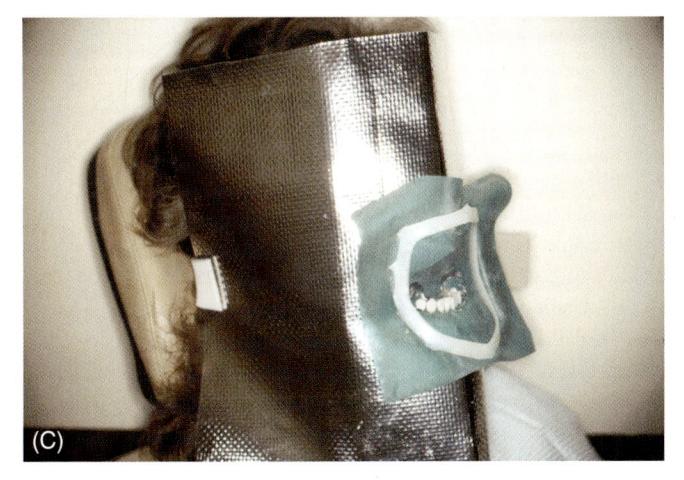

Figure 12.1 **(C)** Due to the excessive heat created by the photoflood lamp, Goldstein developed a bleaching shield that protected the patient's face.

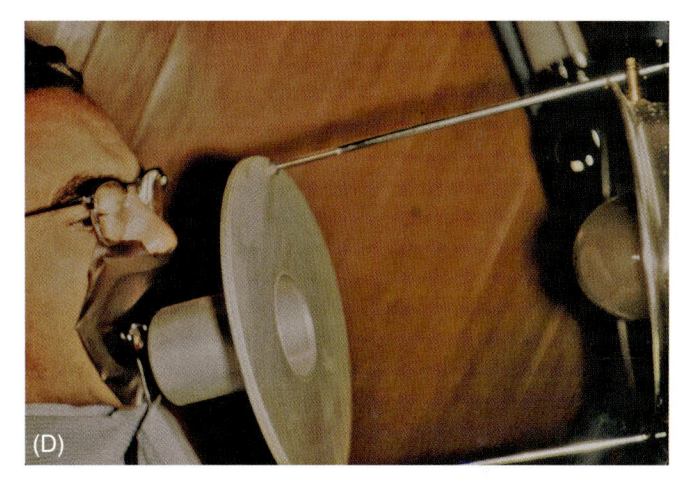

Figure 12.1 **(D)** Goldstein later modified the bleaching light to better isolate the heat and light into a narrower zone for bleaching individual teeth.

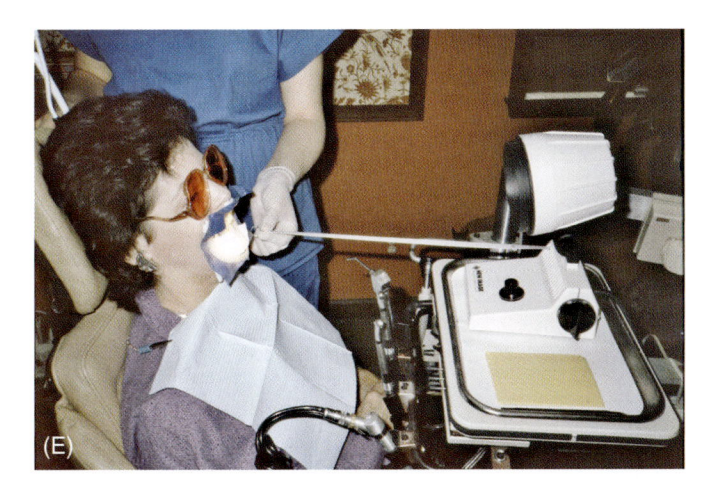

Figure 12.1 **(E)** Later, more directed beam commercial lights were developed by Goldstein with Union Broach Company.

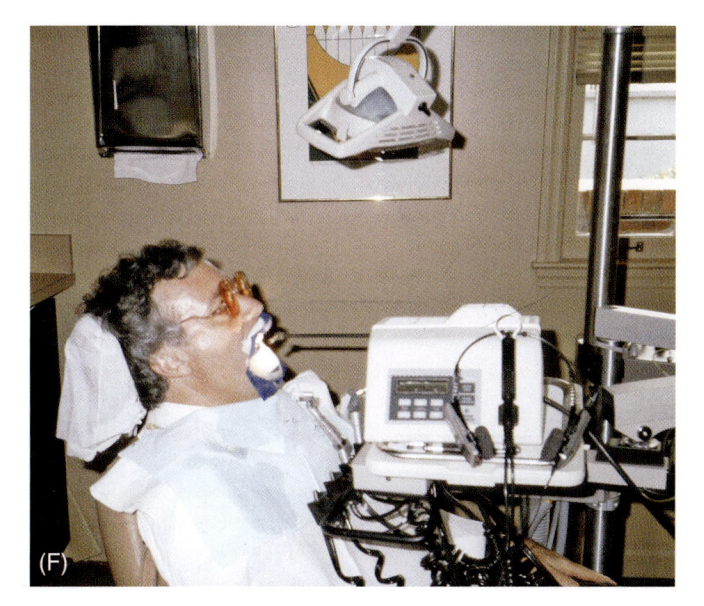

Figure 12.1 **(F)** A later version bleaching light had digitally controlled heat and light, as well as an individual instrument for bleaching single teeth.

Etiology of discoloration

Extrinsic stains

Extrinsic discoloration is caused by the accumulation of stains on the enamel surface and can be accentuated by pitting or irregularities of the enamel, salivary composition, salivary flow rates, and poor oral hygiene.[6] Various types of discoloration ranging from orange, green, brown, and black can be observed and are mostly a result of highly colored beverages or food. In combination with poor oral hygiene stains can be associated with chromogenic bacteria which can be easily removed by dental prophylaxis. Nicotine stains start as tenacious extrinsic stains, but over time absorb into the tooth and become an intrinsic stain that tend to be more difficult to bleach.[7] Drug-related tooth discoloration can be either extrinsic or intrinsic. The most common drugs causing extrinsic discoloration include chlorhexidine[8] oral iron salts in liquid form, essential oils,[9] and co-amoxiclav.[10]

Intrinsic stains

Unlike extrinsic discolorations that can be more easily removed by prophylaxis and bleaching, intrinsic discolorations are due to stain molecules within the enamel and dentin, incorporated either during tooth formation or after eruption.[11] Dental fluorosis is the most common cause of intrinsic discoloration because of the wide range of availability from multiple sources.[12] It was first reported by Black and McKay[13] in 1916, although the role of fluoride in causing these defects was not discovered for another 15 years. Histologic examination of the affected teeth will show a hypomineralized, porous subsurface enamel below a well-mineralized surface layer. This hypoplasia is termed endemic enamel fluorosis or mottled enamel.[14] The nature and severity depend on the dosage, duration of exposure, stage of ameloblast activity, and individual variation in susceptibility. Clinically, fluorosis presents as localized areas of white, yellow, or orange discolorations and in severe cases is accompanied with surface pitting or severe surface defects.[6] Bleaching is a good indication for fluorosis with brown pigmentation on a smooth enamel surface (Figure 12.2A and B). Localized white spots frequently seen in fluorosis have an unpredictable prognosis.[15] Bleaching will lighten the surrounding tooth color which may make the white spots less noticeable. However, in many cases the white spots tend to stand out even more. In such cases and in cases with surface defects, bleaching should be performed as an adjunctive treatment prior to esthetic restorative treatments including bonding or veneering. How the stain occurs is a significant factor in understanding and evaluating bleaching techniques.

Tetracycline stain

The success of bleaching for the yellow or brown stains caused by tetracycline discoloration was key to its place in the emerging field of dental esthetics. The devastating effect on tooth formation of as little as 1 g of tetracycline was recognized in the late 1950s,[16] with the first certain identification reported by a study of cystic fibrosis patients by Shwachman et al.[17] In 1970, Cohen and Parkins published a method for bleaching the discolored dentin of young adults with cystic fibrosis who had undergone tetracycline treatment.[18] The results were promising, and dentists concerned with esthetics began applying bleaching procedures to other stains and discolorations.

Teeth are most susceptible to tetracycline discoloration during their formation; that is, during the second trimester in utero to roughly 8 years of age. It is believed that the tetracycline particles are incorporated into the dentin during calcification of the teeth. Mello[19] reports that the probable mechanism by which tetracycline molecules bind to dentin involves chelation with calcium, which forms tetracycline orthophosphate, the cause of tooth discoloration. When tetracycline-stained teeth are exposed to sunlight, they gradually turn to shades of dark gray or brown. Cohen and Parkins[18] suggest that the reason the labial surfaces of the incisors darken while the molars remain yellow for a longer period of time is because of the different exposure to light.

Although the US Food and Drug Administration (FDA) issued a warning about the use of such antibiotics for treating pregnant women and children, unfortunately tetracycline cases are still seen.

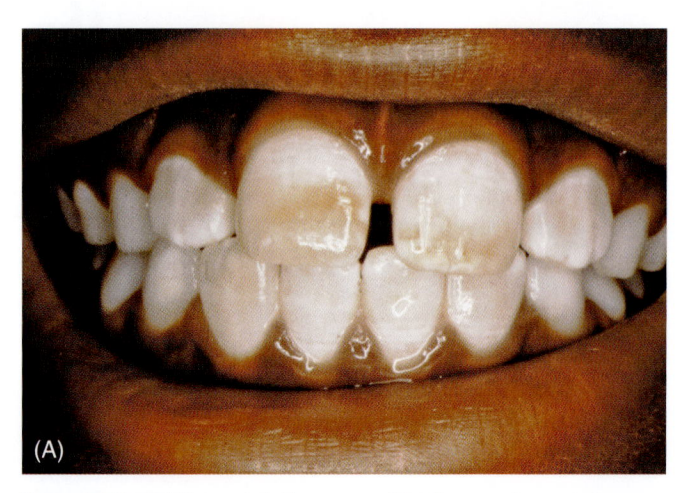

Figure 12.2 **(A)** Fluorosis is the cause of this brown pigmentation.

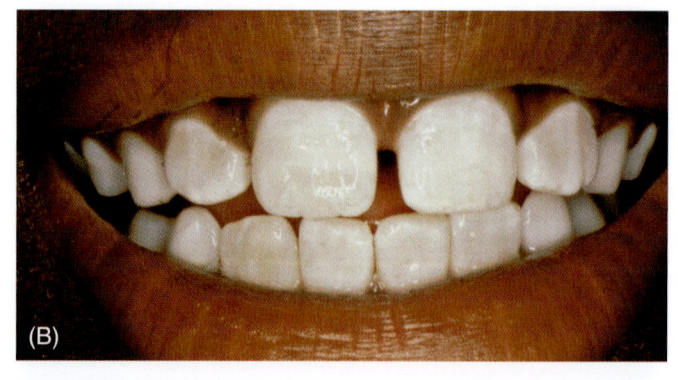

Figure 12.2 **(B)** Individual in-office tooth bleaching was effective in eliminating the stain and producing a more pleasing smile.

The severity of the stains depends on the time and duration of the drug administration and the type of tetracycline administered (more than 2000 variants have been patented). Because of these factors, tetracycline staining is extremely variable in its extent, coloration, depth, and location. Fluorescence is necessary for precise diagnosis and description but most cases fall into the three major categories of tetracycline involvement first proposed by Jordan and Boksman[20] in 1984. Each category has a different prognosis for successful bleaching.

1. First-degree tetracycline staining is a light yellow or light gray staining, slight but uniformly distributed throughout the crown without banding, or concentrated in local areas. It is highly amenable to vital bleaching, with good results usually in fewer than four sessions of office bleaching or one series of dentist-monitored home bleaching (Figure 12.3A and B).
2. Second-degree tetracycline staining is a darker or more extensive yellow or gray staining without banding. Although this type is responsive to vital bleaching, it may take five or more in-office treatments to obtain a satisfactory result. A combination of in-office/home matrix bleaching is the preferable technique (Figure 12.4A and B). Home bleaching alone may take 2–6 months.
3. Third-degree tetracycline staining produces severe staining, characterized by dark gray or blue coloration, usually with banding. Although bleaching may lighten these teeth to some degree, the bands may remain evident following even extensive treatment. Veneering techniques with opaquers are often necessary to achieve satisfactory esthetic results (Figure 12.5A and B).
4. Fourth-degree tetracycline, while not one of the original categories proposed by Jordan and Boksman,[20] includes those stains that some dentists believe are too dark to attempt vital bleaching[14] (Figure 12.6). However, these stains may not be too dark to try bleaching unless there is blue-gray stain at the gingivae.

Minocycline stain

Because tetracycline is incorporated in the dentin during calcification of the teeth, adults whose teeth have already formed appear to be able to use the antibiotic without risk of discoloration. However, recently a semisynthetic derivative of tetracycline has been found to cause staining on the teeth of adolescents who were being given the drug for severe acne.[21] Unlike tetracycline, minocycline is absorbed in the gastrointestinal tract and combines poorly with calcium. Researchers believe the tooth pigmentation occurs because of minocycline's ability to chelate with iron and form insoluble complexes. A study by Dodson and Bowles[22] suggests the minocycline pigment produced in tissues is the same or very similar to that produced by UV radiation. Since minocycline is used for a variety of infections as well as for acne, you should expect to see rising numbers of cases of this

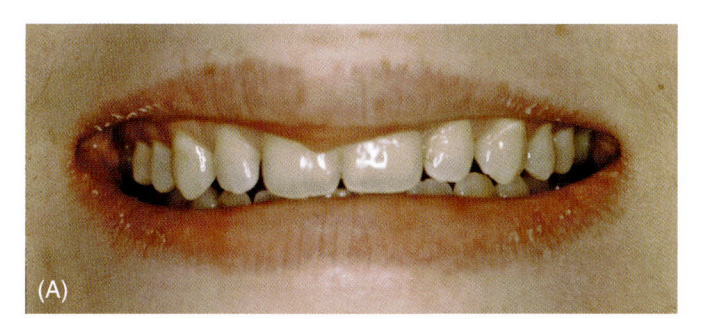

Figure 12.3 **(A)** This is a good example of first-degree tetracycline stain, which is usually light yellow or gray, and slight and uniformly distributed throughout the crown with no banding or localized heavy concentration.

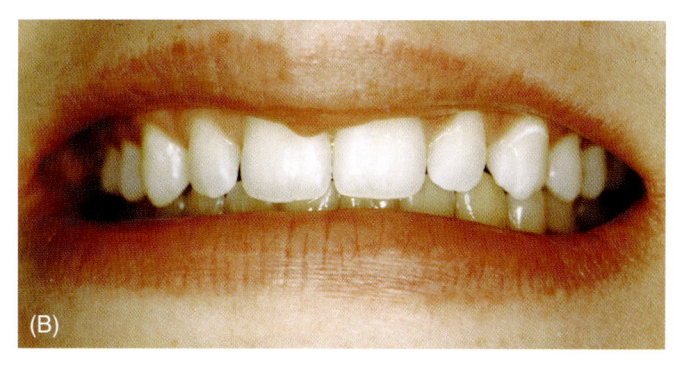

Figure 12.3 **(B)** Bleaching a first-degree tetracycline stain usually produces a good result like the one shown here, which is a combination of one in-office treatment plus home bleaching for 3 weeks.

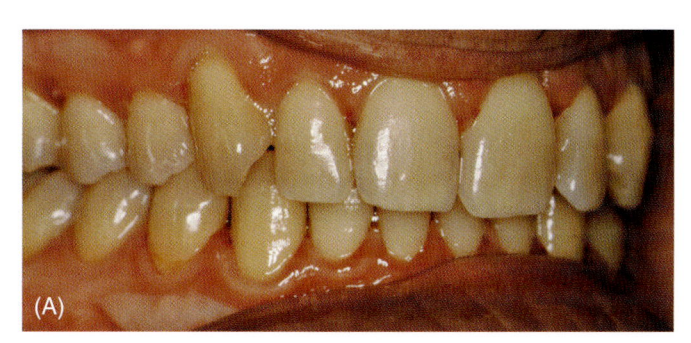

Figure 12.4 **(A)** The darker and more extensive yellow stain seen here is typical of second-degree tetracycline stain.

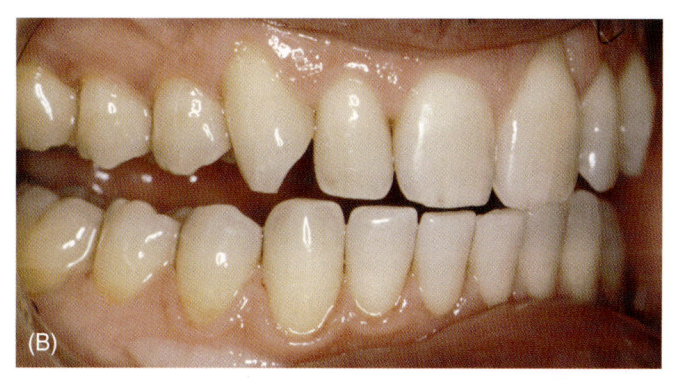

Figure 12.4 **(B)** Although responsive to vital bleaching, second-degree tetracycline stain generally takes five or more in-office treatments, as this one did, to obtain a good result.

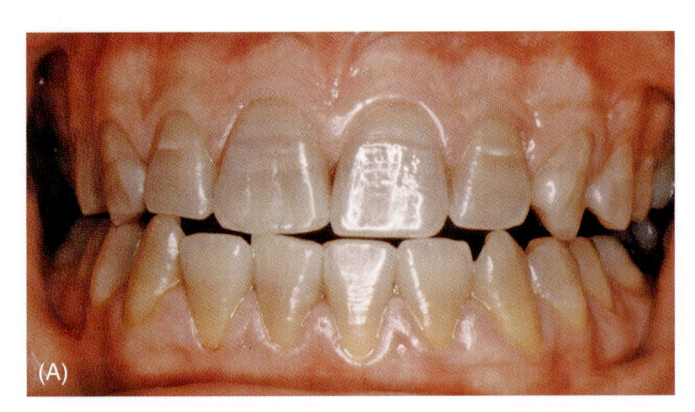

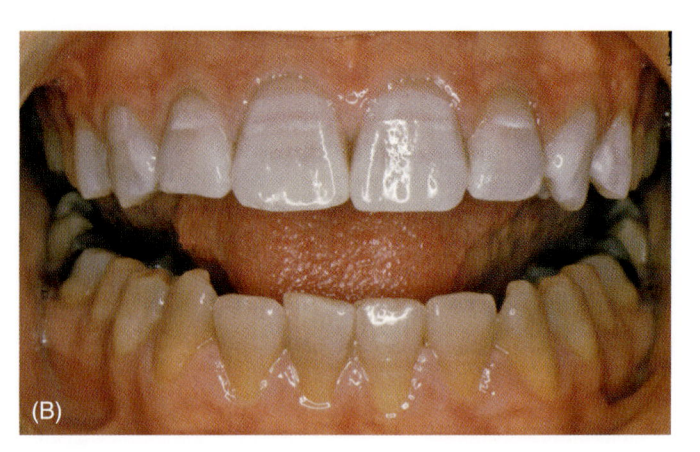

Figure 12.5 **(A)** Third-degree tetracycline stain generally does not respond well to bleaching. Depending on the patient's needs, a better result would be achieved with porcelain laminates. **(B)** This is an example of what can be achieved with multiple in-office visits. Although bleaching did lighten these teeth to some degree, the bands are still evident and the overall color would not be satisfactory to most patients. Nevertheless, there will be some patients who will prefer their own teeth lightened as much as possible rather than veneering.

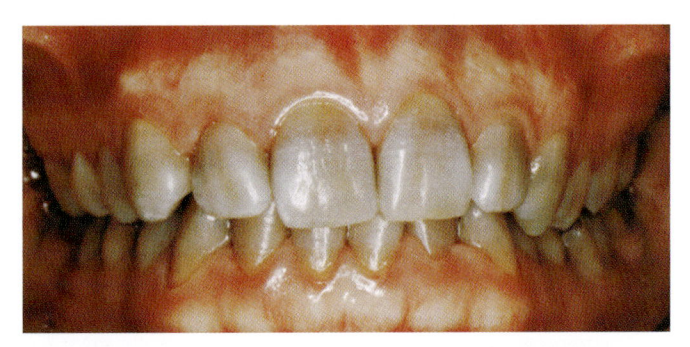

Figure 12.6 This is a good example of what has been termed fourth-degree tetracycline stain, which is so dark that bleaching may not respond enough to please the patient. Patients can be persuaded to seek one of the veneering methods to accomplish tooth lightening.

discoloration and questions regarding its use should be included in the medical history of patients. Although these stains may be responsive to bleaching, severe banding of the stains may suggest laminating for a satisfactory result. In each situation, the treatment depends on the degree of lightening desired by your patient.

Several adult patients have presented with stained teeth similar to the patient seen in Figure 12.7A. In each instance, the patients stated that the teeth had severely discolored after they began taking minocycline. Although the stain is somewhat amenable to bleaching, there is no guarantee that the final result will match the patient's previous tooth color. As a case in point, the patient in Figure 12.7B did achieve a light shade. Nevertheless, she ultimately decided to have her teeth veneered so she could obtain a much lighter color.

Stain from dental conditions or treatments

Dental caries are a primary cause of pigmentation and may be seen as an opaque, white halo, or a gray discoloration. An even deeper brown to black discoloration can result from bacterial degradation of food debris in areas of tooth decay or decomposing fillings. Such problems should be corrected before bleaching is attempted. In some cases, repair and proper cleaning may negate the need for bleaching.

Restorations also frequently cause discolorations. Degraded tooth-colored restorations such as acrylics, glass ionomers, or composites can cause teeth to look grayer and discolored. Metal restorations, such as amalgams, even silver and gold, can reflect discoloration through the enamel and should be replaced with less visible materials such as composite resin before bleaching.[23] Restorative materials that have leaking margins may allow debris or chemicals to enter and discolor the underlying dentin. Again, in some cases, bleaching may then not be necessary once such changes are made. If amalgams cannot be replaced, however, bonding or veneering may be preferable alternatives.

Oils, iodines, nitrates, root canal sealers, pins, and other materials used in dental restorations can cause discoloration. The length of time these substances have been allowed to penetrate the dentinal tubules will determine the amount of residual discoloration and will, consequently, affect the success of bleaching. Metallic stains are the most difficult to remove. Endodontic materials and sealers have various staining potentials that cause intrinsic discoloration of the root canal filled tooth over time.

Stain from systemic conditions

Developmental defects of enamel or dentin can be associated with amelogenesis imperfecta, dentinogenesis imperfecta, and enamel hypoplasia. Amelogenesis imperfecta is a hereditary disorder of enamel formation involving both the primary and permanent dentition.[24] Discolorations associated with amelogenesis imperfecta tend to aggravate with time as the rough surfaces allow stains to accumulate more easily. Dentinogenesis imperfecta is a hereditary disorder affecting both dentitions, exhibiting abnormal dentin formation. Affected teeth exhibit slender roots, small or obliterated pulp chambers and root canals with enamel that easily chip away from the dentin.[25] Enamel hypoplasia is incomplete or defective formation of enamel matrix induced by systemic or local factors. Hematologic disorders cause a deposition of blood pigments in the dentin or enamel resulting in discoloration of the tooth structure. Bleaching can

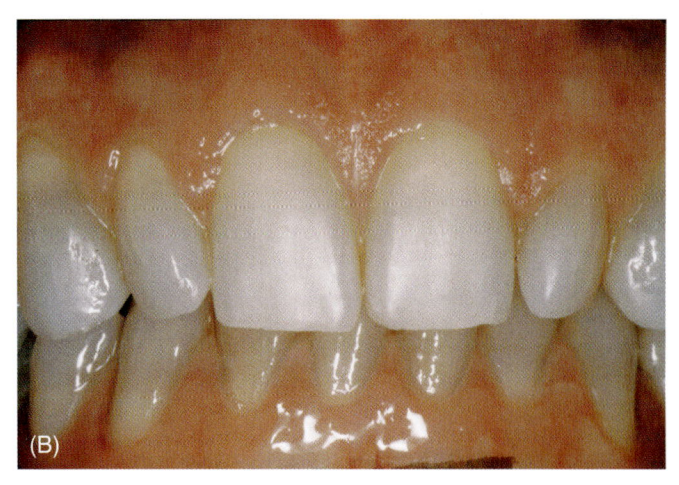

Figure 12.7 **(A)** This female took several doses of the antibiotic minocycline for her facial complexion. Shortly after, she began to notice some darkening of the teeth, which continued until they reached the color shown. She states that she had "white" teeth up until that time. **(B)** Six in-office treatments plus 1 month of home matrix treatments were used to obtain this result.

be quite effective for the discoloration caused by infusion of the dentin during development. Some examples are as follows:

- The bluish-green or brown primary teeth seen in children who suffered severe jaundice as infants. The stains are the result of postnatal staining of the dentin by bilirubin or biliverdin.
- The characteristically brownish teeth caused by destruction of an excessive number of erythrocytes in the blood cells that occurs in erythroblastosis fetalis, a result of Rhesus factor incompatibility between mother and fetus.
- The purplish-brown teeth color of persons with porphyria, an extremely rare condition that causes an excess production of pigment.

Other illnesses cause discoloration of the teeth by interfering with the normal matrix formation or calcification of the enamel.[26] Hypoplasia or hypocalcification can occur with genetic conditions like amelogenesis imperfecta and clefting of the lip and palate or with acquired illnesses such as cerebral palsy, serious renal damage, and severe allergies. Brain, neurological, and other traumatic injuries also can interfere with the normal development of the enamel. Deficiencies of vitamins C and D, and calcium, and phosphorus can cause enamel hypoplasia if they take place during the formative period. Bleaching is usually a less appropriate treatment than bonding, veneering, or crowning for these problems involving the structure of enamel.

Discoloration due to aging

With the aging population, an increasing number of your patients will be older. We no longer expect to lose our teeth as we age as our great grandparents did, nor do most persons in our youth-oriented society easily accept the changes in color, form, and texture of teeth that almost inevitably accompany aging. The type and degree of such changes will depend on a mixture of genetics, use and abuse, and habits. Years of smoking and coffee drinking have a cumulative staining effect, and these and other stains become even more visible because of the inevitable cracking and other changes on the surface of the tooth, within its crystalline structure, and in the underlying dentin and pulp. In addition to wear and trauma on the teeth, amalgams and other restorations placed years ago may begin to degrade.

Even with the most careful avoidance of or attention to such problems, our teeth are likely to become more discolored as we age, from both natural wear and exposure to normal environmental contaminants. The first change to occur is usually a thinning of the enamel. This may cause the facial surface of the tooth to appear flat with a progressive shift in color due to a loss of the translucent enamel layer. At the same time the enamel begins to thin, secondary dentin formation begins through a natural tooth protective mechanism in the dentin and pulp. This larger mass of dentin also begins to darken. The combination of thinned enamel and darkened dentin creates an older-looking tooth. For these types of problems, veneering will produce a better long-term result (Figure 12.8A and B).

For many of the discolorations seen in older patients, home matrix bleaching can be a safe, effective treatment option. Additionally, unless the enamel is too badly worn, in-office or combined bleaching can be an effective treatment. For many older patients, the short time required in the dental chair, relatively low cost, and lack of trauma involved, make bleaching an especially appealing treatment. Another reason why bleaching can be such an effective treatment for older patients is that in most instances the pulp has shrunk back, making it possible to use higher bleaching temperatures.

Contraindications to bleaching of vital teeth using in-office techniques

The following problems may suggest the use of other methods of esthetic improvement or may be more appropriate for dentist-monitored home bleaching:

- extremely large pulps, which may increase sensitivity
- other causes of hypersensitivity, such as exposed root surfaces or the transient hyperemia associated with orthodontic tooth movement

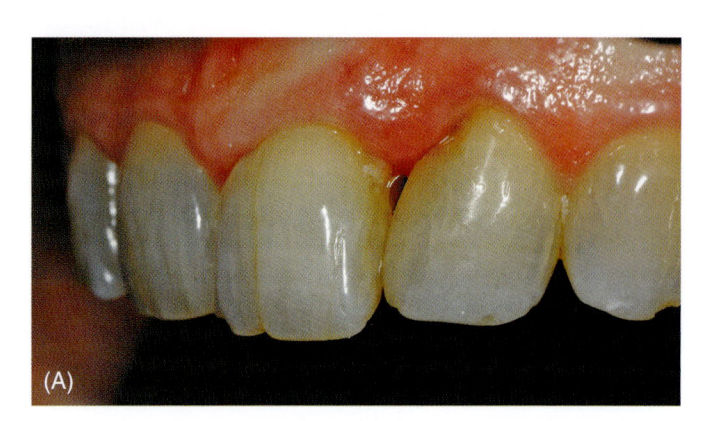

Figure 12.8 **(A)** The combination of thinned enamel and darkened dentin creates older-looking teeth.

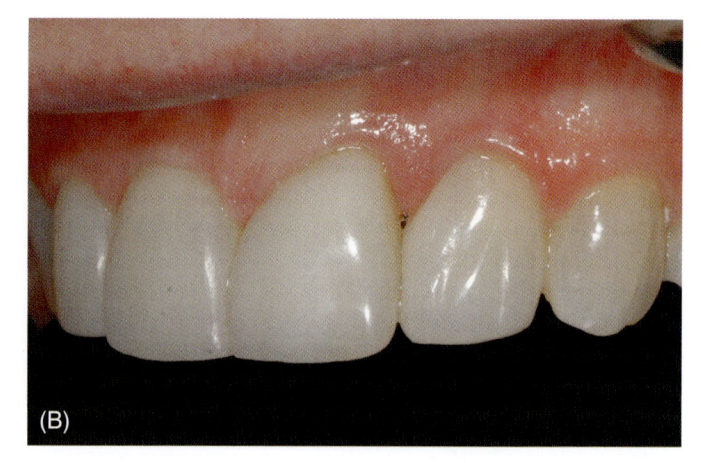

Figure 12.8 **(B)** In this case, bleaching was followed by direct composite resin restorations for better long-term results.

- severe loss of enamel due to attrition, abrasion, or erosion
- teeth exhibiting gross or microscopic enamel cracking
- extremely dark teeth, and severe tetracycline staining, especially those with marked banding
- teeth with white or opaque spots: although bleaching will not eradicate these spots, the process can lighten the surrounding tooth structure and then the white spots can be eliminated with microabrasion or with bonding
- teeth in which there are restorations that must be matched or, especially, teeth that have been bonded or veneered
- extensive restorations: Koa et al.[27] suggest strongly that bleaching materials never come in contact with restorative materials. Their study of bleaching chemicals found some roughening on contact with all tooth-colored restorative materials, the greatest damage done to glass ionomer, the least to porcelain. (See also various studies referenced in the section on matrix bleaching in which the teeth have a longer exposure to the chemicals, although the chemicals are less invasive.)
- patients who are perfectionists: bleaching is not perfect, in the way veneers can be. This is especially true for severe stains. With darker tetracycline stains, for example, the majority of the bleaching will occur on the incisal one-half of the teeth. The remaining surfaces can only be partially helped by a selective bleaching solution and heat application.

For these patients, and others, you may find that a combined bleaching approach and restorative procedures like bonding, veneering, or crowning are indicated. For example, patients with Class V lesions which are eroded and sensitive may find there is too much discomfort with the bleaching process, either in the office or at home. In these instances, an alternative is to cover the sensitive areas with a dam substitute or temporize with a temporary filling while bleaching, and to bond the cervical after the color has been stabilized and the bond strength fully recovered.

Level of expectation

The "perfectionist" type of patient may not be happy unless the teeth resemble the concept of the "Hollywood star." However, others may enjoy and appreciate only a slight lightening of tooth shade (Figure 12.9A and B). It is essential that you thoroughly understand the color level your patient expects. Computer imaging can be of considerable help in this regard.

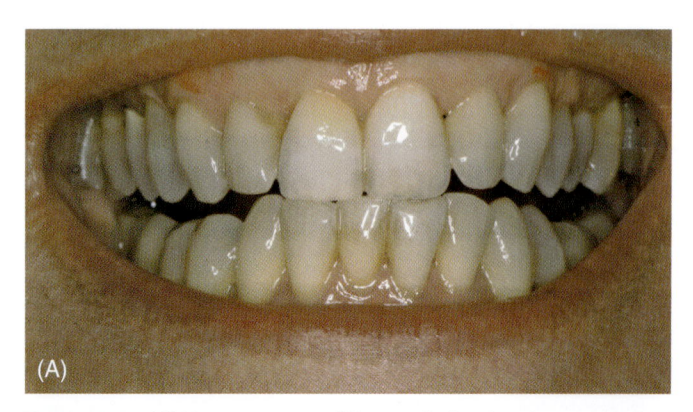

Figure 12.9 **(A)** Many patients will be satisfied with only a minimal result.

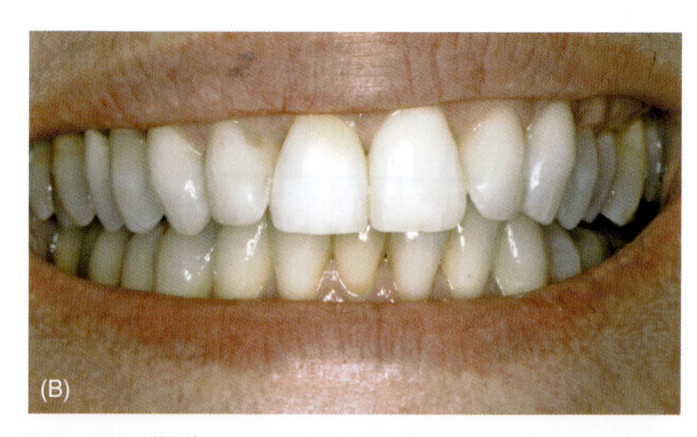

Figure 12.9 **(B)** The patient was happy after two in-office bleaching treatments.

Sequence of treatment

Simple discoloration generally can be effectively treated with in-office bleaching. An individual tooth discoloration would usually require an in-office individual bleaching instrument whereas generalized discoloration would need a comprehensive in- and/or out-of-office treatment. Classification should be based on the type of discoloration and whether it is generalized or individualized.

Teeth that have staining in one or more areas are usually treated differently than generalized staining. Although tooth contouring can sometimes make stains disappear if they are only in the first cell layers of enamel, bleaching the darker stain with repeated short treatments is generally the treatment of choice. Selective tooth isolation with the rubber dam is the best method for treating this problem (Figure 12.10). Teeth that have had traumatic injury can sometimes be bleached in-office, either by itself or combined with matrix bleaching, or by matrix bleaching alone. Selective placement can also be effective with traumatically involved teeth (Figure 12.11A–C).

Teeth that are yellowing due to heredity or age can usually be improved with both in-office and matrix bleaching. In most instances, bleaching teeth should be attempted before any other treatment is undertaken, with the exception of soft tissue management. In general, treat one arch at a time. This provides a good comparison of just how effective your treatment is

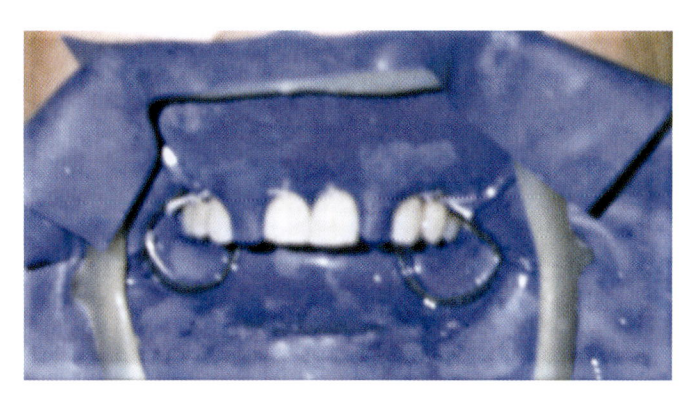

Figure 12.10 Rubber dam placement: in-office selective bleaching can be accomplished by carefully applying the rubber dam to expose only the teeth that require bleaching.

(Figure 12.12A–C). However, certain patients have limited time or want to maximize their dental appearance, so consider bleaching both arches simultaneously.

Combined bleaching and restorative dentistry

When combining bleaching with restorative dentistry, estimate the number of bleaching treatments in the office or at home before an acceptable result will be obtained, in order to calculate how long afterwards the restorative treatment could begin. Generally, this occurs 2–6 weeks after the last bleaching

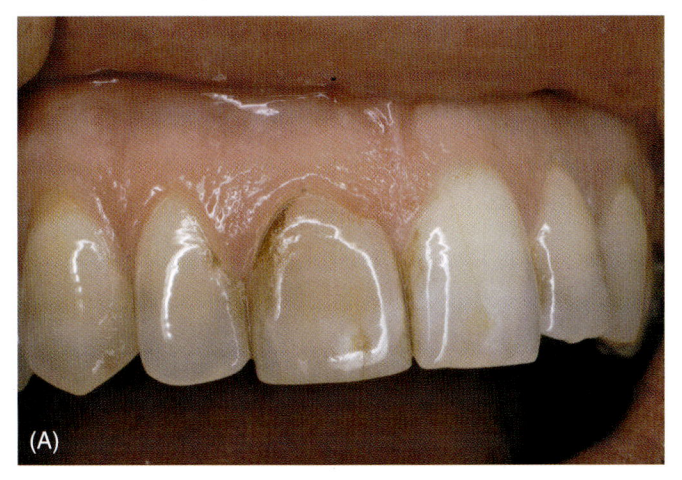

Figure 12.11 **(A)** This female patient presented with a cervical stain on this previously traumatized yet still vital tooth.

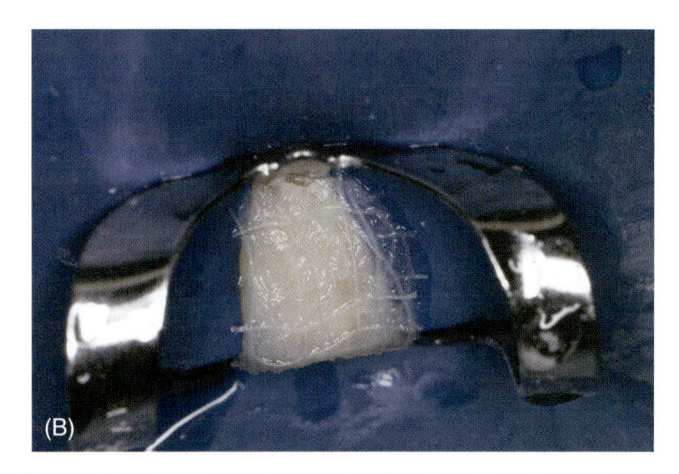

Figure 12.11 **(B)** The tooth was isolated with a rubber dam and treated with 35% hydrogen peroxide combined with a heat wand.

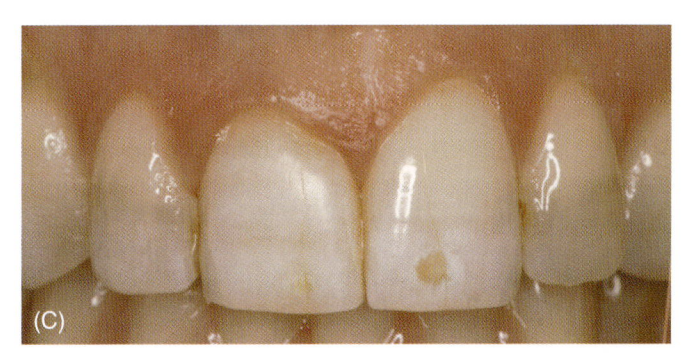

Figure 12.11 **(C)** Polishing with coarse pumice and external surface bleaching with heat successfully restored the patient's tooth color.

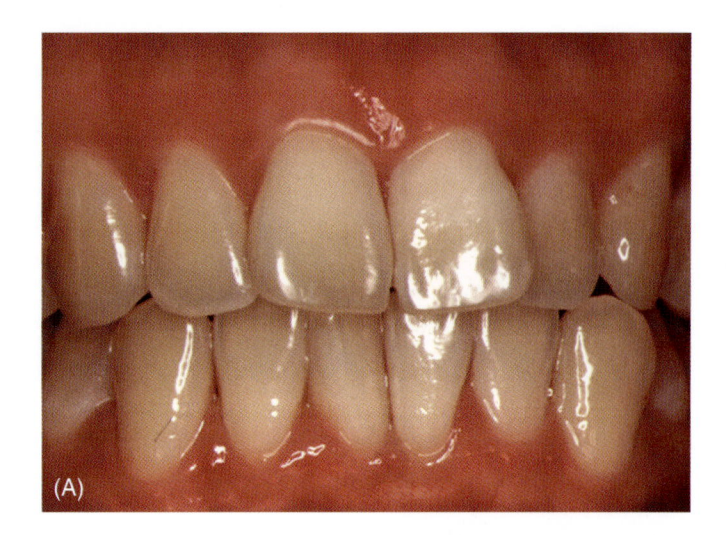

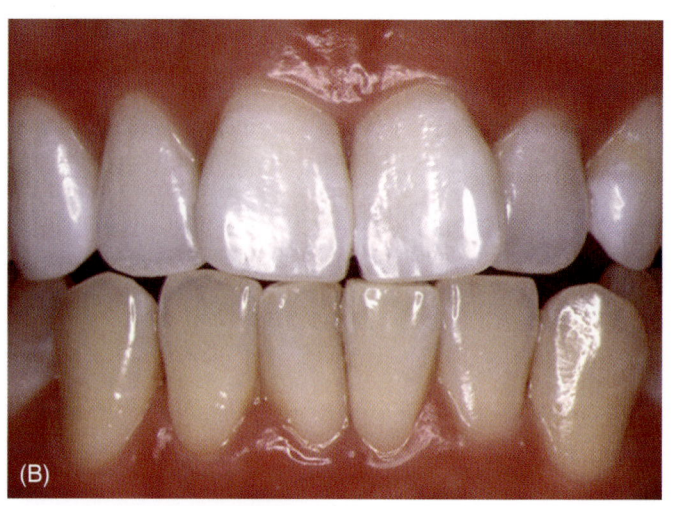

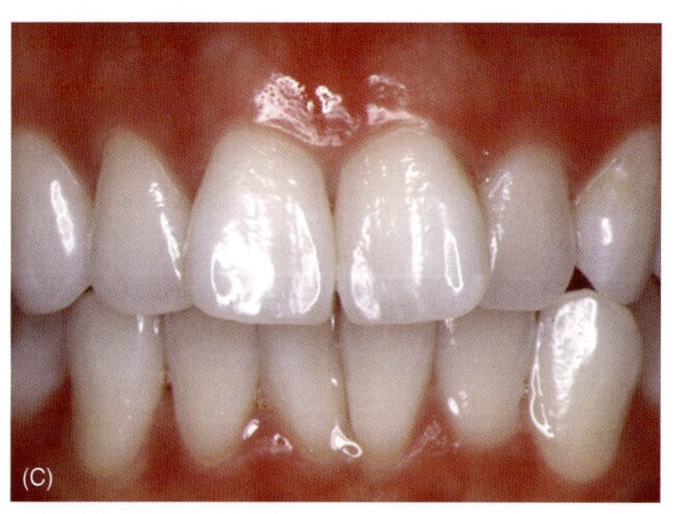

Figure 12.12 **(A–C)** In general, treat one arch at a time. This provides a good comparison of just how effective your treatment is.

treatment: for in-office bleaching alone, it is about 2 weeks but if at-home treatments are included then add an additional 4 weeks. Eight weeks from the onset of this combined bleaching approach is usual. Some patients are happy with the bleaching regimen alone but others will desire bonding or veneering as the total treatment.

Bleaching combined with minor restorative treatment

Many times bleaching will be combined with simple composite resin bondings, veneers, or all-ceramic crowns to meet the expectations of the patient regarding a beautiful smile. Bleaching should be the starter treatment and restorative procedures should be postponed to 2–3 weeks after the last bleaching to select the shade for matching the final restoration and to wait for the recovery of the bonding strength to tooth structure.[7] In the event you must take a shade prior to seeing the final bleaching result, choose a lighter shade, and be prepared to darken the crown if necessary to match the final color. The patient should be warned that additional matrix or in-office bleaching may be necessary from year to year or after several years in order to keep the adjacent teeth matched to the new crown or crowns.

Bleaching combined with orthodontics

It is generally preferred to bleach teeth before orthodontia is initiated if ceramic or metal brackets will be bonded to the teeth because the bonding impregnates the enamel and thus makes it more difficult to bleach. However, it is acceptable to straighten the teeth first, remove the brackets, and clean the teeth of all bonding materials before bleaching. In this case, a Prophy-Jet (Dentsply) should be used, followed by a mild etching before the first bleaching treatment to make sure there is no bonding material remaining on the teeth.

It is also possible to do a combined technique when a removable orthodontic positioner is being used to move the teeth (Figure 12.13A). The bleaching solution can be added to one or both arches in the clear orthodontic positioner. A breathing space can also be created in the splint between the arches (Figure 12.13B). When minor therapy with removable appliances or invisalign is underway, bleaching can also be done simultaneously.

Figure 12.13 **(A)** Bleaching solution is added to this removable orthodontic positioner.

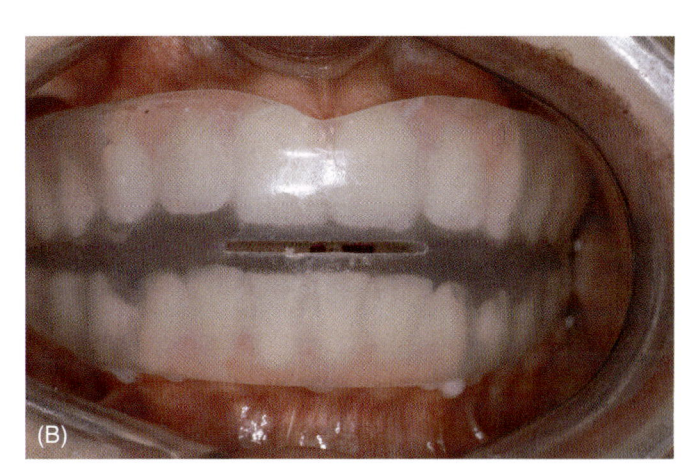

Figure 12.13 **(B)** If both arches are being straightened and bleached, a breathing space can be created in the combined matrix/retainer. This special dual-therapy appliance represents a real time saver for the patient.

Bleaching in patients with multiple caries, abrasion, and erosion

Deep cavities in the esthetic zone that require tooth-colored restorations should be addressed prior to bleaching. Deep caries lesions should be removed and filled temporarily with glass-ionomer fillings. The final tooth-colored restoration can be placed after bleaching to provide a natural color match. Abrasion and erosion areas that need bonded restorations should be bleached first. If home bleaching is performed, the custom-fitted tray can be adjusted so that the bleaching gel will not contact the abraded or eroded area. During in-office bleaching the protective resin barrier can be placed over the affected area, so that the highly concentrated bleaching gel will be applied only on sound tooth surfaces. Once the teeth have lightened Class V composite resin restorations can be placed to match the lightened teeth. Recently, the use of home bleaching for the prevention of cervical caries lesions due to dry mouth has been suggested.[28]

Bleaching combined with periodontics

Generally, bleaching follows oral disease control and management of any periodontal disease. If there is evident periodontal inflammatory disease or gingival hyperplasia that covers the cervical enamel, bleaching should be postponed until the swelling has subsided to expose the healthy clinical crown. If the sequence is reversed, a color differential may result in the subgingival unbleached area. However, if advanced bone loss is present and surgery will mean raising the tissue well onto the root surface, it may be advisable to perform an in-office power bleach with adequate rubber dam protection before periodontal therapy is undertaken. This would make it easier for the tissue to hold the dam in place at the cementoenamel junction, rather than having the cervical root surfaces being exposed to the bleaching solution.

In the event that the patient already has root exposure, you may need to mask those areas with artificial dam material (Ultradent or Den-Mat) and seal the defects with composite resin to prevent any leakage of the bleaching solution from damaging these areas.

Bleaching for children

Children with discolored teeth may be good candidates for bleaching especially if trauma has taken place, but there are several caveats. The larger pulps of children can lead to greater sensitivity when office bleaching is performed and one should be especially careful to avoid irritation of the pulp, including not using heat. If a child has an adequate number of teeth to hold a matrix in place, dentist-monitored home bleaching may be preferable (Figure 12.14A and B). However, you will need to make the child understand that less-than-perfect home care will tend to leave plaque on teeth, diminishing the effect of bleaching. It is imperative that the teeth be clean before bleaching at home. Disclosing tablets or solutions may be effective tools in helping less-than-meticulous brushers see what they are missing. And you must forewarn the child and parents that bleaching will need to be repeated as new teeth erupt.

Bleaching for elderly patients

Older patients are excellent candidates for bleaching, especially to improve the yellowing that can occur with age, but their teeth must be basically free of defects and restorations. In fact, since the pulps often have receded, there usually will be little or no sensitivity present during the bleaching process. This means you will be able to use photooxidation or heat as a method of choice. Older patients can withstand higher heat when the illuminator (Union Broach) or bleaching light or even laser is used, which should permit faster results.

Office bleaching will most often be the technique chosen by the elderly who wish to have lighter teeth. Although they may have more time for home or matrix bleaching, their patience with all the ramifications of matrix bleaching may not be sufficient. In addition, if there is any problem with the intraoral tissues, matrix bleaching could be contraindicated. Dry mouth syndrome, periodontal disease, or advanced bone loss are all conditions that may influence the choice of bleaching technique. If you find that your patient's soft tissues become irritated with matrix bleaching, switch to resin barrier protected office

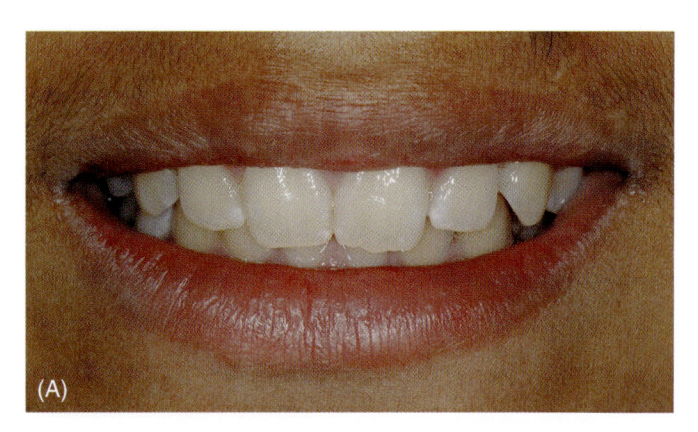

Figure 12.14 **(A)** This child had an adequate number of teeth to hold a matrix in place.

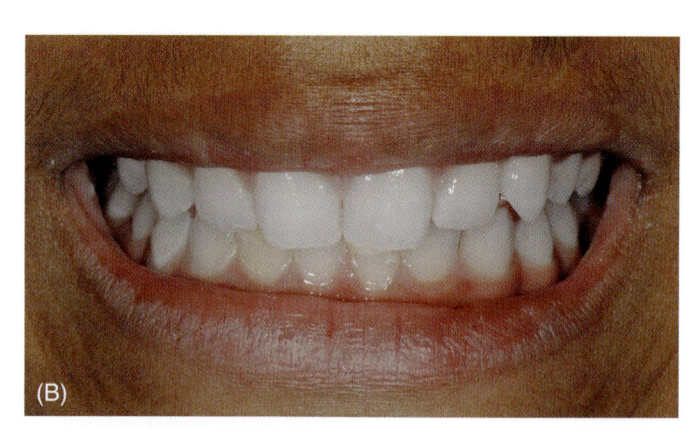

Figure 12.14 **(B)** Dentist-monitored home bleaching was performed for good results.

bleaching. For many older patients, the short time required in the dental chair, relatively low cost, and lack of trauma involved make bleaching an especially appealing treatment.

Recording the baseline color

The baseline color should be recorded and can be accomplished with the use of shade guides or special electronic devices for color measurement. There are many shade guides available, and the decision on which to use should be according to the ease of use and the purpose of color evaluation. The VITA classical introduced to the dental profession in 1956 is still the most widely used because of its ease of use and broad availability. The major drawback of the VITA classical guide is that there are no uniform distribution between the individual color tabs and the lack of lighter shade tab than B1. The VITA Toothguide 3D-Master shade guide has facilitated the matching of color by evaluating three components of color—value, chroma, and hue—separately into three steps. However, the 3D system has caused confusion for the dentists who have adjusted to the linear system over such a long time. In 2007, Paravina[29] introduced a new linear bleached shade guide for the purpose of monitoring color change during bleaching. The advantages of this system are that it is easy to use, there is uniform color distribution between the tabs, and there are very light bleaching shade tabs available. Regardless of the shade guide system used, the most common way to record the baseline color is to take a picture with an intraoral camera with the shade guide tab as a reference next to the tooth. With the advancement of technology special devices for color measurement have become available which are not influenced by the human eye, environment, or light source, and which produce reproducible data. Shade systems include spot measurement devices like Shade Eye-NCC (Shofu) and Easyshade (Vita), as well as complete tooth measurement devices such as the Spectro Shade Micro (MHT Optic Research), ShadeScan (Cynovad), Shade Vision (X-Rite), and the Crystaleye. The benefit of using complete tooth measurement devices in tooth bleaching is the ability to print out a smile analysis that can effectively motivate the patient into the treatment (Figure 12.15A–D). However, the color measurement procedure has to be performed tooth by tooth, making it time consuming, and the cost has limited its use to a limited range of dentists.

Techniques for in-office bleaching of vital teeth

Discolored vital teeth can be successfully bleached with highly concentrated hydrogen peroxide gels at the chair side. In-office whitening provides an alternative to home bleaching, especially when patients desire faster results and demonstrate low compliance in wearing a tray at home. In-office whitening can be performed on selective teeth, on one arch or even on both arches where speedy treatment is desired. Generally, the whitening effect is noticed immediately after a single session. However, generally a single session is not enough to achieve optimal results and for maximum bleaching several appointments are required. Ideally, in-office bleaching can be combined with home bleaching to obtain faster and whiter results. No matter which form of concentrated hydrogen peroxide or bleaching apparatus is used, it is essential to protect the tissue.

Preparation and application of bleaching material

See Figure 12.16A–M.

1. Record the baseline color with a shade guide and take a photograph with the selected tab next to the teeth to be bleached. This provides an excellent data baseline and record of pretreatment that will be useful in determining needed follow-up. Because bleaching can be incremental with a gradual change, patients easily forget their initial shade and are surprised to see how their teeth actually were.

2. Free the teeth of all surface stains and plaque with a Prophy-Jet (Dentsply) or similar cleaning device. Special attention should be given to patients who have recently completed orthodontic treatment. Remnants of bonding materials might interfere with the penetration of bleaching materials and adversely affect the bleaching result.

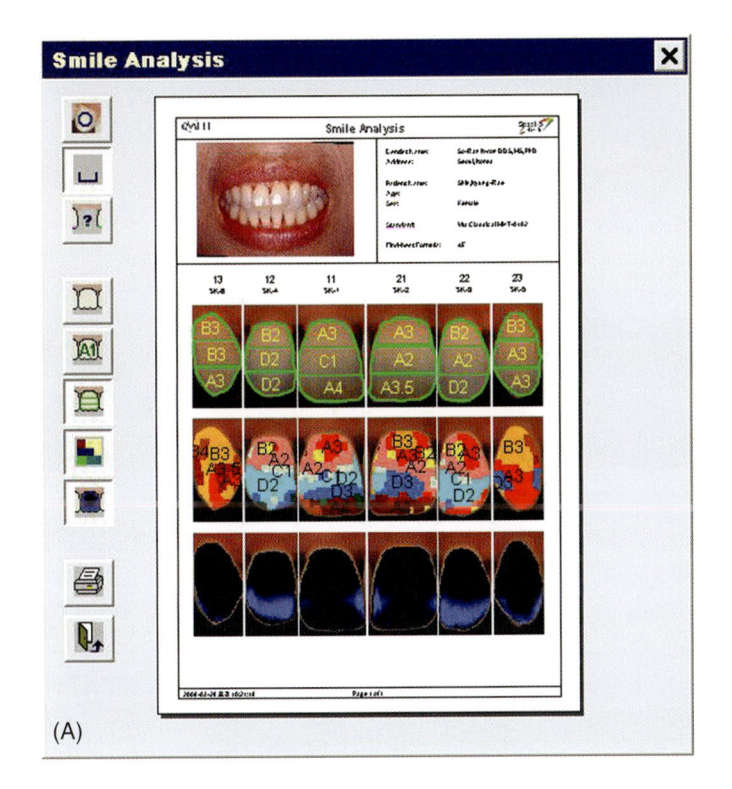

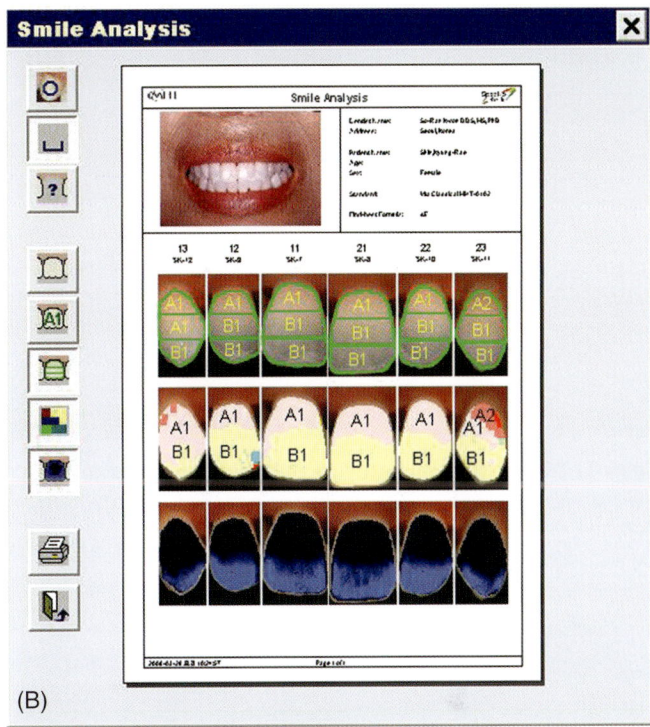

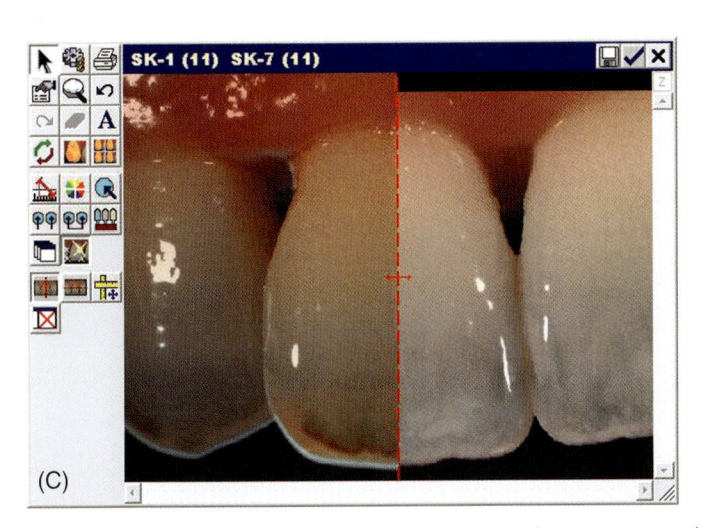

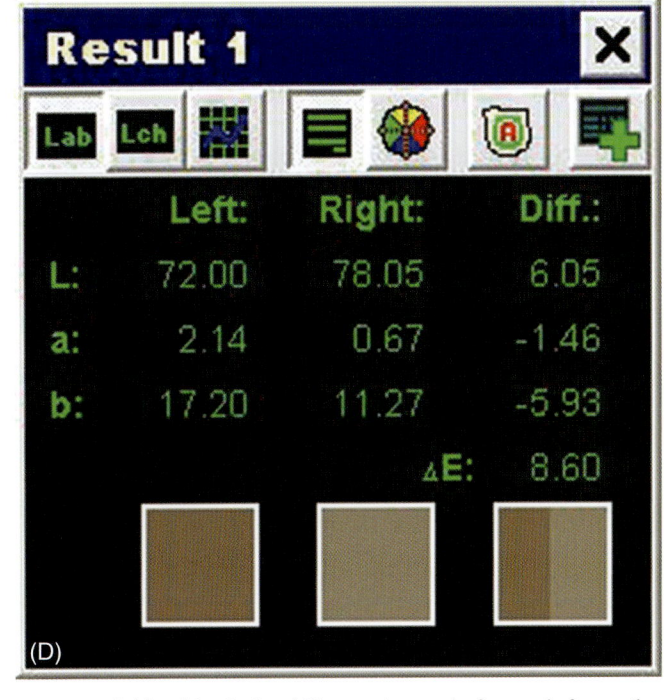

Figure 12.15 (A–C) The benefit of using complete tooth measurement devices in tooth bleaching is the ability to print out before and after smile analyses that can effectively motivate the patient into the treatment. The before and after images can also be synchronized. (D) Measuring the color change as expressed as ΔE.

3. Take steps to protect the patient from bleaching materials, light, and/or heat used. Explain in detail the necessity of the patient to protect their eyes with safety glasses until they are told to remove them.
4. Select the proper size of cheek retractors to protect and stretch the cheek and lips. The conventional rubber dam has been replaced by the use of cheek retractors and gingival protectors, due to the use of hydrogen peroxide gels or paste that can be easily localized onto the tooth surface.
5. Place cotton rolls, gauze, and saliva absorbent triangles to maintain a dry field. Dry the mucosa and place a resin

Esthetic Treatments

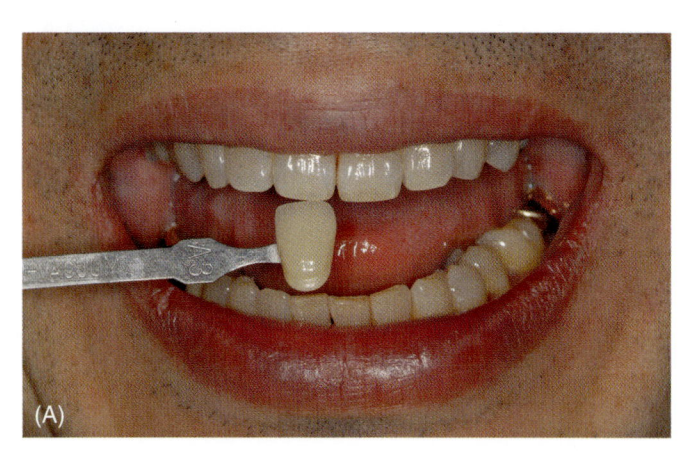

Figure 12.16 (A) Record the baseline color with a shade guide and take a photograph with the selected tab next to the teeth to be bleached.

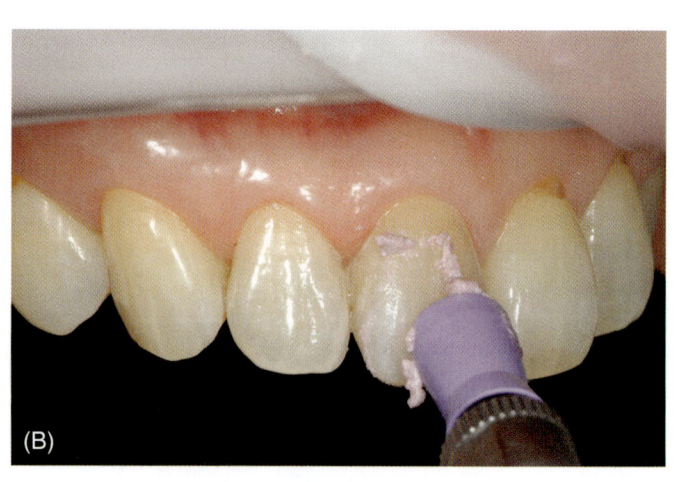

Figure 12.16 (B) Free the teeth of all surface stains and plaque.

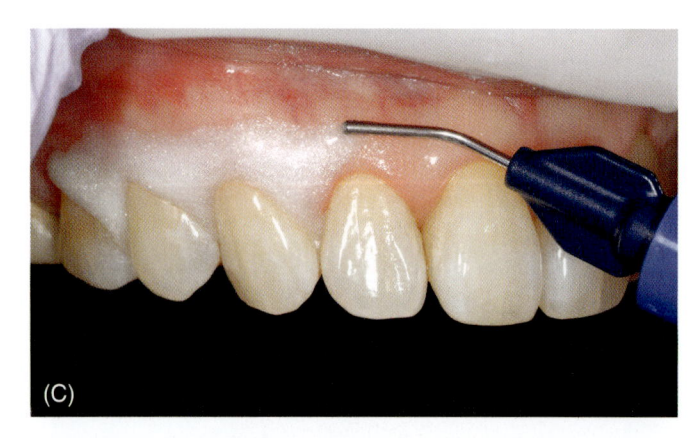

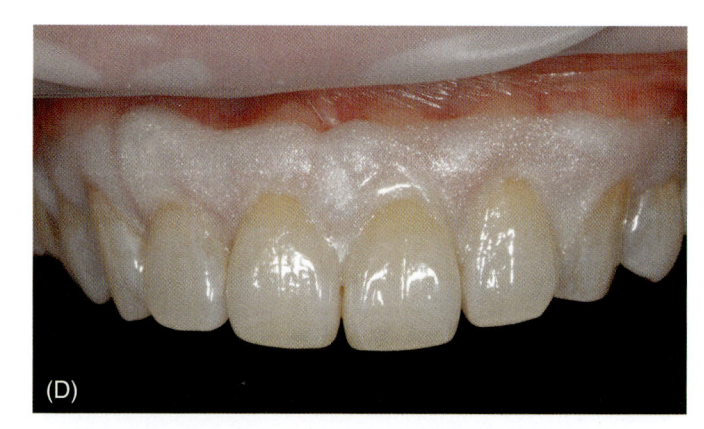

Figure 12.16 (C, D) Dry the mucosa and place a resin barrier (Opal Dam, Ultradent) to cover approximately 0.5 mm of the cervical area of the tooth and extend 2–3 mm onto the gingiva.

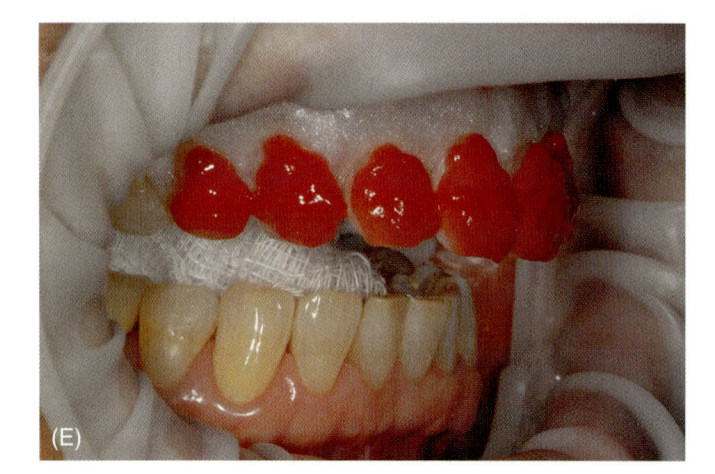

Figure 12.16 (E) Apply the highly concentrated bleaching material homogeneously onto the tooth (Opalescence Boost, Ultradent).

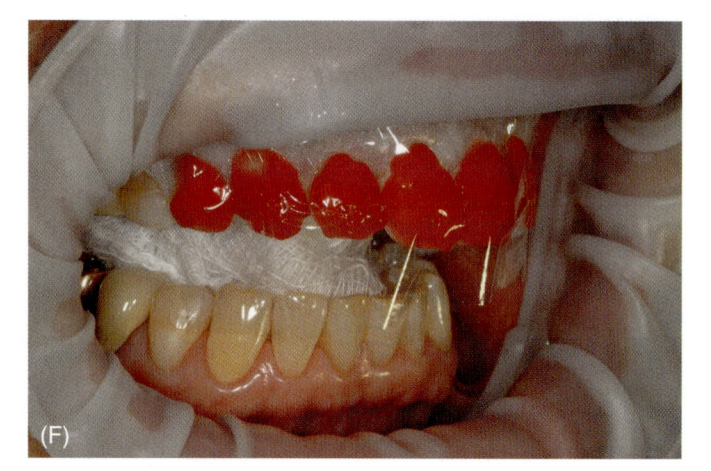

Figure 12.16 (F) Place a precut linear low-density polyethylene wrap (Saran wrap) onto the teeth to prevent evaporation of the active material and create a good seal.

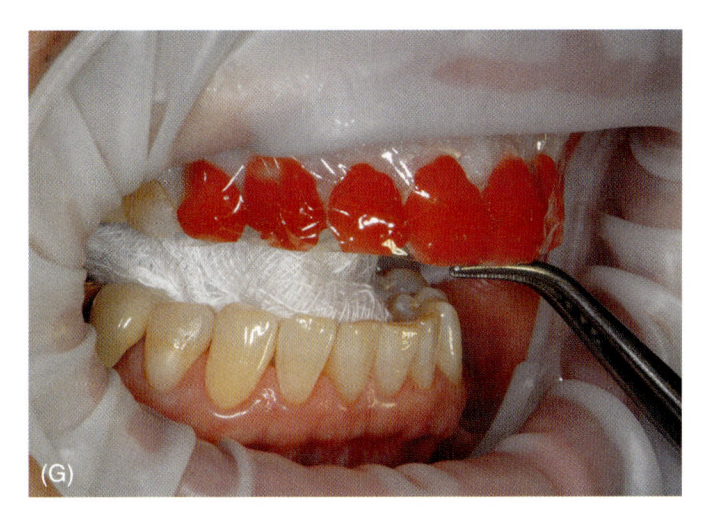

Figure 12.16 **(G)** Use cotton pliers to seal the wrap around the incisal edges.

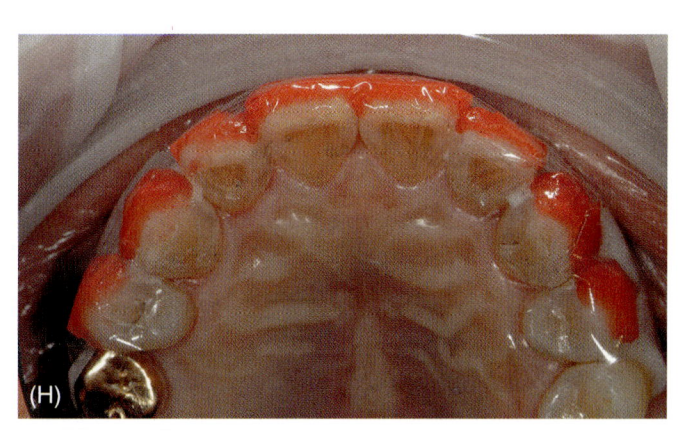

Figure 12.16 **(H)** Double check whether there are areas allowing any leakage of the bleaching material applied.

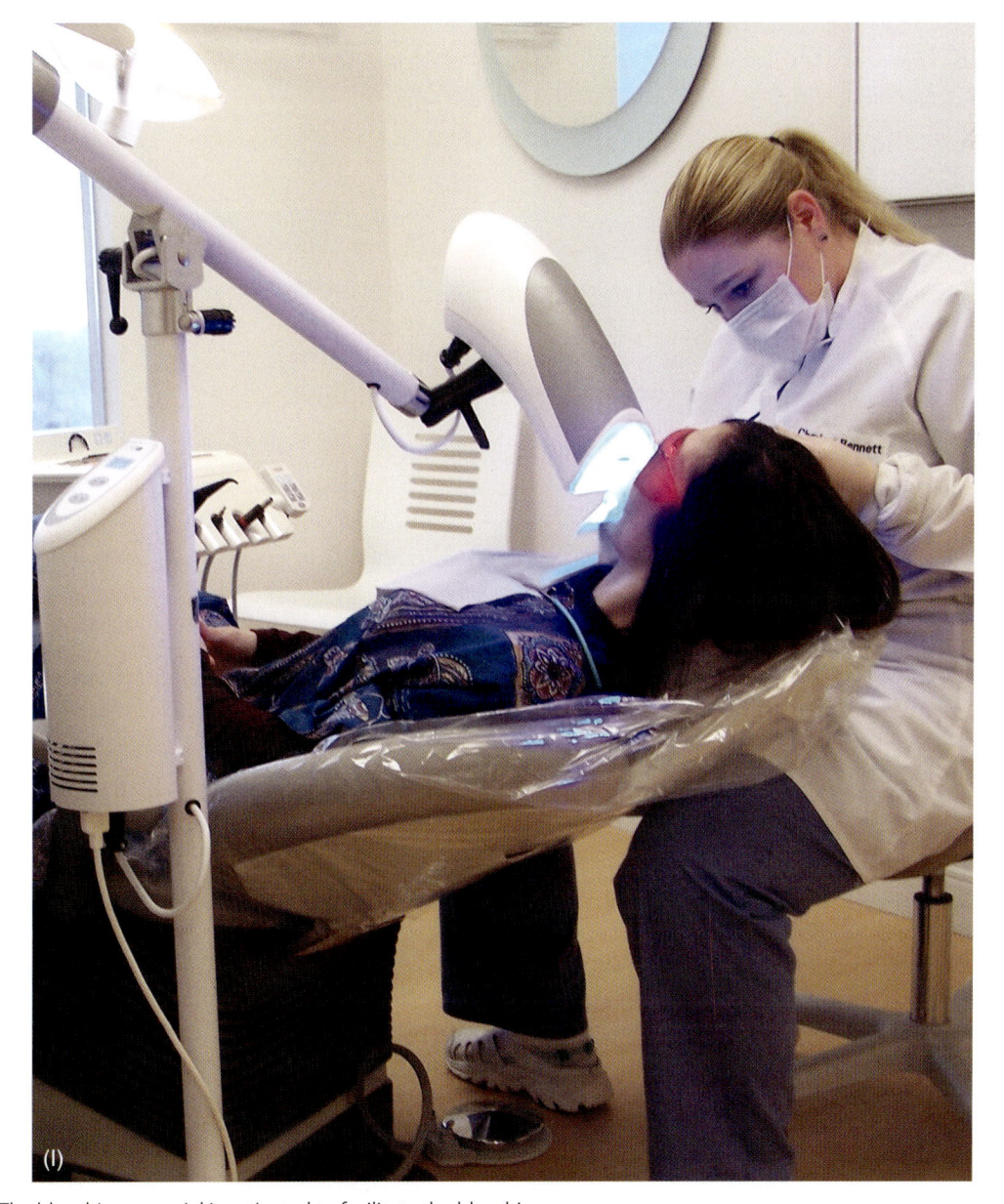

Figure 12.16 **(I)** The bleaching material is activated to facilitate the bleaching process.

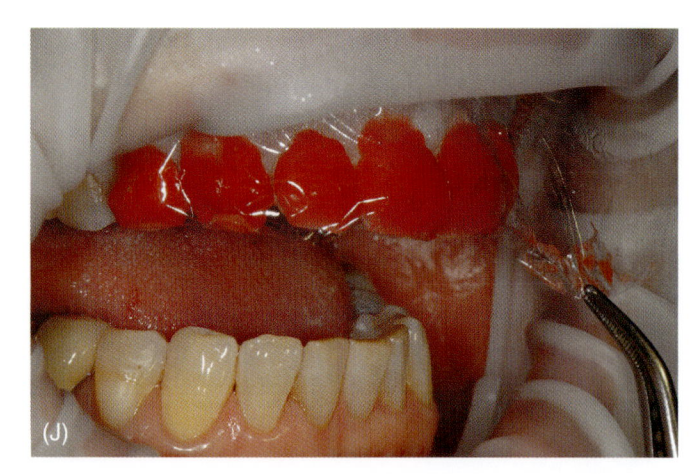

Figure 12.16 (J) Remove the wrap and the bleaching material after 40–60 min.

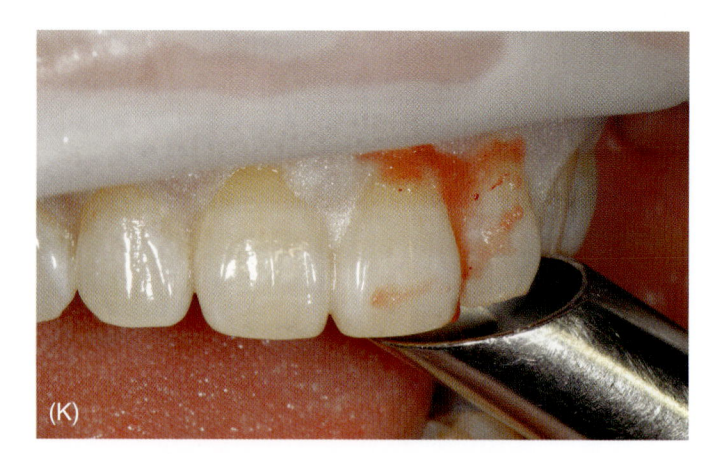

Figure 12.16 (K) Remove the remaining bleaching material with a high-suction tip and rinse the teeth with copious amounts of lukewarm water.

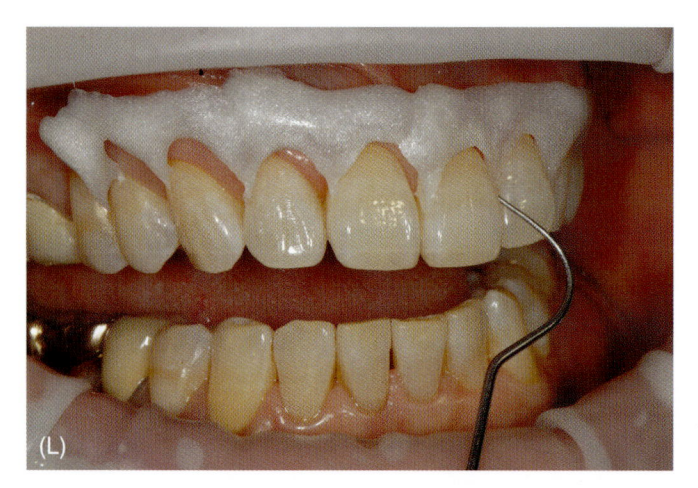

Figure 12.16 (L) Remove the resin barrier with the explorer tip.

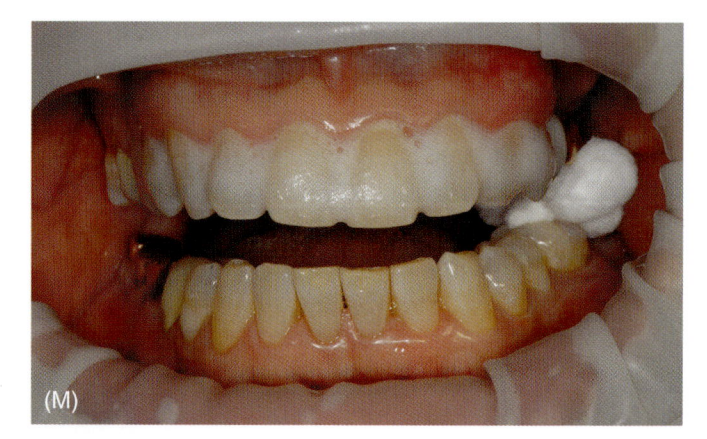

Figure 12.16 (M) Finish with a 2% neutral sodium fluoride gel for 5–10 min.

barrier to cover approximately 0.5 mm of the cervical area of the tooth and extend 2–3 mm onto the gingiva. Confirm with mirrors that there are no exposed areas of gingival and that all embrasure areas are protected. Light-cure the resin barrier and double check whether there are areas allowing any leakage of the bleaching material to be applied.

6. Apply the bleaching material homogeneously onto the tooth. Place a precut linear low-density polyethylene wrap (Saran wrap) onto the teeth to prevent evaporation of the active material and create a good seal.[41] Activate with light according to the manufacturer's directions.

7. Remove the bleaching material with a high-suction tip and rinse the teeth with copious amounts of lukewarm water. Depending on the severity of the discoloration new bleaching material can be applied and repeated several times to achieve maximum bleaching results.

8. Finish the in-office bleaching session with a 2% neutral sodium fluoride gel for 5–10 min to minimize sensitivity and remineralize the superficial enamel layer that might have been affected by bleaching. It is always best to whiten the upper and lower arches separately so that the patient can see the color change. For maximum bleaching another bleaching session can be scheduled with an interval of a week, or bleaching can be continued at home with a matrix in which case in-office bleaching would serve as a jump-start treatment to speed-up the whole process.

Apart from the dentist's decision to use a heating or light catalyst device, which is a matter of preference, there are several differences in the actual bleaching procedure to consider, depending on the etiology and severity of the discoloration as follows:

- The number of treatments required will differ. For teeth stained by coffee, tea, or other substances, a dramatic difference can appear in only one or two visits. This is also true for many cases of fluorosis-stained teeth. For tetracycline-stained teeth, three or more visits are generally required even if combined with an out-of-office matrix technique. We believe it is psychologically advantageous to prepare the patient for a longer sequence and to check carefully as the treatment proceeds, treating every 2–4 weeks.
- The solution itself will vary, depending on the severity of the stain. For most bleaching, a 30–35% concentration of hydrogen peroxide is used.

The patient needs to be told that the teeth may appear chalky because of dehydration and that they will darken over the next

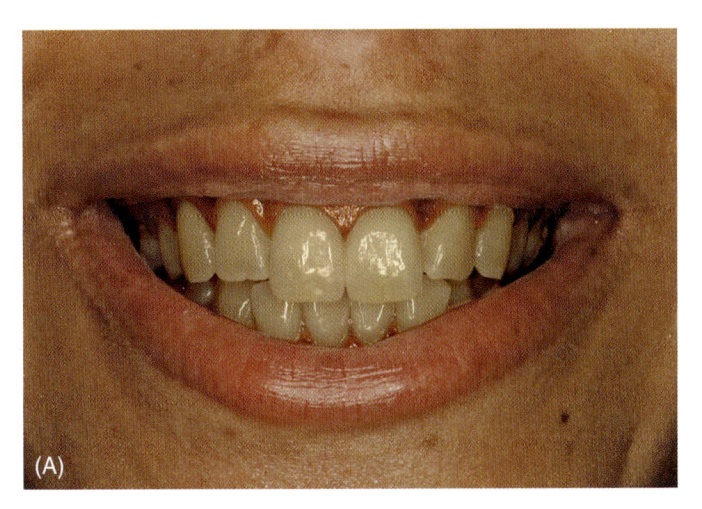

Figure 12.17 **(A)** Before in-office bleaching.

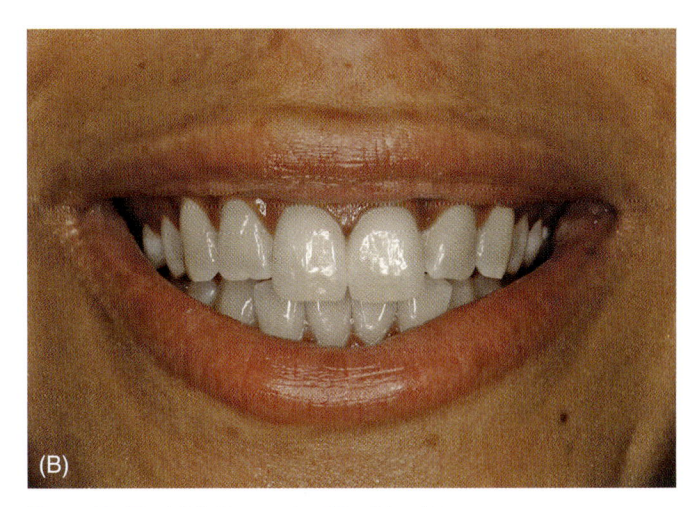

Figure 12.17 **(B)** Following in-office bleaching treatment.

few days after treatment, although to a shade lighter than the previous one. Some patients experience heightened sensitivity to cold for 1–2 days and should avoid cold weather and cold drinks or food. Most patients are able to alleviate any discomfort in this period by taking two acetylsalicylic acid, acetaminophen, or ibuprofen tablets every 4–6 h. Caution patients that an annual "touch-up" bleach usually will be recommended for the removal of any new accumulated stain.

The longevity of tooth color change has been found to vary widely between patients.[30] This may be in part because of the inability of patients to remember change. Rosenstiel et al.[31] report only 1 of 10 young adults who received one vital bleaching treatment were able to see the effects of the treatment past 1 month, although colorimetry could still detect change. The best clinical evidence that color change is taking place is to check the upper to lower cuspid areas. Before-treatment photographs are especially important so these areas can be compared for both the patient's and your use in determining color change (Figure 12.17A and B).

Microabrasion

In cases of severe enamel stains on isolated teeth, you can use a microabrasion slurry (Prema, Premier, Opalustre, Ultradent), a combination of hydrochloric acid (muriatic acid) and pumice with mechanical abrasion, which will etch the enamel slightly to facilitate stain removal (Figure 12.18A–C). Another alternative is to use air abrasive technology (American Dental Technologies, Sunrise, or Kreativ). Although several seconds with air abrasive can remove certain stains, you must be prepared to bond the enamel surface if the technique is not successful. You can also use "macro-abrasion" as per Bodden and Haywood,[32] with friction grip diamonds or carbides with Soflex disk polishing.

Matrix bleaching (nightguard vital bleaching)

Matrix bleaching refers to bleaching procedures that the patient uses outside the dental office. Wearing a matrix fabricated by the dentist, the patient is able to apply bleaching material to the affected teeth while at his or her office, exercise facility, driving a car, or almost any place in daily life.

Nightguard vital bleaching has proven to be quite successful, with 9 out of 10 patients experiencing a lightening of their teeth in 2–6 weeks' application time.[5] There are three basic forms of matrix bleaching, involving different levels of dentist participation and supervision. Many patients who desire a rapid and effective result prefer a combined approach in which in-office bleaching is bolstered and continued by matrix bleaching sessions, enabling close monitoring of the process by the dentist. However, some patients prefer to use matrix bleaching only, still relying on the dentist's diagnostic and monitoring abilities. And finally, there is a growing trend toward whiteners sold over the counter that are intended for home use by unsupervised individuals. These three forms of matrix bleaching are discussed below.

Power and monitored matrix bleaching: a combined approach

The combination approach of one in-office bleaching session, using the stronger bleaching solutions with a heat/light device to speed the chemical reaction, and a sequence of matrix treatments controlled by the patient provides the most effective result seen to date.[33] With optimal patient selection, treatment, and compliance, the results of the dentist-monitored power/matrix bleaching provides the most predictable of all the bleaching techniques. The power bleach achieves immediate results. The creation of a matrix to fit the patient's own mouth increases the efficiency and safety of the home bleach sessions. The continuous nature of the matrix bleaching sessions with a milder solution permits refreshing of the bleaching when the brightening effect begins to regress, as occurs in all bleaching processes.

The Kor whitening system follows a very specific protocol, with both an in-office and an at-home whitening component. The first step requires home bleach trays to be made in Kor's lab in California, USA. Once delivered, the patient uses the trays to apply both bleach and desensitizer for 2 weeks. After the 2 week

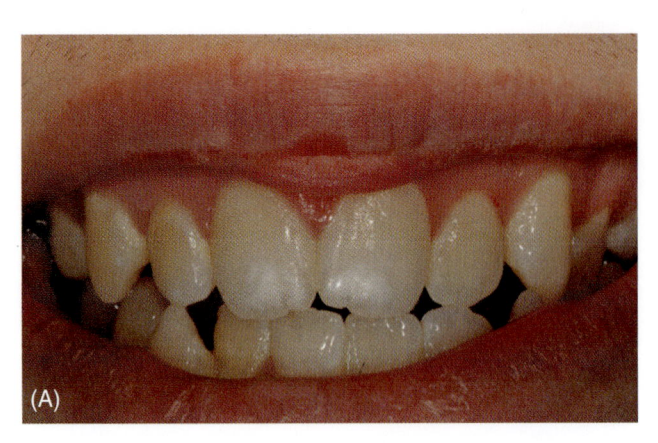

Figure 12.18 **(A)** This 16-year-old boy was concerned about the hypocalcification in his maxillary central incisors.

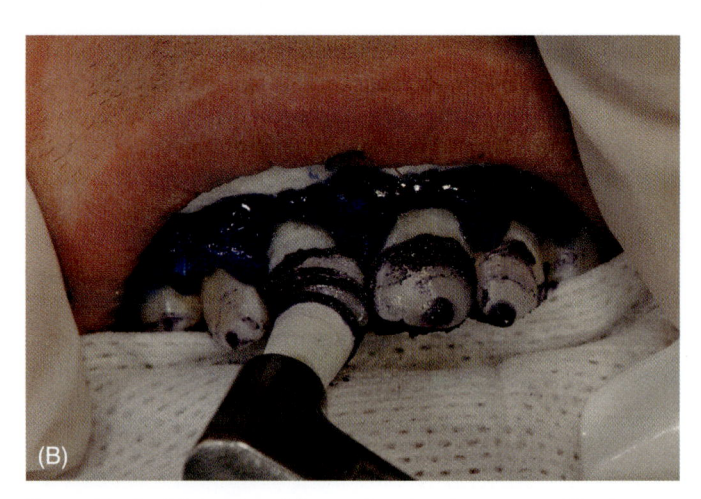

Figure 12.18 **(B)** A series of three microabrasion sessions (Opalustre, Ultradent) was sufficient to remove the hypocalcification.

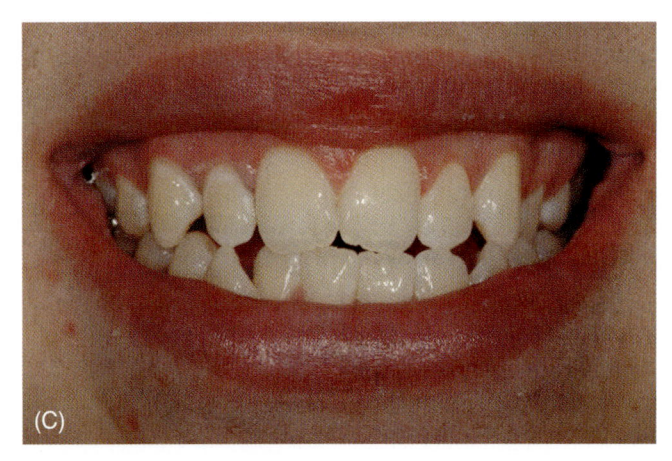

Figure 12.18 **(C)** The patient was pleased with his new, improved smile.

time period, the patient will undergo one or two sessions (depending on the severity of the stain) with Kor's in-office material.

Indications for power/matrix bleaching of vital teeth

Many of the conditions for which in-office bleaching has been appropriate are also appropriate for the power/matrix bleaching, although the patient must recognize that the matrix bleaching segment of the treatment depends on a milder bleaching solution. Compliance with the prescribed regimen is essential for success. The indications for which matrix bleaching is most often suggested are as follows:

- yellowed or discolored teeth in first degree and moderate second degree
- moderate yellow and/or brown tetracycline stains, and intrinsic stains (brown and yellow, as well as light to moderate gray), although the success depends on the severity and the ability of the teeth to absorb rebleaching as well as patient compliance
- patients who are not candidates for in-office bleaching because of hypersensitive teeth, time restrictions, financial considerations, or psychological objection to rubber dam placement.

Contraindications for power/home bleaching of vital teeth

- Extremely hypersensitive teeth as described in contraindications for bleaching, but also transient hypersensitivity that may occur with prolonged application. For example, in certain patients a potentiated 15% urea peroxide or a 10% hydrogen peroxide can lead to tooth sensitivity if worn more than 1–3 h per day. Instead, substitute with a lower concentration of carbamide peroxide (5–10%).
- Other hypersensitivity reactions, such as burning sensations, sore throat, nausea, irritation, or edema. These may indicate allergic reactions.
- Lack of compliance, whether through inability or simple unwillingness to wear the appliance the necessary 1–3 h per day.
- Severe discoloration, including cases for which all bleaching is assumed to be ineffective except as an adjunctive therapy.
- Teeth with extensive restorations may be contraindicated as well. Several studies have suggested in-office and matrix bleaching products cause degradation of resin composite surfaces,[27,34–36] although others disagree.[37] The costs of replacement may be an additional factor.

Preparing the patient for matrix-monitored bleaching

First use the appropriate procedure above for diagnosis, and preparation, for bleaching of the discolored teeth.

1. Take color photographs to provide a standard for comparison against the initial session. This will be especially useful since the patient has more control over deciding when renewal is needed.

2. An impression of the arch to be treated is made with an alginate or other accurate material, and a cast of durable stone is poured and trimmed. With the appropriate trimming of the cast, the vacuum-formed matrix will adapt completely over the cast with minimal creasing. Modeling clay or block-out compound may be used to block out significant undercuts. In addition, you may wish to incorporate a die spacer to create a reservoir.

3. A plastic nightguard-like matrix is used to completely cover all teeth to be treated and minimize the exposure of the gums to bleaching solution. It is constructed on a vacuum-forming machine. According to Haywood,[39] the best prosthetic material is a 0.9 mm clear soft material (Soft-Tray, Ultradent). Thin materials also diminish chances for a temporomandibular joint or occlusal problem.

4. Again, appropriate trimming is necessary to minimize injury to the soft tissue. In particular, the palatal portion and the majority of the matrix covering the gingival tissue must be removed with a scalpel or hot knife while the material is still on the model and with scissors, diamond disc, or a carbide acrylic trimming bur once it is removed from the model. Further adjustments must be made at the time of patient try-in. Trim the gingival margins as close as possible to the cervical margin of the teeth. The objective is to keep bleaching material in contact with the tooth surface and away from the tissue. Selective bleaching can also be accomplished by carefully trimming the matrix to include only the teeth to be bleached (Figure 12.19A and B).

5. Instruct the patient to place a drop of solution in the appropriate space around each tooth corresponding to the areas to be lightened, as in the written instructions given to the patient. The most common regimen is between 1 and 4 hours daily use from 4 weeks to 6 months (for tetracycline stain). Some companies recommend wearing the matrix up to 20 hours per day with the bleaching gel changed every 2–4 hours, but such long-term exposure of the soft tissue to bleaching materials has not yet been researched adequately. Most dentists, however, suggest 1–3 hours daily with one application or changing the solution once during that time. One suggested regime is to arrange the first session on the same evening as the power bleaching, with subsequent sessions every night for 3 weeks. Another is to have the gel worn every other night for 6 weeks (for laboratory procedures for bleaching tray fabrication see Figure 12.20A–H).

Most matrix bleaching uses 10–15% carbamide peroxide rather than the 35% hydrogen peroxide used in in-office procedures. However, several companies manufacture a three-tier bleaching approach beginning with a 5 or 6% solution and followed a week or so later with a solution percentage increased to 10 or 12%, and finally to a 15–17% solution. The advantage is to reduce possible patient sensitivity by beginning with lesser concentrations of hydrogen peroxide. The greater the concentration of urea peroxide and the thicker the material, the quicker the results will be and the less wearing time will be necessary. In our experience, more viscous solutions work best; they stay in the tray better and appear to provide the necessary time for the H_2O_2 to diffuse into the tooth, since the viscosity seems to prevent the saliva from breaking down the H_2O_2. The total diffusion into the enamel may allow for the tooth to be bleached more effectively from deeper within this enamel layer. In summary, 15% solutions work faster than a 5% solution, thicker gels generally work better than thinner ones, and dispersants with pigment are superior to those without.

The combination of power bleach and continued home treatment by the patient means there is little or none of the usual degradation of the lightening effect usually observed after the first in-office bleach since the home bleaching begins immediately and continues over the next 2 weeks. The costs of in-office bleaching with multiple appointments are lowered, the patient has control over when the bleaching is to be enhanced, and there is minimal exposure of the tissue to the bleaching agent.

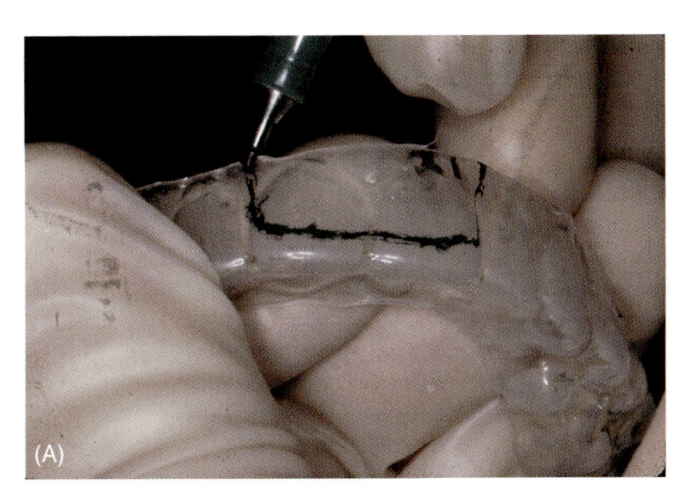

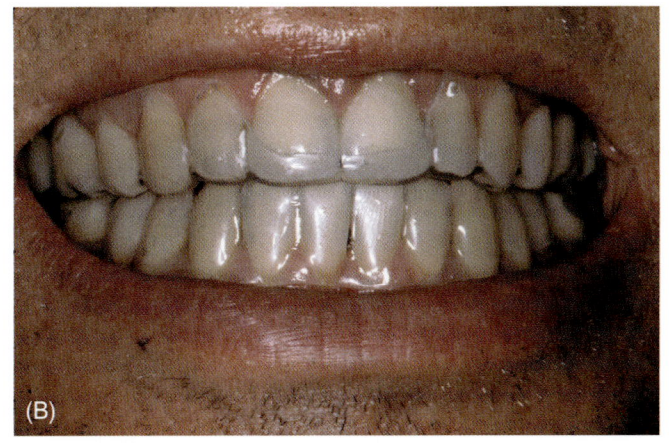

Figure 12.19 (A, B) Selective bleaching can also be achieved with matrix bleaching by removing specific areas in the matrix.

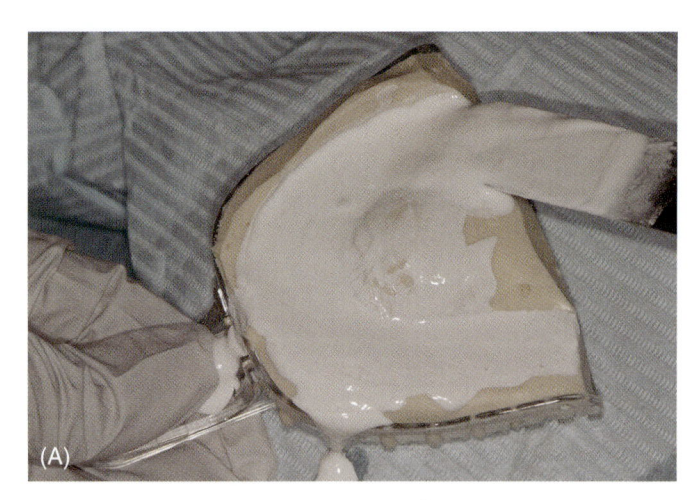

Figure 12.20 **(A)** An alginate impression of the arch to be treated is made, and stone is poured carefully to avoid any bubble or void formation.

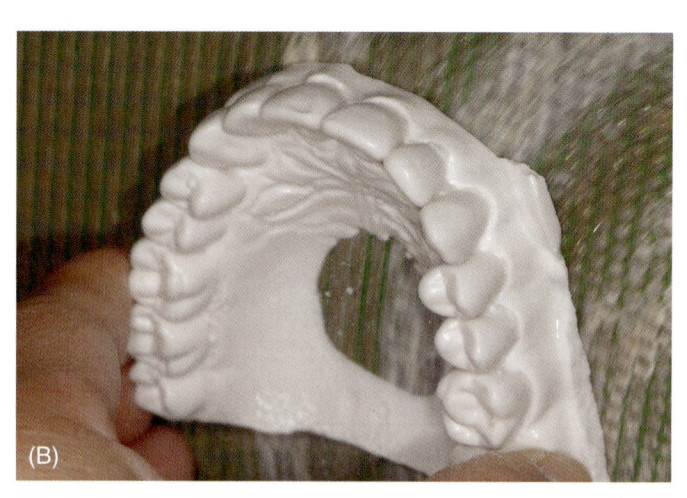

Figure 12.20 **(B)** The stone model is trimmed so that the base is flat and parallel to the occlusal plane.

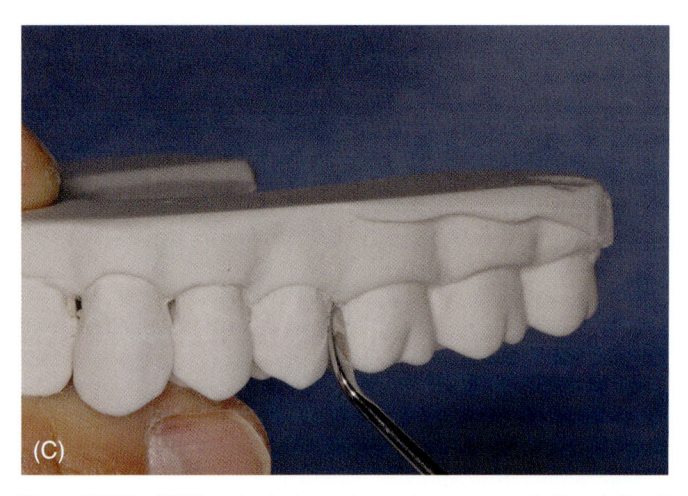

Figure 12.20 **(C)** The gingival margin on the stone model is redefined with a sharp instrument to create a better seal around the tray margin.

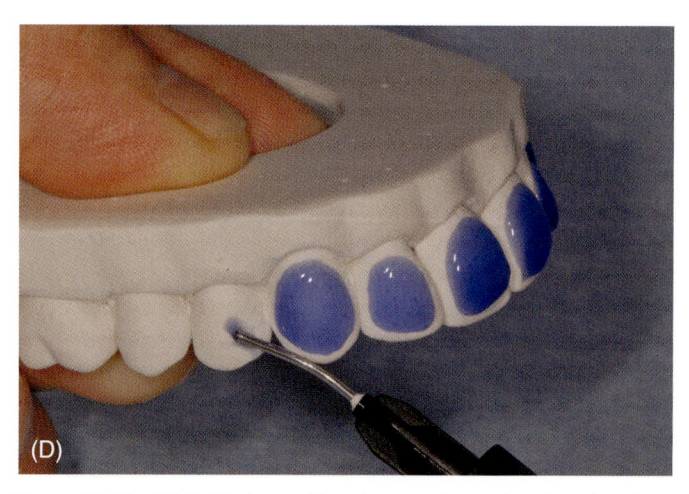

Figure 12.20 **(D)** A thin layer of block-out resin can be placed on the buccal surface as a reservoir for the bleaching material.

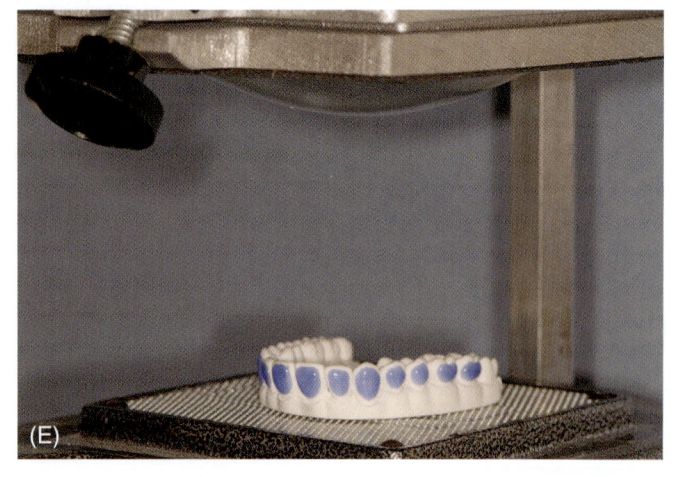

Figure 12.20 **(E)** A soft and thin sheet is heated in a vacuum-forming unit until it sags 12 mm.

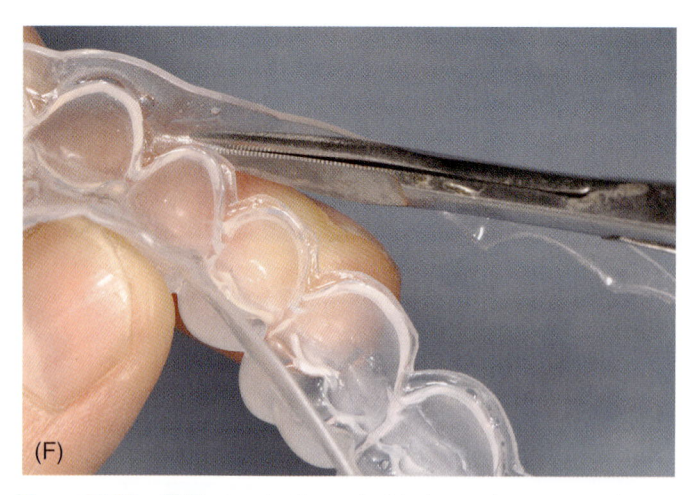

Figure 12.20 **(F)** The tray is trimmed with sharp scissors approximately 0.5 mm away from the gingival margin to create a scalloped pattern on the buccal surface.

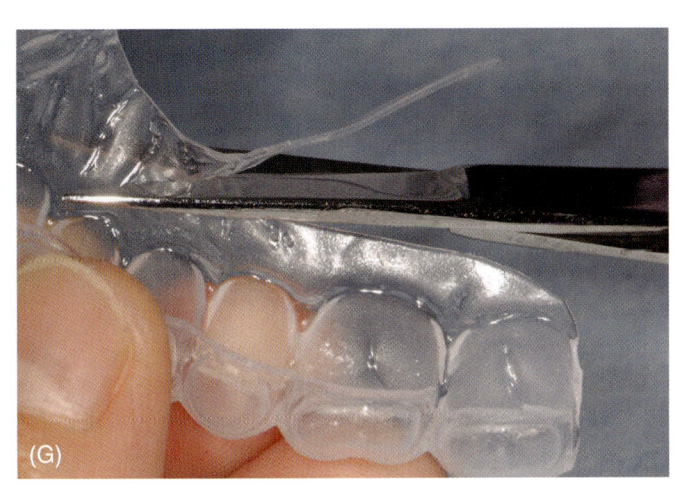

Figure 12.20 **(G)** The lingual border is extended 2 mm from the gingival margin in a straight pattern.

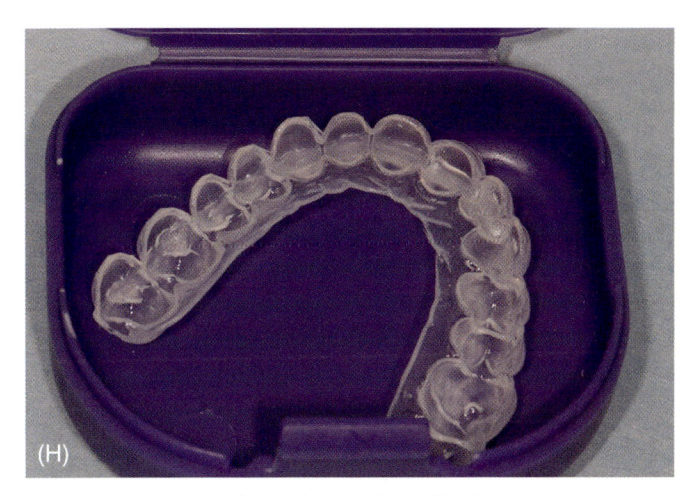

Figure 12.20 **(H)** The finished tray is cleaned and stored in a tray case until delivery to the patient.

Home bleaching without dental supervision (over-the-counter systems)

When the mouthguard vital bleaching technique burst upon the scene in the late 1980s, product claims often exceeded the proof of research or clinical experience. As Haywood outlines in a detailed history of the FDA's influence on home bleaching,[5] before the FDA stepped in to attempt to control home bleaching products intended for over-the-counter sales, there was virtually no control on ethical advertising to the public. People were buying various kits and products that in many cases were contraindicated for the very problem they were trying to solve. Although some people asked the advice of their dentists before embarking on their purchased treatment package plan, many did not.

The controversy over home bleaching has been an interesting, and in many ways helpful, time for dentistry. In 1991, the FDA ruled that the use of carbamide peroxide in the form advocated for home bleaching constituted a new drug use and hence was subject to new drug approval process. The agency did not make a distinction between the home bleaching provided by dentists and the home bleaching kits the consumer could pick up in a department store. (Thirty-five percent hydrogen peroxide used for in-office bleaching was considered to be "grandfathered" because of its long time use for this purpose.) Because of this ruling, manufacturers were forced to submit evidence to back up their claims of the efficacy of bleaching materials, or to demonstrate these materials' safety. Consequently, many small manufacturers faced closure because they lacked the resources to do so, and inferior products were more likely to be taken off the market. The ruling also forced manufacturers of materials sold directly to dentists to examine whether their products could meet the new drug standards.

The FDA appears to have reconsidered its position, especially concerning distinctions between home-bleaching agents meant for use under dental supervision and those meant for sale to the general public. Possible negative effects would include a restricted supply market to the dentist, with the removal of adequate but less costly materials. However, there have been many positive effects already, including a public made more aware of the risks of unsupervised home bleaching, increased funding for research in this area, a recognition by many general dentists that they must stay current with laboratory and clinical research literature for the good of their patients, and a greater involvement by the dental organizations in the federal and public arenas.

The earlier sections have described the advantage of having a dentist involved in home bleaching, with the correct diagnosis and decision on appropriate treatment, the recognition and management of side effects, and the use of more potent or highly viscous materials. Other reasons, as outlined by Haywood,[5,40] include the following:

- A thinner, softer, better fitting mouthguard can be constructed, increasing patient comfort and minimizing side effects due to tissue or tooth irritation.
- Not subjecting the person to the dangers of using boiling water in the self-fabrication of the mouthguard.
- Adjustment of the occlusion on the mouthguard to minimize any potential temporomandibular joint problems.

Tooth sensitivity during vital bleaching

Tooth sensitivity during bleaching is the most prevalent side effect to treatment, and the dental office should be prepared to offer treatment options. Tooth sensitivity experienced during bleaching can be treated actively or passively by the dentist. Passive treatment consists of reducing either the duration of each treatment (fewer hours) or the frequency of treatment (skip days). Originally, the only active treatment cited was the use of a neutral fluoride gel placed in the tray at the onset of sensitivity. Some current bleaching products now incorporate a neutral fluoride with no apparent compromise of the bleaching process (15% opalescence with fluoride, Ultradent). The mechanism of action of fluoride is as a tubular blocker.

Another active approach to treating sensitivity involves the use of 5% or less concentrations of potassium nitrate applied in the bleaching tray. Potassium nitrate is generally found in desensitizing toothpastes, which are applied via brushing.

This application technique generally takes 2 weeks to see results. Because the application of toothpaste in a bleaching style can cause gingival irritations in some patients, dental companies have now introduced products of potassium nitrate with and without fluoride in a base barrier (Desentize, DEN-MAT; UltraEZ, Ultradent; Relief, Discus Dental). The mechanism of action of potassium nitrate is different from that of fluoride. Potassium nitrate is thought to act to chemically depolarize the nerve to inhibit refiring[7] and is a good adjunct for any type of chronic sensitivity, as well as bleaching sensitivity.

Maintaining bleaching results

Although both in-office and matrix techniques can produce effective results, the advantage of the latter technique is that it will allow for touch-ups or retreatment as necessary. As long as the matrix continues to fit properly, new solution can be given to the patient for an additional series of bleaching treatments every few years or as needed. Generally it may be 3 years before retreatment is desirable.[40,41]

In-office bleaching of nonvital teeth

The pulpless tooth is frequently an excellent candidate for bleaching. The fact that the pulp is already nonvital immediately removes one of the major concerns of in-office bleaching; that is, the intense heat will cause damage to the pulp. While you should remain within the upper limits of the normal range of heat due to possible internal or external resorption, the ability to use higher temperatures without causing the patient discomfort will enable you to increase the rate at which the bleaching agent is effective. However, for many patients, custom-designed matrix bleaching trays may be used.

Garretson[42] first bleached nonvital teeth at the turn of the twentieth century. The presence of a pulpless chamber inspired dentists such as Pearson[43] to use chemicals with both bleaching capability and oxygen-releasing capability to provide the same activation of bleaching as heat does in bleaching for nonvital teeth. He left his bleaching agent, Superoxol, in the pulp chamber for 3 days. Nutting and Poe's "walking bleach" technique[44] went another step: Superoxol and sodium perborate are sealed in the pulp chamber for as long as a week. A range of choices is important in treating nonvital teeth since the discoloration can range from mild to extreme.

Etiology of discoloration

Although nonvital teeth are subject to external and other stains, the primary discoloration of the nonvital tooth is likely to come from within the pulp chamber itself, resulting from pulp degeneration, with or without hemorrhage. Pulp hemorrhage is more likely to cause pronounced discoloration than pulp degeneration not accompanied by hemorrhage. In fact, according to Ingle,[45] the greatest amount of discoloration seen is in the traumatized anterior tooth. Nutting and Poe[44] also list necrotic pulp tissue with pulp hemorrhage as the factor most frequently responsible for tooth discoloration. Trauma severe enough to cause pulp death also causes the rupture of blood vessels into the pulp chamber. The blood from the ruptured vessels is driven into the dentinal chamber where the red blood cells undergo hemolysis, exuding hemoglobin. This released hemoglobin is further degraded, releasing iron, which forms a black compound by combining with hydrogen sulfide to become iron sulfide. The resultant necrotic tissue contains various protein degradation products that create the familiar grayish-black discoloration of the tooth.

After pulp necrosis, the most frequent cause of discoloration is an incomplete root canal in which pulpal debris is left in the tooth. Pulp remnants, residual tissue in the pulp horns, filling material, and medicaments all can lead to discoloration. Spasser[47] has noted that color changes also may be caused by a root canal sealer containing eugenol, Canada balsam, or precipitated silver. Since nonvital teeth are deprived of tissue fluid, fluid may penetrate them more easily than vital teeth.

Whatever the cause, the degree of discoloration is directly related to the length of time between pulp death and treatment. The longer the discoloring compounds are in the chamber, the deeper the penetration into the dentinal tubules and the greater the discoloration. Discoloration of long duration presents the greatest challenge to successful treatment.

Contraindications to bleaching of pulpless teeth with concentrated hydrogen peroxide (35%)

It remains as true as when Nutting and Poe first stated it more than 50 years ago:[44] prudent case selection is vital to a successful esthetic result. The primary requirement for bleaching is the existence of an adequate root canal filling. Contraindications include the following:

- small amount of remaining dentin
- extensive restorations: there may not be sufficient tooth structure to make bleaching worthwhile
- restorations with composite or acrylic resins, since as Cohen and Parkins[18] point out, the bleaching technique probably causes temporary dehydration; however, this may only be a problem if your patient does not want or need to replace his or her restorations following bleaching
- cracks and hypoplastic or severely undermined enamel
- discoloration by metallic salts, particularly silver amalgam; the dentinal tubules of the teeth are virtually saturated with the alloys and no amount of bleaching with available products will significantly improve the esthetic quality of these teeth.

Techniques for bleaching pulpless teeth

The choice of techniques employed for bleaching pulpless teeth will depend on the degree of discoloration and patient compliance. In all procedures, the purpose is to allow the bleaching agent to release oxygen in a concentration high enough to

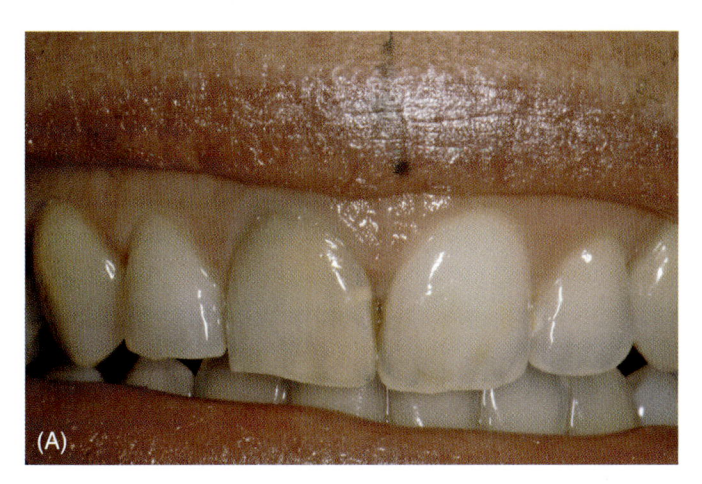

Figure 12.21 **(A)** This young woman was self-conscious about her discolored central incisor.

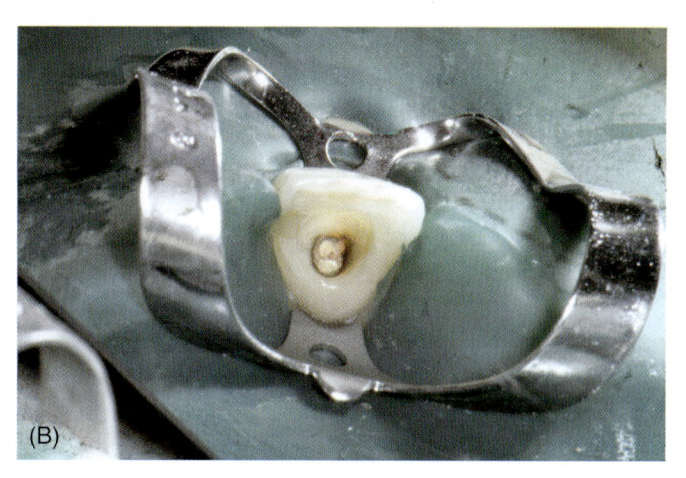

Figure 12.21 **(B)** After an adequately sized access opening was made, gutta percha is removed to slightly below the gingival line.

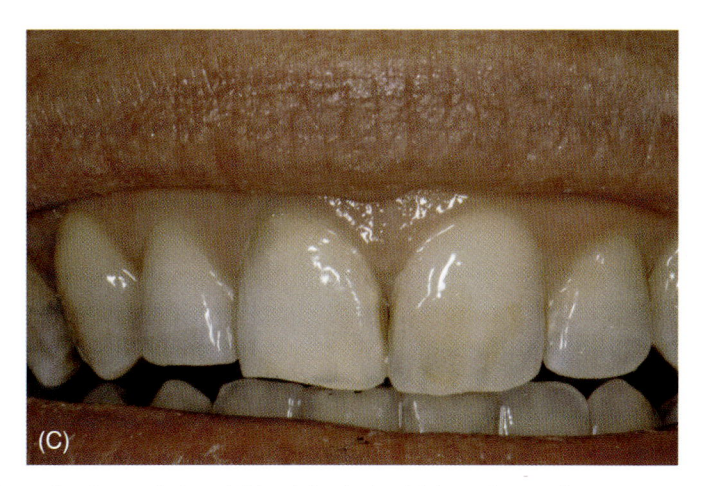

Figure 12.21 **(C)** After bleaching, the patient's nonvital tooth blends in nicely with her other teeth.

penetrate the stained dentinal tubules and neutralize the discoloration (Figure 12.21A).

Preparation

Preparatory procedures are similar whether in-office or walking bleach techniques are to be used.

1. Isolate the tooth or teeth. To protect the patient's tissues from the highly concentrated bleaching material, use a well-fitted rubber dam of heavy material. The size of the hole punched is also important; too small a hole will cause the dam to tear. Since tears can allow leakage, a torn dam should be removed and the cause for the tear found and corrected. A ligature may be placed around the tooth if desired but this is not usually necessary. Before placing the dam, the gingivae should be coated with Oraseal (Ultradent) as a precaution against damaging the periodontal tissue if some of the bleaching material should seep through the dam. After the dam is sealed, the lubricant may be applied with a cotton applicator on the labial and lingual surfaces. Meticulous care must be taken to ensure the tissue is completely protected. When the dam is in place, additional lubricant can be used in the interdental spaces by using a small plastic instrument. Extreme caution also must be used to ensure that the solution does not come in contact with the lip, which could result in an unsightly disfiguring lesion with extensive edema. (However, these lesions generally heal without scarring.)

2. After isolation, the tooth is meticulously cleaned. Any caries in the crown should be excavated and any leaky or washed out restorations replaced.

3. Establish a lingual opening of sufficient size to secure proper access to the entire pulp chamber and orifice of the root canal. B. Seidler (personal communication to R.E. Goldstein) suggests using a #8 round bur for initial entry into the chamber and for removal of the necrotic tissue. A smaller bur should be used in lower anteriors and in those teeth in which pulp recession would be evident radiographically.

4. Remove all debris and the surface layer of dentin within the pulp chamber with a slow-rotation bur. The freshened dentin permits easier penetration of the bleaching material. Since the dentin will be bleached as well as the enamel, the more mature the tooth and the greater the amount of dentin present, the longer the effect will be retained following bleaching. For this reason, preserve as much dentin as possible.

5. In endodontically treated teeth, the root canal filling material should be removed to a depth of 2–3 mm apical to the cervical line. This distance may be extended if the gingival recession has been severe. Ingle[45] recommends that the root canal filling be removed to a level well below the height of the labial gingivae, although Grossman[47] recommends that the root canal filling extend only to the gingival margin (Figure 12.21B).

6. Remove any surface stains visible on the inside of the preparation with a bur. The apical seal should be checked and secured at this time.

7. The entire preparation should be swabbed with acetone or xylol to dissolve any fatty material and facilitate the penetration of the bleaching agent into the tubules. The chamber should then be blown dry.

8. Cover the root canal filling with zinc phosphate cement, polycarboxylate cement, glass ionomer, or Cavit, 2 mm thick, since bleaching agents may affect the root canal sealer. Bleaching should never be attempted on any tooth without a complete seal in the root canal since the agent could escape through a porous root canal filling and cause the patient extreme discomfort. If this should occur, heavy sedation will be required to mask the pain, and removal of the bleaching agent and the root canal filling may be required to restore comfort.

Some improvements can be obtained in difficult cases by sealing H_2O_2 or sodium perborate wetted with H_2O_2 on a cotton pellet inside the pulp chamber between bleaching appointments. Bleach the teeth a little higher than the final shade desired to compensate for anticipated slight darkening (Figure 12.21C).

Inside-outside tray bleaching technique

This technique was described by Settembrini and Liebenberg[48] in 1997 to bleach the discolored tooth from the inside as well as from the outside with a 10% carbamide peroxide solution retained in a custom-fitted tray. The major advantage of this technique is that the nonvital discolored tooth can be bleached together with the adjacent vital teeth. However, the periodic insertion of whitening material and cleaning of the access cavity can be burdensome. There is also possibility of tongue irritation from the margins of the open access cavity. The preparation for the inside–outside bleaching technique is the same as for the walking bleaching technique up to the placement of the barrier material.

1. Deliver a custom-fitted tray and 10% carbamide peroxide solution to the patient.
2. Give instructions on how to insert the bleaching gel into the cavity and into the tray.
3. Show the patient how to clean the open access cavity with the use of an empty syringe.
4. Have the patient return to the office, once the teeth have whitened.

Out-of-office bleaching technique (or walking bleach)

Follow the same preparation techniques given earlier.

1. On a glass mixing slab, prepare a bleaching paste of peroxyborate monohydrate (Amosan) or sodium perborate and enough 35% hydrogen peroxide to form a thick white paste.
2. Fill the entire preparation with the bleaching paste, leaving adequate space to place a temporary restoration and sealer (Figure 12.22). Make certain that the seal is effective as moist paste can damage tissue if it leaks into the pulp chamber. One method is to carefully apply a solvent (Prep Dry, PrimaDry [Ultradent]) around the enamel margin and flow a medium-stiff mix of Cavit to close the area. If the patient experiences a burning on the tongue, rinse until the sensation is gone.

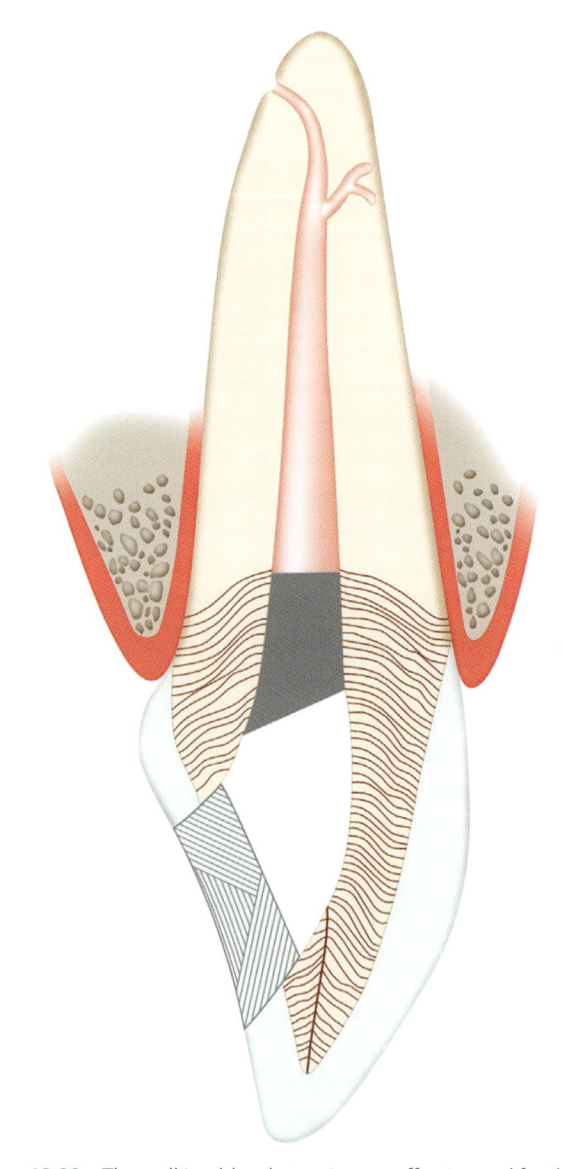

Figure 12.22 The walking bleach requires an effective seal for the bleaching paste to remain active. From reference 61.

3. Have the patient return in 3–5 days. If the degree of bleaching is not sufficient, repeat the entire procedure. Again, a slight overbleaching is desirable since teeth tend to darken slightly after the final bleach.

Finishing

On return to the office after completion of the inside–outside or conventional walking bleaching technique, the orifice to the nonvital tooth is debrided and temporarily sealed for 2 weeks with a noneugenol-containing temporary cement. A noneugenol-containing material is used to avoid future contamination of the acid-etched composite restoration, which will be used to close the orifice to the canal and make any final minor color adjustments by varying the composite color internally. Placement of the final restoration is delayed for 2 weeks to allow the oxygen generated during bleaching to dissipate from the tooth and the shade to stabilize. The presence of residual oxygen in the tooth results in the reduction of bond strengths[7] and an artificially light shade. Two weeks after termination of bleaching, the bond strength potential will have returned to normal,[7] and the shade will have stabilized. This shade stabilization (a slight darkening) is thought to occur from the change in optical qualities of the tooth after residual oxygen generated during the oxidation process of bleaching has diminished. Two weeks after a completion of bleaching, the temporary stopping is removed, and the orifice is occluded using an acid-etched composite as follows:

1. Remove the cotton or bleaching paste and swab the preparation throughout with acetone or xylol.
2. Air dry internally and throughout the bleached crown to penetrate and seal the dentinal tubules and to maintain the tooth's translucency. Use several coats of a clear dentin bonding agent to prevent recurrent coronal stain.
3. Etch the marginal walls with 35% phosphoric acid to assure good mechanical bonding. The entire restoration is placed at one time and finished properly to assure good marginal adaptation.
4. Apply a dental bonding agent and cure before filling the cavity with composite resin restorative materials of the lightest shade esthetically compatible with the tooth. Use a composite with a good dentin bonding agent, being careful to etch the enamel walls before restoring the final area. A microfill or polishable hybrid is the best material to use because it allows a polished surface to blend with the adjacent enamel surface. A typical result is seen in Figure 12.23A and B.

Planning for continued treatment

You must use your clinical judgment to decide if rebleaching would effect greater improvement. If the tooth shows significant improvement, then the solution chosen obviously contained the solvent for the stain and rebleaching is likely to continue improvement. Conversely, if results are not obtained, bleaching out the discoloration may not be possible. It may be advantageous to employ one or two parts of HCl in such instances as an added solvent before abandoning the procedure as ineffective. Try at least three to four visits.

You also must use your clinical judgment about the length of time a tooth is likely to remain bleached. Spasser[46] notes that the determining factors include the amount and depth of the external enamel cracks and the integrity of the marginal seal of the restoration. Hayashi[51] reports that discoloration may also recur in time from penetration of pigments in the saliva into the dentinal tubules. To help prevent pigment penetration into the dentin, Grossman[47] recommends putting silicone oil in the cavity after bleaching. Silicone oil will not evaporate and has a low surface tension which will help the dentin retain it. If the discoloration occurs one to three years after the initial treatment, you can retreat using dentist-monitored home treatment.

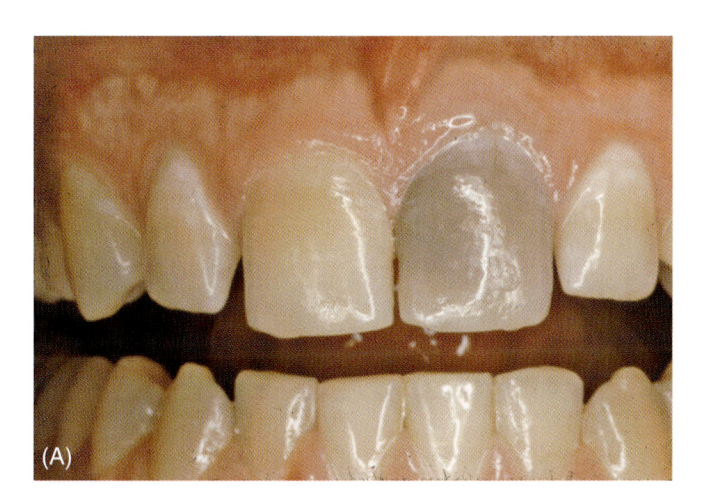

Figure 12.23 **(A)** This severely gray-brown nonvital tooth is a good candidate for bleaching.

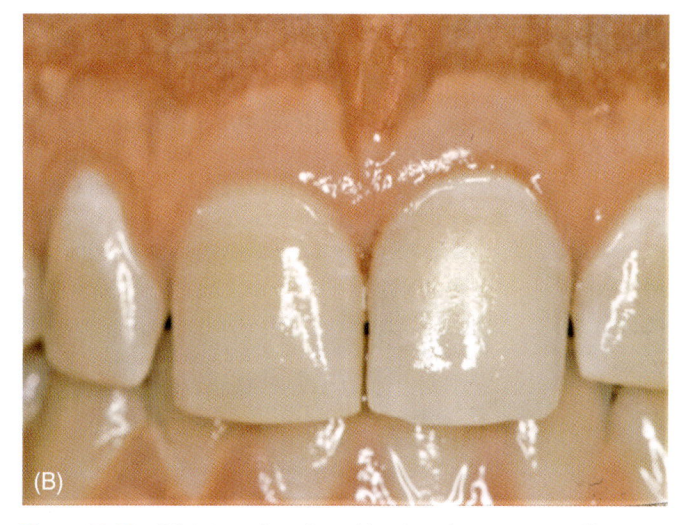

Figure 12.23 **(B)** A 3 week walking-bleach technique was sufficient to regain the original tooth color for this man.

Complications and risks

Cervical root resorption

Cervical root resorption related to intracoronal bleaching is a complication that was first reported by Harrington and Natkin in 1979.[52] Heithersay analyzed cervical resorption cases and reported that 24.1% were caused by orthodontic treatment, 15.1% by dental trauma, 5.1% by surgery, and 3.9% by intracoronal bleaching.[53] The combination of bleaching and history of trauma seems to be the most important predisposing factor for cervical resorption.[53] Several theories have been proposed to explain the mechanism of cervical root resorption. It has been postulated that the bleaching material may diffuse into the periodontal ligament and initiate an inflammatory reaction, denaturation of dentin proteins, or a decrease in pH, thereby activating osteoclastic activity leading to resorption.[54-56] Consequently, there is a special risk factor in young patients with relatively wide open dentinal tubules and in patients with a natural anatomic defect between the cementum and enamel at the level of cemento-enamel junction.[57] Application of heat leads to widening of dentinal tubules and facilitates the diffusion of hydrogen peroxide into dentin.[58] Higher risk of cervical root resorption associated with the thermocatalytic bleaching technique has reduced its use in intracoronal bleaching.[59]

Cervical root resorption is usually detected on follow-up radiographs and may present clinical symptoms as gingival swelling and sensitivity to percussion. Remineralization can be attempted at the early stage but if the resorption has progressed, exposure of the lesion with a crown lengthening procedure or forced eruption followed by an appropriate filling is required.

Color relapse

Optimal color match with adjacent teeth can be achieved after intracoronal bleaching. However, color relapse can be observed occasionally, which is presumably caused by the penetration of staining substances through marginal gaps between the tooth and the restoration.[60]

The future of bleaching

The history of bleaching has been one of continued improvements in bleaching materials, delivery systems, and devices to activate the bleaching action. In order to develop the ideal bleaching agent that is indicated for a specific discoloration, there needs to be more accurate ways to assess, quantify, and describe the discoloration. There also needs to be better understanding on the mechanism of bleaching so that dentists can better predict for which patient it will be most successful. The mechanism of color regression needs further investigation. Researchers and clinicians do not know why some patients' teeth remain stable over extended periods, while other patients' teeth regress in color. It is also not known whether the color regression is a result of recolorizing of the oxidized stain molecule or whether it results from the combination of new stains and the aging process.

And finally, the sudden surge of bleaching kits intended to be used with little or no dentist monitoring makes the need for more research into the long-term safety and effects of such materials imperative. Dentistry must maintain control of both research and treatment for maximum patient protection and success rates. As scientists learn more about bleaching efficacy, safety, and longevity, the technique will no doubt continue to be at the top of the list of esthetic modalities.

References

1. Dzierzak J. Factors which cause tooth color changes protocol for in-office "power" bleaching. *Pract Periodontics Aesthet Dent* 1991;3(2):15–20.
2. Zaragoza VMT. Bleaching of vital teeth: technique. *Estomodeo* 1984;9:7–30.
3. Friedman J. Variability of lamp characteristics in dental curing lights. *J Esthet Dent* 1989;1(6):189–190.
4. Hodosh M, Mirman M, Shklar G, Povar M. A new method of bleaching discolored teeth by the use of a solid state direct heating device. *Dent Dig* 1970;76(8):344–346.
5. Haywood VB. The food and drug administration and its influence on home bleaching. *Curr Opin Cosmet Dent* 1993;12–18.
6. Hattab FN, Qudeimat MA, Al-Rimawi HS. Dental discoloration: an overview. *J Esthet Dent* 1999;11:291–310.
7. Haywood United States, IL. VB. *Tooth Whitening: Indications and Outcomes of Nightguard Vital Bleaching*. Chicago, IL: Quintessence; 2007.
8. Addy M, Roberts WR. Comparison of the bisbiguanide antiseptics alexidine and chlorhexidine. II. clinical and in vitro staining properties. *J Clin Periodontol* 1981;8(3):220–230.
9. Addy M, Moran J, Newcombe R, Warren P. The comparative tea staining potential of phenolic, chlorhexidine and anti-adhesive mouthrinses. *J Clin Periodontol* 1995;22(12):923–928.
10. Garcia-Lopez M, Martinez-Blanco M, Martinez-Mir I, Palop V. Amoxycillin-clavulanic acid-related tooth discoloration in children. *Pediatrics* 2001;108(3):819.
11. Dahl JE, Palleson U. Tooth bleaching: a critical review of the biological aspects. *Crit Rev Oral Biol Med* 2003;14(4):292–304.
12. Burt BA. The changing patterns of systemic fluoride intake. *J Dent Res* 1992;71(5):1228–1237.
13. Black GV, McKay FS. Mottled teeth, an endemic developmental imperfection of the enamel of the teeth here-to-fore unknown in the literature of dentistry. *Dent Cosmos* 1916;58:129.
14. Goldstein R, Garber D. *Complete Dental Bleaching*. Chicago, IL: Quintessence; 1995.
15. Bailey RW, Christen AG. Effects of a bleaching technic on the labial enamel of human teeth stained with endemic dental fluorosis. *J Dent Res* 1970;49(1):168–170.
16. Arens D. The role of bleaching in esthetics. *Dent Clin North Am* 1989;33(2):319–336.
17. Shwachman H, Fekete E, Kulezychi L, Foley G. The effect of long-term antibiotic therapy in patients with cystic fibrosis of the pancreas. *Antibiot Annu* 1958–1959;6:692–699.
18. Cohen S, Parkins FM. Bleaching tetracycline-stained vital teeth. *Oral Surg Oral Med Oral Pathol* 1970;29(3):465–471.
19. Mello HS. The mechanism of tetracycline staining in primary and permanent teeth. *J Dent Child* 1967;34(6):478–487.

20. Jordan RE, Boksman L. Conservative vital bleaching treatment of discolored dentition. *Compend Contin Educ Dent* 1984;5(10):803–805, 807.
21. Bowles W. Teeth discolored by minocycline. *Dent Today* 1986;5(2):4.
22. Dodson D, Bowles W. Production of minocycline pigment by tissue extracts. *J Dent Res* 70(Sp. Issue April): 424
23. Bailey SJ, Swift EJ Jr. Effects of home bleaching products on composite resins. *Quintessence Int* 1992;23(7):489–494.
24. Stewart RE, Witkop CJ, Bixler D. *Pediatric Dentistry: Scientific Foundations and Clinical Practice*. St Louis, MO: C.V. Mosby; 1982.
25. Faunce F. Management of discolored teeth. *Dent Clin North Am* 1983;27(4):657–670.
26. Berman LH. Intrinsic staining and hypoplastic enamel: etiology and treatment alternatives. *Gen Dent* 1982;30(6):484–488.
27. Koa E, Peng P, Johnston W. Color changes of teeth and restorative materials exposed to bleaching (abstract 2436). *J Dent Res* 1991;70:570.
28. Lazarchik DA, Haywood VB. Use of tray-applied 10 percent carbamide peroxide gels for improving oral health in patients with special-care needs. *J Am Dent Assoc* 2010;141(6):639–646.
29. Paravina RD, Johnston WM, Powers JM. New shade guide for evaluation of tooth whitening—colorimetric study. *J Esthet Restor Dent* 2007;19(5):276–283; discussion 283.
30. Haywood V, Leonard R, Nelson C. Nightguard vital bleaching longevity and side effects: 13-25 months data. *J Dent Res* 1993;72:208.
31. Rosenstiel SF, Gegauff AG, Johnston WM. Duration of tooth color change after bleaching. *J Am Dent Assoc* 1991;122(4):54–59.
32. Bodden MK, Haywood VB. Treatment of endemic fluorosis and tetracycline staining with macroabrasion and nightguard vital bleaching: a case report. *Quintessence Int* 2003;34(2):87–91.
33. Garber DA, Goldstein RE, Goldstein GE, Schwartz CG. Dentist monitored bleaching: a combined approach. *Pract Periodontics Aesthet Dent* 1991;3(2):22–26.
34. Barghi N, Godwin JM. Reducing the adverse effect of bleaching on composite-enamel bond. *J Esthet Dent* 1994;6(4):157–161.
35. Barkhordar RA, Pontejos J, Machado S, Watanabe LG. The effect of a bleaching agent on leakage of composite resin (abstract 2437). *J Dent Res* 1991;70:570.
36. Burger KM, Cooley RL. Effect of carbamide peroxide on composite resins (abstract 2431). *J Dent Res* 1991;70:570.
37. Friend G, Jones J, Wamble S, Covington J. Carbamide peroxide tooth bleaching: changes to composite resins after prolonged exposure (abstract 2432). *J Dent Res* 1991;70:570.
38. Haywood VB. Bleaching of vital and nonvital teeth. *Curr Opin Dent* 1992;2:142–149.
39. Haywood V, Houck V, Heymann H. Nightguard vital bleaching: effects of varying pH solutions on enamel surface texture and color changes. *Quintessence Int* 1991;22:775–782.
40. Haywood VB. Achieving, maintaining, and recovering successful tooth bleaching. *J Esthet Dent* 1996;8(1):31–38.
41. Kwon S, Ko S, Greenwall L. *Tooth Whitening in Esthetic Dentistry*. Germany: Quintessence; 2009.
42. Garretson J. *A System of Oral Surgery*, 6th edn. Philadelphia, PA: J.B. Lippincott Co.; 1895.
43. Pearson H. Bleaching of the discolored pulpless tooth. *J Am Dent Assoc* 1958;56(1):64–68.
44. Nutting EB, Poe GS. A new combination for bleaching teeth. *J S Calif State Dent Assoc* 1963;31:289–291.
45. Ingle J. *Endodontics*. Philadelphia, PA: Lea and Febiger; 1967.
46. Spasser HF. A simple bleaching technique using sodium perborate. *N Y State Dent J* 1961;27:332–334.
47. Grossman LI. *Endodontic Practice*. Philadelphia, PA: Lea and Febiger; 1970.
48. Settembrini L, Gultz J, Kaim J, Scherer W. A technique for bleaching nonvital teeth: Inside/outside bleaching. *J Am Dent Assoc* 1997;128(9):1283–1284.
49. Torneck CD, Titley KC, Smith DC, Adibfar A. The influence of time of hydrogen peroxide exposure on the adhesion of composite resin to bleached bovine enamel. *J Endod* 1990;16(3):123–128.
50. Torneck CD, Titley KC, Smith DO, Adibfar A. Effect of water leaching the adhesion of composite resin to bleached and unbleached bovine enamel. *J Endod* 1991;17(4):156–160.
51. Hayashi K, Takamizu M, Momoi Y, et al. Bleaching teeth discolored by tetracycline therapy. *Dent Surv* 1980;56(3):17–25.
52. Harrington GW, Natkin E. External resorption associated with bleaching of pulpless teeth. *J Endod* 1979;5(11):344–348.
53. Heithersay GS. Invasive cervical resorption: an analysis of potential predisposing factors. *Quintessence Int* 1999;30(2):83–95.
54. Lado EA, Stanley HR, Weisman MI. Cervical resorption in bleached teeth. *Oral Surg Oral Med Oral Pathol* 1983;55(1):78–80.
55. Madison S, Walton R. Cervical root resorption following bleaching of endodontically treated teeth. *J Endod* 1990;16(12):570–574.
56. Montgomery S. External cervical resorption after bleaching a pulpless tooth. *Oral Surg Oral Med Oral Pathol* 1984;57(2):203–206.
57. Trope M. Cervical root resorption. *J Am Dent Assoc* 1997;128(suppl):56S–59S.
58. Pashley DH, Thompson SM, Stewart FP. Dentin permeability: effects of temperature on hydraulic conductance. *J Dent Res* 1983;62(9):956–959.
59. Rotstein I, Zalkind M, Mor C, et al. In vitro efficacy of sodium perborate preparations used for intracoronal bleaching of discolored non-vital teeth. *Endod Dent Traumatol* 1991;7(4):177–180.
60. Feiglin B. A 6-year recall study of clinically chemically bleached teeth. *Oral Surg Oral Med Oral Pathol* 1987;63(5):610–613.
61. Cohen S, Burns R, eds. *Pathways of the Pulp*, 6th edn. St. Louis, MO: Mosby; 1994.

Additional references

Al-Harbi A, Ardu S, Bortolotto T, Krejci I. Effect of extended application time on the efficacy of an in-office hydrogen peroxide bleaching agent: an in vitro study. *Eur J Esthet Dent* 2013;8:226–228.

Briso ALF, Goncalves RS, Almeida de Azevedo F, et al. Transenamel and transdentinal penetration of H_2O_2 in restored bovine teeth. *J Adhes Dent* 2015;17:529–534.

Croll TP, Donly KJ. Tooth bleaching in children and teens. *J Esthet Restor Dent* 2014;26:147–150.

Dietschi D. Nonvital bleaching: general considerations and report of two failure cases. *Eur J Esthet Dent* 2006;1:52–61.

Haywood VB, Cordero R, Wright K. Brushing with a potassium nitrate dentifrice to reduce bleaching sensitivity. *J Clin Dent* 2005;16:17–22.

Higashi C, Dall'Agnol AL, Hirata R. Association of enamel microabrasion and bleaching: a case report. *Gen Dent* 2008;56:244–249.

Lee YK, Powers JM. Color and optical properties of resin-composites for bleached teeth after polymerization and accelerated aging. *Am J Dent* 2001;14:349–354.

Loyola-Rodriguez JP, Pozos-Guillen Ade J, Hernandez-Hernandez F. Effectiveness of treatment with carbide peroxide and hydrogen peroxide in subjects affected by dental fluorosis: a clinical trial. *J Clin Pediatric Dent* 2003:28;63–67.

Machado LS, Anchieta RB, Henrique dos Santos P, et al. Clinical comparison of at-home and in-office dental bleaching procedures: a randomized trial of a split-mouth design. *Int J Periodontics Rest Dent* 2016;36:251–260.

Martin J, Vildosola P, Bersezio C, et al. Effectiveness of 6% hydrogen peroxide concentration for tooth bleaching - a double-blind, randomized clinical trial. *J Dent* 2015;43:965–972.

Strassler HE, Griffin A, Maggio M. Management of fluorosis using macro- and micro abrasion. *Dent Today* 2001;30:94–96.

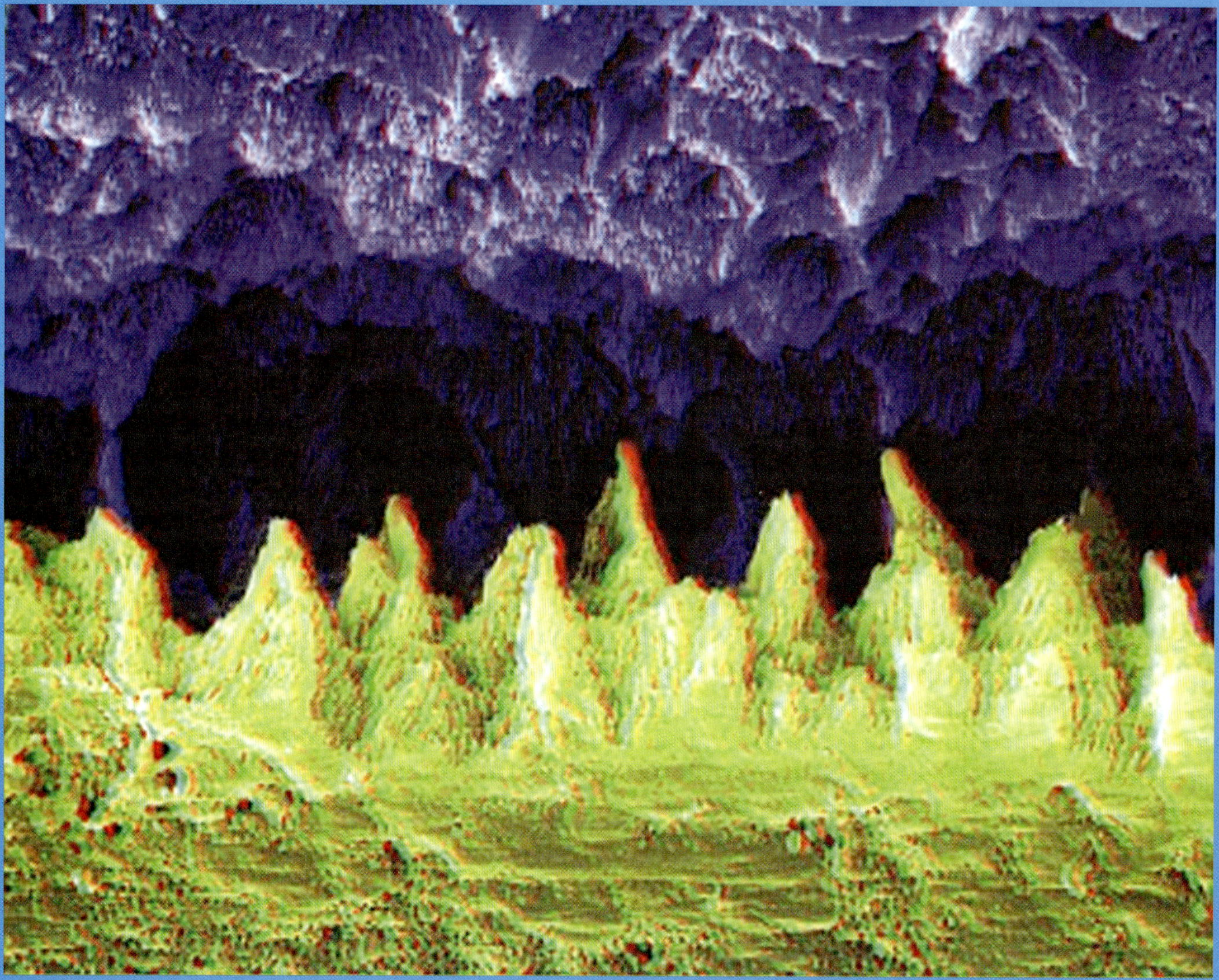

Chapter 13 Adhesion to Hard Tissue on Teeth

Roland Frankenberger, DMD, PhD, Uwe Blunck, DDS, and Lorenzo Breschi, DDS, PhD

Chapter Outline

Introduction	355	Universal adhesives	361
Basics about adhesion	356	Dark-curing adhesives	361
Definitions	356	Filled adhesives	362
Prerequisites	356	Valuation of adhesives	363
Enamel bonding	356	Biocompatibility of adhesives	363
Adhesion mechanisms to enamel	356	Aging of the adhesive interface	363
Conditioning with phosphoric acid	356	Reliability and degradation of etch-and-rinse adhesives	364
Self-etch adhesives	357	Reliability and degradation of self-etch adhesives	365
Historical development	358	Technique sensitivity: a problem and its solution	365
Adhesion to dentin	358	Etch-and-rinse adhesives	365
Adhesion mechanism to dentin	359	Self-etching adhesives	365
Conditioning with phosphoric acid	359	Postoperative hypersensitivities	366
Self-etch adhesives	360	Failure prevention: clinical application	367
Priming of the collagen network	360	Recommendations for using etch-and-rinse adhesives	367
Stabilizing by bonding agents	360	Recommendations for using self-etching adhesives	368
Classification of adhesive systems	360		

Introduction

Resin composites do not adhere to enamel and dentin by themselves like, for example, glass ionomer cements. Therefore, after polymerization, marginal gaps would be the logical consequence. These would even be deteriorated by different coefficients of thermal expansion (tooth/restorative) and mechanical load.[1–12] Without appropriate pretreatment, strength, and durability, adhesion is impaired (Figure 13.1); therefore, adhesive retention is a fundamental prerequisite for resin composites.

Recurrent caries is still estimated to be one of the main reasons for resin composite restoration failure, especially in stress-bearing areas. The integration of adhesion concepts led to a breakthrough for the clinical use of resin composites.[13–26]

Adhesive dentistry gained considerable importance within the field of modern restorative dentistry and it is meanwhile established as daily routine. Only with durable adhesion to tooth

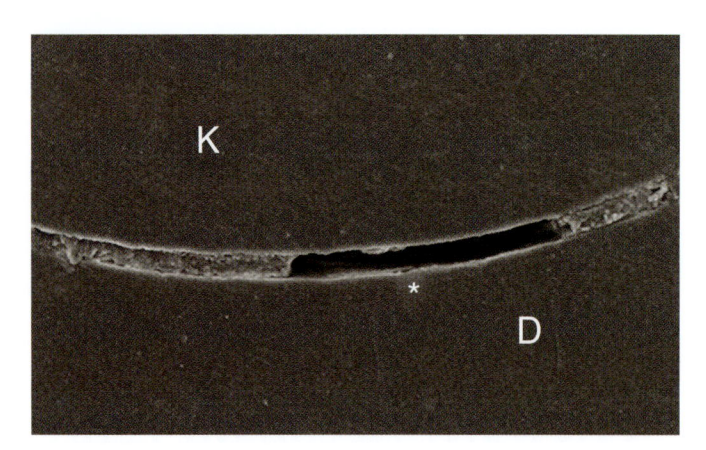

Figure 13.1 A gap under the scanning electron microscope (SEM; 1:500). K, resin composite; D, dentin.

hard tissues is it possible to reach the goal of true minimally invasive restorative therapy. Today, adhesive dentistry is based on minimum loss of hard tooth substrate by rotary burs during preparation and treatment of recurrent caries in the case of adhesive failure.

Basics about adhesion

Definitions

Adhesion means "bonding of different substances in tight contact." Molecular adhesion forces cause this when two bodies are close together. In most of these cases, there is a solid adhesive substrate and a liquid phase called adhesive.[27]

There are different explanations for adhesion phenomena. Rough and porous surfaces lead to mechanical and microretentive adhesion, while adhesive and substrate are able to act via chemical bonding such as ionic bonding, covalent bonding, hydrogen bonds, and van der Waals forces.[27–30] The majority of studies in the field of dentistry assume that the resin-enamel and resin-dentin bond are of a micromechanical nature mainly because chemical interactions have seldom been reported.[31–33]

Prerequisites

Tight contact (0.1 nm) is the main factor for adhesion. Bodies and surfaces, however, have direct contact only in special areas; therefore, a liquid phase must fill remaining spaces as a guarantee for increased wettability.[34–36] Ideally, the adhesion substrate provides high surface energy and the adhesive low viscosity (i.e. surface tension). Additionally, surface roughness is another important factor for adhesion by resulting in increased surface area. Micromechanical interlocking is caused by filling the gaps and irregularities between substrates.[12,37–39]

Chemical bonding exists when two atoms use the same electrons. Hydrogen bonds and attraction of polar groups are physical adhesion phenomena. To allow for chemical adhesion, distances of <0.7 nm have to be provided.[39]

Durable, tight contact is the most important prerequisite for strong bonds. Because it is not possible to bring two bodies into 100% tight contact, liquid phases ("adhesives") with good wettability are used to compensate for differing distances. In order to level this discrepancy, low-viscosity materials are used. An additional advantage is the combination of a substrate with high surface energy and an adhesive with low viscosity. When irregularities of bonded surfaces are more or less completely filled, micromechanical attachment is obtained. It is primarily of mechanical nature and based on rheological and geometrical effects.

Roughening of dental surfaces must be generated by appropriate pretreatment. Micromechanical interlocking is based on physical attachment of adhering parts and provided by filling of voids and irregularities.

Enamel bonding

The fundament of dental adhesion was published in 1955 with the introduction of the enamel etch technique by Dr Michael Buonocore.[40] Although Dr Oskar Hagger reported something similar[41] in 1948, the actual invention of enamel etching dates back to Buonocore.[34–36]

Adhesion mechanisms to enamel

Conditioning with phosphoric acid

With regard to clinical success, adhesion to enamel via phosphoric acid etching is estimated positively. It creates an ideal surface morphology (Figure 13.2) for micromechanical attachment of resin composites. Due to the different solubility of enamel prisms in their center and periphery, a rough structure is created and penetrated by unfilled or filled adhesives then bonded by polymerization. The resulting adhesion is sufficient to counteract the polymerization stresses of resin composites under clinical conditions. Furthermore, stabilization of previously weakened tooth structures occurs.[36–43]

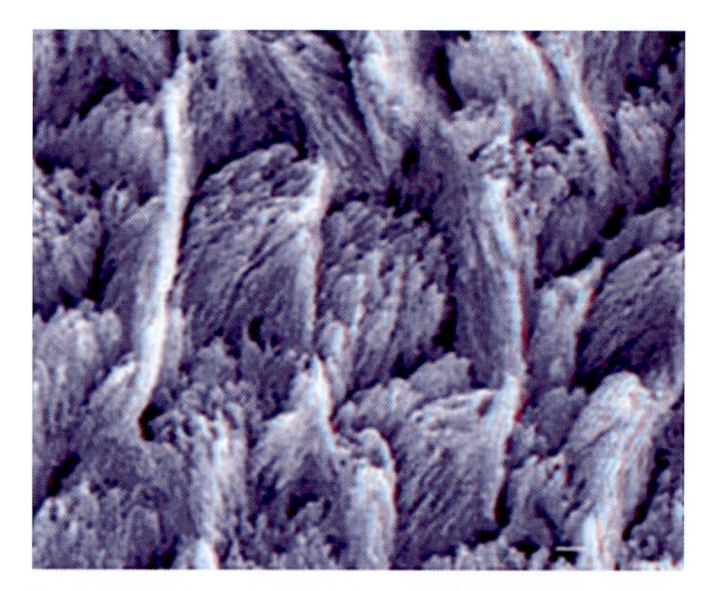

Figure 13.2 Etch pattern (bevelled enamel after 15 s etching with phosphoric acid, SEM, 1:3000).

Enamel consists of 98% inorganic material by weight, i.e. hydroxyapatite crystals. Crystallites form prisms, which differ in solubility by acids in various areas, providing a typical etching pattern. Prismless enamel is detectable only in very outer and not abraded layers (e.g. in pits and fissures). Etching time has to be prolonged to 60 s in order to dissolve prismless enamel areas. Phosphoric acid irreversibly removes about 10 μm enamel with a roughness of 50 μm underneath, the so-called etch pattern.[44]

The retentive etching pattern provides high surface energy allowing good wettability of etched enamel. Phosphoric acid products are normally provided as gel in concentrations of 35–40% applied for 15–60 s followed by rinsing with air/water spray to remove both acid and precipitates formed during acid etching. Shorter etching times are possible on prepared enamel. To guarantee successful wetting of the etched enamel surface, appropriate isolation has to be obtained during treatment to avoid contamination with blood, saliva, sulcus fluid, or oil. Any contamination impedes penetration of low-viscosity adhesives into the retentive surface and corroborates retention.

The optimum utilization of differently soluble enamel surfaces is possible when they are cut rectangularly during bevelling of cavosurface margins (Figure 13.3). With enamel prisms being cut longitudinally, the adhesive may only penetrate into the laterally loosened enamel parts.[44] The necessity of enamel bevels, especially in posterior teeth, was always controversial. Although several in vitro reports describe a positive effect,[45] there is no clinical proof for this paradigm.[25]

The concentration of phosphoric acid is of some importance, with 30–40% as the most effective concentration. Three-dimensional etching depth is increased up to 40%; however, higher concentrations dissolve less calcium and cause shallower etching patterns. Concentrations of <27% have less soluble precipitates. These concentrations are not gentle or as effective as higher concentrations, despite the claims of some advertisements. The ideal mix is 37% and 30 s.[46,47]

The actual bond to enamel is obtained by functional adhesives based on bis-GMA, sometimes diluted with triethylene glycol dimethacrylate (TEGDMA). Resin tags guarantee micromechanical interlocking. Another way in which micromechanical interlocking is guaranteed is by intercrystallite retention.[34–36,46,47]

In any case, separately applied primers have to be brushed no longer than 15 s on previously etched enamel in order to avoid any destruction of the fragile etch pattern.[42]

Self-etch adhesives

Having been actually developed for gentle conditioning of dentin, self-etch adhesives are also routinely used for enamel bonding. Based on market data these adhesives are the most popular in the world. These adhesives contain acidic primers or acidic monomer mixtures providing pH values of between <1 and 2. These adhesives are classified according to their acidity (Table 13.1).

Etching effects of these adhesives are normally less pronounced than after phosphoric acid etching, and enamel bevels are more mandatory than with etch-and-rinse adhesives. Both efficacy and durability of bonding to enamel, generated by self-etch adhesives, are debated in the literature. Our own results

Table 13.1 pH Values of Self-Etching Primers and Universal Adhesives

Strong (pH <1)	Adper Prompt L-Pop (3 M Espe)
	AquaPrime & Monobond (Merz Dental)
	Xeno III (Dentsply)
Moderate (pH ≈ 1.5)	AQ-Bond (Morita)
	Bond Force (Tokuyama)
	Clearfil Liner Bond 2 V (Kuraray)
	Clearfil SE Bond (Kuraray)
	Clearfil Protect Bond (Kuraray)
	Clearfil Tri-S Bond (Kuraray)
	G-Bond Plus (GC)
	Hybrid Bond (Morita)
	iBond GI (Kulzer)
	One Coat SE Bond (Coltène)
	Unifill Bond (GC)
	Xeno V (Dentsply)
	Peak Universal Adhesive (Ultradent))
Mild (pH ±2)	Contax (DMG)
	Futurabond U (Voco)
	iBond Self Etch (Kulzer)
	Optibond Solo Plus SE (Kerr)
	One-up Bond F (Tokuyama)
	Revolcin One (Merz)
	Prime&Bond Elect (Dentsply)
	Scotchbond Universal (3M Espe)
Ultra-mild (pH >3)	All-Bond Universal (Bisco)
	Adhese Universal (Vivadent)

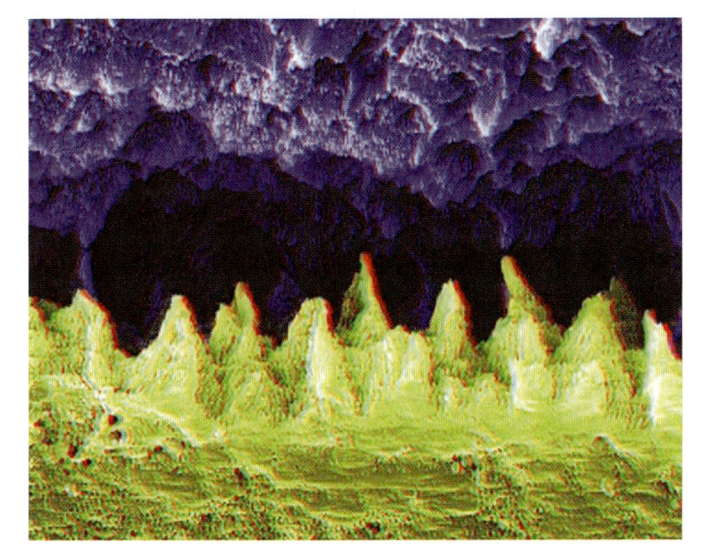

Figure 13.3 Micromechanical interlocking of resin tags (yellow) with etched enamel (blue) (SEM; 1:3000).

have always been worse for self-etch adhesives compared to etch-and-rinse adhesives.[5] Studies from Berlin reported marginal quality of Class I restorations and clearly showed similar results. Other studies also confirm these findings. Several authors showed that the efficiency of self-etch adhesives in enamel may be increased by selective phosphoric acid etching of enamel margins.[27,48–52]

Phosphoric acid etching, however, can compromise the efficiency of self-etching adhesives on dentin.[53] Therefore it may be better to completely avoid dentin etching or at least limit it to 10 s or less.[54] This aspect will be discussed later together with the effect of phosphoric acid etching on dentin cavity walls.

Historical development

The first- and second-generation adhesives never reached clinically relevant efficacies because they only bonded to smear layers;[12,35,36,38,55,56] however, the adhesion of smear layers to underlying dentin was too low to counteract polymerization shrinkage of resinous materials. The first documented clinical success was accomplished with so-called third-generation adhesives such as Gluma (Bayer Dental), Syntac (Ivoclar Vivadent), or A.R.T. Bond (Coltène Whaledent). In this scenario, prepared enamel is selectively conditioned with 30–40% phosphoric acid[57,58] followed by the application of primers providing acidic monomer mixtures for smear layer dissolution on dentin. Under clinical circumstances selective enamel etching is nearly impossible. Therefore, simultaneous etching of enamel and dentin was desirable and was realized by the fourth generation including a simultaneous etching of enamel and dentin with phosphoric acid, which is removed by rinsing. After conditioning of enamel and dentin with phosphoric acid, the application of first a hydrophilic primer followed by a more hydrophobic adhesive is a characteristic of these fourth-generation adhesives.

Dentists' wishes for more simplification led to the development of the fifth generation as "one bottle bonds." Although the literature in the field mainly reflects inferior results with this generation,[59–68] its easier handling guaranteed marketing success. Phosphoric acid etching the dentin always has one central problem: the collagen network exposed after phosphoric acid etching must be penetrated by hydrophilic monomers and therefore the fibrils must not collapse; otherwise, penetration is insufficient.

To avoid this problem in general, sixth-generation adhesives were developed, without phosphoric acid etching, called self-etch adhesives, containing primer having acidic pH values. They allowed demineralization of enamel and dentin while simultaneously penetrating the demineralized structures, providing a depth of demineralized dentin identical to that of the penetrated area. The applied acidic components are intentionally not rinsed off to guarantee appropriate function of the priming parts. After the self-etching primer, a conventional adhesive is applied. Due to problems regarding chemical stability of monomers in acidic environments, earlier products had to be mixed before application. The primers of the more recent products are premixed, containing short-chain self-etch monomer mixtures that stay hydrolytically stable even in acidic pH environments.

Even more simplification was introduced with the seventh generation of adhesives, with self-etch systems being available with only one liquid. This consists of mixtures of hydrophilic and hydrophobic monomers, which are so acidic that they are able to act as etchant, primer, and adhesive in one. Earlier products were mixed; recent adhesives are non-mix versions.

Adhesion to dentin

It took a considerably long time to achieve first success in dentin bonding (Figure 13.4).[1,4,13,34,55,61,69–72] This was due to two major problems:

- Dentin provides a moist structure with tubules filled with liquid, resulting in considerable hydrophilicity. Therefore, it is difficult to bond hydrophobic resins to hydrophilic dentin surfaces.[14,16,44,57,65,73–86]

- After rotary treatment of dentin, a smear layer prohibits direct contact to underlying dentin.[4,13,30,55,87]

The transfer of an etch-and-rinse technique from enamel to dentin was initially unsuccessful.[34,88] As a result, the first clinical consequence from failures was to cover all dentin areas with liners and/or cements. This situation, however, provided only limited adhesion areas, especially for stress-bearing restorations. Therefore, in order to utilize the whole cavity surface, successful dentin bonding was desirable. The first success stories were recounted decades later. The development of different classes and stages of adhesive systems can be recognized in so-called generations, which have recently been displaced by functional classifications and numbers of steps.

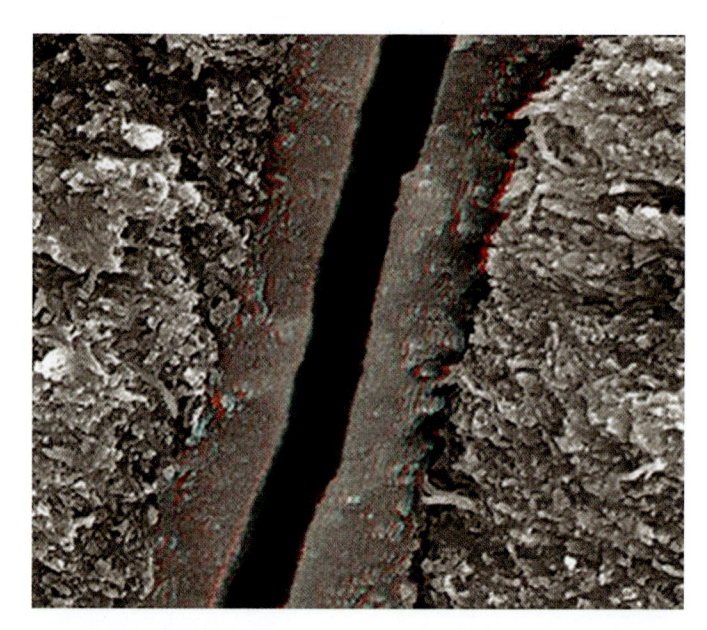

Figure 13.4 Dentin in a fractured specimen (SEM, 1:5000). The higher mineralized peritubular dentin is clearly visible; the intertubular dentin is less dense.

Adhesion mechanism to dentin

For strong and durable adhesion, hydrophilicity of the dentin substrate and the smear layer have to be handled. To remove the smear layer, two main approaches are available:

- application of phosphoric acid for about 15 s or
- application of acidic monomer mixtures.

Conditioning with phosphoric acid

It took a long time until it was accepted that phosphoric acid be applied not only to enamel but also to dentin. This technique was previously called 'total etching' because the entire cavity was etched by acid. More accurate is the term "etch and rinse" because self-etch adhesives also etch totally, emphasizing that phosphoric acid is removed by rinsing.

For the etch-and-rinse technique, colored 35–40% orthophosphoric acid gels are used. The acid penetrates along the dentinal tubules that have been opened by the acid (Figure 13.5).

The smear layer is completely removed; demineralization depth is around 5 µm.

The intertubular dentin is demineralized to 3–10 µm. The average irreversible dentin loss is 10 µm and the overall penetration is 20 µm; that is, altogether 30 µm without damage to the dentinal structures per se.[89,90]

The duration of phosphoric acid etching leads to different demineralization depths being additionally dependent on acid agitation during application.[91] After 10 s without agitation almost no dentin demineralization was found. With agitation, it increased to 3 µm. Sixty seconds with agitation result in 13 µm. In general, an application time of 15–20 s is recommended. Prolonged etching times lead to deeper demineralization and possibly suboptimal infiltrated areas[92] (Figure 13.6).

These deeper areas of nonpenetrated collagen are especially prone to biodegradation processes. Prolonged etching therefore may reduce dentin bonding performance.[68] With a thorough rinse step for 15 s the etch-and-rinse approach is finished.

Now the exposed collagen network has to be safely penetrated by monomers. Due to a low surface energy of etched dentin, surface-active components (primers) have to be meticulously applied.

To visualize the effect of enamel etching, at least the margins of the cavity have to be dried. This alone results in almost dry dentin in adjacent areas. So the collagen fibers may collapse and are consequently less receptive to penetration. The term "wet bonding" is directly derived from this particular clinical problem because wet or moist dentin after phosphoric acid etching avoids collagen collapse. It also guarantees better penetration and intact hybrid layers by sufficiently filling interfibrillar spaces.[93–95] However, the wet bonding issue has to be discussed relating to different solvents being present in primers or priming adhesives. Solvents act as monomer carriers bringing amphiphilic molecules to their place of action on the dentin surface. Possible solvents are water, alcohol, and acetone. The actual term wet bonding results from studies having been carried out with acetone-based adhesives only (e.g. Prime&Bond NT, Dentsply).[93–95] When acetone is used as solvent, it is true that exclusively moist dentin works as an adhesion substrate after phosphoric acid etching. Under clinical circumstances this is almost impossible to perform because etched enamel should be controlled for its frosty appearance to confirm appropriate etching. Therefore, the best way is first to dry and to guarantee good enamel etching and proper isolation against contamination, and second to rewet the surface with water to re-expand the previously collapsed collagen fibrils. This explains why ethanol- or acetone-based primers fall short on dry dentin.[66,68,93–95] From the clinical point of view, it is timely that *tert*-butanol was recently introduced as a less technique-sensitive solvent in XP Bond (Dentsply). Nevertheless, some rewetting is also recommended here.

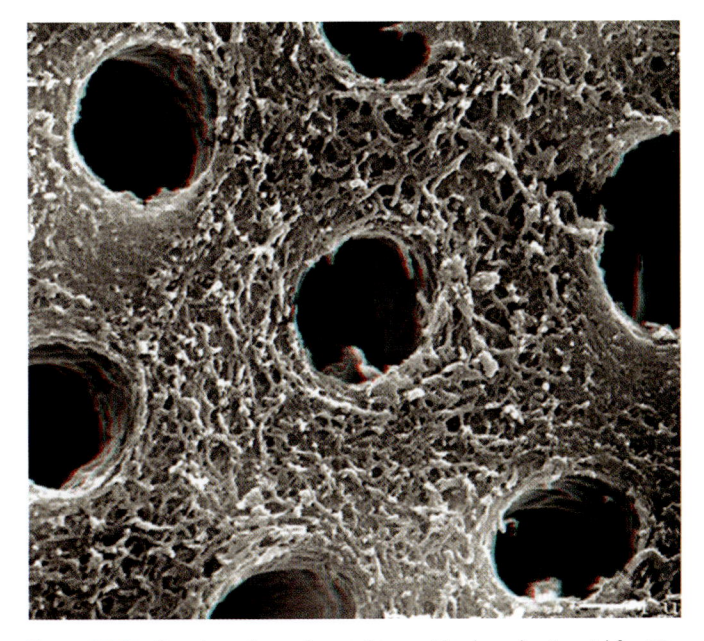

Figure 13.5 Dentin surface after etching with phosphoric acid for 15 s (SEM; 1:5000).

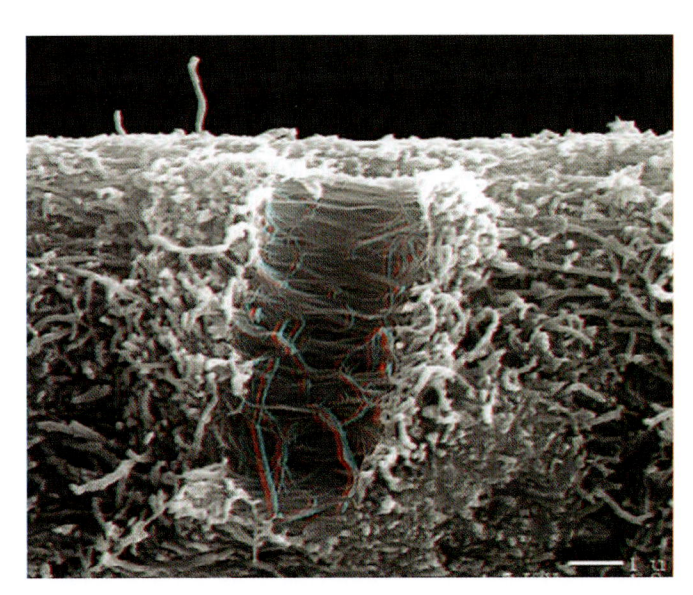

Figure 13.6 Fractured specimen from Figure 13.5 after critical point drying (SEM; 1:7000). Collagen fibrils are exposed by phosphoric acid etching.

Deficient primer penetration means that unfilled areas remain around some deeper areas of the demineralized matrix. This is referred to as "nanoleakage."[4,81,97] The incidence of postoperative hypersensitivities is of clinically higher relevance and is also a sign of incomplete resin penetration, allowing for fluid movement inside the dentinal tubules.

Less prone to the described wet bonding problem are water-based systems (Adper Scotchbond Multi-Purpose, 3M Espe) and water-/alcohol-based adhesives (OptiBond FL, Kerr), because the contained water obtains acceptable rehydration even in the absence of rewetting.[4,5,81,97,98] A simpler view shows that all multistep adhesives with separate primers and adhesives contain water. In contrast, all simplified two-step etch-and-rinse systems do not or do not sufficiently (<1%) contain water for incorporated rewetting.

Self-etch adhesives

The main advantage of self-etch adhesives is that incomplete penetration of previous demineralization should not occur. By making primers acidic with maleic acid or polyacrylic acid they are able to superficially demineralize enamel and dentin without prior etching with phosphoric acid. There are dentin-conditioning primers and enamel-/dentin-conditioning agents.

According to their ability to dissolve hydroxyapatite, the self-etch systems are classified (Figure 13.7) as strong or aggressive (pH <1), moderate (pH ≈ 1.5), or mild (pH ±2) (Table 13.1).[55] Neither dentin bonding nor enamel adhesion can be derived from the pH itself.[48–50,55]

The solvent of these self-etch agents must contain at least some water, because dissociation of acid is, in most of the cases, only possible in the presence of water. The acidic action is terminated by dissolved hydroxyapatite, evaporation of the solvent, and finally photo-polymerization. Demineralization depth and penetration depth are more or less the same here in order to remove excess solvent. These primers are solely air-dried, not rinsed off. To emphasize this aspect, some authors call these adhesive systems "etch-and-dry" systems. Since the applied monomer mixture is not rinsed off, parts of the dissolved smear layer, as well as dissolved parts of dentin, are integrated into the hybrid layer, i.e. as a hybrid complex.[57,58]

Priming of the collagen network

Application of acids exposes an instable collagen "sponge." Primers always contain amphiphilic molecules with a hydrophilic end to penetrate the moist collagen network and a hydrophobic end for copolymerization with other monomers. Typical amphiphilic monomers are hydroxyethyl methacrylate (HEMA) or TEGDMA. These molecules impregnate the collagen parts by penetration and amphiphilic action.

Stabilizing by bonding agents

Primers consist of short chains for optimized penetration, while adhesives require longer, cross-linking monomers for stabilization of the whole interface. Reaching the interfibrillar pore volumes, all previously removed parts are replaced by the adhesive. Classical bonding agents, i.e. unfilled resins, consist of bis-GMA and urethane dimethacrylate (UEDMA), viscosity-decreasing TEGDMA and HEMA, and photo initiators for light-curability. The complex interface of previously demineralized dentin and resinous materials is called hybrid layer.[8,96,99,100]

Furthermore, adhesives flow into dentinal tubules generating resin tags. This leads to the effective sealing of the dentin. Unfilled resins need some time for appropriate penetration in previously generated pore volumes (10s). Light curing of the unfilled adhesive resin is mandatory.

Adhesives with hydrophilic monomers working as primers are so-called primer-adhesives. Self-etching primer-adhesives are now called all-in-one adhesives because they act as etchant, primer, and bonding agent in one application step.

Classification of adhesive systems

Generally, four different working steps are present with adhesives to generate adhesion to tooth hard tissues (Figure 13.8):

1. enamel conditioning with phosphoric acid or self-etch primer mixtures
2. dentin conditioning with phosphoric acid or self-etch primer mixtures for exposure of the collagen network
3. dentin priming (application of short-chain, hydrophilic monomers for dentin wettability) for penetration of the exposed collagen network to generate the hybrid layer
4. application of a cross-linking adhesive for stabilization of the interfaces to enamel and dentin.

These different steps are differently covered by different adhesive approaches (Table 13.2).

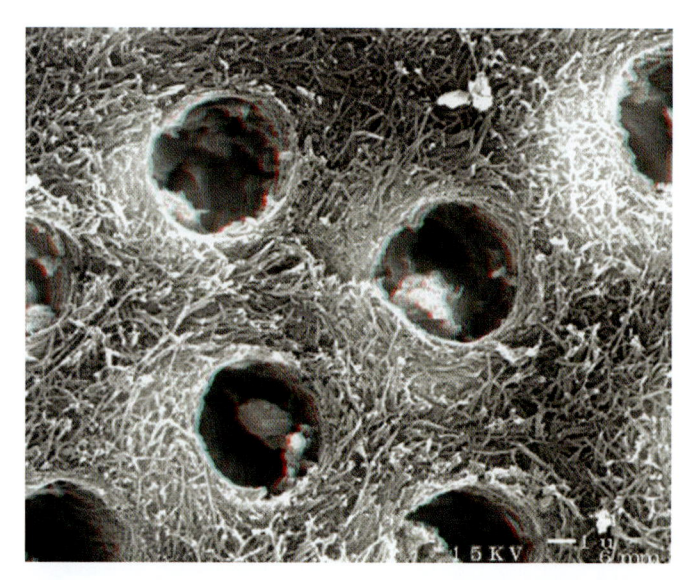

Figure 13.7 Etching effect of a self-etch adhesive on dentin (SEM, 1:4000): the intertubular dentin is demineralized to 1 μm, the orifices of the dentinal tubules are partially clogged with remnants of the smear layer.

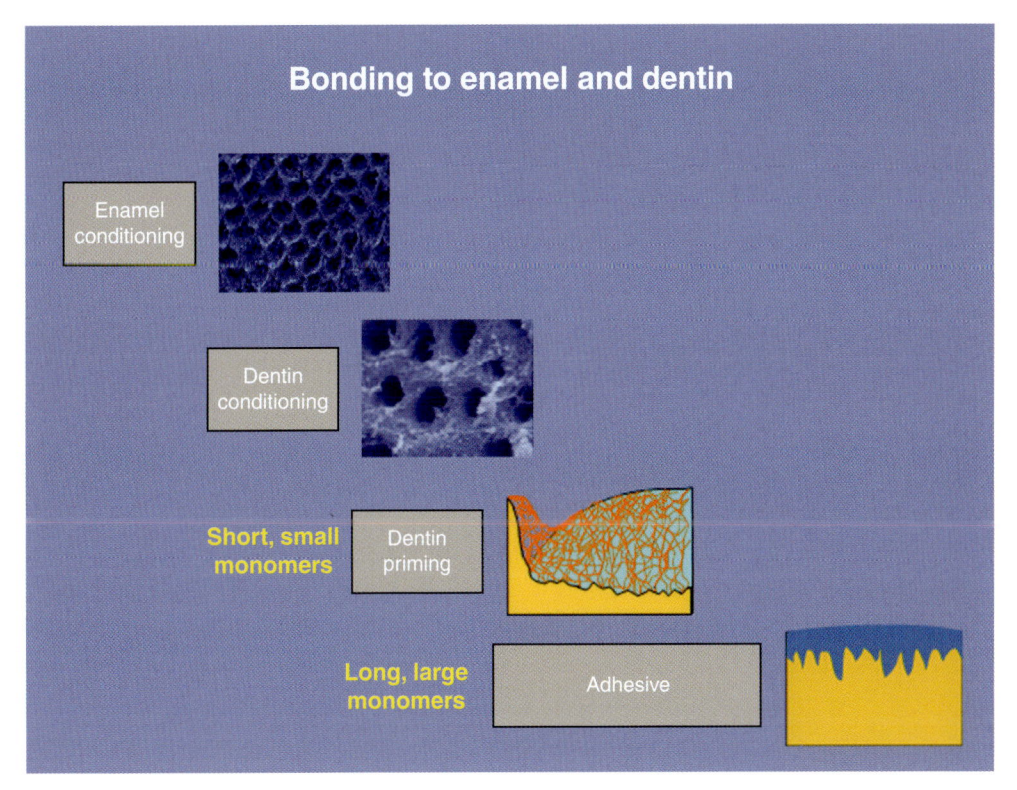

Figure 13.8 Fundamental steps for bonding to enamel and dentin.

Universal adhesives

The latest developments are so-called "universal adhesives." The idea behind these adhesives is to combine universal primers (e.g. Clearfil Ceramic Primer, Monobond Plus) with primers for conditioned enamel and dentin surfaces.

Universal primers are applied to ceramic surfaces like HF-acid-etched glass-ceramic, airborne Al_2O_3-particle pretreated oxide ceramics, as well as tribochemically pretreated ceramic or metal surfaces, either precious or nonprecious. The mixture of different monomers is able to enhance bonding to all mentioned surfaces after surface roughening by different approaches. This is a tremendous advantage in repairing insufficient restorations when it is not exactly known what kind of ceramic was used or if different material surfaces are affected at one site.[101]

Another—and the most important—approach of universal adhesive is to use the adhesive as an etch-and-rinse system, even on dried or on moist dentin surfaces, as well as a self-etching primer at the same cavity in order to facilitate handling in daily situations when adhesives are used. As mentioned before, it has been shown that the performance of self-etch adhesives in enamel may be increased by selective phosphoric acid etching of enamel margins.[27,48,49,51,52] However, it cannot always be totally avoided that phosphoric acid is also applied to dentin, which can cause some adhesives to show a decrease in efficiency.[53,54,102] Universal adhesives are developed to promote bonding to dentin as etch-and-rinse adhesive, independently of whether the phosphoric acid-etched surface is kept moist or dry, and as a self-etch adhesive. The first clinical data[102,103] as well as in vitro evaluations[104–107] show rather promising results. Today, MDP is incorporated into most universal adhesives, which was shown to be effective in reducing aging effects, primarily in self-etch mode,[33,108] which was attributed to nanolayering as well as chemical bonding to calcium in dentin.[108] However, most recent studies are also indicating that universal adhesives are also prone to hydrolytic degradation, primarily when used as etch-and-rinse adhesives.[108] So here the combination of selective enamel etching and using a universal adhesive in self-etch mode is recommended.[33,108]

Dark-curing adhesives

Bonding agents can be classified not only by working steps and kind of conditioning, but also in relation to the initiation of polymerization (Table 13.3). The majority of available adhesives are light-cured, and the predominant initiator is camphorquinone. Radicals for further cross-linking are part of the light-curable adhesive. Primers normally do not contain photoinitiators.

However, for some dual-curing (i.e. chemically initiated by addition of catalysts) build-up composites or luting composites, special dual-polymerizing adhesives are available (e.g. Clearfil New Bond, XP Bond + SCA). Before or after priming, these systems involve sulfuric acid salts for cross-linking of primer monomers. The adhesives contain benzoylperoxide which reacts with tertiary amines of dual-curing resin composites for luting. These systems gain more importance in the adhesive luting of root canal posts.

Table 13.2 Groups of Adhesives

Multi-bottle etch-and-rinse adhesives
Syntac Classic
A.R.T. Bond
Solobond Plus
Adper Scotchbond MP
Gluma Solidbond
Ecusit Primer/Mono
OptiBond FL
Solobond Plus

Single-bottle etch-and-rinse adhesives
Admira Bond
Adper Scotchbond 1
Cumdente Adhäsiv
Fantestic Flowsive
Excite F
iBond Total Etch
One Coat Bond
OptiBond Solo Plus
PQ1
Prime & Bond NT
Solobond Mono
Teco
XP Bond

Two-step self-etch adhesives
AquaPrime & Monobond
Clearfil SE Bond
One Coat SE Bond
OptiBond XTR

One-step self-etch adhesives
Adper Prompt L-Pop
Futurabond DC
Xeno III
AdheSE One F
Adper Easy Bond
Bond Force
iBond Self Etch
Futurabond M
Geanial-Bond
One Coat 7.0
OptiBond All in One
Tri-S-Bond
Xeno V+

Universal adhesives
Adhese Universal
All-Bond Universal
Clearfil Universal Bond
Futurabond M+
Futurabond U
G-Premio Bond
iBond Universal
One Coat 7 Universal
Peak Universal Bond
Scotchbond Universal
Xeno Select

Table 13.3 Dual-Curing Adhesives

Etch and rinse	Self-etch	Universal adhesive
Clearfil New Bond	Clearfil Liner Bond 2V	Clearfil Universal Bond
Excite DSC	OptiBond Solo Plus SE	Futurabond M+
Adper Scotchbond MP	Fantestic Flowsive SE	Futurabond U
Ambarino Bond	Futurabond DC	Scotchbond Universal
Clearfil Photobond	Hybrid Bond	
Cosmedent Complete		
CumDente Adhäsiv		
EnaBond		
Fantestic Flowsive		
LuxaBond		
One Coat 7		
OptiBond Solo Plus		
Prime & Bond NT		
XP Bond		

All-in-one adhesives must contain acidic components for conditioning of hard tissue surfaces. These acids neutralize the basic tertiary amine, which is important for sufficient initiation of dual-polymerizing resin composites. This leads to compromised bond strength of core materials to tooth substrate if all-in-one adhesives are used in combination with dual-cured resin composites.[8,109]

All-in-one adhesives create semipermeable membranes that enhance fluid penetration from the dentinal tubules through the adhesive layer and create droplets within minutes, risking interference with the hydrophobic composite resin.

Filled adhesives

Irrespective of the affiliation to different classes, there is one special modification of adhesives. By adding considerable amounts of filler particles (e.g. 48% in OptiBond FL Adhesive and 26% in OptiBond Solo Plus, Kerr) it was possible to increase adhesive performance.[13,44]

The resulting thicker, potentially elastic adhesive layer is reported to be beneficial for gap prevention in vitro (Figure 13.9). A similar effect is obtained with the so-called lining technique by use of flowable resin composites.[13,44] According to my own in-vitro results (R. Frankenberger) it is sufficient to apply one component (i.e. filled adhesive or a flowable). With a special focus on OptiBond FL, it must be stated that maybe this particular adhesive is also effective without fillers (Figure 13.10).[110] Film thickness and homogeneity may be enhanced with the addition of filler (Clearfil SE Bond, Fuji Bond LC, OptiBond FL, Gluma Solid Bond). An important point in this context is that filled adhesives with thicker adhesive layers have to provide sufficient radiopacity.[111] Whether additional fluoride release would increase adhesive effectiveness further and prevent recurrent caries is unknown.

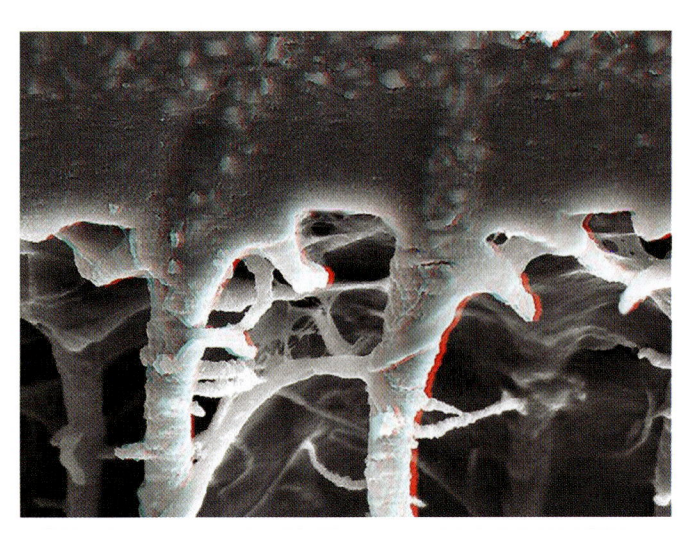

Figure 13.9 Resin–dentin interface of OptiBond FL (SEM; 1:5000). The filled adhesive penetrates the dentinal tubules and lateral branches.

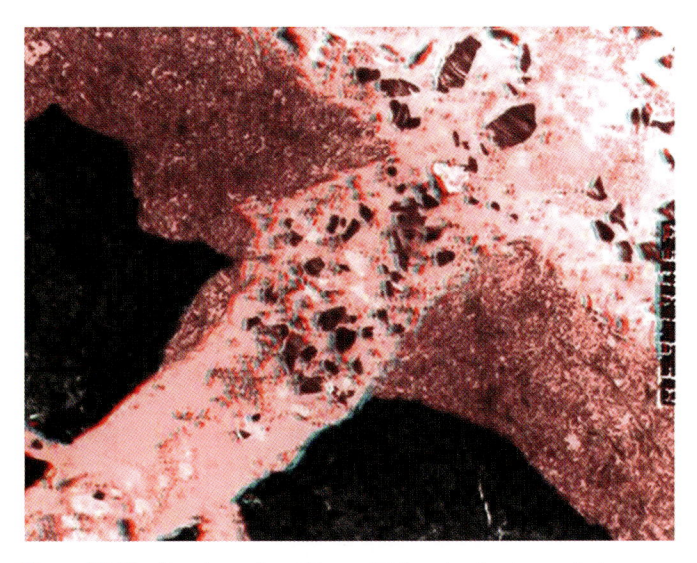

Figure 13.10 Specimen from Figure 13.8 under the transmission electron microscope (1:8000).

Valuation of adhesives

Figure 13.11 displays results of the author´s (R. Frankenberger's) own marginal quality evaluations in vitro during 1994–2013. It is clearly shown that many recent adhesives show diminished performance compared to the established ones.

The main findings were:

1. Simplification leads to less effectiveness.
2. Self-etch adhesives are overestimated regarding their enamel bonding performance.

These results are confirmed in the literature with the highest bond strengths and best marginal qualities with old-fashioned multistep adhesives.[103,112–114]

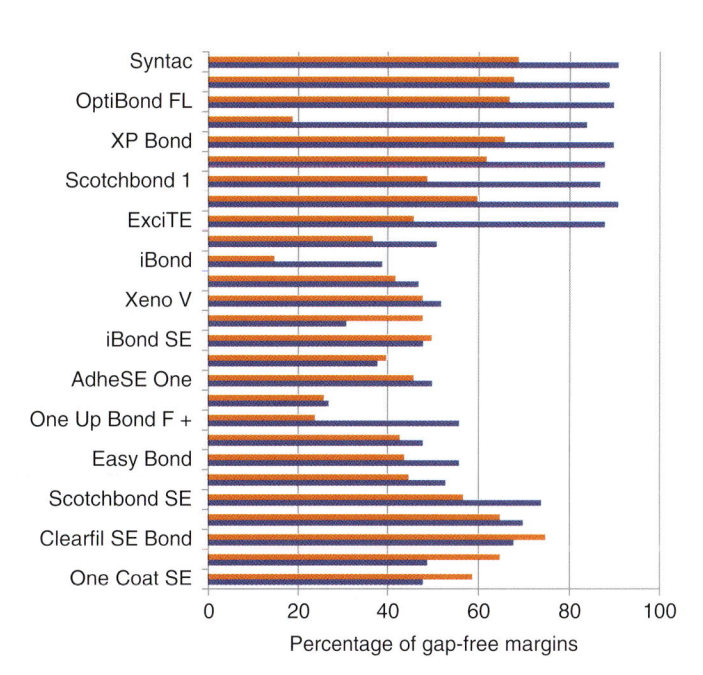

Figure 13.11 Percentage of gap-free margins after thermomechanical loading in vitro. Blue bars, enamel; orange bars, dentin.

Biocompatibility of adhesives

It is still believed that phosphoric acid etching increases dentin permeability and consequently the danger of damage to vital pulp tissues; however, the increase of permeability is related to cavity depth. Shallow cavities providing residual dentin thicknesses of >500 μm are not relevant for higher permeability.[115] Therefore, in these cavities some phosphoric acid etching is not detrimental. In the clinical setting, pulp damage is not caused by penetration of toxic substances from the resin. Pulpal inflammation is usually triggered by bacterial contamination in marginal gaps;[115,116] therefore, adhesives primarily protect the dentin by sealing it appropriately.

Deep cavities (<200 μm remaining dentin thickness) suffer a significant increase of dentin permeability, also potentially allowing for penetration of toxic monomers from primers or bonding agents. Furthermore, primers may be permanently thinned with dentinal liquid.[115,116] Clinically, <200 μm means already glimmering pulp tissues; therefore, a conventional calcium hydroxide lining is recommended (e.g. Kerr Life) covered by a resin-impregnated glass ionomer cement (e.g. Vitrebond).

Facing components of modern restorative resin composites, their biocompatibility is questionable on first sight.[117] The most important issue here is their correct use and a no-touch policy for dental personnel to avoid allergic reactions.[117]

Aging of the adhesive interface

Marginal discolorations, poor marginal adaptation, and loss of the restoration are frequent clinical findings related to exposed bonded margins.[118] In fact, despite excellent immediate and short-term bonding effectiveness for most of the dentin-bonding systems, the durability and stability of resin/dentin bonded interfaces created by some bonding agents (particularly the simplified ones) still remain questionable.[119–121] Interestingly, the new simplified adhesives exhibit not only the lowest bond strength values, but also the least predictable clinical performance when compared with multistep etch-and-rinse and self-etch systems.[30,122]

While enamel margins are more stable over time, the stability of the dentin–adhesive interface is strictly related to the intrinsic stability of the hybrid layer. Clinically, the aging of the hybrid layer involves both physical (occlusal chewing forces, and repetitive expansion and contraction related to temperature)[123] and chemical factors such as dentinal fluid, saliva, food and beverages, and bacterial products.[39,99,124] All these factors affect the single components of the hybrid layer: dentin organic matrix, hydroxyapatite, resin monomers, and residual solvents.

Different degradation patterns have been described, mainly related to the bonding approach: etch-and-rinse versus self-etch strategy.

Reliability and degradation of etch-and-rinse adhesives

Bonding with etch-and-rinse adhesive systems is achieved with the impregnation of the resin monomers into the demineralized substrate created by the etching agent that is rinsed away.[30,125,126] As previously mentioned, one of the major problems related to this approach is the incomplete infiltration of the adhesive into the demineralized dentin collagen network that frequently occurs due to several factors: collagen collapse, insufficient flowability of the primer/bonding agents, and presence of residual water that cannot be displaced within the collagen fibrils.[30,83,127–136] This suboptimal adhesive impregnation on the dentin surface (which is typical for the etch-and-rinse systems) determines nanoleakage formation; that is, presence of tracer along the interface at a nanoscale level (Figure 13.12).

This phenomenon is particularly evident in two-step etch-and-rinse adhesives versus the three-step systems due to the higher hydrophilicity of the primer and bonding agent that results in increased permeability, even after polymerization.[136–140] Interestingly, the higher permeability of the two-step etch-and-rinse systems was correlated with incomplete polymerization of these adhesives,[136–140] while better curing (and reduced permeability) can be obtained with the three-step systems that include a solvent-free and relatively hydrophobic resin coating as the last step of the bonding procedure.[141]

Additionally, the reduced polymerization and higher hydrophilicity of two-step etch-and-rinse systems determine increased water sorption[141] compared to the three-step systems. The presence of water within the hybrid layer determines hydrolysis, which is the primary reason for resin degradation within the hybrid layer created by two-step etch-and-rinse systems.[142] The disruption of covalent bonds between polymers in contact with water finally results in the loss of resin mass. This correlates well with the clinical performance of most hydrophilic two-step etch-and-rinse systems that show lower stability over time compared with the corresponding non-simple hydrophobic three-step systems.[129]

The presence of water additionally affects the stability of the adhesive interface due to degrading phenomena occurring to the collagen fibrils that are not fully encapsulated by the resin. This causes disorganization and further disruption of the dentin collagen fibrils, finally affecting the integrity of the hybrid layer.[143] It has been described that the breakdown of the collagen matrices can be attributed to host-derived proteinases, called matrix metalloproteinases (MMPs), incorporated within mineralized dentinal matrix during tooth development.[140–143]

The phosphoric acid application of 35% phosphoric acid (pH 0.7–1), typical of the etch-and-rinse approach, seems to be able to expose pro-MMPs trapped within the mineralized dentin.[118] Then the application of the adhesive blend reactivates the quenched collagenolytic/gelatinolytic activities of the endogenous enzymes contributing to the degradation of the collagen fibrils poorly impregnated within the hybrid layer.[133,144–146] An indirect confirmation of the role of endogenous MMPs in the degradation of the adhesive interface has been reported by using an MMP inhibitor to stabilize the bond over time. Interestingly, when used on acid-etched dentin as an additional therapeutic primer during the bonding procedure, an antibacterial agent with MMP-inhibiting properties called chlorhexidine resulted in the maintenance of the hybrid layer's collagen integrity over

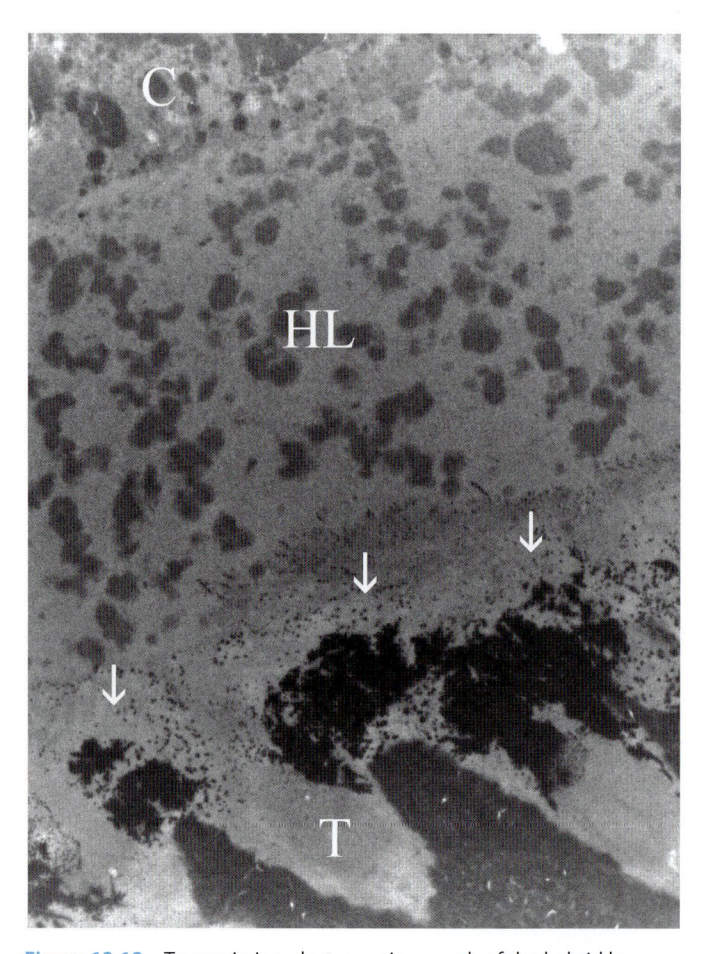

Figure 13.12 Transmission electron micrograph of the hybrid layer created by Adper Scotchbond 1XT (3M ESPE) aged for 2 years in artificial saliva. Extensive nanoleakage expression is shown (arrows). T, dentin tubule; HL, hybrid layer; C, composite resin.

time. This effect is used by rewetting the phosphoric acid-etched dentin after rinsing and drying with a 2% chlorhexidine solution. Similarly, promising preliminary results have been reported using collagen cross-linking agents to stabilize the collagen network. This approach showed not only increased immediate bond strength values but also improved bond stability over time, probably due to MMP inhibition.[145–147]

Reliability and degradation of self-etch adhesives

In self-etch adhesive systems, demineralization and infiltration of the acidic resin blends occur simultaneously,[148] thus no discrepancy between demineralization and infiltration (typical of the etch-and-rinse approach) has been described. Additionally, due to the lack of rinsing after etching, residual hydroxyapatite crystals remain available on the dentinal collagen. For this reason, the number of denuded collagen fibrils within the hybrid layer should be significantly less than in the etch-and-rinse system. However, some strong and aggressive one-step self-etch systems showed continuous etching after curing, leading to exposed collagen and accelerated bond degradation.

Similar to etch-and-rinse adhesives, self-etch systems (particularly the most simplified one-step systems) exhibit high permeability correlated with a low degree of curing and increased water sorption. As previously described for two-step etch-and-rinse systems, all these degrading phenomena seem to be strictly correlated with the high hydrophilicity of one-step systems and the difficulties with getting them to properly polymerize.[126,133,138,145]

Technique sensitivity: a problem and its solution

Etch-and-rinse adhesives

In contrast to enamel bonding, dentin bonding is considerably more technique-sensitive.[149] Bouillaguet et al. reported a different outcome of the same adhesives with different operators.[150] Peschke et al. simulated application errors with OptiBond FL, while Frankenberger et al. showed similarly catastrophic effects of errors for Syntac and Prime&Bond NT.[114,149] Any deviation from the recommendations for use decreased clinical performance. These errors were:

- overetching of dentin
- overdrying of previously etched dentin
- shortcuts in application protocols.

Overetching of dentin results in deeper demineralization zones, and potentially insufficient impregnation by primers. With time, these areas of naked collagen are subjected to biodegradation and hydrolysis. The first hints of insufficient interface forming are postoperative hypersensitivities.

During clinical use of etch-and-rinse adhesives, the problem becomes easily apparent: the whole cavity is etched with phosphoric acid. However, ideal etching times are 15 s for dentin and 30 s for enamel. When an uncontrolled flush of acid is applied many times a day, this idea is not achievable. Therefore, it makes sense to reduce the overall etching time to 15–20 s for both adhesive substrates without any decrease in performance.[151]

Overdrying of etched dentin causes collagen fiber collapse and should, therefore, be avoided. This is easily written but hard to realize. For an image of the frosty appearance of etched enamel, a certain drying process is necessary. This always leads to some dried areas on adjacent dentin. These areas are the only ones close to the pulp in proximal boxes of Class II cavities. Rewetting is the only solution of this particular problem. A microbrush is either sprayed with air/water mix from 25 cm away in order to generate some hoar frost or dipped into water or—as mentioned before—into a 2% chlorhexidine solution and dabbed on a paper tissue resulting in a moist but not dripping wet tuft of the microbrush. This microbrush is applied to the cavity, creating a slightly shiny surface in dentin. It can even be accepted that water also contaminates enamel margins. This is not crucial because primer solvents remove the water equally just like the interfibrillar spaces in dentin do. Water-based primers are easier to handle. They consist of 50% water, which is able to re-expand the collagen meshwork by itself. Therefore, water- and water/ethanol-based adhesives provide less technique sensitivity because rewetting is not as mandatory as with ethanol- and acetone-based systems.[66,96] Also, with less-technique-sensitive adhesives, rewetting is not forbidden. However, as mentioned before, rewetting can also be managed by chlorhexidine, which supports the longevity of etch-and-rinse adhesives. When working with water-containing components, it is fundamentally important to dry primers instead of gentle blowing them because the water must be safely evaporated. In contrast, it is easier with ethanol and acetone due to their higher vapor pressures.[66,96]

Air thinning of unfilled resins is also restricted due to technique sensitivity. The unfilled resin also needs some time to penetrate, and it should not be overly thinned by air due to the presence of an oxygen-inhibition zone that may counteract light curing. On the other hand, thicker layers of unfilled resins should also be avoided because, due to their lack of radiopacity, these zones may be misinterpreted as gaps in bitewing radiographs.

General problems with wet bonding and its transfer to the clinical situation still result in a remarkable amount of postoperative hypersensitivity with this class of adhesives. The reason is not primarily the presence of some aggressive phosphoric acid, but improper moisture management after the actual etching process.

Self-etching adhesives

All-in-one adhesives represent a revolutionary simplification because only one liquid needs to be applied. Nevertheless, technique sensitivity is not completely absent.[41,44,53,84,139,152–156] For example, most of the products must be repeatedly applied to generate measurable bonding,[5] which means that the timesaving aspect is almost gone.

The major issue with all-in-one adhesives is their permeability against water. Several publications have shown that these adhesives are permeable membranes even after polymerization.[5,23,97,157] The more hydrophilic the adhesive is, the less clinically promising its prognosis. Conventional adhesives with separate primers and separate hydrophobic bonding agents still prevail.[44,60,98]

Two-step self-etch adhesives also avoid phosphoric acid etching; however, they have separate liquids for priming and bonding. Today, this class of adhesives is estimated to be the most promising for durable dentin bonds with low rates of postoperative hypersensitivity.

Where dentin bonding is favorable with self-etch systems, effective enamel adhesion is still questionable. A viable solution is selective enamel etching with conventional phosphoric acid, followed by a self-etch adhesive. Dentin etching was beneficial with Syntac and A.R.T. Bond, though proved detrimental with AdheSE and Clearfil SE Bond.[157]

Recent all-in-one adhesives contain complex monomer mixtures that are able to etch, prime, and bond. This results in phase separation in many cases.[158] To avoid this, some all-in-one adhesives have to be strongly air-dried, although this may again lead to insufficient polymerization, as described above.[52] It is surprising that mechanical properties of adhesive mixtures have a stronger impact on performance than acidity itself.[48–51]

Light microscopy shows droplet formation with all-in-one adhesives being dependent on their hydrophilicity.[52,159] For example, HEMA-free G-Bond results in phase separation, while HEMA-containing Clearfil Tri-S-Bond and Xeno III showed droplet formation by osmotic blistering. Hybrid Bond, Absolute and iBond Self Etch exhibited both phenomena. OptiBond AIO revealed cluster formation of filler particles.[52]

This leads to special recommendations for use with this class of adhesives. Some adhesives allow evaporation of the solvent by gentle air stream (One Coat 7.0, "gently light air-stream"), while others require maximum air pressure (G-Bond). Finally, some adhesives must be air-thinned with increasing pressure (Bond Force).

Another clinically relevant problem is application time. This may be interesting from the marketing point of view; however, 5–10 s for G-Bond seems to be unrealistically short for thorough penetration (Figures 13.13 and 13.14). The resin–dentin interface improves considerably with multiple applications of adhesive (Figure 13.13) when compared to a single coating (Figure 13.14). It has to be taken into account that not only does dentin need to be treated during that period, but so does a thick smear layer of dentin after rotary bur preparation. Therefore, active application under continuous rubbing is recommended.[160,161] Altogether it can be stated that easier handling does not automatically mean less or no technique sensitivity.

Postoperative hypersensitivities

Postoperative hypersensitivities are mainly caused by fluid movement in dentinal tubules which irritates odontoblast processes.[120,122] This is mainly attributed to an insufficient adhesive dentin seal and not to cavity depth because hypersensitivities

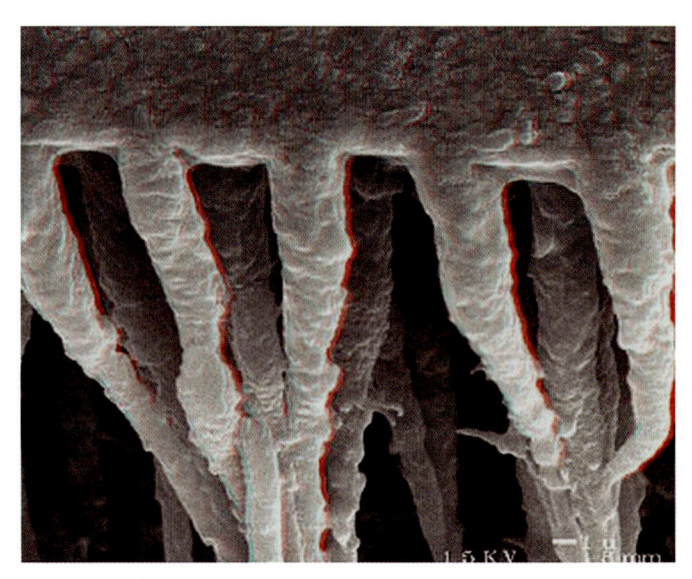

Figure 13.13 Resin–dentin interface of an all-in-one-system with five coats (SEM; 1:4000).

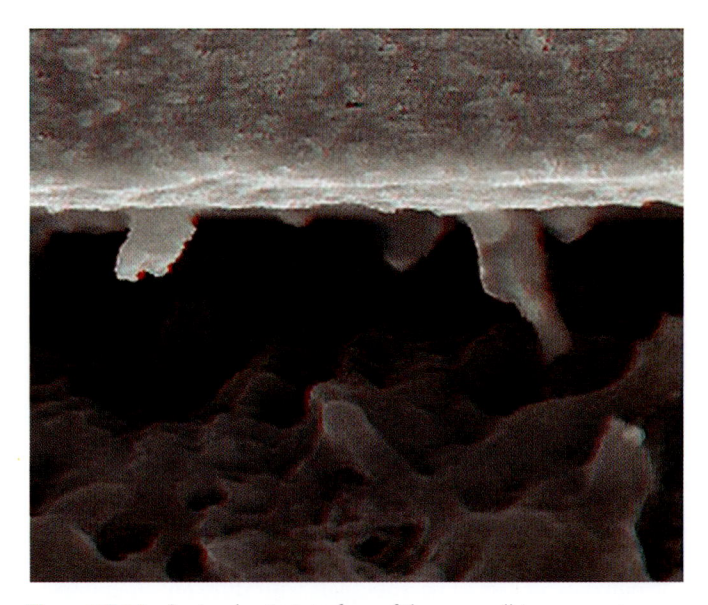

Figure 13.14 Resin–dentin interface of the same all-in-one-system as in Figure 13.13 with one coat (SEM; 1:4000).

also occur in shallow cavities. The main reasons for postoperative hypersensitivities with etch-and-rinse adhesives are:

- overetching of dentin with phosphoric acid
- overdrying of dentin after phosphoric acid etching
- overwetting of previously phosphoric acid-etched dentin
- no or insufficient light curing of the adhesive.

Also self-etch adhesives may fail, this is mainly due to:

- smear layers too thick
- application times too short for smear layer removal
- insufficient evaporation of the solvent.

Under strict adherence to the adhesive's instructions for use and prevention of common treatment errors, enamel and dentin may be effectively pretreated, providing a tight and durable seal. The dentin seal is better than any cement linings use previously. Subjective contentment of patients is good; clinical outcomes are excellent.

Failure prevention: clinical application

Beside biological parameters like tubular sclerosis or caries-affected dentin, handling is a fundamental point in adhesive dentistry. Therefore, practical transfer is very important to guarantee a well-functioning seal of enamel and dentin.

Various clinical procedures were proposed to increase the immediate bond strength and reduce aging:

1. **Use of a hydrophobic coating**: since hydrophilicity of the simplified adhesives (two-step etch-and-rinse and one-step self-etch adhesives) has been shown to increase water sorption and bond instability, the use of nonsimplified bonding systems, such as three-step etch-and-rinse and two-step self-etch adhesives characterized by an hydrophobic coating with a nonsolvated bonding layer, should be preferred.
2. **Increased application time**: prolonged application times (beyond the manufacturer's recommendations) increase monomer penetration and favor solvent evaporation before light curing; this increases the immediate and long-term bonding of most adhesives.[51,160]
3. **Active application**: a continuous and active rubbing motion has shown higher strength and improved stability of the bond, particularly for two-step etch-and-rinse adhesives.[161]
4. **Enhanced solvent evaporation**: the adhesive layer must be carefully air-thinned because if residual solvent remains within the polymer network it could plasticize the polymer,[162] further affecting the adhesive's properties.[157]
5. **Extended polymerization time**: resin permeability and monomer elution are related to suboptimal polymerization of the bonding. When curing times (particularly of simplified adhesives) are extended beyond those recommended by the manufacturer, improved polymerization can be achieved with reduced permeability.[147,162,163] This contributes to stabilizing the bond over time.[30,133,148]
6. **Use of MMP inhibitors**: MMP inhibitors, such as chlorhexidine, used as a rewetting solution (e.g. 2%), stabilize the bond over time, this inhibiting the activation of endogenous dentin enzymes especially when using etch-and-rinse adhesives.

When using adhesives in a clinical setting the following steps should be followed:

- read the manufacturer's manual
- shake bottles before use
- all steps must be carried out under proper isolation, ideally with a rubber dam.

Recommendations for using etch-and-rinse adhesives

According to the results of a huge number of in vitro and in vivo tests the following products can be recommended as the so-called gold standard: OptiBond FL, Syntac, and Scotchbond MP.[59,70,162]

Nevertheless, correct handling has an important impact on long-term success in adhesive techniques:

- It is important to control the penetrability of the cannula of the etch gel prior to intraoral use. Otherwise uncontrolled flushes occur.
- The application of phosphoric acid always starts at the enamel margins and ends on dentin. When this is not possible, the whole cavity should be etched for 15–20 s.
- The acid, the precipitates, and dissolved tooth substrate must be rinsed off thoroughly for 15 s.
- The cavity-drying process has to be carried out with caution to prevent collagen collapse. Short air streams help to visualize the frosty appearance of etched enamel and prevent over-drying of adjacent dentin. *Rewetting is mandatory for adhesives without water addition.*
- Primers need time (30 s) to act on dentin. Rubbing accelerates chemical processes by continually supporting its activity with fresh monomer. Etched enamel should not be excessively rubbed. The solvent has to be evaporated but not overly dried (Figures 13.15 and 13.16).
- Unfilled resins should get some time (10 s) to penetrate into enamel and dentin. Also this layer should not be overly thinned.
- The adhesive has to be light-cured for 20 s with a sufficient light-curing unit.

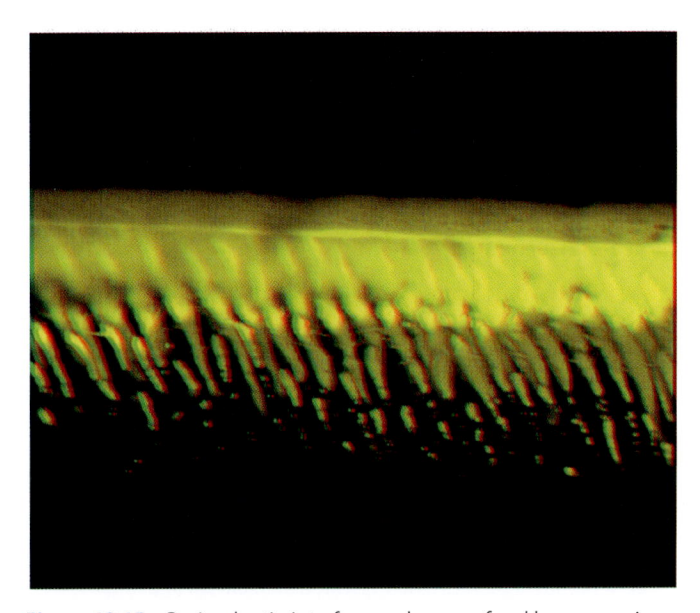

Figure 13.15 Resin–dentin interface under a confocal laser scanning microscope (CLSM; 1:2000). Hybrid layer and sufficient tubular penetration are visible.

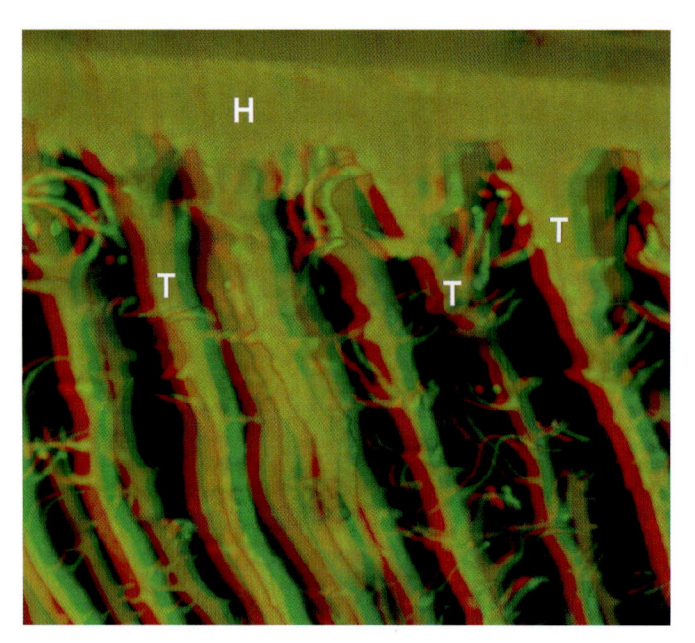

Figure 13.16 Resin tags (T) and hybrid layer (H) under a CLSM (1:3000).

Recommendations for using self-etching adhesives

According to the results of a huge number of in vitro and in vivo tests the following products can be recommended as the so-called gold standard: Clearfil SE Bond, and OptiBond XTR.[44,59,70,168]

Nevertheless, self-etching adhesives also need to be applied carefully in order to improve their performance:

- Systems which involve mixing need to be mixed sufficiently.
- The applied primers should be agitated (30 s) on enamel and dentin to enhance chemical reactions.
- The solvent has to be evaporated accordingly. Then the cavity has to provide a glossy appearance, indicating that no dry spots with insufficient wetting are present.
- In systems with separate unfilled resins, the bonding agent should not be overly thinned.
- The adhesive needs to be light cured for 20 s with a sufficient light-curing unit.

References

1. Abdalla AI, Davidson CL. Marginal integrity after fatigue loading of ceramic inlay restorations luted with three different cements. *Am J Dent* 2000;13:77–80.
2. Ausiello P, Rengo S, Davidson CL, Watts DC. Stress distributions in adhesively cemented ceramic and resin-composite Class II inlay restorations: a 3D-FEA study. *Dent Mater* 2004;20:862–872.
3. Bortolotto T, Onisor I, Krejci I, et al. Effect of cyclic loading under enzymatic activity on resin-dentin interfaces of two self-etching adhesives. *Dent Mater* 2008;24:178–184.
4. Frankenberger R, Pashley DH, Reich SM, et al. Characterisation of resin-dentine interfaces by compressive cyclic loading. *Biomaterials* 2005;26:2043–2052.
5. Frankenberger R, Perdigao J, Rosa BT, Lopes M. "No-bottle" vs "multi-bottle" dentin adhesives–a microtensile bond strength and morphological study. *Dent Mater* 2001;17:373–380.
6. Frankenberger R, Sindel J, Kramer N, Petschelt A. Dentin bond strength and marginal adaptation: direct composite resins vs ceramic inlays. *Oper Dent* 1999;24:147–155.
7. Peumans M, Hikita K, De Munck J, et al. Bond durability of composite luting agents to ceramic when exposed to long-term thermocycling. *Oper Dent* 2007;32:372–379.
8. Peumans M, Kanumilli P, De Munck J, et al. Clinical effectiveness of contemporary adhesives: a systematic review of current clinical trials. *Dent Mater* 2005;21:864–881.
9. Tay FR, Pashley DH. Dentin bonding–is there a future? *J Adhes Dent* 2004;6:263.
10. Tay FR, Pashley DH, Garcia-Godoy F, Yiu CK. Single-step, self-etch adhesives behave as permeable membranes after polymerization. Part II. Silver tracer penetration evidence. *Am J Dent* 2004;17:315–322.
11. Van Meerbeek B, Inokoshi S, Braem M, et al. Morphological aspects of the resin-dentin interdiffusion zone with different dentin adhesive systems. *J Dent Res* 1992;71:1530–1540.
12. Van Meerbeek B, Vanherle G, Lambrechts P, Braem M. Dentin- and enamel-bonding agents. *Curr Opin Dent* 1992;2:117–127.
13. Frankenberger R, Kramer N, Lohbauer U, et al. Marginal integrity: is the clinical performance of bonded restorations predictable in vitro? *J Adhes Dent* 2007;9 Suppl 1:107–116.
14. Frankenberger R, Lohbauer U, Taschner M, et al. Adhesive luting revisited: influence of adhesive, temporary cement, cavity cleaning, and curing mode on internal dentin bond strength. *J Adhes Dent* 2007;9 Suppl 2:269–273.
15. Krämer N, Ebert J, Petschelt A, Frankenberger R. Ceramic inlays bonded with two adhesives after 4 years. *Dent Mater* 2006;22:13–21.
16. Krämer N, Frankenberger R. Compomers in restorative therapy of children: a literature review. *Int J Paediatr Dent* 2007;17:2–9.
17. Krämer N, Lohbauer U, Frankenberger R. Restorative materials in the primary dentition of poli-caries patients. *Eur Arch Paediatr Dent* 2007;8:29–35.
18. Kreulen CM, van Amerongen WE, Akerboom HB, Borgmeijer PJ. Two-year results with box-only resin composite restorations. *ASDC J Dent Child* 1995;62:395–400.
19. Manhart J, Chen H, Hamm G, Hickel R. Buonocore Memorial Lecture. Review of the clinical survival of direct and indirect restorations in posterior teeth of the permanent dentition. *Oper Dent* 2004;29:481–508.
20. Manhart J, Garcia-Godoy F, Hickel R. Direct posterior restorations: clinical results and new developments. *Dent Clin North Am* 2002;46:303–339.
21. Manhart J, Neuerer P, Scheibenbogen-Fuchsbrunner A, Hickel R. Three-year clinical evaluation of direct and indirect composite restorations in posterior teeth. *J Prosthet Dent* 2000;84:289–296.
22. Van Landuyt KL, Snauwaert J, De Munck J, et al. Systematic review of the chemical composition of contemporary dental adhesives. *Biomaterials* 2007;28:3757–3785.
23. Van Meerbeek B, De Munck J, Yoshida Y, et al. Buonocore memorial lecture. Adhesion to enamel and dentin: current status and future challenges. *Oper Dent* 2003;28:215–235.
24. Van Meerbeek B, Kanumilli P, De Munck J, et al. A randomized controlled study evaluating the effectiveness of a two-step

self-etch adhesive with and without selective phosphoric-acid etching of enamel. *Dent Mater* 2005;21:375–383.
25. Van Meerbeek B, Perdigao J, Lambrechts P, Vanherle G. The clinical performance of adhesives. *J Dent* 1998;26:1–20.
26. Van Meerbeek B, Peumans M, Gladys S, et al. Three-year clinical effectiveness of four total-etch dentinal adhesive systems in cervical lesions. *Quintessence Int* 1996;27:775–784.
27. Driessens FC. Chemical adhesion in dentistry. *Int Dent J* 1977;27:317–323.
28. Asmussen E, Uno S. Adhesion of restorative resins to dentin: chemical and physicochemical aspects. *Oper Dent* 1992;Suppl 5:68–74.
29. Hickel R, Kaaden C, Paschos E, et al. Longevity of occlusally-stressed restorations in posterior primary teeth. *Am J Dent* 2005;18:198–211.
30. Van Meerbeek B, Yoshihara K, Yoshida Y, et al. State of the art of self-etch adhesives. *Dent Mater* 2011;27:17–28.
31. Eick JD, Robinson SJ, Byerley TJ, Chappelow CC. Adhesives and nonshrinking dental resins of the future. *Quintessence Int* 1993;24:632–640.
32. Eliades G, Palaghias G, Vougiouklakis G. Surface reactions of adhesives on dentin. *Dent Mater* 1990;6:208–216.
33. Takamizawa T, Barkmeier WW, Tsujimoto A, et al. Influence of different etching modes on bond strength to dentin using universal adhesive systems. *Dent Mater* 2016;32:e9–e21.
34. Buonocore MG. Principles of adhesive retention and adhesive restorative materials. *J Am Dent Assoc* 1963;67:382–391.
35. Buonocore MG, Matsui A, Gwinnett AJ. Penetration of resin dental materials into enamel surfaces with reference to bonding. *Arch Oral Biol* 1968;13:61–70.
36. Buonocore MG. Retrospections on bonding. *Dent Clin North Am* 1981;25:241–255.
37. Van Meerbeek B, Braem M, Lambrechts P, Vanherle G. [Adhesion of composite to dentin. Mechanical and clinical results]. *Ned Tijdschr Tandheelkd* 1993;100:489–494
38. Van Meerbeek B, Lambrechts P, Inokoshi S, et al. Factors affecting adhesion to mineralized tissues. *Oper Dent* 1992;Suppl 5:111–124.
39. De Munck J, Van Meerbeek B, Yoshida Y, et al. Four-year water degradation of total-etch adhesives bonded to dentin. *J Dent Res* 2003;82:136–140.
40. Buonocore MG. A simple method of increasing the adhesion of acrylic filling materials to enamel surfaces. *J Dent Res* 1955;34:849–853.
41. Hagger O. New catalyst for polymerization of ethylene at room temperature. *Helv Chim Acta* 1948;31:1624–1630.
42. Frankenberger R, Kramer N, Petschelt A. Long-term effect of dentin primers on enamel bond strength and marginal adaptation. *Oper Dent* 2000;25:11–19.
43. Frankenberger R, Petschelt A, Kramer N. Leucite-reinforced glass ceramic inlays and onlays after six years: clinical behavior. *Oper Dent* 2000;25:459–465.
44. Frankenberger R, Tay FR. Self-etch vs etch-and-rinse adhesives: effect of thermo-mechanical fatigue loading on marginal quality of bonded resin composite restorations. *Dent Mater* 2005;21:397–412.
45. Opdam NJ, Roeters JJ, Kuijs R, Burgersdijk RC. Necessity of bevels for box only Class II composite restorations. *J Prosthet Dent* 1998;80:274–279.
46. Gwinnett AJ. Histology of normal enamel. IV. Microradiographic study. *J Dent Res* 1966;45:870–873.
47. Gwinnett AJ, Matsui A. A study of enamel adhesives. The physical relationship between enamel and adhesive. *Arch Oral Biol* 1967;12:1615–1620.
48. Kanemura N, Sano H, Tagami J. Tensile bond strength to and SEM evaluation of ground and intact enamel surfaces. *J Dent* 1999;27:523–530.
49. Knobloch LA, Gailey D, Azer S, et al. Bond strengths of one- and two-step self-etch adhesive systems. *J Prosthet Dent* 2007;97:216–222.
50. Perdigao J, Gomes G, Gondo R, Fundingsland JW. In vitro bonding performance of all-in-one adhesives. Part I–microtensile bond strengths. *J Adhes Dent* 2006;8:367–373.
51. Sadek FT, Goracci C, Cardoso PE, et al. Microtensile bond strength of current dentin adhesives measured immediately and 24 hours after application. *J Adhes Dent* 2005;7:297–302.
52. Van Landuyt KL, Mine A, De Munck J, et al. Are one-step adhesives easier to use and better performing? Multifactorial assessment of contemporary one-step self-etching adhesives. *J Adhes Dent* 2009;11:175–190.
53. Frankenberger R, Lohbauer U, Roggendorf MJ, et al. Selective enamel etching reconsidered: better than etch-and-rinse and self etch? *J Adhes Dent* 2008;10:339–344.
54. Blunck U, Kwauka C, Martin P, et al. *Long-Term Water-Storage Class-V Margin Integrity using All-in-One-Adhesives on Phosphoric-Acid-Etched Dentin*. IADR Meeting 2010.
55. De Munck J, Van LK, Peumans M, et al. A critical review of the durability of adhesion to tooth tissue: methods and results. *J Dent Res* 2005;84:118–132.
56. Tay FR, Carvalho R, Sano H, Pashley DH. Effect of smear layers on the bonding of a self-etching primer to dentin. *J Adhes Dent* 2000;2:99–116.
57. Krejci I, Besek M, Lutz F. Clinical and SEM study of Tetric resin composite in posterior teeth: 12-month results. *Am J Dent* 1994;7:27–30.
58. Krejci I, Krejci D, Lutz F. Clinical evaluation of a new pressed glass ceramic inlay material over 1.5 years. *Quintessence Int* 1992;23:181–186.
59. Frankenberger R, Garcia-Godoy F, Lohbauer U, et al. Evaluation of resin composite materials. Part I: in vitro investigations. *Am J Dent* 2005;18:23–27.
60. Frankenberger R, Kern M. Dentin adhesives create a positive bond to dental hard tissue. *Int J Comput Dent* 2003;6:187–192.
61. Frankenberger R, Strobel WO, Lohbauer U, et al. The effect of six years of water storage on resin composite bonding to human dentin. *J Biomed Mater Res B Appl Biomater* 2004;69:25–32.
62. Manhart J, Chen HY, Mehl A, Weber K, Hickel R. Marginal quality and microleakage of adhesive class V restorations. *J Dent* 2001;29:123–130.
63. Nikolaenko SA, Lohbauer U, Roggendorf M, et al. Influence of c-factor and layering technique on microtensile bond strength to dentin. *Dent Mater* 2004;20:579–585.
64. Perdigao J, Frankenberger R, Rosa BT, Breschi L. New trends in dentin/enamel adhesion. *Am J Dent* 2000;13:25D–30D.
65. Perdigao J, Lambrechts P, Van MB, et al. Morphological field emission-SEM study of the effect of six phosphoric acid etching agents on human dentin. *Dent Mater* 1996;12:262–271.
66. Perdigao J, Van MB, Lopes MM, Ambrose WW. The effect of a re-wetting agent on dentin bonding. *Dent Mater* 1999;15:282–295.
67. Aksornmuang J, Nakajima M, Foxton RM, Tagami J. Regional bond strengths of a dual-cure resin core material to translucent quartz fiber post. *Am J Dent* 2006;19:51–55.
68. Armstrong SR, Vargas MA, Fang Q, Laffoon JE. Microtensile bond strength of a total-etch 3-step, total-etch 2-step, self-etch 2-step, and a self-etch 1-step dentin bonding system through 15-month water storage. *J Adhes Dent* 2003;5:47–56.

69. Bottino MA, Baldissara P, Valandro LF, et al. Effects of mechanical cycling on the bonding of zirconia and fiber posts to human root dentin. *J Adhes Dent* 2007;9:327–331.
70. Breschi L, Mazzoni A, Pashley DH, et al. Electric-current-assisted application of self-etch adhesives to dentin. *J Dent Res* 2006;85:1092–1096.
71. Goracci C, Tavares AU, Fabianelli A, et al. The adhesion between fiber posts and root canal walls: comparison between microtensile and push-out bond strength measurements. *Eur J Oral Sci* 2004;112:353–361.
72. Lopes GC, Baratieri LN, Monteiro Jr S, Vieira LC. Effect of posterior resin composite placement technique on the resin-dentin interface formed in vivo. *Quintessence Int* 2004;35:156–161.
73. Lutz F, Krejci I, Imfeld T, Elzer A. [The hydrodynamic behavior of dentinal tubule fluid under occlusal loading]. *Schweiz Monatsschr Zahnmed* 1991;101:24–30.
74. Manhart J, Schmidt M, Chen HY, et al. Marginal quality of tooth-colored restorations in class II cavities after artificial aging. *Oper Dent* 2001;26:357–366.
75. Monticelli F, Osorio R, Tay FR, et al. Resistance to thermo-mechanical stress of different coupling agents used as intermediate layer in resin-fiber post bonds. *Am J Dent* 2007;20:416–420.
76. Naumann M, Preuss A, Frankenberger R. Reinforcement effect of adhesively luted fiber reinforced composite versus titanium posts. *Dent Mater* 2007;23:138–144.
77. Tay FR, Frankenberger R, Krejci I, et al. Single-bottle adhesives behave as permeable membranes after polymerization. I. In vivo evidence. *J Dent* 2004;32:611–621.
78. Tay FR, Gwinnett AJ, Pang KM, Wei SH. Variability in microleakage observed in a total-etch wet-bonding technique under different handling conditions. *J Dent Res* 1995;74:1168–1178.
79. Tay FR, Gwinnett AJ, Wei SH. Ultrastructure of the resin-dentin interface following reversible and irreversible rewetting. *Am J Dent* 1997;10:77–82.
80. Tay FR, Pashley DH. Have dentin adhesives become too hydrophilic? *J Can Dent Assoc* 2003;69:726–731.
81. Tay FR, Pashley DH. Water treeing–a potential mechanism for degradation of dentin adhesives. *Am J Dent* 2003;16:6–12.
82. Van Meerbeek B, Peumans M, Verschueren M, et al. Clinical status of ten dentin adhesive systems. *J Dent Res* 1994;73:1690–1702.
83. Van Meerbeek B, Van Landuyt KL, De Munck J, et al. Technique-sensitivity of contemporary adhesives. *Dent Mater J* 2005;24:1–13.
84. Frankenberger R, Pashley DH, Reich SM, et al. Characterisation of resin-dentine interfaces by compressive cyclic loading. *Biomaterials* 2005;26:2043–2052.
85. Buonocore MG, Quigley M. Bonding of synthetic resin material to human dentin: preliminary histological study of the bond area. *J Am Dent Assoc* 1958;57:807–811.
86. Pashley DH. The influence of dentin permeability and pulpal blood flow on pulpal solute concentration. *Int J Periodont Rest Dent* 1979;16:355–361.
87. Pashley DH. The effects of acid etching on the pulpodentin complex. *Oper Dent* 1992;17:229–242.
88. Wang Y, Spencer P. Effect of acid etching time and technique on interfacial characteristics of the adhesive-dentin bond using differential staining. *Eur J Oral Sci* 2004;112:293–299.
89. Pioch T, Stotz S, Buff E, et al. Influence of different etching times on hybrid layer formation and tensile bond strength. *Am J Dent* 1998;11:202–206.
90. Kanca J, III. The all-etch bonding technique/wetbonding. *Dent Today* 1991;10:58, 60–58, 61.
91. Kanca J, III. Resin bonding to wet substrate. 1. Bonding to dentin. *Quintessence Int* 1992;23:39–41.
92. Kanca J, III. Wet bonding: effect of drying time and distance. *Am J Dent* 1996;9:273–276.
93. Perdigao J, Frankenberger R. Effect of solvent and rewetting time on dentin adhesion. *Quintessence Int* 2001;32:385–390.
94. Tay FR, Frankenberger R, Krejci I, et al. Single-bottle adhesives behave as permeable membranes after polymerization. I. In vivo evidence. *J Dent* 2004;32:611–621.
95. Frankenberger R, Lohbauer U, Tay FR, et al. The effect of different air-polishing powders on dentin bonding. *J Adhes Dent* 2007;9:381–389.
96. Nakabayashi N, Kojima K, Masuhara E. The promotion of adhesion by the infiltration of monomers into tooth substrates. *J Biomed Mater Res* 1982;16:265–273.
97. Pashley DH, Carvalho RM, Tay FR, et al. Solvation of dried dentin matrix by water and other polar solvents. *Am J Dent* 2002;15:97–102.
98. Pashley DH, Tay FR, Carvalho RM, et al. From dry bonding to water-wet bonding to ethanol-wet bonding. A review of the interactions between dentin matrix and solvated resins using a macromodel of the hybrid layer. *Am J Dent* 2007;20:7–20.
99. Perdigao J, Lambrechts P, Van MB, et al. Field emission SEM comparison of four postfixation drying techniques for human dentin. *J Biomed Mater Res* 1995;29:1111–1120.
100. Perdigao J, Lopes L, Lambrechts P, et al. Effects of a self-etching primer on enamel shear bond strengths and SEM morphology. *Am J Dent* 1997;10:141–146.
101. Kimmich M, Stappert CF. Intraoral treatment of veneering porcelain chipping of fixed dental restorations: a review and clinical application. *J Am Dent Assoc* 2013;144:31–44.
102. Loguerico AD, de Paula EA, Hass V, et al. A new universal simplified adhesive: 36-month randomized double blind clinical trial. *J Dent* 2015;43:1083–1092.
103. Perdigão J, Kose C, Mena-Serrano A, et al. A new universal simplified adhesive: 18-month clinical evaluation. *Oper Dent* 2014;39:113–127.
104. De Munck J, Luehrs AK, Poitevin A, et al. Fracture toughness versus micro-tensile bond strength testing of adhesive-dentin interfaces. *Dent Mater* 2013;29:635–644.
105. Hattan MA, Pani SC, Alomari M. Composite bonding to stainless steel crowns using a new universal bonding and single-bottle systems. *Int J Dent* 2013;2013:607405.
106. Muñoz MA, Luque I, Hass V, Reis A, et al. Immediate bonding properties of universal adhesives to dentine. *J Dent* 2013;41:404–411.
107. Perdigão J, Sezinando A, Monteiro PC. Laboratory bonding ability of a multi-purpose dentin adhesive. *Am J Dent* 2012;25:153–158.
108. Yoshihara K, Yoshida Y, Hayakawa S, et al. Nanolayering of phosphoric acid ester monomer on enamel and dentin. *Acta Biomater* 2011;7:3187–3195.
109. Tay FR, Suh BI, Pashley DH, et al. Factors contributing to the incompatibility between simplified-step adhesives and self-cured or dual-cured composites. Part II. Single-bottle, total-etch adhesive. *J Adhes Dent* 2003;5:91–105.
110. Armstrong SR, Keller JC, Boyer DB. The influence of water storage and C-factor on the dentin-resin composite microtensile bond strength and debond pathway utilizing a filled and unfilled adhesive resin. *Dent Mater* 2001;17:268–276.
111. Kemp-Scholte CM, Davidson CL. Marginal integrity related to bond strength and strain capacity of composite resin restorative systems. *J Prosthet Dent* 1990;64:658–664.

112. Garcia-Godoy F, Tay FR, Pashley DH, et al. Degradation of resin-bonded human dentin after 3 years of storage. *Am J Dent* 2007;20:109–113.
113. Pashley DH, Tay FR, Yiu C, et al. Collagen degradation by host-derived enzymes during aging. *J Dent Res* 2004;83:216–221.
114. Peschke A, Blunck U, Roulet JF. Influence of incorrect application of a water-based adhesive system on the marginal adaptation of Class V restorations. *Am J Dent* 2000;13:239–244.
115. Schmalz G, Hiller KA, Nunez LJ, et al. Permeability characteristics of bovine and human dentin under different pretreatment conditions. *J Endodont* 2001;27:23–30.
116. Bergenholtz G, Cox CF, Loesche WJ, Syed SA. Bacterial leakage around dental restorations: its effect on the dental pulp. *J Oral Pathol* 1982;11:439–450.
117. Schweikl H, Hiller KA, Bolay C, et al. Cytotoxic and mutagenic effects of dental composite materials. *Biomaterials* 2005;26:1713–1719.
118. Heintze SD, Ruffieux C, Rousson V. Clinical performance of cervical restorations–a meta-analysis. *Dent Mater* 2010;26:993–1000.
119. Breschi L, Mazzoni A, Ruggeri A, et al. Dental adhesion review: aging and stability of the bonded interface. *Dent Mater* 2008;24:90–101.
120. De Munck J, Van Landuyt K, Coutinho E, et al. Micro-tensile bond strength of adhesives bonded to Class-I cavity-bottom dentin after thermo-cycling. *Dent Mater* 2005;21:999–1007.
121. Pashley DH, Tay FR, Breschi L, et al. State of the art etch-and-rinse adhesives. *Dent Mater* 2011;27:1–16.
122. Hashimoto M. A review–micromorphological evidence of degradation in resin-dentin bonds and potential preventional solutions. *J Biomed Mater Res* 2010;92:268–280.
123. Hashimoto M, Ohno H, Sano H, et al. Degradation patterns of different adhesives and bonding procedures. *J Biomed Mater Res* 2003;66:324–330.
124. Van Meerbeek B, Mohrbacher H, Celis JP, et al. Chemical characterization of the resin-dentin interface by micro-Raman spectroscopy. *J Dent Res* 1993;72:1423–1428.
125. Breschi L, Prati C, Gobbi P, et al. Immunohistochemical analysis of collagen fibrils within the hybrid layer: A FEISEM study. *Oper Dent* 2004;29:538–546.
126. Eliades G, Vougiouklakis G, Palaghias G. Heterogeneous distribution of single-bottle adhesive monomers in the resin-dentin interdiffusion zone. *Dent Mater* 2001;17:277–283.
127. Sano H, Yoshiyama M, Ebisu S, et al. Comparative SEM and TEM observations of nanoleakage within the hybrid layer. *Oper Dent* 1995;20:160–167.
128. Tay FR, Pashley DH. Aggressiveness of contemporary self-etching systems. I: Depth of penetration beyond dentin smear layers. *Dent Mater* 2001;17:296–308.
129. Hashimoto M, Ohno H, Sano H, et al. In vitro degradation of resin-dentin bonds analyzed by microtensile bond test, scanning and transmission electron microscopy. *Biomaterials* 2003;24:3795–3803.
130. Breschi L, Cadenaro M, Antoniolli F, et al. Polymerization kinetics of dental adhesives cured with LED: correlation between extent of conversion and permeability. *Dent Mater* 2007;23:1066–1072.
131. Cadenaro M, Antoniolli F, Sauro S, et al. Degree of conversion and permeability of dental adhesives. *Eur J Oral Sci* 2005;113:525–530.
132. Cadenaro M, Breschi L, Antoniolli F, et al. Degree of conversion of resin blends in relation to ethanol content and hydrophilicity. *Dent Mater* 2008;24:1194–1200.
133. Tay FR, Pashley DH, Suh BI, et al. Water treeing in simplified dentin adhesives–déjà vu? *Oper Dent* 2005;30:561–579.
134. Mazzoni A, Carrilho M, Papa V, et al. MMP-2 assay within the hybrid layer created by a two-step etch-and-rinse adhesive: biochemical and immunohistochemical analysis. *J Dent* 2011;39:470–477.
135. Mazzoni A, Mannello F, Tay FR, et al. Zymographic analysis and characterization of MMP-2 and -9 forms in human sound dentin. *J Dent Res* 2007;86:436–440.
136. Mazzoni A, Nascimento FD, Carrilho M, et al. MMP activity in the hybrid layer detected with in situ zymography. *J Dent Res* 2012;91:467–472.
137. Mazzoni A, Pashley DH, Tay FR, et al. Immunohistochemical identification of MMP-2 and MMP-9 in human dentin: correlative FEI-SEM/TEM analysis. *J Biomed Mater Res A* 2009;88:697–703.
138. Carrilho MRO, Carvalho RM, de Goes MF, et al. Chlorhexidine preserves dentin bond in vitro. *J Dent Res* 2007;86:90–94.
139. Mazzoni A, Pashley DH, Nishitani Y, et al. Reactivation of inactivated endogenous proteolytic activities in phosphoric acid-etched dentine by etch-and-rinse adhesives. *Biomaterials* 2006;27:4470–4476.
140. Tjäderhane L, Nascimento FD, Breschi L, et al. Optimizing dentin bond durability: Control of collagen degradation by matrix metalloproteinases and cysteine cathepsins. *Dent Mater* 2013;29:116–135.
141. Breschi L, Cammelli F, Visintini E, et al. Influence of chlorhexidine concentration on the durability of etch-and-rinse dentin bonds: a 12-month in vitro study. *J Adhes Dent* 2009;11:191–198.
142. Breschi L, Mazzoni A, Nato F, et al. Chlorhexidine stabilizes the adhesive interface: a 2-year in vitro study. *Dent Mater* 2010;26:320–305.
143. Carrilho MRO, Geraldeli S, Tay F, et al. In vivo preservation of the hybrid layer by chlorhexidine. *J Dent Res* 2007;86:529–533.
144. Cova A, Breschi L, Nato F, et al. Effect of UVA-activated riboflavin on dentin bonding. *J Dent Res* 2011;90:1439–1545.
145. Bedran-Russo AKB, Vidal CMP, Santos Dos PH, Castellan CS. Long-term effect of carbodiimide on dentin matrix and resin-dentin bonds. *J Biomed Mater Res* 2010;94:250–255.
146. Carvalho RM, Chersoni S, Frankenberger R, et al. A challenge to the conventional wisdom that simultaneous etching and resin infiltration always occurs in self-etch adhesives. *Biomaterials* 2005;26:1035–1042.
147. Tay FR, Hashimoto M, Pashley DH, et al. Aging affects two modes of nanoleakage expression in bonded dentin. *J Dent Res* 2003;82:537–541.
148. Wang Y, Spencer P. Continuing etching of an all-in-one adhesive in wet dentin tubules. *J Dent Res* 2005;84:350–354.
149. Frankenberger R, Kramer N, Petschelt A. Technique sensitivity of dentin bonding: effect of application mistakes on bond strength and marginal adaptation. *Oper Dent* 2000;25:324–330.
150. Bouillaguet S, Degrange M, Cattani M, et al. Bonding to dentin achieved by general practitioners. *Schweiz Monatsschr Zahnmed* 2002;112:1006–1011.
151. Barkmeier WW, Erickson RL. Shear bond strength of composite to enamel and dentin using Scotchbond Multi-Purpose. *Am J Dent* 1994;7:175–179.

152. Itthagarun A, Tay FR, Pashley DH, et al. Single-step, self-etch adhesives behave as permeable membranes after polymerization. Part III. Evidence from fluid conductance and artificial caries inhibition. *Am J Dent* 2004;17:394–400.
153. Tay FR, King NM, Chan KM, Pashley DH. How can nanoleakage occur in self-etching adhesive systems that demineralize and infiltrate simultaneously? *J Adhes Dent* 2002;4:255–269.
154. Tay FR, Pashley DH, Suh BI, et al. Single-step adhesives are permeable membranes. *J Dent* 2002;30:371–382.
155. Tay FR, Lai CN, Chersoni S, et al. Osmotic blistering in enamel bonded with one-step self-etch adhesives. *J Dent Res* 2004;83:290–295.
156. Van Landuyt KL, De Munck J, Peumans M, et al. Bond strength of a mild self-etch adhesive with and without prior acid-etching. *J Dent* 2006;34:77–85.
157. Van Landuyt KL, De Munck J, Snauwaert J, et al. Monomer-solvent phase separation in one-step self-etch adhesives. *J Dent Res* 2005;84:183–188.
158. Chan KM, Tay FR, King NM, et al. Bonding of mild self-etching primers/adhesives to dentin with thick smear layers. *Am J Dent* 2003;16:340–346.
159. Velasquez LM, Sergent RS, Burgess JO, Mercante DE. Effect of placement agitation and placement time on the shear bond strength of 3 self-etching adhesives. *Oper Dent* 2006;31.
160. Reis A, Ferreira SQ, Costa TRF, et al. Effects of increased exposure times of simplified etch-and-rinse adhesives on the degradation of resin-dentin bonds and quality of the polymer network. *Eur J Oral Sci* 2010;118:502–509.
161. Cadenaro M, Breschi L, Rueggeberg FA, et al. Effects of residual ethanol on the rate and degree of conversion of five experimental resins. *Dent Mater* 2009;25:621–628.
162. Frankenberger R, Kramer N, Petschelt A. Fatigue behaviour of different dentin adhesives. *Clin Oral Invest* 1999;3:11–17.

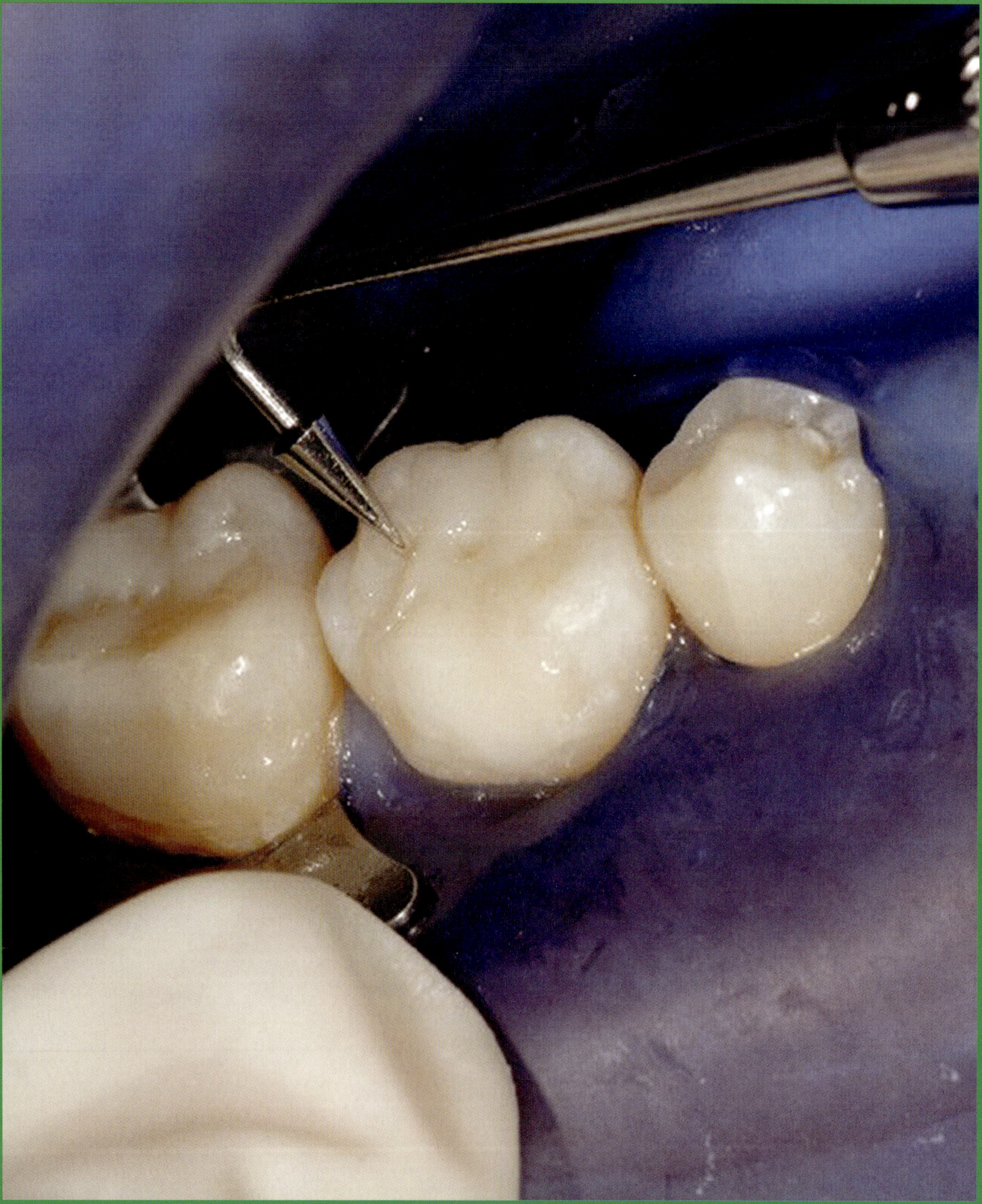

Chapter 14 Composite Resin Bonding

Ronald E. Goldstein, DDS and Marcos Vargas, DDS, MS

Chapter Outline

Basic categories of bonding in use today	377	Bonding techniques	396
Restorative uses	379	Shade selection	396
Class I restorations	379	Clinical procedure for shade selection	397
Class II restorations	382	Tooth preparation	398
Indirect posterior composite restorations	382	Enamel bonding and acid etch	401
Class III restorations	382	Dentin bonding	403
Class IV restorations	384	Polymerization	403
Class V restorations	385	Finishing the restoration	406
Labial veneer	385	Texturing your bonded restoration	407
Repairs of existing restorations	392	Problems in finishing	408
Provisional treatment	392	Interproximal finishing	409
Direct and indirect inlays	393	Maintaining the restoration	409
Materials	393	Bonding protection	413
Microfilled composites	394	Homecare	415
Small-particle macrofilled composites	395	Recall visits	415
Hybrid, microhybrids, and nanohybrid composites	395	Pit and fissure stain	416
		Use of air-abrasive technology	417
Nanofilled composites	396	The future	421

Whether it is used to replace an unsightly metal filling, to mend fractured teeth, to restructure badly spaced or crowded teeth, or to cover a series of discolored teeth, bonding remains the single fastest transformation of the mouth available to you as a dentist (Figure 14.1A and B). The patient walks in afraid to smile, with a hand in front of his or her mouth, and walks out more attractive, self-confident, and happy.

Development of the acid-etched enamel technique by Buonocore[1] and the BIS-GMA-based composite resin by Bowen[2,3] made possible the direct bonding of composite resin to the facial surface of stained, malposed, fractured, and other teeth requiring esthetic and functional improvement. As Phillips[4] said, the development of dental polymers and the technology for their use were the principal factors opening up the era of esthetic dentistry and improving and expediting the delivery of dental care. Esthetic dentistry accounts for almost half of gross dental income. Approximately 72% of restorations that replace existing restorations use composite resins.[5]

Bonding has been termed the most important discovery since the high-speed drill. Certainly bonding was the first of what

Ronald E. Goldstein's Esthetics in Dentistry, Third Edition. Edited by Ronald E. Goldstein, Stephen J. Chu, Ernesto A. Lee, and Christian F.J. Stappert.
© 2018 John Wiley & Sons, Inc. Published 2018 by John Wiley & Sons, Inc.

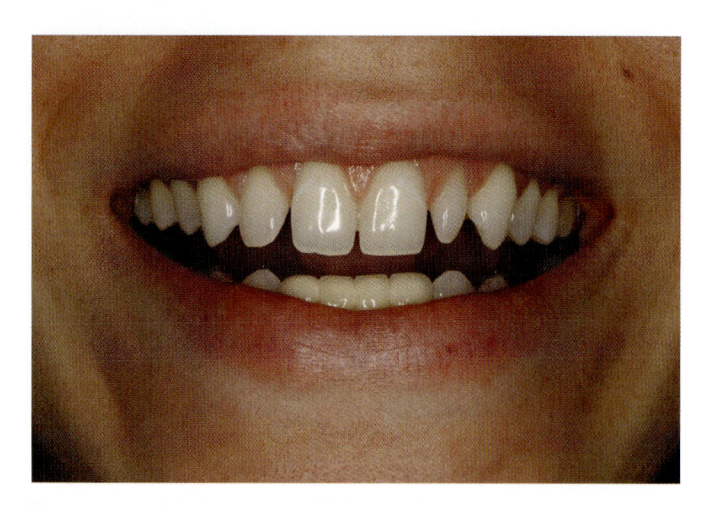

Figure 14.1 **(A)** This 28-year-old dentist disliked smiling because of the spaces in her teeth.

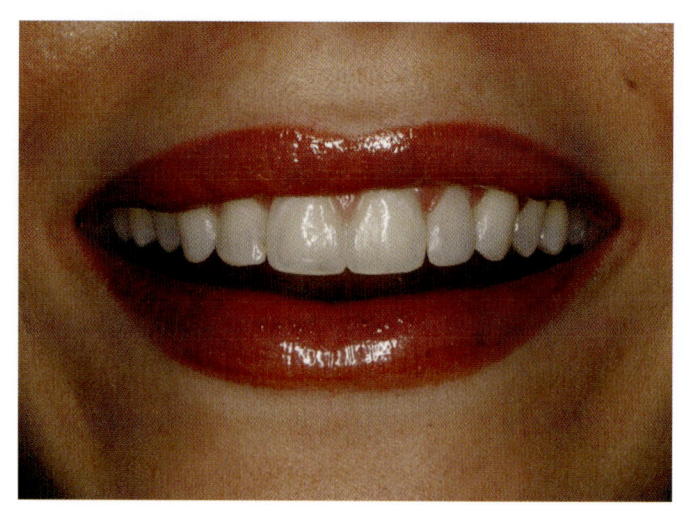

Figure 14.1 **(B)** Not only were the spaces closed, but better shapes for the central incisors were also accomplished in the one-appointment smile makeover.

since have become numerous painless techniques in restorative dentistry, requiring no anesthesia and generally producing little or no discomfort. The technique has the additional advantages of minimal tooth reduction and reversibility. Furthermore, it remains one of the most economic restorative techniques in esthetic dentistry.

But most importantly for the field of esthetic dentistry, the esthetic success of bonding—its ability to change the shape of teeth as well as their color—encouraged dentists to move from a focus on individual teeth to the comprehensive consideration of the appearance of the smile and mouth. For the first time dentists began to share fully their patients' concern with not just how the teeth functioned but how they looked. Dentists concerned with esthetic restorations, and increasingly with esthetic improvements on what the patient might have been dealt genetically, became diagnosticians of facial anomalies.

Bonding has evolved through the years; its various roles in esthetic dentistry have changed dramatically. To some extent, bonding has undergone some of the same shift in emphasis as crowning underwent earlier. Teeth that would have been reduced and crowned without question in the 1960s were instead bonded with one of the new composite resins in the 1970s, especially after the introduction of high-intensity light curing to both control and strengthen the bond. Now, in the 21st century, porcelain veneers are being used for many of the same problems for which bonding previously appeared to be such a "miracle solution" (see Chapter 15). Porcelain veneers have many of the same advantages: minimal tooth reduction, little or no discomfort resulting in less need for anesthesia, and fairly rapid transformation since two rather than one appointments are necessary. Their increased expense, time requirement, and relative fragility must be weighed against their superior esthetic effect and longer esthetic life.

Yet no text that purports to cover esthetic dentistry as it is practiced today can relegate bonding to history. Bonding remains the treatment of choice for many conditions—and for many patients. As is true for bleaching, its lower cost has been one of the routes by which esthetic dentistry has become important and feasible for great numbers of people. The superior handling properties of today's composites, and new techniques that permit good adhesion to biologic structure as well as to dental materials, make bonding the treatment of choice in many circumstances where an esthetic improvement might otherwise not be achievable.

Furthermore, the new composite resins are substantially more resistant to wear than their predecessors. Placed under appropriate conditions and monitored routinely, many restorations can be expected to last a decade or more;[6,7] Bayne and his colleagues found that the failure rate of 899 composite posterior restorations—sometimes raised as reason to use other treatments than bonding—was in fact less than half that of conventional amalgams at 5 years, suggesting that even posterior composites can provide excellent long-term clinical service.[8] In fact, Maitland[9] (Figure 14.2A and B) has said that many of the failings sometimes ascribed to bonding can be avoided by attention to patient selection, material used, and techniques of preparation and finishing. Additionally, proper placement and careful attention to adhesive procedures is a must for the success of bonding.

There are several excellent books to which you can turn for detailed instructions on applying the technique to various situations.[10-17] This chapter makes no effort to duplicate those, but concentrates on some points that may enhance the esthetic effects of your own techniques. This chapter reviews briefly the categories of bonding in use today, based on the adhesive nature, the basic uses, and the materials and techniques that have broadened the use of bonding in esthetic dentistry. The description of the bonding procedure emphasizes an overlay technique that these authors have used for more than 40 years and found to overcome some of the difficulty in maintaining a long esthetic life for bonded teeth. And finally, the chapter concludes with the simplest and yet most overlooked role in esthetic dentistry: education of the patient in the maintenance of his or her new appearance through prevention, care, and an attentive eye to how dental professionals such as hygienists should approach the bonded teeth.

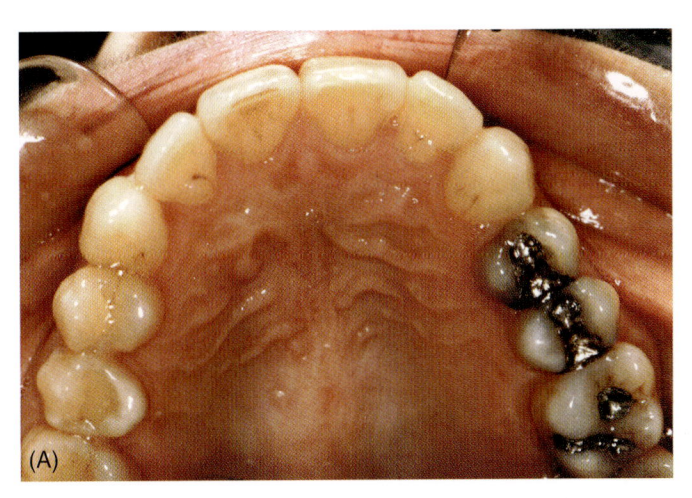

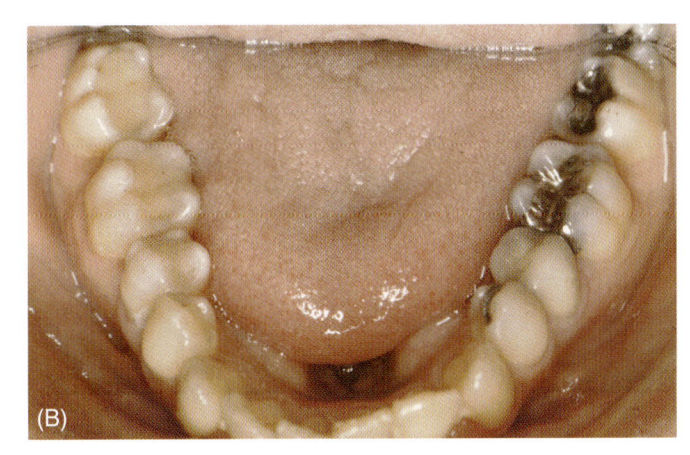

Figure 14.2 (A, B) These pictures depict a 10-year status of posterior composite restorations on one side and amalgam restorations that were placed on the other side at the same time. All restorations continue to be functional.

Basic categories of bonding in use today

The major reason that bonding is so useful in terms of conservative operative dentistry is that composite materials are directly bondable to tooth structure.[18] While bonding to enamel is by far the most frequently used, reliable, and predictable of all bonding procedures,[19] as can be seen in the listing of basic uses to follow, the ability of the newer materials to bond to all hard tissue and to dental materials continues to broaden the uses for bonding. Basic categories are as follows:

- bonding composite resin to enamel
- bonding composite resin to dentin
- bonding composite resin to other composites, glass ionomer, and porcelain
- bonding glass ionomer to dentin and enamel
- bonding porcelain to enamel and dentin
- bonding composite resin to metal.

Bonding is a highly esthetic method of obtaining both functional and esthetic restoration of individual teeth, using one or more of the above categories. Patients who appear to be difficult to please may be good candidates for bonding, since it is reversible.[20] This allows the flexibility of redoing or altering the shade for the types of patients who may find it difficult to accept an unchangeable porcelain laminate once it is irreversibly bonded into place. Bonding can be used as a transitional step to more complex procedures or drastic changes that be done through crowns or porcelain veneers or as a means to evaluate occlusal changes. Lately, this is called "transitional bonding;" it has the advantage to simulate complex procedures and test the definitive treatment plan. Bonding is also an excellent choice for closure of interdental spaces with mesial or distal composite resin augmentation because composite resin can be added for cosmetic purposes without any tooth reduction.[21] It has proved beneficial following orthodontic treatment to obtain proximal contact between adjacent teeth to improve retention. A possible contraindication for composite restorations would be in the patient who wishes to replace existing posterior amalgams and exhibits a high caries index and/or consistently demonstrates poor oral hygiene.[22] The esthetic effect, even more than the clinical success, will be based on the proper choice of materials and techniques used. With this in mind, bonding can be used in all five classifications of restorations as well as in repairs of chipped or fractured porcelain.

Specific requirements are that first, and most important, the esthetic need of the patient must be determined. This need filters down to the individual or requirement of specific teeth. It should be further based on a tooth-to-tooth analysis, upper-to-lower arch comparison, and examination of tooth and soft tissue, the smile, or a combination of all the above.

The esthetic need of a patient is determined by considering several parameters as follows:

1. Do you need to make the tooth or teeth more opaque, or develop a depth of color? (Figure 14.3A–E). Depth can be achieved by bonding the darker, more chromatic shade first, then adding incremental veneered layers of lighter or transparent shades.
2. What do you need to do to obtain your best color? This often means mixing and blending composites, or even tints or opaques, from different manufacturers.
3. For what purpose is the composite being used? For facial bonding? Occlusal pits? Class V? The composite(s) you select must, at best, be capable of withstanding the long-term functional stress placed on it by the intended restorations.

Available composite systems generally fall into the following categories:

- Those formulated to match a few shades most commonly found in the general public.
- Those manufactured in various opacities, "dentin-like" materials to replace dentin, "enamel-like" materials to replace enamel, and incisal or translucent shades to replace translucent areas or to provide translucent areas to the restoration. On certain occasions tints and opaquers help to create more difficult, multicolored shading (Figure 14.4A–C).

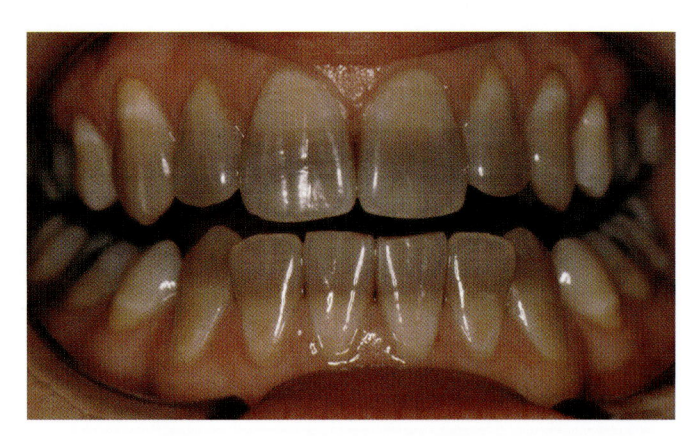

Figure 14.3 (A) Extremely dark tetracycline-stained teeth provide the most difficult challenge for direct resin full-veneer bonding. This 24-year-old student wanted a conservative and economical solution to her esthetic problem without reducing her enamel surface.

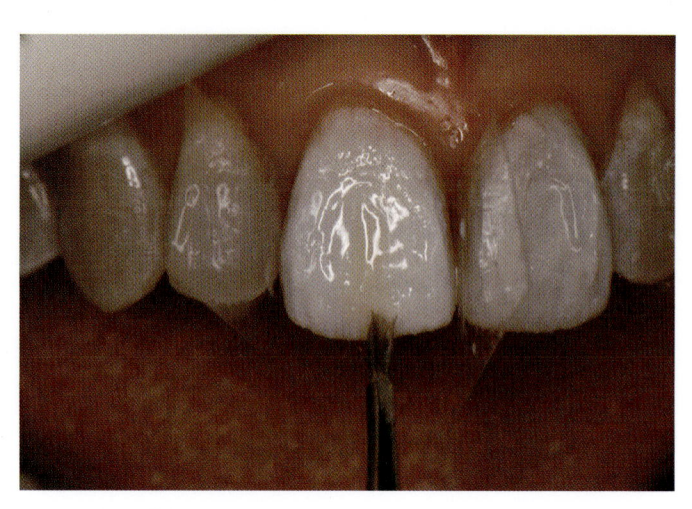

Figure 14.3 (B) To obtain the best natural-looking polychromatic tooth color, first mask the tetracycline discoloration with multiple layers of opaque (Cosmedent, Chicago, IL, USA). Next, orange/brown stain is applied as a thin stripe down the center of the labial surface to give the appearance of underlying dentin.

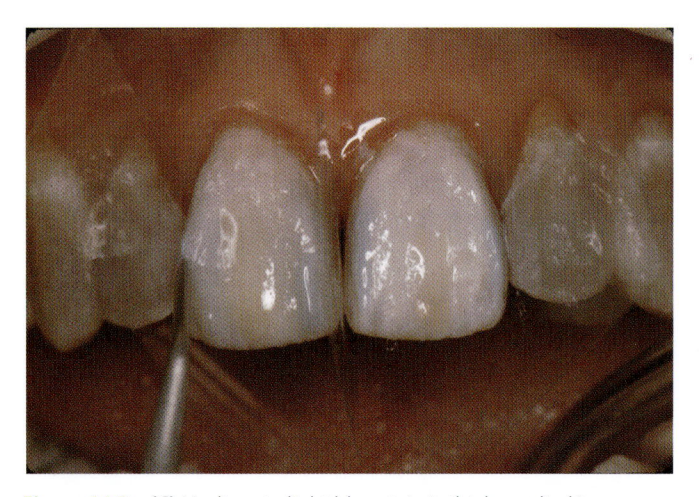

Figure 14.3 (C) Medium to light blue stain is thinly applied in a vertical stripe at both mesial and distal line angles to help simulate the appearance of enamel.

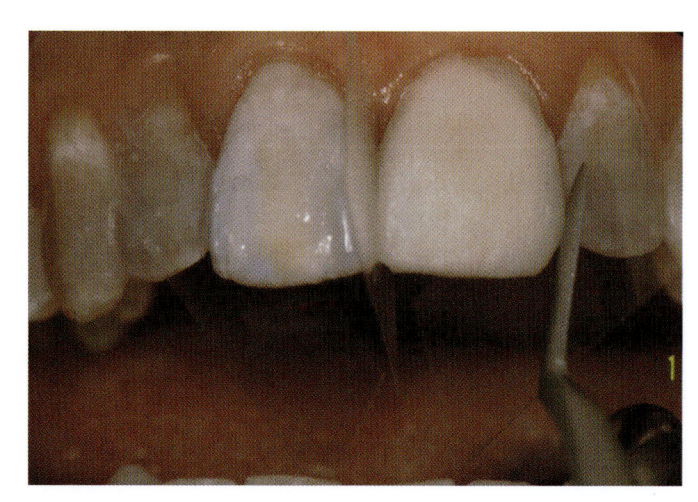

Figure 14.3 (D) Next, the preselected body shade is uniformly applied over the opaque and stained layers with the anodized aluminum GC3 instrument (Hu-Friedy).

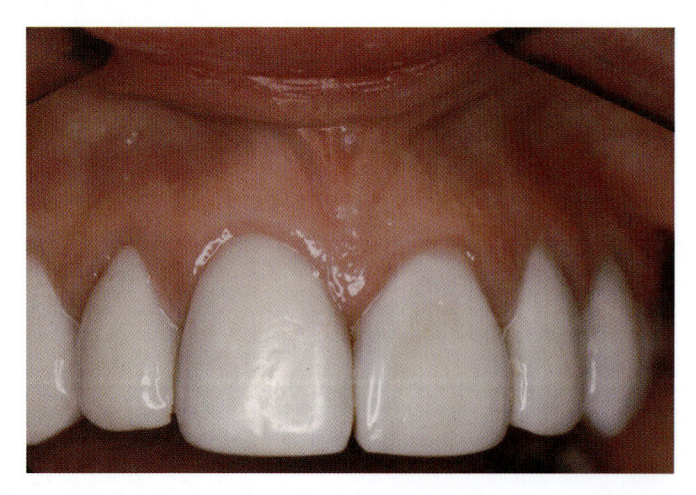

Figure 14.3 (E) The final view of the polished restorations shows how the layered colors increase the appearance of naturalness. Over time, these restorations can be refinished and polished as necessary, which will renew their luster and layered colors.

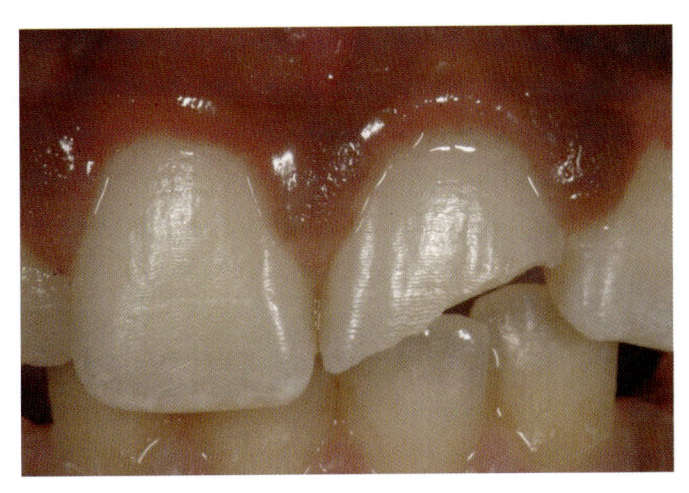

Figure 14.4 **(A)** This 12-year-old boy presented with an emergency of a fractured left central incisor. Note the adjacent central incisor had an opaque incisal stain.

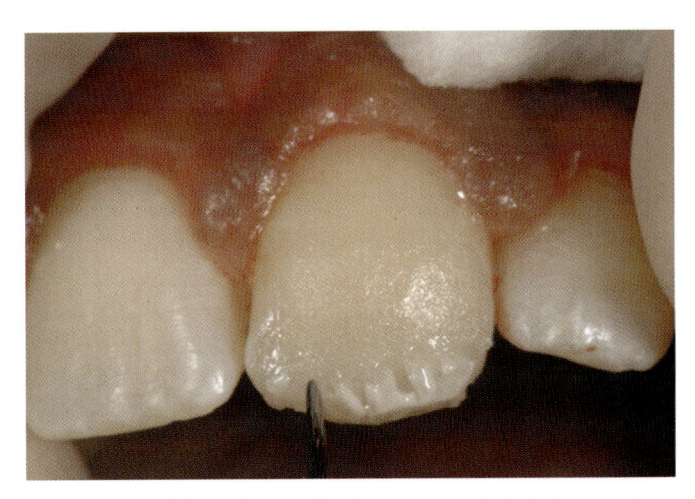

Figure 14.4 **(B)** After the initial body layer is applied, slight space is left for opaque incisal stains, to be followed by a translucent layer.

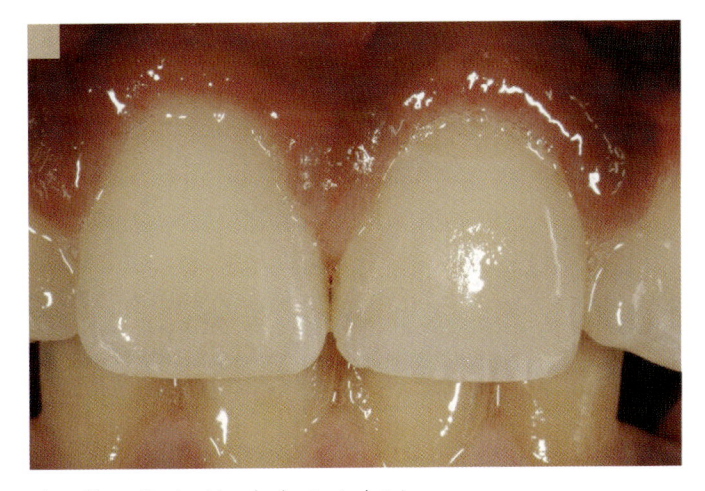

Figure 14.4 **(C)** The final result shows the effect of color blend, plus incisal stains.

Restorative uses

Class I restorations

These include pits and fissures that can be easily, quickly, and esthetically restored by composite resins with almost exclusive removal of decay, without the need for removal of sound tooth structure for mechanical retention. As an added bonus, the bonding of small grooves, defects, or pits in individual teeth is an excellent means of preventing either initial or further caries with little or no risk of tooth discoloration, as may be the case with amalgam.[23] Life expectancy is the longest in this category, with 10 or more years not being uncommon.

When matching an exact shade is important to your patient, be sure to make your shade selection before placing a rubber dam. In the event the tooth is discolored due to an old amalgam restoration, it may be necessary to select the shade from the adjacent tooth or remove the amalgam first. Then make your color selection.

Use a "stock" shade guide supplied by the manufacturer only to select several of the closest shades with which to do your actual shade trial bonding. To achieve the closest match, remove all of the old restorative material plus any stained tooth surface that might mar your esthetic result. Have all your materials ready, including a mylar strip and GCI#3 (Hu-Friedy). Place a small amount of composite resin on the tooth to be matched. Quickly apply the mylar strip using more pressure on one end of the composite so you will achieve a good range of color from thick to thin on the labial surface after polymerization. Then let the tooth regain its moisture until its normal color has returned. Make your shade comparison as quickly as possible, avoiding any long periods of tooth desiccation.

Typical Class I composite resin restorations on average last 5–8 years but the patient's occlusal wear may dictate less than ideal longevity. However, the authors have had composite restoraations lasting well over 15 years in many instances. The advantage of the direct composite restoration is the ability to see microleakage in the form of marginal stain (Figure 14.5A–J). Although early detection of the stain can mean use of air abrasion and resealing the margin, if the patient does not schedule hygiene visits frequently enough (three–four times yearly) replacement of the restoration may be necessary.

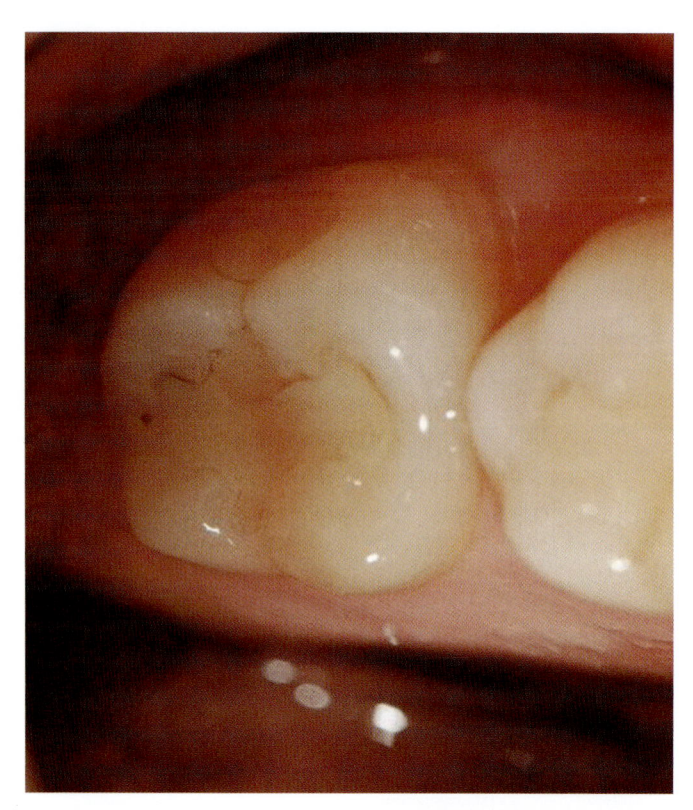

Figure 14.5 (A) The defective existing composite resin restorations in the lower first and second molars have microleakage at the margins, fractures, and secondary decay. These restorations were functional for over 10 years.

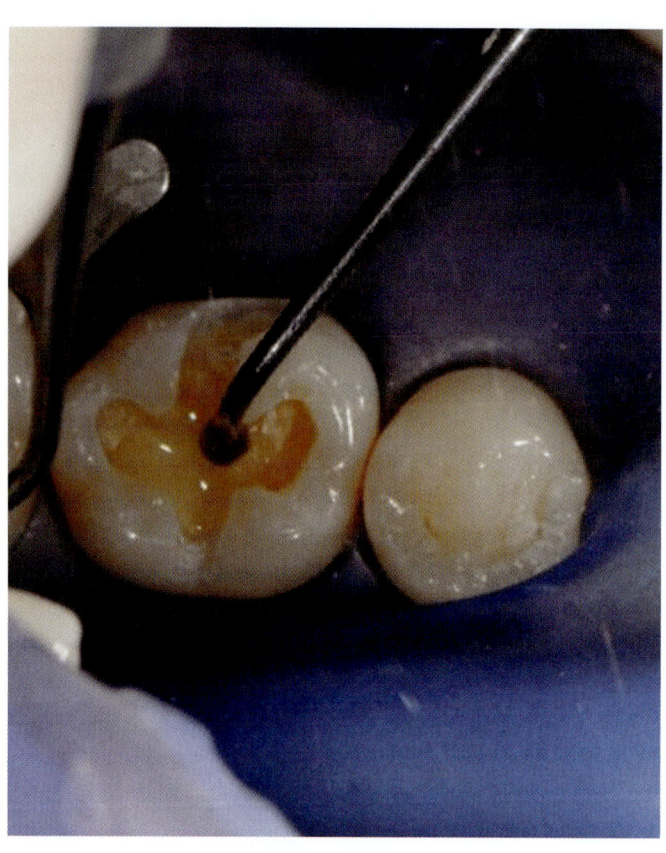

Figure 14.5 (B) After removal of the defective restorations and secondary caries, a cavity cleanser is used, followed by a glass ionomer liner/base (Vitrebond, 3 M).

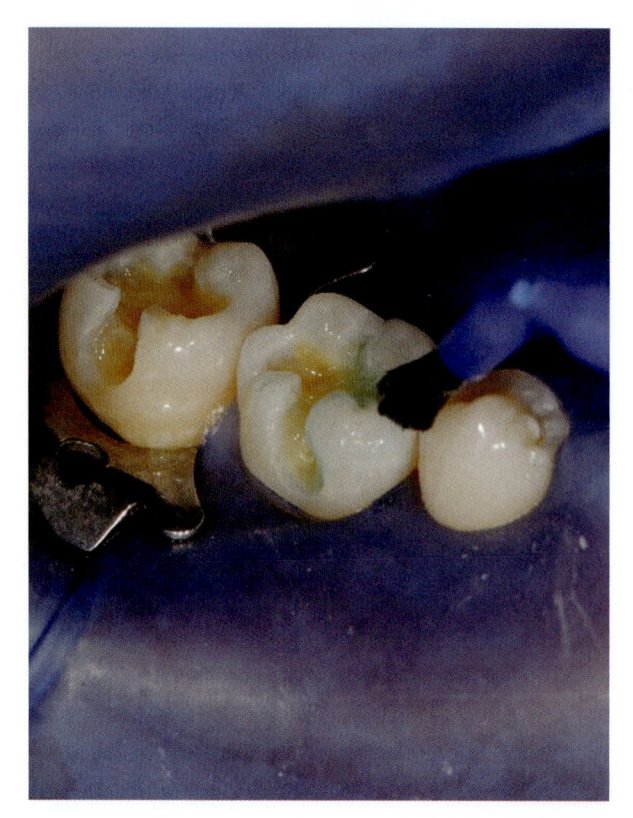

Figure 14.5 (C) Here a 37% phosphoric acid etch being placed on the enamel margins, which will be followed by a thorough washing with air/water syringe.

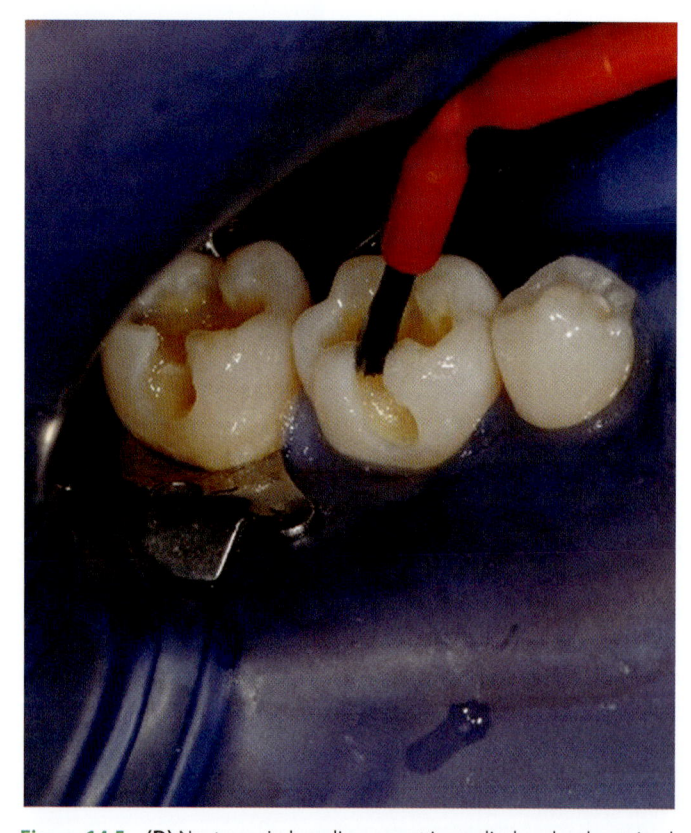

Figure 14.5 (D) Next a resin bonding agent is applied and polymerized.

Chapter 14 Composite Resin Bonding

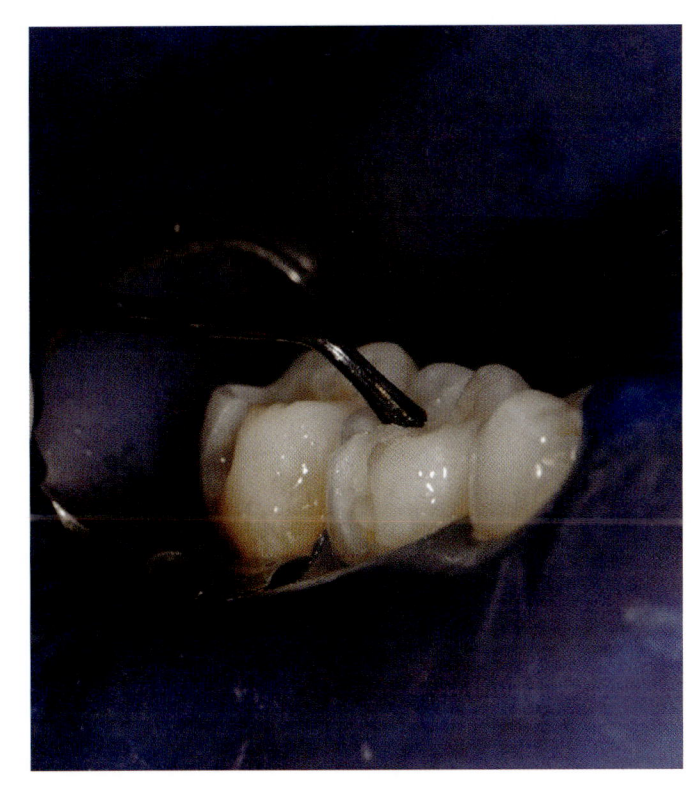

Figure 14.5 **(E)** Layers of the chosen shade of microhybrid composite resin (Venus Diamond, Heraeus) are bonded individually with appropriately sized condensing instruments (#1 TNCIGFTI and #2 TNCIGFT2, Hu-Friedy).

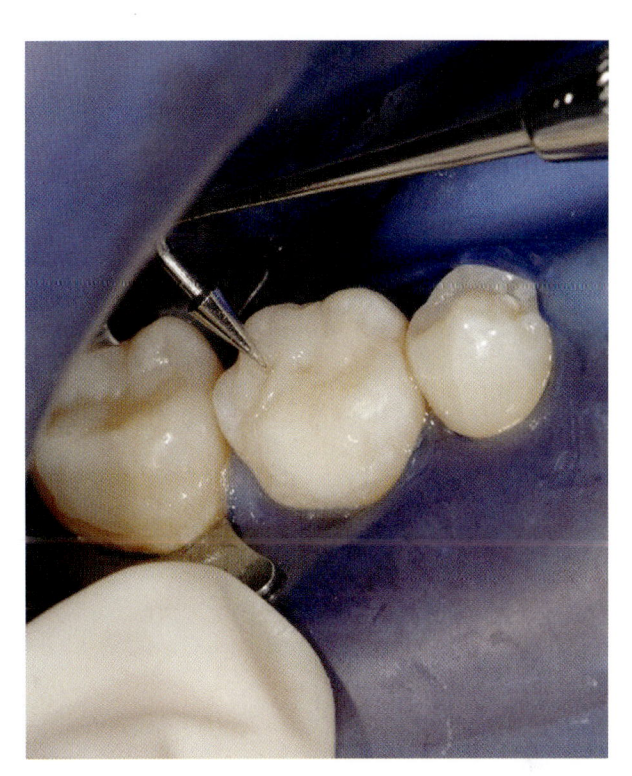

Figure 14.5 **(F)** A reverse-ended carver is ideal for placing anatomy into the composite before final polymerization (#6 Composite Carver TNCIGFT6, Hu-Friedy).

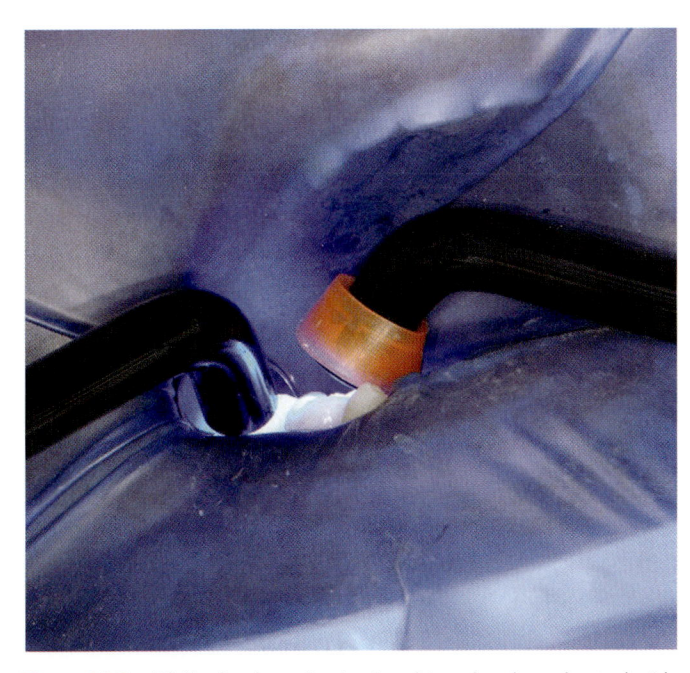

Figure 14.5 **(G)** Final polymerization is achieved and accelerated with a dual-light technique.

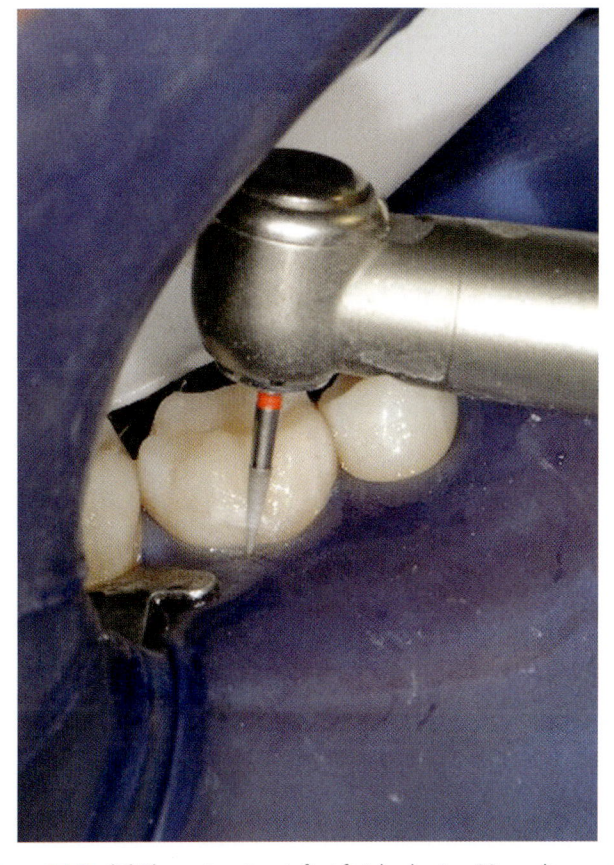

Figure 14.5 **(H)** The restoration is first finished using 30 μm diamond (ET6, Brasseler USA), to be followed by finishing burs of the same size.

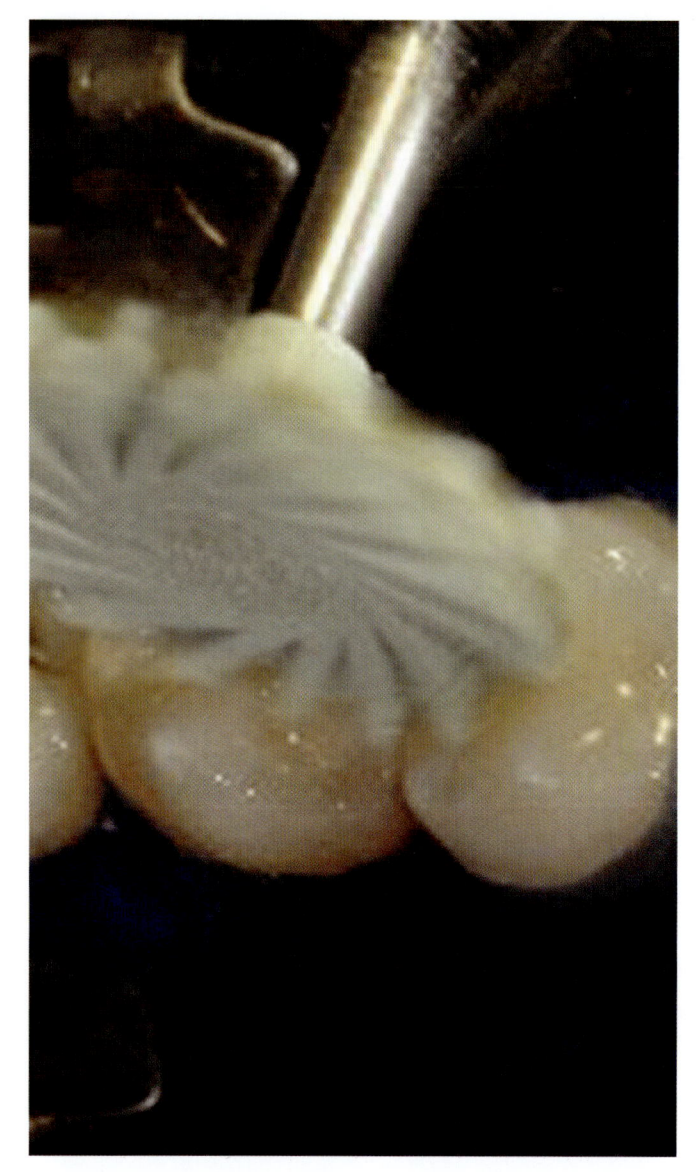

Figure 14.5 (I) The final restorations have been polished with impregnated finishers (Diacomp Featherlite, Brasseler USA).

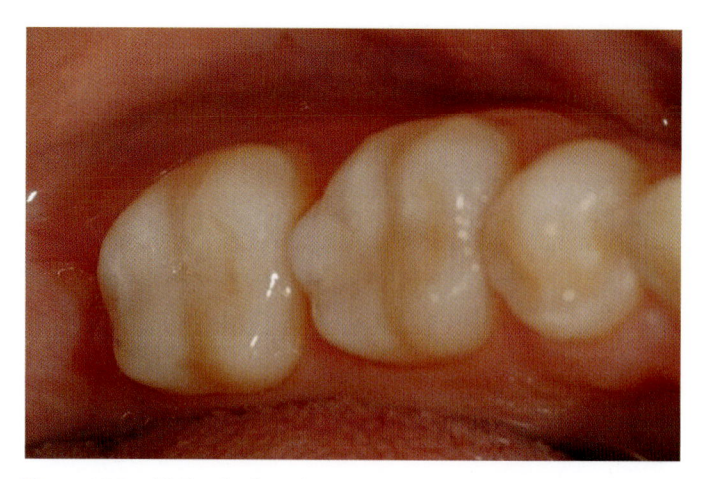

Figure 14.5 (J) The final result.

Class II restorations

If conservative, these can be achieved, both functionally and esthetically, through composite resins. Tunnel preparations are ideal for composite resin or glass ionomer restorations. Functionally try to salvage as much tooth structure as possible. It is esthetically easier to blend in a composite to existing enamel instead of creating a new color. In addition to conserving tooth structure, Douvitas[24] notes that gap formation between resin and enamel occurs most visibly in the cervical wall of Class II restorations, which may be minimized by using a spherical, rather than rectangular, cavity preparation. This class illustrates quite well the role bonding often plays in making esthetic dentistry (as opposed to dentistry for function only) economically available to a larger number of patients. At times, there will be need for larger Class II restorations, especially on the mesial aspect of bicuspids where the labial margin would show if it were amalgam or gold and the patient wants to keep the cost lower than that for a porcelain inlay. This is permissible, provided the patient understands that the life expectancy may be considerably shorter for other restorative options.

Patients' main objection to amalgam restorations has been either the "silver," "black," or "metal" color of restoration and the darker-appearing enamel associated with these restorations. Esthetically, the Class II restoration can present special problems, especially with a large mesiolabial wall that needs restoring. The shade that blends well with the occlusal portion may not match the proximal wall. You may need to bevel the cavosurface margin of this wall or use a more translucent shade or blend a slight blue or violet tint into the proximal portion to obtain a better match (Figure 14.6A–E).

Indirect posterior composite restorations

Emphasis on bonding, esthetics, and tooth conservatism has prompted research for the optimal material for use in posterior tooth-colored restorations. Dental porcelain has basic problems including questionable wear of the opposing dentition, difficulty with modification and polishing in the oral cavity, and an inherently brittle nature. Polymer-based systems of the past, on the other hand, have lacked sufficient strength and wear resistance. Recent advances in polymer ceramic technology combined with new fiber developments have generated an entire genre of metal-free restorative materials.

These systems may provide the esthetics, biocompatibility, and enamel wear similar to an ideal resin material while encompassing the flexural strength and fracture resistance of metal-reinforced restorations for anterior and posterior areas.[25]

Although these materials are used frequently for posterior inlays and onlays, for the purpose of this book they are discussed in Chapter 15.

Class III restorations

These are the major use for composite resins today. Composite resin materials have become the most popular material for Class III, as well as Class IV and Class V, restorations.[26] These cavity classifications are excellent examples of the use of bonding for

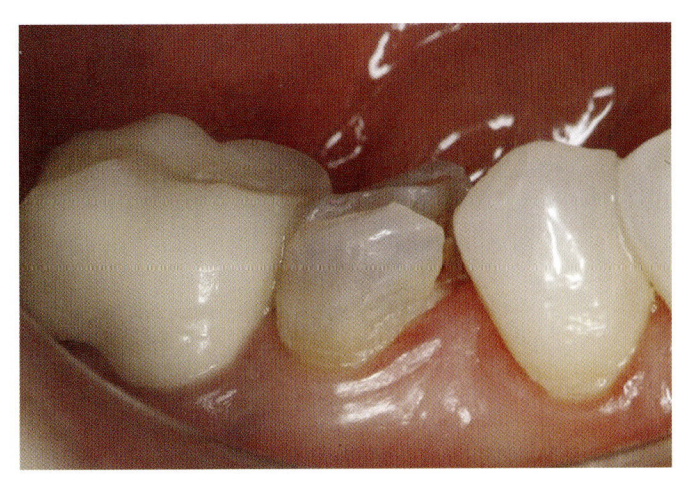

Figure 14.6 **(A)** This lady fractured her previous bonded restoration. Due to the minimal amount of remaining enamel, it was decided to proceed with a direct bonded restoration rather full or partial ceramic coverage.

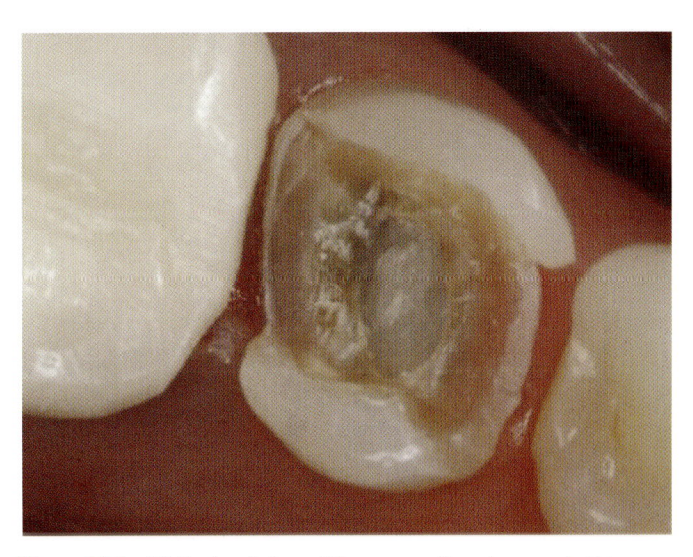

Figure 14.6 **(B)** Occlusal view of the preparation shows only thin labial and lingual walls of enamel remain.

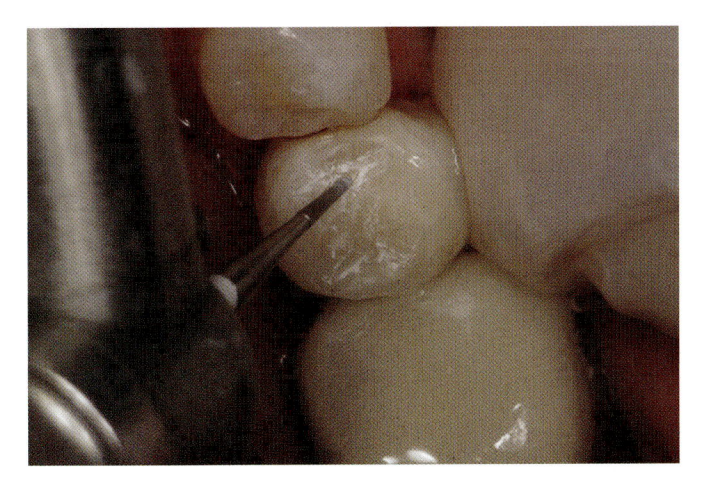

Figure 14.6 **(C)** After a direct bonded Class II composite restoration was placed, final carving was completed with a 30-blade carbide (ETOS2, Brasseler USA).

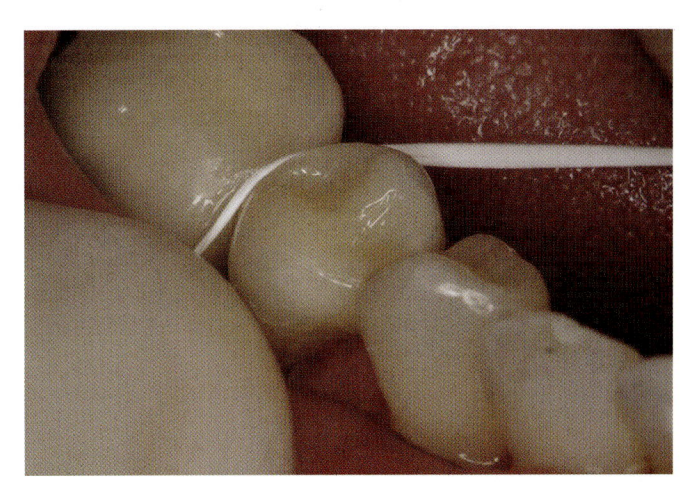

Figure 14.6 **(D)** Tight contact was achieved by use of heavy wedging.

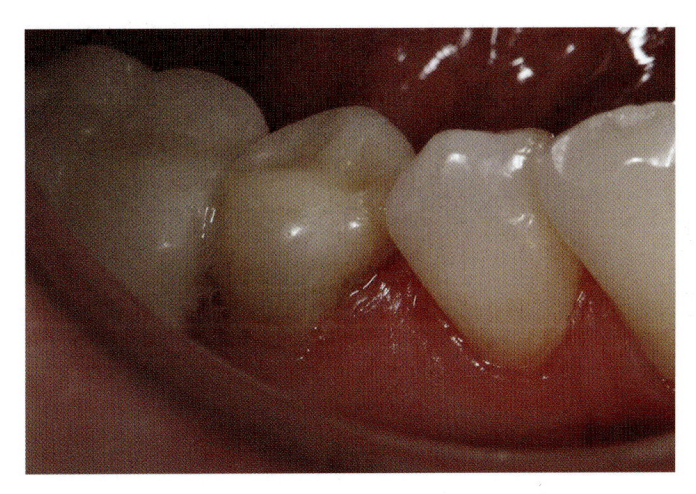

Figure 14.6 **(E)** The final restoration after finishing and polishing.

esthetic superiority as well as its economic pluses. As Croll and Donly[27] point out, when bonded composite resin restorations are placed, finished, and polished correctly, and a suitable shade and translucency of composite resin is used, Class III restorations can simulate perfectly the appearance of natural enamel and dentin, and they last for many years (Figure 14.7A–N). Composites come in almost every shade, range, translucency, and opacity. Acid etching seals the composite to the enamel for functional soundness. However, you may need to purchase additional shades from several different manufacturers to cover a complete range of color options. Shade selection for the Class III composite can be both time consuming and frustrating. The major problem is choosing a shade that will actually match after you have inserted and finished the restoration. Typically, the first thing you do is place a sample of the intended material on the tooth to be restored. The difficulty is to anticipate the correct amount of material thickness so the final result will match. A good method of accomplishing this is to vary the thickness of the sample by pressing harder on one end with the mylar strip so you will get a gradation of color and, therefore, get a better indication of just how close your shade will match with the estimated thickness.

Class IV restorations

These, including chipped or fractured teeth, are one of the main reasons for using composite resin. Frequently, bonding is the ideal solution, providing both the immediate answer to an esthetic emergency and a long-term, low-cost restoration. There is no reason to crown a tooth that has minor chips or a slight

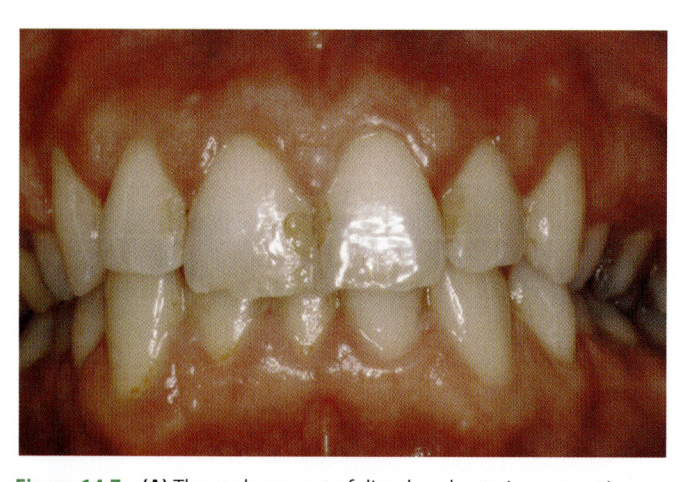

Figure 14.7 **(A)** The replacement of discolored anterior restorations with composite resin comprises one of the largest percentages of esthetic restorative dentistry.

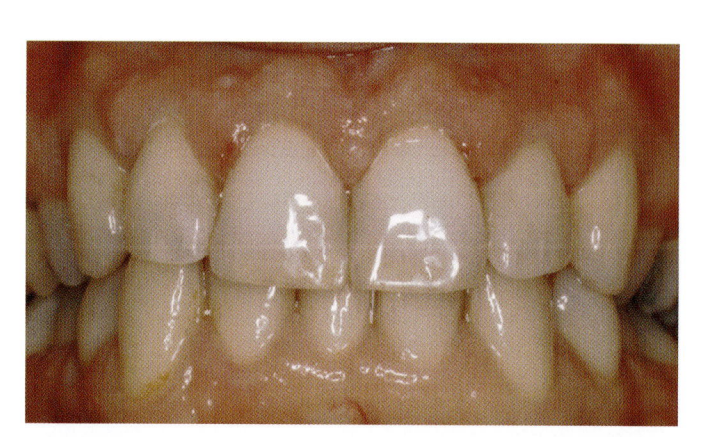

Figure 14.7 **(B)** The objective of replacement is to obtain invisible margins and a blending of color to match existing tooth structure.

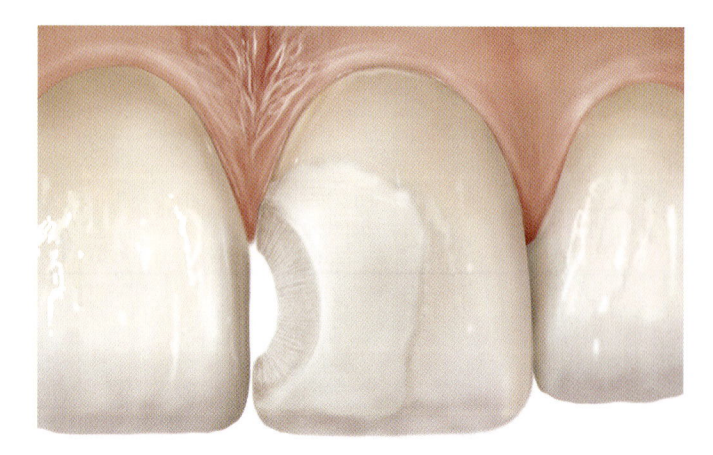

Figure 14.7 **(C)** The basic tooth preparation for the Class III restoration consists of a reverse bevel and an overlaid margin that extends several millimeters past the bevel. This provides extended restoration longevity and a better color blend.

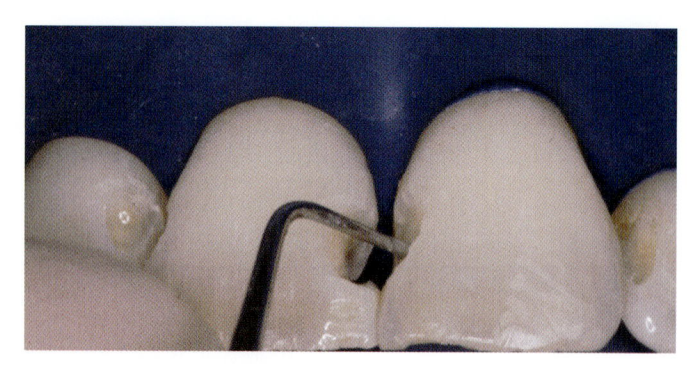

Figure 14.7 **(D)** After the old restorative material is removed and a reverse bevel is placed, light-polymerized glass ionomer liners are inserted with a Novatech PINT I I (Hu-Friedy).

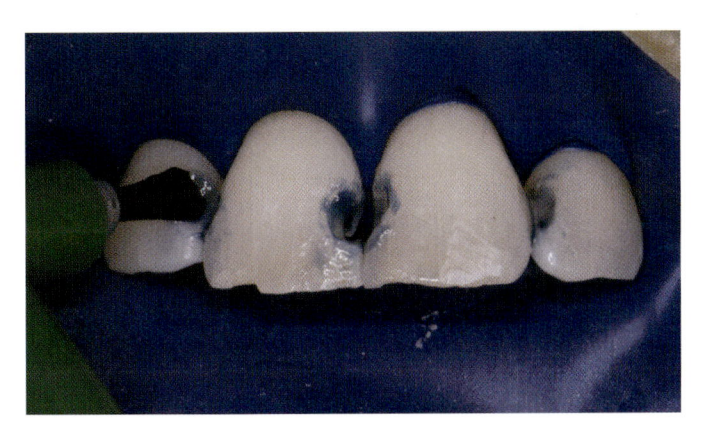

Figure 14.7 **(E)** Acid etching should be accomplished for 10–30 s depending on the composition of the tooth structure that is being etched.

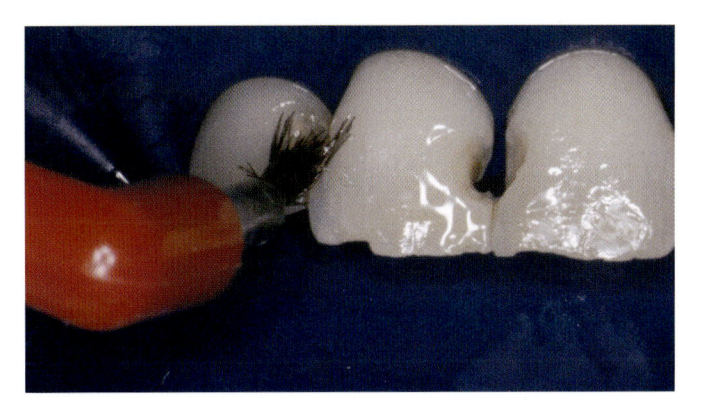

Figure 14.7 **(F)** Use different-colored brush handles (Centrix) to apply the various agents used in the bonding process. Here, a red brush is used to apply the final bonding agent, which is then polymerized.

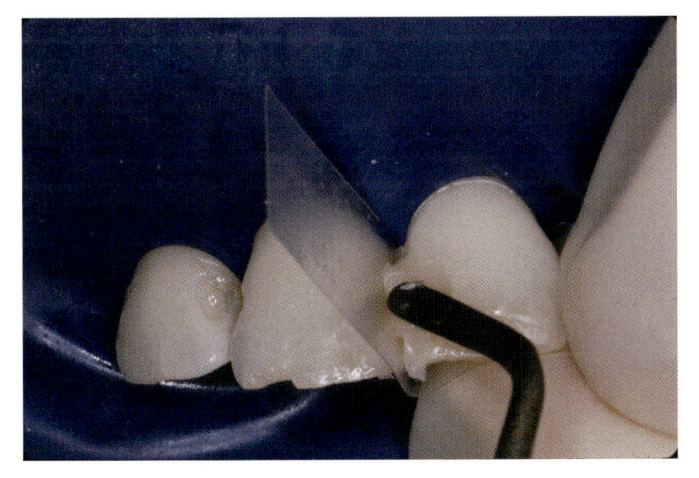

Figure 14.7 **(G)** The preselected shade of microfill composite resin is applied with a thin-bonded, nonstick composite instrument (#3 Extra-Flex TNCIGFT3, Hu-Friedy) in small increments and polymerized layer by layer. To increase the depth of color, consider using a slightly darker shade initially, followed by a lighter one, rather than one shade for the entire restoration.

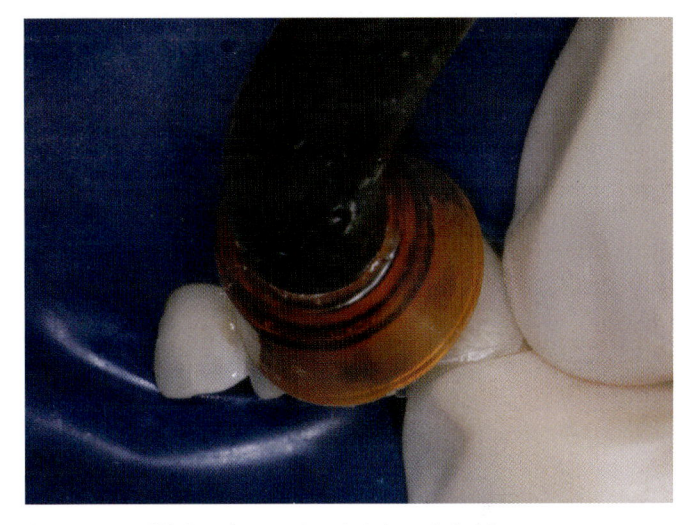

Figure 14.7 **(H)** A mylar matrix strip is loosely held to ensure separation and adequate thickness for proper finishing to occur. Polymerize each layer both labially and lingually for the time specified by the manufacturer as each increment of composite resin is applied.

fractured piece missing when a direct-fill light-polymerized composite restoration is more economic and equally functional and esthetic (Figure 14.8A–H). Minor chips of anterior and posterior teeth also can be repaired easily with composite resin with predictable success (Figure 14.9A and B).

Class V restorations

Caries and even large, eroded defects are generally handled with a microfill highly polished restoration, which is the treatment of choice. However, new materials with improved polishability, color stability, resistance to wear, and extended range of shades are suitable for Class V restorations. One possible disadvantage of microfilled composite, as stated by Davidson and Kemp-Scholte,[28] is its tendency to undergo hygroscopic expansion, which produces marginal overhangs. In the less-motivated patient, this may result in excessive staining and recurrent caries. When making a shade selection for Class V restorations, first note your patient's lip line. This is particularly important for patients with a medium lip line where the incisal-most margin will show during a wide smile. Remember there is a shadow created by the lip line that tends to emphasize the gray shades. Therefore avoid gray or translucent shades if possible, and select the more opaque shades for better blending (Figure 14.10A–J).

Labial veneer

As previously stated in this chapter, the quickest and most economic method of obtaining an esthetic tooth transformation is through the direct resin labial veneer. Although esthetic perfection may be more easily obtained with the porcelain veneer, the extra time and laboratory costs involved may make the procedure economically difficult for many patients. Therefore, composite resin bonding becomes the restoration of choice for these patients. The best candidate for the direct resin veneer is the monochromatic shaded tooth, since multicolored restorations are much more easily constructed in the laboratory (Figure 14.11A–D). However, if you take the extra amount of time and have developed the skill to master inlaid shades and stains, you will certainly be able to match almost any tooth with direct composite resin bonding (Figure 14.11E–J).

A potential dilemma arises when tooth deformity exists on approximately half of the tooth. Is it better to restore one half of the tooth and attempt to blend a potentially revealing margin or veneer the entire labial surface and extend the margin subgingivally? One instance where the veneer would be preferred is with the patient who wants to avoid periodic showing of a Class III margin. It is a better choice to veneer the entire labial surface and completely mask the tooth/composite margin. When doing so, consider improving the smile line by extending the labial surface in a buccal direction.

The bonded composite veneer also can be used with porcelain veneers or full crowns when economics is a problem. A good example of this technique would be to either use crowns or

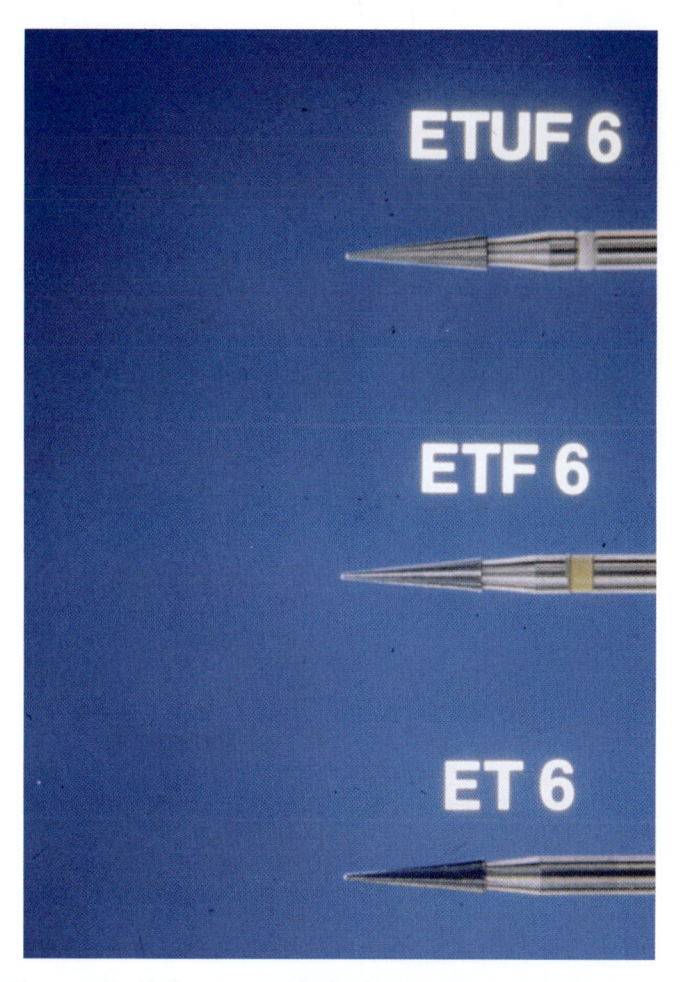

Figure 14.7 (I) The sequence for finishing requires an entry-level instrument of 8-, 16-, or 30-blade carbide (E.T. Burs, Brasseler USA) depending on the amount of excess composite present.

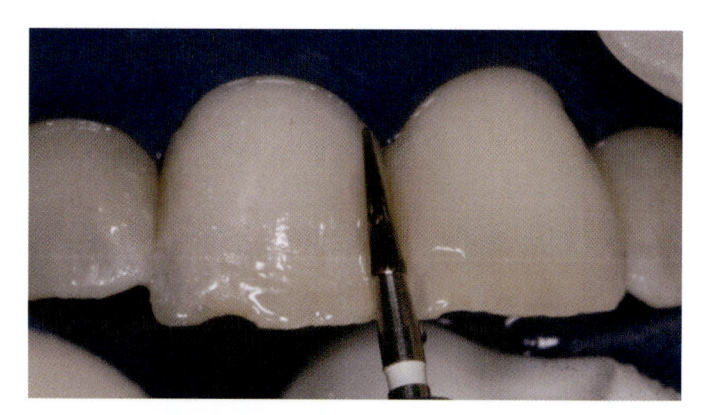

Figure 14.7 (J) Final labial finishing is done with the ET6UF 30-bladed carbide (Brasseler USA).

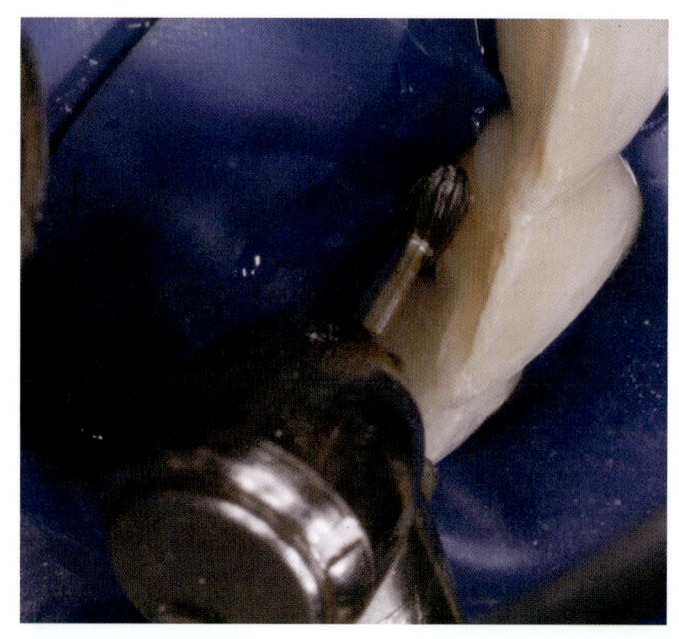

Figure 14.7 (K) The OS-1 finishing bur (E.T. Burs, Brasseler USA) is the perfect shape for lingual contouring.

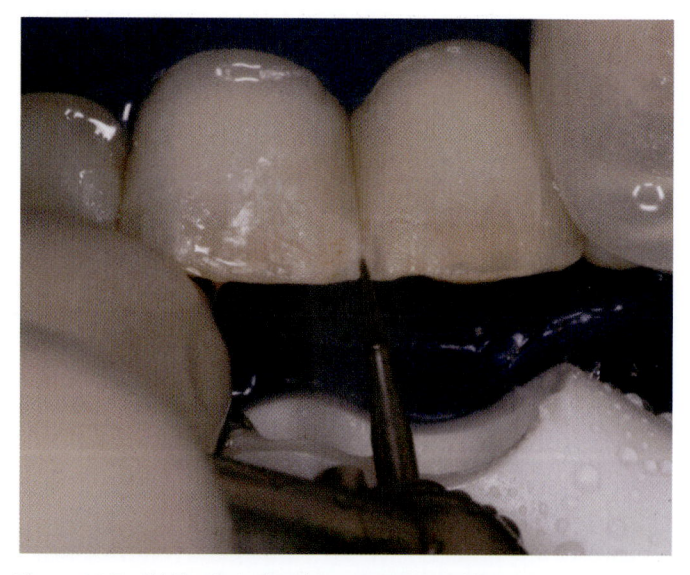

Figure 14.7 (L) The incisal embrasure is opened by an E.T. "cutting bur" (Brasseler 132-A).

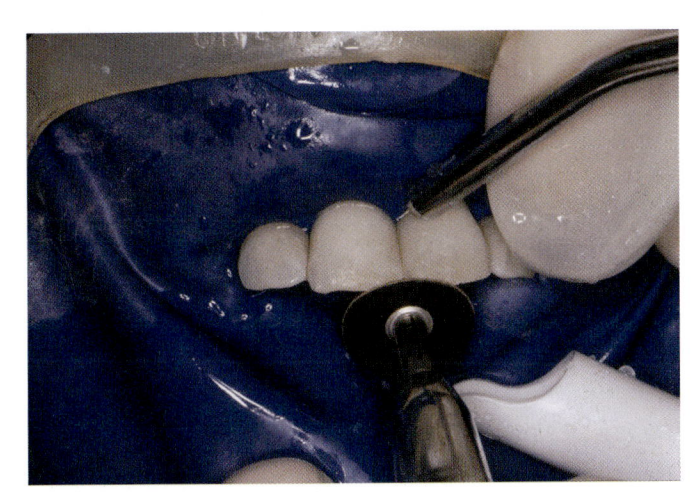

Figure 14.7 **(M)** A series of flexible sandpaper disks are useful for leveling and final polish (Sof-Lex, 3M).

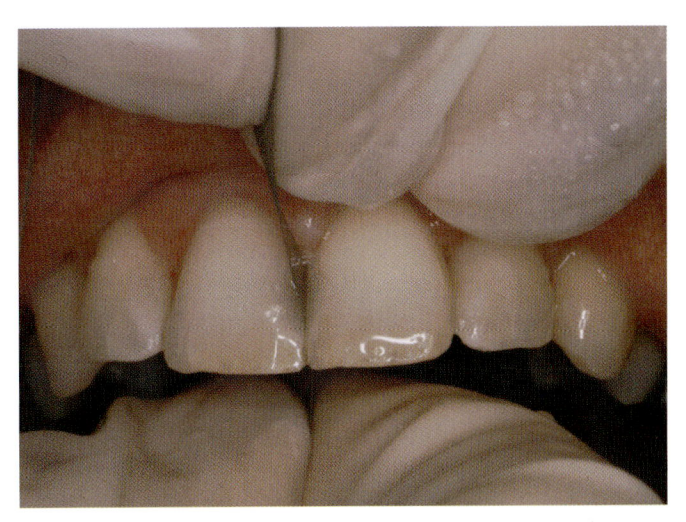

Figure 14.7 **(N)** If contact is too tight, an extra-thin abrasive diamond strip can be used to make it easier for the patient to floss (Premier Dental Products, Cosmedent, 3M, Shofu, Brasseler USA).

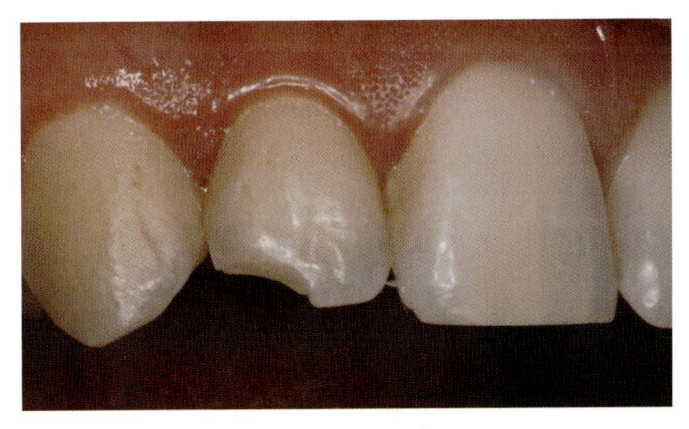

Figure 14.8 **(A)** This 18-year-old fractured his right lateral incisor in a sports accident.

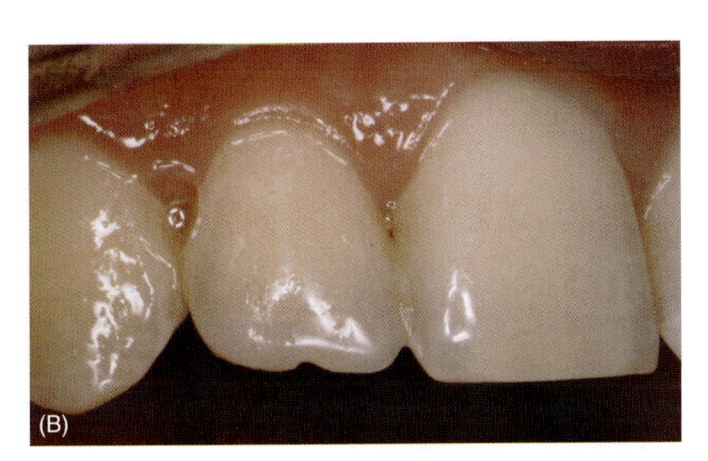

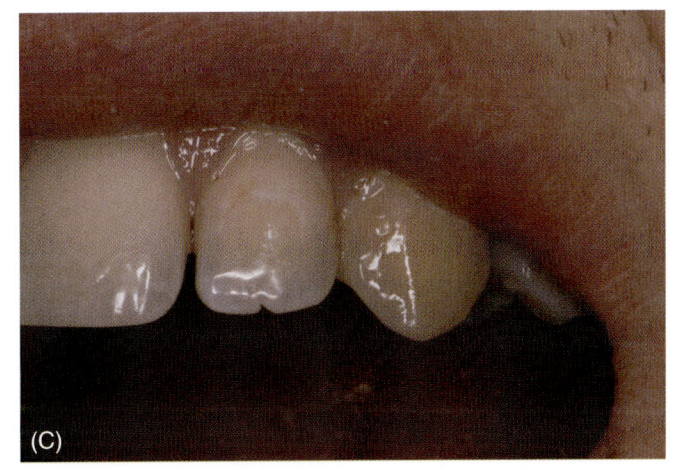

Figure 14.8 **(B and C)** The final bonded result shows a microhybrid composite resin with a color blend that successfully masks the restoration margin. Note the maxillary left lateral reveals an incisal notch that was also incorporated into the restoration of the right lateral.

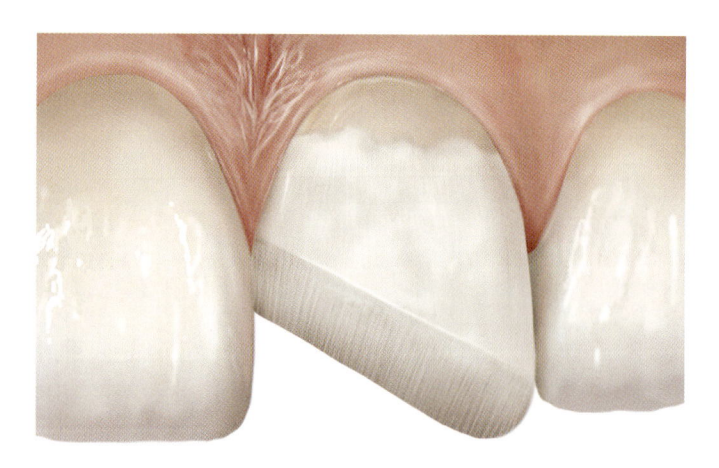

Figure 14.8 **(D)** The overlay technique is used to repair the fractured tooth and includes a long bevel and a margin that extends well past the bevel. This technique is described in greater detail in this chapter.

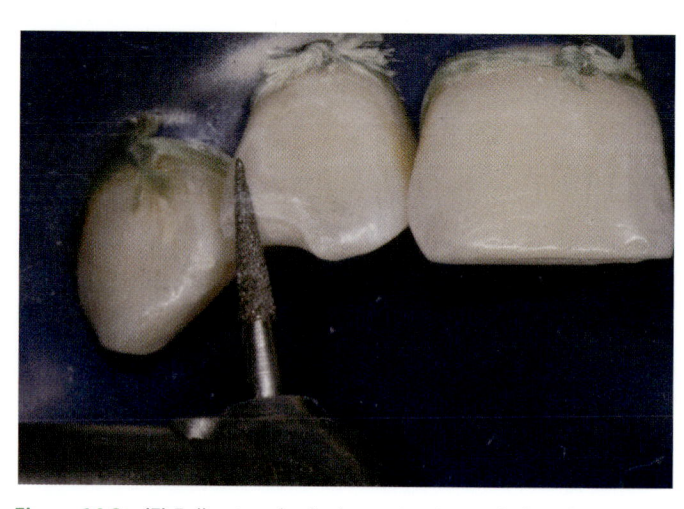

Figure 14.8 **(E)** Following shade determination and after placing the rubber dam, a long bevel is created using an extra-coarse diamond (AC2, Brasseler USA). It is also useful to roughen the enamel surfaces that will be bonded to increase surface retention.

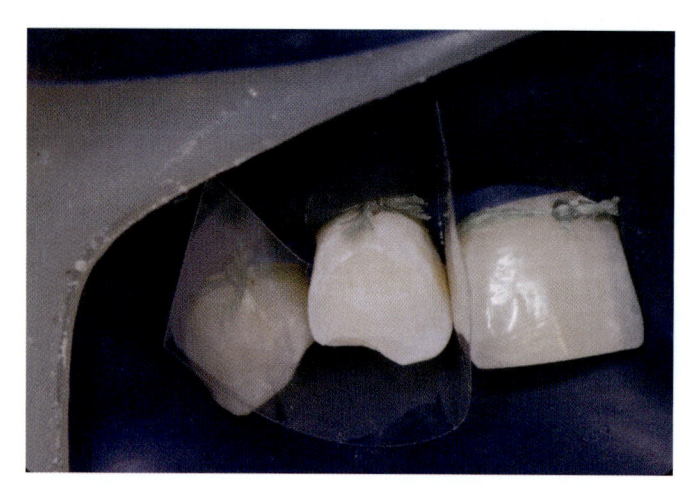

Figure 14.8 **(F)** The entire facial and lingual surface are etched with 37% phosphoric acid etch and rinsed thoroughly.

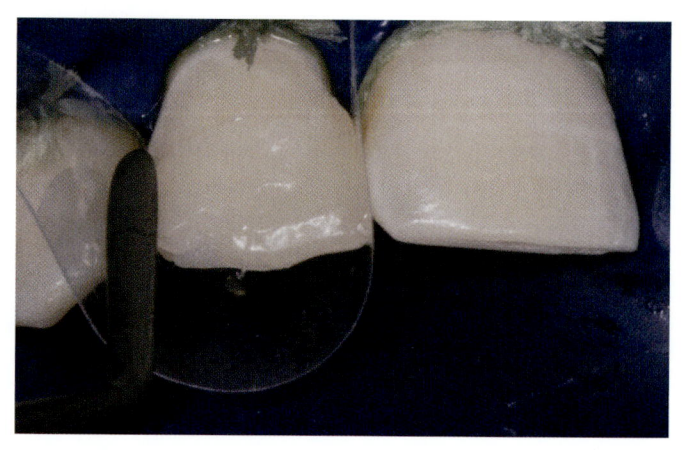

Figure 14.8 **(G)** Initial increments of the darker shade are placed, followed by an incisal overlay. The #3 Extra-Flex (TNCIGFT3, Hu-Friedy) is used in a patting, sweeping motion.

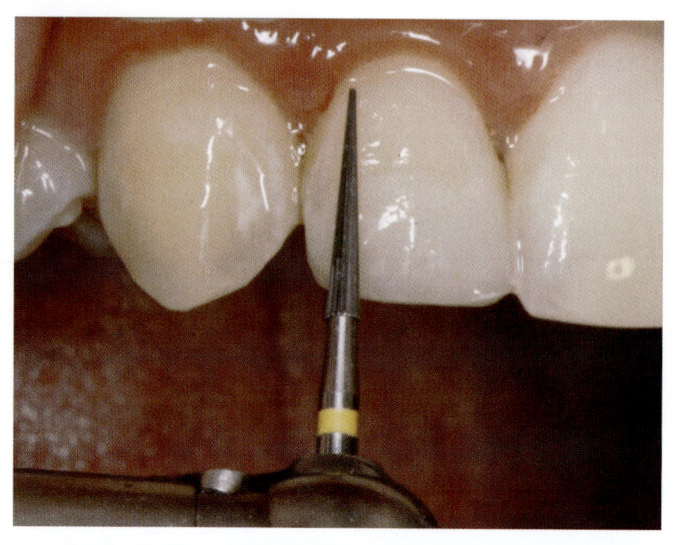

Figure 14.8 **(H)** Final contouring was completed with the 16-bladed ET9F (Brasseler USA), followed by finishing and texturing with the ET9UF 30-bladed carbide (Brasseler USA).

Chapter 14 Composite Resin Bonding

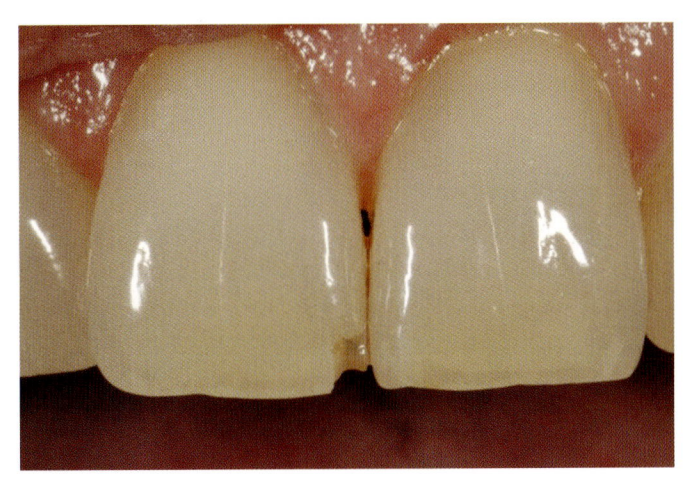

Figure 14.9 **(A)** This lady fractured her right central incisor while eating.

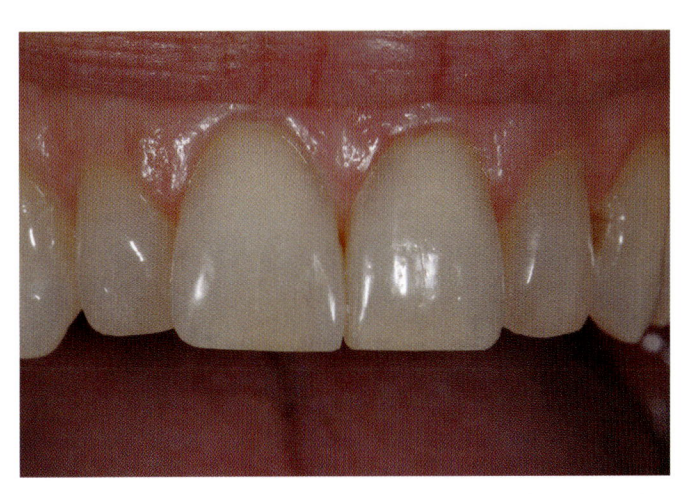

Figure 14.9 **(B)** A microfilled composite resin was used to restore the tooth to its original contours.

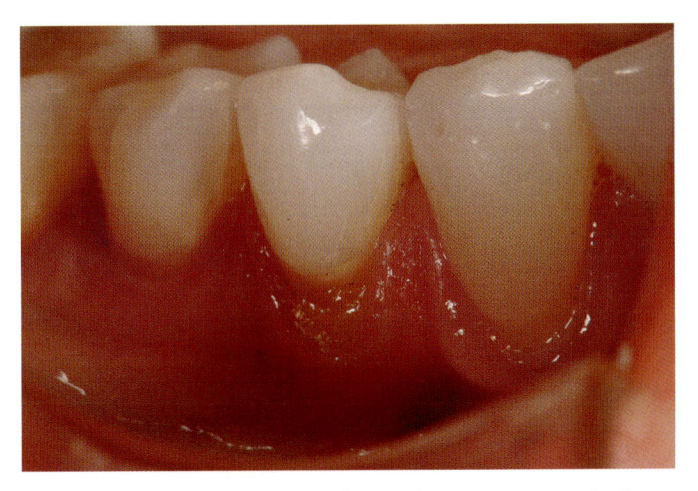

Figure 14.10 **(A)** These Class V abfraction lesions were a result of occlusal trauma.

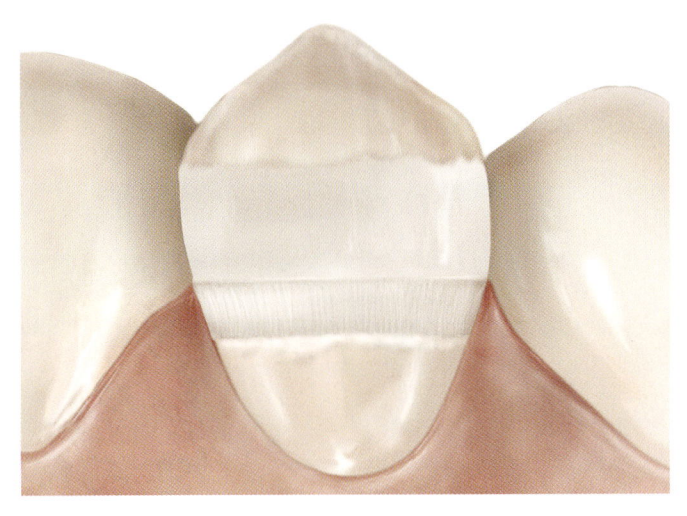

Figure 14.10 **(B)** A medium-to-long bevel is cut from the eroded surface into fresh enamel. The labioincisal or labio-occlusal margin extends to the point where there is a slight lingual inclination which will help match the tooth color.

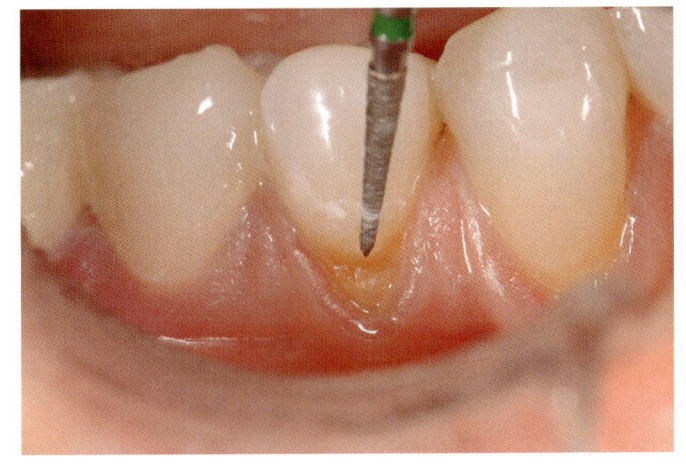

Figure 14.10 **(C)** A long bevel is added with an extra-coarse diamond (AC2, Brasseler USA).

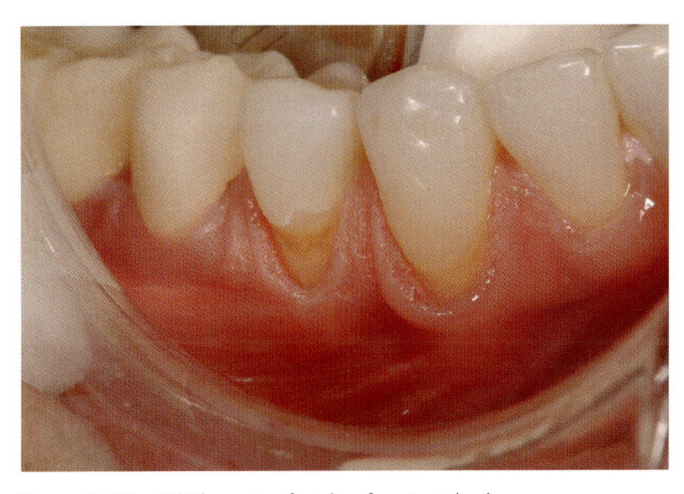

Figure 14.10 **(D)** The entire facial surface is etched.

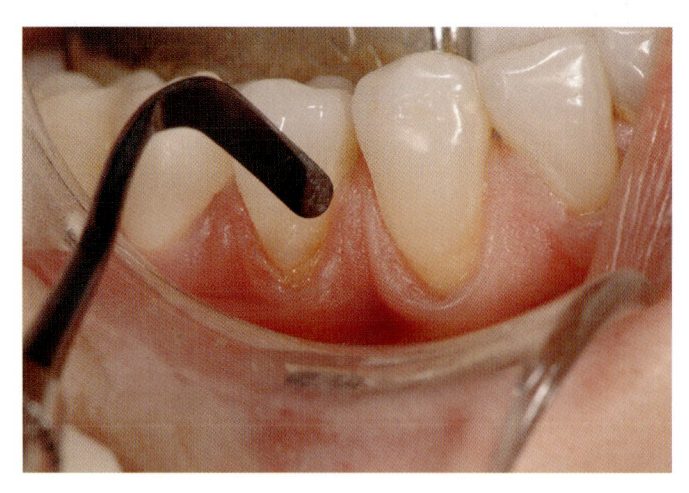

Figure 14.10 **(E)** After bonding agent is applied and polymerized, composite resin is applied in increments (TNCIGFT4, Hu-Friedy).

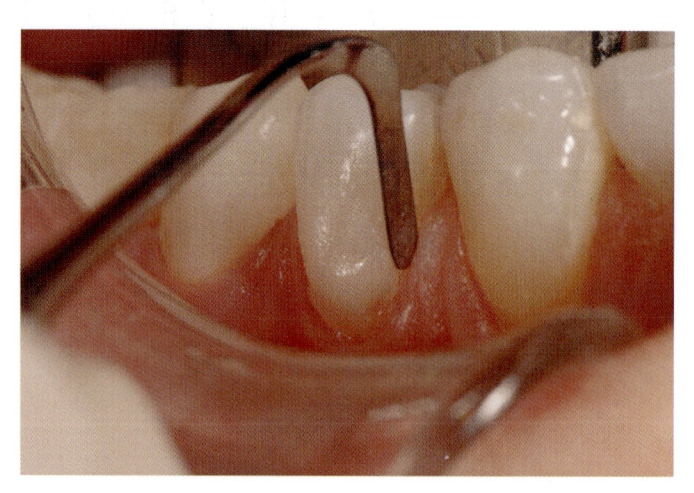

Figure 14.10 **(F)** An extra-thin composite instrument (TNCIGFT4, Hu-Friedy) is used to finalize subgingival margins without causing bleeding.

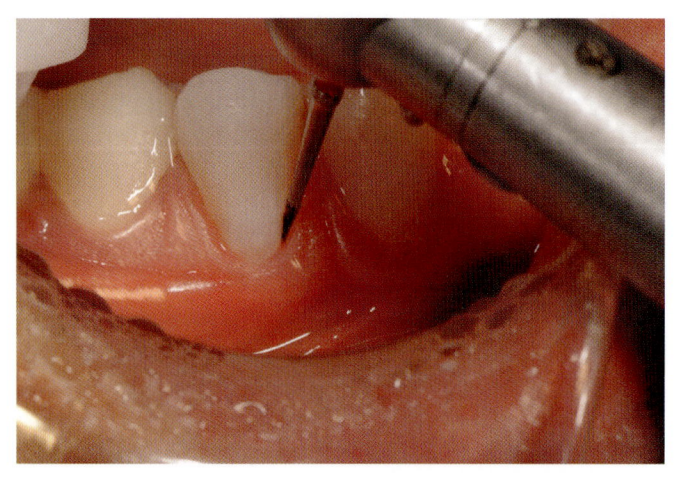

Figure 14.10 **(G)** An 8-bladed finishing carbide (ET4, Brasseler, USA) is used to help contour the gingival aspect of the Class V.

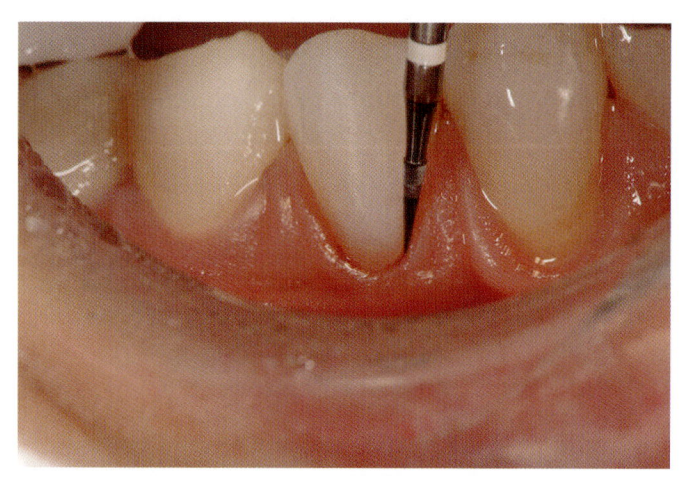

Figure 14.10 **(H)** A 30-bladed carbide (ET4UF, Brasseler USA) provides a final finish to the restoration.

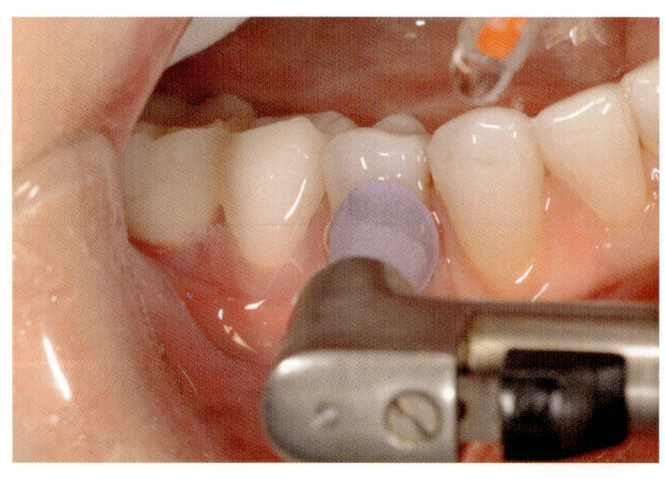

Figure 14.10 **(I)** Polishing is done with silicone rubber polishing cup (Illustra, Brasseler USA).

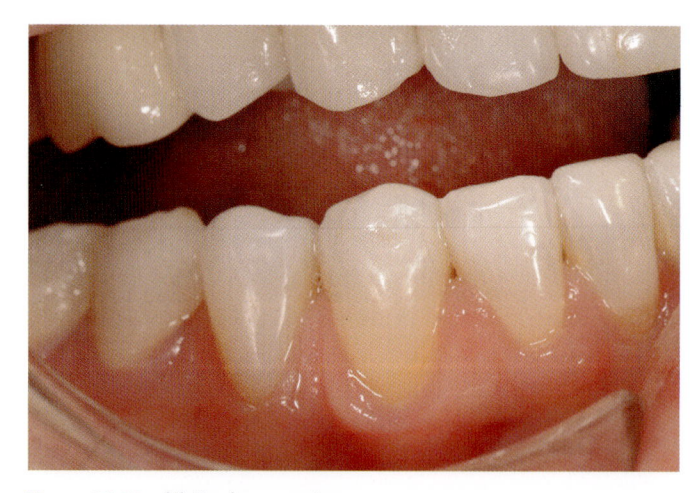

Figure 14.10 **(J)** Final restoration.

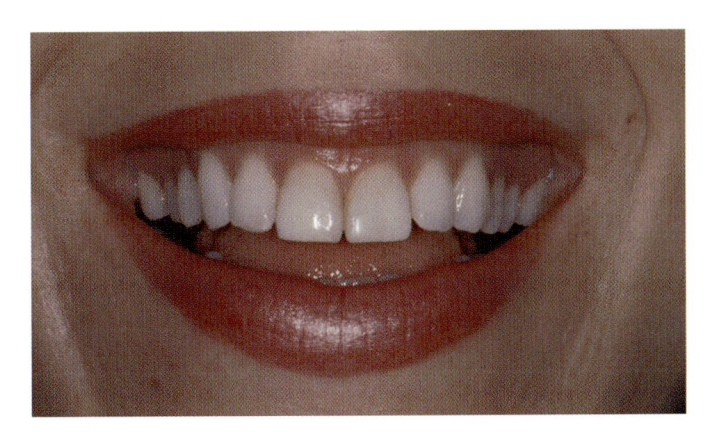

Figure 14.11 **(A)** This beauty contestant wanted a brighter, but more prominent smile.

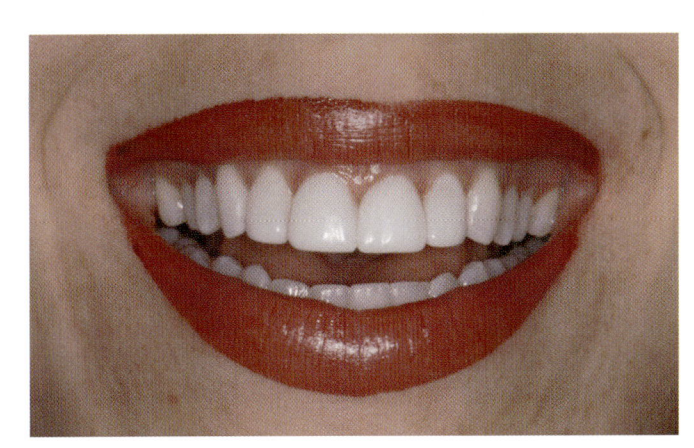

Figure 14.11 **(B)** The final result was achieved utilizing a minimally invasive technique of direct composite bonding. Her newly confident smile may have helped her win the pageant, but more importantly she won a successful career.

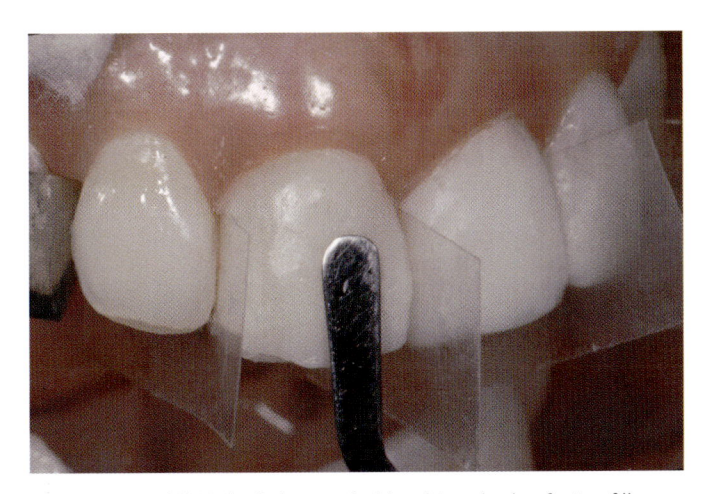

Figure 14.11 **(C)** Multiple layers of a bleaching shade of microfill composite resin was used.

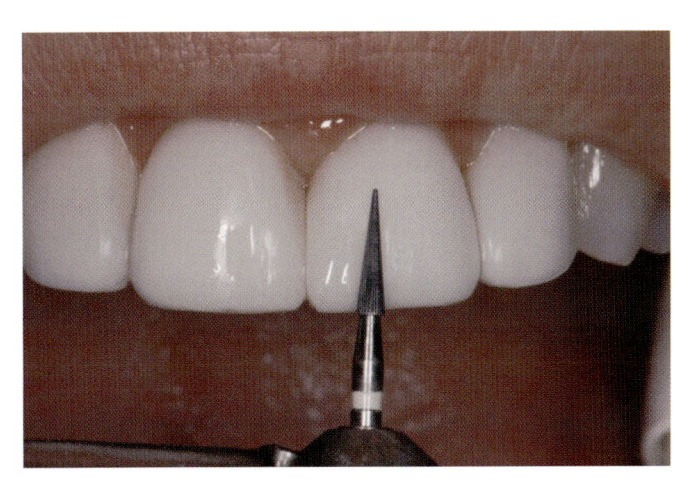

Figure 14.11 **(D)** Final surface texture was achieved using a 30-blade carbide finishing bur (ET6UF, Brasseler USA).

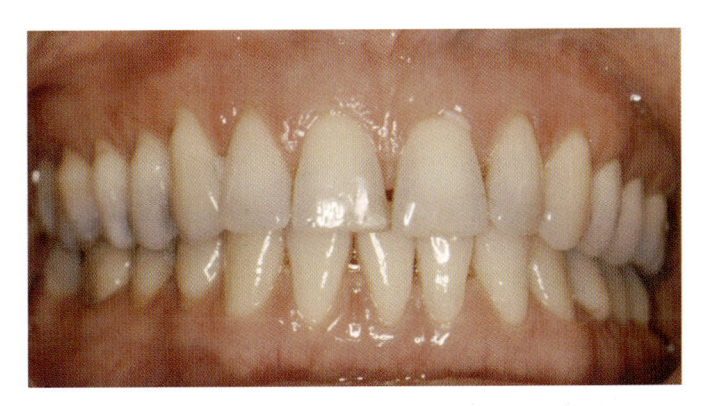

Figure 14.11 **(E)** This 46-year-old businesswoman was concerned about the wear and the loss of interdental tissue between the central incisors. Composite resin bonding was chosen as a conservative, reversible, one-appointment restoration.

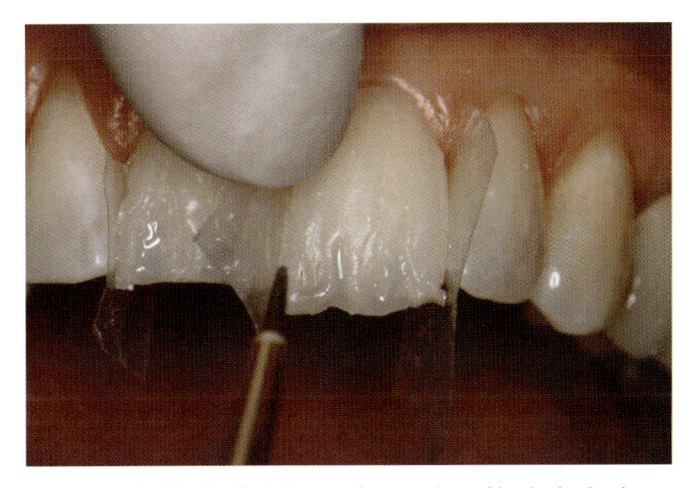

Figure 14.11 **(F)** After building up the preselected body shade, the incisal portion was serrated with a GCI 3 (Hu-Friedy). Next, medium blue stain was placed and polymerized in the serrated areas to help simulate incisal translucency.

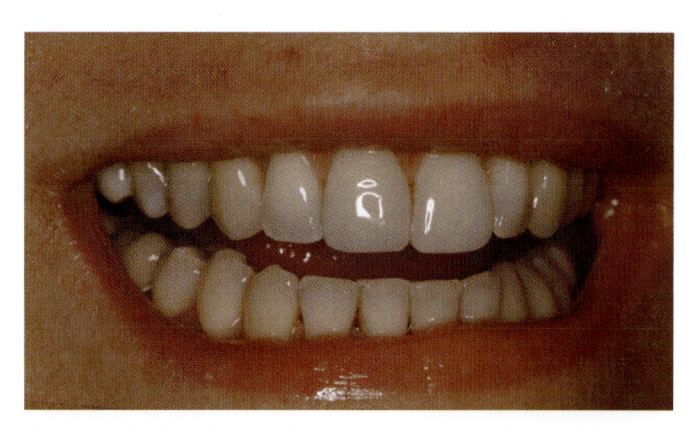

Figure 14.11 **(G)** The completed restorations provided a younger-looking smile line as well as closing the previously open gingival embrasure. Although there is the appearance of a small amount of incisal translucency, it can be enhanced by additional labial finishing.

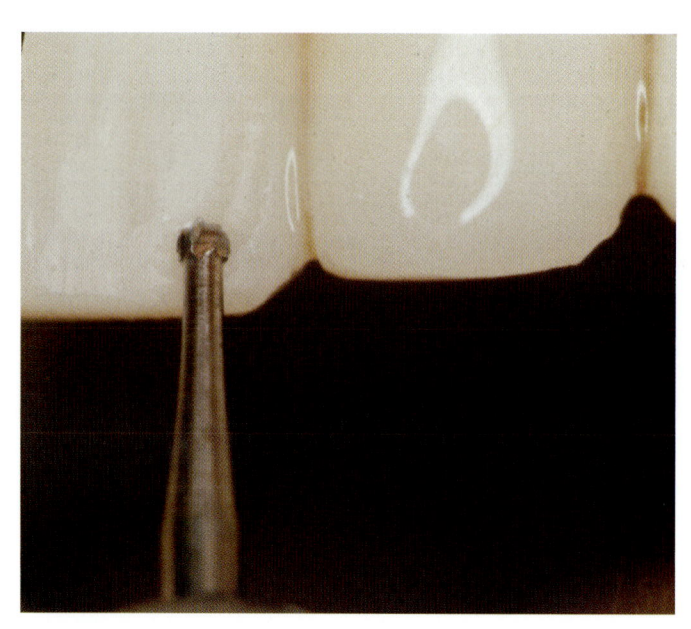

Figure 14.11 **(H)** A more precise method of achieving spot staining can be obtained by slightly cutting back the finished composite restoration.

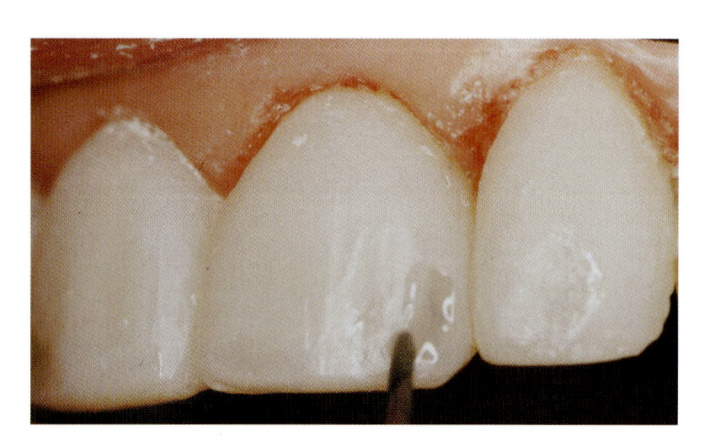

Figure 14.11 **(I)** A mild gray stain is placed and polymerized to help simulate a subtle translucency. Either body- or incisal-colored composite resin is applied and polymerized over the stained area.

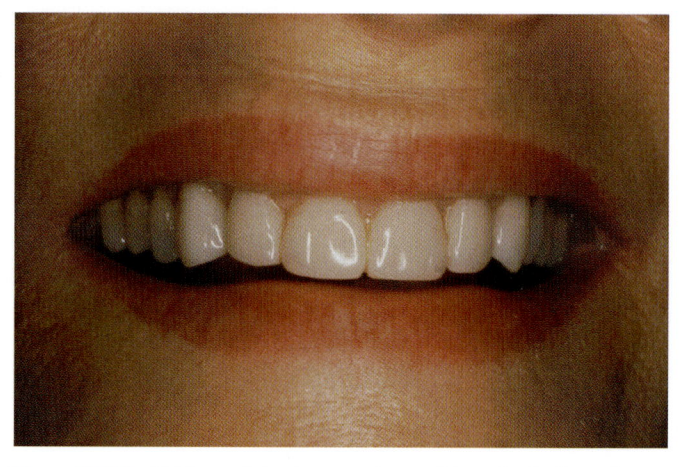

Figure 14.11 **(J)** The polished restorations achieve the feeling of slight translucency. If a more intense translucency is desired, use a darker gray or blue stain.

porcelain veneers on the anterior teeth for maximum longevity and esthetics, while using direct resin veneers on the bicuspids, and even on the first molars if necessary (Figure 14.12A–C).

Repairs of existing restorations

Chipped or fractured porcelain can be repaired quickly and esthetically with composite resin, using direct intraoral porcelain etching procedures. The esthetic life of this type of repair may be considerably shorter than for a normal bonded restoration, however, ranging anywhere from 6 months to several years. And as with most composite restorations, there will be marginal staining, especially in an anterior porcelain repair, necessitating more frequent maintenance and earlier repeat repairs. To improve the bond to porcelain, use one of the air-abrasive systems with medium pressure and a fine abrasive. See Chapter 38.

Provisional treatment

Creation of anterior guidance or posterior rehabilitation during occlusal therapy for patients with bruxism-associated myofascial pain can be achieved using bonding.[20] A hybrid composite is usually the material of choice.

Bonding is an excellent treatment selection for young persons who will have continued facial growth since it is likely that passive eruption will leave unsightly lines or the gingival margins of any veneer. But with direct-bonded veneers, the veneer can be replaced or repaired when growth is finished with either composite resin bonding or porcelain laminate veneering.[29]

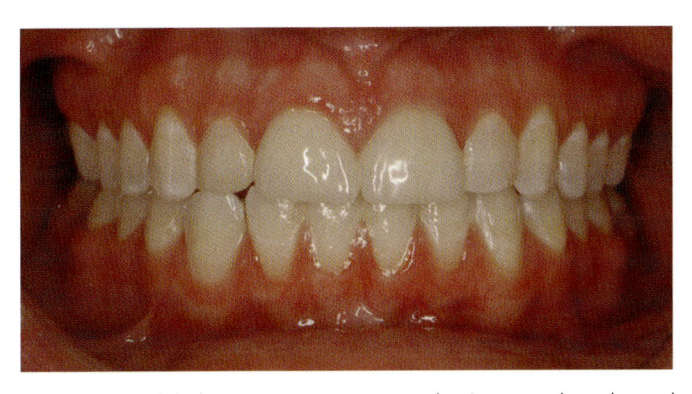

Figure 14.12 (A) This young woman wanted to improve the color and shape of her teeth.

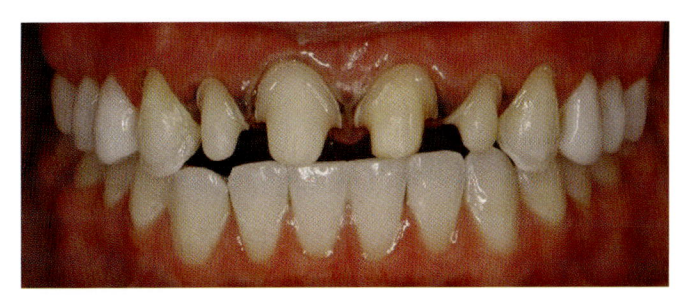

Figure 14.12 (B) For reasons of tooth preservation and economics, a treatment plan was developed that included a combination of ceramic restorations as well as direct composite resin bonding.

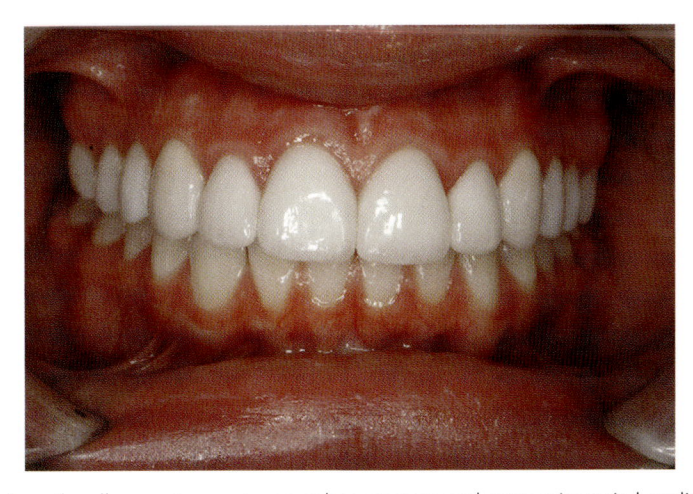

Figure 14.12 (C) Final result shows how the all-ceramic crowns, porcelain veneers, and composite resin bonding blend together.

Direct and indirect inlays

There are several methods of constructing the posterior inlay. Direct resin inlays can be cured initially in the mouth for shaping, then cured again in the laboratory, and only then bonded into the tooth preparations with resin cements. As Christiansen[30] outlines clearly, this restoration solved some of the problems seen with resin restorations cured directly in the tooth. The shrinkage during polymerization takes place in the oven, and there is less shrinkage in the marginal areas. These restorations are time consuming, but they have excellent appearance and lasting power. They also have the advantage of being "custom made," signifying quality and personalization to many patients.[31] One trade-off that must be respected is that indirect curing causes resins to become more brittle and less forgiving under occlusal loads.[32] Indirect inlays that are constructed in the laboratory have been slowly gaining acceptance. They have the same strength and wear characteristics as the direct resin inlays and onlays, but do require laboratory technicians and, thereby, greater cost. The best method of constructing posterior inlays or onlays is with a computer-assisted manufacturing apparatus, which is covered in Chapter 15 (Figure 14.13A–C).

Materials

The technique of bonding is heavily material-dependent. Bonding materials were the first esthetically substantial products used in dental restorations that were simultaneously free of mercury, resistant to corrosion, thermally nonconductive, and without galvanic reactions.[33] The availability of new materials for use in bonding has been the major player in the balancing act between esthetics and strength. Excessive rate of wear was the most serious physical limitation of early dental composite resins, limiting their use, for example, in Class I and II cavities where they are subjected to greater occlusal loads and abrasive actions.[34] However, the wear rate of posterior composites sealed with a surface-penetrating modified bisphenol A-glycidyl methacrylate (BIS-GMA) resin was reduced 50%, as reported by Dickinson et al.[35] Recently, new materials have shown improved wear resistance very similar to that of amalgam.[36,37]

The continuing improvement in bonding technology has created materials that are lasting and can be polished to a porcelain, tooth-like appearance. Earlier bonding materials had a tendency to stain, especially at the edges, and to wear. This is less true of the newer materials, especially when close attention is paid to preparation, application, and finishing.

As Jordan and Gwinnett[38] pointed out, composite materials consist primarily of resin-binding matrix and inorganic filler phases. The resin-bonding matrix is fairly consistent, with Bowen's BIS-GMA resin constituting the resin matrix of most composite materials (although urethane dimethacrylate is occasionally used in some). Composite materials differ primarily in the inorganic filler type and size of particles, and it is these differences that will determine the strength of the bonding—and, inversely, the degree to which the materials can be polished for esthetic appeal, and resistance to discoloration. The ideal composite material is highly polishable, so that the finished restoration would have the smoothness and reflective quality of enamel. It also needs to be highly resistant to chipping or fracture, with maximum durability in stress-bearing areas. Newer microhybrid and nanofilled materials have shown excellent qualities and durability. These new materials are very strong, have nice optical properties, and are able to maintain their luster.

In general, the different composites have different roles to play. When restorations are in high-stress areas, the greater filler loading of microhybrids gives them an advantage. When an enamel-like polished surface is required, microfilled composites are the material of choice.[39] However, the introduction of microhybrids, nanohybrids, and nanofilled composites have shown a great potential to be universal materials. They can be used in the posterior and anterior parts of the mouth.

Concise and extremely detailed comparative summaries of available resins and their recommended uses can be found in newsletters like *The Dental Advisor* (published by Dental Consultants, Ann Arbor, MI, USA), *Reality* (Houston, TX, USA), or *CRA Newsletter* (Provo, UT, USA), and in current journal literature. Although a few commercially available products have various degrees of shades with ranges of opacity, you will find that certain manufacturers tend to place more opacity in their composites than others. Since most BIS-GMA composites are compatible, you may choose to purchase a composite kit with the broadest possible shade range and then add additional individual shades of another brand that may have more or less opacity as you need to have the full range of shades.

Microfilled composites

The inorganic filler in most microfilled composite materials is colloidal silica, a fine white powder with a particle size of 0.04 μm. When the inorganic filler particle is this small in diameter, it is highly polishable. With proper finishing, the surface is smooth and highly reflective, much as natural enamel. However, the particle size means that the composite will not hold a large amount of inorganic filler. The maximum inorganic loading with a microfilled material may be half that of other composite materials.[11,38,40] The microfilled materials, therefore, do best in protected clinical situations such as Class III and Class V labial veneer restorations and small Class IV situations in which the occlusion can be carefully adjusted and controlled.[11] However, full labial bonded direct resin veneers are perfect for microfill composites due to their high polishability (Figure 14.14A–D).

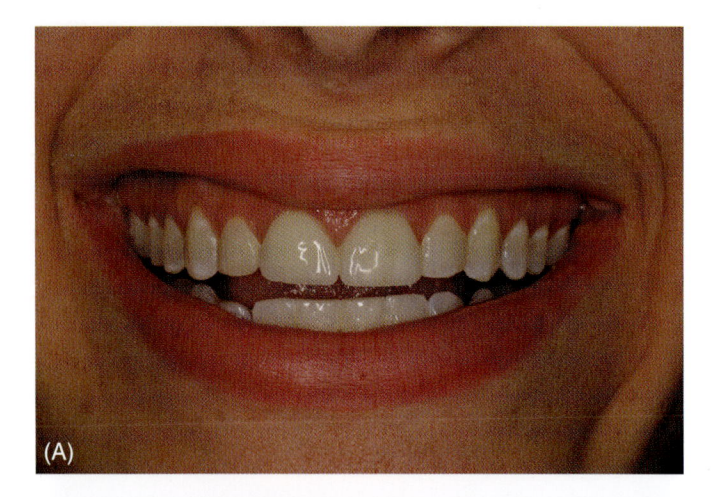

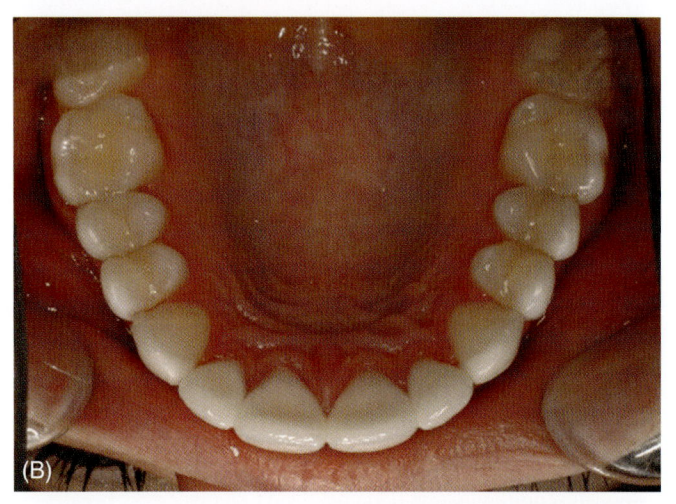

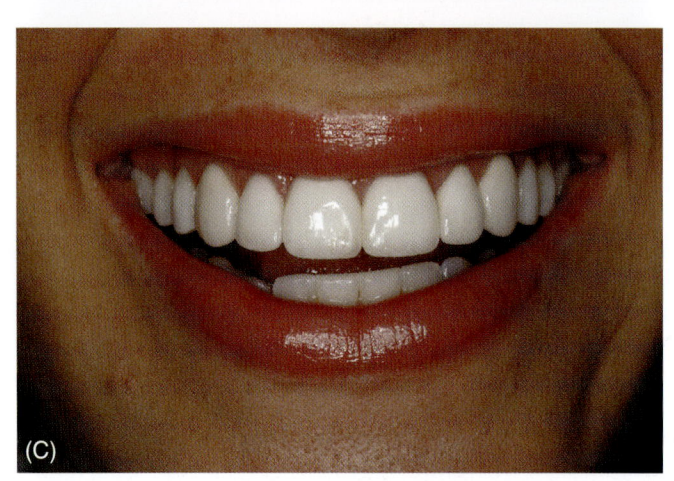

Figure 14.13 **(A)** This young woman was unhappy with her smile due to extra-large central incisor crowns, plus her discolored teeth. Since she could not afford a treatment plan based on full crowns and porcelain veneers, a compromised plan was created which included all-ceramic crowns, porcelain veneers, and direct composite resin bonding. **(B)** The occlusal view shows all-ceramic crowns on centrals and laterals, porcelain veneers on the cuspids, and direct composite resin bonding on the bicuspid and first molars. **(C)** The final smile is the whitest shade possible to please the patient.

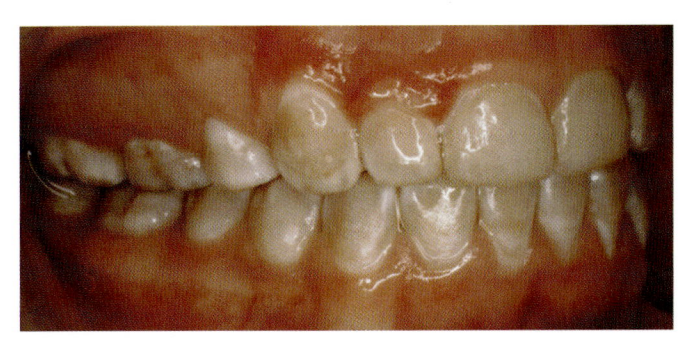

Figure 14.14 **(A)** This 14-year-old student was unhappy with her previous bonding which attempted to mask her tetracycline stain. Note how inflamed the right central, lateral, and cuspid gingival tissue was due to overhanging margins.

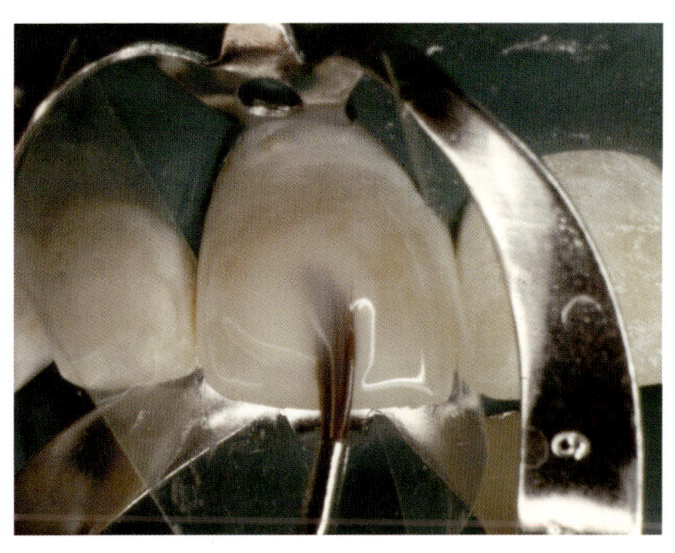

Figure 14.14 **(B)** Due to tissue inflammation, a rubber dam was placed and each tooth was individually clamped before it was bonded. Here the first of multiple layers of opaquer are applied and then polymerized.

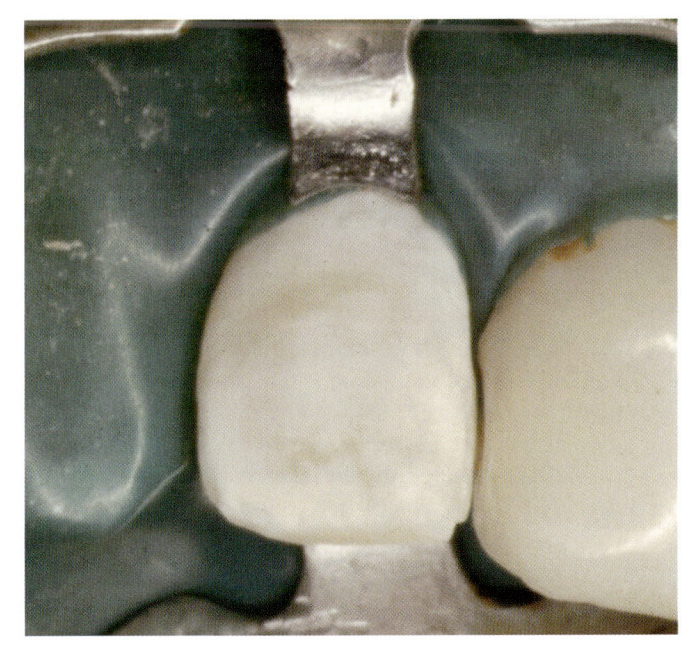

Figure 14.14 **(C)** After multiple layers of the lighter shade of microfill composite resin are applied, polymerized, and finished on the right central, the right lateral is treated.

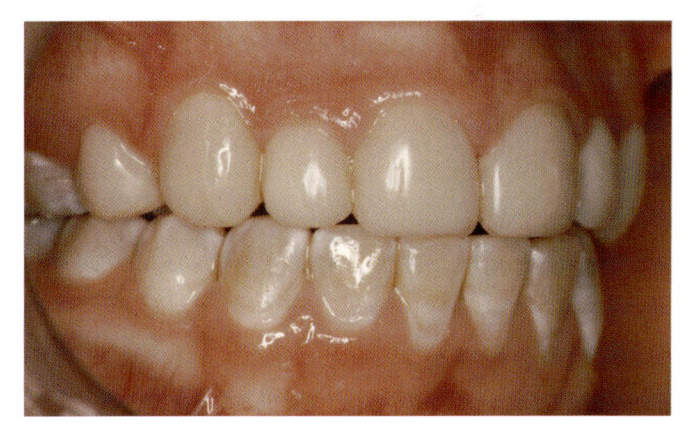

Figure 14.14 **(D)** After 2 weeks, note the final result shows a more favorable color and an improved tissue response to properly finished margins.

Small-particle macrofilled composites

Composite materials in which the size of the inorganic filler particles is between 1 and 8 μm are only semipolishable, with a duller, less reflective surface after finishing. They are more resistant to fracture, however. This makes them highly appropriate in Class IV situations exposed to heavy occlusal loads. These types of materials are obsolete for use in modern bonding where strength and polishability are essential, especially in the anterior region.

Hybrid, microhybrids, and nanohybrid composites

These composite materials address the trade-off between esthetics and strength, combining reasonable polishability with increased resistance to fracture. Average particle size for these materials is about 1 μm. Clinical trials have provided data on the long-term effectiveness of these composites, so they were widely used. In fact, the trend in composite resin technology has been toward smaller average particle size and higher filler loadings.[6] The dental industry has improved the processing of materials which permit high loading and finer particle texture to be achieved together.[41] Advances in technology have allowed a reduction of the particle size used in the fabrication of composites. Thus the average particle size has decreased to a submicron size (about 0.4 μm). Because of the submicron size the new generation of hybrid materials received the name "microhybrids." These materials with enhanced properties and improved appearance have been the workhorse of the profession for the last 15 years. In more recent years the incorporation of even smaller fillers with the purpose of changing handling properties has resulted in naming some of these materials "nanohybrids." These "microhybrids" and "nanohybrids" have good physical properties, polish well, and are esthetic and strong enough to be used universally.

Nanofilled composites

This category of material indicates a new development in resin composites technology. These materials incorporate silanated silica and very small zirconia particles as well as agglomerates or clusters of zirconia and silica. The particle size for these materials varies between 80 and 20 nm. The cluster or agglomeration behaves as a large particle filler, providing strength. Because of the small particle of the agglomerate they can be polished to a high luster.

Bonding techniques

The underlying aim of bonding techniques, just as for the selection of materials, is to achieve an esthetic effect while creating a strong retention of the composite material to the surface and especially the margins of the area to which it has been applied. Not only must the bonded material hold up under stress, but it must eliminate marginal leakage which can destroy your esthetic results.

As with any clinical esthetic procedure, the first step is to make photographic records prior to even cleaning the teeth. This provides the "before" for your restorative "after" photos, and it also provides information about the patient's oral hygiene and stain-forming habits that may threaten the esthetic effect you are about to create. This photographic documentation can prove invaluable if later a question arises about what you did and why you did it. Remember, even the best of patients can have a short memory. Only after the photographs are made should you pumice the area thoroughly and take all steps to provide a thoroughly clean surface. As noted by Paquette,[42] failure to remove all debris from every surface of the tooth to be restored may result in a "peeling" of the composite, especially interproximally. It is probably not a good idea to appoint a patient for resin placement on the same day as a recall prophylaxis because crevicular weeping/hemorrhage can undermine every step of the bonding technique. Instead, allow soft tissue to heal and be certain that your patient is maintaining good home care. Miura et al. have demonstrated that a prophylactic cleaning of enamel raised bond strength by approximately 50%. No wonder Gwinnett called the interface between resin and tissue the potentially weakest link between restorative resin and enamel. He advocated a thorough dental prophylaxis to remove deposits (including calculus) from the enamel to allow the acidic conditioning agent, namely phosphoric acid, to exert its optimal effect.[18,43] Gwinnett also reported that the use of ethanol to remove any residual water from the etched enamel enhances the ability of resin monomers to penetrate the surface irregularities.[18]

An optimal working field can be achieved through careful isolation of the teeth, usually with a rubber dam, after pumicing and rinsing. Do not use prophylactic pastes which contain glycerin and fluoride, however, since these will act as barriers to etching solutions.[10] Brockmann[44] has demonstrated that air abrasion prior to etching a tooth for occlusal sealants creates an enhanced retentive surface. Air abrasion increases the number of enamel "tags," thereby permitting more saturation of the resin.

Possible limitations of routinely using an air-abrasion instrument may be that the force of the spray can cause gingival hemorrhage or crevicular weeping when close to the gingival sulcus. Goldstein has also advocated using an extra-course diamond bur on enamel surface prior to etching (AC2 diamond, Brasseler USA), especially if the surface may have been previously bonded. Then follow up with air abrasion.

Shade selection

This step of the procedure merits a significant amount of time to test and consider a complex mix of factors. Recognize that there can be a marked difference, one noticeable to the naked eye, between color shades and resin samples, especially for the incisal colors and the deep and dark colors.[45] Compounding the difficulty of shade selection are, according to Makinson, color changes that develop during curing. He found that, in general, all become lighter, with some becoming more opaque and some transparent. It therefore follows that a cured try-in of the shade(s) that you have selected offers a good idea of the color of the final restoration.[46] These factors include color of the dentin and enamel and, as discussed previously, the color of the liner. Custom composite shade guides may somewhat improve shade matching.[47]

Prior to shade selection the operator needs to consider several factors as follows:

1. **Teeth need to be clean.** Use a rubber cup and pumice to clean the tooth to be restored and adjacent teeth. It is quite often that a shade needs to be selected from the adjacent tooth, such is the case of a discolored restoration in a central incisor to be restored. In this case the shade needs to be selected from the contralateral incisor to achieve shade match and symmetry between the central incisors.

2. **Avoid dehydration.** Dehydration has proven to make teeth whiter and more opaque. It is a good idea to ask the patient to keep the teeth wet during shade selection.

3. **Use good light.** It is recommended that the operatory environment is properly illuminated in amount of light and type. Color-corrected fluorescent lights with a temperature of 5500 K and a color rendering index (CRI) of at least 90 is the best suited for shade determination. It is recommended that operatory light unit light be turned off because most units use incandescent light which emits orange-red hues.

4. **Remove any surrounding strong color** like lipstick and cover colorful clothing with the patient napkin.

5. **Be brief when selecting shades.** The response time of the rods and cones to differentiate color is short. A determination between shades should be limited to 4–5 s.

6. **If possible, use a shade guide made of the resin composite to be utilized.** It is beneficial to have a shade guide made from the brand of resin composite of choice by the clinician. Most manufacturers of resin composite use nomenclatures based on the Vitapan Classical shade guide. Unfortunately, resin composite shades do not always match those of the Vitapan shade and furthermore the shades among manufacturers do not match each other.

Regardless of whether you have operatory lights that are color-corrected, getting the right amount of color-corrected light into the oral cavity can be challenging. One of the most efficient ways to clearly delineate between tooth and resin shade is by using a specially designed light source that allows you to evaluate your intended shade with different color-corrected light (Figure 14.15).

Clinical procedure for shade selection

Organize the custom shade guide, from lightest to darkest. Position the patient in the chair at eye level, retract the lips, and run the whole shade guide parallel to the incisal edges of the teeth to be restored. Select three or four of the closest shades. Repeat the process with these fewer shades until the closest shade is selected. This process of elimination is usually very reliable for shade selection (Figure 14.16A–G).

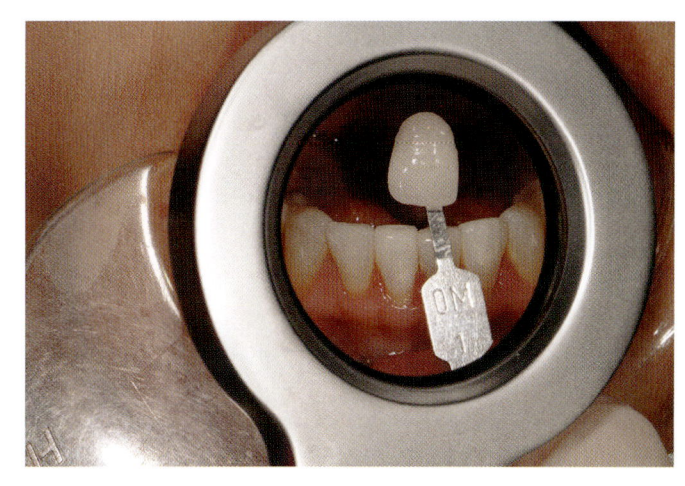

Figure 14.15 An accurate, close-up source of color-corrected light is important in shade selection (Rite-Lite, AdDent).

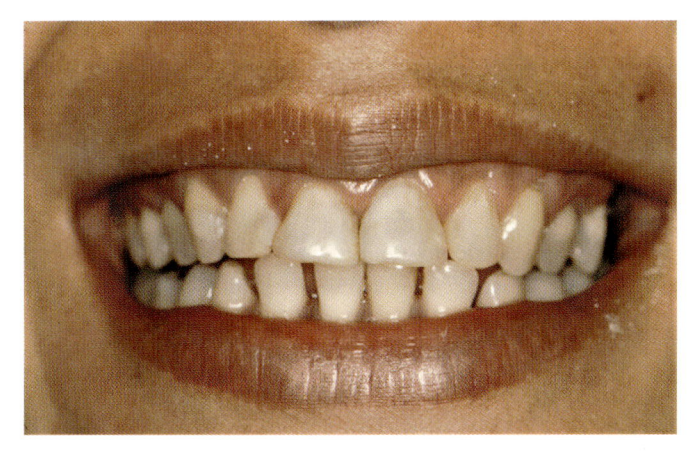

Figure 14.16 **(A)** This 37-year-old prima ballerina was dissatisfied with her discolored, protruding, and spaced teeth. Although orthodontics was the strongly suggested treatment of choice, composite resin bonding was chosen instead as an economic and quick compromise solution to her esthetic problem.

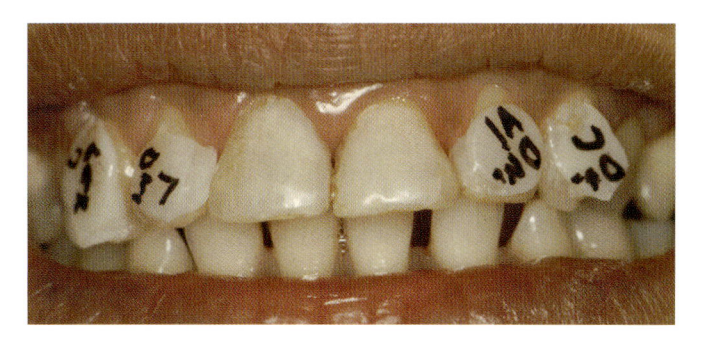

Figure 14.16 **(B)** Multiple shades of composite resin from different manufacturers were applied and polymerized to help determine which shade to use.

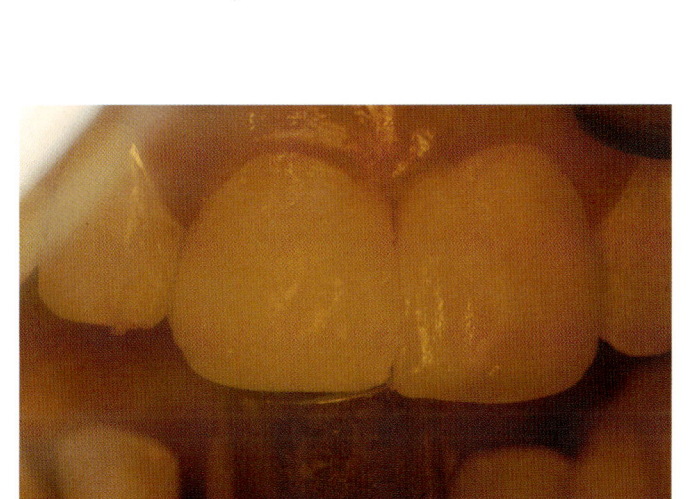

Figure 14.16 **(C)** Composite resin is applied in incremental layers on the central incisors first. During polymerization, a protective eye shield is used.

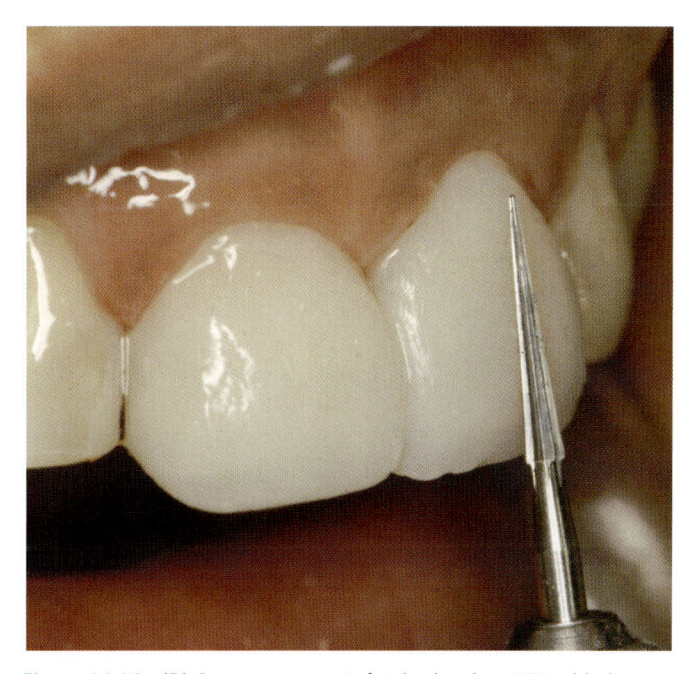

Figure 14.16 **(D)** Composite resin is finished with an ET9 8-blade carbide (Brasseler USA).

In choosing the color, obviously the choice will be the closest shade possible to the tooth that is available with your brand of composite resin. It may be necessary to use a combination of two or even more shades to arrive at the proper depth of color. If so, always use the darker shade first to achieve a depth of color that will look more natural in the mouth. However, for a Class III restoration in a tooth with multiple shades, the lighter (matching the incisal value) composite should be inserted first, and then layered with the shades that match the gingival portion. You may also perform a cutback and then use stains or darker shades, like the repair technique, to provide the most esthetic result.

Once you have chosen a shade, or better yet, a combination of shades or tints/opaques cotton dry the tooth, and place a small amount of composite resin on the tooth. Using a mylar strip to hold the material in place, polymerize with your curing light. Isolation tends to desiccate the tooth, making it appear lighter than it actually will be under normal circumstances, and there is danger in assuming the shade will match if the tooth has been kept dry too long. Therefore, do this step of the shade selection phase of treatment as rapidly as possible. Avoid using cotton rolls and save the tooth drying until the last moment; even then, complete the polymerizing as rapidly as possible. If you anticipate difficulty in matching your patient's tooth color, consider making a separate appointment to spend the necessary time to properly complete this important step. This extra appointment should definitely be considered if your patient's shade is not going to be an easy one to match.

Tooth preparation

Most dentists have been taught standard preparation designs intended to conserve tooth structure and preserve natural tooth contacts whenever possible. A 90° angle of exit is often used when maximum conservation of tooth structure is desired.[10] A chamfer in enamel also allows for a 90° angle of exit, which provides a more durable margin, but it is the least conservative design and most dentists turn to it only when maximum retention is necessary. Modern concepts of cavity preparation for resin composite calls for caries removal followed by a bevel if necessary for esthetics or to increase bonding surface area. The most commonly used finish line for resin composites is a 45° bevel on the enamel. This bevel conserves much of the tooth structure and provides more exposure to the ends of the enamel rods while providing a superior seal to enamel, particularly at the gingival margins.[48,49]

Myers and Butts believe that a bevel of the cavosurface enamel provides increased surface area for resin bonding, reduces microleakage, and improves esthetics in restorations of permanent teeth with acid-etch composite resin.[50] Moore and Vann found that beveling the margin of posterior composite resins reduces microleakage.[51]

The overlay method

For the past 30 years, Goldstein has used a preparation design, which he called the overlay technique: it is a procedure that greatly enhances the esthetic appeal of the bonding without sacrificing stability. A 4–5 mm long finish line is placed past the bevel of the cavosurface margin of a Class III, IV, or V restoration. Although in normal circumstances undercutting will not be necessary, some roughening of the enamel can enhance the

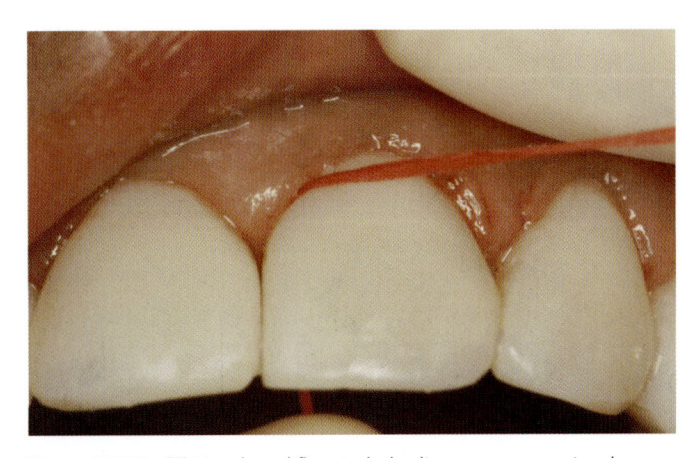

Figure 14.16 **(E)** Use dental floss to help discover any previously undetected overhangs.

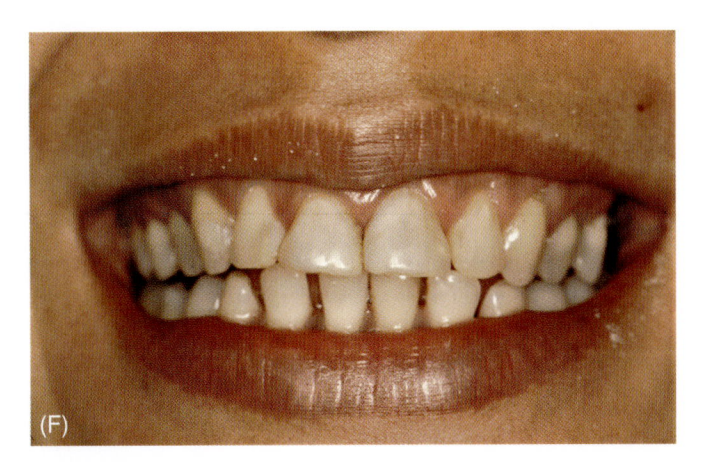

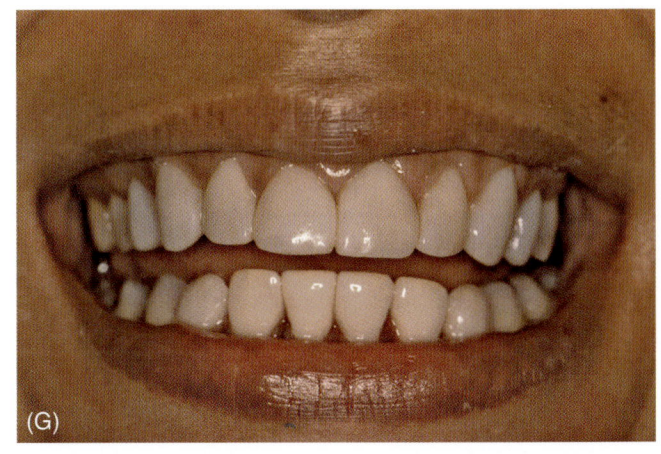

Figure 14.16 **(F and G)** Before and after treatment demonstrate the patient's greatly enhanced smile with improved proportions and lighter tooth shade.

color blend as well as surface retention. It is helpful to round the ending of the enamel bevel to produce a so-called "infinite bevel" to improve blending of the resin composite over enamel. Scalloping of the bevel could prove beneficial in several instances where the preparation is in a straight line, like in a fracture of the incisal edge due to trauma. The scalloping allows for a nonlinear bevel which enhances blending (Figure 14.17A–H).

This overlay technique means that the actual margin of the new restoration overlays the beveled and roughened tooth surface. Remember to etch the enamel involved in the overlay technique and take it even further to ensure adequate enamel preparation and seal. This has several advantages. Esthetic restorations often are trade-offs between beauty and strength—or perhaps more accurately between esthetic appeal the day the patient leaves the office and esthetic appearance some months or years later. The overlay technique provides the best esthetic result today and yet also greatly enhances the durability and esthetic life of the restoration for the future.

First, the overlay technique enhances the color blend from the gingival to the incisal or occlusal part of the labial or lingual surface. With a variable margin, there is a natural transition to and through the different colors of your patient's enamel.

Second, the overlay technique has an extremely important function as a method for tooth lengthening. Figure 14.18A–I illustrate the technique of beveling the labioincisal surfaces of mandibular anterior incisors or shortening the entire incisal surface to allow for the lengthening of the maxillary anterior teeth. The decision of whether to bevel or shorten is dependent largely

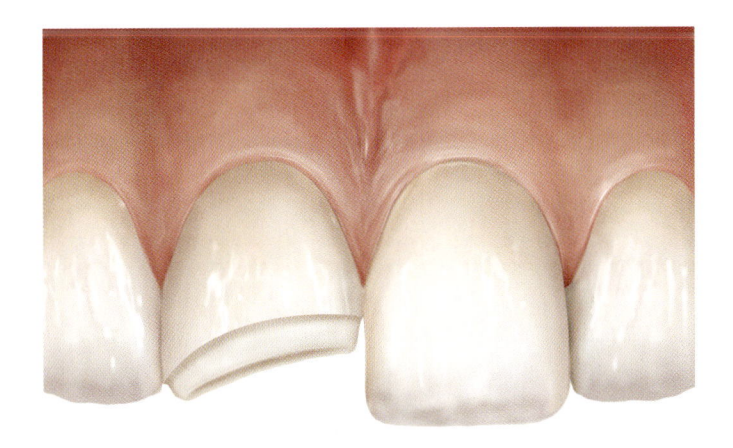

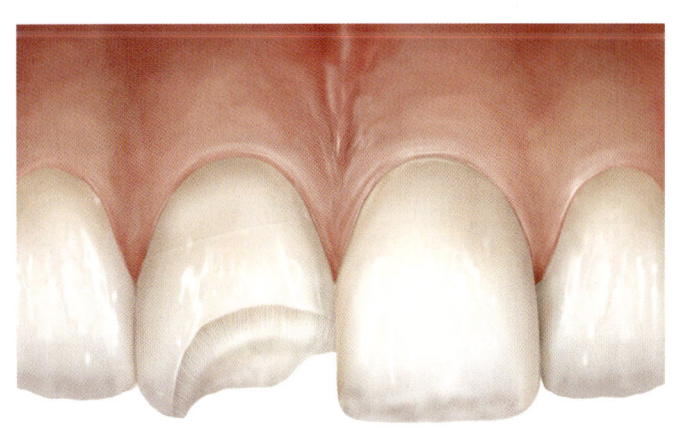

Figure 14.17 **(A)** The fractured right central incisor requires repair with composite resin. Two major repair options are chamfer-shoulder and overlay techniques.

Figure 14.17 **(B)** This illustrates the chamfer-shoulder preparation. Note the margin is situated just above the fracture site.

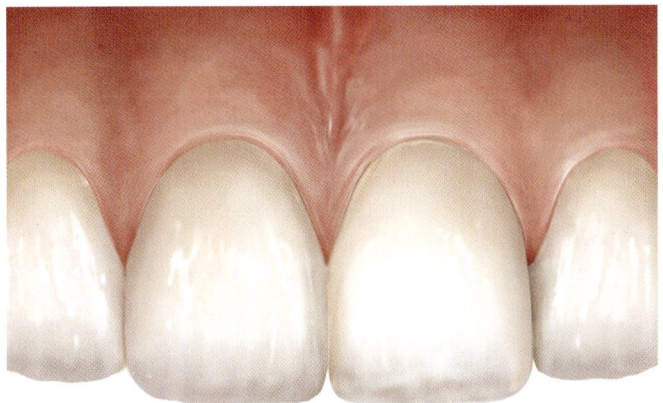

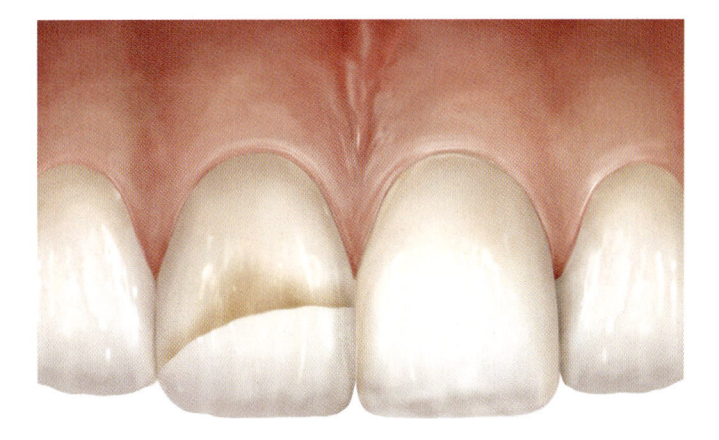

Figure 14.17 **(C)** The overlay technique requires a long bevel and an overlaid margin that extends into the cervical portion of the labial surface and in many instances, subgingivally.

Figure 14.17 **(D)** If performed correctly, both techniques can produce an esthetic result with invisible margins.

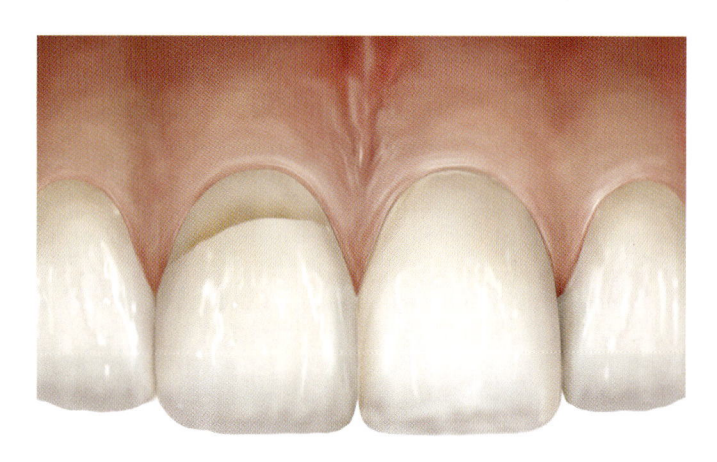

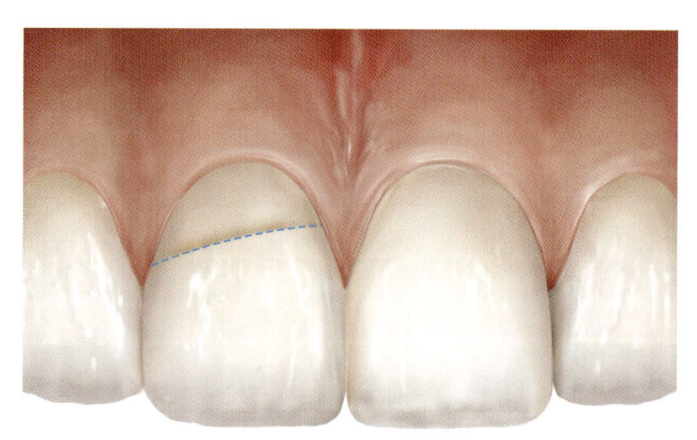

Figure 14.17 **(E)** When inevitable staining occurs, it appears at the marginal junction between the tooth and composite resin. Here stain is seen at the labial margin of the chamfer-shoulder technique. A repair procedure is required to remove the stain.

Figure 14.17 **(F)** With the overlay technique, stain usually appears closer to the cervical margin and is much easier to eliminate using a simple polishing procedure.

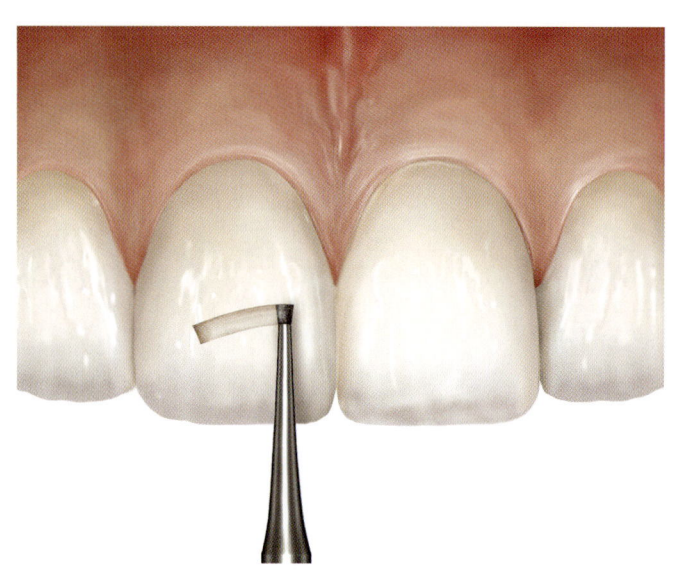

Figure 14.17 **(G)** Since simple polishing would result in a concavity, the chamfer-shoulder technique requires a cut-and-patch repair to eliminate stain.

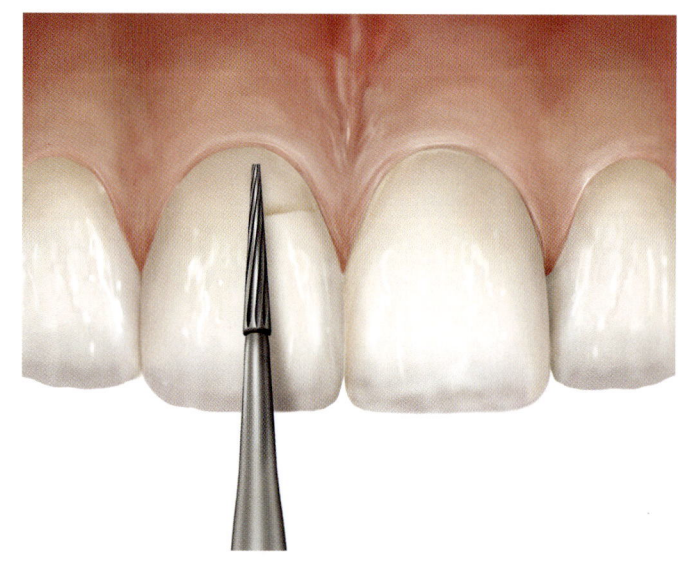

Figure 14.17 **(H)** In the overlay technique, stain can be removed simply by finishing with a 30-blade carbide bur and repolishing, thus achieving a more conservative and economic solution. These advantages, plus ability to achieve a good color blend, make the overlay method the technique of choice.

upon the incisal plane and the arc of the mandibular anterior teeth. Although orthodontic therapy is generally the treatment of choice, many patients elect the restorative compromise. Further, composite resin overlay can extend the longevity of the restoration by providing resiliency as a measure of protection against possible future fracture.

Third, depending on the patient's lip line, staining is less likely to be objectionable because margins are usually placed out of sight either subgingivally or high enough to be concealed by the lip line. A major esthetic problem with any composite restoration is the staining that almost invariably occurs at the margin of tooth and composite. The overlay technique provides the restoration a longer esthetic life without having to pursue a repair technique; staining can usually be corrected by merely polishing the stain away to a new margin further up or down the enamel surface. Figure 14.17 illustrates how much easier it is to freshen a tooth with an overlay technique versus the chamfer-shoulder method, thus avoiding replacing or even repairing the restoration.

Fourth, it also is a more forgiving preparation. With its gentle lines and lack of precise margins, it becomes an easier restoration to complete.

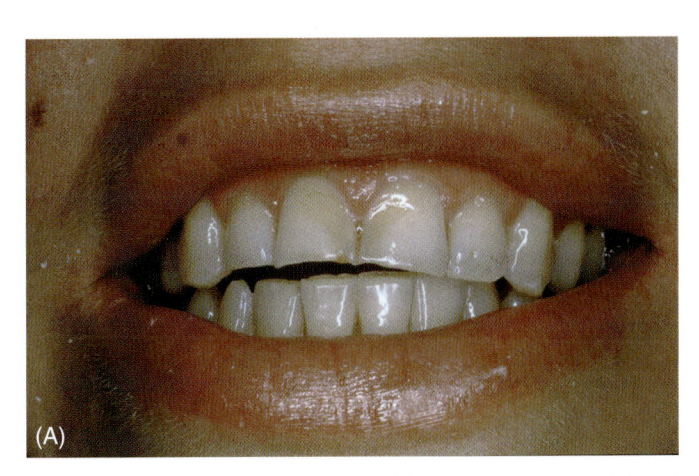

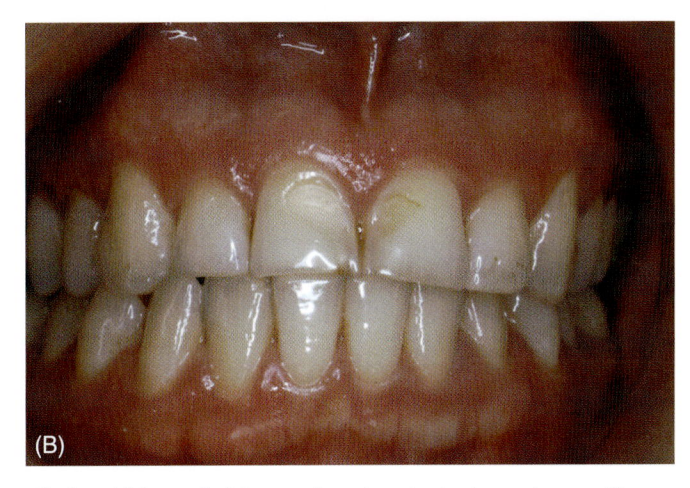

Figure 14.18 **(A and B)** This 23-year-old dancer was concerned about her smile. In addition to facial enamel erosion, she had worn her maxillary anterior teeth so much from bruxism that it made her smile appear deformed.

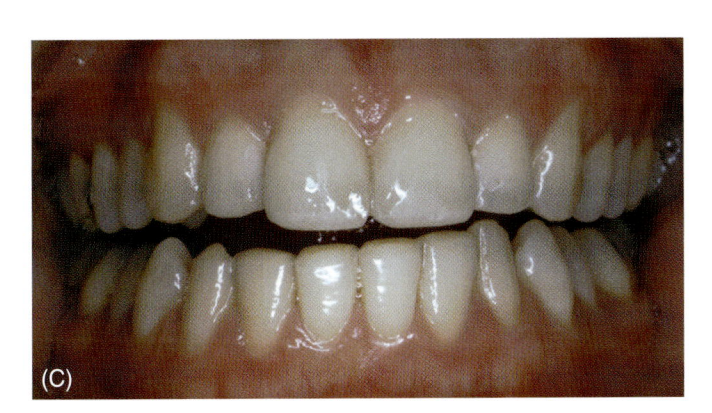

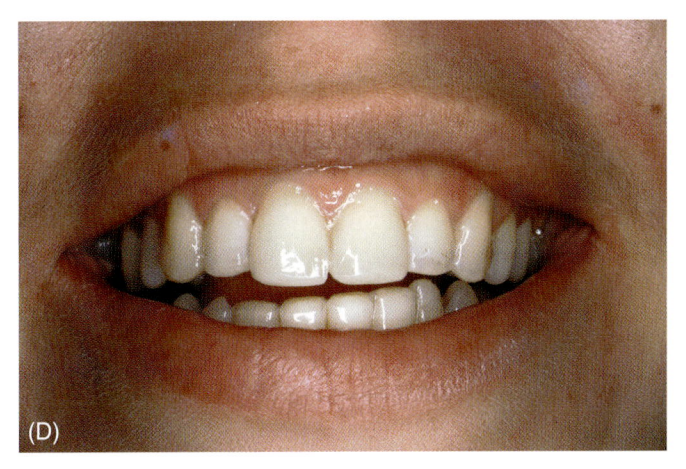

Figure 14.18 **(C and D)** The patient chose an economical and immediate result using composite resin bonding to restore the normal length of her anterior teeth. The incisal edges of the mandibular incisors were cosmetically contoured to compensate for the new length of the maxillary anterior incisors.

Enamel bonding and acid etch

As Phillips pointed out,[4] there are two basic mechanisms for bonding. The purely mechanical can be illustrated by acid-etching of enamel to provide resin tag formation into the surface roughnesses. Adhesive bonding implies molecular attraction between the adhesive and the substrata and is the basis of dentin-bonding agents and polyacrylic acid cements.

The significance of bonding materials to tooth structure is not, of course, purely esthetic. They also serve to protect enamel rods and dentinal tubules, which are inherently opened during preparation, from the effects of bacterial contamination by saliva. In fact, they must protect in order to obtain a satisfactory long-term esthetic and functional result. If microleakage occurs because of lack of a true seal of the restoration, then acids and microorganisms may penetrate from the margins down along the interface, which can lead to stain or even secondary caries.[52] If leakage progresses down and across the floor of the preparation, it also can produce pulpal irritation.[4] However, studies would indicate that restorative materials produce pulpal reactions only when there is bacterial leakage and little or no irritation if bacterial influences are effectively controlled.[53] Cariostatic fluoride-releasing composites or planning a resin-modified glass ionomer base may serve to limit recurrent caries, as proposed by Temin et al.[54] Resin-bonded inlay restorations can provide superb marginal seal, especially at the cervical restoration–dentin interface.[32]

If both enamel and dentin are involved, it is best to etch the enamel with a gel since the gel causes localized penetration that is deeper and wider.[55] It is also self-limiting. It remains exactly where you place it, instead of "running all over the place" on tissue or adjacent teeth or even on unwanted same tooth surface. A 15–30 s gel application should be sufficient to etch the enamel. Although it is not necessary to etch glass ionomer, some clinicians feel a 5 s final etch on just this portion will condition any remaining tooth structure as well as the base itself. However, it is important to consider the individual tooth. Young teeth generally etch more quickly than older teeth. The fluoride content of the teeth also affects etching time, as does whether or not the enamel has been freshly cut. Freshly cut enamel etches faster than unprepared enamel.[10]

(E) (F)

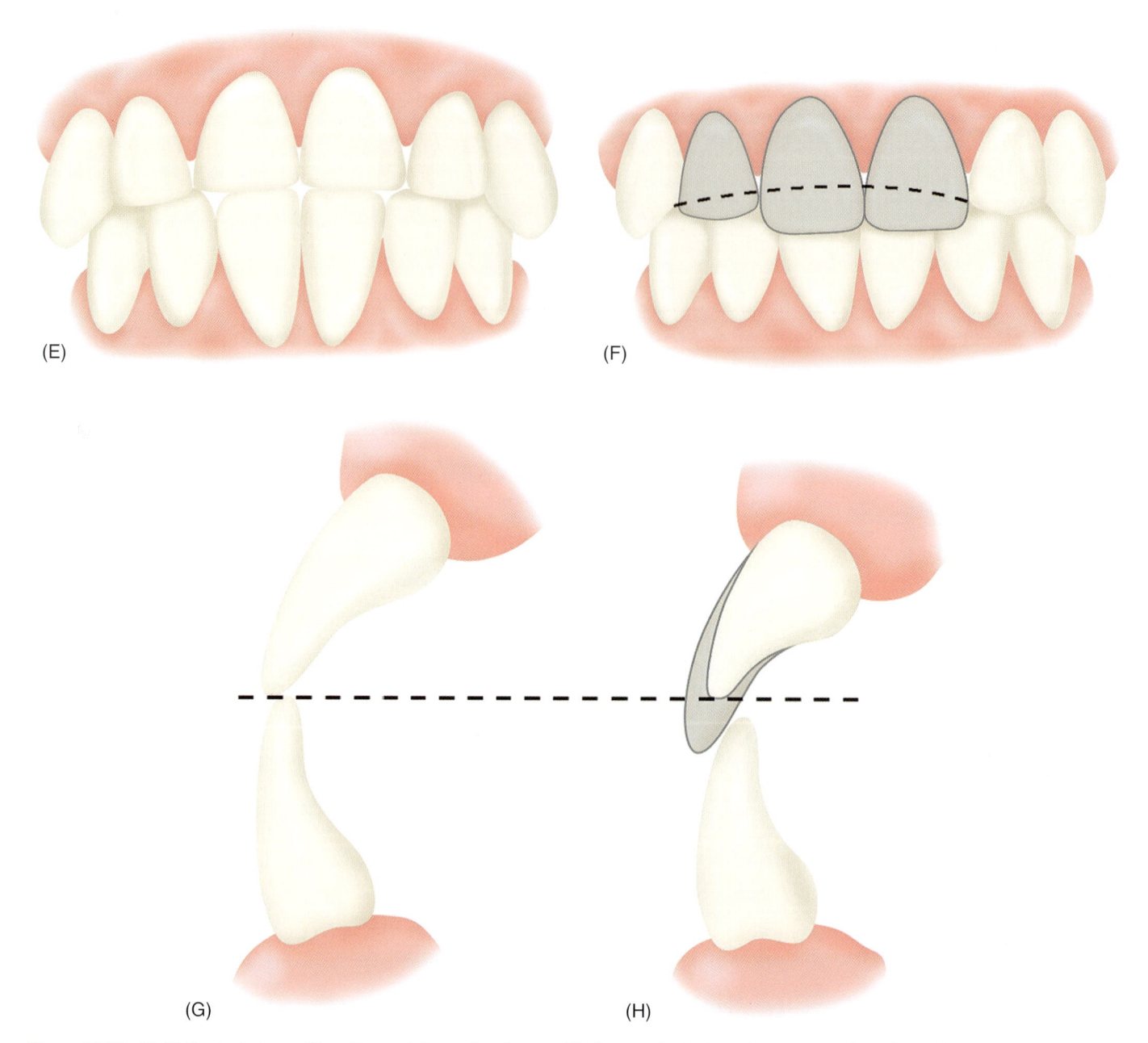

(G) (H)

Figure 14.18 **(E–H)** The technique of beveling and shortening the mandibular anterior incisors demonstrates how the occlusion is compensated for, which allows the bonded maxillary teeth to function virtually parallel to the original lateral and protrusive pathways.

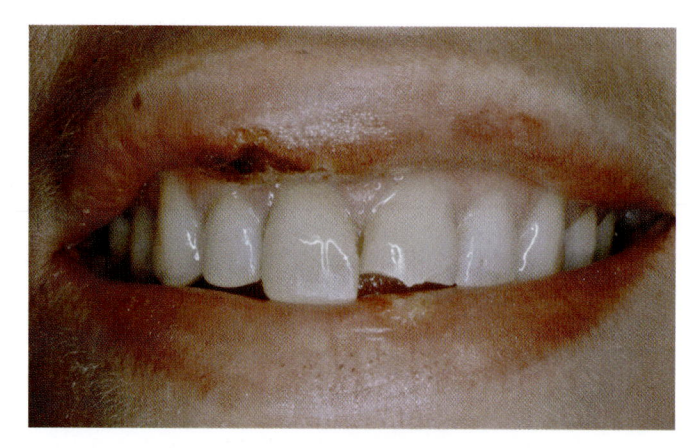

Figure 14.18 **(I)** Five years after treatment was completed, the patient fell down a concrete stairway, fracturing the bonding of one tooth, but not the enamel. Note that the composite resin seemed to act as a "shock absorber" to the natural enamel, which remained intact and required only a 1 h repair technique.

Dentin bonding

An important consideration when bonding to dentin should be to carefully follow the manufacturer's directions. A myriad of bonding systems are available in the market today. Bonding systems can be classified as "total-etch" or "self-etch." "Total-etch" are the bonding agents that use phosphoric acid to create micromechanical retention in enamel and dentin. Self-etch systems do not require the use of an etchant because the primer is acidic. Furthermore, these two categories can be divided by the number of steps involved in their use. "Total-etch" can be used in a three-step approach, with etching, priming, and adhesive application; or a two-step approach where the primer has been combined with the adhesive into one component. Self-etch can be used in a two-step or a one-step approach. The two-step method applies a self-etching primer followed by an adhesive. The one-step approach incorporates all steps into one. Recently, the concept "selective etching" has been suggested for self-etching adhesives. With this technique, the enamel margins are etched with a phosphoric acid and rinsed, while the dentin remains untreated.[56]

Another consideration should be based on the individual's sensitivity after dental procedures, especially if there is an abundance of freshly cut deep dentin or a large pulp. Attaining reliable adhesion to deep dentin is difficult due to the large size and number of dentinal tubules. The use of glass ionomer liners is thus recommended to cover these deep dentin areas before adhesive procedures.

Lastly, self-etch bonding agents are being used to decrease sensitivity (cervical abrasion, for example) and usually do not call for the removal of the smear layer.

McLean and others[57] described what is called the "sandwich technique" using composite resin on the glass ionomer-coated dentinal surface of a cavity preparation (Figure 14.19A–E). The newer glass ionomer liners are presently highly suited materials to use as liners and bases under almost any restorative materials. They provide an adequate amount of opacity and have the added advantages of bonding to dentin or resin, releasing fluoride, and not causing harm to the pulp,[10] and even reducing sensitivity.[58,59] Most recently they have been used in preventive restorations such as small occlusal cavities where carious lesions have extended into dentin.[60] Hembree[61] found that less microleakage occurred at gingival margins of Class II restorations when a glass ionomer cement was used as a liner. The liner should be close to the color of the dentin (not opaque white, which is difficult to mask). The exception is when replacing an amalgam that has left a stain; in this case, the liner may need to be somewhat lighter to cover the dark stain.

If a "total-etch" approach is selected the enamel should be etched for at least 15–30 s, and the dentin no longer than 10 s; this differential timing suggests the application of etchant to the enamel first followed by a brief application to dentin. Immediately rinse thoroughly with an air/water spray, for 10–15 s, and remove excess water to leave a moist surface. It should be noted that Gwinnett advocated an extra 10 s of air/water rinsing if a gel etch is used to prevent its cellulose vehicle from becoming a contaminant which may reduce bond strength.[62] It is also essential to have an oil-free air and air/water spray to prevent contamination that diminishes bond strength. If overdrying occurs, dab the preparation with a moistened cotton pledget to create a uniform amount of "wetness." Alternatively, a specialized rewetting agent can be applied (Aqua-Prep F, Bisco). Next, apply multiple coats of primer or a combination primer/adhesive. Different products require different drying and solvent evaporation protocol, so a careful reading of the manufacturer's instructions is essential.

The overlay technique described earlier provides a broader surface for the bonding process to achieve its primary function: to eliminate the gap that often results at the enamel boundary when the enamel interface contracts from polymerization shrinkage. The phosphoric acid etching before the resin materials are placed helps to eliminate this gap at the enamel boundary, thus enhancing the marginal seal.

Polymerization

All bonding materials are produced to be polymerized either chemically—known as self-curing—or by light. Other composite resins are dual-cure, that is, when the base and catalyst pastes are mixed together, they can be light cured, allowed to self-cure, or both light- and self-cured together. For most dentists today, light curing has become the method of choice because a higher degree of polymerization is possible.[23,63,64] Phillips summarizes these advantages succinctly: the single paste formulations do not require mixing, so there is less porosity in the restoration, making it more resistant to wear. The surface should be perfectly smooth, enamel-like, and free of irregularities. Photocuring provides sufficient working time for more precise and esthetic insertion of the materials. This works especially well with resins used incrementally for color match and improved margin adaptation. The cure is faster and more complete; margins can be feather-edged without concern that the thin, frail marginal areas will be insufficiently cured.[65]

Complete polymerization of composite resin in deep preparations, such as the proximal box of Class II restorations, has long been a concern. Rueggeberg found that for most modern curing systems and composite systems a depth of cure could not be reached beyond 2 mm.[66] Different clinical techniques have been developed to address this issue. The most common is the incremental layering technique.[67] With this technique, a thin layer of composite resin is placed and cured. For stress reasons, these layers are most often placed obliquely rather than horizontally.[17] Lutz introduced the "three-sited light-curing technique," which utilizes translucent matrices and light-reflecting wedges to improve the light's access to the interproximal box.[68]

Other clinicians utilize a flowable composite (Sure-Fil SDR flow Dentsply) as a base or liner to cover the floor of the preparation, including the floor of the proximal box. It has been suggested that this may improve the issues of microleakage and stress resulting from polymerization.[69,70]

While esthetics may be the primary reason for bonding, the trade-off is usually between superb esthetic restoration the day the patient leaves the office and a sometimes less than excellent result that endures and is likely to be esthetically appealing for more years. Good polymerization does not involve such a

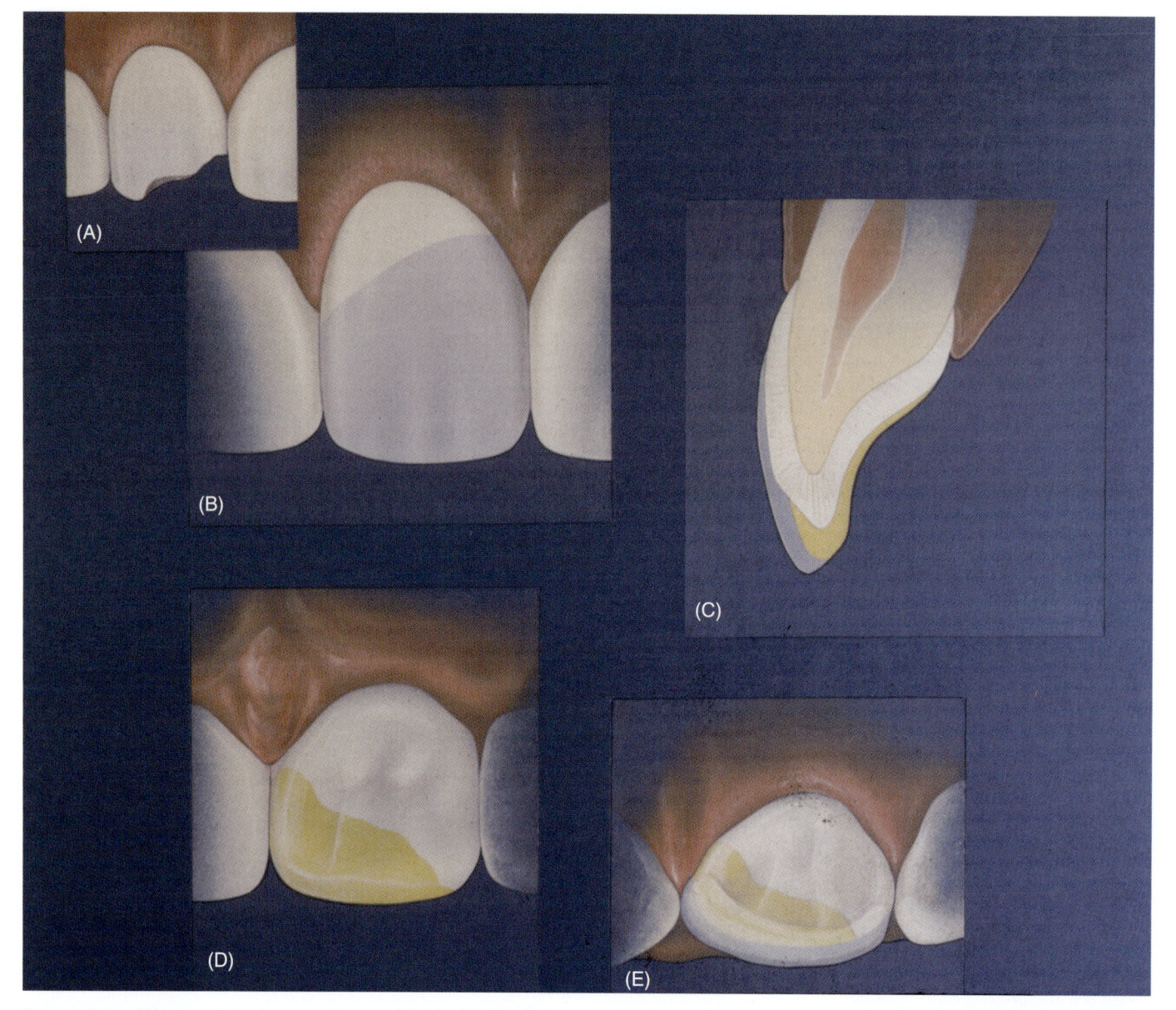

Figure 14.19 **(A)** Fractured right central incisor. **(B)** A highly polishable microfill labial veneer has been placed by using the overlay technique with margins extended to the cervical third of the labial surface. **(C)** The lingual view shows the restoration with a stronger and more durable hybrid composite. **(D)** A sagittal view that shows the "sandwich" outline of both composites in their relative positions. **(E)** The blend of the two composites from the incisal view.

trade-off. Maximum polymerization is important to the clinical as well as the esthetic success of the restoration, and in fact a 20 s repolymerization of the restoration following final finish can provide an *even stronger and long-lasting finish*. After final etching and conditioning, thoroughly dry the preparation and apply the bonding agent on both dentin and enamel.[62] Some agents will require more than one coat, as will be described in the manufacturer's directions. The bonding agent should not be allowed to pool because it may be mistaken for recurrent caries on a radiograph, as demonstrated by Hardison et al.[71] He advocates gently blowing the bonding resin after its application to a thin, even coat. Thinning the bonding agent, however, is best determined by following the manufacturer's instructions. Some are not to be thinned as shown in the research of Hilton et al., who found lowered bond strengths in three agents that were tested with air-thinning.[72] However, Schvaneveldt et al. reported significantly higher bond strengths when an agent was polymerized in a nitrogen environment.[73] Heymann feels that while the issue of air-thinning is material-specific because, for example, some adhesives are filled, the degree of air-thinning is a factor where excessiveness can lower bond strengths (HO Heymann, personal communication, 1998).

Polymerize with the light of your choice for the specified time (Figure 14.20). Both exposure time and light-tip composite distance are important variables, and Jordan[11,38,40] has recommended that the time be a minimum of 40 s and the distance from the light tip to the composite surface should be as close as possible to zero. Be sure to *periodically test your light* to make

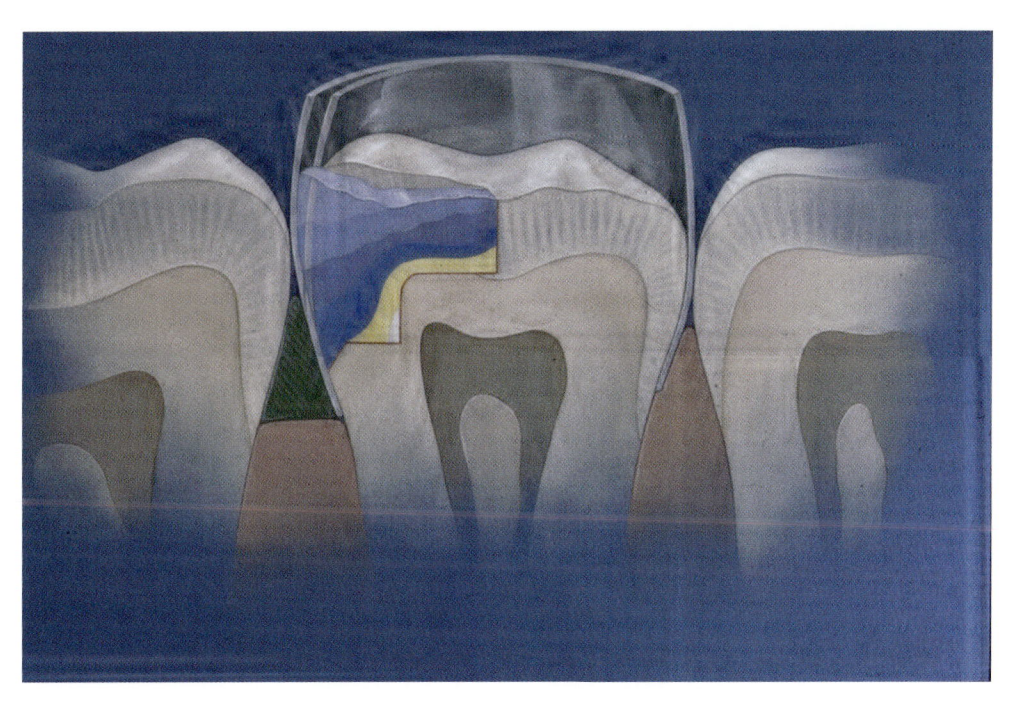

Figure 14.20 This schematic drawing illustrates the layering technique used to construct a properly contacting Class II restoration. After optional pulp protection (white) a glass ionomer liner/base protective layer (yellow) is used to offer the benefits of fluoride (Vitrebond, 3 M). The deep-to-light layers of blue indicate the layering technique by polymerizing the layers one at a time. Note also the tight seal offered by wedging that initially aids in gingival margin closure. After sealing the gingival margin, relax the ultrathin dead-soft matrix band to obtain maximum contact with the adjacent tooth.

certain it is still strong enough to accomplish deep polymerization. Apply no more than 2 mm increments of your chosen shade and polymerize again with your visible light. The extent of polymerization will depend on several factors including the depth reached by the light, catalyst concentration, and composition of the material. The darker shades usually require differing illumination times.[74] Color modifiers also may be mixed with composite restoratives, although this has the disadvantage of weakening the materials and making the curing process somewhat longer and less predictable.[10]

Antonson and Benedetro, Friedman, and others have studied the variability of the longitudinal intensity of visible light-curing units, stating that these findings may have an overlooked impact on complete polymerization of critical margin areas or even the polymerization of dentin-bonding materials.[75,76]

There are two main types of curing lights on the market today: quartz-tungsten-halogen (QTH) bulbs with a broad light spectrum of 400–500 nm, and light-emitting diode (LED) bulbs with a spectrum of 450–490 nm.[77] Plasma arc curing (PAC) lights are also available, but have fallen out of favor in recent years. While studies show QTH and LED units to be similar in their effectiveness,[78–80] LED units tend to be more user-friendly than QTH units. LED units do not require a filter or ventilating fan, so they tend to be smaller and less cumbersome than QTH units. QTH units suffer a decrease in output over time, which may be attributed to lamp filament burnout, bulb blackening or frosting, and reflector degradation, all of which, says Friedman, mandate lamp replacement at least every 6 months.[76] Additionally, LED units tend to maintain their power output for longer periods, consume less energy, and are often cordless, powered by rechargeable batteries. Because of this, LED units are growing in popularity.

If your light does not have a built-in light meter, then purchase one (Figure 14.21), such as L.E.D. Radiometer, Demetron (Ker), or Bluephase Meter (Ivocalr Vivadent), to monitor each curing unit periodically for the manufacturer's recommended output. Other simple measures call for cleaning the end of the curing tip and/or replacing it, inspecting and cleaning the filter/reflector, inspecting the bulb and replacing it, and doubling the curing time if using an older curing light.

All composite resins contract, causing dimensional changes, during polymerization, and this shrinkage can cause separation between the composite resin mass and adjacent tooth structure. The average shrinkage is about 2–3%.[81] This can create defects that welcome bacteria and may cause stress on cusps, resulting in sensitivity, occlusal disharmony, or even delayed fracture.[9]

Polymerization shrinkage coupled with technique sensitivity can lead to a risk of an open margin, especially in situations where the enamel is thin. These open margins then lend themselves to stain. Since too much polymerization shrinkage can reduce the restoration life expectancy, it is much better to take additional time in curing the composite by adding three to five layers of material, making sure the final layer is over the entire restoration, to avoid microscopic composite margins that may attract additional stain. Another advantage in building the restoration in this fashion is that you will be able to vary the shade as you add each layer of composite from gingival to the incisal or occlusal margin. Incremental placement, or layering,

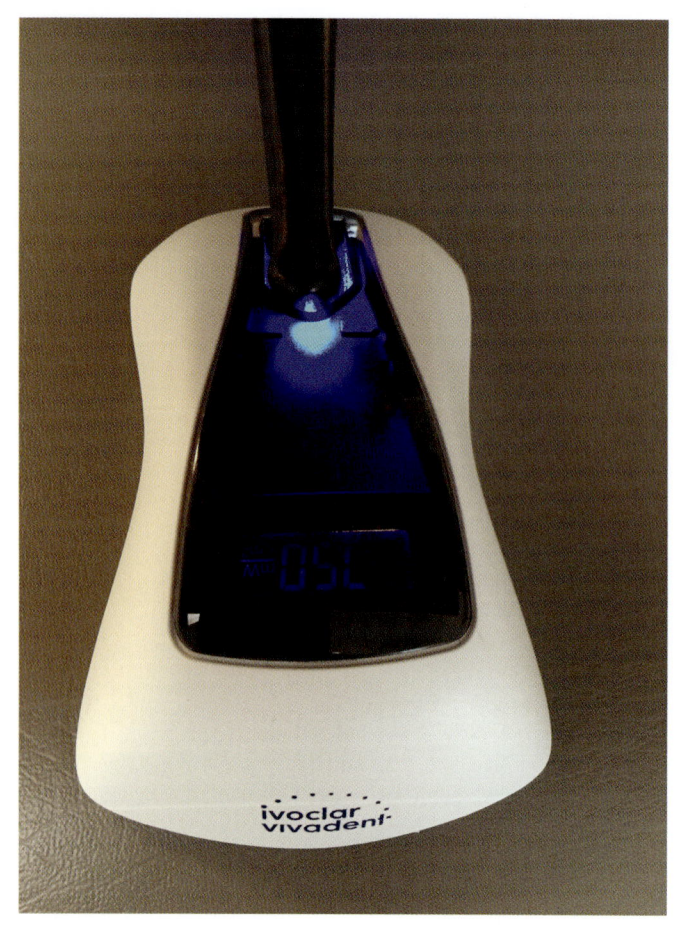

Figure 14.21 Light tips must be kept clean and your light source periodically checked with one of several diagnostic testing devices Bluephase Meter (Ivocalr Vivadent).

of light-activated composites also produces a bond strength that compares with, even exceeds, the cohesive strength of the material used.[82] For these reasons, incremental placement of composite resins, especially in Class V cervical restorations, is the most desirable mode of placement, followed by margin seal procedures.[83,84]

Finishing the restoration

Proper finishing of a restoration *cannot* make up for inadequate preparation or any other step necessary for successful esthetic and functional restorations. It *can*, however, make the difference between an ordinary and an extraordinary esthetic appearance. The objectives of a thorough, well-planned finishing are to improve and finalize restoration margins and contours to help make the restoration biocompatible with both tooth and tissue, and to develop maximum surface luster to enhance esthetics, reduce stain and plaque retention, and minimize wear and fracture potential. You will know you have achieved these objectives if the finished restoration has the following qualities:

- well-finished margins, with no overhang, void, or extension of restorative material that could interfere with tissue health
- a sufficiently smooth surface that will not attract bacterial plaque or food stains
- suitable surface texture that blends in or matches adjacent or opposing natural teeth
- color matching that of the existing adjacent, opposing, or preselected tooth shade
- a surface finish devoid of too obvious contour, finishing bur, or diamond scratches.

As with etching, numerous articles provide detailed instructions on finishing. But the following provides a brief outline of steps of special significance to an esthetic finish. Roulet and his colleagues recommend using a diamond bur with an abrasive particle size of 15–40 μm to contour the facial surface of the restoration.[16,25] Goldstein suggests you begin with either an ET 6 or 9 30 μm diamond or 8-blade carbide (Brasseler USA) for gross contouring (Figure 14.22). Although Greiff, Burgess, Davis, and Theobald[85] report no difference between wet and dry polishing, Goldstein has not found this to be the case. All instruments should be used wet to contain the inevitable dust which can produce an extremely bitter taste for the patient.[84] In addition, Collard, Ladd, and Vogel fear that dental personnel are at a high risk for developing respiratory silicosis if the dust is not minimized, and they recommend the use of face masks during composite finishing.[86] The wet finish also avoids frictional heat that may tend to pull up the margin.[38] Continuing to polish dry after the margin is opened sweeps the composite dust under the margin, producing a "white line." Also, Mazer feels that the initial cracking of a posterior composite is probably caused by the surface and finishing process.[35] If diamonds are used, finish with the ET fine (15 μm diamond) in the same size as above. As reported in a comparison of finishing instruments by Pratten and Johnson,[87] an extra-fine diamond with 15 μm particles (ET yellow band) produces a surface smoothness superior to white stone and similar to that produced with a carbide bur and rubber point. Diamond finishing with a slow speed produces a somewhat smoother finish than with a high speed. For ultrafine diamond finishing, use an 8 μm diamond (DETUF) or a 30-blade carbide (UF Brasseler USA).

If carbides are being used, final contouring should be done with the 16-bladed carbides in the same number (ET fine). Once the final labial contour is completed, make sure the gingival margins also are contoured correctly with the 3 or 4 mm DET in the same sequence. The final instrument subgingivally should be the 30-blade carbide or 8 μm diamond (DETUF; Figure 14.23), usually the 3 or 4 mm. It is important to use the safe-ended ET so the cementum is protected while finishing in this area.

The necessity for careful choice of instrumentation, and the care in finishing, is well illustrated in a clinical study conducted by Ratanapridakul, Leinfelder, and Thomas.[88] The authors found that after the first 30 days, resistance to wear was significantly higher for an unfinished group of teeth as compared to those that received a conventional finish. The authors attributed this to possible microcracks generated by the rapidly rotating blades of the finishing instrument. Similar concerns have been expressed by Watson.[89] This is why it is best to use either an 8-bladed carbide or a 30 μm diamond only for bulk reduction. As soon as possible, switch to a 16-bladed carbide or 15 μm diamond for final contouring and initial finishing. The final finishing will be

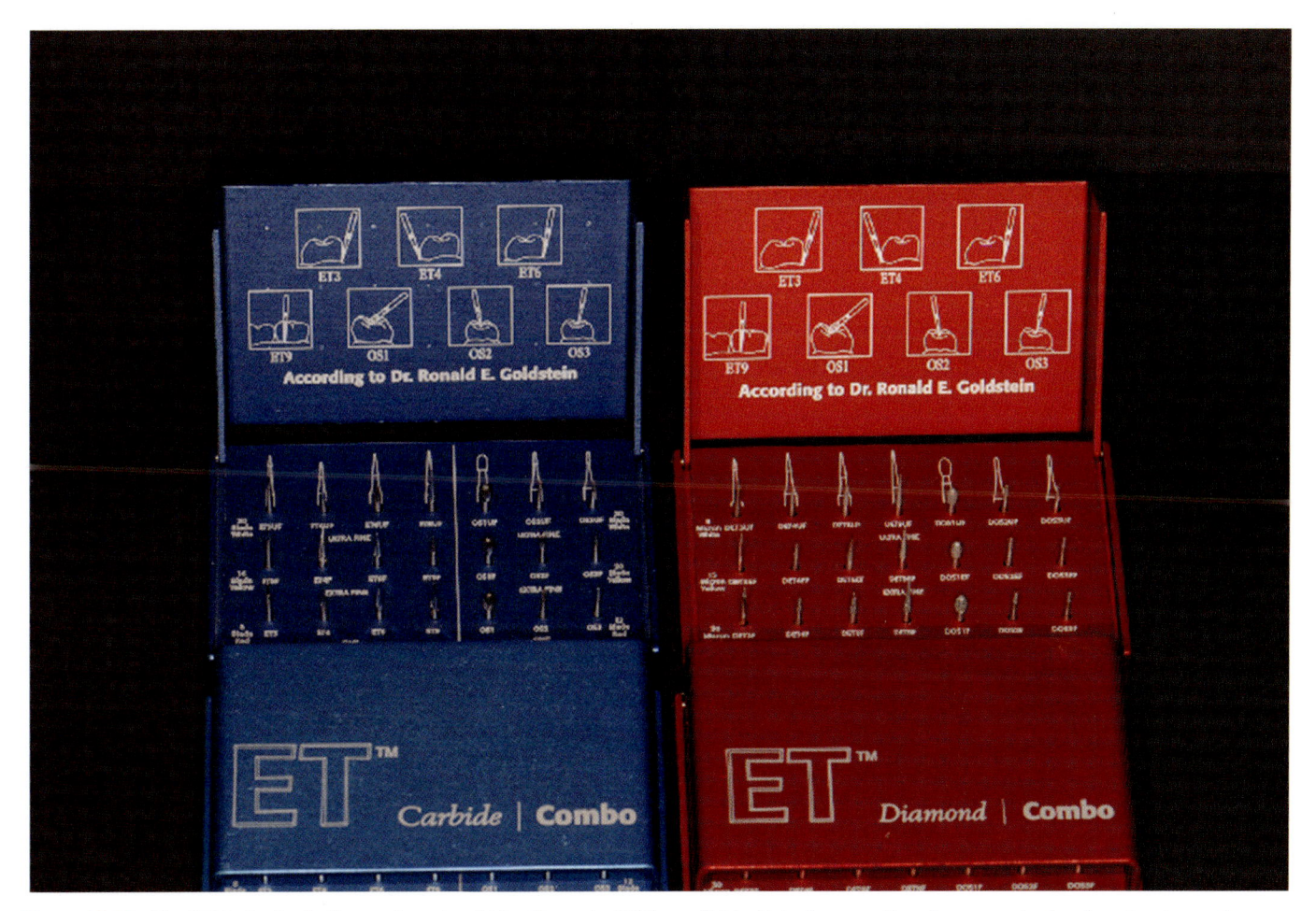

Figure 14.22 The ET kits for both diamonds and carbides (Brasseler USA) are divided into three sections for easy entry-level contouring and finishing. Each kit contains both anterior and posterior finishing burs for specific blade or grit size.

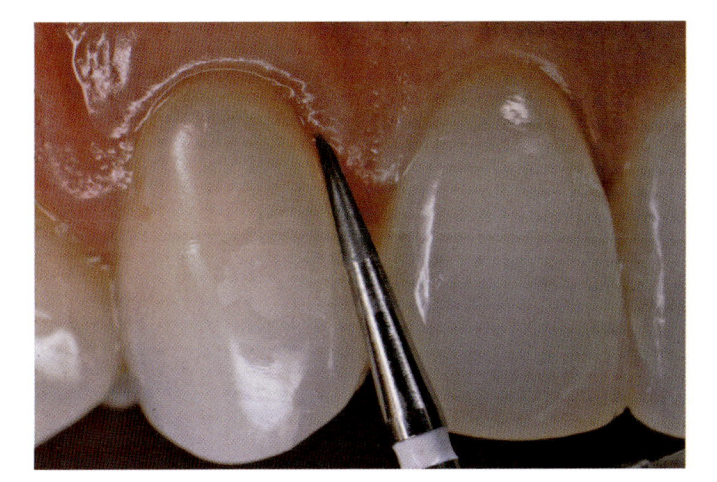

Figure 14.23 Since there is a straight emergence profile as the tooth erupts from the sulcus, the design of the ET3 or ET4 (Brasseler USA) makes them excellent choices for subgingival finishing. Here, a DET4UF (Brasseler USA) diamond bur puts the final finish of the cervical margin on the maxillary right cuspid. This 8 μm diamond is especially helpful to reduce gingival irritation (see Figure 14.27A).

accomplished with either a 30-blade carbide or an 8 μm diamond. Figure 14.24A–C shows the type of surface achieved by using 8-, 16-, and 30-bladed carbides. There are times when an endcutting ET bur is useful. For instance, opening or restoring incisal embrasures can be easily accomplished using the ET3A "cutting" bur (H132A Brasseler) (Figure 14.25).

Polishing will be done by one of the disc systems (3M, Brasseler USA, Cosmedent, Shofu,) for maximum luster. These discs can produce the smoothest polished surfaces.[22,90] Final polishing can also be accomplished with silicon- or diamond-impregnated rubber cups and points or DiaComp composite Feather Lite polishers (Brasseler USA). These should also be used wet and copiously rinsed between grits (Figure 14.26A–H).

Texturing your bonded restoration

If you desire to either mimic adjacent tooth texture or create your own pattern or texture, you will need to alter the finishing procedure slightly. First, perform your labial and gingival contours using the previously described system. Second, begin disc finishing with the first two coarse discs if using a four-disc finishing system. Third, choose either an ET6UF or ET9UF 30-bladed carbide or DET6UF or DET9UF 8 μm diamond to place your desired texture. Be careful to not "ditch" the composite cuts too deep. Make both vertical and horizontal cuts in an asymmetrical pattern. Fourth, following your placement of the textured surface you are now ready to polish with the DiaComp Feather Lites (Brasseler USA) in sequence. Be sure to polish wet

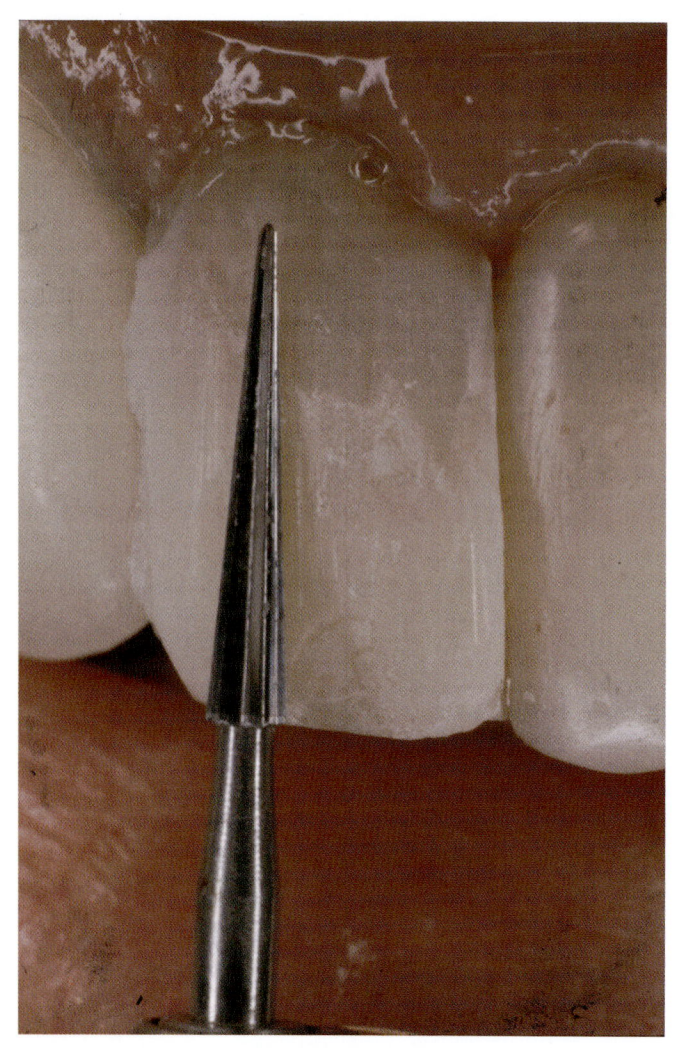

Figure 14.24 **(A)** The ET9 8-bladed carbide (Brasseler USA) should be used on the labial surface when there is considerable bulk present (see Figure 14.27B).

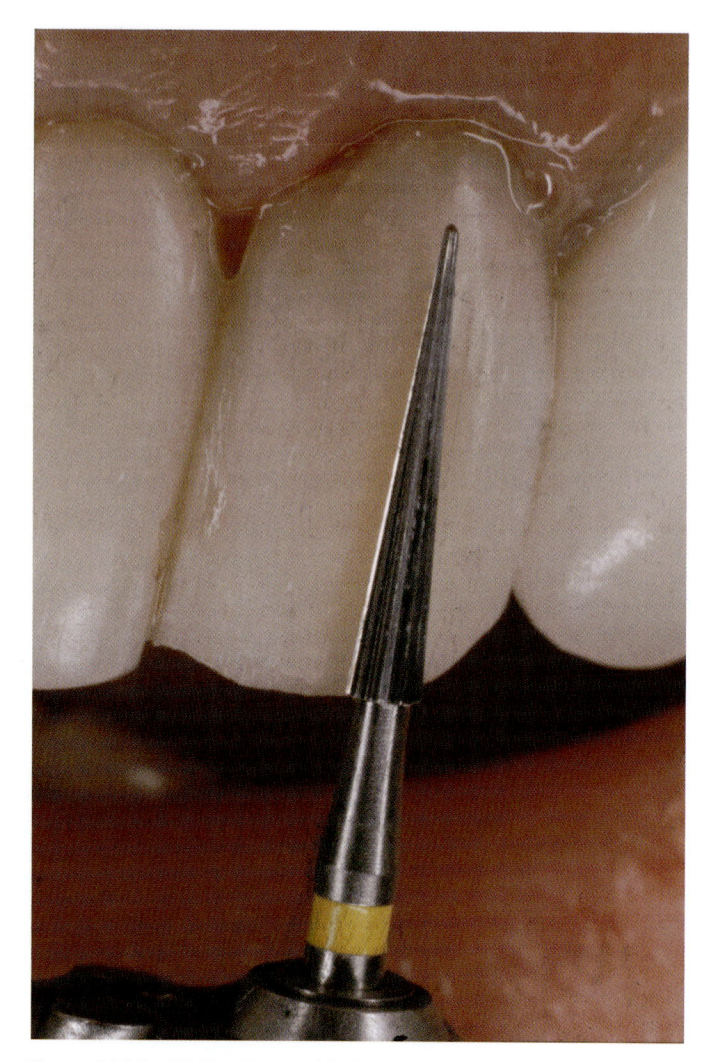

Figure 14.24 **(B)** The ET9F 16-bladed carbide (Brasseler USA) allows you to do more detailed carving while producing a smoother surface.

and vary your polishing angles. The final result should give your bonded restoration a natural-appearing light-reflective surface.

Problems in finishing

Beware of using an inappropriate-sized finishing instrument. For instance, using an ET9 is appropriate for the labial surface of a central incisor. However, it may not be suitable to finish the gingival margin because of the angle of finish and the necessary amount of torque required. Figure 14.27A shows how finishing should utilize most of the finishing instruments' blades. Figure 14.27B shows how maximum utilization of the longer burs is in the body of the anterior teeth whereas just using the tip would result in lack of support, possibly making a bur fracture more likely (Figure 14.27C).

A microfill composite resin is the ideal restorative material to use in restoring Class V tooth defects. Use the overlay technique to restore facial surfaces because it will provide longer esthetic life to the restoration. One not uncommon defect in certain patients is shown in Figure 14.28A–E.

The Class V overlay restoration should be overfilled to allow for two-plane finishing. Use an ET3 or 4 to define the gingival emergence contour. An ET6 or ET9 held parallel to the long facial axis establishes the facial height of the contour.

If there has been a significant amount of gingival recession, you may opt to duplicate the existing anatomy, or reestablish the facial height of contour at a level closer to the receded gingival margin. This is especially true for the patient who has a high lip line, and whose smile displays the roots of the anterior teeth. Using a darker shade on the roots of these teeth minimizes their "long" appearance.

After the final polish, allow the patient to rinse, then dry the teeth and inspect from different views with the dental light reflecting at varied angles. The surface should have enamel reflectivity and the veneer should have depth of color that closely mimics teeth. You are looking for small areas that may be insufficiently polished and thus will show scratches. These should be refinished until the restoration is free from surface scratches and other defects. The finished composite restorations should have margins that are not detectable to floss or a sharp explorer.

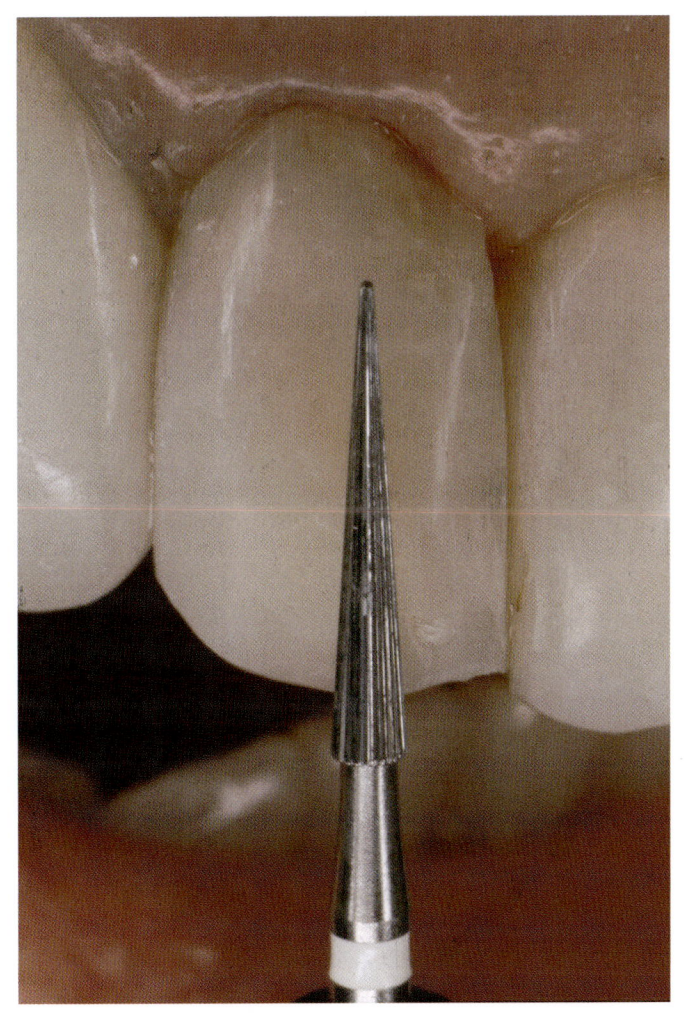

Figure 14.24 (C) The ET9UF 30-bladed carbide (Brasseler USA) accomplishes final texturing and an extra-smooth surface. This will be followed by either a 3 or 4 mm ETUF 30-blade carbide (Brasseler USA) as a final step in contouring and finishing.

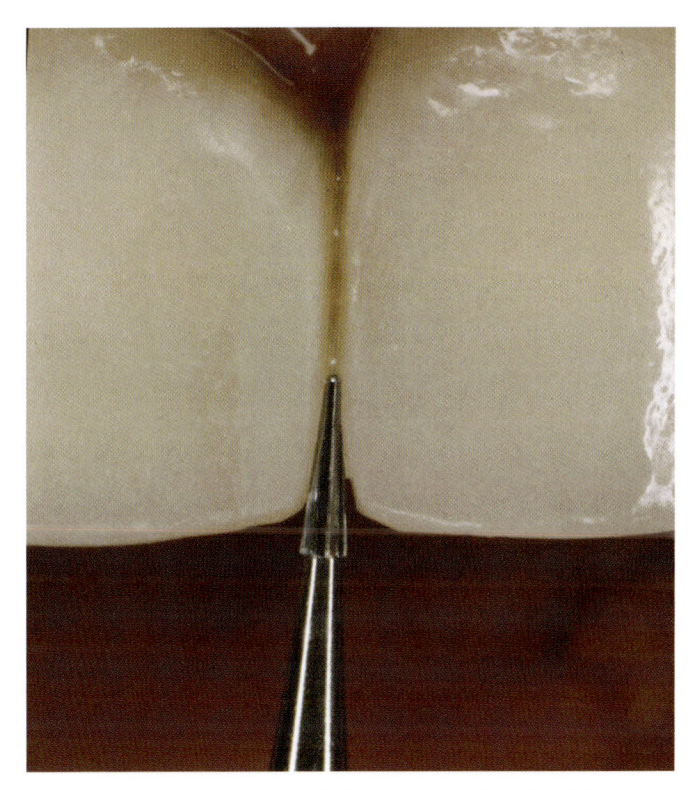

Figure 14.25 The non-safe-ended ET3A "cutting" bur (H132A, Brasseler USA) is a 3 mm carbide that is an excellent design for opening and shaping incisal embrasures as well as removing excess interproximal resin cement.

Posterior finishing requires a special technique because of the occlusal anatomy. As mentioned previously, using a composite carving instrument (TNCIGFT 8 Instrument Series, Hu Friedy) makes final finishing much easier (Figure 14.29A–K).

Interproximal finishing

The last phase of finishing involves interproximal polishing with abrasive strips. Depending on how much is necessary, your choice to begin may be an extremely thin diamond abrasive strip. In certain circumstances a #12 scalpel blade is useful to remove any excess material by scraping or shaping the excess. Following the sequence of a more- to a less-abrasive strip results in a smooth transition when flossing. When interproximal finishing is complete there should be no fraying of the floss.

Note the different width strips. A wide one will reduce the contact area between the teeth whereas the narrow ones can be slipped between the teeth using the nonabrasive center part of the strip and placed exactly where stripping is needed. This will prevent unwanted removal of the contact area which could conceivably leave an unsightly space between the newly bonded teeth.

Maintaining the restoration

The most often overlooked means of extending the life and attractiveness of bonding frequently occurs at this point, when you hand the patient the mirror to admire the new look. This is when you or your assistant should provide instructions to the patient, preferably written, on what to do and what to avoid to insure that the bonding surface is less likely to stain or fracture. Some dentists[91] believe that use of less-forgiving restorative materials should be limited to patients who are "well motivated to high standards of oral hygiene." To clean the bonded surface, patients should pay extra attention to oral hygiene—with brushing and careful flossing, with the floss being pulled through the teeth horizontally, not vertically. Also warn your patients about the potential damage of "guillotining" the papilla (refer to Chapter 25, on oral habits). This occurs when patients, anxious to clean both sides of the proximal surface, do it so fast that they clean one side then forget to return to the height of contour before cleaning the other tooth. Instead they clean one side and rush the floss to the adjacent tooth surface without realizing they are injuring the interdental papilla.

Mouthwashes with high alcohol content should be avoided because they can soften composites. Coffee, tea, and cola drinks

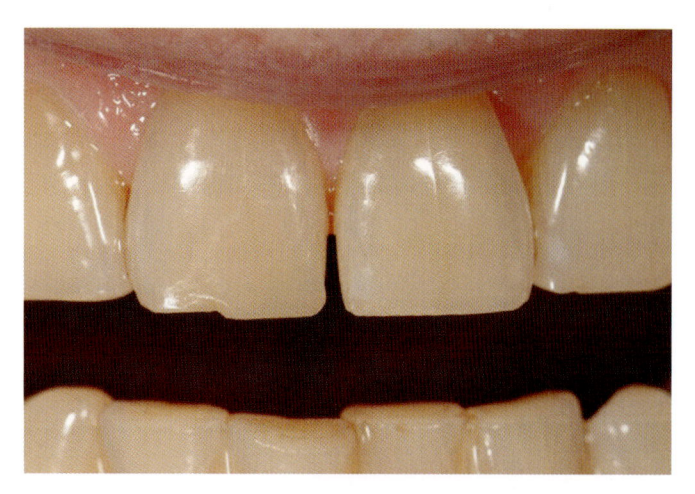

Figure 14.26 **(A)** This man chipped his front tooth from grinding and was advised to have the tooth bonded rather than contour to maintain the tooth's length and width proportion.

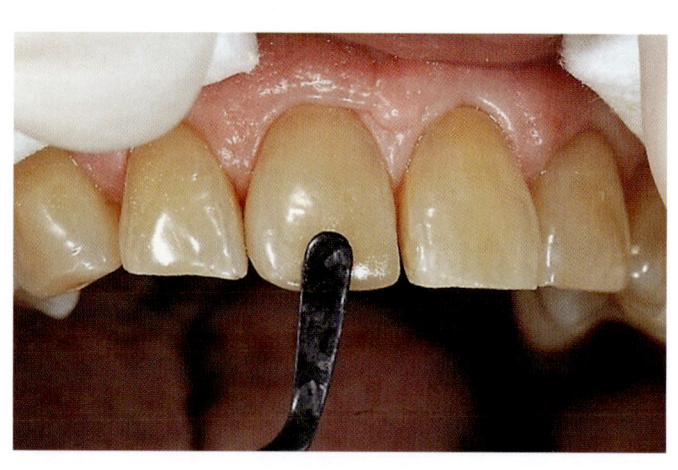

Figure 14.26 **(B)** A microhybrid composite resin was placed to restore the incisal length (Venus Diamond, Heraeus).

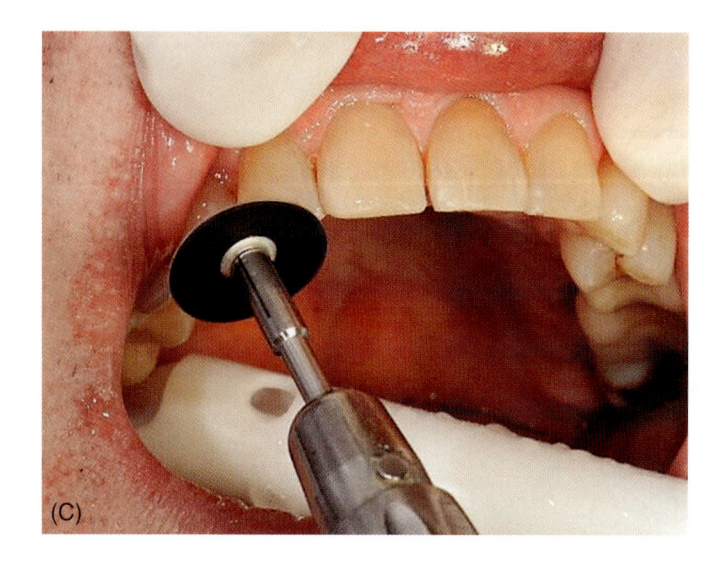

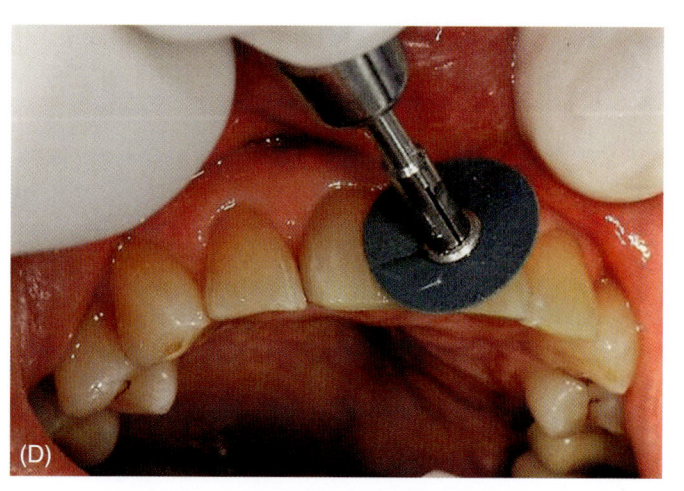

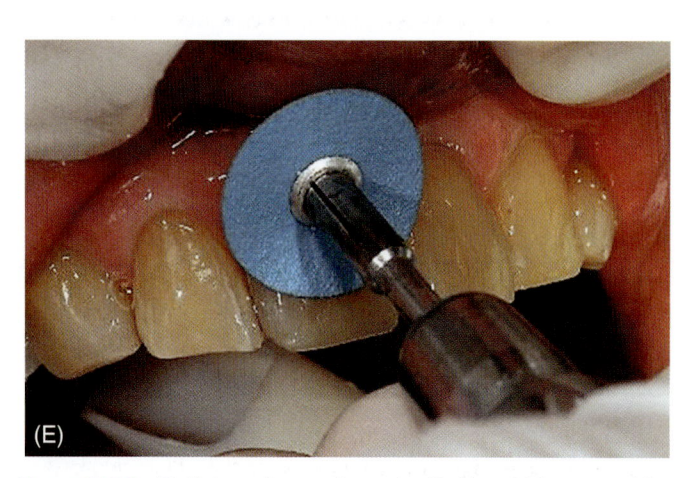

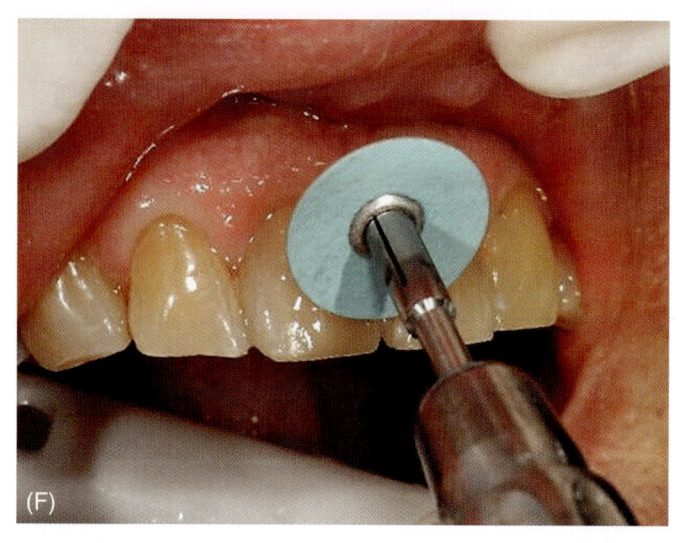

Figure 14.26 **(C–F)** A sandpaper disc series (Sof-Lex, 3M) was used from coarsest to finest, rinsing well between each disc.

Chapter 14 Composite Resin Bonding

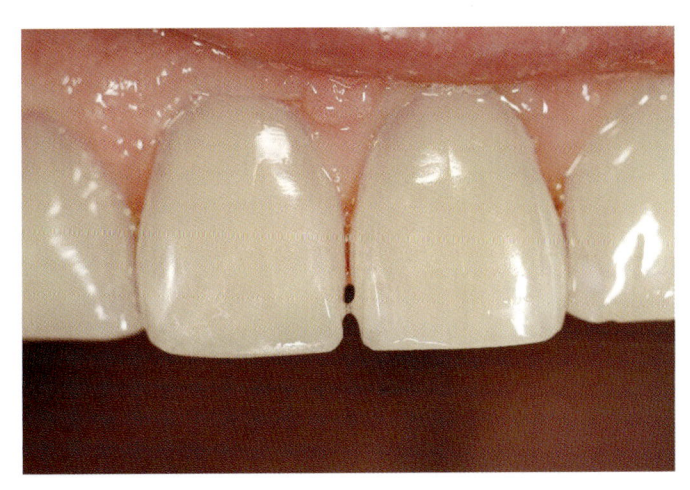

Figure 14.26 (G) The finished restoration, with shine and luster matching the adjacent teeth.

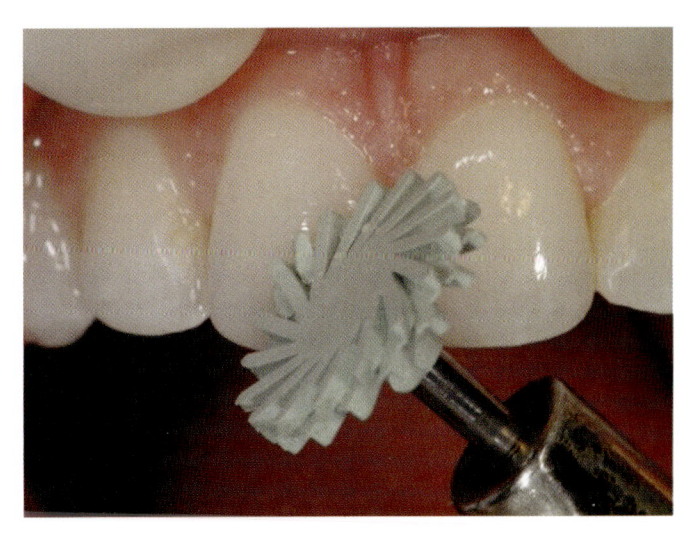

Figure 14.26 (H) Final polish is accomplished with DiaComp Feather Lite intra-oral composite polishers (Brasseler USA)

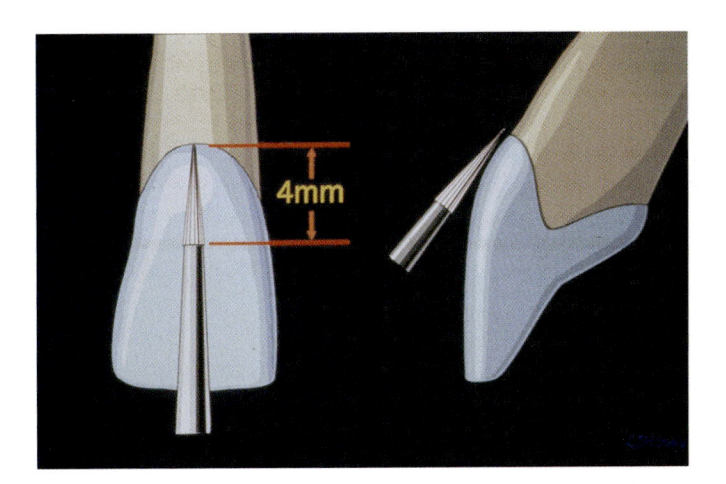

Figure 14.27 (A) This drawing illustrates the correct-length bur for trimming the gingival margin.

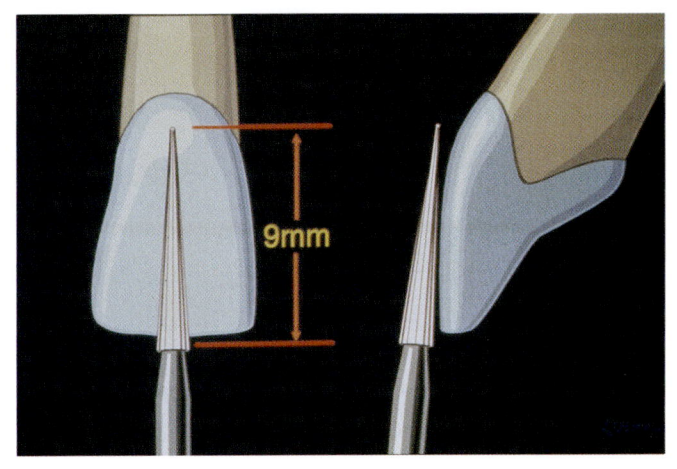

Figure 14.27 (B) The long facial surface is best served by a 6 or 9 mm finishing bur to make a consistent, smooth, and precise cut.

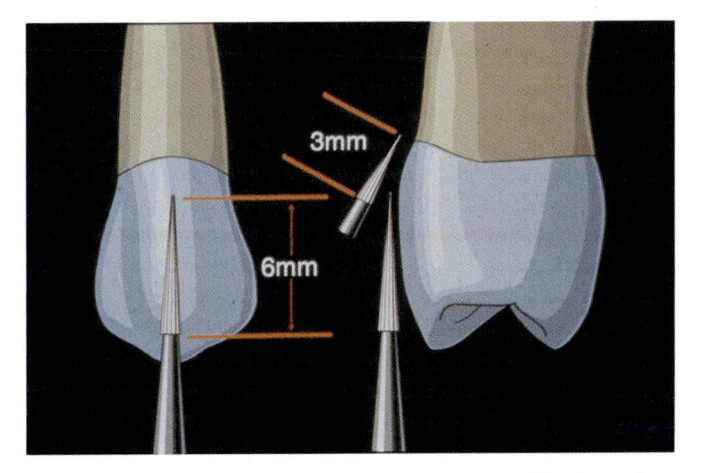

Figure 14.27 (C) This drawing shows the proper length and shape burs to use for contouring and finishing of posterior restorations.

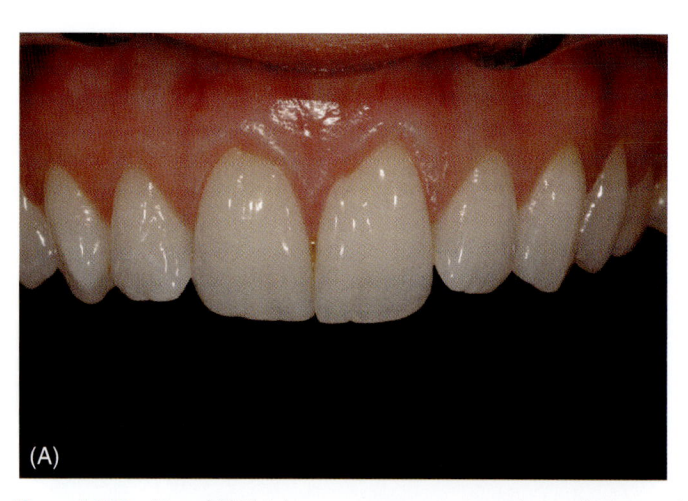

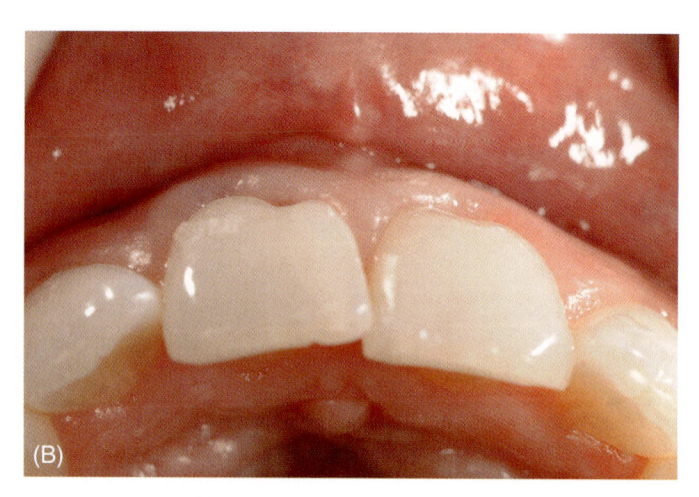

Figure 14.28 (A and B) This beauty contestant wanted to make her smile as attractive as possible. Note the tooth defects in the cervical third of her teeth, which also affected the shape of her gingival contours.

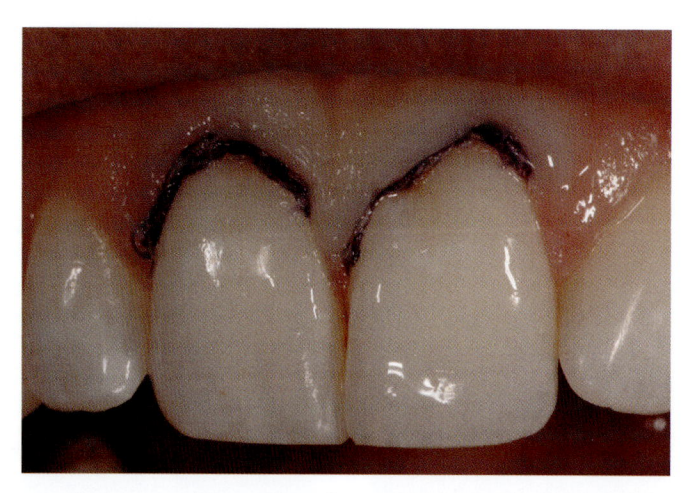

Figure 14.28 (C) Gingival displacement with cotton cord was used to allow access for the subgingival repair.

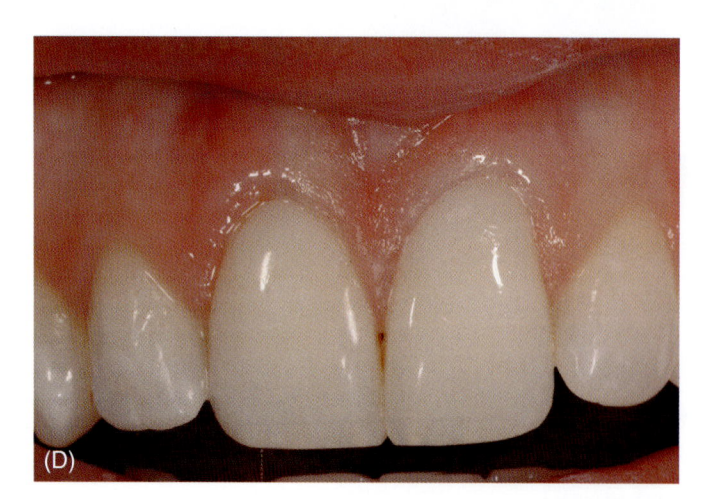

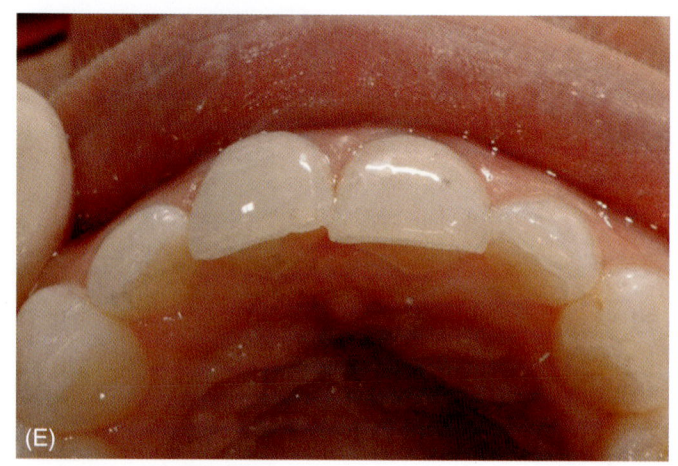

Figure 14.28 (D and E) Final restorations show how restoring the tooth defect helped achieve normal gingival architecture.

can stain the bonded areas even more quickly than original enamel. Should your patients smoke, this is also an excellent time for you to reinforce what the patient's physician doubtless has been telling him or her about cigarette smoking or other tobacco use. Its deleterious effect on the appearance of the teeth, as well as the health of the oral cavity, is yet another reason to quit. The patient should avoid foods that are likely to stain the teeth. Much of the advice is pure common sense, although Chapter 25 outlines in detail some of the ways patients sabotage their restorations by chewing, biting, grinding their teeth, holding objects in the mouth, or even just using hard toothbrushes and abrasive toothpaste.[68,92] Make the patient aware of these harmful habits by asking which habits they have that might cause damage to their restorations. Ask your patients to review the last chapter in *Change Your Smile*,[93] which includes a patient habit questionnaire dealing with these problems.

Bonding protection

Unless your patient has an open bite or a protective occlusion that would prevent unfavorable stress on his/her anterior restorations, consider constructing a special mouthguard to be worn during sleeping or other times of patient need. The most comfortable appliance is one with a hard acrylic outside and soft acrylic inside to provide a "cushion" seat. This appliance is generally made for the maxillary arch (Figure 14.30). Make certain the appliance is occlusally well balanced so that there are no interferences and all teeth have occlusal stops to prevent eruption.

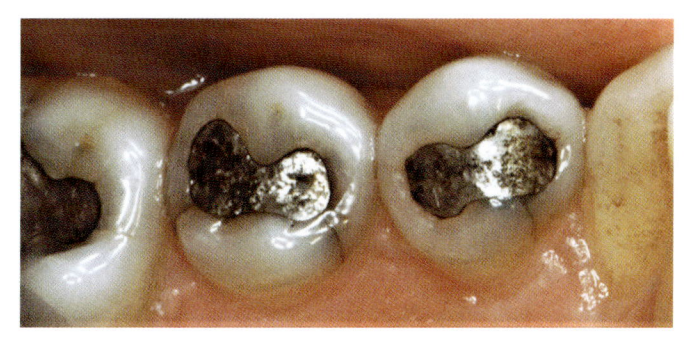

Figure 14.29 **(A)** This 50-year-old man required replacement of his aging amalgam restorations due to defective margins and stained fracture lines, which were the causing facial surface discoloration.

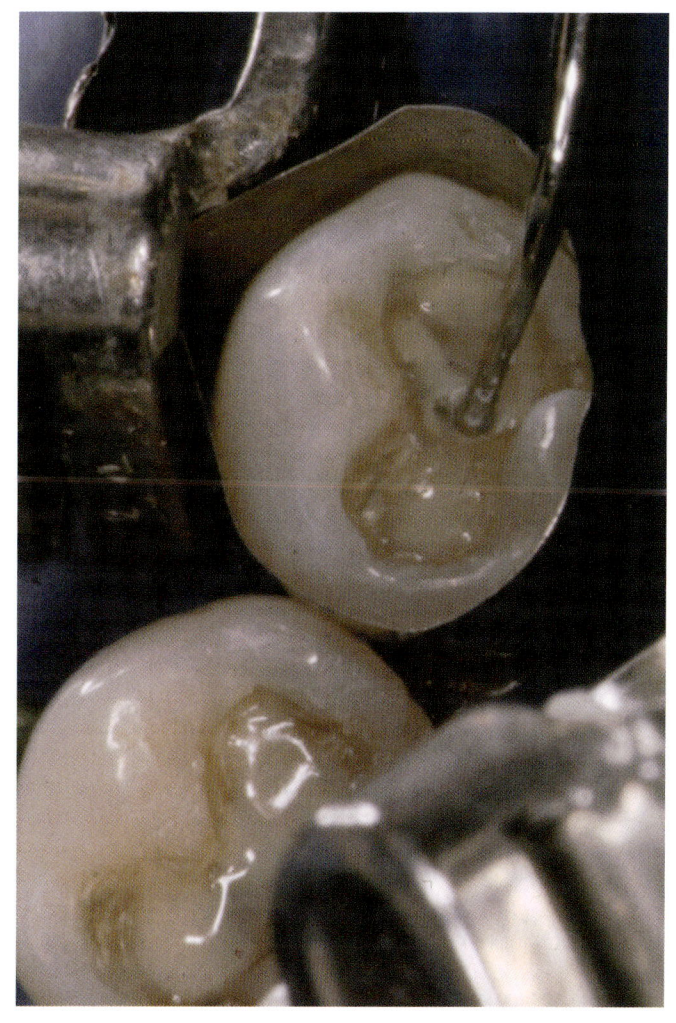

Figure 14.29 **(B)** A glass ionomer layer is applied using a Novatech PINT 11 instrument (Hu-Friedy), then polymerized.

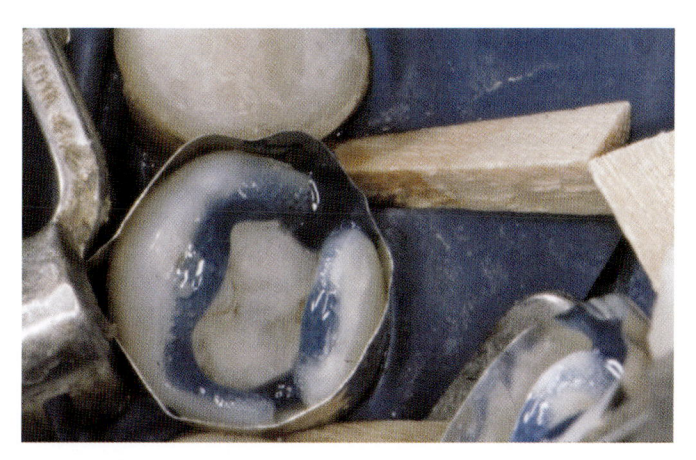

Figure 14.29 **(C)** A semisoft gel etch is used to etch the enamel areas for 15–20 s, and is then washed with a simultaneous combination water/air spray for approximately 5–10 s.

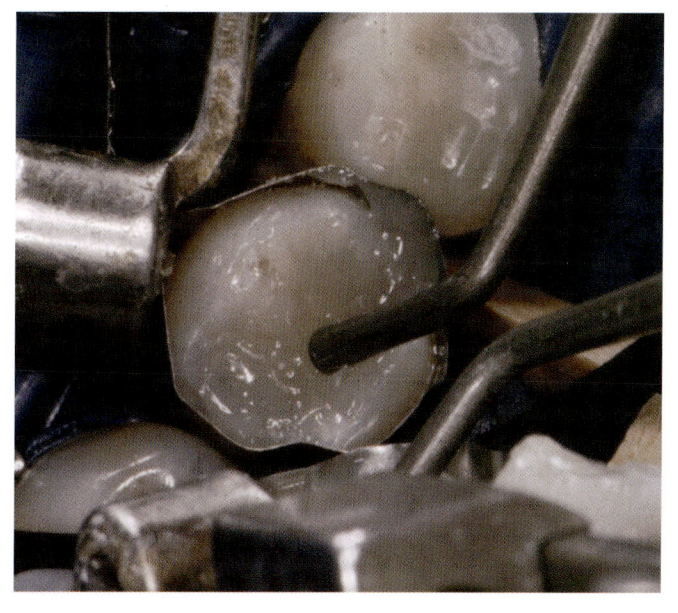

Figure 14.29 **(D)** Each layer of composite resin is placed using the appropriate-sized round-end anodized aluminum or stainless steel instrument TNCIGFTI (Hu-Friedy).

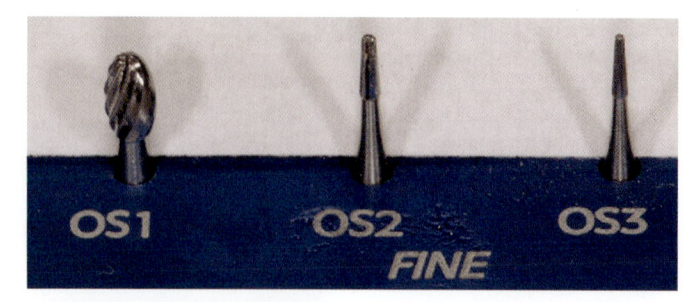

Figure 14.29 **(E)** Initial trimming and finishing cuts are done with the OS 1-, 2-, or 3-carbide burs (Brasseler USA).

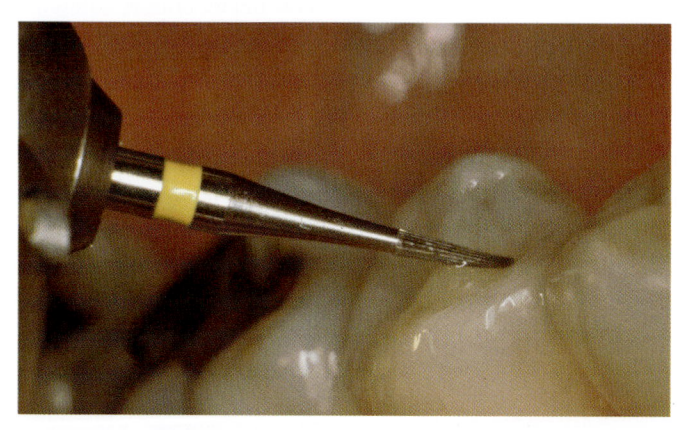

Figure 14.29 **(G)** Initial grooves and fissures are carved with an OS2F (Brasseler USA) 16-bladed instrument.

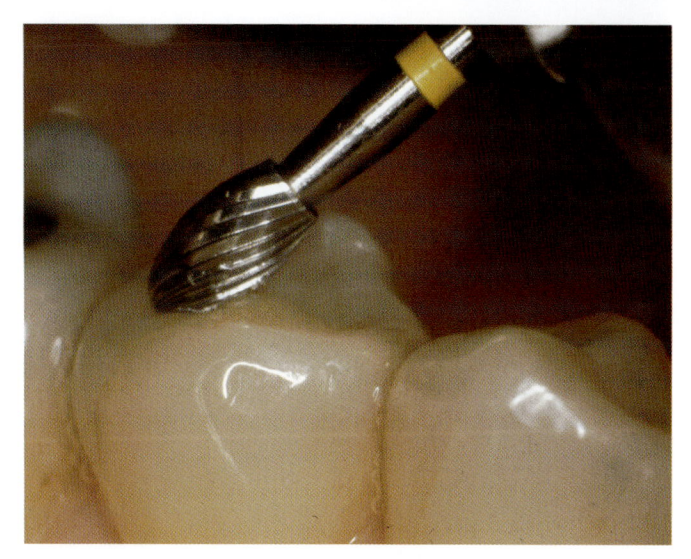

Figure 14.29 **(F)** Initial occlusal anatomy is placed using an ET OSIF 16-bladed carbide (Brasseler USA).

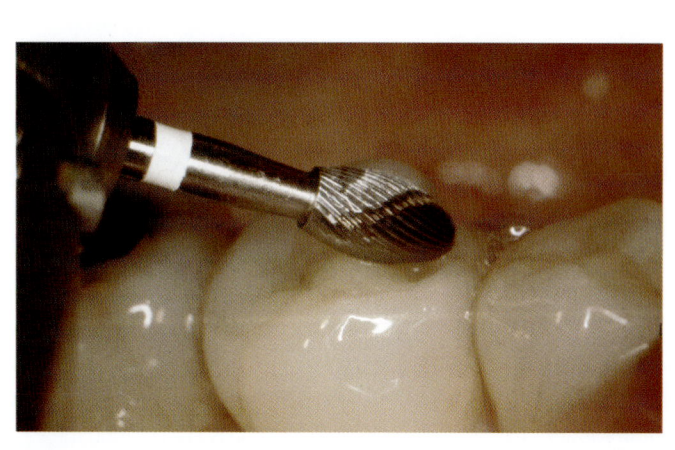

Figure 14.29 **(H)** Final occlusal finishing is done with a 30-bladed OSIUF (Brasseler USA) carbide.

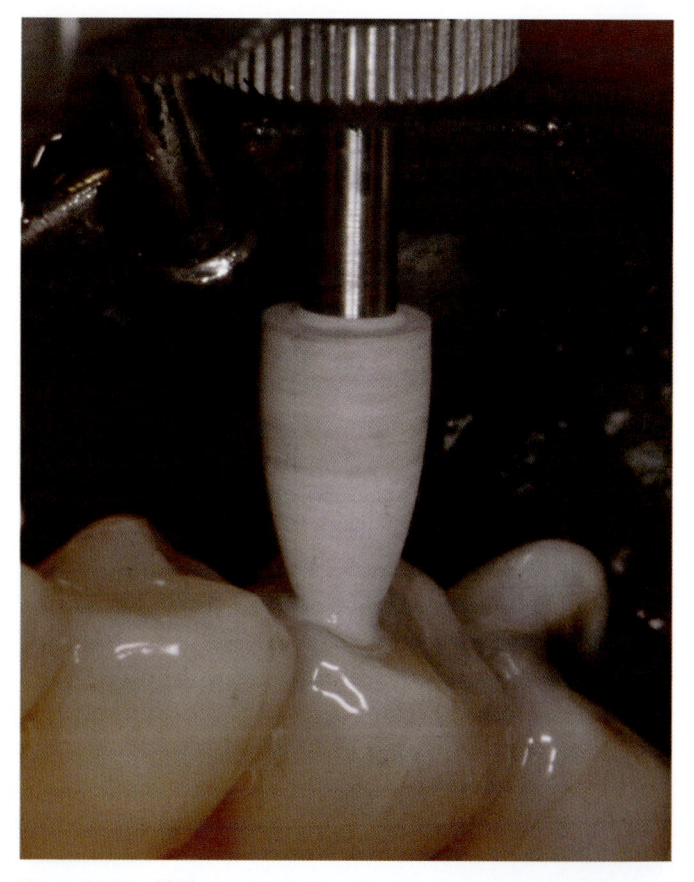

Figure 14.29 **(I)** The tapered point abrasive impregnated polisher (Brasseler USA) can be used to polish the occlusal anatomy.

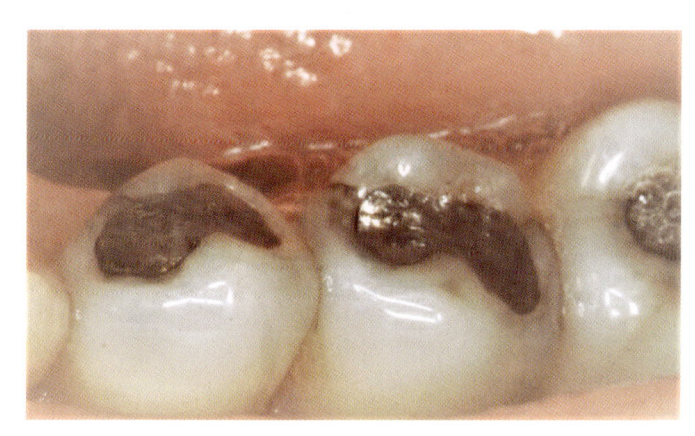

Figure 14.29 **(J)** The before occlusal view of the defective amalgam restorations.

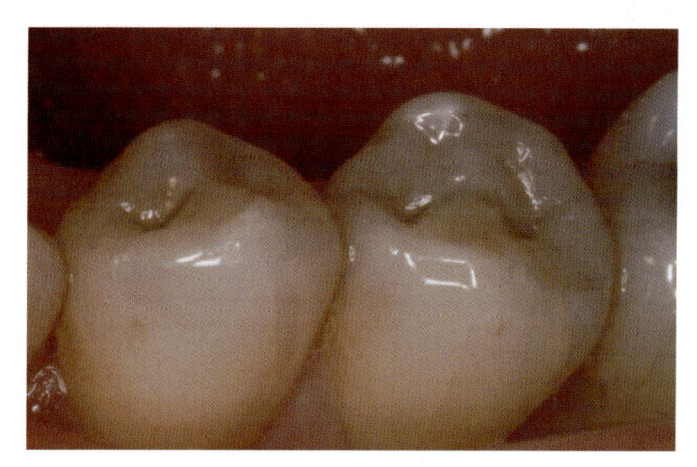

Figure 14.29 **(K)** Occlusal view of the final restorations.

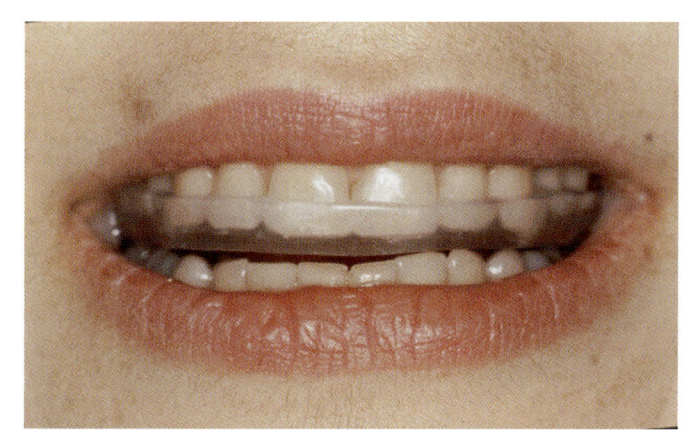

Figure 14.30 After bonding, this patient was fitted for a protective night appliance with hard acrylic outside and soft acrylic inside which she could wear during sleeping and times of possible stress.

An alternative to the full occlusal mouthguard is the nociceptive trigeminal inhibition tensions suppression system (NTI-TSS) appliance. However, a possible limitation to this type of appliance is the necessary torque that may be required to both seat and unseat the appliance. If your anterior bonding consists of tooth lengthening this could be a problem. An alternative would be an anterior guard that covers only the six maxillary anterior teeth (such as the Bite Soft from TriDent Dental Laboratories). This can be made, as previously described, with a soft interior and hard exterior surface.

Beware of the patient who emphatically states "I don't clench or grind." Instead, look for craze lines and wear facets on the teeth and remember that almost everyone can have stressful sleep at times. It only takes one instance of clenching in eccentric positions to damage your patient's bonded restorations. A good way for you and your patient to visualize potential wear patterns is through the use of an intraoral camera. However, the very best way for you to see exactly what is taking place and to communicate it to your patient is through the use of a surgical or operative microscope (Global Surgical). The stereoscopic view as seen by the dentist is outstanding. When connected to a video recorder and monitor both you and your patient can discover exact habit patterns, making it so much easier for you to suggest preventive measures. Consider imposing limitations on your office warranty if your patient does not accept your recommendations for wearing a protective appliance (Figure 14.30).

Homecare

The immediate homecare of the patient should emphasize the most gentle, but thorough, cleaning. During this time, a chemotherapeutic agent, such as Peridex (3M) or Listerine (Johnson & Johnson), can help control plaque. Dipping a Rotadent (Den-Mat) brush tip in the mouthwash before using is an excellent way to apply the solution and obviates some of the staining problems associated with the mouthwash.[94]

Although a sizeable portion of the population is capable of adopting good hand brushing habits, using a rotary cleaning device (ProDentec) can make a dramatic difference for most people. Otherwise, patients may miss important areas where plaque can build up, resulting at the very least in unattractive stain. It is essential for the patient to receive proper instructions on how to use the device. For instance, a close grip to the actual tooth surface will result in better and easier control (Figure 14.31A and B).

Recall visits

In this mobile society where your patient may be receiving follow-up care on the other side of the country next year, he or she also needs to be sure that the new dentist or hygienist knows about the proper professional care of bonded teeth. Hygienists should avoid scaling against the margin of bonded teeth; instead, do hand scaling with a lateral movement to remove any calculus without a counterforce that could dislodge the restoration. Use of a Cavi-jet (Dentsply) or air powder abrasive instruments also pose potential damage to composite restorations,[95,96] as can ultrasonic and sonic instrumentation.[97] Certain polishing pastes can also be harmful.[98] Acidulated fluoride pastes are to be avoided; Miller advocates aluminum oxide polishing paste applied with a wet rotating rubber cup.[99] Remind patients to always make any dentist or dental hygienist (or for that matter, any physician or anesthesiologist who will be working around the mouth) aware that esthetic dental restorations have been done that could be damaged.

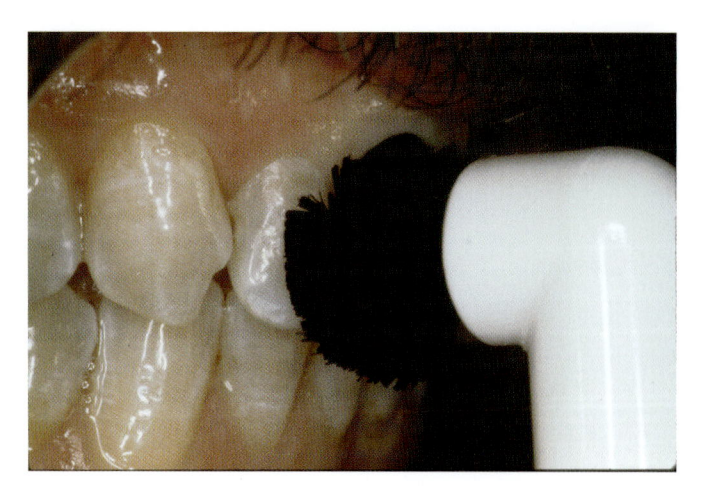

Figure 14.31 **(A)** An individual rotary cleaning device (Rotadent, Den-Mat) provides the patient with an excellent means for maintaining the subgingival margin of this bonded veneer.

Ideally, the patient should return for a postoperative visit within 1–2 weeks to make certain that soft tissue is healing properly. Some additional finishing may need to be done at that time to conform to the patient's emergence profile in order to achieve the highest esthetic and functional gingival margin possible. Until you have evidence of excellent tissue response, continue to have the patient return for periodic postoperative visits.

Most patients with esthetic restorations should be asked to return for inspection and hygiene recall within 3 months, in order for you to detect any problems, to make certain that the patient is caring for his or her mouth properly, and to ensure that there are no habits that could esthetically or functionally shorten the normal life span of a restored tooth. Use this recall to look especially at the margins of Class V composite resin restoration since water absorption in restorations without perfect margin seals may begin to cause a cervical overhang within 3 months.[84] If this happens, refinishing at that time may be required to avoid plaque retention and gingival irritation.

The life expectancy of most bonding may be more than 10 years now, as suggested by Drake et al.[5] However, *Change Your Smile*[93] gives a more conservative forecast of 5–8 years, depending upon the type of restoration and the patient's cooperation in maintaining it. The following point should be made: dentists or treatment coordinators should always remember that patients have a right to expect indefinite life of the bonding *unless* the dental professional enlightens them as to a definite range of life expectancy. Dentists may overestimate the patient's awareness of this. In a study by Goldstein and Lancaster,[100] almost one in three persons said they believed bonding to be permanent. More recently, Davis et al. found a similar lack of information in the general public concerning the strength of composite resins for posterior restorations.[101]

Pit and fissure stain

"It's just stain" is a typical comment made to patients by dentists when patients inquire about a darkly pitted or stained tooth. No longer is it necessary or even wise to allow these types of stained areas to exist in teeth. As Goldstein and Parkins suggest in their

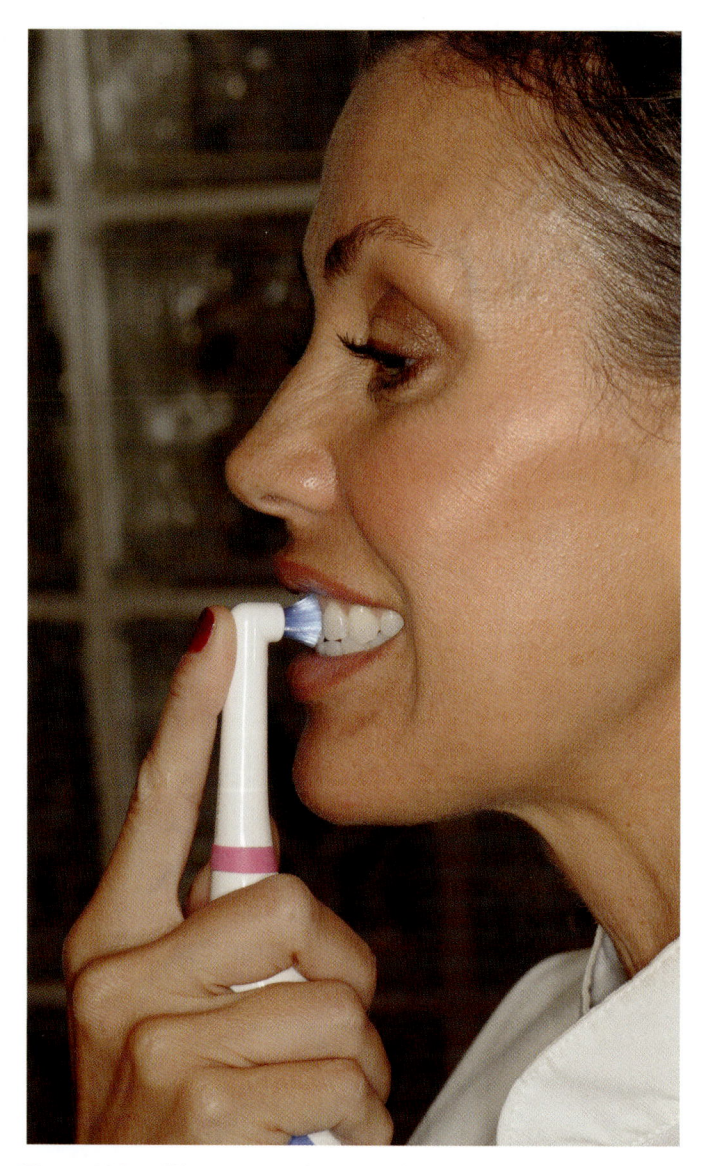

Figure 14.31 **(B)** It is essential to properly instruct your patient on the use of this cleaning device. Note that the closer the patient's forefinger is to the brush tip, the more control and thus cleaning efficiency he or she will have.

article in the *Journal of the American Dental Association*, changing patterns of dental caries suggest the need for a new emphasis on diagnosing and treating pit and fissure caries.[102] Although occlusal surfaces represent only 12% of the total permanent dentition surface area, occlusal surfaces account for more than 50% of reported caries in school-age children. This would suggest a need to focus on pit and fissure stain. In a National Institute of Dental Research (NIDR) study from 1980 to 1987 it was found that decay in pits and fissures had reduced by only 31% while caries in other surfaces dropped by 51–59%. Pit and fissure caries accounted for 80% of total caries in nonfluoridated water areas and 90% in fluoridated water areas.

Our clinical experience has shown 70–75% of these stained areas are involved into the dentin and, in fact, the great majority of them are actually carious lesions. Re-evaluation of the methods used to detect pit and fissure lesions has led to questioning

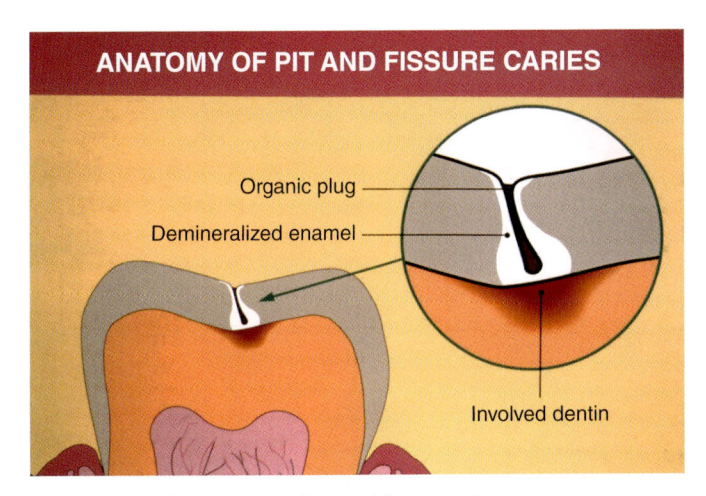

Figure 14.32 **(A)** Anatomy of pit and fissure caries.

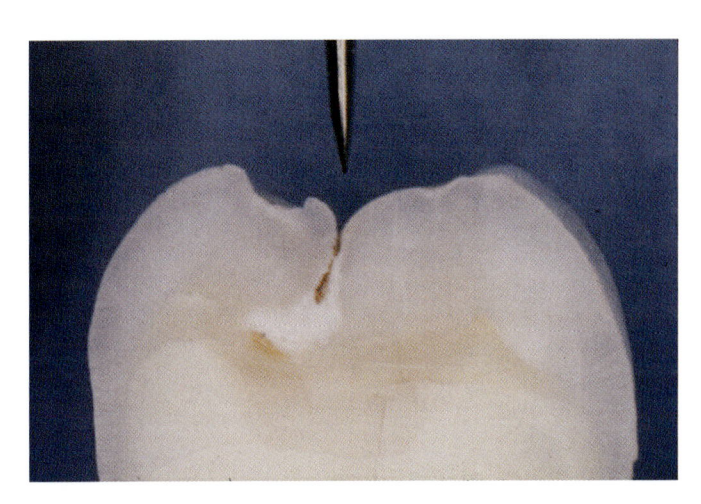

Figure 14.32 **(B)** The explorer is often of limited use in the diagnosis of pit and fissure caries since fissures are frequently narrower than the explore tip. This tool would not have aided in the diagnosis of this lesion. Therefore, the only sure way of knowing if a stained pit or fissure is carious is to "spray" it out with air-abrasive technology. Reproduced from Paterson et al.[103] courtesy of Quintessence Publishing Co, Inc.

the traditional use of the explorer to probe for caries. Enamel that is undermined with caries but strengthened by fluoride makes decay difficult to detect. A sticky fissure detected by the wedging of an explorer tip is no longer considered the only method for detecting pit and fissure caries (Figure 14.32A and B). In fact, probing of pits and fissures also has been deemphasized because of its potential for damaging enamel. It is also interesting to note that few of these lesions are actually seen on radiographs as decay, although intraoral video cameras can facilitate the viewing of caries in grooves that are too narrow for the penetration of an explorer tip. However, difficulty in distinguishing a stain on the surface from a darker-colored organic plug within the pit or fissure that can promote caries also contributes to the diagnostic dilemma (Figure 14.32A). Instead, use either a laser detection device or AC impedance spectroscopy technique which can be quite helpful in determining if a pit or fissure is carious or just stain (Diagnodent, Kavo, Cariescan pro) (Figure 3.5B and C).

The traditional placement of sealants in pits and fissures without removing the stain or organic plug, and possible underlying caries, is *seriously questioned*. Shrinkage and marginal wear often lead to undetected marginal leakage. Paterson et al. report that if such leakage occurs over active dentinal caries, it may not be detected before pulpal involvement or extensive undermining of enamel and/or cuspal fracture occurs.[103]

Use of air-abrasive technology

According to Goldstein and Parkins,[102] air-abrasive technology (PrepStart by Danville) (MicroPrep, Lares; Mach 5, Kreativ) offers options in caries diagnosis and treatment. The air-abrasive system uses a narrowly focused particle stream that abrades tooth structure in proportion to the particle size, air pressure, and nozzle distance employed. The key issue for this newly revived technology is that it provides a more conservative approach to both diagnosis and treatment of pit and fissure caries than conventional methods. After observing suspiciously stained pits or fissures, one or more short bursts of alpha alumina powder from the air-abrasive system can be used to remove both the stain and organic plug for a more accurate evaluation of the presence of caries. If this is simply stain or the organic plug, the abrasive action will eliminate it while leaving all but a few micrometers of healthy tooth structure intact. This examination is especially facilitated by the use of an intraoral camera or operative microscope. Several intraoral cameras also have caries detection ability (Figure 3.9A–F featuring Kodak CS1600, CareStream, Soprolife, Acteon). If there is no decay, the air-abrasively prepared pit or fissure can then be sealed or restored with resin materials.

If underlying caries is detected, further bursts of the abrasive powder stream may be used to completely eradicate the lesion, preserving the maximum amount of healthy tooth structure. (Hand or rotary instruments may be used as well if the area of decay is large.) The air-abrasive technique roughens the tooth surface, leaving it ready for direct bonding techniques with or without acid etching.[104–109] The preparation can be restored immediately with either filled or unfilled composite resin. A combined sealant and bonding technique may be considered: if tooth structure has been removed or the anatomy is irregular, restore those areas with a bonded filled resin. The smaller, secondary grooves may then be covered with a sealant, creating a preventive resin restoration (Figure 14.33A–E). With the introduction of flowable composite resins, this procedure can be accomplished in a single step.

Patients like the fact that abrasive technology does not usually require an anesthetic, and therefore an "uncomfortable" injection and associated numbness are often eliminated.[3] This also saves time for the dentist because he or she can begin immediately with a happier patient, not waiting for an anesthetic to take effect. The unpleasant heat, pressure, and bone-conducted noise and vibration associated with most "drilling" is minimized. This gentleness is confirmed by histologic studies demonstrating that this technology is much kinder to the pulp.[84]

The esthetic advantage of using air-abrasive technology is the ability to easily eliminate stained and/or carious areas without

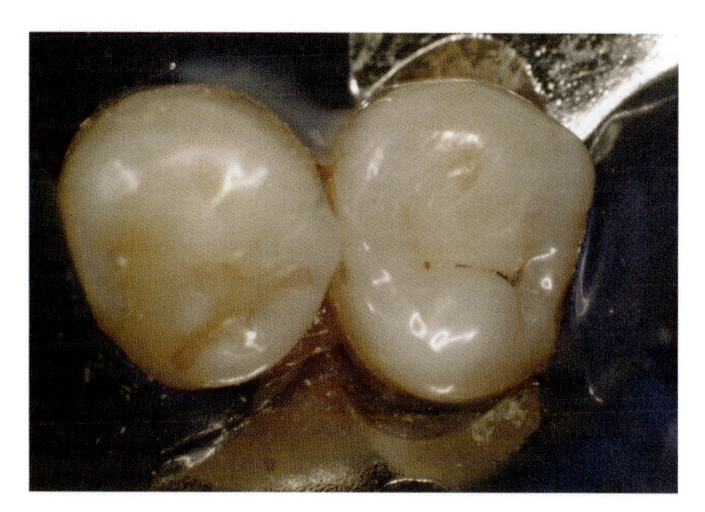

Figure 14.33 **(A)** This lower bicuspid reveals a stain.

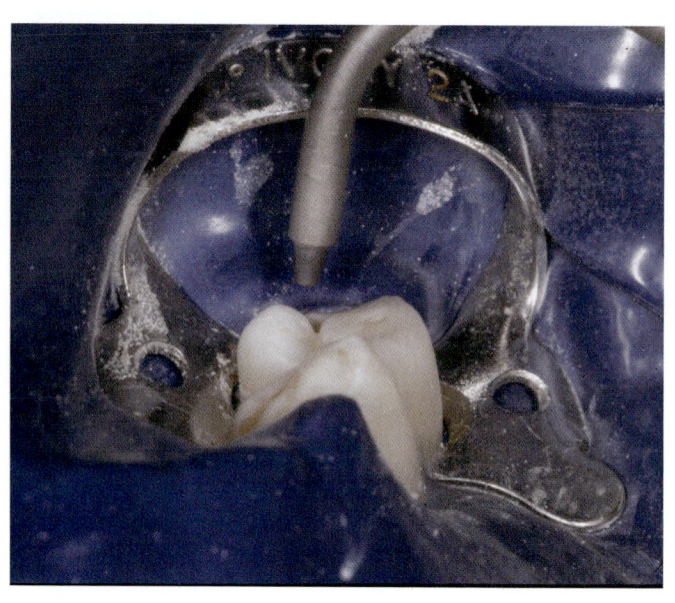

Figure 14.33 **(B)** A 3 s burst by an air-abrasive system (PrepStart, Danville) helps determine if the problem is caries or just stain.

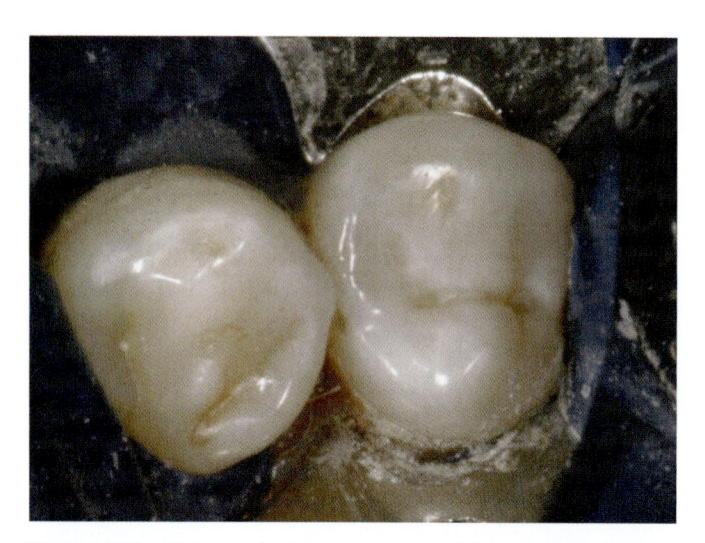

Figure 14.33 **(C)** Using the intraoral camera with caries detection ability helps to ensure that all caries is removed.

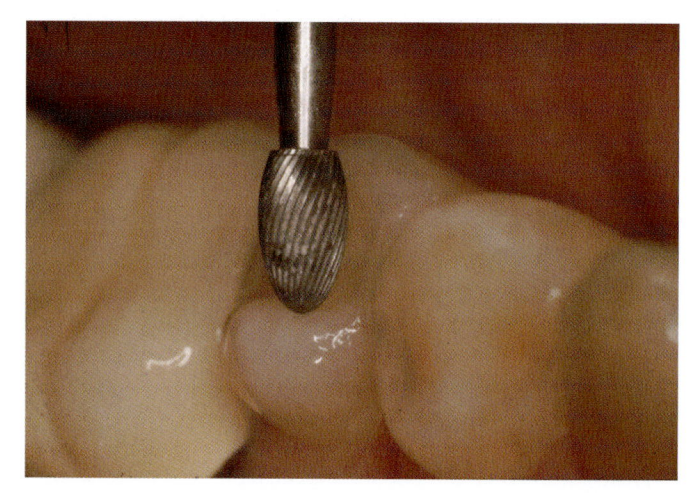

Figure 14.33 **(D)** Once all caries are removed, the tooth is restored with a hybrid composite. The final finish is achieved with a 30-bladed carbide finishing bur (OSIUF, Brasseler USA).

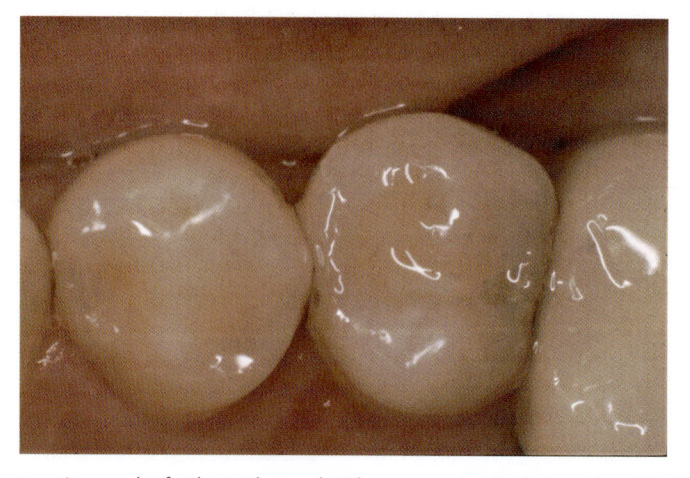

Figure 14.33 **(E)** The final bonded restoration can be further enhanced with a composite surface sealant (Fortify, Biscover).

cutting into the tooth with a rotary handpiece. Patient acceptance is so high that it is a definite practice builder. Psychologically, patients also may feel better about maintaining teeth that have been restored to a natural, healthy appearance, rather than restored teeth that retain unsightly stains around the restoration. Further, patients appreciate the concept of maximizing the conservation of healthy tooth structure by attacking decay at the earliest possible moment. Preliminary studies of shear bond strength also suggest that the roughened surface created by air-abrasive technology may enhance bonding, especially bonding to dentin.[109]

Other techniques of eliminating pit and fissure caries are use of special ultrathin diamonds or burs or hard tissue lasers. Goldstein has also used the ET3 30 μm to enter previously diagnosed carious pit and fissures. However, use of a diamond bur makes it necessary to use a restorative technique to keep out the lesion, whereas the use of air abrasion may eliminate the stain and no further treatment may be necessary.

A major advantage in using the hard tissue laser is the ability to perform most procedures without injectable anesthesia (Solea CO_2) (Figure 14.34A–I). This means children and young adults may never have to have injections for restorative dental treatment. Specifically, defective or carious pits and fissures plus interproximal decay can easily be done with the hard tissue laser that also anesthetizes the tooth being treated.

Another major use of air-abrasive technology is the repair of composite resin and porcelain restorations. Until now, no satisfactory method had been devised to etch the existing composite resin when new composite resin was to be added as in a repair or even esthetic enhancement of a discolored composite. By first preparing the surface of the composite with the air-abrasive

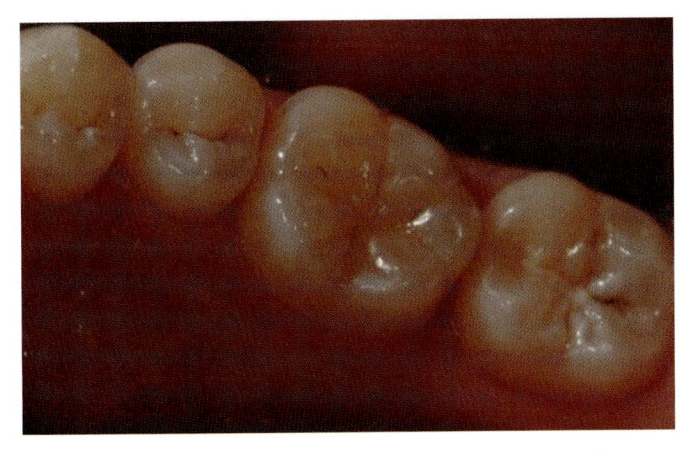

Figure 14.34 **(A)** The second bicuspid revealed a 2.5 LED reading (Kavo, USA). It was decided to follow out the stain to verify that caries were present.

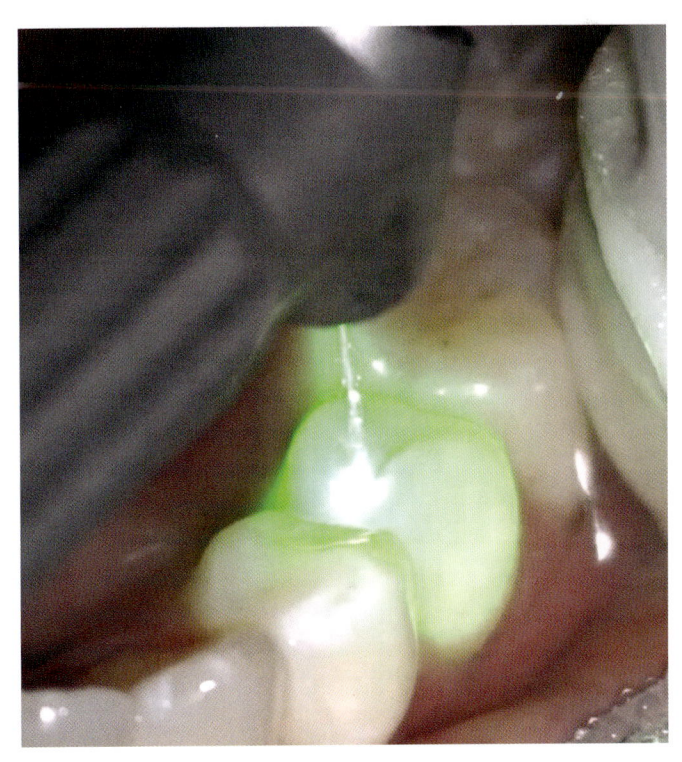

Figure 14.34 **(B)** A CO_2 laser (Solea, Convergent) hard tissue laser was selected so no local anesthesia would be necessary.

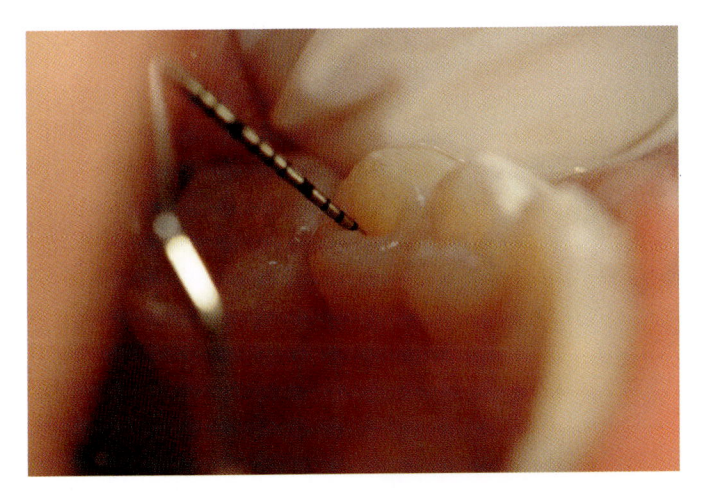

Figure 14.34 **(C)** The probe showed almost 2 mm depth to the carious lesion after it opened up in the dentin.

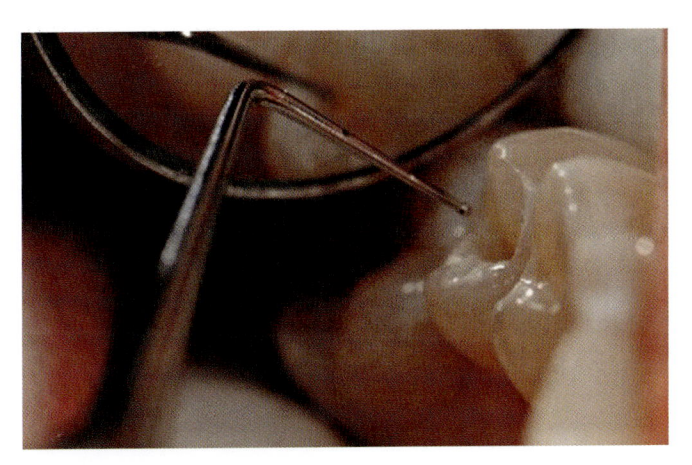

Figure 14.34 **(D)** One advantage of the laser is to keep the opening as narrow as possible. Therefore, a very thin placement instrument is used to place the inner base (Vitrebond), plus light-curing glass ionomer, (3 M).

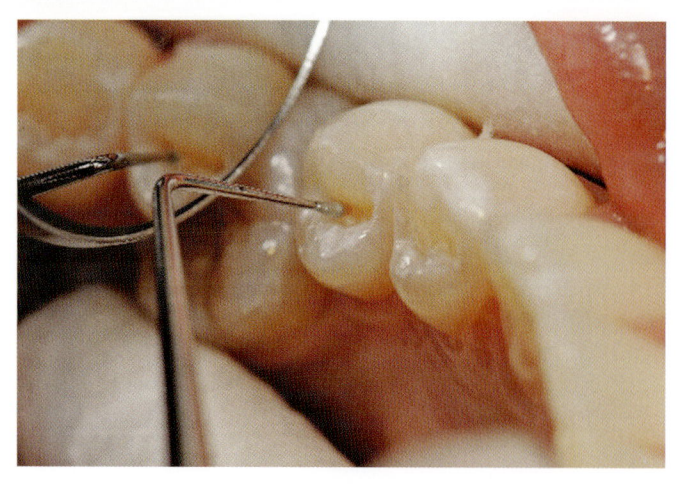

Figure 14.34 **(E)** Note how the special end of the Goldstein micro placement instrument (Hu-Friedy TMGPI) can carry and place a very small amount of liner/base into the preparation without even touching the walls of the cavity.

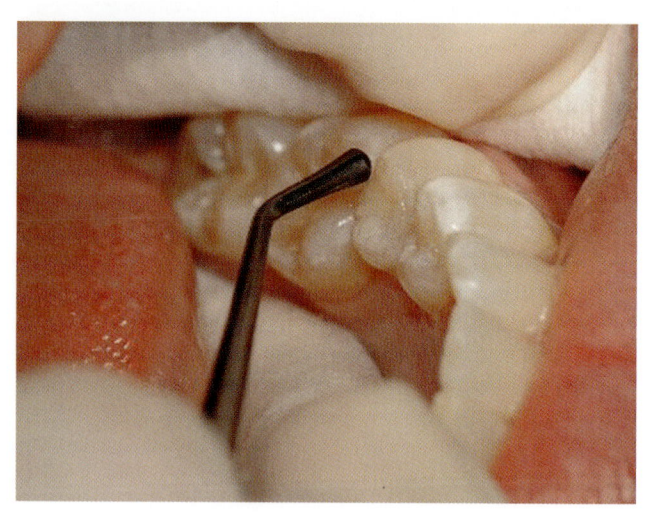

Figure 14.34 **(F)** The final layer of micro-hybrid composite is condensed by an aluminum titanium nitride-coated double-ended condenser (TNCIGFT 2, Hu-Friedy).

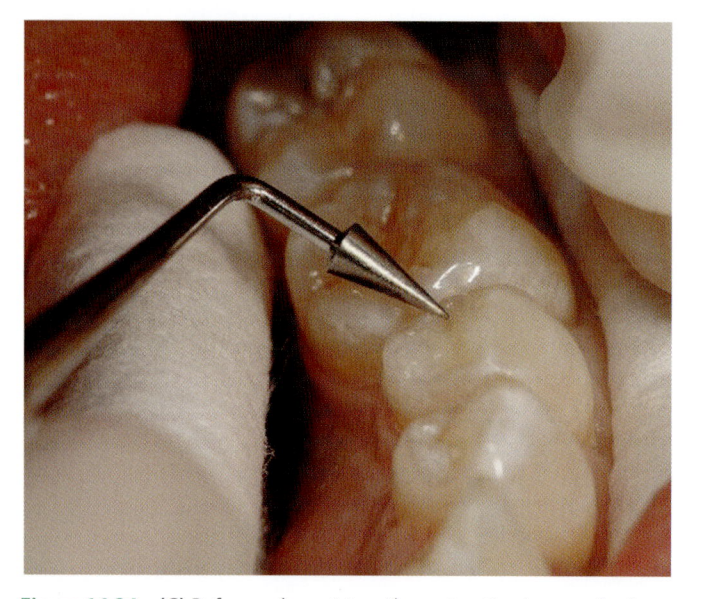

Figure 14.34 **(G)** Before polymerizing, the restorative is carved using a satin steel XTS composite carver (#5-TNCIGFT 5, Hu-Friedy).

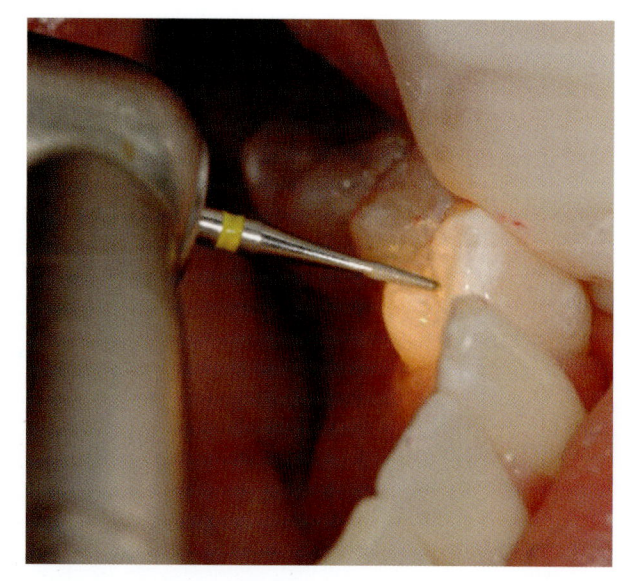

Figure 14.34 **(H)** After polymerization, the occlusal anatomy is smoothed using either a 15 μm diamond (DOS3, Brasseler USA) or a 30-blade carbide (OS3UF, Brasseler USA).

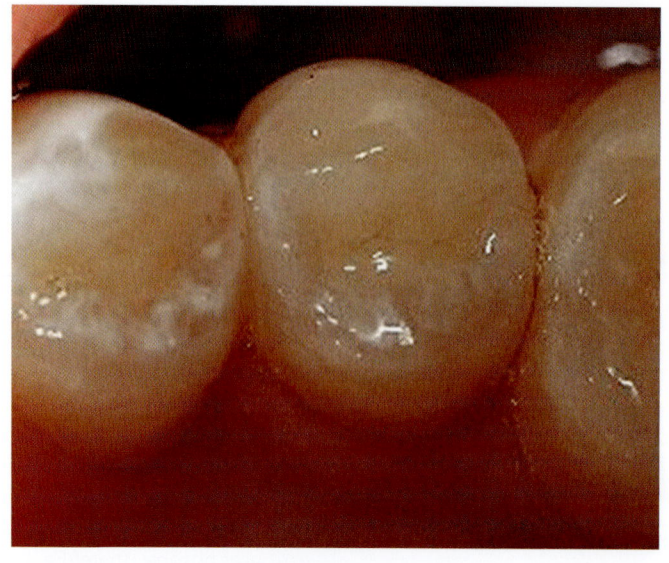

Figure 14.34 **(I)** The final restoration after polishing with the Feather Lite polisher (Brasseler USA), and a 10 s polymerization to reinforce surface hardness.

system, an excellent etched surface exists to help gain greater retention of the newly bonded composite resin. A study by Chen et al. also showed that a 120 s air abrasion provided the highest bond strength of composite resin to porcelain.[110]

The future

McLean doubted that the ideal restorative material will be achieved until well into the 21st century,[111] but it is clear that bonding will continue to improve through both materials and technique. The use of erbium:YAG lasers for tooth preparation and etching as well as argon and other lasers, some of which feature subsecond polymerization, may result in shorter procedural time and increased restoration strength.[57] New strength, new direct and indirect materials, and perhaps even decreasing costs will bring bonding to larger numbers of people. Furthermore, if current findings continue to hold true, composites will not only become more valuable for esthetics but also for reducing caries,[4] in combination with glass ionomers and other similar compounds.

References

1. Buonocore MG. A simple method of increasing the adhesion of acrylic filling materials to enamel surfaces. *J Dent Res* 1955;34:849–853.
2. Bowen RL. *Development of a Silica-Resin Direct Filling Material. Report 6333.* Washington, DC: National Bureau of Standards; 1958.
3. Bowen R. Properties of a silica-reinforced polymer for dental restorations. *J Am Dent Assoc* 1963;66:57–64.
4. Phillips RW. Era of new biomaterials in esthetic dentistry. *J Am Dent Assoc* 1987;Special Issue:7E–13E.
5. Drake CW, Maryniuk GA, Bentley C. Reasons for restoration replacement: differences in practice patterns. *Quintessence Int* 1990;21:125–130.
6. Leinfelder KF. Posterior composite resins. *J Am Dent Assoc* 1988;Special Issue:21-E–26-E.
7. Wilson MA, Wilson NHF, Smith GA. A clinical trial of a visible light-cured posterior composite resin restorative: two year results. *Quintessence Int* 1986;17:151–155.
8. Bayne SC, Taylor DF, Roberson TM, et al. Long term clinical failures in posterior composites. *J Dent Res* 1989;68.
9. Maitland RI. Director posterior composites. *Esthet Dent Update* 1990;1:49–52.
10. Albers H. *Tooth Colored Restoratives Principles and Techniques,* 9th edn. Ontario, Canada: BC Decker Inc.; 2002.
11. Jordan RE. Resin-enamel bonding. In: Jordan RE, ed. *Esthetic Composite Bonding: Techniques and Materials,* revised edn. Philadelphia, PA: B.C. Decker; 1988.
12. Mount GJ. Changes in operative dentistry - beyond G.V. Black. In: Roulet JF, Vanherle G, eds. *Adhesive Technology for Restorative Dentistry.* London: Quintessence; 2005.
13. Baratieri LN. *Inspiration People, Teeth and Restorations.* New Malden, UK: Quintessence; 2012.
14. Baratieri LN, Monteiro Jr S, Spezia de Melo T. *Routes for Excellence in Restorative Dentistry, vols 1 and 2.* Hanover Park, IL: Quintessence; 2014.
15. Baratieri LN, Araujo Jr EM, Monteiro Jr S. *Composite Restorations in Anterior Teeth.* São Paulo, Brazil: Quintessence; 2005.
16. Roulet J, Vanherle G. *Adhesive Technology for Restorative Dentistry.* New Malden, UK: Quintessence; 2005.
17. Dietschi D, Spreafico R. *Adhesive Metal-Free Restorations: Current Concepts for the Esthetic Treatment of Posterior Teeth.* Chicago, IL: Quintessence; 1997.
18. Gwinnett AJ, Matsui A. A study of enamel adhesives: the physical relationship between enamel and adhesive. *Oral Biol* 1967;12:1615.
19. Jordan RE, Suzuki M, Gwinnett AJ. Conservative applications of acid etch resin techniques. *Dent Clin North Am* 1981;25:307.
20. Ford RT, Douglas W. The use of composite resin for creating anterior guidance during occlusal therapy. *Quintessence Int* 1988;19:331–337.
21. Goldstein RE. Diagnostic dilemma: to bond, laminate, or crown? *Int J Periodontics Restorative Dent* 1987;8:8–29.
22. Weinstein AR. Anterior composite resins and veneers: treatment planning, preparation, and finishing. *J Am Dent Assoc* 1988;Special Issue:38E–45E.
23. Cooley RL, Barkmeier WW, Matis BA, Siok JF. Staining of posterior resin restorative materials. *Quintessence Int* 1987;18:823–827.
24. Douvitas G. Effect of cavity design on gap formation in Class II composite resin restorations. *J Prosthet Dent* 1991;65:475–479.
25. Roulet JF, Hirt T, Lutz F. Surface roughness and marginal behavior of experimental and commercial composites: an in vitro study. *J Oral Rehabil* 1984;11:499–509.
26. Mopper KW. The subtleties of anterior direct-bonded Class III restorations. *Pract Periodontics Aesthet Dent.* 2(6):17–20.
27. Croll TP, Donley KJ. Imperceptible bonded composite resin Class III restoration using labial access. *Quintessence Int* 1990;21:795–799.
28. Davidson CL, Kemp-Scholte CM. Shortcomings of composite resins in Class V restorations. *J Esthet Dent* 1989;1:1–4.
29. Goldfogle M. Case selection: expert shares tips on direct bonding. *Cosmet Dent GPs* 1990;1:6–7.
30. Christensen GJ. Veneering of teeth. State of the art. *Dent Clin North Am* 1985;29:373–391.
31. Levin RP. Composite inlays as management tools in dental practice. *J Esthet Dent* 1989;1:38–40.
32. Shortall AC, Baylis RI, Baylis MA, Grundy JR. Marginal seal comparisons between resin-bonded Class II porcelain inlays, posterior composite restorations, and direct composite resin inlays. *Int J Prosthodont* 1989;2:217–222.
33. Valentine CW. Composite resin restoration in esthetic dentistry. *J Am Dent Assoc* 1987;Special Issue:55E–61E.
34. Mohd Z, Aziz R. Wear of materials used in dentistry: a review of the literature. *J Prosthet Dent* 1990;63:342–349.
35. Dickinson GL, Leinfelder KF, Mazer RB, Russell CM. Effect of surface penetrating sealant on wear rate of posterior composite resins. *J Am Dent Assoc* 1990;121:251–255.
36. Yip KH, Smales RJ, Kaidonis JA. Differential wear of teeth and restorative materials: clinical implications. *Int J Prosthodont* 2004;17:350–356.
37. Lutz F, Imfeld T, Meier CH, et al. Composite resins versus amalgam—comparative measurements of in vivo wear resistance. 1-year report. *Quintessence Int* 1979;3(3):77–87.
38. Jordan RE, Gwinnett AJ. Methods and materials. In: Jordan RE, ed. *Esthetic Composite Bonding: Techniques and Materials,* revised ed. Philadelphia, PA: B.C. Decker; 1988.
39. Dunn JR. Microfills retain importance. *Dentist* 1990;68:29–32.
40. Jordan RE, Suzuki M. Direct hybrid composite inlay technique. *J Esthet Dent* 1988;(1):57–60.
41. Pintado MR. Characterization of two small-particle composite resins. *Quintessence Int* 1990;21:843–848.

42. Paquette DE, Vann WF, Oldenberg TR, Leinfelder KF. Modified cavity preparation for composite resins in primary molars. *Pediatr Dent* 1983;5:246–251.
43. Gwinnett AJ. Bonding of restorative resins to enamel. *Int Dent J* 1988;38:91–96.
44. Brockmann SL, Scott RL, Erick JD. A scanning electron microscopic study of the effect of air polishing of the enamel-sealant surface. *Quintessence Int* 1990;21:201–206.
45. Hosoya Y, Goto G. Color differences between light cured composite resins and shade guides. *J Dent Res* 1990;69.
46. Makinson OR. Color changes on curing light-activated anterior restorative resins. *Dent Abstracts* 1989;34:467.
47. Pink FE. Use of custom composite shade guide for shade determination. *J Dent Res* 1989;69.
48. Crim GA. Influence of bonding agents and composites on microleakage. *J Prosthet Dent* 1989;61:571–574.
49. Hinoura K, Stecos JC, Phillips RW. Cavity design and placement techniques for class 2 composites. *Oper Dent* 1988;13:12–19.
50. Myers DR, Butts MB. Surface topography of the cavosurface enamel bevel following acid etching in primary teeth. *J Pedod* 1985;10:63–67.
51. Moore DH, Vann WF. The effect of a cavosurface bevel on microleakage in posterior composite restorations. *J Prosthet Dent* 1988;59:21–24.
52. Jefferies SR, Smith RL, Barkmeier WW, Gwinnett AJ. Comparison of surface smoothness of restorative resin materials. *J Esthet Dent* 1989;1:169–175.
53. Anusavice KJ. *Quality Evaluation of Dental Restorations: Criteria for Placement and Replacement*. Chicago, IL: Quintessence; 1989.
54. Temin SC, Csuros Z, Mellberg JH. Fluoride uptake form a composite restorative by enamel. *Dent Mat* 1989;5(1):64–65.
55. Baharav H, Cardash HS, Helft M, Langsam J. Penetration of etched enamel by bonding agents. *J Prosthet Dent* 1988;59:33–36.
56. Van Meerbeek B, et al. A randomized controlled study evaluating the effectiveness of a two-step self-etch adhesive with and without selective phosphoric-acid etching of enamel. *Dent Mat* 2005;21:375–383.
57. McLean JW, Powis DR, Prosser HJ, Wilson AD. The use of glass-ionomer cements in bonding composite resins to dentine. *Br Dent J* 1985;158:410–414.
58. Kanca J. Bonding to tooth structure: a rationale for a clinical protocol. *J Esthet Dent* 1989;1:135–138.
59. Kanca J. Composite resin luting materials: a rationale for the '90s. *J Esthet Dent* 1989;1:105–109.
60. Garcia-Godoy F, Draheim RN, Titus HW. Preventive glass ionomer restorations. *Am J Dent* 1988;1:97–99.
61. Hembree JH. Microleakage at the gingival margin of Class II composite restorations with glass ionomer liner. *J Prosthet Dent* 1989;61:28–30.
62. Mixson JM, Eick JD, Tira DE, Moore DL. The effects of variable wash times and techniques on enamel-composite resin bond strength. *Quintessence Int* 1988;19:279–285.
63. Leinfelder KF. The amalgam restoration. *Dent Clin North Am* 1983;27:685–696.
64. Lloyd CH. Resistance to fracture in posterior composites. *Br Dent J* 1983;155:411.
65. Phillips RW. Changing trends of dental restorative materials. *Dent Clin North Am* 1989;33:285–291.
66. Rueggeberg FA, Ergle JW, Mettenburg DJ. Polymerization depths of contemporary light curing units using microhardness. *J Esthet Dent* 2000;12:340–349.
67. Roberson TO, Heymann HO, Ritter AV. Introduction to composite restorations. In: Roberson TO, Heymann HO, Swift EJ, eds. *Sturtevant's Art and Science of Operative Dentistry*, 5th edn. St. Louis, MO: Elsevier Mosby; 2005: 498–524.
68. Lutz F, Krejci I, Oldenburg TR. Elimination of polymerization stresses at the margins of posterior composite resin restorations: a new restorative technique. *Quintessence Int* 1986;17:777–784.
69. Sadhegi M, Lynch CD. The effect of flowable materials on the microleakage of Class II composite restorations that extend apical to the cemento-enamel junction. *Oper Dent* 2009;34(3):306–311.
70. Deliperi S, Bardwell DN. An alternative method to reduce polymerization shrinkage in direct posterior composite restorations. *J Am Dent Assoc* 2002;133:1387–1398.
71. Hardison JD, Rafferty-Parker D, Mitchell RJ, Bean LR. Radiolucent alos associated with radiopaque composite resin restorations. *J Am Dent Assoc* 1989;118:595–597.
72. Hilton TJ, Schwartz RS. The effect of air thinning on dentin adhesive bond strength. *Oper Dent* 1995;20:133–137.
73. Schvaneveldt SL, Rozmajzl WF Jr, Barkmeier WW, Latta MA. Bond strength of an adhesive polymerized under nitrogen. *Am J Dent* 1996;9:157–160.
74. Beard CC, Donaldson K, Clayton JA. A comparison of articulator settings to age and sex. *J Prosthet Dent* 1986;56:551–554.
75. Antonson DE, Benedetro MD. Longitudinal intensity variability of visible light curing units. *Quintessence Int* 1986;17:819–820.
76. Friedman J. Variability of lamp characteristics in dental curing lights. *J Esthet Dent* 1987;1:189–190.
77. Strassler H. Light-curing guidelines. *Inside Dent* 2012;8(1):70–74.
78. Yazici AR, et al. Effects of different curing light units/modes on the microleakage of flowable composite resins. *Eur J Dent* 2008;2:240–246.
79. Camphreger UB, Samuel SM, Fortes CB, et al. Effectiveness of second-generation light-emitting diode (LED) light curing units. *J Contemp Dent Pract* 2007;8(2):35–42.
80. Hasler C, et al. Curing capability of halogen and LED light curing units in deep class II cavities in extracted human molars. *Oper Dent* 2006;31(3):354–363.
81. Donly KJ, Dowell A, Anixiadas C, Croll TP. Relationship among visible light source, composite resin polymerization shrinkage, and hygroscopic expansion. *Quintessence Int* 1990;21:883–886.
82. Terkla LG, Brown AC, Hainisch AP, Mitchem JC. Testing sealing properties of restorative materials against moist dentin. *J Dent Res* 1987;66:1758–1764.
83. Kemp-Scholte CM, Davidson CL. Marginal sealing of curing contraction gaps in Class V composite resin restoration. *J Dent Res* 1988;67:841–845.
84. Laurell K, Carpenter W, Daugherty D, Beck M. Histopathologic effects of kinetic cavity preparation for the removal of enamel and dentin. An in vivo animal study. *Oral Surg Oral Med Oral Pathol Oral Radiol Endod* 1995;80:214–225.
85. Greiff RM, Burgess JO, Davis RD, Theobald WD. Wet and dry finishing techniques for composite resin. *J Dent Res* 1989;68.
86. Collard S, Vogel J, Ladd G. Respirability, microstructure, and filler content of composite dusts. *Am J Dent* 1991;4:143–152.
87. Pratten DH, Johnson GH. An evaluation of finishing instruments for an anterior and a posterior composite. *J Prosthet Dent* 1988;60(2):154–158.
88. Ratanapridakul K, Leinfelder KF, Thomas J. Effect of finishing on the in vivo wear rate of a posterior composite resin. *J Am Dent Assoc* 1989;118:333–335.

89. Watson TF. High speed dental burr/tooth cutting interactions and their implications for adhesive restorative materials. *J Dent Res* 1989;69.
90. Chen RCS, Chan DCN, Chan KC. A quantitative study of finishing and polishing techniques for a composite. *J Prosthet Dent* 1988;59:292–297.
91. Toffenetti F. Considerations about esthetics of composite resin restorations. *J Esthet Dent* 1989;1:62–66.
92. Strassler H, Serio F, Litkowshi L, Moffitt W. Effect of toothpastes on polished composite resin surfaces. *J Dent Res* 1987;66:211.
93. Goldstein RE. *Change Your Smile*, 4th edn. Chicago, IL: Quintessence; 2009.
94. Goldstein RE, Garber DA, Schwartz CG, Goldstein CE. Patient maintenance of esthetic restorations. *J Am Dent Assoc* 1992;123:61–66.
95. Cooley RL, Lubow RM, Brown FH. Effect of airpowder abrasive instrument on porcelain. *J Prosthet Dent* 1988;60:440–443.
96. Reel DC, Abrams H, Gardner SL, Mitchell RJ. Effect of a hydraulic jet prophylaxis system on composites. *J Prosthet Dent* 1989;61:441–445.
97. Bjornson E, Collins DE, Engler WO. Surface alteration of composite resins after curette, ultrasonic, and sonic instrumentation: an in vitro study. *Quintessence Int* 1990;21:381–389.
98. Serio R, Litkowski L, Strasseler H, Krupa C. The effects of polishing pastes on polished composite resin surfaces. *J Dent Res* 1987;66:211.
99. Miller DL, Hodges KO. Polishing the surface: a comparison of rubber cup polishing and airpolishing. *Probe* 1991;25(3):103, 105–109.
100. Goldstein RE, Lancaster JS. Survey of patient attitudes toward current esthetic procedures. *J Prosthet Dent* 1984;52:775–780.
101. Davis EL, Laura JC, Joynt RB, Wieczkowski G. Determination of demand for posterior resin restorations. *J Prosthet Dent* 1988;59:242–248.
102. Goldstein RE, Parkins F. Using air-abrasive technology to diagnose and restore pit and fissure caries. *J Am Dent Assoc* 1995;126:761–765.
103. Paterson RC, Watts A, Saunders WP, Pitts NB. *Modern Concepts in the Diagnosis and Treatment of Fissure Caries*. Chicago, IL: Quintessence; 1991:14–16.
104. Doty WD, Pettey D, Holder R, Phillips S. KCP 2000 enamel etching abilities tested. *J Dent Res* 1994;73(Special issue):411, Abstract 2474.
105. Eakle WS, Goodis HE, White JM, Do HK. *J Dent Res* 1994;73 (Special Edition):131, Abstract 239.
106. Fahl Jr N. A solution for everyday direct restorative challenges-Part 1. *J Cos Dent* 2010;26(3):56–68
107. Fahl Jr N. Step-by-step approaches for anterior direct restorative challenges. *J Cos Dent* 2010;26(4):42–55.
108. Keen DS, von Fraunhofer JA, Parkins FM. Air-abrasive etching bond strengths. *J Dent Res* 1994;73 (Special Issue):131, Abstract 238.
109. Laurell K, Lord W, Beck M. Kinetic cavity preparation effects on bonding to enamel and dentin. *J Dent Res* 1993;72(Special Issue):273, Abstract 1437.
110. Chen JH, Matsumura H, Atsuta M. Effect of different etching periods on the bond strength of a composite resin to a machinable porcelain. *J Dent* 1998;28:53–58.
111. McLean JW. Long-term esthetic dentistry. *Quintessence Int* 1989;20:701–708.

Additional resources

Abdalla AI, Alhadainy HA. 2-year clinical evaluation of class I posterior composites. *Am J Dent* 1996;9(4):150–152.

Abdalla AI, Davidson CL. Effect of mechanical load cycling on the marginal integrity of adhesive class I resin composite restorations. *J Dent* 1996;24:87–90.

Abdalla AI, Davidson CL. Shear bond strength and microleakage of new dentin bonding systems. *Am J Dent* 1993;6:295–298.

Albers HF, Alternatives for Class li restorations (results of clinical trial of 21 materials at 3 years). *CRA Newsletter* 1994;May.

Alharbi A, Rocca GT, Dietschi D, Krejci I. Semidirect composite onlay with cavity sealing: a review of clinical procedures. *J Esthet Restor Dent* 2014; 26 97–106.

Alshali RZ, Salim NA, Satterthwaite JD, Silikas N. Long-term sorption and solubility of bulk-fill and conventional resin-composites in water and artificial saliva. *J Dent* 2015;43:1511–1518.

Andreasen JO, Andreasen FM. *Textbook and Color Atlas of Traumatic Injuries to the Teeth*. St. Louis, MO: Mosby; 1994.

Anzai M, Yoshihashi R, Kobori M, Ohashi M. Synthesis of monomer for radiopaque composite resin and their properties. *J Dent Res* 1989;68.

Applequist EA, Meiers JC. Effect of bulk insertion, per polymerized resin composite balls, and beta-quartz inserts on microleakage of class V resin composite restorations. *Quintessence Int* 1996;27:253–258.

Arcoria CJ, Vitasek BA, Ferracane JL. Microleakage of composite resin restorations following thermocycling and instrumentation. *Gen Dent* 1990;38:129–131.

Arends J, Ruben J. Fluoride release from a composite resin. *Quintessence Int* 1988;19:513–514.

Arends J, van der Zee Y. Fluoride uptake in bovine enamel and dentin from a fluoride-releasing composite resin. *Quintessence Int* 1990;21:541–544.

Arends J, Ruben J, Dijkman A. The effect of fluoride release from a fluoride-containing composite resin on secondary caries: an in vitro study. *Quintessence Int* 1990;21:671–674.

Asmussen E, Munksgaard EC. Bonding of restorative resins to dentine: status of dentine adhesives and impact on cavity design and filling techniques. *Int Dent J* 1988;38:97–104.

Bader JD, Graves RC, Disney JA, et al. Identifying children who will experience high caries increments. *Community Dent Oral Epidemiol* 1986;14:198–201.

Bader JD, Brown JP. Dilemmas in caries diagnosis. *J Am Dent Assoc* 1993;124:48–50.

Baratieri LN, Coral Neto AC, Monteiro Jr S, et al. The sandwich technique, an alternative for tetracycline-stained teeth: a case report. *Quintessence Int* 1991;22:929–933.

Baratieri LN. *Dentistica: Procedimentos Preventivos e Restauradores*. São Paulo, Brazil: Quintessence; 1992.

Baratieri LN. *Estetica: Restauracoes Adesivas Diretas em Dentes Anteriores Fraturados*. São Paulo, Brazil: Quintessence; 1995.

Baratieri LN, Monteiro S Jr, de Albuquerque FM, et al. Reattachment of a tooth fragment with a new adhesive system: a case report. *Quintessence Int* 1994;25:91–96.

Barnes DM, Holston AM, Strassler HE, Shires PJ. Evaluation of clinical performance of twelve posterior composite resins with a standardized placement technique. *J Esthet Dent* 1990;2:36–43.

Barnwell S, Cooley R, Dodge W, Dale R. The effect of wet and dry finishing on composite resin surfaces. *J Dent Res* 1989;68.

Baum L. *Principles and Practice of Operative Dentistry*, 3rd edn. 1988.

Beaudreau DE. *Atlas of Fixed Partial Prosthesis*. Springfield, IL: Charles C. Thomas; 1975.

Behery H, El-Mowafy O, El-Badrawy W, et al. Cuspal deflection of premolars restored with bulk-fill composite resins. *J Esthet Restor Dent* 2016; 28:122–130.

Berman G, Linden L. The action of the explorer on incipient caries. *Svensk Tandlaek Tidskr* 1969;62:629–634.

Berry EA III, Berry LL, Powers JM. Bonding of hybrid ionomer to air-abraded enamel and dentin. *J Dent Res* 1994;73 (Special Issue):183, Abstract 654.

Bertschinger C, Paul SJ, Luthy H, et al. Dual application of dentin bonding agents: effect on bond strength. *Am J Dent* 1996;9:115–119.

Biederman JD. Direct composite resin inlay. *J Prosthet Dent* 1989;62:249–253.

Black RB. Application and re-evaluation of air abrasive technic. *J Am Dent Assoc* 1955;50:408–414.

Blankenau RJ, Barkmeier WM, Powell GL, Kelsey WP. Enhancement of physical properties of resin restorative materials by laser polymerization. *Lasers Surg Med* 1989;9:623–627.

Blomgren J, Axell T, Sandahl O, Jontell M. Adverse reactions in the oral mucosa associated with anterior composite restorations. *J Oral Pathol Med* 1996;25:311–313.

Boghosian A. Clinical evaluation of a filled adhesive system in class 5 restorations. *Compend Contin Educ Dent* 1996;17:750–752, 754–757.

Boksman L, Jordan RE, Suzuki M, et al. Etched porcelain labial veneers. *Ont Dent* 1985;62:15–19.

Bouschlicher MR, Vargas MA, Denehy GE. Effect of desiccation on microleakage of five class 5 restorative materials. *Oper Dent* 1996;21:90–95.

Bowen RL. Properties of a silica-reinforced polymer for dental restorations. *J Am Dent Assoc* 1963;66:57–64.

Brockmann SL, Scott RL, Eick JD. The effect of an airpolishing device on tensile bond strength of a dental sealant. *Quintessence Int* 1989;20:211–217.

Browning WD, Dennison JB. A survey of failure modes in composite resin materials. *Oper Dent* 1996;21:160–166.

Brunelle JA. *U.S. Department of Public Health and Human Services. Oral Health of United States Children, National and Regional Findings*. NIH publication no. 89-2247; 1989.

Bullard RH, Leinfelder KF, Russel CM. Effect of coefficient of thermal expansion on microleakage. *J Am Dent Assoc* 1988;116:871–874.

Burbach G. Micro-invasive cavity preparation with an air-abrasive unit. *GP* 1993;2(4):55–58.

Burgess JO, Norling BK, Rawls HR, Ong JL. Directly placed esthetic restorative materials—the continuum. *Compend Contin Educ Dent* 1996;17:731–732.

Burgoyne AR, Nicholls JI, Brudvik JS. In vitro two-body wear of inlay/onlay composite resin restoratives. *J Prosthet Dent* 1991;65:206–214.

Burke FJT, Wilson NHF, Watts DC. The effect of cuspal coverage on the fracture resistance of teeth restored with indirect composite resin restorations. *Quintessence Int* 1993;24:875–880.

Cahen PM, Obry-Musset AM, Grange D, Frank RM. Caries prevalence in 6-to 15-year-old French children based on the 1987 and 1991 national surveys. *J Dent Res* 1993;72:1581–1587.

Calamia JR, Simonsen RJ. Effect of coupling agents on bond strength of etched porcelain. *J Dent Res* 1984;63:162–166.

Calamia JR. Etched porcelain veneers: the current state of the art. *Quintessence Int* 1985;16:5.

Carvalho RM, Pereira JC, Yoshiyama M, Pashley DH. A review of polymerization contraction: the influence of stress development versus stress relief. *Oper Dent* 1996;21(1):17–24.

Chalifoux PR. Checklist to aesthetic dentistry. *PP&A* 1990;2:9–12.

Chalifoux PR. Aesthetic guidelines for posterior composite restorations. *Pract Periodontics Aesthet Dent* 1996;8:39–48.

Chan DCN. Current methods and criteria for caries diagnosis in North America. *J Dent Educ* 1993;57:422–427.

Chan KC, Swift Jr EJ. Marginal seal of new-generation dental bonding agents. *J Prosthet Dent* 1994;72:420–423.

Chappell RP, Spencer P, Eick JD. The effects of current dentinal adhesives on the dentinal surfaces. *Quintessence Int* 1994;25:851–859.

Chiba K, Hosoda H, Fusayama T. The addition of an adhesive composite resin to the same material: bond strength and clinical techniques. *J Prosthet Dent* 1989;61:669–675.

Christiansen GJ. A new technique for restoration of worn anterior teeth. *Oral Health* 1996;86:25–27.

Christensen GJ. Tooth sensitivity related to class I and II resin restorations. *J Am Dent Assoc* 1996;127:497–498.

Ciamponi AL, Del Portillo Lujan VA, Santos JFF. Effectiveness of reflective wedges on the polymerization of composite resins. *Quintessence Int* 1994;25:599–602.

Coli P, Brannstrom M. The marginal adaptation of four different bonding agents in class II composite resin restorations applied in bulk or in two increments. *Quintessence Int* 1993;24:583–591.

Costa TR, Reis A, Loguercio AD. Effect of enamel bevel on the clinical performance of resin composite restorations placed in non-carious cervical lesions. *J Esthet Restor Dent* 2013; 25(5):346–356.

Cozean C, Arcoria CJ, Pelagalli J, Powell GL. Dentistry for the 21st century? Erbium: YAG laser for teeth. *J Am Dent Assoc* 1997;128:1–8.

Craig RG. *Restorative Dental Materials*, 10th edn. St. Louis, MO: Mosby; 1996.

Craig RG, O'Brien WJ, Powers JM. *Dental Materials: Properties and Manipulation*, 6th edn. St. Louis, MO: Mosby; 1996.

Crispin BJ. *Contemporary Esthetic Dentistry: Practice Fundamentals*. Tokyo: Quintessence; 1994.

Croll TP. Bonded resin sealant for smooth surface enamel defects: new concepts in 'microrestorative' dentistry. *Quintessence Int* 1987;18:5–10.

Croll TP. Bonded composite resin crown restoration without enamel reduction. *Quintessence Int* 1987;18:753–757.

Croll TP. *Enamel Microabrasion*. Chicago, IL: Quintessence; 1991.

Cross TP, Cavanaugh RR. Augmentation of incisor width with bonded composite resin: another look. *Quintessence Int* 1990;21:637–641.

da Costa J, Fox P, Ferracne J. Comparison of various resin composite shades and layering technique with a shade guide. *J Esthet Restor Dent* 2010;22:114–124.

Davis EL, Joynt RB, Yu X, Wieczkowski Jr G. Dentin bonding system shelf life and bond strength. *Am J Dent* 1993;6:229–231.

Degrange M, Roulet JF. *Minimally Invasive Restorations with Bonding*. Chicago, IL: 1997.

Denehy GE, Cobb DS. A direct composite resin approach to anterior tooth alignment. *Contemp Esthet Rest Pract* 1998;2:10–22.

Dickerson WG. A functional and esthetic direct resin technique. *Pract Periodont Aesthet Dent* 1991;3:43–47.

Dickerson W. The effect of a dentin primer on enamel bond strength. *Esthet Dent Update* 1994;5:63–64.

Dickinson PT, Powers JM. Evaluation of fourteen direct-bonding orthodontic bases. *Am J Orthod* 1980;78:630–639.

Dietschi D. Free-hand bonding in the esthetic treatment of anterior teeth: creating the illusion. *J Esthet Dent* 1997;9:156–164.

Dietschi D. Layering concepts in anterior composite restorations. *Adhes Dent* 2001;3:71–80.

Donly KJ, Gomez C. In vitro demineralization-remineralization of enamel caries at restoration margins using fluoride-releasing composite resin. *Quintessence Int* 1994;25:355–358.

Douglas WH. The esthetic motif in research and clinical practice. *Quintessence Int* 1989;20:739–745.

Duarte Jr S, Perdigão J, Lopes M. Composite resin restorations; natural aesthetics and dynamics of light. *Pract Proced Aesthet Dent* 2003;15:657–664.

Duke ES, Robbins JW, Schwartz RS, Summitt JB. Clinical and interfacial laboratory evaluation of a bonding agent in cervical abrasions. *Am J Dent* 1994;7:307–311.

Eick JD, Fenn H. Polymerization shrinkage of posterior composite resins and its possible influence on postoperative sensitivity. *Quintessence Int* 1986;17:103–111.

Eli I, Liberman R, Levi N, Haspel Y. Bond strength of jointed posterior light-cured composites: comparison of surface treatments. *J Prosthet Dent* 1988;60:185–188.

Ericson D, Derand T. Increase of in vitro curing depth of class II composite resin restorations. *J Prosthet Dent* 1993;70:219–223.

Fahl Jr N. A solution for everyday direct restorative challenges-mastering composite artistry to create anterior masterpieces-Part I. *J Cosmetic Dent* 2010; 26:56–68.

Fahl Jr N. Coronal reconstruction of a severely compromised central incisor with composite resins: a case report. *J Cosmetic Dent* 2010; 26:92–113.

Fahl Jr N. A polychromatic composite layering approach for solving a complex Class IV/direct veneer-diastema combination: part I. *Pract Proced Aesthet Dent* 2006;18:641–5.

Fahl Jr N. A polychromatic composite layering approach for solving a complex Class IV/direct veneer-diastema combination: part II. *Pract Proced Aesthet Dent* 2007;19:17–22.

Fahl Jr N. Optimizing the esthetics of class IV restorations with composite resins. *J Can Dent Assoc* 1997;63(2):108–111, 114–115.

Fahl Jr N. Predictable aesthetic reconstruction of fractured anterior teeth with composite resins: a case report. *Pract Periodont Aesthet Dent* 1996;8:17–31.

Farah JW, ed. Anterior and posterior composites. *Dent Advisor* 1991;8:4.

Faunce FR, Myers DR. Laminate veneer restoration of permanent incisors. *J Am Dent Assoc* 1976;93:790–792.

Feigenbaum N. Class IV technique overcomes snags in frailty, esthetics. *Dentist* 1990;68:38–39.

Feigenbaum N, Mopper KW. *A Complete Guide to Dental Bonding.* Johnson and Johnson; 1984.

Fell WP. One-visit composite and amalgam bonding for strong, aesthetic posterior restorations. *J Am Dent Assoc* 1996;127:1656–1658.

Ferraccane JL. Resin composite-state of the art. *Dent Mater* 2011;27:29–38.

Ferrari M. The micromorphologic relationship between resin and dentin in class V restorations: an in vivo and in vitro investigation. *Quintessence Int* 1994;25:621–625.

Ferrari M, Davidson CL. Sealing capacity of a resinmodified glass-ionomer and resin composite placed in vivo in class 5 restorations. *Oper Dent* 1996;21:69–72.

Ferraris, F. Diamantopoulou, S. Acunzo, R. Aicidi, R. Influence of enamel composite thickness on value, chroma, and translucency of a high and a non-high refractive index resin composite. *Int J Esthet Dent* 2014;9:382–400.

Filler SJ, Lazarchik DA, Givan DA, et al. Shear bond strengths of composite to chlorhexidine-treated enamel. *Am J Dent* 1994;7:85–88.

Fitchie JG, Reeves GW, Scarbrough AR, Hembree JH. Microleakage of two new dentinal bonding systems. *Quintessence Int* 1990;21:749–752.

Foreman FT. Sealant prevalence and indication in a young military population. *J Am Dent Assoc* 1994;125:182–186.

Friedl KH, Schmalz G. Placement and replacement of composite restorations in Germany. *Oper Dent* 1995;20:34–38.

Fritz UB, Finger WJ, Uno S. Resin-modified glass ionomer cements: bonding to enamel and dentin. *Dent Mater* 1996;12:161–166.

Fusayama A, Kohno A. Marginal closure of composite restorations with the gingival wall in cementum/ dentin. *J Prosthet Dent* 1989;61:293–296.

Fusayama T. Gingival irritation of restoration margins. *Quintessence Int* 1987;18:215–222.

Fusayama T. Optimal cavity wall treatment for adhesive restorations. J Esthet Dent 1990;2:95–99.

Garber DA, Goldstein RE. *Porcelain and Composite Inlays and Onlays: Esthetic Posterior Restorations*. Chicago, IL: Quintessence; 1994.

Garcia EJ, Mena-Serrano A, Andrade A, et al. *Eur J Esthet Dent* 2012;7:154–162.

Garcia-Godoy F, Draheim RN, Titus HW. Shear bond strength of a posterior composite resin to glass ionomer bases. *Quintessence Int* 1988;19:357–359.

Gilpatrick RO, Johnson W, Moore D, Turner J. Pulpal response to dentin etched with 10% phosphoric acid. *Am J Dent* 1996;9:125–129.

Godder B, Zhukovsky L, Trushkowsky R, Epelboym D. Microleakage reduction using glass-ceramic inserts. *Am J Dent* 1994;7:74–76.

Gondo R, Monteiro S Jr, Andrada MAC, Baratieri LN. Influence of cavosurface configuration on the esthetic of composite restorations. *J Dent Res* 2005;84 (Special Issue A):417.

Goldstein RE. *Esthetics in Dentistry*. Philadelphia, PA: J.B. Lippincott; 1976.

Goldstein RE. Communicating esthetics. *N Y State Dent J* 1985;15:477–479.

Goldstein RE. Finishing of composites and laminates. *Dent Clin North Am* 1989;33:305–318.

Goldstein R, Parkins F. Air-abrasive technology: its new role in restorative dentistry. *J Am Dent Assoc* 1994;125:551–557.

Greggs TS. *Method for cosmetic restoration of anterior teeth*. United States Patent Number: 4,473,353. Filled April 15, 1983. Date of patent: September 25, 1984.

Gregory WA, Berry S, Duke E, Dennison JB. Physical properties and repair bond strength of direct and indirect composite resins. *J Prosthet Dent* 1992;68:406–411.Hallett KB, Garcia-Godoy F, Trotter AR. Shear bond strength of a resin composite to enamel etched with maleic or phosphoric acid. *Aust Dent J* 1994;39:292–297.

Handelman SL, Washburn F, Wopperer P. Two-year report of sealant effect on bacteria in dental caries. *J Am Dent Assoc* 1976;93:967–970.

Hardin JF. *Clark's Clinical Dentistry, 1997 Update*. St. Louis, MO: Mosby; 1997.

Herschfeld J. The progress of esthetic restorations in dentistry. *J Phil Cty Dent Soc* 1991;56:10–13.

Heymann HO. Indirect composite resin veneers: an alternative. In: Garber DA, Goldstein RE, Feinman RA, eds. *Porcelain Laminate Veneers*. Chicago, IL: Quintessence; 1988:126–133.

Hicks MJ. The acid-etch technique in caries prevention: pit and fissure sealants and preventive resin restorations. In: Pinkham JR, ed. *Pediatric Dentistry: Infancy Through Adolescence*, 2nd edn. Philadelphia, PA: W.B. Saunders; 1994:451–482.

Hilton TJ, Schwartz RS. The effect of air thinning on dentin adhesive bond strength. *Oper Dent* 1995;20:133–137.

Hinoura K, Onose H, Moore BK, Phillips RW. Effect of the bonding agent on the bond strength between glass ionomer cement and composite resin. *Quintessence Int* 1989;20:31–35.

Hilton T, Ferracane J, Broome J. *Summitt's Fundamentals of Operative Dentistry*, 4th edn. Hanover Park, IL: Quintessence; 2013.

Hirata R. Tips. São Paulo, Brazil: Artes Medicas; 2011.

Horn HR. Porcelain laminate veneers bonded to etched enamel. *Dent Clin North Am* 1983;27:671–684.

Hornbrook DS. Optimizing form and function with the direct posterior composite resin: a case report. *Pract Periodont Aesthet Dent* 1996;8:405–411.

Hosoya Y. Resin adhesion to the primary enamel: influence of light—irradiation times. *J Clin Pediatr Dent* 1995;19:185–190.

Hoyle P. Indirect resin systems. *Reality* 1993;8:121–124.

Hugo B. *Esthetics with Resin Composite*. New Malden, Surrey, UK: 2008.

Hume WR, Gerzia TM. Bioavailability of components of resin-based materials which are applied to teeth. *Crit Rev Oral Biol Med* 1996;7:172–179.

Ibsen RL, Strassler HE. An innovative method for fixed anterior tooth replacement utilizing porcelain veneers. *Quintessence Int* 1986;17:455.

Ironside JG, Makinson OF. Resin restorations: causes of porosities. *Quintessence Int* 1993;24:867–873.

Ishioka S, Caputo AA. Interaction between the dentinal smear layer and composite bond strength. *J Prosthet Dent* 1989;61:180–185.

Jaarda MJ, Wang RF, Lang BR. A regression analysis of filler particle content to predict composite wear. *J Prosthet Dent* 1997;77:57–67.

Janda R, Roulet JF, Kaminsky M, Steffin G, Latta M. Color stability of resin matrix restorative materials as a function of the method of light activation. *Eur J Oral Sci* 2004;112:280–285.

Janus J, Fauxpoint G, Arntz Y, et al. Surface roughness and morphology of three nano-composites after two different polishing treatments by a multi-technique approach. *Dent Mater* 2010;26:416–425.

Jensen OE, Handelman SL. Effect on autopolymerizing sealant on viability of microflora in occlusal dental caries. *Scand J Dent Res* 1980;88:382–388.

Jeronimus DJ, Till MJ, Sveen OB. Reduced viability of microorganisms under dental sealants. *J Dent Child* 1975;42:275–280.

Jordan RE. *Esthetic Composite Bonding: Techniques and Materials*, 2nd edn. St. Louis, MO: 1993.

Jordan RE, Suzuki M. *Clinical Evaluation of Concept as a Posterior Composite Restorative Material in an Indirect Inlay/Onlay Technique*. St. Louis, MO: Mosby; 1993.

Joynt RB, Davis EL, Wieczkowski G, Williams DA. Fracture resistance of posterior teeth restored with glass ionomer-composite resin systems. *J Prosthet Dent* 1989;62:28–31.

Kanca J. Maximizing the cure of posterior light-activated resins. *Quintessence Int* 1986;17:25–27.

Kanca J. The effect of thickness and shade on the polymerization of light-activated posterior composite resins. *Quintessence Int* 1986;17:809–811.

Kanca J. Visible light-activated composite resins for posterior use: a comparison of surface hardness and uniformity of cure. *Quintessence Int* 1985;10:687–690.

Kanka J III. Microleakage of five dentin bonding systems. *Dent Mater* 1989;5:63–64.

Kanka J III. Resin bonding to wet substrate. I. Bonding to dentin. *Quintessence Int* 1992;23:39–42.

Kanca J. Improving bond strength through acid etching of dentin and bonding to wet dental surfaces. *J Am Dent Assoc* 1992;123:35–43.

Kaplan BA, Goldstein GR, Vijayaraghavan TV, Nelson IK. The effect of three polishing systems on the surface roughness of four hybrid composites: a profilometric and scanning electron microscopy study. *J Prosthet Dent* 1996;76:34–38.

Khokhar ZA, Razzog ME, Yaman R. Color stability of restorative resins. *Quintessence Int* 1991;22:733–737.

Kidd EA, Beighton D. Prediction of secondary caries around tooth-colored restorations: a clinical and micro-biological study. *J Dent Res* 1996;75:1942–1946.

Kildal KK, Ruyter IE. How different curing methods affect the degree of conversion of resin-based inlay/onlay materials. *Acta Odontol Scand* 1994;52:315–322.

Kinzer RL. Aesthetic factors. In: Clark JW, ed. *Clinical Dentistry IV*. New York: Harper and Row; 1976: ch. 32.

Kilpatrick NM, Murray JJ, McCabe JF. A clinical comparison of a light cured glass ionomer sealant restoration with a composite sealant restoration. *J Dent* 1996;24:399–405.

Khokhar Z, Razzoog M, Yaman P. Color stability of restorative resins. *Quintessence Int* 1991;22:733–737.

Knight GT, Berry TG, Barghi N, Burns TR. Effects of two methods of moisture control on marginal microleakage between resin composite and etched enamel: a clinical study. *Int J Prosthodont* 1993;6:475–479.

Krejci I, Besek M, Lutz F. Clinical and SEM study of tetric resin composite in posterior teeth: 12-month results. *Am J Dent* 1994;7:27–30.

Krishnan VK, Bindhu DB, Manjusha K. Studies on microleakage associated with visible light cured dental composites. *J Biomater Appl* 1996;10:348–359.

Kugel G. Classification and application of cementation alternatives. *Signature* 1997;4:8–11.

Kumbuloglu O, Ozcan M. Clincial survival of indirect, anterior 3-unit surface-retained fibre-reinforced composite fixed dental prosthesis: up to 7.5-years follow up. *J Dent* 2015;43:656–663.

Lacy AM. An effective technique for extended proximal contacts in composite resin restorations. *Pract Periodont Aesthet Dent* 1996;8:287–293.

Lacy AM. Application of composite resin for single-appointment anterior and posterior diastema closure. *Pract Periodont* 1998;10:279–286.

Lambrechts P, Braem M, Vanherle G. Evaluation of clinical performance for posterior composite resins and dentin adhesives. *Oper Dent* 1987;12:53–78.Larson TD, Phair CB. The use of a direct bonded microfilled composite resin veneer. *J Am Dent Assoc* 1987;115:449–452.

Latta Jr GH. The light-cured composite restoration: an adjunct to removable partial prosthodontics. *Compend Contin Educ Dent* 1996;17:164.

Laurell K, Carpenter W, Beck M. Pulpal effects of air-brasion cavity preparation in dogs. *J Dent Res* 1993;72(Special Issue):273, Abstract 1360.

Lawson N, Robles A. Bulk-fill composites for class ii restorations. *Inside Dent* 2015; 43–48.

Leinfelder KF. Evaluation of criteria used for assessing the clinical performance of composite resins in posterior teeth. *Quintessence Int* 1987;18:531–536.

Leinfelder KF. Posterior composite resins: the materials and their clinical performance. *J Am Dent Assoc* 1995;126:663–676.

Leinfelder KF. Wear patterns and rates of posterior composite resins. *Int Dent J* 1987;37:152–157.

Leinfelder KF, Wilder AD, Teixeira LC. Wear rates of posterior composite resins. *J Am Dent Assoc* 1986;112:829–833.

Leinfelder KF. Indirect posterior composite resins. *Compend Contin Educ Dent* 2005;26:495–503.

Li SH, Kingman A, Forthofer R, Swango P. Comparison of tooth surface-specific dental caries attack patterns in U.S. school children from two national surveys. *J Dent Res* 1993;72:1398–1405.

Li X, Pongprueksa P, Meerbeek BV, Munck JD. Curing profile of bulk-fill resin-based composites. *J Dentistry* 2015;43:664–672.

Liberman R, Gorfil C, Ben-Amar A. Reduction of microleakage in class II composite resin restorations using retentive pins. *J Oral Rehabil* 1996;23:240–243.

Liebenberg WH. Intracoronal bleaching of nonvital dis-colored mandibular incisors. *Pract Proced Aesthet Dent* 2007;19:47–53.

Liebenberg WH. Occlusal index-assisted restitution of esthetic and functional anatomy in direct tooth-colored restorations. *Quintessence Int* 1996;27:81–88.

Liebenberg WH. Successive cusp build-up: an improved placement technique for posterior direct resin restorations. *J Can Dent Assoc* 1996;62:5501–5507.

Los SA, Barkmeier WW. Effects of dentin air abrasion with aluminum oxide and hydroxyapatite on adhesive bond strength. *Oper Dent* 1994;19:169–175.

Lussi A. Comparison of different methods for the diagnosis of fissure caries without cavitation. *Caries Res* 1993;27:409–416.

Lutz F, Krejci I, Luescher B, Oldenburg TR. Improved proximal margin adaptation of Class II composite resin restorations by use of light-reflecting wedges. *Quintessence Int* 1986;17:659–664.

Lutz FU, Krejci I, Oddera M. Advanced adhesive restorations: the post-amalgam age. *Pract Periodont Aesthet Dent* 1996;8:385–394.

Magne P, Dietschi D, Holz J. Esthetic restorations for posterior teeth: practical and clinical considerations. *Int J Periodont Rest Dent* 1996;16:104–119.

Magne P, Holz J. Stratification of composite restorations: systematic and durable replication of natural aesthetics. *Pract Periodont Aesthet Dent* 1996;8:61–68.

Manauta J, Salat A. *Layers*. Milan: Quintessence; 2012.

Marcondes M, Souza N, Manfroi FB, et al. Clinical evaluation of indirect composite resin restorations cemented with different resin cements. *J Adhes Dent* 2016;18:59–67.

Mathewson RJ, Primosch RE. *Fundamentals of Pediatric Dentistry*, 3rd edn. Chicago, IL: Quintessence; 1995.

Matsumura H, Leinfelder KF, Kawai K. Three-body wear of light-activated composite veneering materials. *J Prosthet Dent* 1995;73:233–239.

McComb D. Adhesive luting cements—classes, criteria, and usage. *Compend Contin Educ Dent* 1996;17:759–762.

McGuire MK, Miller L. Maintaining esthetic restorations in the periodontal practice. *Int J Periodont Rest Dent* 1996;16:230–239.

McLaughlin G. Porcelain fused to tooth—a new esthetic and reconstructive modality. *Compend Contin Dent Edu* 1985;5:430–435.

McLean JW. Limitations of posterior composite resins and extending their use with glass ionomer cements. *Quintessence Int* 1987;18:517–529.

Mednick GA, Loesche WJ, Corpron RE. A bacterial evaluation of an occlusal sealant as a barrier system in humans. *J Dent Child* 1974;41:356–360.

Meiers JC, Shook LW. Effect of disinfectants on the bond strength of composite to dentin. *Am J Dent* 1996;9:11–14.

Meryon SD, Johnson SG. The effect of smear layer removal on the in vitro cytotoxicity of four dental restorative materials. *J Dent* 1989;16:22–26.

Meskin LH. *The 1996 Year Book of Dentistry*. St. Louis, MO: Mosby; 1996.

Meskin LH. *The 1997 Year Book of Dentistry*. St. Louis, MO: Mosby; 1997.

Meyerowitz JM, Rosen M, Cohen J, Becker PJ. *J Dent Assoc S Afr* 1994;49:389–392.

Millar BJ, Robinson PB, Inglis AT. Clinical evaluation of an anterior hybrid composite resin over 8 years. *Br Dent J* 1997;182:26–30.

Miller LM. Maintaining hybrid and microfill composites. *J Esthet Dent* 1990;2:109–113.

Miller MB, Castellanos IR, Vargas MA, Denehy GE. Effect of restorative materials on microleakage of class II composites. *J Esthet Dent* 1996;8:107–113.

Miserendino LJ, Pick RM. *Lasers in Dentistry*. Chicago, IL: Quintessence; 1995.

Mitchem JC. The use and abuse of aesthetic materials in posterior teeth. *Int Dent J* 1988;38:119–125.

Mjor IA. Repair versus replacement of failed restorations. *Int Dent J* 1990;43:466–472.

Mjor IA. The reasons for replacement and the age of failed restorations in general dental practice. *Acta Odontol Scand* 1997;55:58–63.

Mjor IA, Jokstad A, Qvist V. Longevity of posterior restorations. *Int Dent J* 1990;40:11–17.

Mjor IA, Quist V. Margin failures of amalgam and composite restorations. *J Dent* 1997;25:25–30.

Morrison AH, Berman L. Evaluation of the airdent unit: preliminary report. *J Am Dent Assoc* 1953;46:298–303.

Myers GE. The air-abrasive technique: a report. *Br Dent J* 1954;97:291–295.

Nash R. A predictable restorative Class V erosion technique. *Pract Periodont Aesthet Dent* 1991;3:39–42.

Nash RW. Cosmetic correction of crowded anterior teeth. *Dent Today* 1991;10:48–49.

Nash RW. Tooth-colored bonded posterior restorations: aesthetic alternatives to amalgam and gold. *Dent Today* 1991;10:34–35.

Nathanson D. Current developments in esthetic dentistry. *Curr Opin Dent* 1991;1:206–211.

Neo J, Chew CL. Direct tooth-colored materials for noncarious lesions: a 3-year clinical report. *Quintessence Int* 1996;27:183–188.

Neo J, Chew CL, Yap A, Sidhu S. Clinical evaluation of tooth-colored materials in cervical lesions. *Am J Dent* 1996;9:15–18.

Nery S, McCabe JF, Wassell RW. A comparative study of three dental adhesives. *J Dent* 1995;23:55–61.

Newbrun E. Tooth morphology and arch form. In: Newbrun E, ed. *Cariology*, 3rd edn. Chicago, IL: Quintessence; 1989:52.

Nixon RL. *The Chairside Manual for Porcelain Bonding*. Wilmington, DE: B.A. Videographics; 1987.

Nixon RL. The advent of metal-free dentistry: a versatile new fiber and polymer-glass system. *Pract Periodontics Aesthet Dent* 1997;9(8):1–7.

O'Brien WJ. *Dental Materials and their Selection*, 2nd edn. Chicago, IL: Quintessence; 1997.

Opdam NJ, Roeters JJ, Peters TC, et al. Cavity wall adaptation and voids in adhesive class I resin composite restorations. *Dent Mater* 1996;12:230–235.

Pagliarini A, Rubini R, Rea M, et al. Effectiveness of the current enamel-dentinal adhesives: a new methodology for its evaluation. *Quintessence Int* 1996;27:265–270.

Pallesen U, Dijken JWVV. A randomized controlled 27 years follow up of three resin composites in Class II restorations. *J Dent* 2015;43:1547–1558.

Paravina RD, Kimura M, Powers JM. Evaluation of polymerization-dependent changes in color and translucency of resin composites using two formulae. *Odontology* 2005;93:46–51.

Pashley DH. In vitro simulations of in vivo bonding conditions. *Am J Dent* 1991;4:237–240.

Pashley DH, Depew DD. Effects of the smear layer, copalite, and oxalate on microleakage. *Oper Dent* 1986;11:95–102.

Pashley EL, Tao L, Mackert JR, Pashley DH. Comparison of in vivo vs. in vitro bonding of composite resin to the dentin of canine teeth. *J Dent Res* 1988;67:467–470.

Penning C, van Amerongen JP, Seef RE, Ten Cate RJ. Validity of probing for fissure caries diagnosis. *Caries Res* 1992;26:445–449.

Perdigao J. Universal Adhesives. *J Esthet Restor Dent* 2015;27:331–334.

Perdigao J, Sezinando A, Monteiro P. Evaluation of a new universal adhesive using different bonding strategies. *J Dent Res* 2012; 91(Special Issue A), Abstract 18.

Perdigão J, Dutra-CorrêaM, Anuate-Netto C, et al. Two-year clinical evaluation of self-etching adhesives in posterior restorations. *J Adhes Dent* 2009;11:149–159.

Peumans M, De Munck J, Van Landuyt KL, et al. A 13-year clinical evaluation of two three-step etch-and-rinse adhesives in non-carious Class-V lesions. *Clin Oral Invest* 2012;16:129–37.

Peyton FA, Henry EE. The effect of high-speed burs, diamond instruments and air abrasive in cutting tooth tissue. *J Am Dent Assoc* 1954;49:426–435.

Pincus CR. Building mouth personality. *J Calif Stud Dent Assoc* 1938;14:125–129.

Pitts NB, Lond FDS. Current methods and criteria for caries diagnosis in Europe. *J Dent Educ* 1993;57:409–413.

Powell GC, Kelsey WP, Blankeneau RJ, Barkmeier WW. The use of an argon laser for polymerization of composite resin. *J Esthet Dent* 1989;1:34–37.

Prati C, Montanari G. Comparative microleakage study between the sandwich and conventional three-increment techniques. *Quintessence Int* 1989;20:587–594.

Price RBT, Felix CA. Effect of delivering light in specific narrow bandwidths from 394–515 nm on the micro-hardness of resin composites. *Dent Mater* 2009;25:899–908.

Puppala R, Hegde A, Munshi AK. Laser and light cured composite resin restorations: in-vitro comparison of isotope and dye penetrations. *J Clin Pediatr Dent* 1996;20:213–218.

Purk JH, Eick JD, DeSchepper EJ, et al. Fracture strength of Class I versus Class II restored premolars tested at the marginal ridge. I. Standard preparations. *Quintessence Int* 1990;21:545–551.

Reel DC, Mitchell RJ. Fracture resistance of teeth restored with Class II composite restorations. *J Prosthet Dent* 1989;61:177–179.

Reinhardt J, Capilouto ML, Padgett CD. Composite resin esthetic dentistry survey. *J Dent Res* 1989;68.

Ripa LW. Occlusal sealants. In: Nitiforuk G, ed. *Understanding Dental Caries. Vol 2: Prevention, Basic and Clinical Aspects*. New York: Karger; 1985:145–173.

Ritter AV, Swift EJ, Heymann HO, et al. An eight-year clinical evaluation of filled and unfilled one-bottle dental adhesives. *J Am Dent Assoc* 2009;140:28–37.

Roeder RA, Berry EA III, You C, Powers JM. Bond strength of composite to air abraded enamel and dentin. *J Dent Res* 1994;73 (Special Issue):131, Abstract 237.

Rosatto CMP, Bicalho AA, Verissimo C, et al. Mechanical properties, shrinkage stress, cuspal strain and fracture resistance of molars restored with bulk-fill composites and incremental filling technique. *J Dent* 2015;43:1519–1528.

Roulet JF. Benefits and disadvantages of tooth-colored alternatives of amalgam. *J Dent* 1997;25:459–473.

Roulet JF. The problems associated with substituting composite resins for amalgam: a status report on posterior composites. *J Dent* 1988;16:101–103.

Rozmajzl WF Jr, Los SA, Albrechtsen LA, Barkmeier WW. Composite to dentin bond strength using a curing unit with nitrogen. *Am J Dent* 1994;7:319–321.

Rueggeberg FA. Exposure times for contemporary composites. *J Esthet Restor Dent* 2013; 25:82–84.

Rueggeberg FA, Caughman WF, Curtis Jr JW. Effect of light intensity and exposure duration on cure of resin composite. *Oper Dent* 1994;19:26–32.

Rueggeberg FA, Cole MA, Looney SW, et al. Comparison of manufacturer-recommended exposure durations with those determined using biaxial flexure strength and scraped composite thickness among a variety of light-curing units. *J Esthet Restor Dent* 2009;21:43–61.

Rueggeberg FA. Composite inlays: a review of concepts, techniques, and limitations. *Georgia Acad Gen Dent* 1990;Winter.

Sabatini C, Campillo M, Aref J. Color stability of ten resin-based restorative materials. *J Esthet Restor Dent* 2012; 24:185–200.

Sasaki RT, Florio FM, Basting RT. Effect of 10% sodium ascorbate and 10% alpha-tocopherol in different formulations on the shear bond strength of enamel and dentin submitted to a home-use bleaching treatment. *Oper Dent* 2009;34:746–752.

Saunders WP, Saunders EM. Microleakage of bonding agents with wet and dry bonding techniques. *Am J Dent* 1996;9(1):34–36.

Schulein TM, Chan DCN, Reinhardt JW. Rinsing times for a gel etchant related to enamel/composite bond strength. *Gen Dent* 1986;34:296–298.

Schwartz R, Summitt J, Robbins W, dos Santos J. *Fundamentals of Operative Dentistry: a Contemporary Approach*. Chicago, IL: Quintessence; 1996.

Schwendicke F, Kern M, Dorfer C, et al. Influence of using different bonding systems and composites on the margin integrity and the mechanical properties of selectively excavated teeth in vitro. *J Dent* 2015;43:327–334.

Sheth PJ, Jensen ME, Sheth JJ. Comparative evaluation of three resin inlay techniques: microleakage studies. *Quintessence Int* 1989;20:831–836.

Shinkai K, Suzuki S, Leinfelder KF, Katoh Y. How heat treatment and thermal cycling affect wear of composite resin inlays. *J Am Dent Assoc* 1994;125:1467–1472.

Shintani H, Satou N, Satou J. Clinical evaluation of two posterior composite resins retained with bonding agents. *J Prosthet Dent* 1989;62:627–632.

Shortall AC. Long-term monitoring of microleakage of composites. Part II: scanning electron microscopic examination of replica patterns of composite tags. *J Prosthet Dent* 1988;60:451–458.

Shortall AC, Wilson HJ. New materials, bonding treatments and changes in restorative practice. *Br Dent J* 1988;164:396–400.

Simonsen RJ. *Clinical Applications of the Acid Etch Technique*. Chicago, IL: Quintessence; 1978.

Simonsen RJ. Conservation of tooth structure in restorative dentistry. *Quintessence Int* 1985;16:15–24.

Simonsen RJ. Editorial: Dentin: to etch, or not to etch. *Quintessence Int* 1990;21:75.

Simonsen RJ. New materials on the horizon. *J Am Dent Assoc* 1991;122(8):25–31.

Simonsen RJ. Pit and fissure sealant: theoretical and clinical considerations. In: Frahm RL, Morris ME, eds. *Textbook of Pediatric Dentistry*, 2nd edn. Baltimore, MD: Williams & Wilkins; 1985:217–234.

Simonsen RJ. Preventive resin restorations: three-year results. *J Am Dent Assoc* 1980;100:535–539.

Simonsen RJ. The acid etch technique and preventive resin restorations. In: Stallard RE, ed. *A Textbook of Preventive Dentistry*, 2nd edn. Philadelphia, PA: Saunders; 1982:322–328.

Simonsen RJ, Calamia JR. Tensile bond strength of etched porcelain. *J Dent Res* 1983;Abstract 1154.

Simonsen RJ, Kanca J. Surface hardness of posterior composite resins using supplemental polymerization after simulated occlusal adjustment. *Quintessence Int* 1986;17:631–633.

Sjodin L, Uusitalo M, van Dijken J. Resin modified glass ionomer cements. In vitro microleakage in direct class V and class II sandwich restorations. *Swed Dent J* 1996;20:77–86.

Soliman S, Preidl R, Karl S, et al. Influence of cavity margin design and restorative material on marginal quality and seal of extended class II resin composite restorations in vitro. *J Adhes Dent* 2016;18:7–16.

Spitznagel F, Horvath SD, Guess PC, Blatz MB. Resin bond to indirect composite and new ceramic/polymer materials: a review of the literature. *J Esthet Restor Dent* 2014; 26:382–393.

Stamm JW, Disney JA, Beck JD, et al. The University of North Carolina caries risk assessment study: final results and some alternative modeling approaches. In: Bowen WH, Tabak LA, eds. *Cariology for the Nineties*. Rochester, NY: University of Rochester Press, 1993:209–234.

Staninec M, Mochizuki A, Tanizaki K, et al. Interfacial space, marginal leakage, and enamel cracks around composite resins. *Oper Dent* 1986;111:14–24.

St-Pierre L, Bergeron C, Qian F, et al. Effect of polishing direction on the marginal adaptation of composite resin restorations. *J Esthet Restor Dent* 2013;25:125–138.

Strassler HE, Buchness GF. The Class III acid-etch light polymerized composite resin restoration. *J Esthet Dent* 1990;2:13–16.

Sturdevant CM, Roberson TM, Heymann HO, Sturdevant JR. *The Art and Science of Operative Dentistry*, 3rd edn. St. Louis, MO: Mosby; 1994.

Sutherland L, Jensen ME, Hawkins BF, Lainson PR. Root caries inhibition using dentin bonding resin and fluoridated varnishes. *J Dent Res* 1989;69.

Suzuki S, Leinfelder KF. An in vitro evaluation of a copolymerizable type of microfilled composite resin. *Quintessence Int* 1994;25:59–64.

Suzuki S, Leinfelder KF. Localized wear and marginal integrity of posterior resin composites. *Am J Dent* 1993;6:199–203.

Swift EJ Jr, Perdigao J, Heyman HO. Bonding to enamel: a brief history and state of the art, 1995. *Quintessence Int* 1995;26:95–110.

Swift EJ Jr, Triolo PT Jr, Barkmeier WW, et al. Effect of low-viscosity resins on the performance of dental adhesives. *Am J Dent* 1996;9:100–104.

Taira Y, Matsumura H, Yoshida K, et al. Adhesive bonding to dentin with ferrous chloride primers and tri-n-butylborane-initiated luting agents. *J Dent Res* 1996;75:1859–1864.

Tay FR, Pashley DH, Suh BI, et al. Single-step adhesives and permeable membranes. *J Dent* 2002;30:371–82.

Terry DA. Color matching with composite resin: a synchronized shade comparison. *Pract Proced Aesthet Dent* 2003;15:515–21.

Terry D, Geller W. *Aesthetic and Restorative Dentistry Material Selection and Technique*, 2nd edn. Hanover Park, IL: Quintessence; 2013.

Tjan AHL, Bergh BH, Lidner C. Effect of various incremental techniques on the marginal adaptation of Class II composite resin restorations. *J Prosthet Dent* 1987;67:62–66.

Tjan AHL, Glancy JF. Interfacial bond strengths between layers of visible light-activated composites. *J Prosthet Dent* 1988;59:27–29.

Triolo PT Jr, Swift Jr EJ, Barkmeier WW. Shear bond strengths of composite to dentin using six dental adhesive systems. *Oper Dent* 1995;20:46–50.

Triolo PT Jr, Swift EJ, Mudgil A, Levine A. Effects of etching time on enamel bond strengths. *Am J Dent* 1993;6:302–304.

Turkun M, Celik EU, Kaya AD, Arici M. Can the hydrogel form of sodium ascorbate be used to reverse compromised bond strength after bleaching? *J Adhes Dent* 2009;11:35–40.

Tyas MJ. Clinical evaluation of five adhesive systems: three-year results. *Int Dent J* 1996;46:10–14.

Tyas MJ. Clinical performance of two dentine adhesives: 2-year results. *Aust Dent J* 1996;41:324–327.

Tyas MJ, Beech DR. Clinical performance of three restorative materials for non-undercut cervical abrasion lesions. *Aust Dent J* 1985;30:260–264.

Unterbrink GL, Muessner R. Influence of light intensity on two restorative systems. *J Dent* 1995;23:183–189.

Van der Laan-Van Dorp CSE, Exterkate RAM, ten Cate JM. Effect of probing on progression of fissure caries. *Caries Res* 1986;20(2):151 (Abstract 9).

Van der Veem HJ, Pilon HJ, Henry PD. Clinical performance of one micro-filled two hybrid anterior composite resins. *Quintessence Int* 1989;20:547–550.

Van Doklen JWV. A 6-year evaluation of a direct composite resin inlay/onlay system and glass ionomer cement-composite resin sandwich restorations. *Acta Odontol Scand* 1994;52:368–376.

Van Meerbeek B, Peumans M, Poitevin A, et al. Relationship between bond-strength tests and clinical outcomes. *Dent Mater* 2010;26:e100–e121.

Vargas MA, Denehy GE, Silberman JJ. Bond strength to etched enamel and dentin contaminated with saliva. *Am J Dent* 1994;7:325–327.

Vanini L. Light and color in anterior composite restorations. *Pract Periodont Aesthet Dent* 1996;8:673–682.

Vanini L, De Simone F, Tammaro S. Indirect composite restorations in the anterior region: a predictable technique for complex cases. *Pract Periodont Aesthet Dent* 1997;9:795–802.

Vanini L. Light and color in anterior composite restorations. *Pract Periodont Aesthet Dent* 1996;8:673–682.

Van Noort R. *An Introduction to Dental Materials*. St. Louis, MO: Mosby; 1995.

Venhoven BA, de Gee AJ, Werner A, Davidson CL. Influence of filler parameters on the mechanical coherence of dental restorative resin composites. *Biomaterials* 1996;17:735–740.

Versluis A, Douglas WH, Cross M, Sakaguchi RL. Does an incremental filling technique reduce polymerization shrinkage stresses? *J Dent Res* 1996;75:871–878.

Villarroel M, Fahl Jr N, Sousa AM, Oliveira Jr OB. Direct esthetic restorations based on translucency and opacity of composite resins. *J Esthet Restor Dent* 2011; 23:73–88.

Wassell RW, McCabe JF, Walls AWG. Wear rates of regular and tempered composites. *J Dent* 1997;25:49–52.

Wei YR, Wang XD, Zhang Q, et al. Clinical performance of anterior resin-bonded fixed dental prostheses with different framework designs: A systemic review and met-analysis. *J Dent* 2016;47:1–7.

Weiner RS. The effect of post-cure heat treatment systems on composite resin restorations. *J Am Dent Assoc* 1997;128:88.

Wendt SL Jr, Ziemiecki TL, Leinfelder KF. Proximal wear rates by tooth position of resin composite restorations. *J Dent* 1996; 24(1–2):33–39.

Winkler MM, Lautenschlager EP, Boghosian A, Greener EH. An accurate and simple method for the measurement of dental composite wear. *J Oral Rehabil* 1996;23:486–493.

Winkler MM, Lautenschlager EP, Boghosian A, Greener EH. Visual versus mechanical wear measurement of dental composite resin. *J Oral Rehabil* 1996;23:494–500.

Worm DA Jr, Meiers JC. Effect of various types of contamination on microleakage between beta-quartz inserts and resin composite. *Quintessence Int* 1996;27:271–277.

Wu J, Weir MD, Melo MAS, et al. Effects of water-aging on self-healing dental composite containing microcapsules. *J Dent* 2016;47:86–93.

Villaroel M, Fahl N, De Sousa AM, De Oliveira Jr OB. Direct esthetic restorations based on translucency and opacity of composite resin. *J Esthet Restor Dent* 2011;23:73–87.

Yaffe A, Hochman N, Ehrlich J. Severe vertical overlap: a modified method of treatment. *J Prosthet Dent* 1989;62:636–641.

Yanagawa T, Chigira H, Manabe A, et al. Adaptation of a resin composite in vivo. *J Dent* 1996;24:71–75.

Yap AU, Pearson GJ, Billington RW, Stokes AN. An in vitro microleakage study of three restorative techniques for class II restorations in posterior teeth. *Biomaterials* 1996;17:2031–2035.

Yoshiyama M, Carvalho RM, Sano H, et al. Regional bond strengths of resins to human root dentine. *J Dent* 1996;24:435–442.

Yuan H, Li M, Guo B, Gao Y, Liu H, Li J. Evaluation of microtensile bond strength and microleakage of a self-adhering flowable composite. *J Adhes Dent* 2015; 17:535–543.

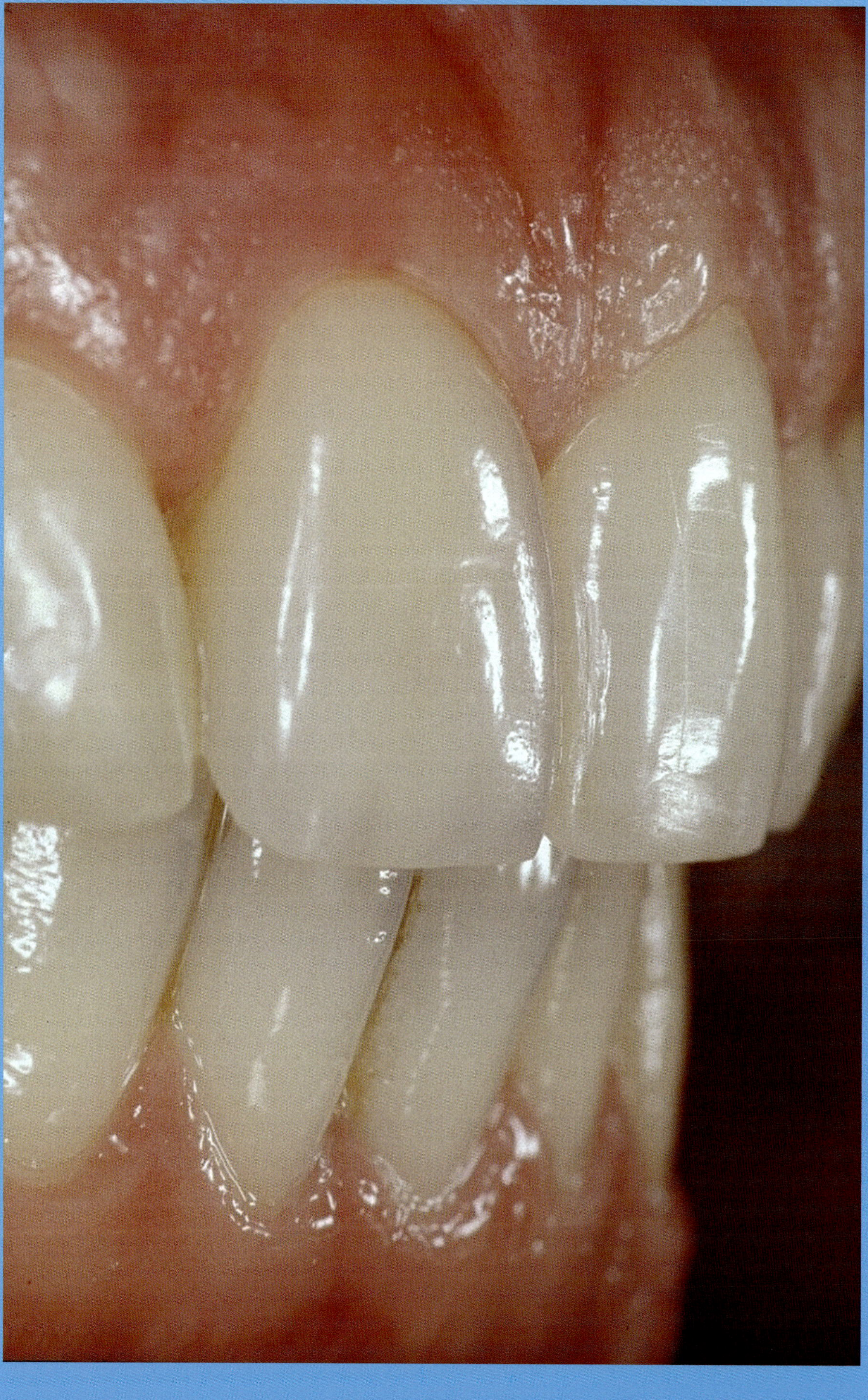

Chapter 15: Ceramic Veneers and Partial-Coverage Restorations

Christian F.J. Stappert, DDS, MS, PhD, Ronald E. Goldstein, DDS, Fransiskus A. Tjiptowidjojo, DDS, MS, and Stephen J. Chu, DMD, MSD, CDT

Chapter Outline

History	434
Traditional porcelain veneers	438
Advantages of porcelain veneers	438
Disadvantages of porcelain veneers	440
Indications for porcelain veneers	440
Contraindications for porcelain veneers	441
Shade selection	441
Classification of tooth preparation for anterior veneers	442
Classic preparation classes	442
Novel preparation classes	447
Mandibular veneers: special considerations	448
To reduce or not	449
Classic veneer preparation technique	456
Novel extended veneer preparation technique	456
Impressions	459
Digital impression	459
Conventional impression	459
Temporaries	460
Classic porcelain veneers: laboratory procedures	461
Making a model	461
Foil versus refractory die	461
Pressable ceramic veneers: laboratory procedures	462
IPS Empress	463
IPS e.max Press	463
Placement of veneers	465
Try-in	465
Final insertion	469
Post-treatment care and instructions	473
Posterior ceramic partial coverage restorations	478
Indications	480
Contraindications	481
Technique: preparation	481
Veneer onlay	482
Impression	482
Insertion	482
Finishing	482
Patient instructions	483
Alternative techniques	483
The CEREC system	483
The Carestream system	490

Ronald E. Goldstein's Esthetics in Dentistry, Third Edition. Edited by Ronald E. Goldstein, Stephen J. Chu, Ernesto A. Lee, and Christian F.J. Stappert.
© 2018 John Wiley & Sons, Inc. Published 2018 by John Wiley & Sons, Inc.

History

In the early part of the 20th century, movie actors frequently had dingy but otherwise healthy anterior teeth reduced for full crowns. Then, in the 1930s, California dentist Charles Pincus developed thin facings of air-fired porcelain that could be fastened in place with adhesive denture powder.[1] While these smiles live on in the film archives and in late-night movies, the veneers themselves were peeled away when the camera was turned off. Nonetheless, with this technique, Pincus had laid the groundwork for a new kind of dentistry, one that considered esthetics, not just articulation and function.

Veneering remained merely another form of cosmetics until the techniques and materials evolved to produce strong veneers that could be mechanically bonded to teeth. In 1955, Buonocore's research into the acid etch technique provided a simple method of increasing the adhesion to enamel surfaces for acrylic filling materials.[2] His discovery was quickly followed by Bowen's work with filled resins.[3,4] Only in the 1970s, however, with the introduction of visible-light-cured composites, did the dentist have the necessary working time to properly shape direct composite veneers.[5,6] Even so, these veneers were difficult to do: they were highly technique-sensitive, required extensive clinical chair time, and were frequently subject to in situ polymerization problems.

In the 1970s, Faunce described a one-piece acrylic resin prefabricated veneer as an improved alternative to direct composite resin bonding.[7,8] The veneer was attached both chemically, with a chemical primer applied to the veneer, and mechanically, with a composite resin to lute the veneer onto the etched tooth. These early indirect veneers and their successors had certain advantages over the direct veneers. Because they were fabricated by a manufacturer or trained technician, the indirect veneers typically displayed greater anatomical accuracy and almost always required less chair time for the patient and the dentist. More completely cured through laboratory processing, they were less likely to shrink during polymerization, and they provided superior shading capabilities and control of facial contours.[9] The indirect veneers had the additional advantage of being more stain-resistant than direct veneers.

Both acrylic resin and microfill resin veneers offer a smooth surface and good masking ability, with very little need for finishing. However, both exhibit poor resistance to abrasion[10] and are restricted to teeth not involving heavy functional contacts.[9] Presently, modern direct composite restorations can offer an alternative midterm solution, if the need of dental correction is limited, and the patient wants to avoid tooth structure preparation or has financial limitations (Figure 15.1A–T).

It was inevitable that the pioneers in veneers would turn to porcelain, one of the most popular and attractive materials in the dental armamentarium. The concept of acid etching porcelain and bonding to a tooth with an acid etch technique was first cited in the dental literature in 1975 with Rochette's description of an innovative restoration of a fractured incisor.[11] Since then, there have been key advances in the development of ceramic veneers and their fabrication and placement.[6,12–21]

The introduction of glass-ceramic and oxide-ceramic materials with enhanced flexural strength offered an alternative to feldspathic porcelain to fabricate dental veneers.[22–25] The new ceramic materials allowed for extension of classic facial veneer preparation designs[16,26] to more defect-oriented partial coverage and full veneer preparations introduced by Stappert et al. in 1999.[21,27] The new flexibility in preparation design based on enhanced ceramic material strength established ceramic veneers as valid alternative to full crown restorations in the anterior

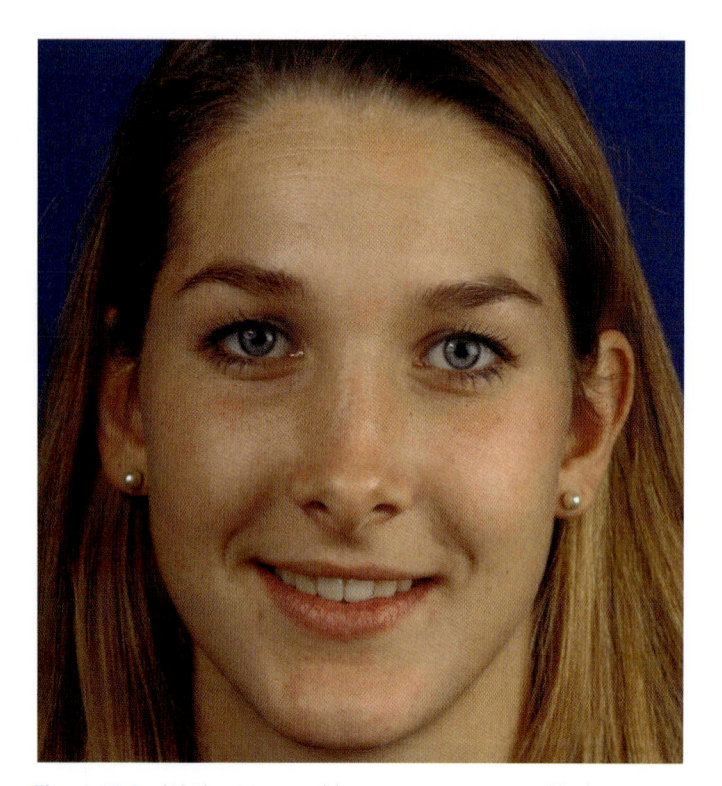

Figure 15.1 **(A)** This 24-year-old patient was concerned by her compromised anterior esthetics. Aged composite restorations showed discoloration at the four maxillary incisors.

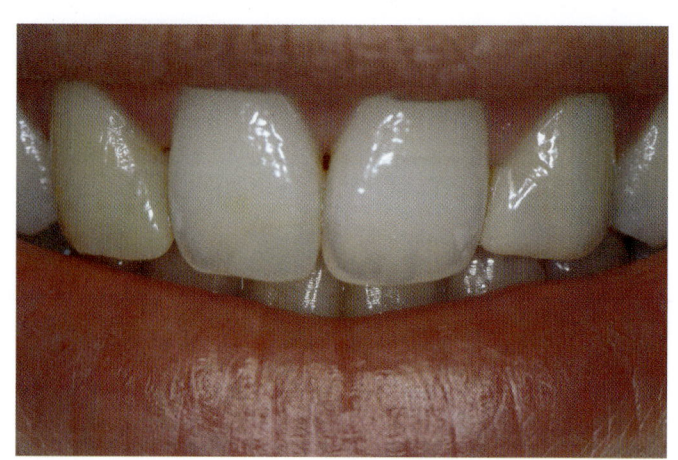

Figure 15.1 **(B)** The lateral incisors showed malformation and were built up by extended composite restorations. The incisal edge of tooth #8 had been replaced.

Chapter 15 Ceramic Veneers and Partial-Coverage Restorations

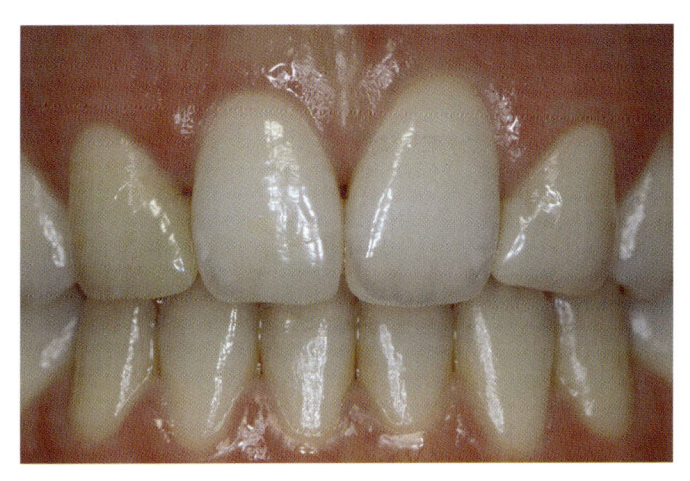

Figure 15.1 (C) Facial interocclusal dental overview demonstrates multiple shades, ranging from A3.5 to A1.

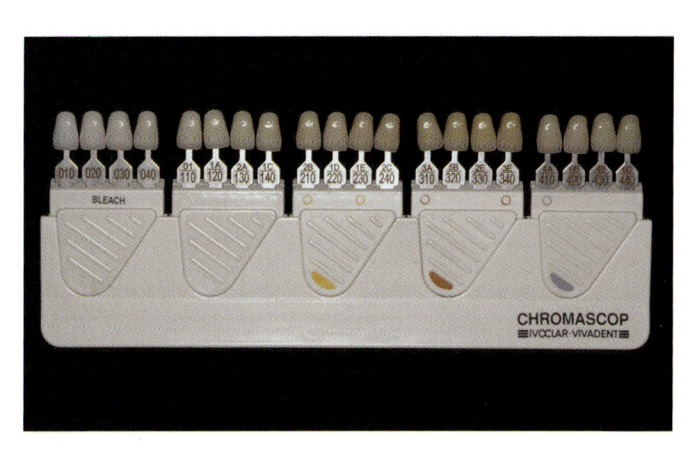

Figure 15.1 (D) To anticipate the bleaching outcome better, a bleaching shade guide was used.

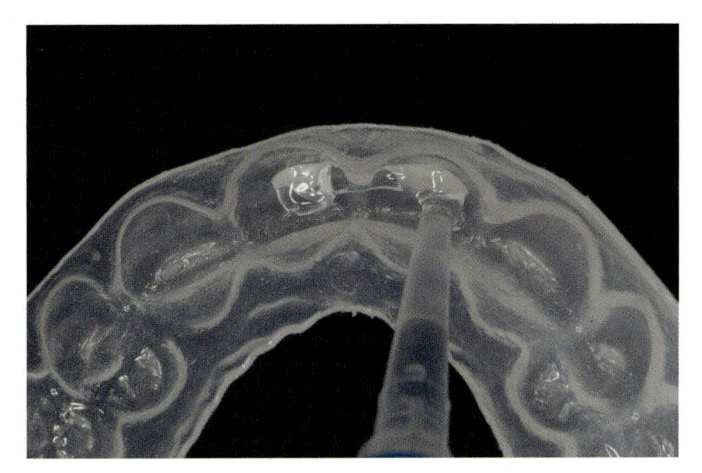

Figure 15.1 (E) Home bleaching was used to allow for customized bleaching periods of individual teeth.

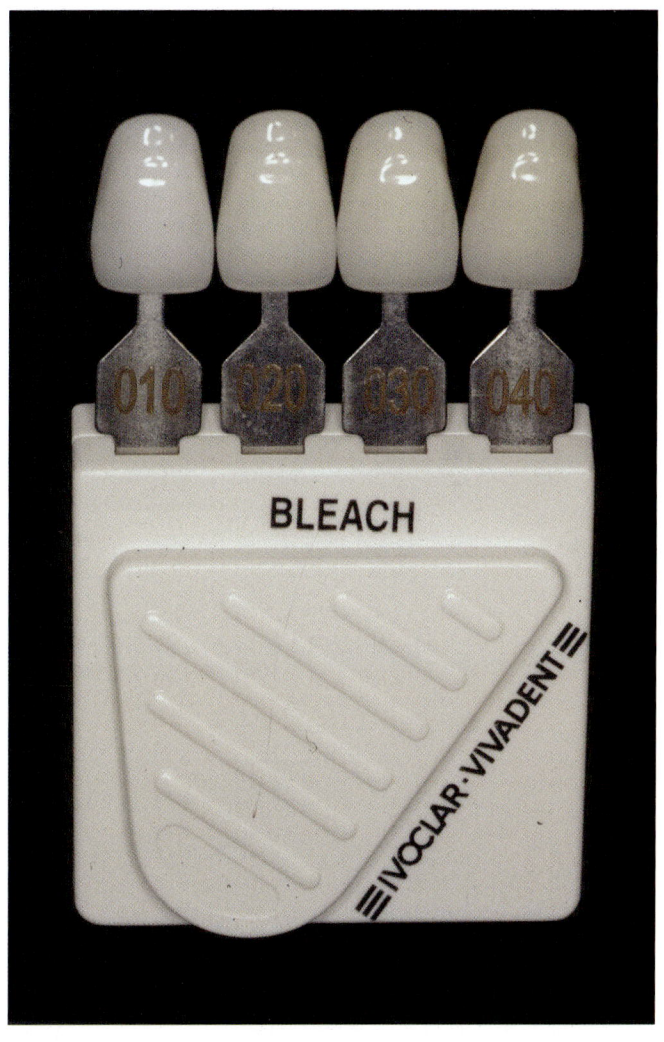

Figure 15.1 (F) A bleaching level of 020 or 030, according to the bleaching guide, was anticipated.

dentition.[28] Anterior veneer restorations require on average only 17–30% coronal tooth structure removal when compared to 60–70% of full coverage restorations.[29]

The further development of physical and biomechanical characteristic of dental ceramics resulted in ceramic material classes, showing significant differences in esthetics, strength, and reliability.[30]

Glass-ceramics and oxide ceramics exceed the fracture toughness and durability of silicate ceramics[31] and can be used even under higher masticatory loads of the posterior dentition.[32,33]

As the demand for esthetic dental services continues to grow, the introduction of stronger indirect ceramic restorations offers new minimal invasive options for both anterior and posterior restorations.

This chapter describes in detail the advantages and disadvantages, the indications and contraindications, and the techniques for using ceramic partial coverage restorations for anterior and posterior teeth, ranging from veneers to partial crowns (Figure 15.2).

Esthetic Treatments

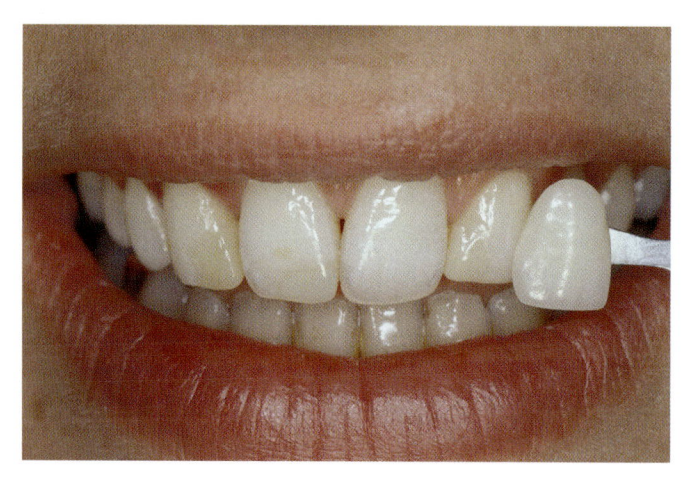

Figure 15.1 **(G)** Bleaching progress was monitored and dental hygiene treatments performed. The previous composite restorations became more visible.

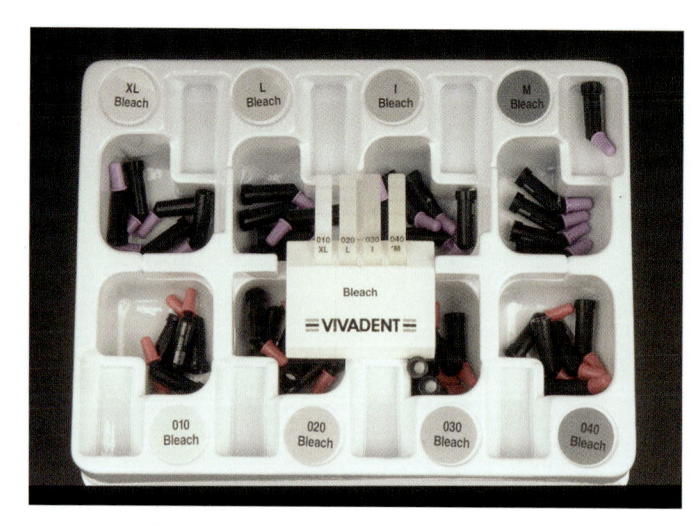

Figure 15.1 **(H)** Following the bleaching shade guide, composite material was used in a multilayer fashion.

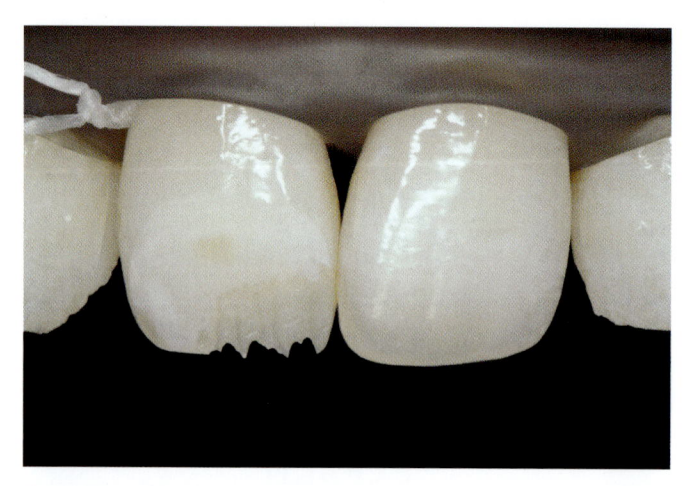

Figure 15.1 **(I)** Rubber dam was applied and composite build-ups in dentin and enamel were performed.

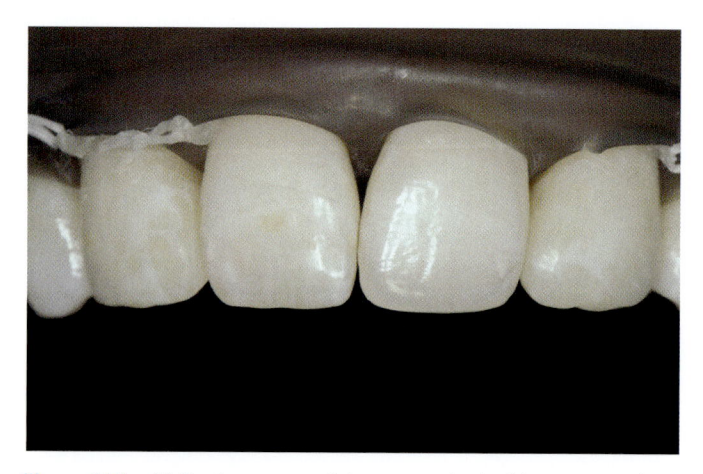

Figure 15.1 **(J)** Final outcome of the composite build-ups on teeth #7, #8 and #9 under dry condition.

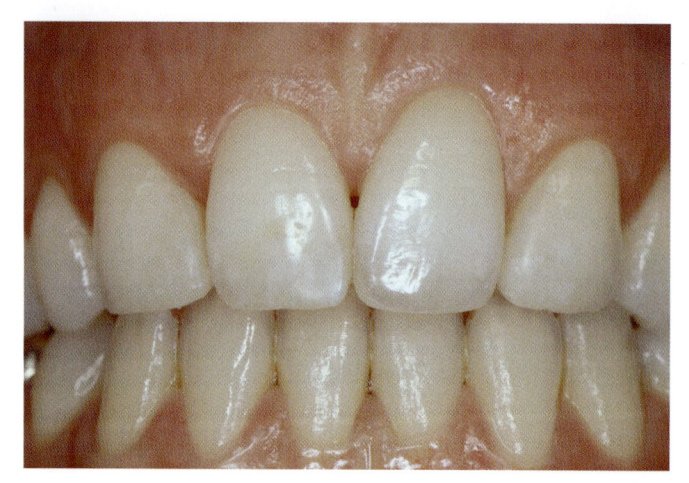

Figure 15.1 **(K)** Facial interocclusal view of the upper and lower dentition. The upper dentition shows a lighter shade than the lower dentition (A1 vs. A2). The patient didn't want to perform further bleaching in the lower dentition due to sensitivity concerns.

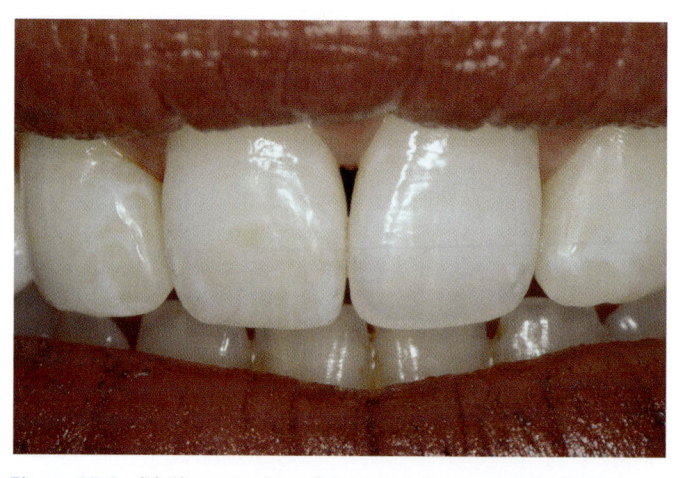

Figure 15.1 **(L)** Close-up view of the upper four restored anterior teeth #7–#10 in relation to the upper and lower lip position.

Chapter 15 Ceramic Veneers and Partial-Coverage Restorations

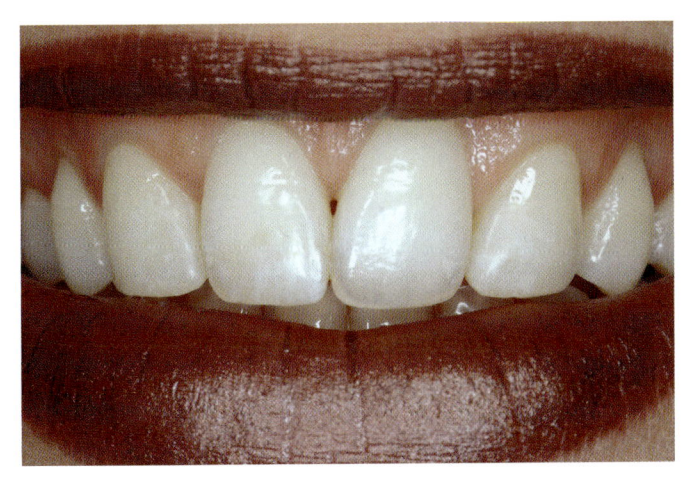

Figure 15.1 **(M)** Facial display of the patient's smile in area #5–#12 in relation to the lower and upper lip line.

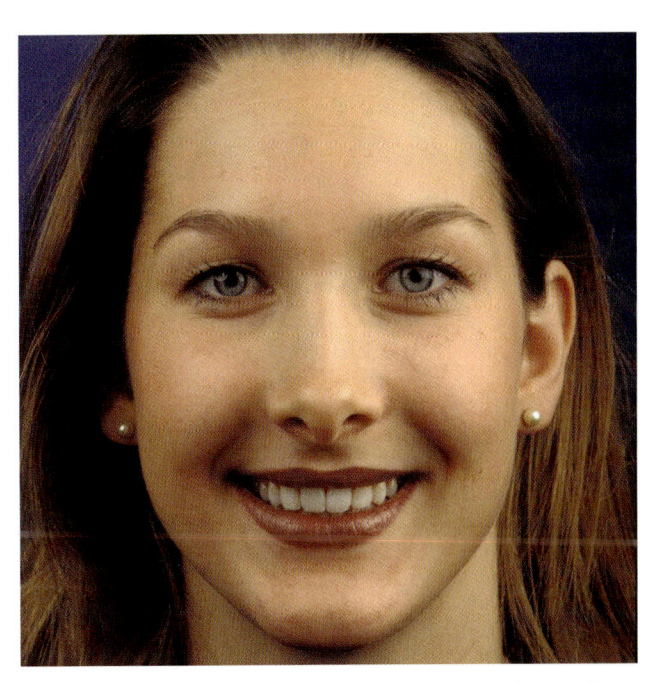

Figure 15.1 **(N)** Patient facial appearance after completion of the composite restorations in the anterior dentition. The patient was very satisfied with the final outcome.

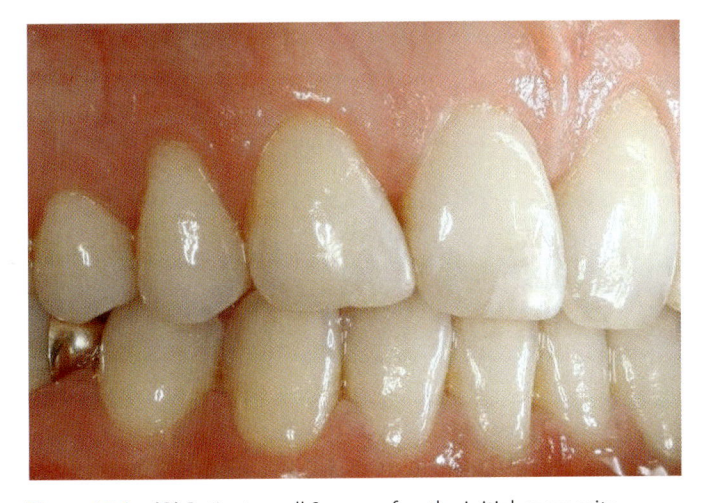

Figure 15.1 **(O)** Patient recall 9 years after the initial composite restorations on teeth #7–#10. The right lateral view demonstrates intact composite restorations with minor discoloration.

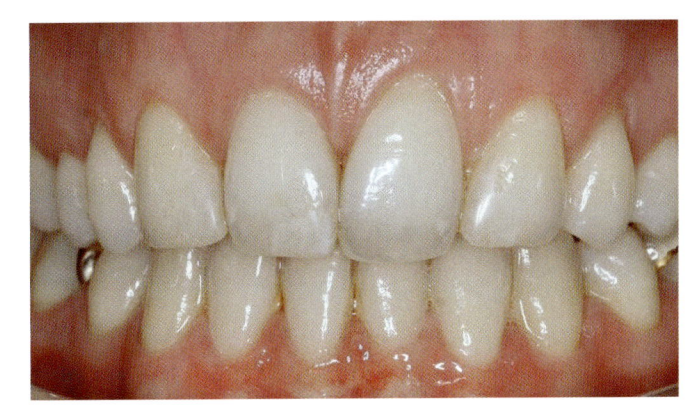

Figure 15.1 **(P)** Facial view of interocclusal relationship demonstrates discoloration of the mesiofacial restoration # 8 and recognition of the filling margins at tooth # 10.

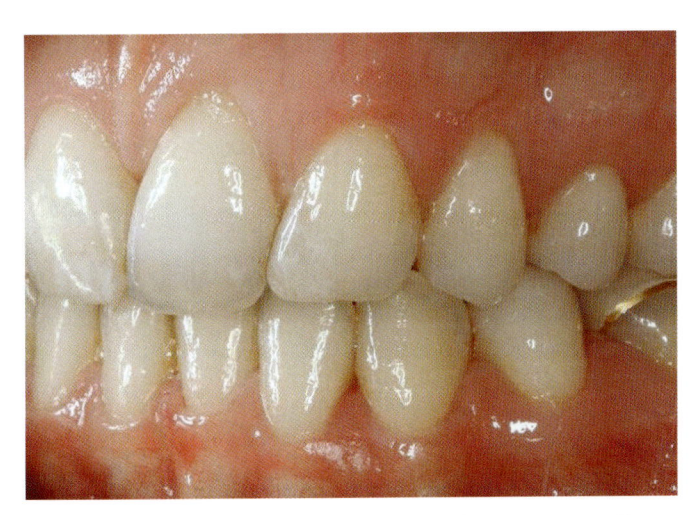

Figure 15.1 **(Q)** The left lateral view does not demonstrate significant discoloration areas.

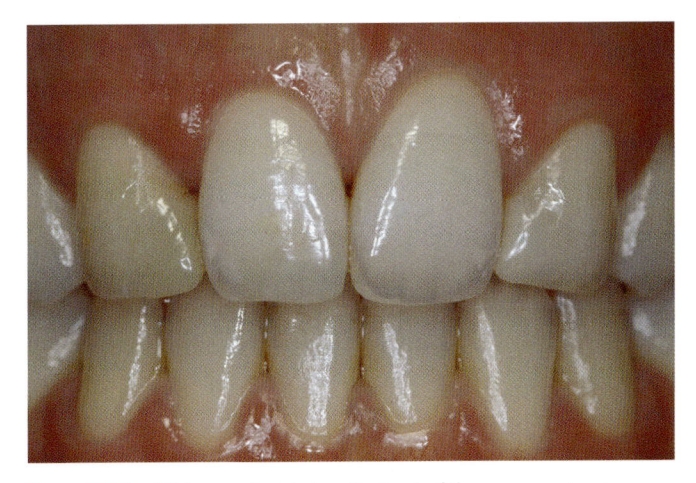

Figure 15.1 **(R)** Pre-op facial view (before) of the upper anterior dentition.

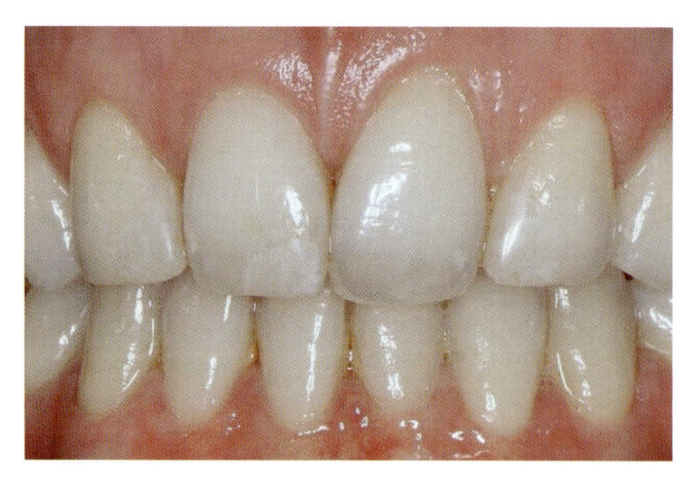

Figure 15.1 **(S)** Post-op facial view (after) of the composite restored upper anterior dentition 9 years later.

Traditional porcelain veneers

Porcelain is generally considered the most esthetic and biocompatible material available for dental restorations.

Advantages of porcelain veneers

1. Natural and stable color. The smooth surface texture and natural color of porcelain are exceptional, and the crystalline structure of porcelain gives it optical refractive properties similar to those of translucent enamel.[34,35] Furthermore, porcelain can be internally stained and the ability to adjust the final color of the veneers during placement allows considerable flexibility in final shade adjustments. Texture also is easily developed on the veneer surface to simulate that of adjacent teeth, and this texture can be maintained indefinitely,[16] as opposed to veneers of

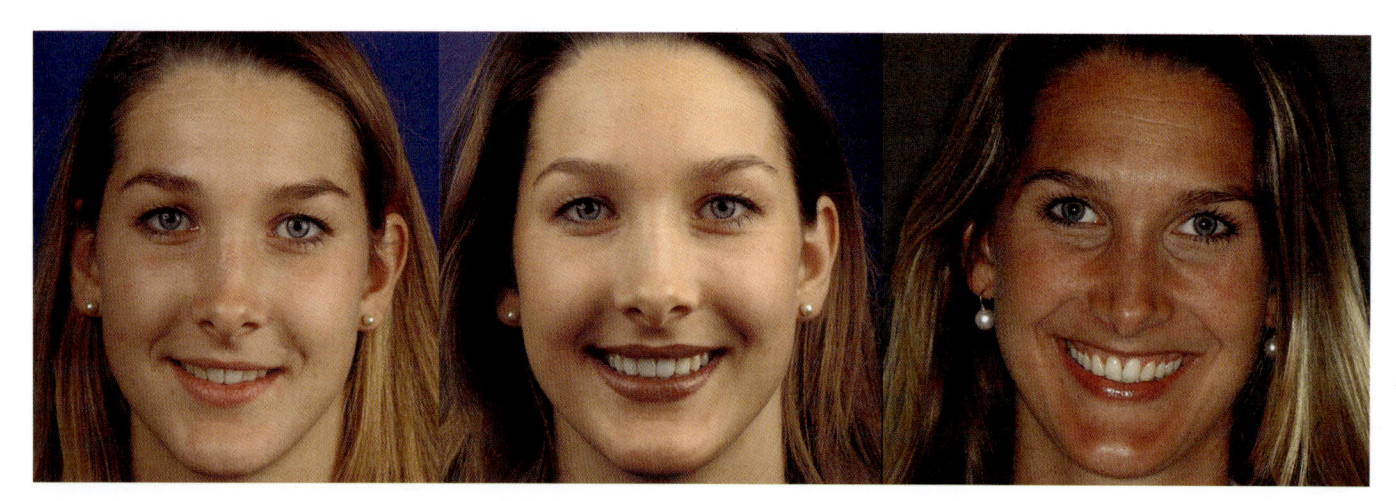

Figure 15.1 **(T)** The patient presents excellent dental hygiene and continues to appreciate her anterior composite restorations.

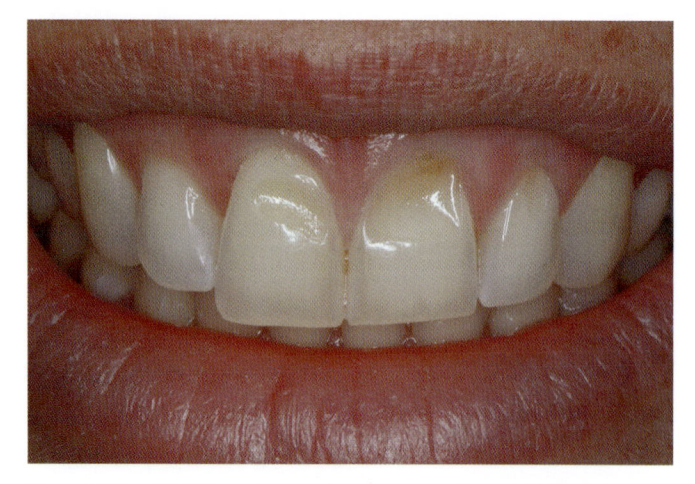

Figure 15.2 **(A)** This patient had a gummy smile and disliked the appearance of her two anterior front teeth. The teeth #8 and #9 appeared darker than the lateral incisors.

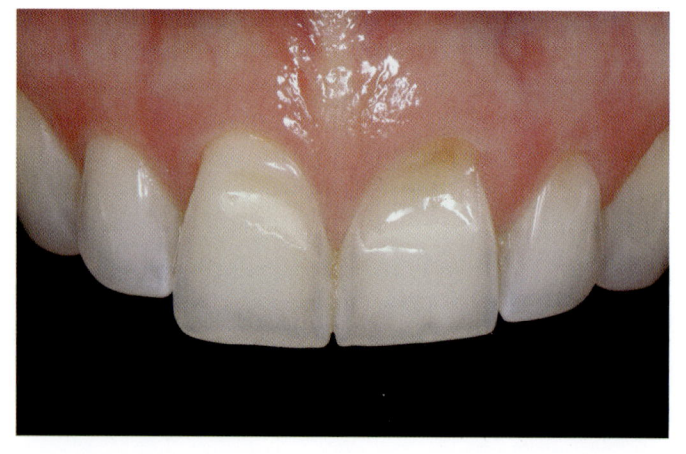

Figure 15.2 **(B)** Strong facial cervical enamel attritions at teeth #8 and #9 on this 30-year-old patient. Gingival conditions of the patient are very favorable. The cervical defects end below the cementoenamel junction close to the gingival margin.

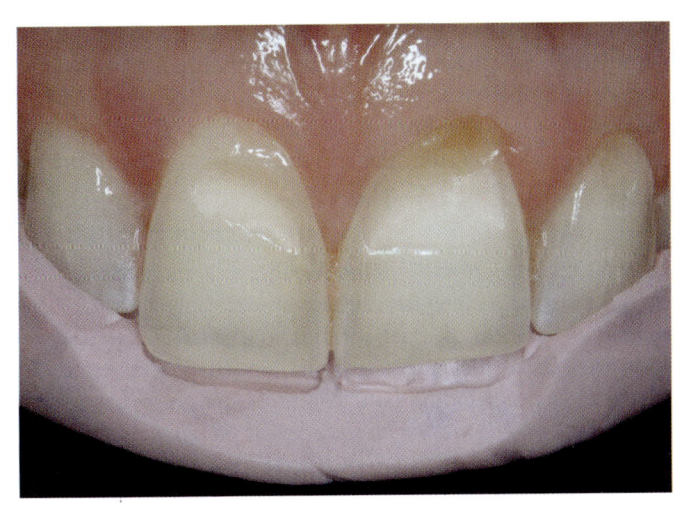

Figure 15.2 (C) Facial smile analysis resulted in a wax-up of the anterior two front teeth. A preparation guide was fabricated, showing the potential new incisal lengths.

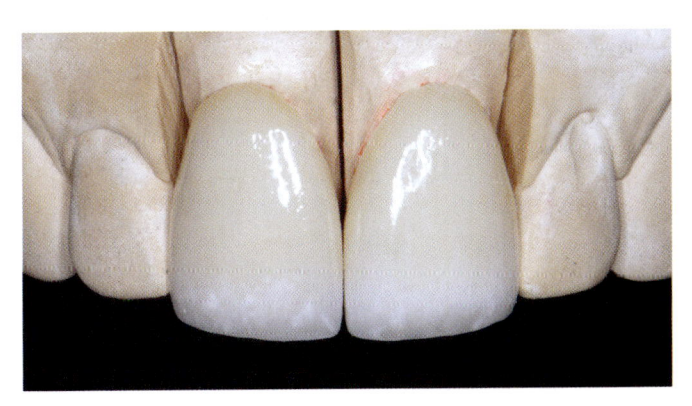

Figure 15.2 (D) Master model shows two very thin 0.4 mm press-ceramic e.max Press veneers for teeth #8 and #9.

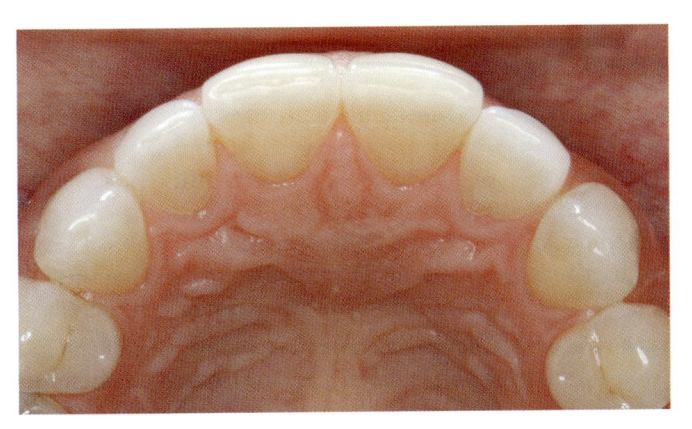

Figure 15.2 (E) Occlusal view of the adhesively bonded two anterior restorations.

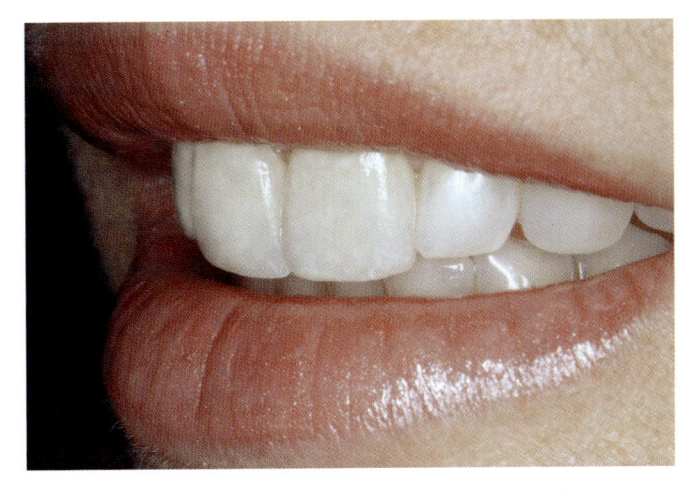

Figure 15.2 (F) Patient smile 6 months after placement of the anterior veneers. The new incisal length implies a more positive smile line.

monolithic pressed glass or computer-aided design/computer-aided manufacture (CAD/CAM) ceramics.[36,37]

2. Highly acceptable tensile bond strength. The bond of etched porcelain veneers to enamel is considerably stronger than that of any other material or veneering system. The resin to silane-treated etched porcelain veneer has bond strengths ranging from 17.9 to 22.1 MPa as compared to composite resin veneer to enamel bond strengths of only 6.2–9.7 MPa.[38,39]

3. Inherent porcelain strength that permits reshaping teeth.[40] Although porcelain veneers are themselves rather fragile once bonded to enamel, the restoration develops high tensile and shear strengths.[38,41,42] Porcelain therefore can be used to increase the length of a given tooth by extending it over the incisal edge. In certain instances, porcelain veneers can also be used to repair ceramometal restorations.[43,44]

4. Extremely good biocompatibility with gingival tissues. The highly glazed porcelain surface is less of a depository area for plaque accumulation as compared to any other veneer system, and it appears that some types of porcelain veneers actually deter plaque accumulation.[45]

5. Long lasting. Once bonded, porcelain veneers develop high tensile and shear strengths and remain in place.[46] For example, a 5 year clinical study of 186 porcelain veneers placed in 61 patients showed a survival rate of 98.4%.[47] Fradeani et al. reported a probability of survival of 182 porcelain veneers of 94.4% at 12 years, with a low clinical failure rate of approximately 5.6%.[48]

6. Exceptional resistance to wear and abrasion.[49,50] Porcelain veneers still look good after many years (Figure 15.3A and B).

7. Resistance to stain. The microscopic porcelein structure reveals only very few voids and irregularities that could accumulate stain. Therefore, the highly glazed porcelain surface is very resistant to stain accumulation.

8. More resistant to deleterious effects of solvents, including alcohol, medications, and cosmetics than any composite resin veneer.[49]

9. Much less absorption of fluids than any other veneering materials.[50] Water absorption of resin veneers leads to a decrease in physical properties and increasing wear and surface changes over time.[51]

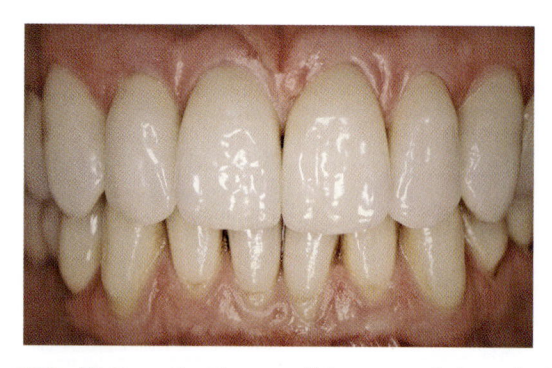

Figure 15.3 **(A)** The patient improved his upper smile by replacing discolored fillings and dental defects with six veneers and four partial coverage ceramic restorations one year ago.

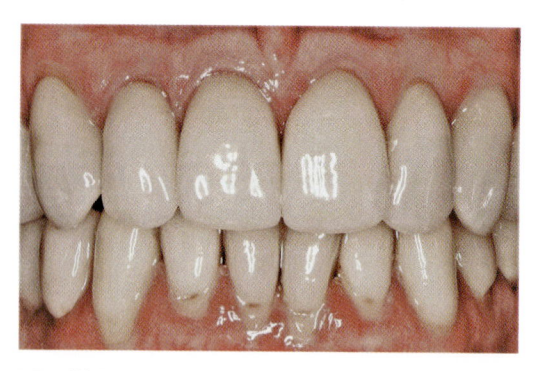

Figure 15.3 **(B)** Ten years after placement, the ceramic veneers and partial coverage restorations still look good despite the presence of some tissue recessions.

10. Surface luster retention. Composite resin tends to lose the initial luster, requiring frequent repolishing. Porcelain retains its glazed luster over the entire life of the restoration.
11. Lack of radiopacity. On radiographs porcelain resembles natural tooth structure, allowing radiographic access to areas that would be shielded by radiopaque restorations.

Disadvantages of porcelain veneers

1. Porcelain veneers can be easily repaired with composite once bonded to the enamel, but the repairs are not long lasting due to staining which tends to occur at the margin of composite resin and porcelain.
2. The color cannot be easily modified once bonded in position.
3. Irreversibility of preparation versus little or no preparation for direct composite resin bonding.
4. Level of difficulty of fabrication and placement, time involved, and expense. The extremely fragile veneers are difficult for the dental laboratory to make and manipulate, and the process requires at least two appointments, plus laboratory fees.
5. Technical difficulties in avoiding overcontours and obtaining closely fitted porcelain/enamel margins. The margins can be especially brittle and difficult to finish.[16]
6. Lower reparability compared to composite veneers. Yet, Kimmich and Stappert point out that porcelain can be repaired using hydrofluoric acid for 1 min or Co-Jet to create surface roughness to bond to porcelain intraorally.[44] The veneers are then silanated and coated with a layer of unfilled resin, followed by a color-matched composite repair. But the disadvantage still remains in terms of time and complexity, and unknown durability of the repair.
7. Susceptibility to pitting by certain topical fluoride treatments. Stannous fluoride paste should not be used with porcelain restorations. Also it is best to avoid air-polishing prophylaxis systems (Prophy Jet, Dentsply, Air Flow S1, Hu-Freidy Prophy Jet, or NSK Prophy Mate L, Hu-Friedy) on the porcelain surface. Finally, hygienists must avoid ultrasound in prophylaxis treatment, especially around gingival margins. Goldstein, Lamba, Lawson, Beck, Oster, and Burgess demonstrated in a clinical study at the University of Alabama at Birmingham that ultrasonic scaling around margins of Class V composite restorations could result in microleakage.

Indications for porcelain veneers

Classic veneer indications are listed here.[40]

Type I: moderate tooth discolorations/color corrections:
  Tetracycline
  Fluorides
  Amelogenesis imperfecta

Type II: anatomical malformations/corrections of position:
  Type IIa   Conoid teeth
  Type IIb   Diastemata
  Type IIc   Incisal edge lengthening

Type III: extensive damage/changes in form:
  Type IIIa   Extensive coronal fractures
  Type IIIb   Congenital and acquired malformations

The covering power of porcelain veneers and their ability to reshape teeth make this procedure almost ideal for many clinical situations including those outlined below.

1. Moderate discolorations, such as tetracycline staining, fluorosis, devitalized teeth, and teeth darkened by age which are not conducive to vital bleaching.[8] Porcelain veneers can be especially useful for single discolored teeth.
2. Teeth with generalized moderate facial discoloration from amalgam shine-through.[52]
3. Surface defects. Small cracks in the enamel caused by aging, trauma, or ice chewing can weaken the enamel and stain darkly. In these situations, porcelain veneers can mask the stains, seal, and strengthen the teeth. Also, teeth with numerous shallow, esthetically compromising restorations on the labial surfaces can be dramatically improved (Figure 15.2A–F).
4. Replacement of missing or fractured parts of the teeth.[19,40] Nixon[52] and Kimmich and Stappert[44] report the use of veneers on porcelain crowns to repair porcelain fractures.

5. Closing of diastemas, single or multiple spaces between the teeth, and improving the appearance of rotated or malpositioned teeth. Persons who have relatively sound teeth but who do not want to undergo orthodontics may be helped with veneers that create the esthetic illusion of straight teeth.

6. Short teeth.[52] These teeth can be lengthened to a more esthetic, appropriate size.

7. Malocclusions or periodontally compromised teeth. Porcelain veneers can restore or change the configuration of the lingual surfaces of anterior teeth to develop increased guidance or centric holding areas. Porcelain veneers can also be used to reshape interproximal embrasure spaces when the gingival tissues have receded.

8. Agenesis of the lateral incisor. When the cuspid erupts adjacent to the central incisor in situations in which there is a missing lateral incisor, porcelain veneers can be used to develop a different coronal form of the cuspid, simulating a lateral incisor. This treatment may have to be combined with veneers on the central incisors to obtain a more ideal ratio in the relative proportion of the teeth, because the cuspid is invariably too wide.

9. Progressive wear pattern. If sufficient enamel remains and the desired increase in length is not excessive, porcelain veneers can be bonded to the remaining tooth structure to restore the shape, color, or function of the teeth. Assuming the parafunctional behavior itself is under control, porcelain veneers even can be used to repair dentitions damaged by the effects of anorexia nervosa or bulimia.

10. Functionally sound ceramometal or all-ceramic crowns with unsatisfactory color.[52] The labial surface of the old porcelain is prepared as you would for a conventional veneer. After an impression, a veneer is constructed in the new shade. The existing crown surface is roughened with air abrasion, and then etched with a buffered intraoral use hydrofluoric acid and silanated.[44] The veneer is then bonded to place with resin cement. However, the cost of this procedure is basically the same as making a new crown, so its use should be limited to those patients not wanting their entire crown or extended fixed dental prosthesis remade.

Contraindications for porcelain veneers

In comparison to other forms of bonding, porcelain veneers have fewer and more forgiving contraindications. Nonetheless, such contraindications do exist.

1. Patients with certain tooth-to-tooth habits such as bruxism or parafunctional habits such as pencil chewing or ice crushing may place undue stress on the porcelain veneers.

2. Ideally, enamel should be around the whole periphery of the veneer, not only for adhesion, but more importantly to seal the veneer to the tooth surface.[25] In addition, there should be sufficient enamel available for bonding, since bonds to dentin are generally less retentive and predictable than bonds to enamel. If the tooth or teeth are composed predominantly of dentin and cementum, extended veneer restorations or crowning with high-strength ceramics may well be the preferable treatment.[26,28] A strict adhesive bonding protocol for dentin bonding should be applied to achieve predictable long-term reliability of the bonding interface.

3. Certain types of occlusion may have problems. These include Class III and end-to-end bites. However, there may still be the possibility of cosmetic treatment by contouring the lower incisors and building out the maxillary incisors. An alternative can be a protective bite appliance for the patient to wear after treatment is completed to protect the veneers from clenching or grinding forces. This appliance would be worn at night or when sleeping, driving, playing sports, etc., as necessary. Still, day clenching or grinding could be a problem.

4. Deciduous teeth and teeth that have been excessively fluoridated may not etch effectively. In order for porcelain veneers to be successful in these cases, special measures such as aggressive roughening of the enamel/dentin surface with an extra-coarse diamond plus air abrasion may be required in combination with last-generation bonding agents. Extreme bleaching-resistant discolorations, such as deep tetracycline or amalgam staining, or discolored devitalized roots and coronal tooth structure, are very difficult to cover with porcelain ceramic restorations. In these cases, the use of more opaque high-strength ceramics such as lithium disilicate,[53,54] aluminum oxide,[55-57] or zirconium oxide[58,59] is indicated.

Shade selection

Shade determination begins at the consultation and examination appointment. This is when an understanding of what exactly the patient wants is needed. How light does the patient envision his or her teeth will be? If the patient is looking for "white" teeth, does that mean opaque white or translucent white? The clinician must determine how much leeway he or she has in arriving at what seems to be appropriate and agreeable color. The easiest way of accomplishing this is to image the patient on a computer so that the clinician and the patient can see how the different colors will look. However, if the patient is a perfectionist, the best method is to have the ceramist construct several trial veneers made from an impression of your patient's teeth. Thus, several samples of different shade choices can be offered and applied directly to the teeth.

If all teeth that show are going to be veneered, then proceed with shade selection as any other ceramic restoration. If, however, some teeth are to be covered with porcelain veneers and others are to be bonded or restored with full crowns, the porcelain veneers should be placed first because of the difficulty in modifying the color of the veneers once they are bonded in place. The adjacent teeth can then be easily matched to the final, bonded porcelain veneer color. If the procedure involves matching one discolored tooth (especially a central incisor) to another, provide the ceramist with extra room with additional depth of tooth preparation to add sufficient opacity to the veneer to mask the darkness before exact matching of the required tooth shade.

One of the most important steps in the entire procedure is deciding when, where, and how to record color or shade. This should be done before beginning treatment, at a session when the teeth have not been dried out for any period of time. It should be done inside the operatory using color-corrected light, outside in daylight, and inside using incandescent light. A good external device to be able to see all three light values is the Rite-Lite 2 shade-matching light (AdDent). Finally, reconsider the shade after the enamel has been prepared. If the prepared tooth has turned much darker than previously anticipated, consider a lighter shade or a shade with more opaquer, or even re-prepare the tooth to gain more porcelain thickness and thereby additional room for both color and opaquer. If this is the situation, the clinician should have a consultation with the ceramist if possible. In the event the technician is not available, a photographic consultation may suffice to record exactly what the color problems are for the ceramist. However, the final impression may be delayed pending a joint decision on which approaches to take.

The available shade guides, such as the VITA porcelain shade guide, may not be ideal for veneers because they are too thick and are composed of several different layers including opaques. It is better for the ceramist to make an individualized shade guide of porcelain veneers exactly as he or she would fabricate them and use this to select a shade. And always, take photos with the shade guides on the same plane as the teeth to be restored.

Classification of tooth preparation for anterior veneers

The following is based on the present evidence-based literature.[20,21,25,26,40,60-63]

Class 0: no preparation (Figure 15.4A–C).

Class 1: window preparation (window) (Figure 15.5A and B). Veneer ends below the incisal edge.

Class 2: feather-edged preparation technique (feather) (Figure 15.6A and B). Veneer extends to the incisal edge; there is no reduction of the incisal edge.

Class 3: bevel preparation (bevel/small butt joint) (Figure 15.7A and B). Buccopalatal bevel; there is reduction of the incisal edge.

Class 4: overlapping preparation of incisal edges (incisal overlap) (Figure 15.8A and B). Reduction of the incisal edge and palatal extension of the preparation.

Class 5: butt joint preparation (Figure 15.9A and B). Incisal reduction of ≥2 mm, 90° lingual marginal finish. Interproximal preparation includes the contact areas.

Class 6: full veneer preparation (complete veneer, ¾ veneer) (Figure 15.10A and B). Interproximal and palatal preparation extension, including palatal deep chamfer or rounded shoulder preparation. Variable defect-oriented preparation; hybrid between veneer and all-ceramic crown.[21,27]

Classic preparation classes

The veneer preparation Classes 0–4 can be considered 'classic.' The preparation guidelines have the following philosophies in common:

1. The main veneer indication groups for these veneer preparation classes are Type I (discoloration), and to a moderate extent Type IIa, b, and c (conoid teeth, diastemata, incisal edge lengthening) indications.

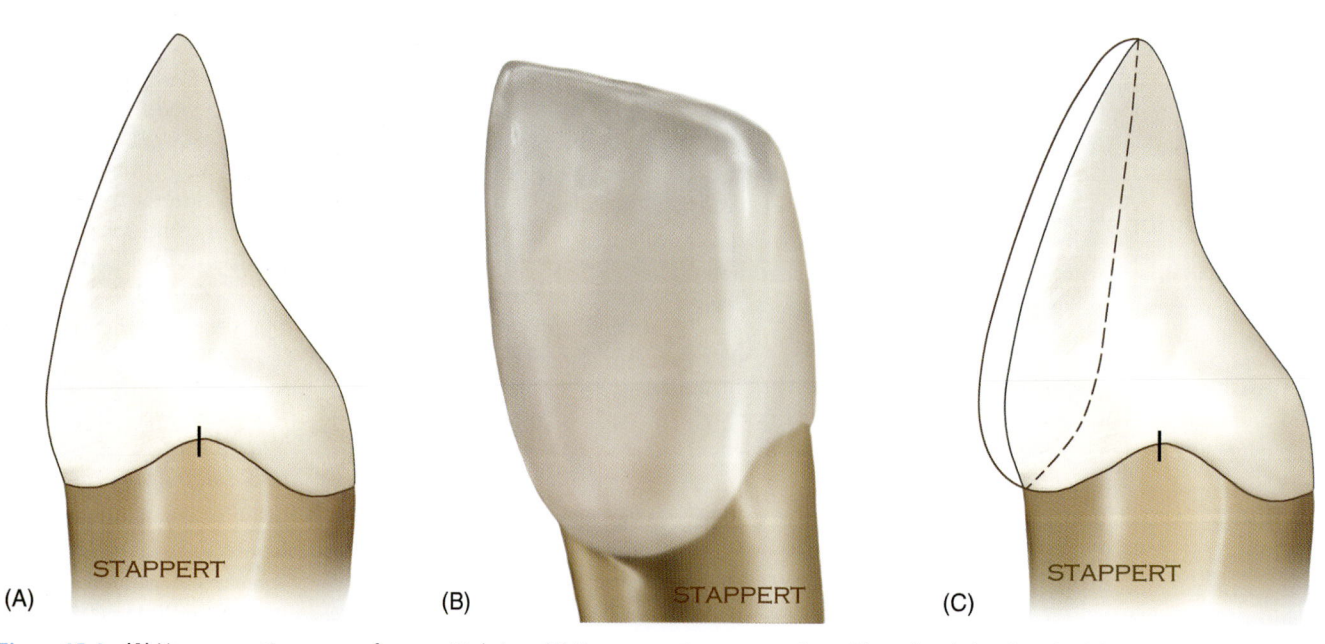

Figure 15.4 (A) No-preparation veneer from sagittal view. (B) No-preparation veneer viewed from facial-distal angle. (C) No-preparation veneer illustrated with future restoration.

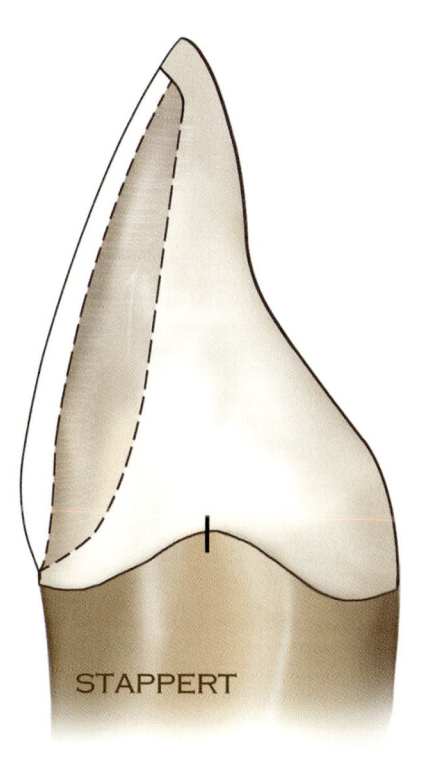

Chapter 15 Ceramic Veneers and Partial-Coverage Restorations

Figure 15.5 **(A)** Window veneer preparation from sagittal view.

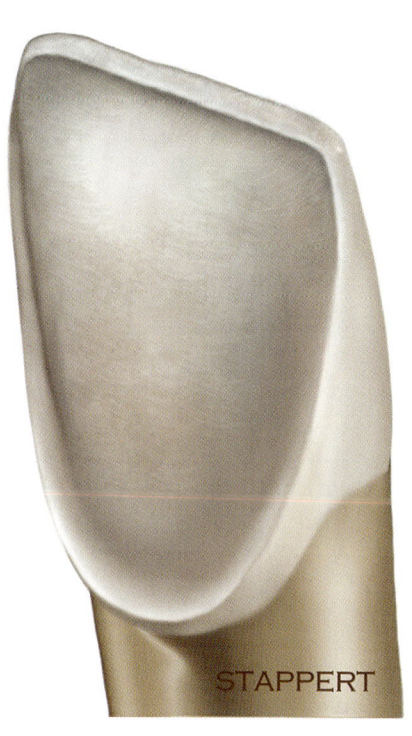

Figure 15.5 **(B)** Window veneer preparation viewed from facial-distal angle. Notice the veneer ends below the incisal edge.

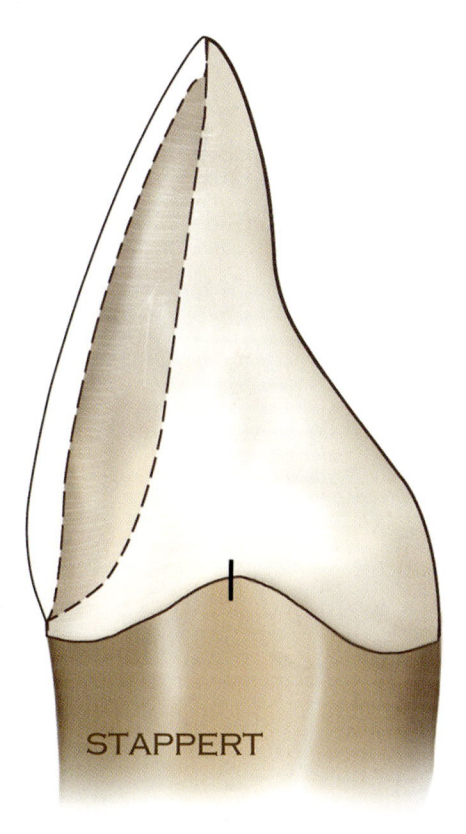

Figure 15.6 **(A)** Feather-edged veneer preparation from sagittal view.

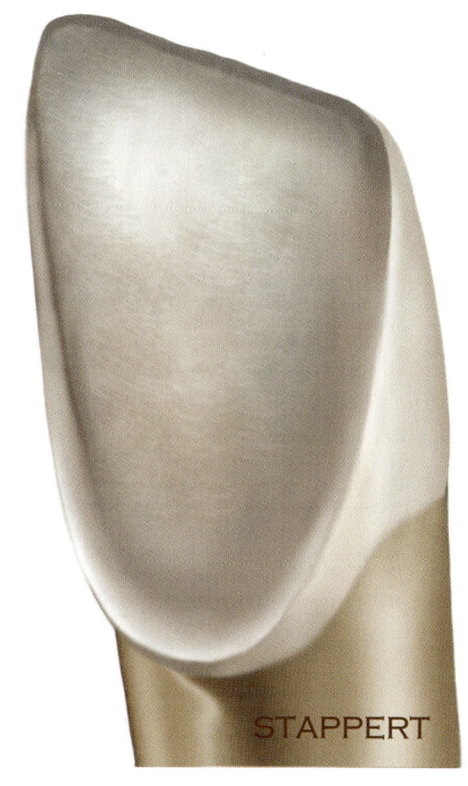

Figure 15.6 **(B)** Feather-edged veneer preparation viewed from facial-distal angle. Notice the veneer extends to the incisal edge with no reduction of the incisal edge.

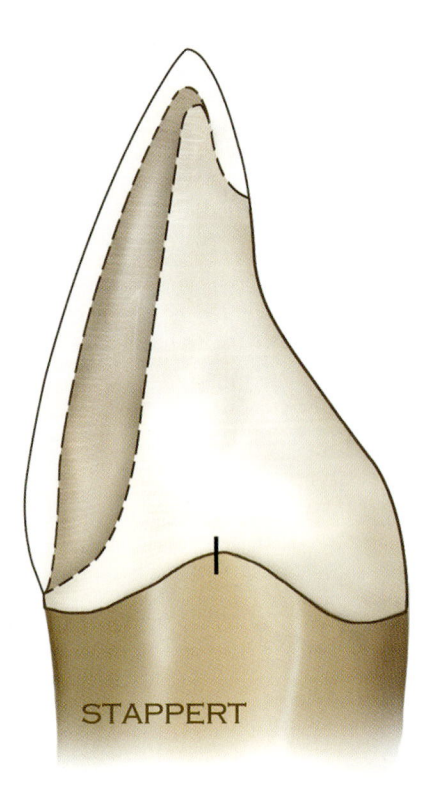

Figure 15.7 **(A)** Bevel veneer preparation from sagittal view.

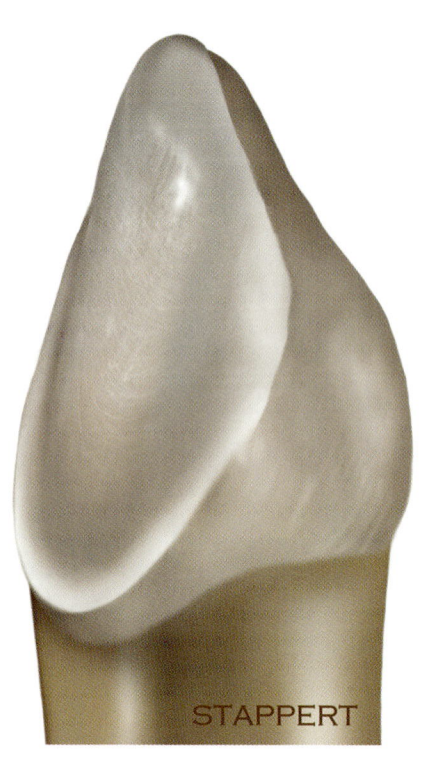

Figure 15.7 **(B)** Bevel veneer preparation viewed from facial-distal angle. Notice buccopalatal bevel/small butt joint reduction of the incisal edge.

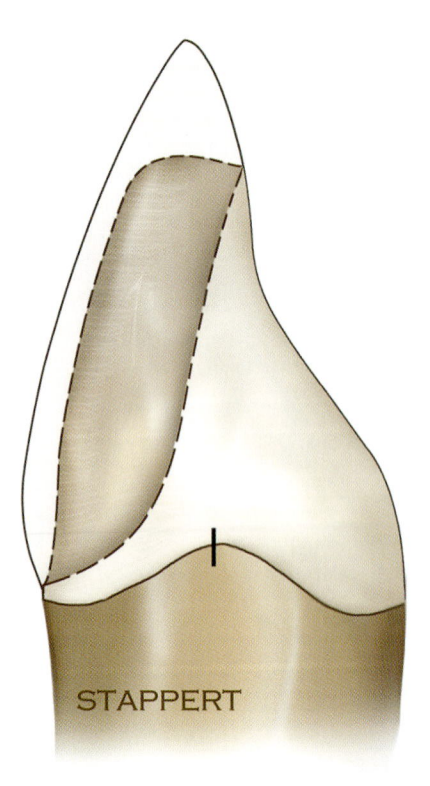

Figure 15.8 **(A)** Overlapping of incisal edges veneer preparation from sagittal view.

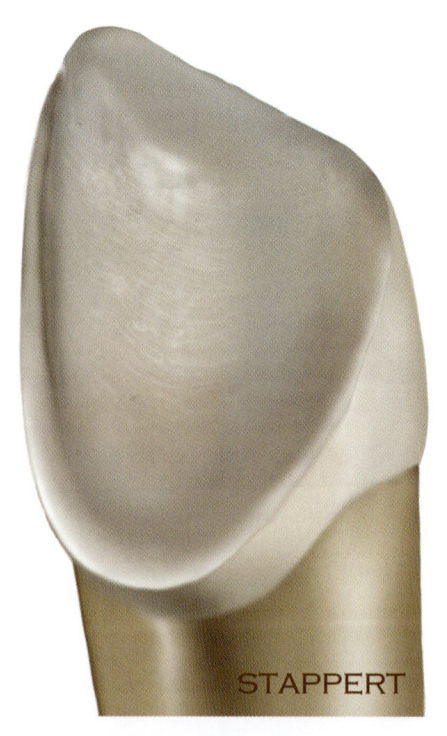

Figure 15.8 **(B)** Overlapping of incisal edges veneer preparation viewed from facial-distal angle. Notice incisal overlap and palatal wraparound extended preparation.

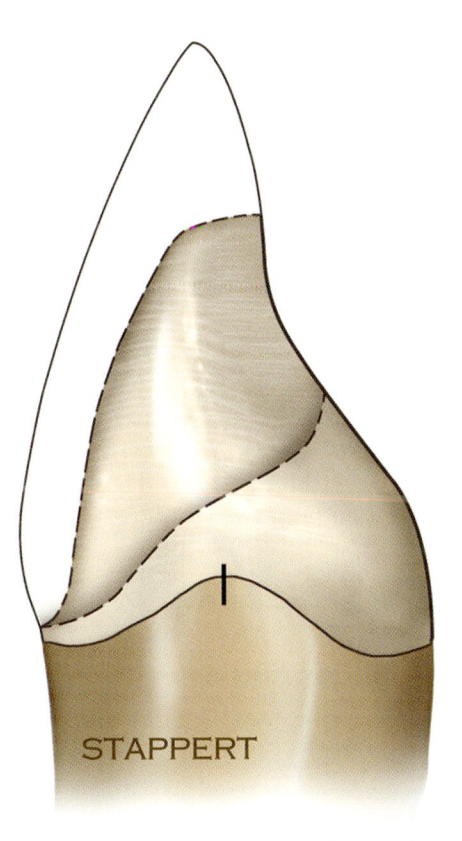

Chapter 15 Ceramic Veneers and Partial-Coverage Restorations

Figure 15.9 **(A)** Butt joint veneer preparation from sagittal view.

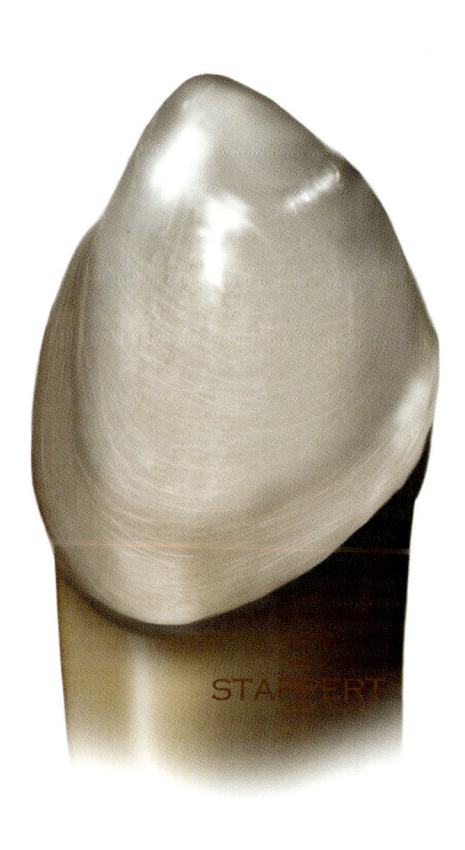

Figure 15.9 **(B)** Butt joint veneer preparation viewed from facial-distal angle. Notice incisal reduction of ≥2 mm with 90° lingual marginal finish.

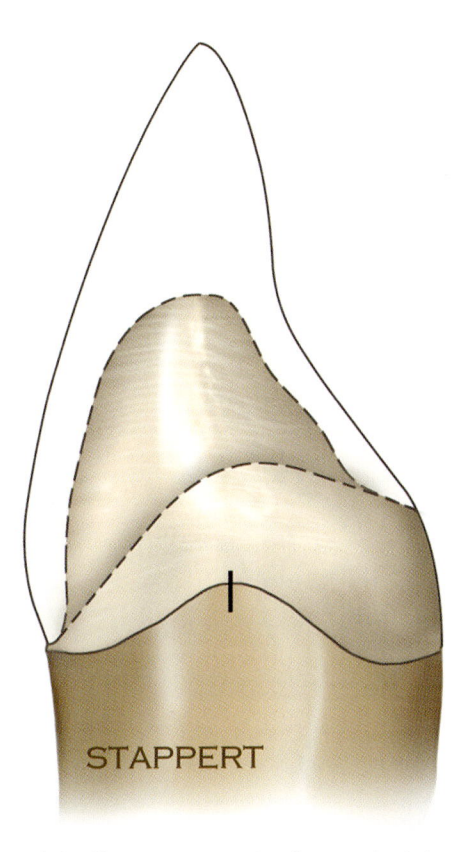

Figure 15.10 **(A)** Full veneer preparation from sagittal view.

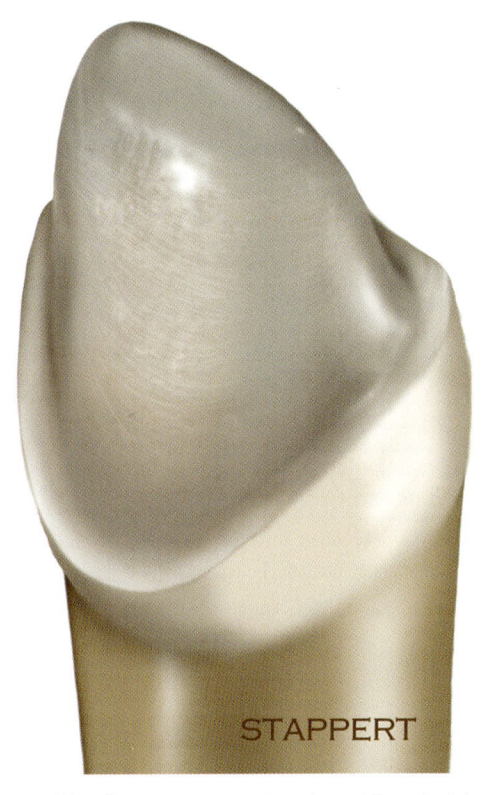

Figure 15.10 **(B)** Full veneer preparation viewed from facial-distal angle. Notice extension of the preparation that resembles hybrid between veneer and all-ceramic crown.

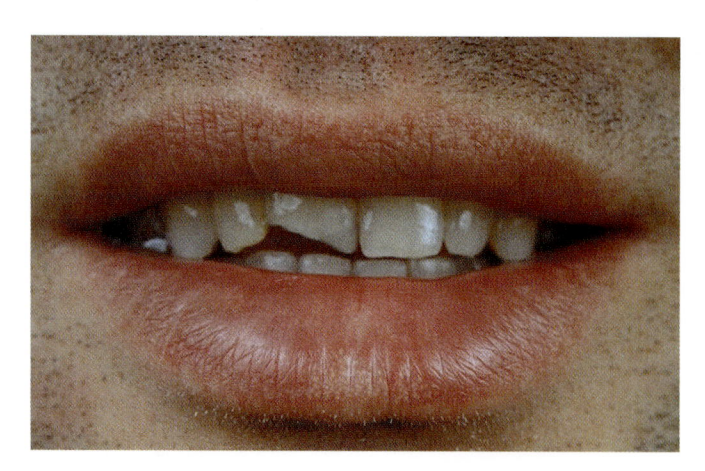

Figure 15.11 **(A)** This 32-year-old male patient presented after a bicycle accident with incisal tooth fracture of tooth #8. Dental evaluation did not demonstrate increased mobility or hypersensitivity. The rehabilitation of tooth #8 was planned with an IPS Empress veneer.

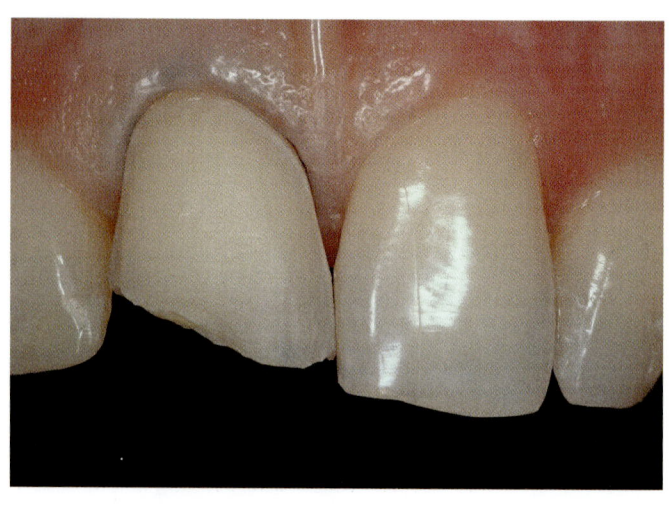

Figure 15.11 **(B)** Facial preparation of tooth #8 with estimated 0.4 mm preparation depth, ending epigingival in a light chamfer. Incisal butt joint preparation provided a 90° finish line at the palatal surfaces.

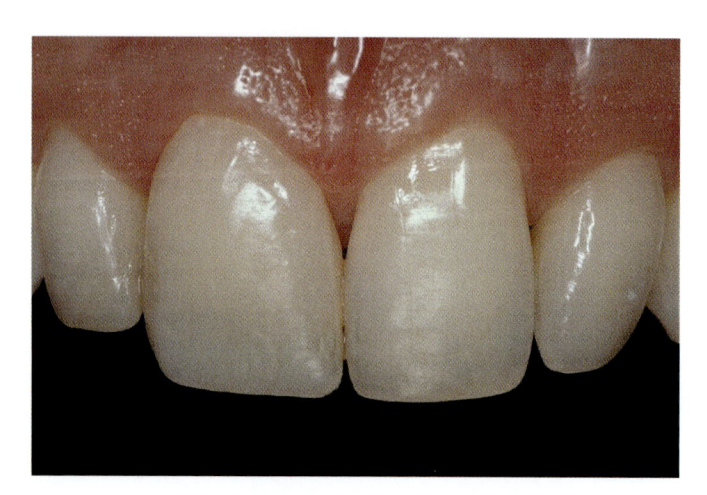

Figure 15.11 **(C)** Fabrication of direct composite veneer as provisional. First the tooth was isolated with glycerin gel to allow later removal of the composite veneer. For fixation, point etching was performed facially and HelioBond was used to bond the restoration temporarily.

2. All of these preparation classes primarily restore the facial aspect of a tooth.
3. The preparation approach is minimally invasive, ideally by maintaining the incisal edge of the restored tooth.
4. Preparation extension into the interproximal contact area or beyond is mostly avoided.
5. Preparation is enamel-sparing and bonding of the veneer restoration relies predominantly on enamel bonding.
6. The most common used material in these classes is feldspathic porcelain.

An example Class 4 preparation is shown in Figure 15.11A–L.

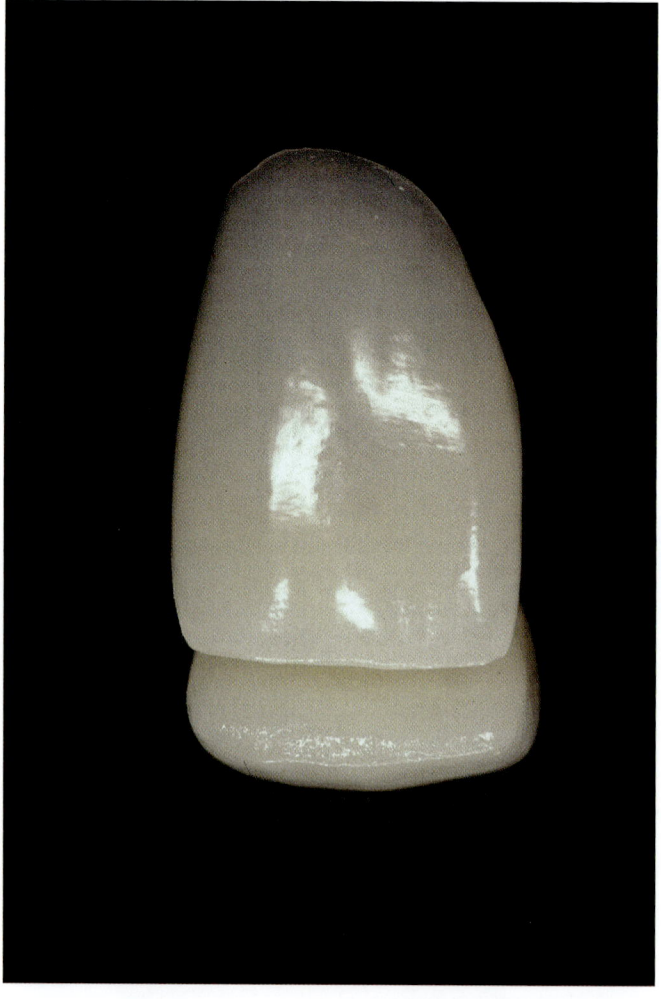

Figure 15.11 **(D)** Final IPS Empress veneer restoration, using the cut-back technique to customize the esthetic outcome.

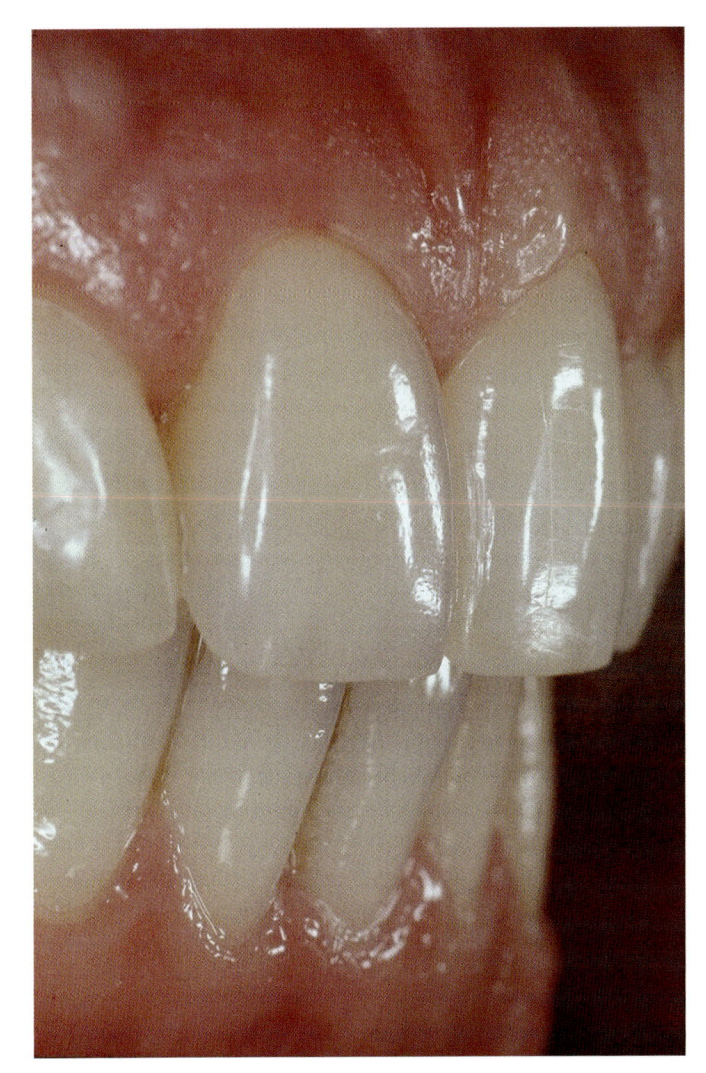

Figure 15.11 (E) Adhesively bonded ceramic veneer at tooth #8. Epigingival placed veneer by using triple-zero retraction cord to catch excess cement.

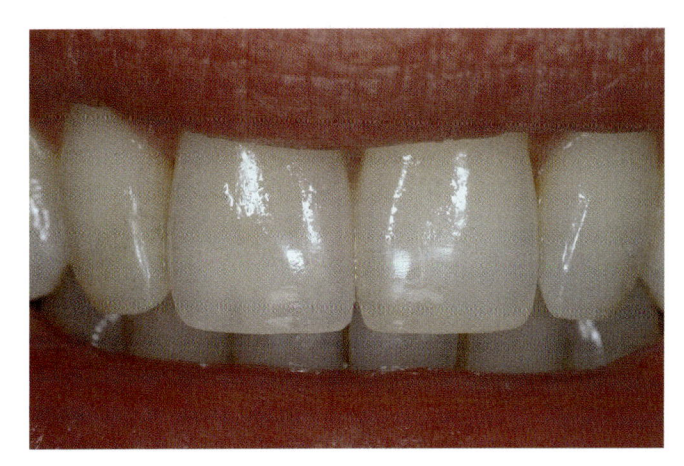

Figure 15.11 (F) Facial view of the bonded ceramic veneer in relation to the smile line. The incisal defect at tooth #7 was treated with a layered composite filling to achieve an enhanced symetrical outcome.

Novel preparation classes

The veneer preparation Classes 5 and 6 can be considered 'novel.' The preparation guidelines aim for the following goals:

1. The main veneer indication groups for these veneer preparation classes are severe Type IIa, b, and c (conoid teeth, diastemata, incisal edge lengthening) and Type IIIa and b (extensive coronal fractures, and congenital and acquired malformation) indications.
2. Preparation includes facial, proximal and palatal dental deficiencies or defects.
3. The preparation is defect-oriented. Enamel preservation and marginal enamel integrity are preferred, yet areas of dentin exposure due to extended dental hard tissue loss are expected, and, due to the path of insertion of the final restoration, unavoidable.

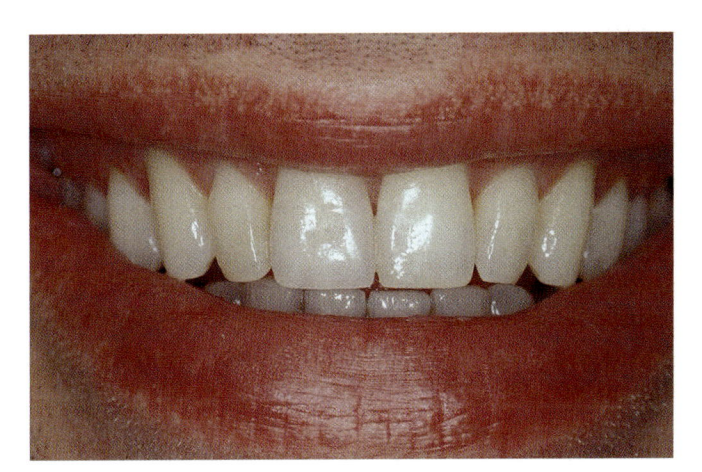

Figure 15.11 (G) Full facial view of the full smile of the patient.

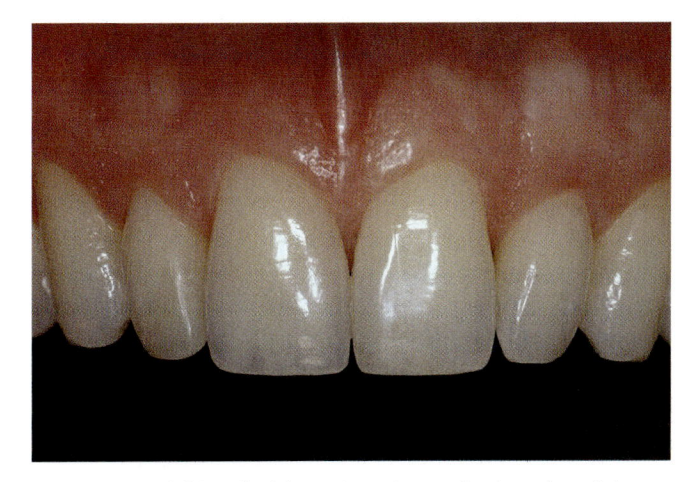

Figure 15.11 (H) Recall of the patient, 1 year after insertion of the ceramic veneer at tooth #8.

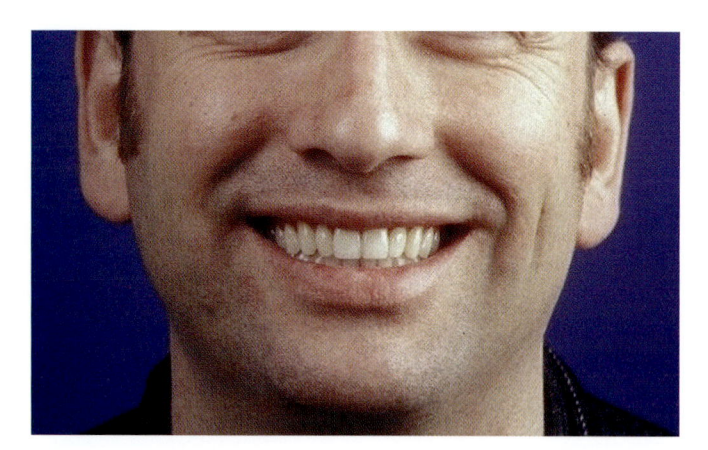

Figure 15.11 **(I)** Facial view of the patient's smile 1 year after insertion of the ceramic restoration.

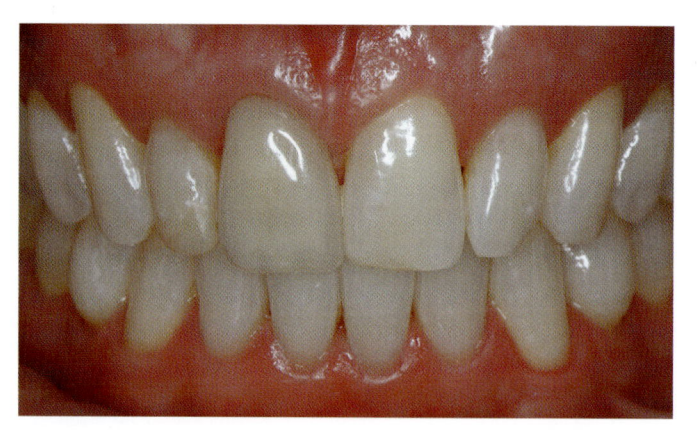

Figure 15.11 **(J)** Recall shows anterior view of veneer tooth #8 14 years after placement.

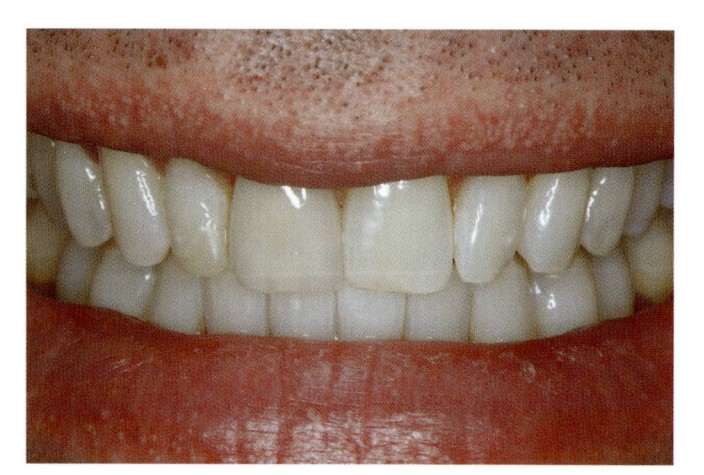

Figure 15.11 **(K)** The smile line of the patient does not expose the light marginal discoloration at the extended veneer restoration.

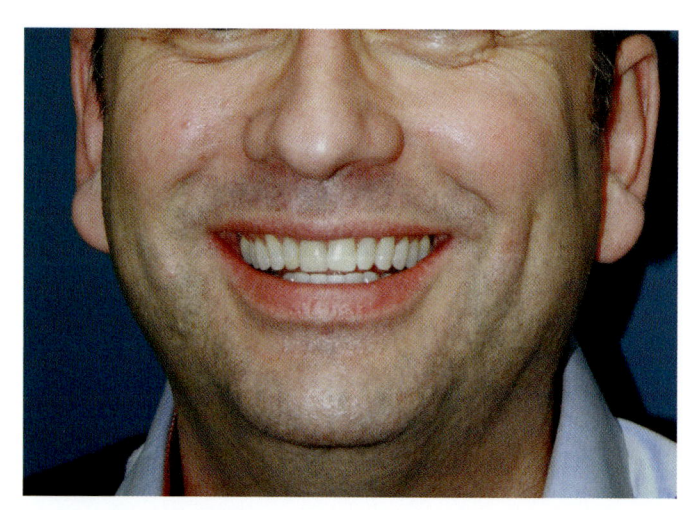

Figure 15.11 **(L)** Patient is still satisfied about his treatment choice to have his tooth restored with an all ceramic veneer (facial view).

4. The preparation includes the interproximal contact areas and extends proximally to the lingual aspect.
5. Incisal reduction or extension depends on the final restorative goals, and preparation depth can vary from 0.4 to 1.0 mm according to diagnostic wax-up and mock-up.
6. Bond strength relies on a combination of enamel and dentin bonding.
7. High-strength ceramics, presently largely lithium-disilicate glass-ceramic, compensates for extended tooth structure loss.

Mandibular veneers: special considerations

From an esthetic standpoint, the mandibular veneer can provide an excellent result in most situations. However, its life expectancy can be drastically compromised unless the patient's occlusion is favorable. The usual problem with preparations for lower veneers is leaving enough tooth structure remaining after the horizontal and vertical reduction. A potentially weak point is at the incisolabial junction, which must always be sufficiently reduced and rounded to allow the veneer to be thick enough in that area to have the strength to resist fracturing when placed under an occlusal load (Figure 15.12A). The possibility of fracturing or cracking means greater maintenance for mandibular veneers in patients with heavy occlusal demands, which includes patients with habits such as severe bruxism or clenching. If this is the situation and if discoloration is the reason for wanting to do mandibular porcelain veneers, it is advised to try bleaching first to see if the teeth will become light enough to satisfy the patient.

Also, the incisal edge of mandibular anteriors is usually the most visible part of the veneer so consider this fact when preparing the tooth. Simply reducing from the labial surface will almost always be insufficient to mask the tell-tale signs of color differences that the veneer has been placed. Sufficient incisal reduction is needed to ensure a normal incisal edge appearance for that patient.

One advantage of the mandibular veneer is that it is seldom necessary to go subgingivally, as with the maxillary veneer, because most people do not show the gingival margin of mandibular anteriors. However, the clinician needs to discuss this with the patient, since there are many individuals who do not want to see a margin or be reminded of the previous discoloration regardless of the fact that he or she is the only one who

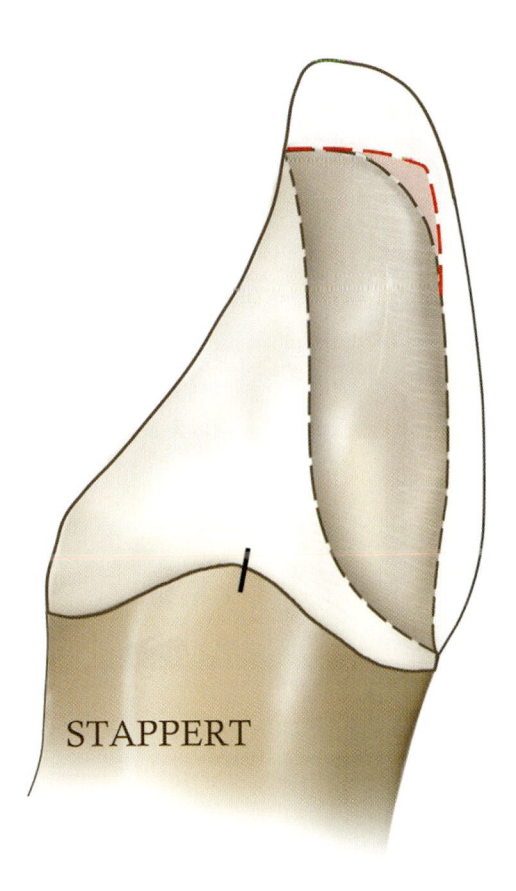

Figure 15.12 **(A)** This illustration shows the proper amount of horizontal and vertical reduction necessary for the average porcelain veneer on a lower incisor. Note that the incisal-facial line angle needs to be rounded to allow for sufficient ceramic thickness of the restoration. A sharp edge preparation (red area marked) will compromise the restoration and can lead to fracture. Interincisal clearance needs to be checked before final impression is performed.

might view the margin (Figure 15.12B–O). Another important consideration is to make sure your patient will agree to wear a nightguard to protect the veneers. This is essential for both maxillary and mandibular veneers. If not, then the patient must understand you will not be responsible for future fractured veneers.

To reduce or not

There are different opinions with regard to how much or how little the teeth need to be prepared—that is, reduced—before the application of porcelain veneers. Some clinicians argue that little or no reduction is required. Teeth that will require building out labially for better appearance are a good example of this. Clinicians at the opposite end of the spectrum argue for a full deep chamfer preparation on the labial aspect of the teeth that extends most or all of the way through the interproximal contact areas. Accordingly, it was reported that high variations in preparations for porcelain veneers exist in general dental practice.[64]

The most practical approach is to evaluate each patient, and indeed each tooth to be veneered, on the basis of (a) the thickness of the veneer needed for covering or reshaping, (b) the degree of anticipated retention of the veneer, considering the receptivity of the tooth to the bonding agent and placement of the veneer, and (c) recognition of how the increased thickness of the veneered tooth will change its appearance, structure, alignment, and function.

Obviously, the ideal would be a technique that requires no preparation and a veneer that is strong, attractive, and functional, with no subsequent adverse periodontal changes. However, that ideal is seldom the case. Most patients need to have about 50% of the labial and some proximal enamel removed in order not to overbuild the teeth being veneered.

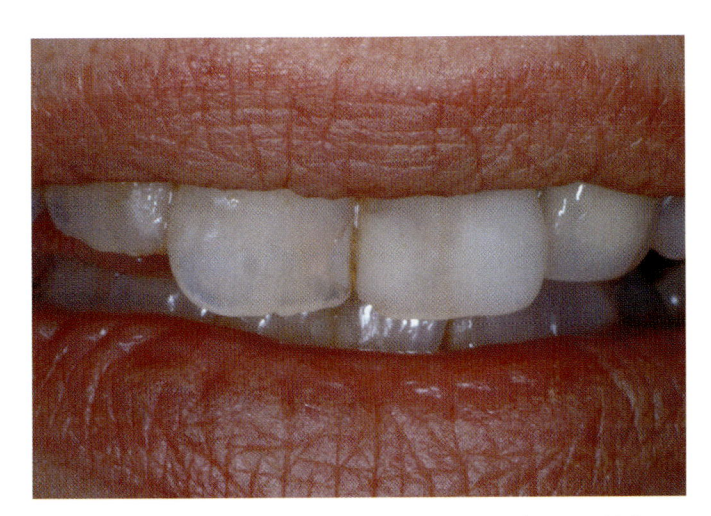

Figure 15.12 **(B)** Pre-op smile picture. Patient is not happy with her smile because of the discolored teeth, irregular shape, and defective old restorations.

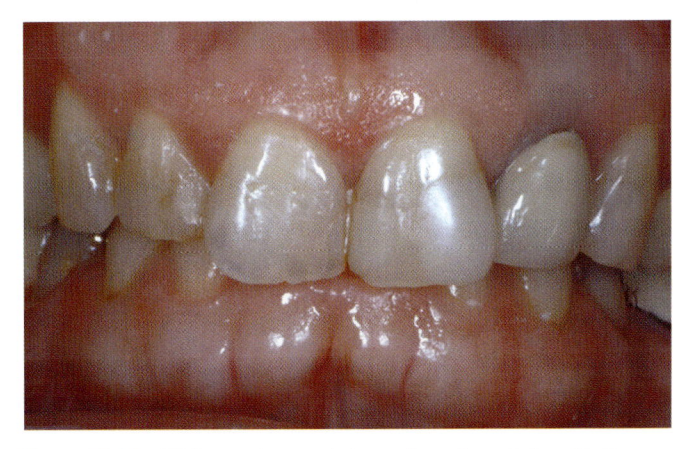

Figure 15.12 **(C)** Pre-op intraoral picture from frontal view. Notice heavy restorations on #8 and #9, old porcelain fused to metal (PFM) crown #10, and deep overbite.

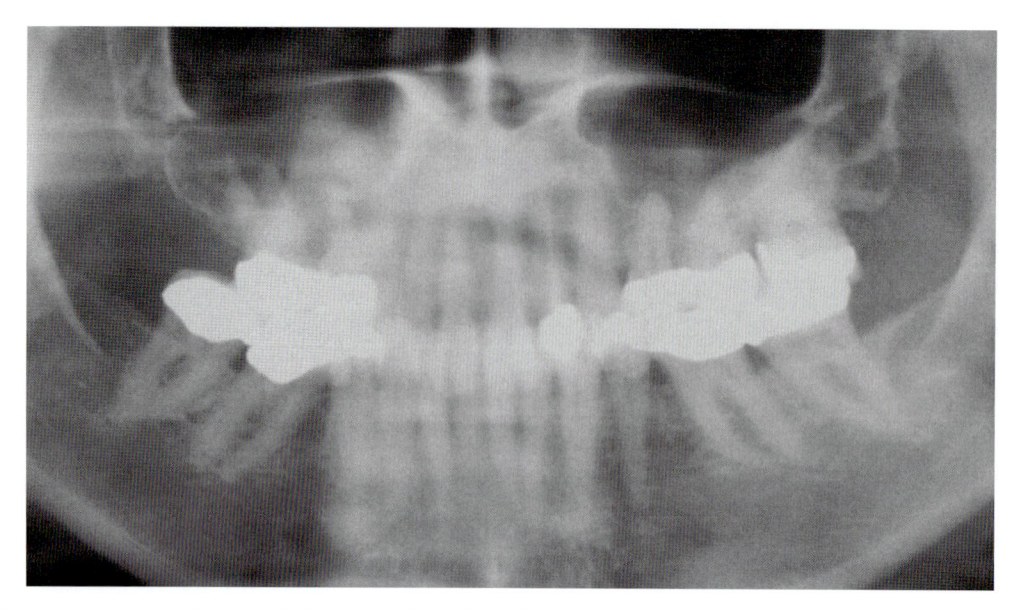

Figure 15.12 **(D)** Pre-op panoramic radiograph. Notice patient has a dental history with multiple restorations and endodontic treatment of tooth #10.

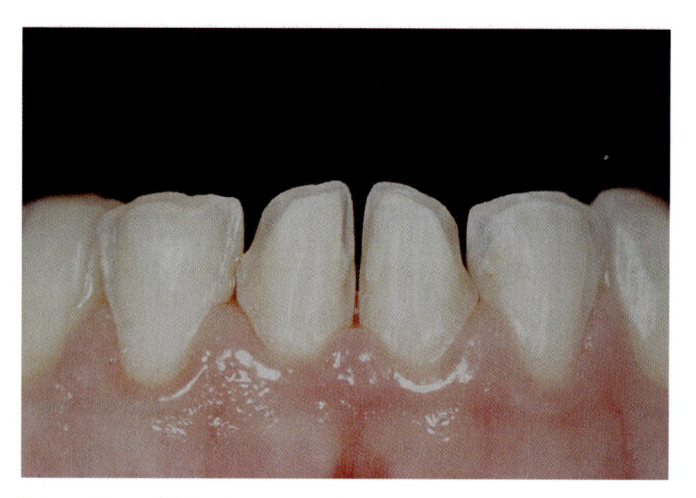

Figure 15.12 **(E)** Teeth #22–#27 show conservative veneer preparations from facial view. Notice #24 and #25 defect-oriented preparation technique due to previous restorations on distal aspects.

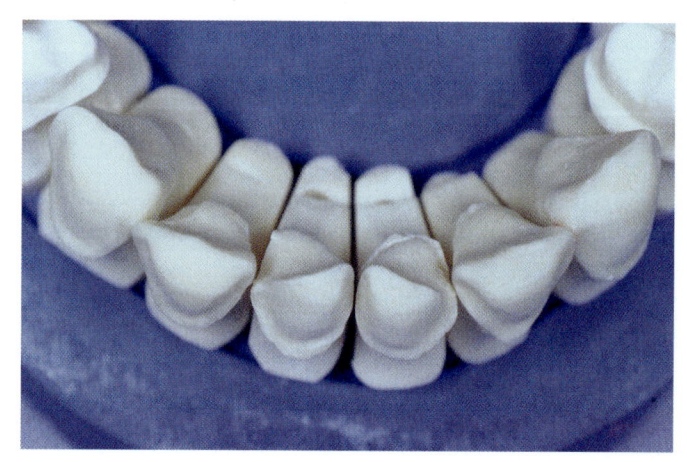

Figure 15.12 **(F)** Preparation design of mandibular lower dentition on master cast with dies from occlusal view.

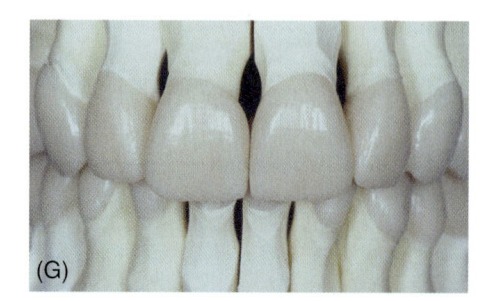

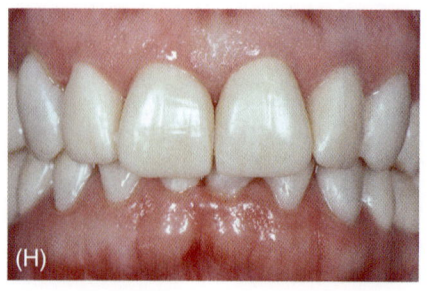

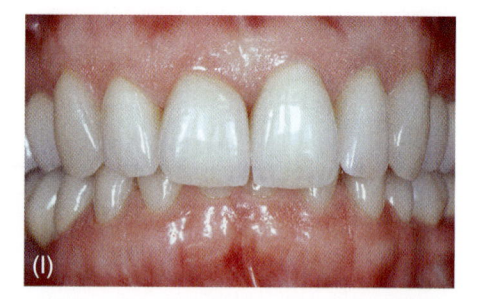

Figure 15.12 **(G)** Wax-up from master casts that can be utilized as a mock-up to evaluate the function and esthetics. **(H)** Mock-up in the mouth utilizing wax-up made from the master casts. Patient has a better appreciation of the final outcome. Wax-up allows for intraoral minor modifications. **(I)** Post-op picture from frontal view: Final leucite reinforced IPS Empress upper and lower restorations after adhesive bonding 4 weeks after insertion.

Chapter 15 Ceramic Veneers and Partial-Coverage Restorations 451

Figure 15.12 **(J)** Post-op close-up picture of the upper anterior dentition: final restorations #7–#10 4 weeks after adhesive bonding.

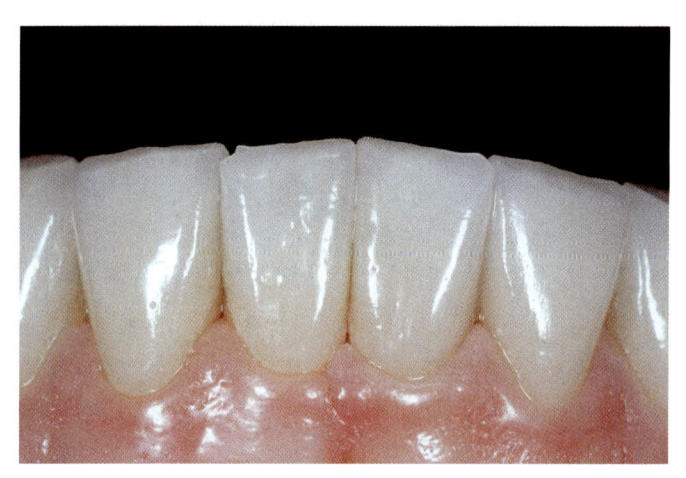

Figure 15.12 **(K)** Post-op picture from close-up view: final IPS Empress restorations #22–#27 4 weeks after final insertion.

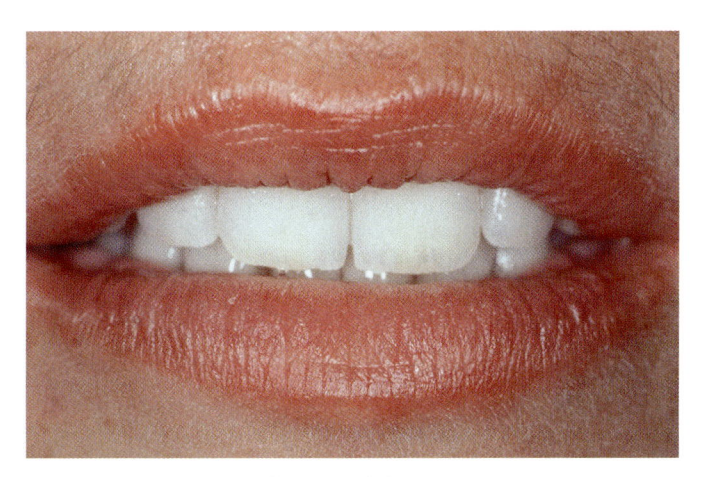

Figure 15.12 **(L)** Post-op final monolithic IPS Empress restorations in relaxed light smile position from a facial view.

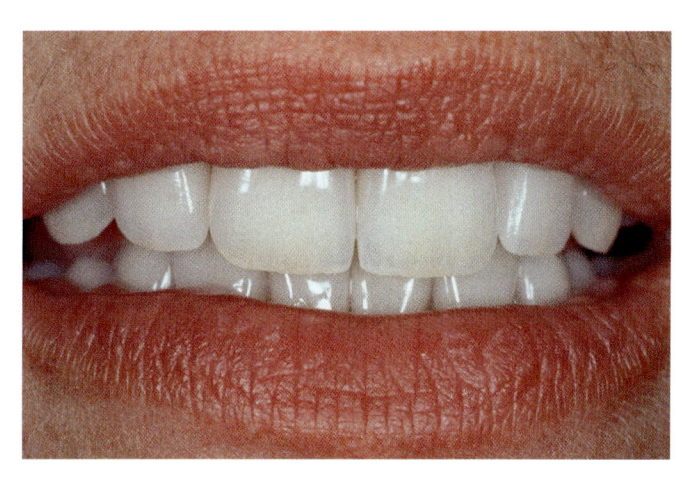

Figure 15.12 **(M)** Post-op final monolithic IPS Empress restorations with wider smile display of upper and lower dentition.

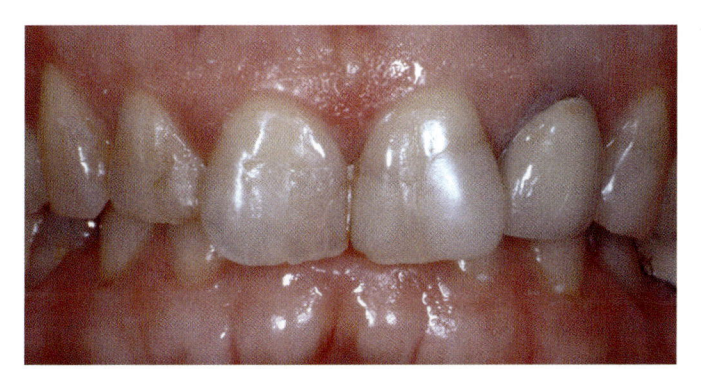

Figure 15.12 **(N)** Facial image of the intermaxillary anterior upper and lower dentition *before* extended ceramic restorations.

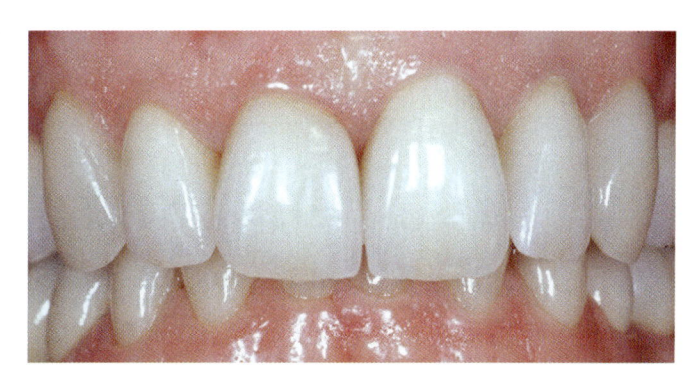

Figure 15.12 **(O)** Facial image of the intermaxillary anterior upper and lower dentition *after* extended ceramic restorations were placed. Case courtesy of Study Group: Doris Zimmer and Christian Stappert.

When to consider reduction

Without reduction, the teeth will be larger and more labially positioned. (In lingually inclined teeth, this may be an advantage.) McLean[65] believes failure to remove proximal enamel can result in the finish line placed too far labially and encroachment on the embrasure areas, resulting in exposure of unsightly porcelain margins that may be difficult to finish. Proceeding without preparation will lead to not only distinct overcontouring at cervical and proximal tooth surfaces, but also to higher clinical failure rates as a result of gingival inflammation and secondary caries due to an increase in microbial plaque accumulation.[66]

1. Remove convexities and provide a path for insertion in those situations where either the incisal or the interproximal areas are to be included in the veneer.[67]
2. Provide space for adequate opaquing or heavier coloring. Darkly stained teeth often require more reduction for opaquing purposes. This will allow for a thicker, more opaque veneer.[50] For veneers on tetracycline-stained teeth, for example, the underlying tooth color will modify its shade dramatically. This is because, in most cases, the veneer is only 0.5 mm thick and rather translucent. As a result, the actual shade of the porcelain has only a nominal influence on the final color of the bonded veneer. By reducing the tooth, usually it will be possible to neutralize the underlying color and create the illusion of a normal tooth color by having the opaque incorporated into the veneer itself.[68] Also, by making room for the application of opaquing layers under the veneer, additional opaquing can be obtained at the cementation appointment by using resin opaquers.
3. Provide a definite seat to help position the veneer during placement.
4. Prepare a receptive enamel surface for etching and bonding the veneer.
5. Allow for a smoother transition from the veneer to the tooth surface, enabling the patient to more easily keep it plaque-free.

Contraindications to reduction include consideration of the following points.

1. The size of the pulp. If young individuals or others with large pulps require laminating, consider an alternative to enamel reduction, especially if there is any indication of irreversible sensitivity by reducing the thickness of the enamel. One alternative is building out each of the teeth slightly to avoid preparation. However, this usually requires including at least 8–10 teeth for a natural result.
2. The patient's psychological state and feelings about tooth reduction or veneers. If the patient is apprehensive and unsure, then it is wise to do no reduction. Then if the patient becomes dissatisfied with the veneer or the slightly overbuilt look, the option will be removing the porcelain veneer and repolishing the enamel, thus returning the patient to a semblance of their pre-veneer state.

Tip: make sure you take precaution to record the exact amount of overbuilding you intend to do. This should include a set of pre- and posttreatment study casts and photographs. The photographs should include incisal views as well so you can clearly show just how much you have built out labially. Also, use of a clear vacuform matrix with both cervical and incisal holes placed will allow you to make sure you have adequate reduction (see Figure 15.18H, below).

If reducing, how much?

As a general principle, the enamel should be reduced just as much as necessary to facilitate the placement of an esthetic restoration. Ideally, one would like to remove the same amount of enamel that will eventually be replaced by the veneer and bonding composite resin.

Decisions about reduction need to take into account the relative position of the tooth in the arch. For example, in treating a crowded or rotated tooth or a tooth in labioversion, it may be advantageous to first bring the offending tooth into alignment with the rest of the arch by reducing its labial contour through cosmetic contouring. The use of mock-ups, followed by a wax model, esthetic pre-evaluative temporaries, and silicone index, provides the best esthetic, phonetic, and functional assessment of necessary tooth preparation for veneers.[69]

To facilitate placement of interproximal extensions, the margin of the porcelain veneer should be hidden within the embrasure area. Proper interproximal extension will provide additional stability and retention, due to the wraparound effect. Yet, it should be considered that placing the finish line in the proximal contact area creates a higher risk of interdental decay, especially with patients of compromised dental hygiene.[70]

Another factor to consider in placement of the interproximal margins is the size of the interdental space. If there is an unsightly gap that needs to be closed, the exact placement of the interproximal margin will vary depending upon the size of the space. The larger the space, the further mesiolingually or distolingually the margin will need to be extended. Otherwise, the resultant contact areas will be bulky and potential food traps.

Decisions about reduction need to take into account the need for a good seal. If at all possible, porcelain veneers should be bonded mainly to enamel,[65] so ideally margins of the preparation should have enough enamel left to ensure an adequate seal. The gingival finish line should be epigingival or ≤0.5 mm subgingival to the gingival margin. Unfortunately, esthetics require any tooth discoloration to be masked, may frequent make it necessary to locate the veneer margins subgingivally, terminating on either dentin or cementum. It is important to remember that while it is sometimes necessary to terminate the veneer on dentin, dentin bonding has at least two disadvantages: it provides less bond strength than enamel bonding, and it is a less effective seal. In general, this is not necessarily a problem since the reliability of dentin bonding has significantly improved.[71] Yet, it is very difficult to achieve ideal dry bonding conditions with rubber dam insulation at subgingival veneer margins. In cases where the preparation margins are expected to be positioned deeper than 0.5 mm subgingivally, an initial surgical crown-lengthening procedure may be indicated.

Reduction considerations should also include the color of the teeth to be veneered. Darkly stained teeth often require more reduction for opaquing purposes. Reid[72] proposed neutralization and use of opaquers at cementation. However, it is the easiest and best solution for the ceramist to build opacity into the veneer itself, thereby eliminating the need to experiment on the tooth for maximum opacity. With tetracycline stains, for example, the finish line must be placed subgingivally to hide the dark discoloration that tends to show through marginal tissue. Tetracycline stains are usually darkest in the cervical region where there is thinner enamel covering the stained dentin, making sufficient enamel reduction more difficult. The tooth also appears darker as the enamel is removed because the underlying stained dentin is more exposed. Actually any tooth in which the cervical area is darker than the intended color of the veneer might require a subgingival margin placement to avoid a visible color change between the new veneer and the existing root color. If this outcome is expected, make sure the patient signs an informed consent documenting acceptance of the intended treatment.

The best alternative for deeply stained teeth is the use of more opaque ceramic materials than porcelain. Monolithic lithium-disilicate offers higher opacity for pressable (e.g. IPS e.max Press)[21,25,73] and CAD/CAM fabricated (e.g. Emax CAD)[74,75] veneer restorations. In extreme discoloration cases, highly opaque zirconium oxide veneers might be an alternative to crowning of the tooth (Figure 15.13A–U).

The last, but important, consideration is the ceramist's needs in terms of fabricating an accurately fitting veneer. It is difficult to work with a porcelain thickness much less than 0.4 mm or to create a veneer that will adjust to a feather edge. This means that the ceramist should be allowed to work with veneers no thinner than 0.4, and a preferable clear chamfer margin or butt joint ending for extended veneer preparations. The latter is significant, since new high strength materials for veneers, mainly glass-ceramics are fabricated by pressing or CAD/CAM, which creates either rounded restoration margins (pressed) or higher risk of chipping of too thin margins by cutting tools (CAD/CAM). A good example of a patient who requires average reduction is seen in Figure 15.14A.

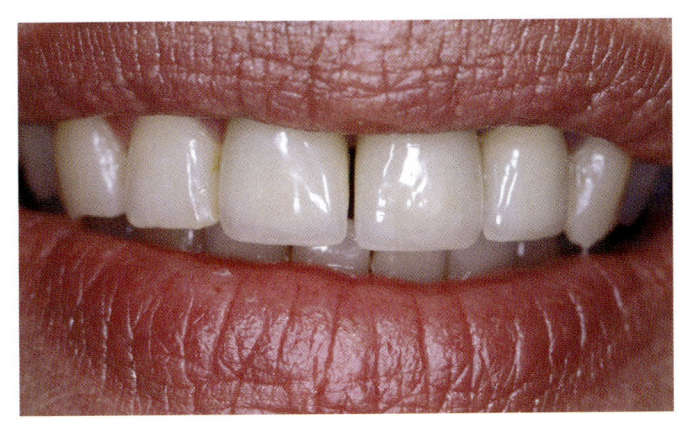

Figure 15.13 **(A)** Pre-op smile picture: patient is not happy with her old restorations and the diastema between #8 and #9.

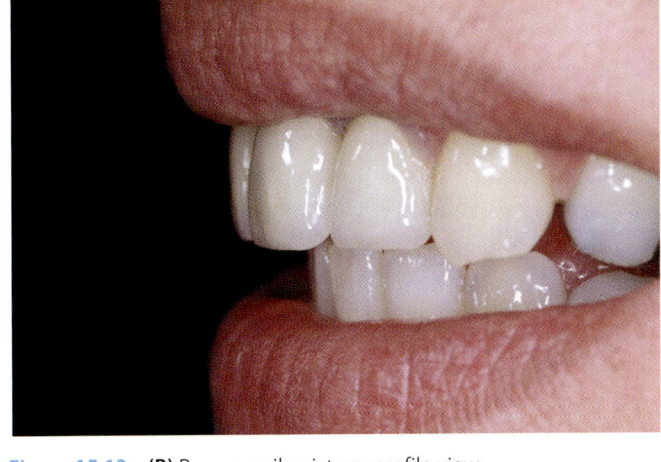

Figure 15.13 **(B)** Pre-op smile picture: profile view.

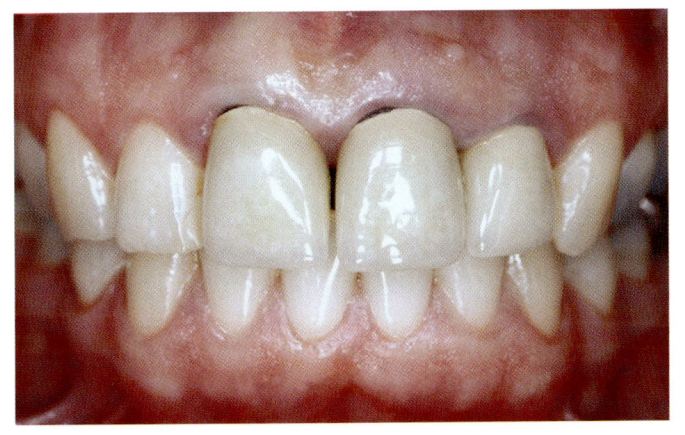

Figure 15.13 **(C)** Pre-op intraoral picture from frontal view. Notice dark gingival color around the cervical areas #8, #9, and #10 due to old PFM restorations. Multiple insufficient composite fillings are present on adjacent anterior teeth.

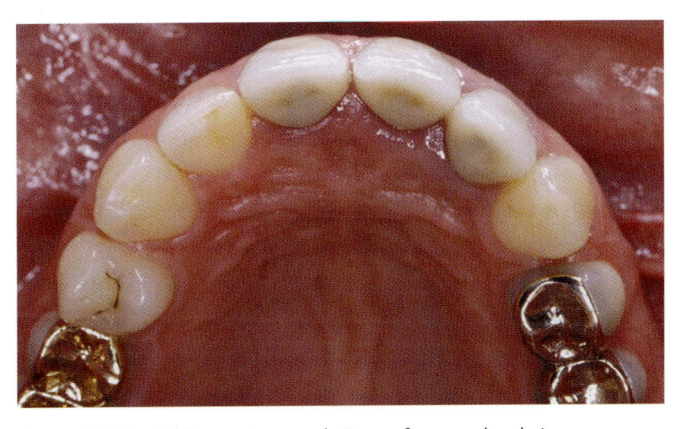

Figure 15.13 **(D)** Pre-op intraoral picture from occlusal view.

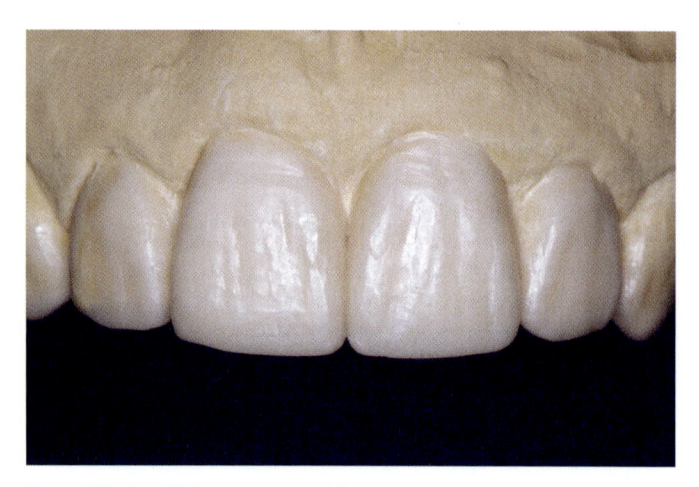

Figure 15.13 **(E)** Diagnostic and functional wax-up to fabricate all ceramic e.max Press restorations from labial aspect.

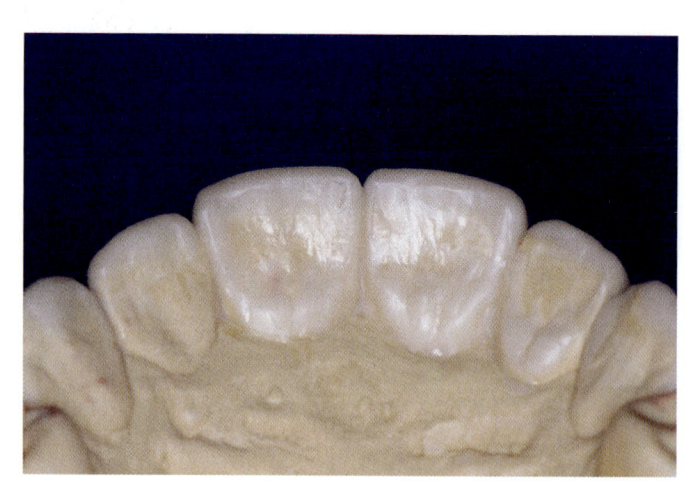

Figure 15.13 **(F)** Diagnostic and functional wax-up from palatal aspect. The wax-up was duplicated and a preparation guide produced by the dental technician.

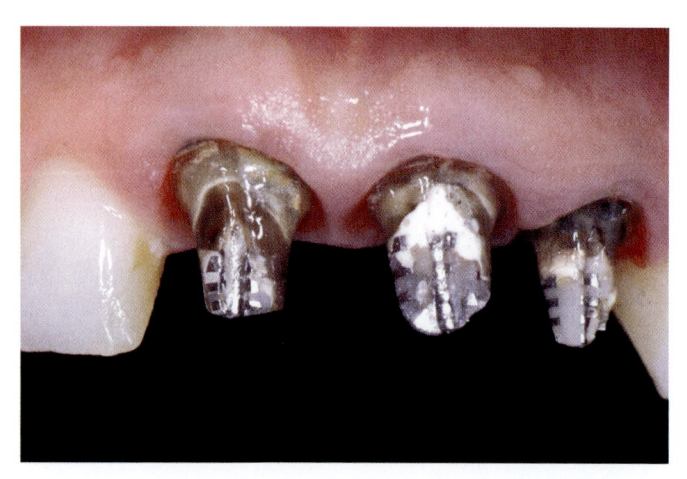

Figure 15.13 **(G)** Teeth #8, 9 and 10 after removing the old PFM crowns. Notice that the dark gingival discoloration around cervical #8 and #9 disappeared immediately.

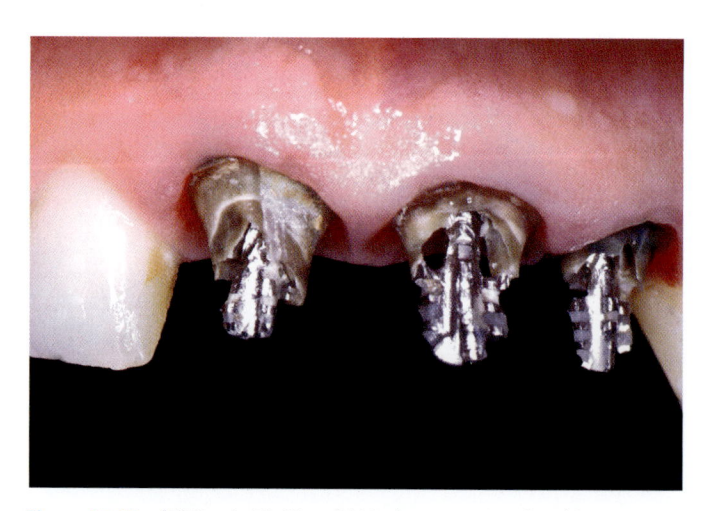

Figure 15.13 **(H)** Teeth #8, #9 and #10 after removing the old core build-up material while maintaining the old prefabricated posts. Attempt to remove the previous posts failed due to increased risk of root fracture.

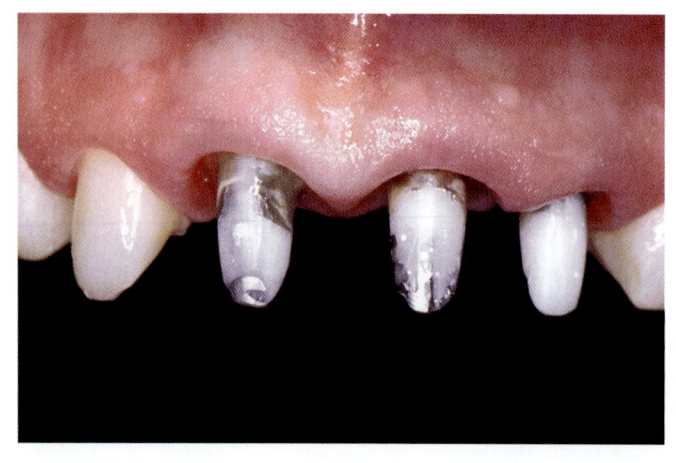

Figure 15.13 **(I)** Teeth #6–#11 show final preparation. Notice #8, #9, and #10 have new opaque core build-up material to mask the dark stump shade.

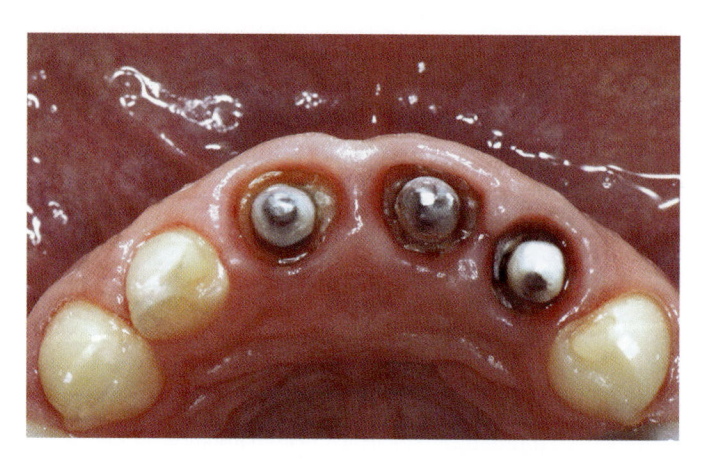

Figure 15.13 **(J)** Teeth #6–#11 demonstrate final preparation from occlusal view.

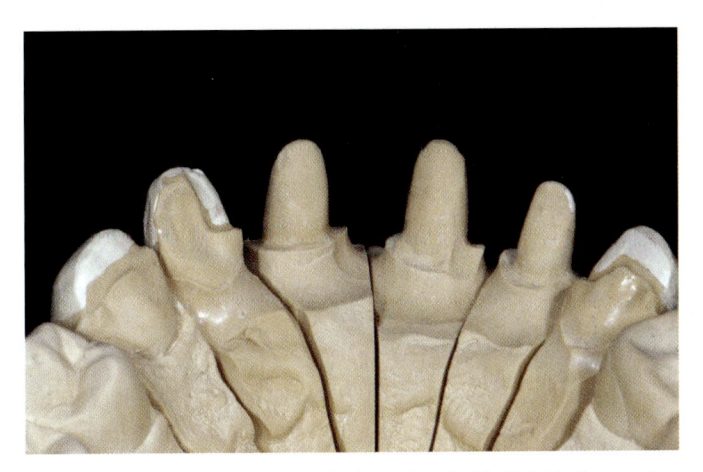

Chapter 15 Ceramic Veneers and Partial-Coverage Restorations

Figure 15.13 **(K)** Master cast with dies of teeth #6–#11. Notice teeth #7 and #11 defect-oriented preparation design due to position of old restorations. All defects needed to be covered by the new ceramic restorations.

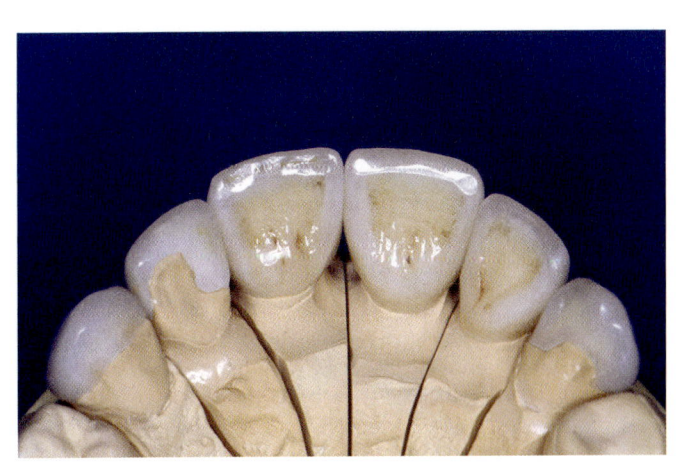

Figure 15.13 **(L)** Teeth #6–#11 show final restorations on master cast from palatal view. Notice tooth #7 and #11 defect-oriented restorations.

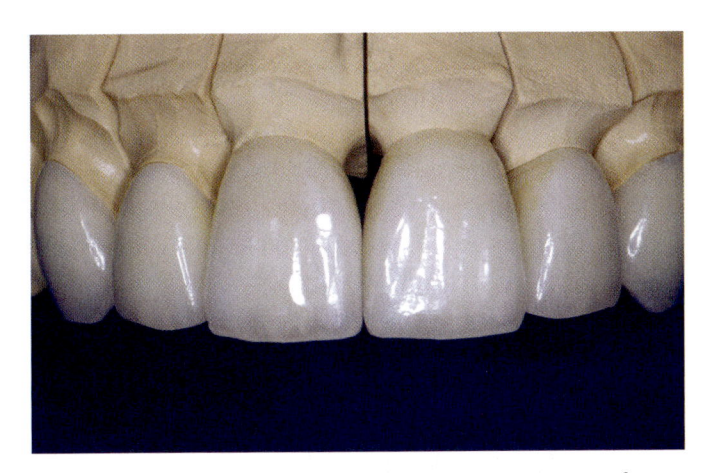

Figure 15.13 **(M)** Final e.max Press restorations on master cast for teeth #6–#11 from labial view.

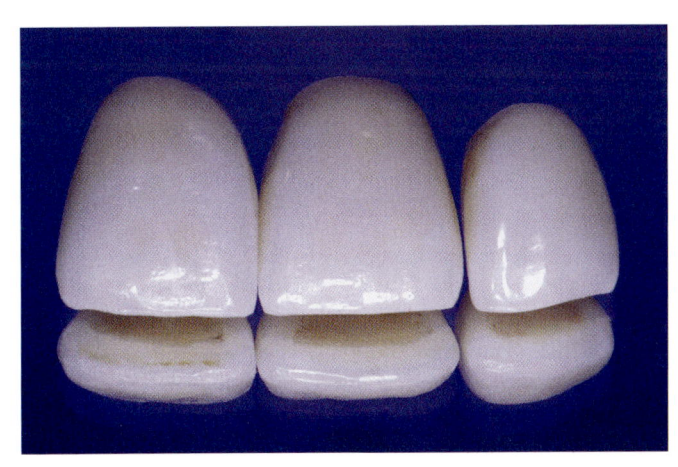

Figure 15.13 **(N)** Teeth #8, #9, and #10 final lithium-disilicate crown restorations. An opaque liner was applied to the intaglio crown surfaces to mask the dark post and core structure and discolored stump shade.

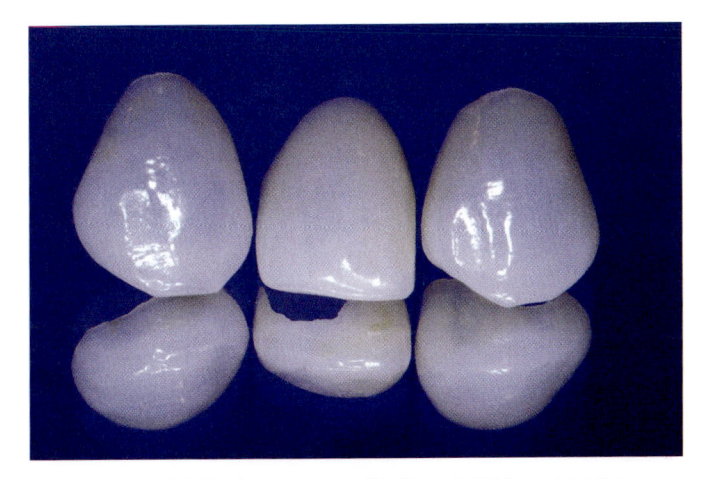

Figure 15.13 **(O)** Final restorations #6, #7, and #11 from labial view. Pay attention to the variation of ceramic thicknesses due to the monolithic application of the press ceramic.

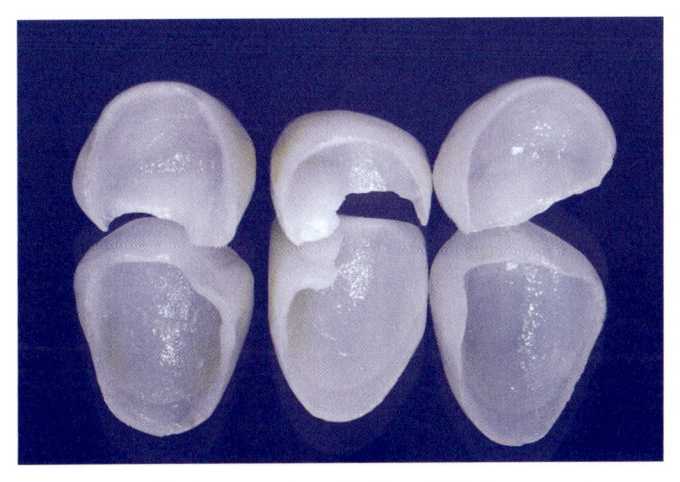

Figure 15.13 **(P)** The restorations #6, #7, and #11 do not require any underlying coping. Therefore, preparation can be minimal invasive and defect-oriented (intaglio surface view).

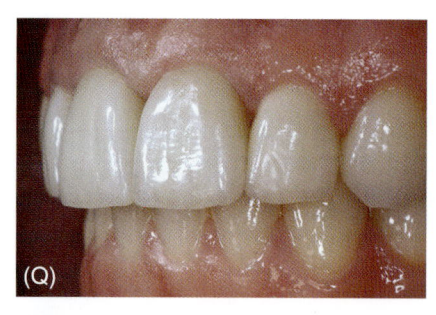

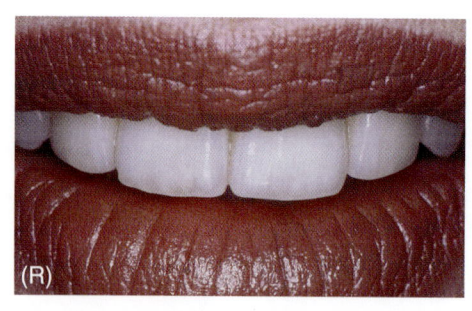

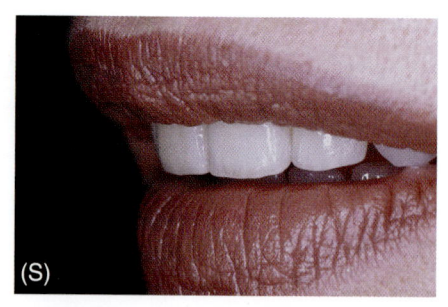

Figure 15.13 **(Q)** Post-op picture: final ceramic restorations 4 weeks after adhesive bonding from lateral view. **(R)** Six months post-op picture: final press ceramic restorations in relation to smile and lip line from frontal view. **(S)** Six months post-op smile picture from lateral profile view. The female patient was very pleased with the outcome. The patient was restored in 2001, and represents one of the first monolithic lithium-disilicate cases documented.

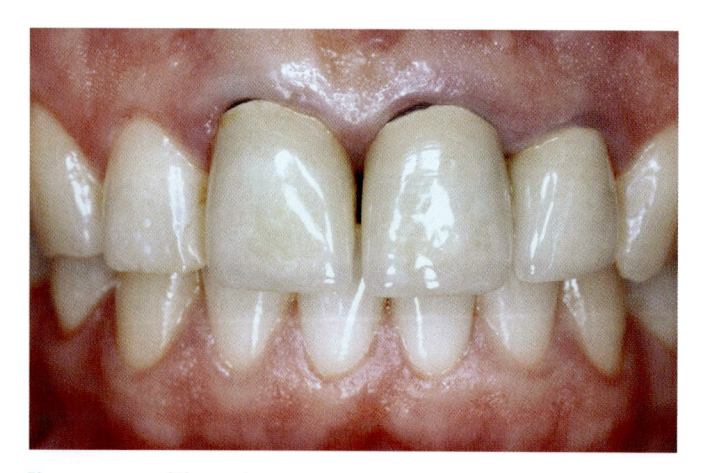

Figure 15.13 **(T)** Initial retracted view of the patient's upper and lower dentition (before).

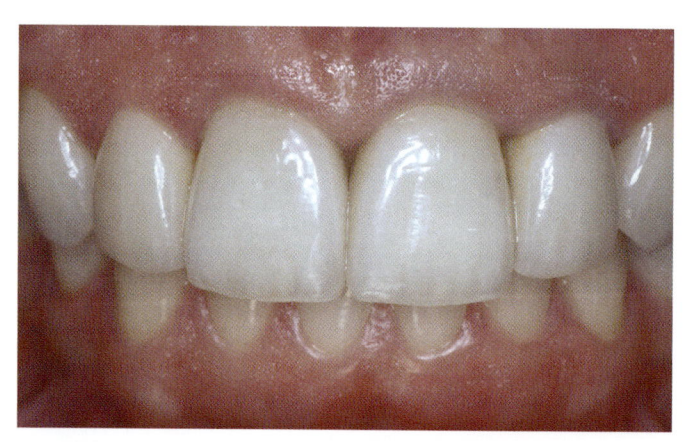

Figure 15.13 **(U)** Follow-up photo of the patient's upper and lower dentition 3 years post-op. Based on present recall results, the restorations are still in place and in full function.

Classic veneer preparation technique

The Goldstein veneer preparation kit (LVS; Brasseler USA) (Figure 15.14B) provides a rapid method of measured reduction for porcelain veneers. First the clinician must decide on the required amount of reduction, using the considerations given previously. In most instances the needed reduction will be 0.5 mm, obtained by using the LVS-1. Small teeth such as the mandibular incisors where the thickness of enamel is considerably less may only require 0.3 mm reduction and you would use LVS-2. The appropriate LVS diamond depth cutter is selected and gently drawn across the labial surface of the tooth from mesial to distal. This will develop the depth cuts as horizontal grooves, leaving a raised strip of enamel in between (Figure 15.14C and D). The depth of the cut is limited by the instrument itself. The remaining enamel is then reduced to the depth of these initial cuts, using a coarse diamond (LVS-3 or -4). The resulting rough enamel surface facilitates retention and refraction of the light reflected back out through the veneer. At the marginal areas, however, it is desirable to use a finer-grit diamond which will create a definitive polished finish line to enhance the seal at the periphery. Thus, the special two-grit LVS-3 or -4 is an ideal instrument to accomplish these tasks (Figure 15.14E and F).

The basic preparation should be completed with only the finishing of the final margins remaining. If the margin is planned to be placed subgingivally, it is best to begin by displacing the tissue for 10 min with retraction cord saturated with a hemostatic agent. Once this step is completed it will be much easier to complete the final margin using the LVS-3 (Figure 15.14G–I). If the teeth are extremely dark, consider using a deep chamfer or modified shoulder. This will give the technician extra depth, and thus extra veneer thickness, to mask the grayness that can show through the gingiva, especially if the gingival tissue is thin and transparent. An initial impression and cast will allow for corrections before the final impression is taken (Figure 15.14J and K).

Novel extended veneer preparation technique

Both, the overlapping incisal edge preparation (modified overlap design; Stappert 1999) and the full veneer preparation design (Stappert 1999) include the proximal tooth surfaces, but differ in palatal extension. The extent of tooth structure defect and the functional and esthetic objectives of the therapy determine the choice of preparation design. The extended veneer preparation kits combine classic crown burs with veneer burs. They are performed initially with rough diamond burs (80 μm)

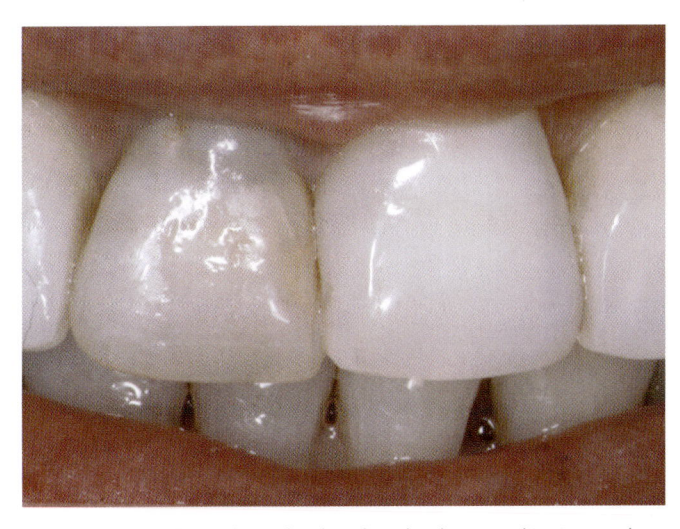

Figure 15.14 (A) Matching the discolored right central incisor to the left central presents one of the most difficult challenges in dentistry.

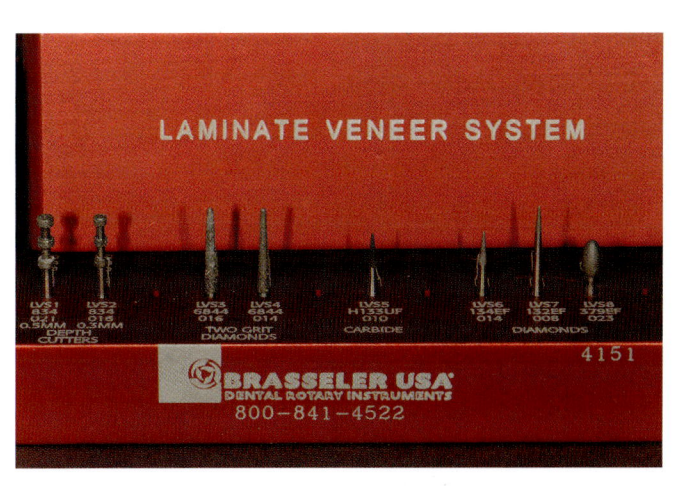

Figure 15.14 (B) This veneer system (Brasseler USA) includes four burs to prepare the tooth and four to finish the veneer.

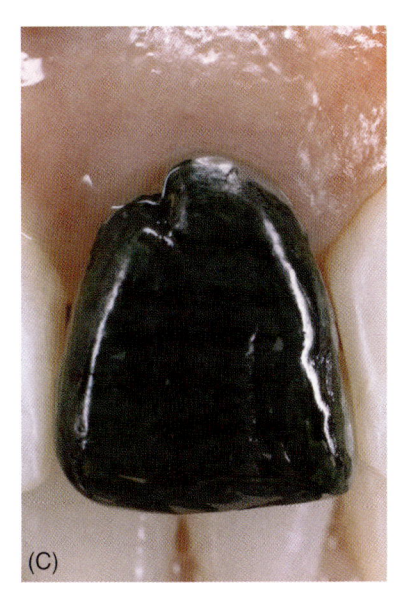

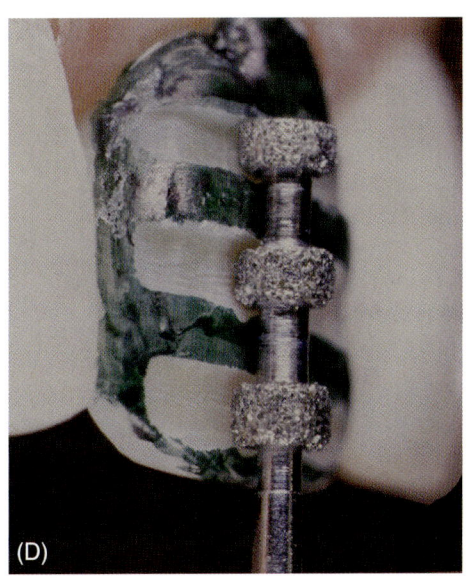

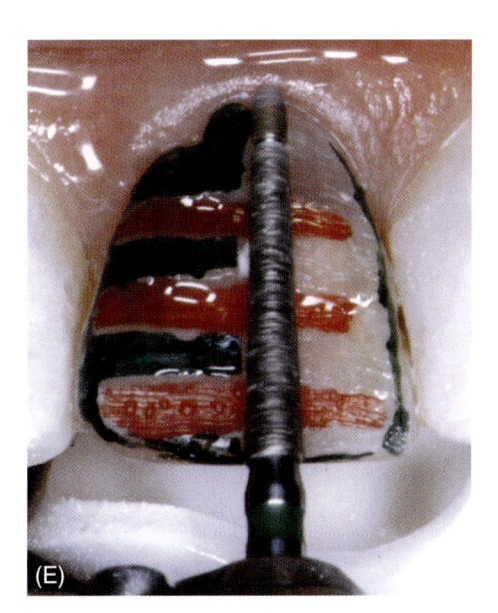

Figure 15.14 (C) The discolored incisor is painted green to help guide the depth cuts. (D) The special three-tier extra-coarse diamond depth cutter (Brasseler USA) comes in 0.5 mm (LVS-1) and 0.3 mm (LVS-2) thicknesses and is so efficient that usually one sweep across the labial surface completes the depth cut. Since the veneer will be approximately 0.6 mm in thickness (up to 0.8 mm in darkly stained teeth), the 0.5 mm bur will generally be the depth cutter of choice unless overbuilding is desired. (E) After completing the depth cut (marked in red for illustrative purposes only), the remainder of the preparation is completed with the two-grit diamond. The body of the diamond contains extra-coarse grit, which leaves a rough finish on the preparation to maximize veneer retention.

(e.g. #837KR.314.012, #878.204.012; Brasseler USA) followed by finer shape-congruent diamond burs (30–40 μm) (e.g. #8837KR.314.012, #8878.204.012; Brasseler USA) for the finishing procedure. The extent of labial and incisal reduction is predetermined for both preparation forms by using a silicone key based on an esthetic functional wax-up. The labial surface is axially reduced by 0.3–0.5 mm. Cervically, a shallow chamfer (0.5 mm) is prepared epigingival. The proximal reduction is 0.5–0.7 mm. The incisal edge is shortened by a minimum of 0.5–1.5 mm for both preparation forms (e.g. #837KR.314.012;

Brasseler USA), depending on the defect size. For the overlapping incisal edge preparation (overlap veneer) the incisal edge is extensively shortened and slightly beveled towards the labial aspect. The angle between labial surface and incisal platform is approximately 110°. On the palatal aspect, a right-angled contour between the incisal and the palatal surface is achieved (butt joint). The palatal centric contact point of all overlap veneers remains on the natural tooth structure. Full veneer restorations differ by preparing an extensive 0.5–0.7 mm deep rounded shoulder in the palatal area. Extension of palatal preparation is

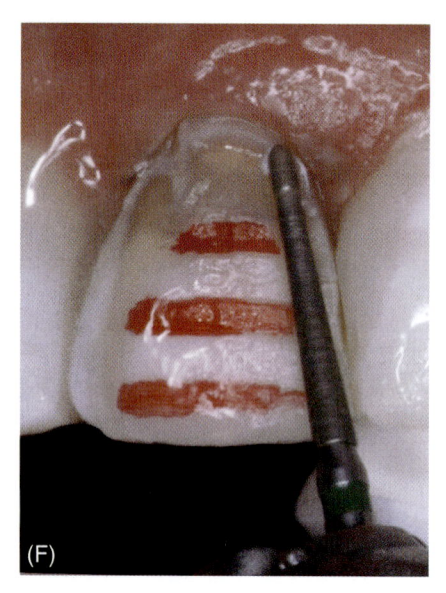

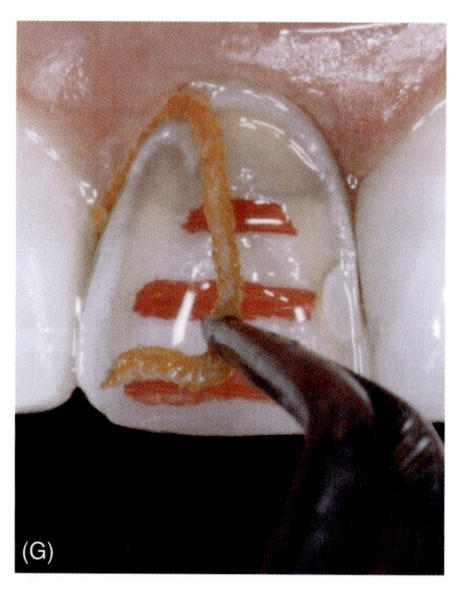

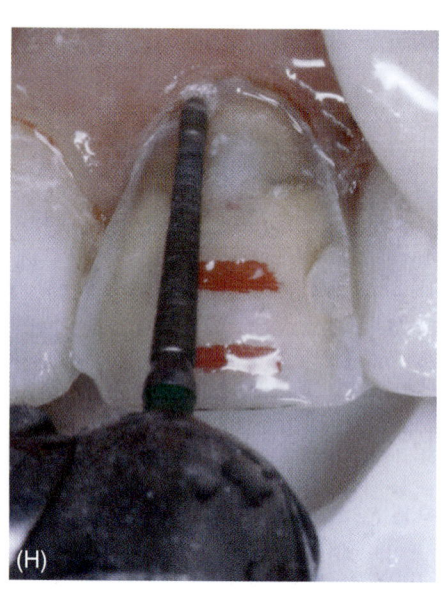

Figure 15.14 **(F)** The tip of the two-grit diamond LVS-3 or -4 (Brasseler USA) has a fine grit for marginal finishing. Note how close the preparation was finished to the base of the depth cut as shown by the remaining illustrative red markings. **(G)** Gingival displacement cord is carefully removed after remaining in the sulcus for approximately 10 min. **(H)** With the tissue displaced, the gingival margin can now be placed just into the gingival sulcus.

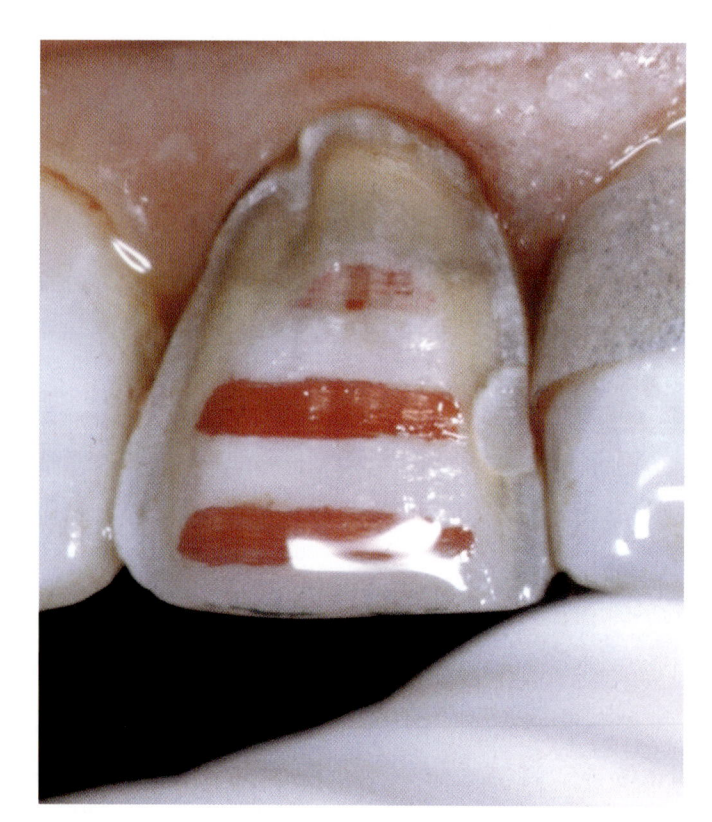

Figure 15.14 **(I)** When using the foil technique for veneer construction (see section on Foil versus refractory die), slight separation between the teeth is obtained by using a diamond strips. The proximal surfaces can then be finished with a sandpaper strip.

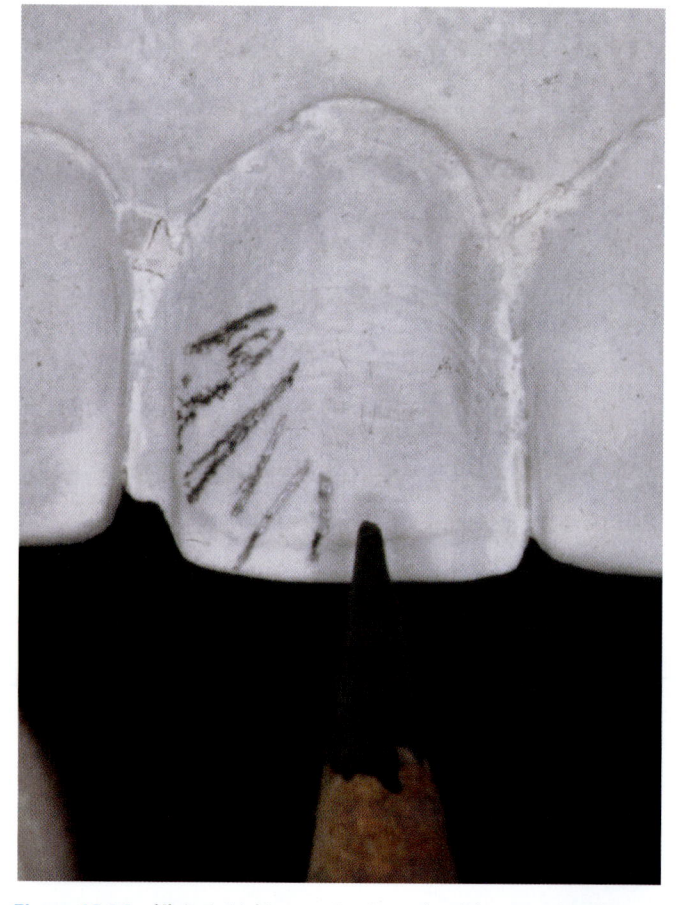

Figure 15.14 **(J)** An initial impression is made of the completed preparations and poured in quick-set plaster or stone to carefully analyze each tooth. Here the distal-labial aspect appears to need slightly more reduction.

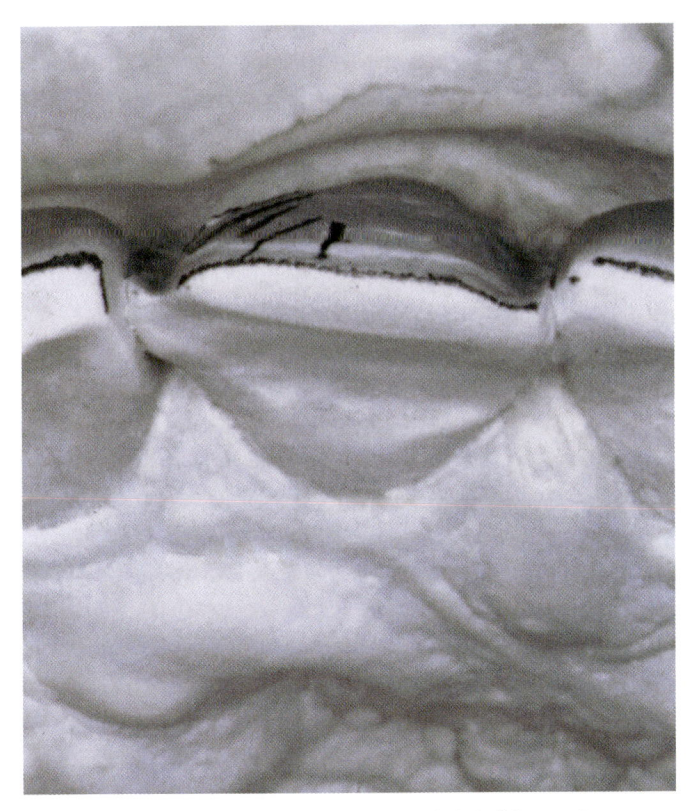

Chapter 15 Ceramic Veneers and Partial-Coverage Restorations

Figure 15.14 **(K)** The incisal view is especially helpful in analyzing whether or not more tooth reduction is necessary. Tilting the study cast from buccal to incisal and mesial to distal allows you to verify that you have not left any sharp line angles.

generally limited to the cingulum area; however, an extension is justified with large tooth defects. Palatal centric contact points on the ceramic surface are avoided, when applicable. All preparation margins should be restricted by enamel. Labial epigingival preparation and controlled preparation depth enable adhesive cementation mainly to enamel. All inner line angles should be rounded. Preparation margins are not beveled. Minimum material thickness (axially at least 0.4 mm and incisally 1.5 mm), should be consistently maintained during preparation. Incisal ceramic thickness of 1.5–2.5 mm is ensured for overlap and full veneer restorations. (See Figure 15.13A–U, and Figures 15.18A–R and 19A–P below.)

Impressions

Although it may be possible to take an impression without further tissue displacement, it is preferable to place a new cotton tissue displacement cord to make certain all margins will be properly recorded. Approximately 5 min should be sufficient to gain enough tissue displacement to capture the "lip" or actual margin plus a bit of tooth structure gingival to the margin. Obtaining an impression with this extra amount of uncut tooth structure guarantees that the technician will be better able to identify the margins and follow the correct tooth contour.

Basically, there are two choices regarding impression types: digital or conventional.

No doubt, most convenient for the patient would be digital, since most patients prefer not having impressions trays in their mouth for several minutes. Plus, scanning techniques have become both accurate and time saving, especially in extended patient cases which often require taking backup impressions chair side.

Digital impression

Intraoral chair side scanners (e.g. CEREC-Sirona Dental Systems, Lava COS-3 M Dental ESPE, iTero, TRIOS-3Shape Dental) allow digital impressions to be taken, yet still the basic principles and preparations of conventional impressions must be followed. Dry field and clear margin with sufficient soft tissue retraction are critical. CAD/CAM systems (such as NobelProcera, CEREC, Lava 3 M) utilize the digital scanning data to fabricate the final restorations directly, whereas other systems offer the option to produce a patient master cast based on the digital impression, which allows a dental technichian to generate restorations in a conventional way or to combine both methods.

Conventional impression

Materials can vary from hydrocolloid, polysulfide, polyethers to polyvinyl siloxane (PVS):

- **Hydrocolloid** impression material is highly hydrophilic. Therefore, moderate wetness during the impression does not reduce the impression accuracy. Yet, hydrocolloid impressions tend to tear into unprepared undercut areas below or between the contact areas. If this material is your first choice, sending off two impressions to fabricate two verification models is recommended. In some cases, it might be required to block out undercuts before taking the impression from the lingual aspect.

- **Polysulfide** impression materials are generally low to moderately hydrophilic and can generate an accurate impression. They reproduce excellent details, but their dimensional stability is only fair. The material is not very rigid; therefore the impressions are easier to remove than polyether or PVS impressions.[76–80] They can capture subgingival margins upon impression without tearing during removal, which is an advantage when compared to PVS. However, polyethers and silicones offer better elastic recovery and accuracy.

- **Polyether** impression materials are moderately hydrophilic; thus they can capture accurate impressions in the presence of some localized saliva or blood. In general, a dry field is required to make an acceptable impression. They produce impressions with excellent details and their dimensional stability allows multiple pours of accurate casts for 1–2 weeks, if there is no tearing of the impression. They are rigid and more difficult to remove than PVS, so cases with short teeth are the easiest to impress with polyether.[79,81] They allow clinicians to get good subgingival detail on removal due to their high tear strength. Common commercial examples are Impregum and Permadyne (3 M ESPE).

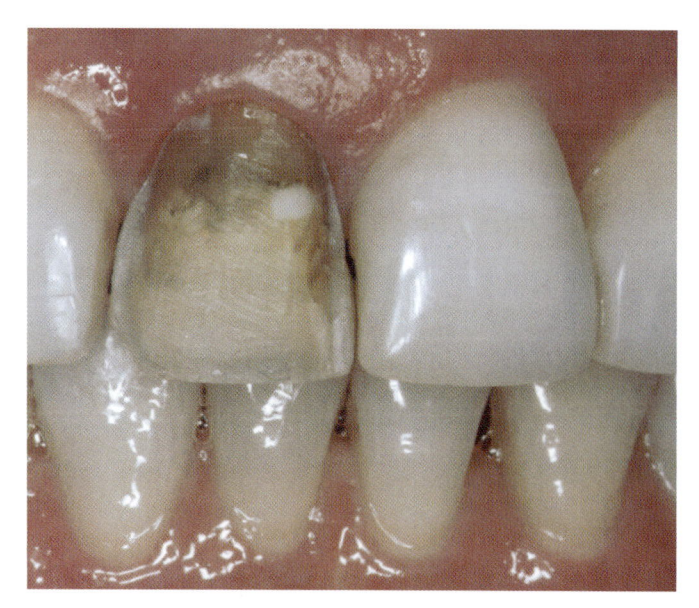

Figure 15.14 (L) The final preparation of this badly discolored central incisor has been completed for the porcelain veneer and an impression will be performed.

- **Polyvinyl siloxane (PVS) or addition silicone** impression materials can be either hydrophobic or hyrophillic. If hydrophobic, moisture presence from saliva or blood can interfere with impression accuracy.[82] This is why the newer hydrophilic impression materials may be easier to use. PVS has the best elastic recovery of all available impression materials.[83,84] It has an excellent ability to reproduce detail and its dimensional stability allows multiple pours of accurate casts for several weeks.[85,86] The material is moderately rigid but less rigid than polyethers. It has good tear strength and it is easier to remove than polyether materials (Figure 15.14 L–N).[83,86]

The choice of impression materials depends mainly on the subjective choice of the operator. It is based on personal preferences, handling, and the impression techniques used. In recent years, dentists have tended to use PVS and polyethers because of their improved physical and mechanical properties. The injection method for PVS is probably the cleanest and easiest conventional impression technique.

Temporaries

Temporaries for classic veneers usually are unnecessary because in many situations only half of the enamel surface is removed, not exposing the dentinal tubules. There should be little or no sensitivity and only minimal esthetic compromise. Temporaries also may cause gingival inflammation unless carefully trimmed and polished.

Situations that require temporaries include those Class 4–6 preparations in which (a) the teeth have been extensively reduced, particularly if dentin is exposed, and/or sensitivity exists, (b) open contacts have been created that could allow movement of the teeth, or (c) the patient finds that the reduced teeth are too esthetically compromised for comfort (see

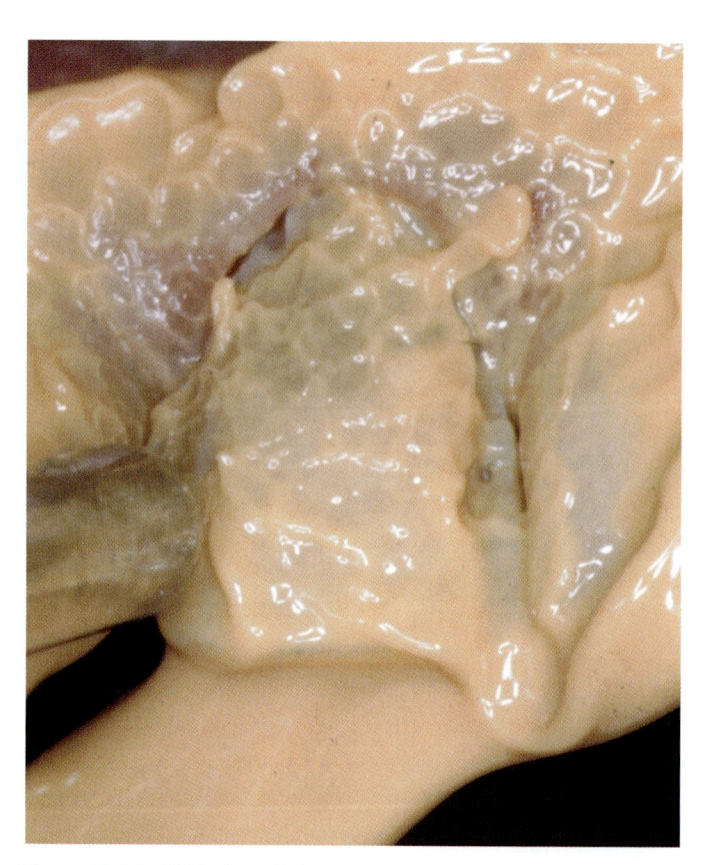

Figure 15.14 (M) Polyvinyl siloxane (PVS) is an excellent material for a final impression. Here, the syringe material has been placed and an air stream gently spreads the material so that you can be assured that the entire preparation has been covered and that no air pockets or bubbles exist.

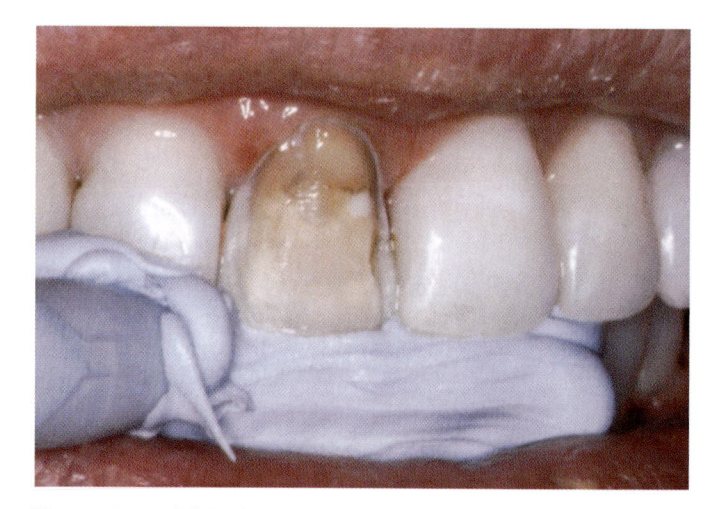

Figure 15.14 (N) Occlusal registration is also made with polyvinyl siloxane paste (Regisil PB, Caulk/Dentsply).

Figure 15.14 L). In these situations, temporaries can be constructed through one of five methods: (1) direct composite veneers, involving the placement of a composite restorative material directly on the non-etched surface of the prepared tooth; (2) direct composite veneers, involving the placement of a composite restorative material directly on a 1–2 mm etched surface of the prepared tooth (Figure 15.14O–S); (3) direct

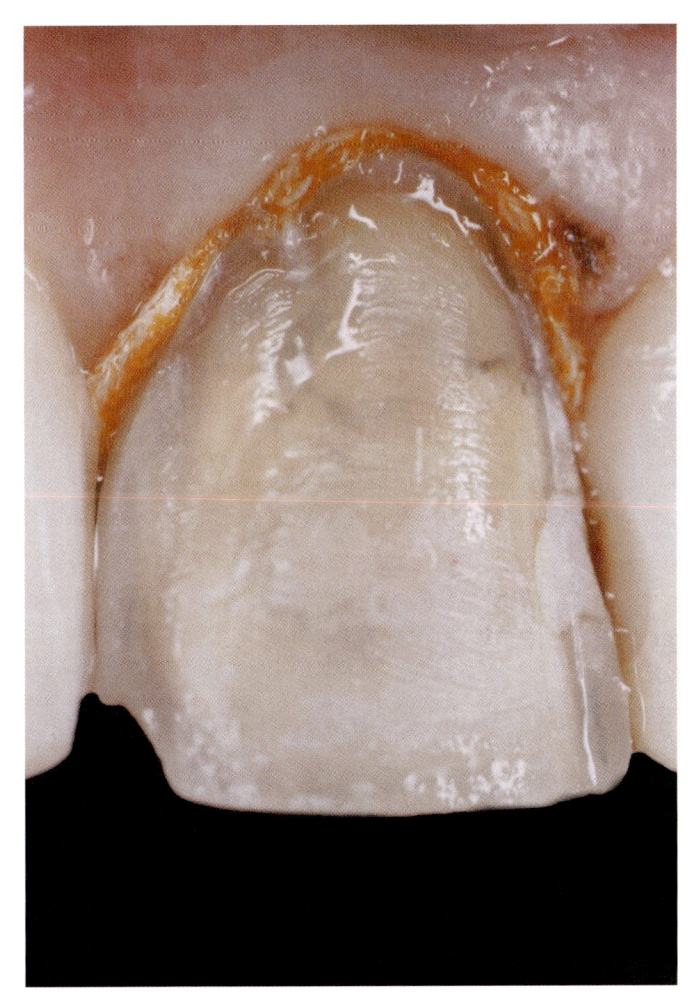

Figure 15.14 **(O)** Tissue displacement with retraction cord for 3–5 min will make it easier to create a more accurate gingival margin for the interim restoration.

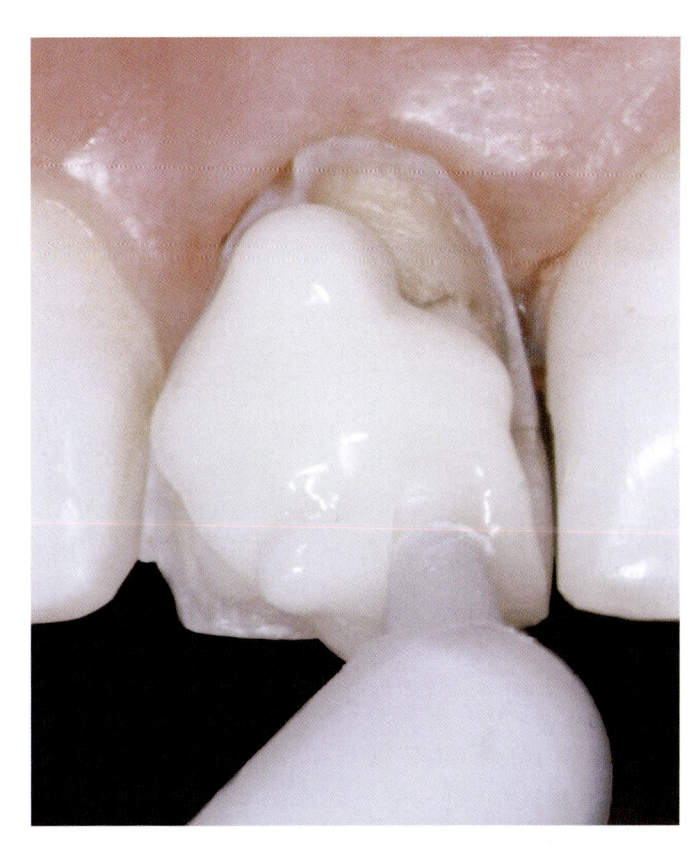

Figure 15.14 **(P)** A direct composite veneer can be used as temporary restoration. First the tooth can be isolated with glycerin gel and point etching can be performed facially to bond the restoration temporarily.

composite veneers using a vacuform or silicone matrix made on a preoperative plaster model of the patient's mouth, or on the duplicate wax-up model if changes are to be made before esthetics or functionality; (4) direct acrylic veneers in which methyl methacrylate self-cure acrylic is mixed into a soupy state, flowed into the buccal aspects of a vacuform matrix or silicone matrix and allowed to reach the "doughy" stage of curing, and then manipulated into position over the prepared teeth; and (5) indirect composite/acrylic temporaries, which are fabricated in the laboratory on a model of the prepared teeth (Figure 15.T–Z).

Classic porcelain veneers: laboratory procedures

Making a model

A master cast that accurately reproduces what exists in the mouth is the necessary next step in the fabrication of veneers. The laboratory veneer fabrication technique, die or foil, may determine the type of impression and the type of model.

Foil versus refractory die

There are two basic techniques for fabrication of porcelain veneers, both of which can produce excellent results. In the platinum foil technique (Figure 15.15A–G), the more conventional of the two methods, porcelain is fired over a 0.0254 mm thick platinum foil matrix. This technique uses individual removable dies on a master cast poured in conventional die stone. Good delineation of each tooth is assured if the contact points in the mouth are modified by stripping with an ultrafine diamond strip (Brasseler USA or, Premier Dental Products) (see Figure 15.14 L).

In the refractory die technique, porcelain is fired directly on a refractory die material. This reduces the cost of construction by eliminating the need for platinum foil. It also avoids some of the shrinkage and distortion that can occur with the more technique-sensitive foil method.

It may be prudent in the refractory die technique to block out lingual-interproximal undercut areas with orthodontic wax before taking the impression. Never do this if the foil technique is being used, however, as the technician will not be able to section the model. Porcelain is an excellent material in terms of color because the amount of opaqueness can be controlled, through both mixture of the ceramic powder components and depth of the veneer.[50] In tetracycline-stained teeth, for example, the clinician usually will neutralize the underlying color and then create the illusion of normal tooth color by having the opaque incorporated into the porcelain veneer, using the

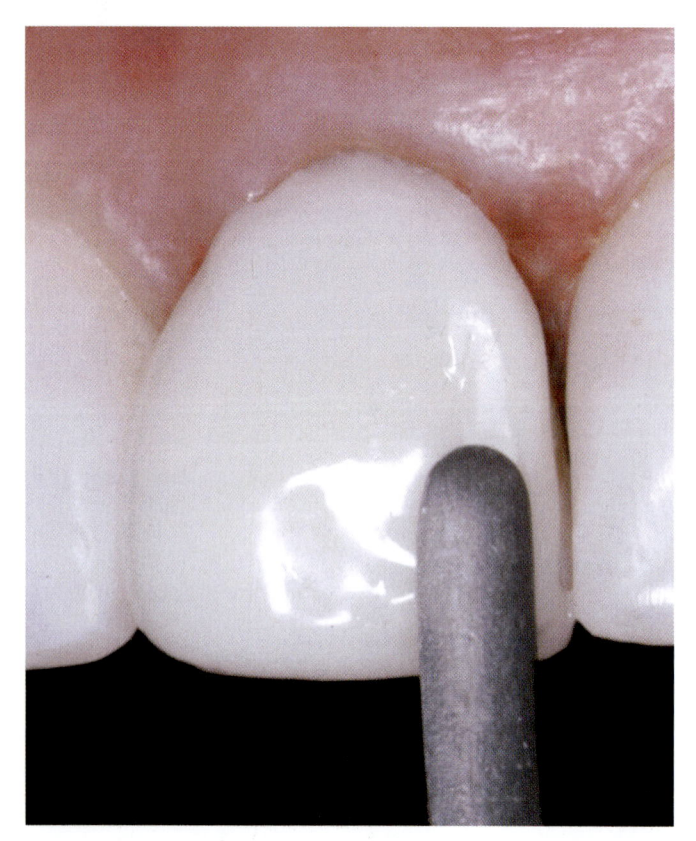

Figure 15.14 **(Q)** The temporary composite resin veneer is carefully shaped with a Goldstein #3 anodized aluminum Flexi-Thin instrument (Hu-Friedy).

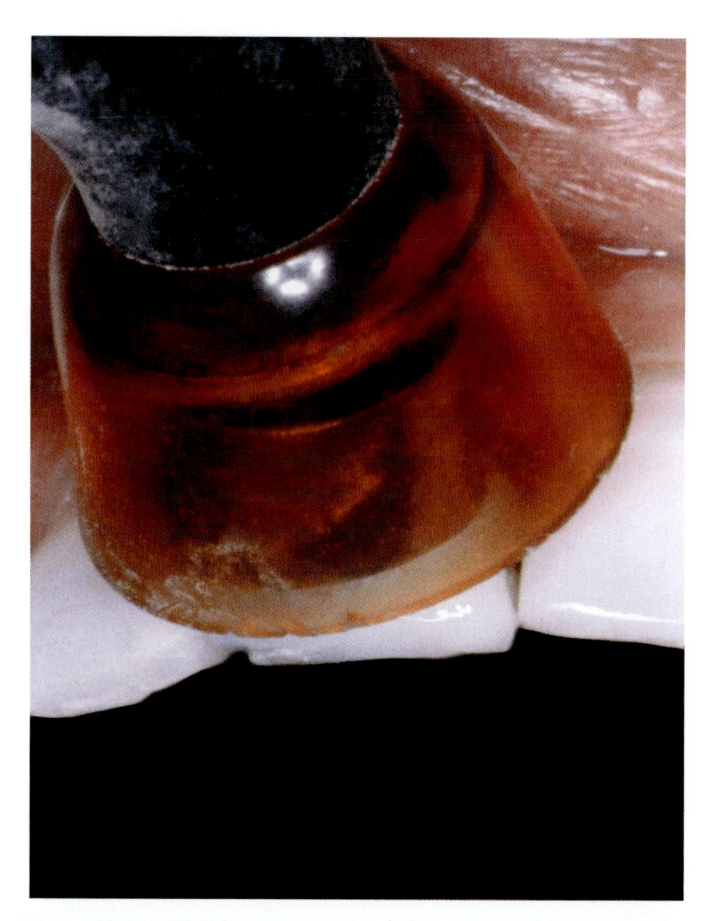

Figure 15.14 **(R)** Polymerization should be completed from both the labial and lingual aspects.

composite cement for additional help if needed. Despite the attractive teeth that can be achieved this way, it is important to remember that the actual shade of the porcelain has only nominal bearing on the bonded final veneer. This is because in most cases the veneer is only 0.5 mm thick and rather translucent. The underlying tooth color and resin can modify its shade dramatically. Fortunately, several systems for opaquing the dark stain exist, one involving the use of opaque powder, another a complex layering.[68,87]

The porcelain veneers are then constructed in the ceramic laboratory, following the prescription of form, fit, and color. Although most any porcelain can be baked and etched for a veneer, some of the current products have been specifically developed for this procedure. They are especially formulated to have increased amount of opacifiers and metallic oxide pigments so that within the 0.5 mm thickness of a veneer, intricate characterization and color effects can be developed.

Pressable ceramic veneers: laboratory procedures

A master cast that accurately reproduces the preparation margins and contact points in the mouth is necessary in the fabrication of glass-ceramic veneers.

Extended veneer restorations can be made of the leucite-reinforced glass-ceramic IPS Empress or lithium-disilicate reinforced e.max Press (Ivoclar Vivadent). This pressable ceramic is processed according to the IPS Empress layering technique using IPS Empress conventional lost-wax method following the manufacturer's instructions. After an ideal wax-up of the extended veneer restoration, the surface is cut back by 0.2–0.4 mm to allow for a layer of veneering porcelain. The wax-up is then embedded in an investment cylinder. The glass-ceramic ingot is pressed into the pre-heated hollow mold (furnace EP 500, Ivoclar Vivadent) at 910–920 °C. Restorations are removed from the molds and cleaned with a steam jet cleaner (EV1 SJ, Silfradent Sync.). Manufacturing individually layered veneer restorations is enabled by fusing IPS Empress dentin, incisal, and transparent veneering porcelain, as well as the IPS Empress glaze material (Ivoclar Vivadent) onto the ceramic core structure (ceramic furnace Programat P90/P95; Ivoclar Vivadent).

Minor corrections of the glazed restorations during trying-in are made at the chair side. Changes to the incisal and labial surfaces can be repolished to a high gloss using ceramic silicone polishers (Dialite Polishing Set Ceramic, Gebr. Brasseler). Veneers requiring major corrections or needing complete revisions will be sent to the dental laboratory. Those restorations receive entirely new coats of ceramic glaze.

Veneers can be created as full contour monolithic structure as well, without cut back of the wax-up for a layer of veneering porcelain. In this case, the level of esthetic individualization and

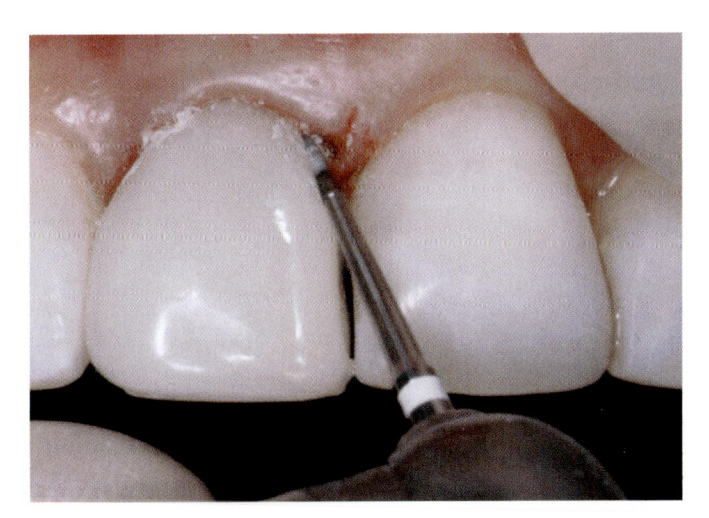

Figure 15.14 (S) Since the temporary veneer restoration is initially contoured close to the desired final form, only slight finishing with a 30-blade carbide (ET3UF, Brasseler USA) is necessary. Additional polishing can be done with a series of impregnated discs (Soflex [3M], Cosmedent, or Brasseler USA).

correction is limited to superficial staining and ceramic glazing procedures. Special emphasis must be given to the right choice of ceramic ingot, matching the right shade and level of translucency of the residual dentition. In many cases, monolithic glass-ceramic veneers can offer a respectable esthetic result, especially when the veneer restorations remain fairly thin (≈0.5 mm) and a chameleon effect is achieved. Yet, once the veneer has been permanently adhesively bonded, incisal or occlusal adjustments need to be avoided, since the superficial staining would be removed at these locations.

The most common pressable glass-ceramic material choices are outlined below.

IPS Empress

In 1990, the high-strength glass-ceramic IPS Empress (Ivoclar) was introduced. It is pressed in a hot, ductile state into a hollow mold. Analogous to Dicor, the restoration is fashioned with the lost-wax technique, and the final coloration is achieved using the staining or the layering technique. In a feldspar glass matrix, leucite crystals with an average diameter of 3–5 μm are homogeneously distributed in a high concentration (40–50 %). Due to the higher thermal expansion coefficient of the leucite crystals, the glass matrix is subjected to compressive stress during cooling, which results in an increase of flexural strength.[88] Data published so far on the suitability of IPS Empress for adhesively inserted inlays, onlays, partial crowns, and veneers allow the conclusion that the procedure is clinically safe.[89] Initially good clinical experiences with adhesively fixed crowns in the posterior tooth area were modified by failure rates of up to 12 % after 6 years.[90]

IPS e.max Press

This ceramic belongs, together with Empress 2, to the group of lithium disilicate glass-ceramics ($2SiO_2 \cdot Li_2O$). IPS e.max Press consists of a high-strength lithium disilicate framework

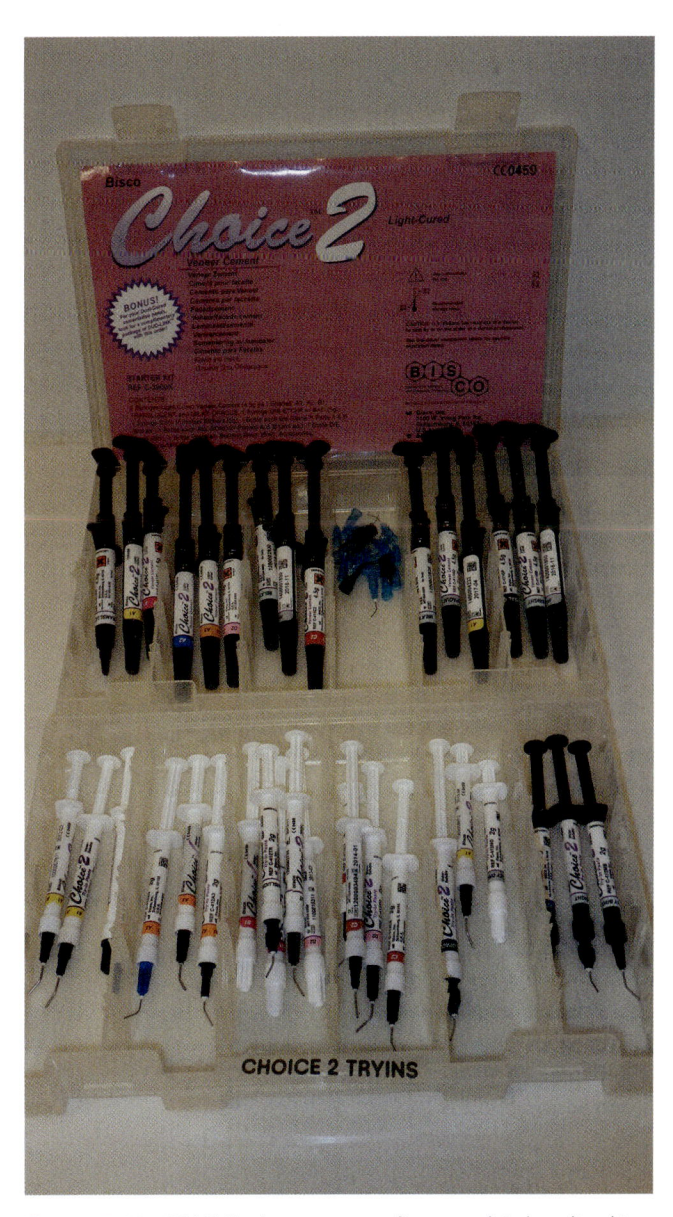

Figure 15.14 (T) While there are many fine porcelain bonding kits available, this is an example of an all-inclusive kit (Choice 2, Bisco).

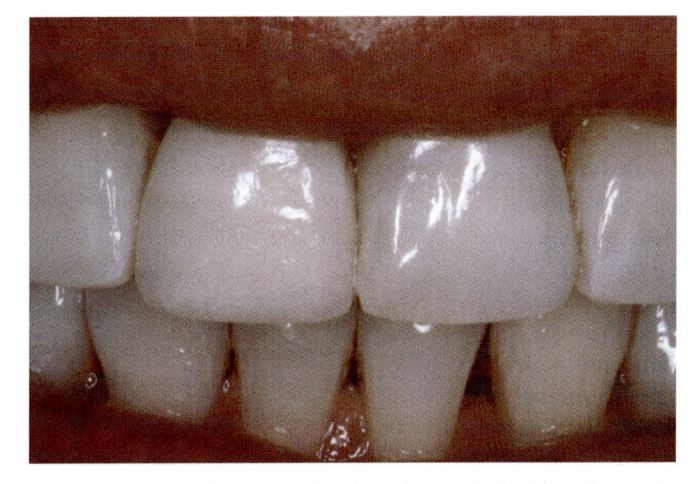

Figure 15.14 (U) The previously selected cement shade used as try-in paste shows the color is slightly too light. A darker tint or opaquer added to the bonding cement is used to adjust the color appropriately.

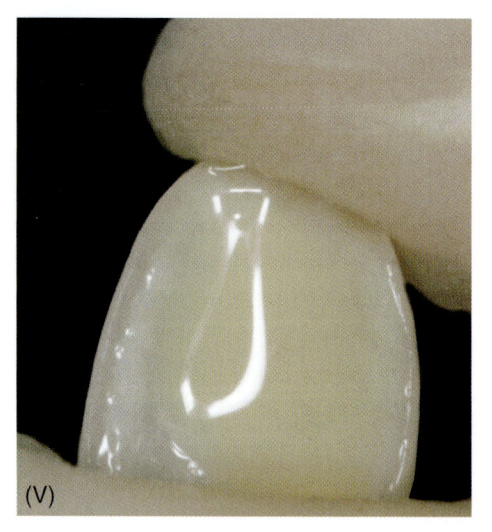

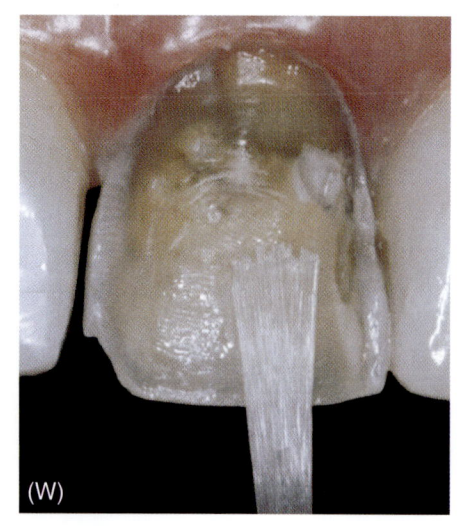

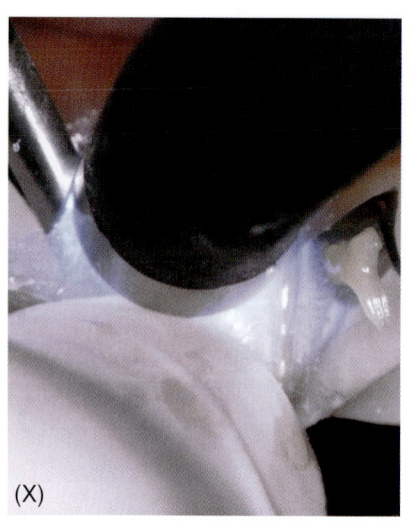

Figure 15.14 (V) After etching and silanizing the interior surface of the porcelain veneer, the tinted cement is added. (W) The prepared tooth is cleaned with coarse pumice and etched with phosphoric acid, treated with primer and adhesive, before the bonding agent is applied. (X) The composite filled veneer is gently pressed to place, and held there with a gloved finger while polymerizing the incisal edge with the light for 5–8 s (stabilizing the veneer in place). Excess cement can be removed with a soft brush or foam pellets before final light curing.

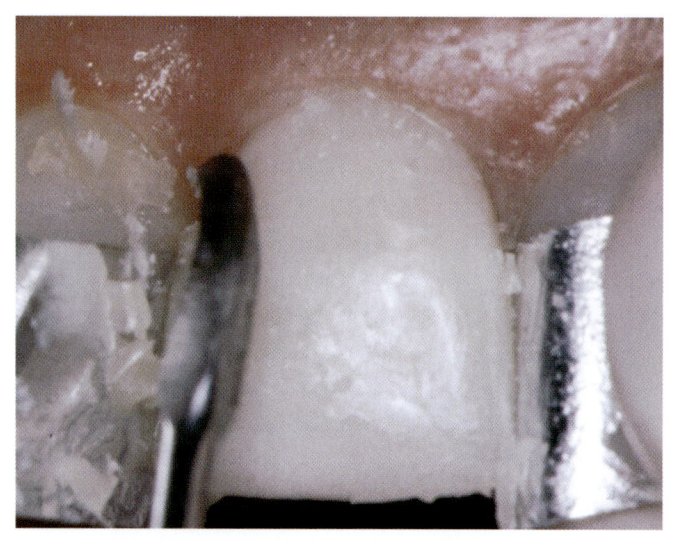

Figure 15.14 (Y) Interproximal excess is removed with the sickle end of the Novatech 12 (Hu-Friedy) and the veneer is then completely cured for 40 s labially and 40 s lingually. Note the ultrathin separation strips.

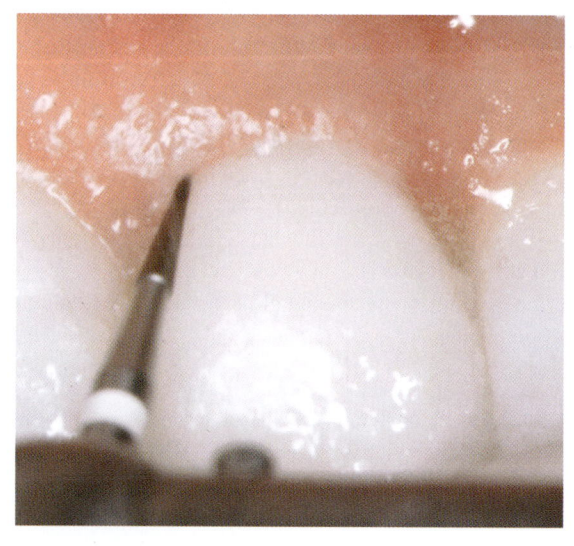

Figure 15.14 (Z) All remaining composite resin cement excess is then removed with the LVS-5 30-blade carbide bur. If contouring is required it can easily be accomplished with the LVS-6, -7, or -8 burs.

material, which may, if required, be veneered with a glass-ceramic containing fluoroapatite. IPS e.max Press is composed of SiO_2 (>57 weight percent), Li_2O, K_2O, MgO, ZnO_2, Al_2O_3, P_2O_5, and other oxides. The main crystalline phase of lithium disilicate consists of lengthy crystals of 0.5–4 µm, which are added to the glass in suitable grinding fineness. According to the manufacturer's indications, the microstructure of IPS e.max Press shall prevent crack propagation. IPS e.max Press resembles the Empress 2 ceramic both in its mechanical and its physical properties. The fabrication procedure of IPS e.max Press corresponds to that of the IPS Empress system. For pressing, the specific furnaces EP 500, EP 600 or EP 600 Combi (Ivoclar Vivadent) are used. The ceramic is pressed in viscous form into hollow molds at 915–930 °C using pneumatic pressers.

By a new fabrication process, the homogeneity of the ceramic ingots seems to be optimized, increasing the strength up to 400 MPa. This strength allows the use of single-tooth monolithic lithium disilicate restorations in the anterior and molar tooth areas.

IPS e.max Press comes as glass-ceramic blanks, which are available in different degrees of opacity. Ingots of medium opacity are suitable for fabrication of restorations on vital or slightly discolored stumps. Ingots of high opacity are used for fabrication

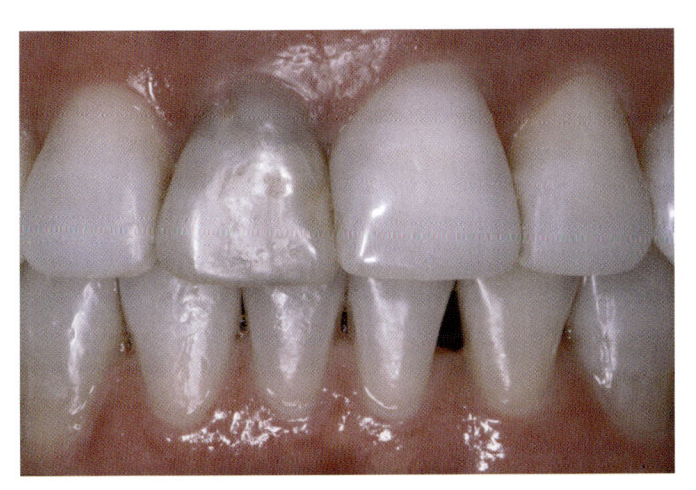

Chapter 15 Ceramic Veneers and Partial-Coverage Restorations

Figure 15.14 (Z1) Pre-op facial view: comparison of discolored tooth #8 and healthy tooth #9 reveal a substantial esthetic compromise.

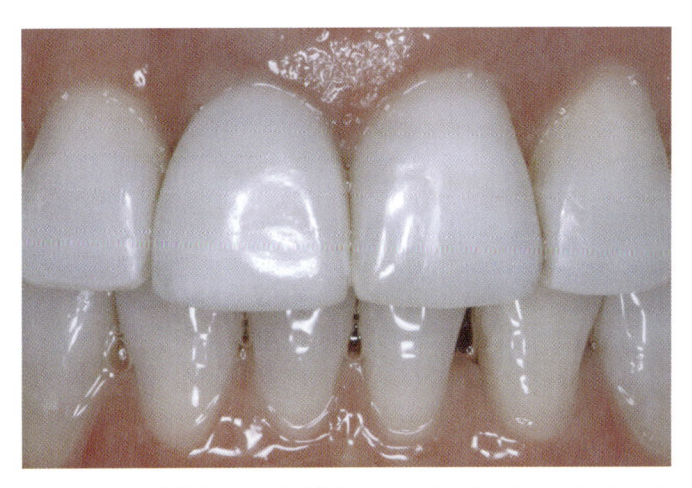

Figure 15.14 (Z2) Post-op facial view: note the closely matched result and healthy tissue response despite the light subgingival margin.

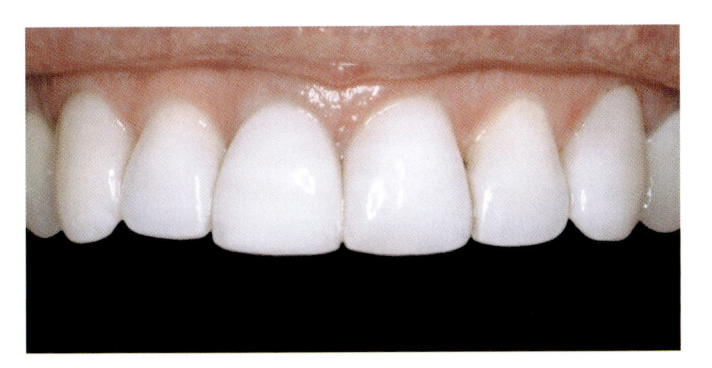

Figure 15.14 (Z3) Smile design and tissue conditions 10 years post veneer treatment of tooth #8.

of crowns on nonvital stumps or for coverage of posts and cores made of metal. The tooth-colored, esthetic lithium disilicate glass-ceramic restorations can be individually veneered with the glass-ceramic IPS e.max Ceram. Individualization is attained by staining and subsequent glaze firing.

Placement of veneers

Try-in

Before the veneers are bonded into place (see Figure 15.14 T–Z3), it is important to go through a try-in stage (see Figure 15.14 T and U), which is a three-phase process:

1. Check the intimate adaptation of each individual porcelain veneer to the prepared tooth surface. The teeth should first be cleaned with a slurry of fine flour of pumice that contains no oils or fluoride. Next, use a fine composite finishing strip to clean the contact areas. Then each of the veneers is tried in individually, beginning with the most distal veneer, with the margins checked carefully. (It may be useful to place a drop of glycerin or water on the etched surface to facilitate temporary adhesion of the veneer to the tooth surface.) If the veneer does not go into place immediately, check for any undercuts and contact point impingements and adjust with a 15 μm diamond bur until it seats easily.

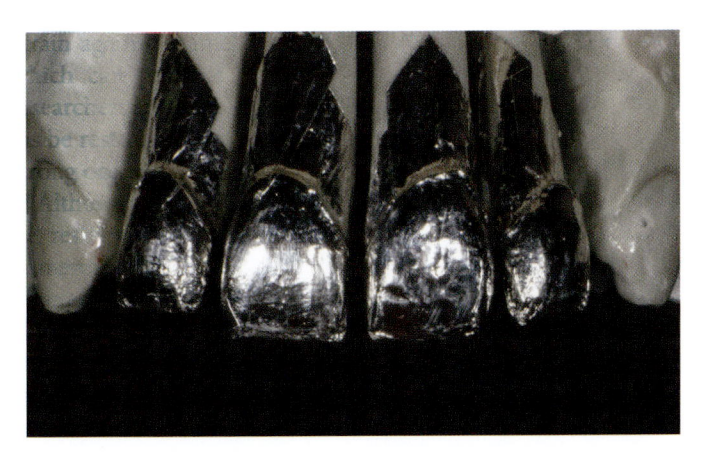

Figure 15.15 (A) Four veneers are being constructed to help close multiple diastemas. Here platinum foil is adapted to each individual tooth on the master model.

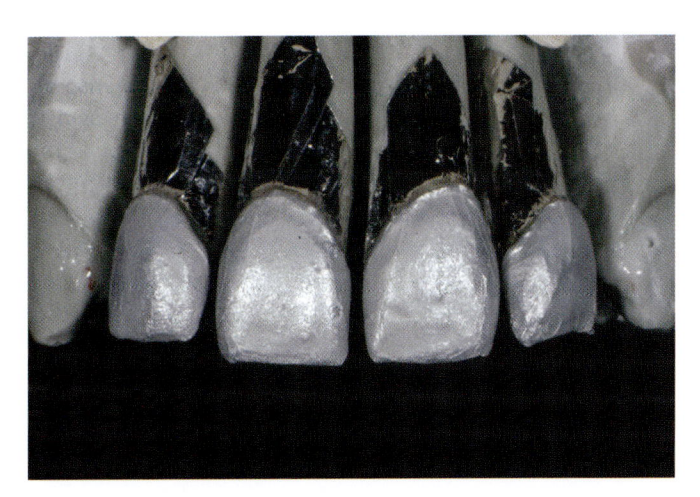

Figure 15.15 (B) The body porcelain is baked and this initial layer is thinned to outline the margins and surfaces on which the ensuing layers of porcelain will be built.

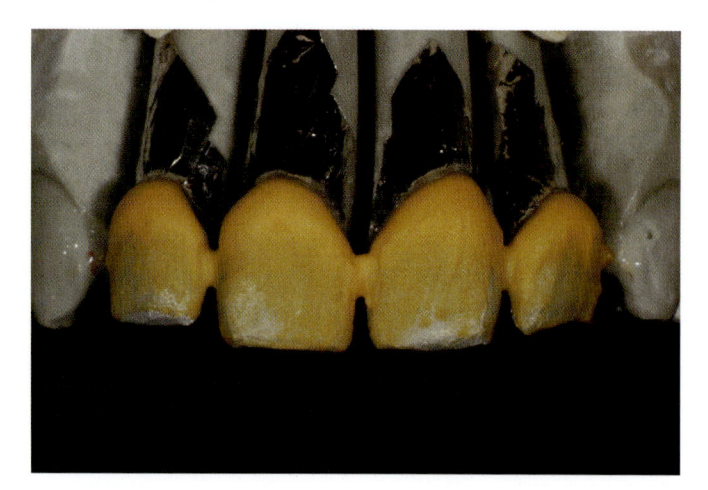

Figure 15.15 **(C)** The yellow build-up represents the cervical color blended with opacious dentin.

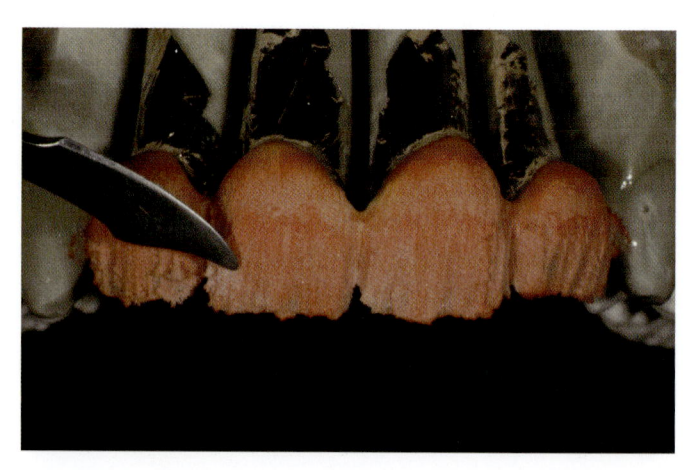

Figure 15.15 **(D)** The orange red layer is the body color. After completing the build-up, the incisal area is cut back for incisal porcelain placement.

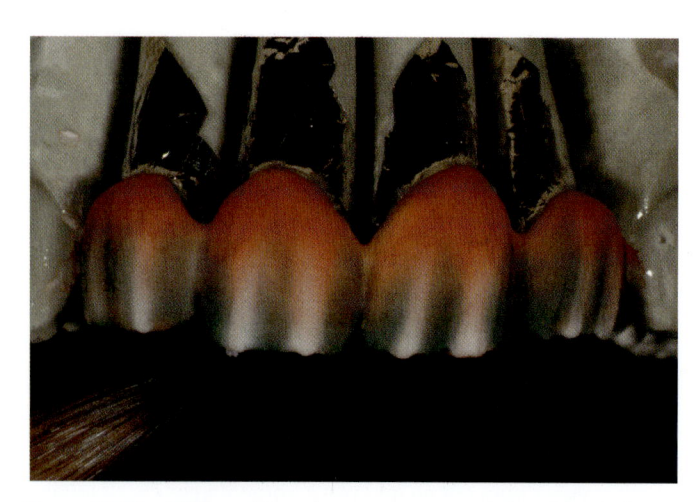

Figure 15.15 **(E)** The white color represents translucent blended porcelain and is placed between the more opaquely colored mamelons.

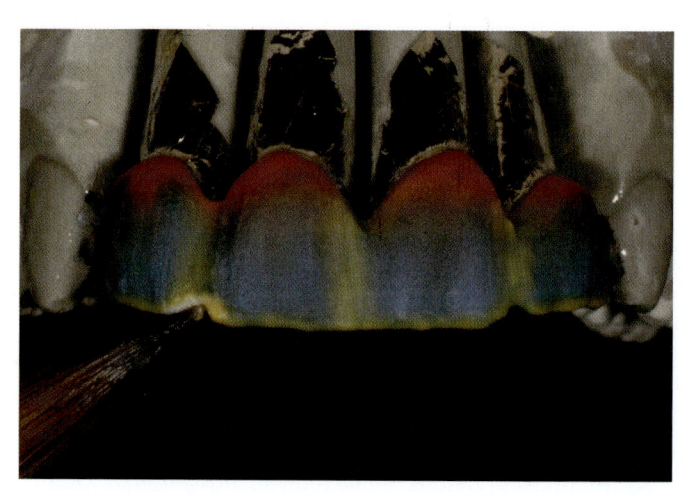

Figure 15.15 **(F)** Finally, the blue represents the outer layer, a blend of 50% translucent and 50% incisal color. The yellow creates the "halo" effect and is a 50% mixture of dentin and incisal porcelains.

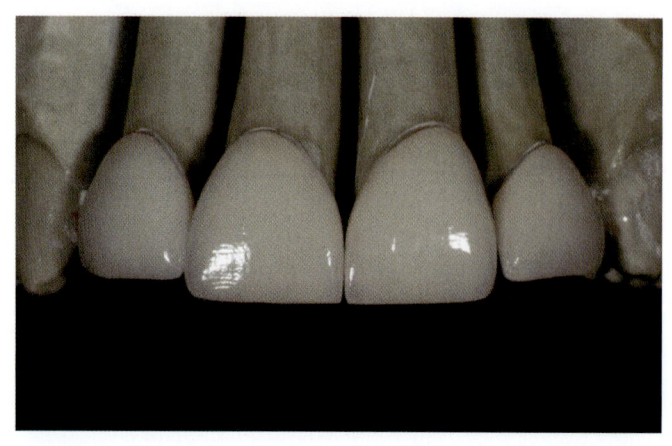

Figure 15.15 **(G)** The finished veneers on the master model with no foil. Reproduced with permission of Pinhas Adar.

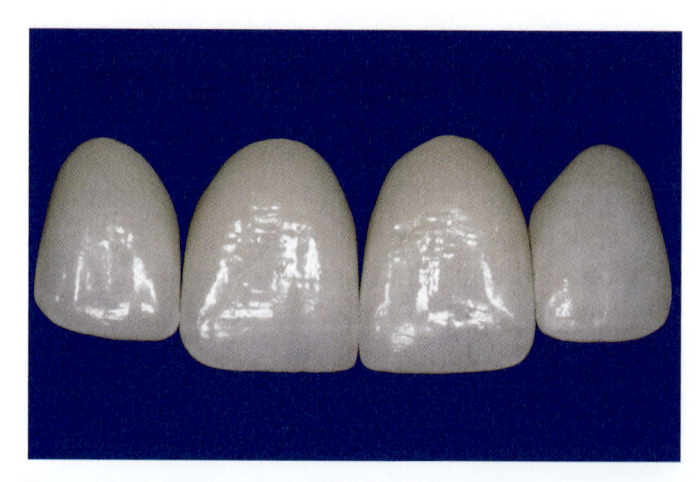

Figure 15.16 **(A)** These four porcelain veneers have been etched and are ready for try-in.

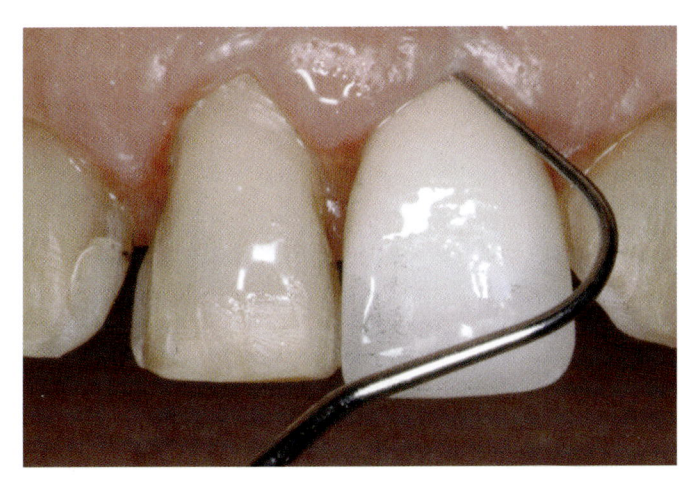

Figure 15.16 (B) Each veneer is individually fitted and checked for marginal accuracy.

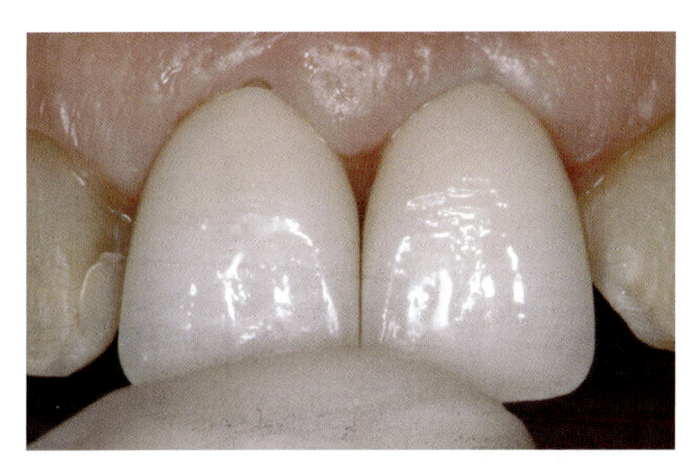

Figure 15.16 (C) Following individual fitting, pairs, then groups of veneers are checked for proper contact until all were properly related to one another.

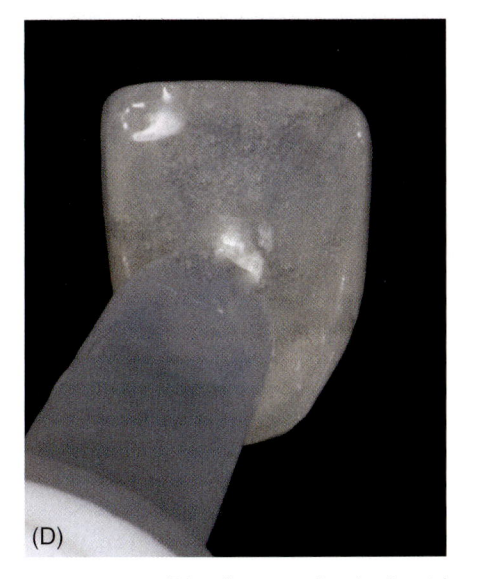

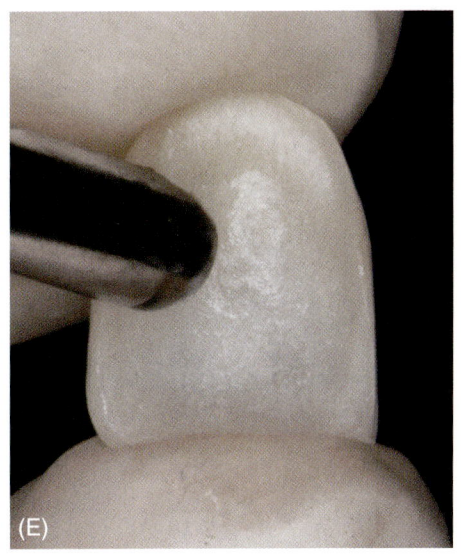

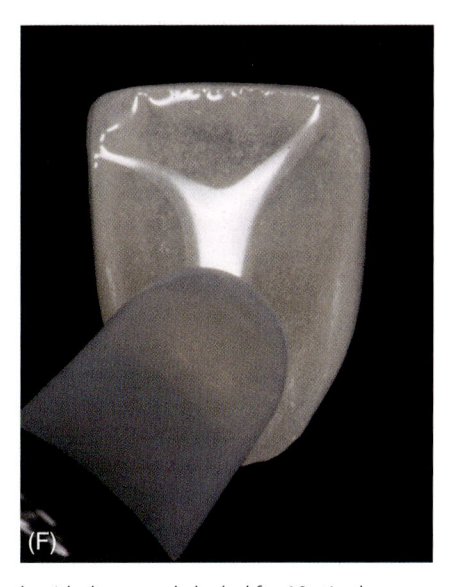

(D) (E) (F)

Figure 15.16 (D) Following color checks with try-in paste, the veneers are cleaned in an ultrasonic bath with denatured alcohol for 10 min then treated with hydrofluoric acid porcelain conditioner for 1 min. (E) Hydrofluoric acid porcelain conditioner is thoroughly washed off and then air dried. (F) Silane primer is applied according to the manufacturer's instructions.

2. After ascertaining individual fit, each veneer should be placed on one by one, until all are in place. Thus you can ascertain if there are any problems with the insertion paths and order of insertion (usually done posterior to anterior, except the centrals and laterals which should be placed centrals first, then laterals). Then check the collective fit and relationship of one veneer to another, especially in the contact areas.

3. Assess the shade and modify it as necessary. Since the prepared tooth color, shade, and opacity of the bonding resin and the veneer itself all contribute to the color of the veneer once in place, this phase of the try-in is essential.

A good initial test is to place one veneer in position with glycerin on the tooth and compare that veneer to a shade tab of the selected shade. If the veneer color is unsatisfactory, use try-in pastes that do not polymerize, or place a small portion

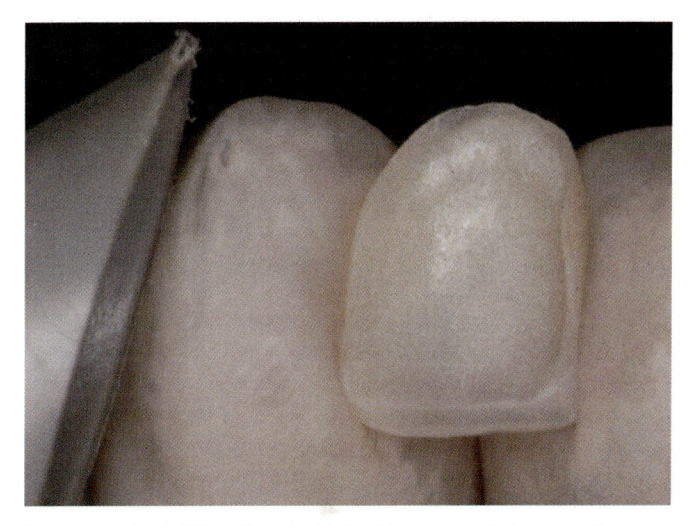

Figure 15.16 (G) The silane is dried with a warm air dryer or oil and moisture-free laboratory or chairside air syringe.

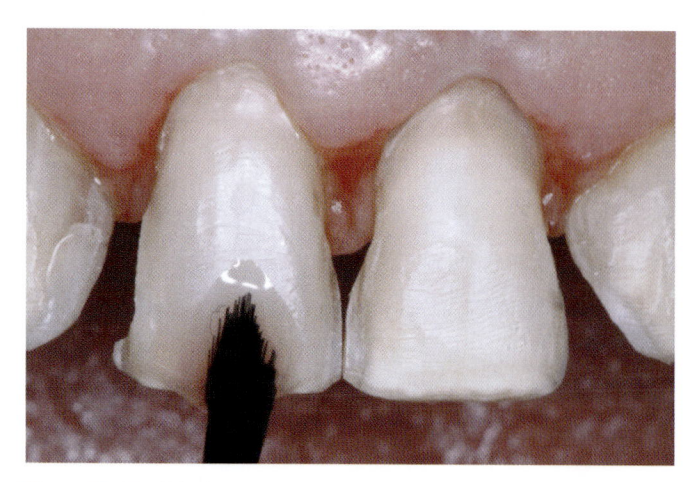

Figure 15.16 **(H)** The two central incisor preparations are etched; 15 s for dentin and 20 s for enamel.

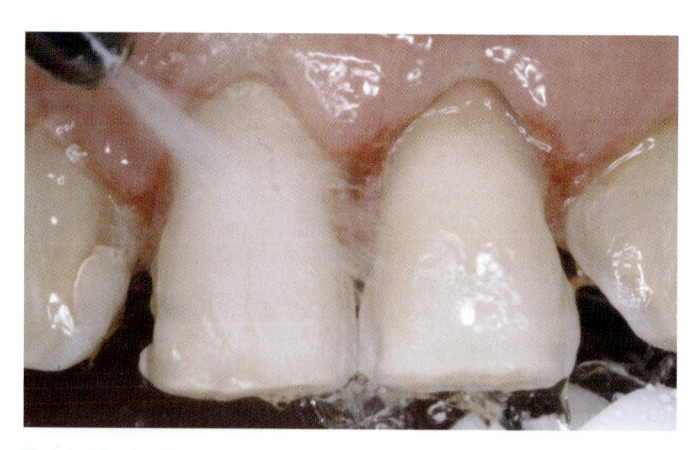

Figure 15.16 **(I)** A 10 s air/water spray as used to wash off the etchant.

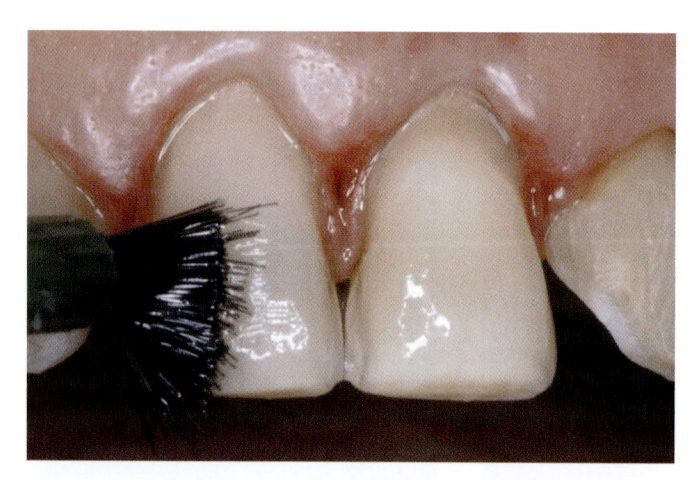

Figure 15.16 **(J)** Multiple coats of dentin/enamel bonding agent are applied and then dried and polymerized. The prepared tooth surface should now be slightly glossy. If not, repeat the process.

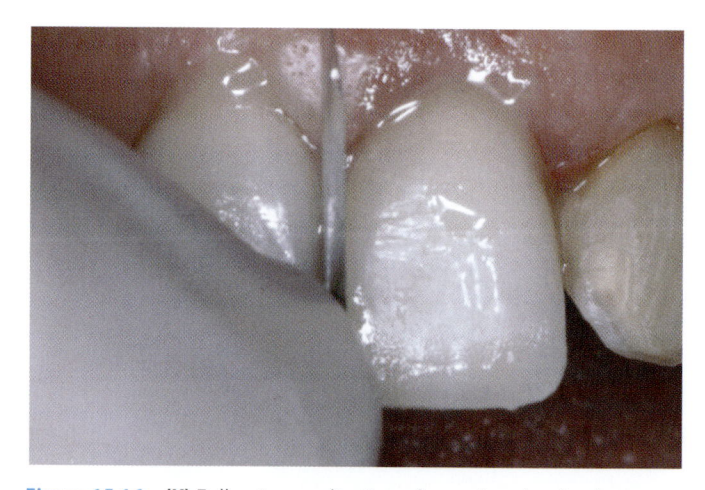

Figure 15.16 **(K)** Following application of a pre-bond resin, the two central veneers, filled with cement, are carefully placed and checked with an explorer to certify correct alignment.

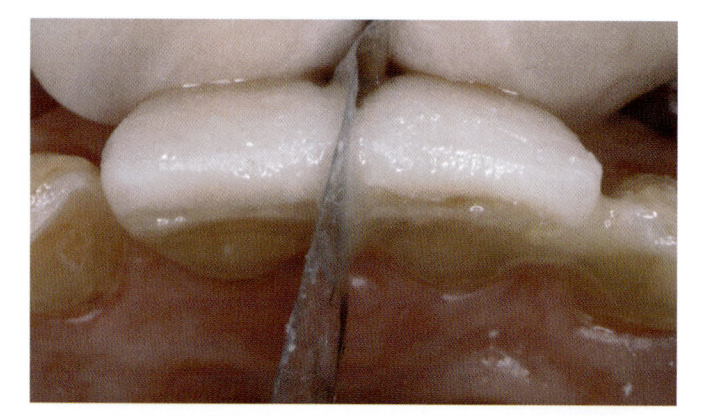

Figure 15.16 **(L)** Holding the veneers in place, make certain the ultrathin (0.002 mm) matrix (Artus) provide adequate separation along the entire contact area.

of the luting composite on the veneer and then reset the veneer on the prepared tooth to check the color. If you or the patient is not happy with the shade, try the veneer with a lighter or darker shade of try-in paste or composite until the right one is found.

There is no absolute method of predetermining the exact shade of the veneer following cementation. However, using try-in pastes that are matched to the final shades can go a long way to satisfying most dentist and patient demands (Bisco Choice 2). Even so, there will almost always be a slight shade shift following polymerization. That shift will generally be towards the darker rather than lighter side. So, if there is a choice, choose the lighter shade cement. If the veneer appears lighter than expected at the trial phase, try adding tints or opaquers.

While it is ideal to have all of the necessary color contained in the porcelain, certain discolorations and problems present in the tooth itself may be too much for the veneer alone to correct, because of its thinness. In these cases, correction can be made for the individual tooth discoloration through the use of resins painted onto the internal surface of the veneer. In others, where the teeth are discolored in strips, lines, or small areas, only these discreet areas may need opaquing. When a satisfactory result is achieved, the veneers then can be bonded in position with the usual composite luting cement. This process allows a better coloration of the finished tooth but it does raise problems of added thickness and possible weakening of the bond. You also may

Figure 15.16 **(M)** Following a 5–8 s initial polymerization, excess cement is trimmed. Next, polymerize each aspect (labial, lingual, and incisal) for 40 s.

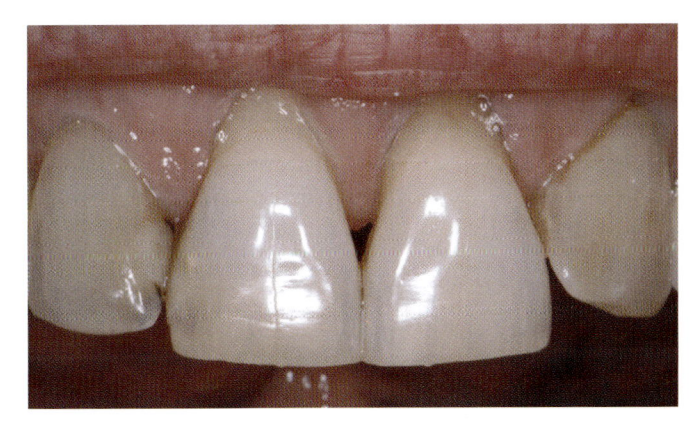

Figure 15.16 **(N)** This 60-year-old woman looked older due to her discolored, worn, and eroded incisors.

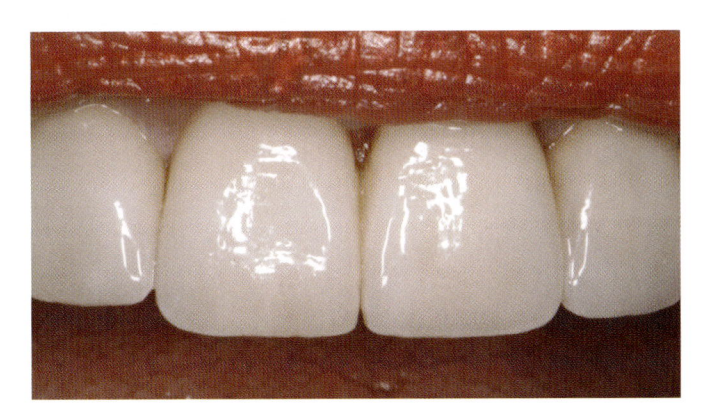

Figure 15.16 **(O)** A younger and more attractive appearance was achieved by four porcelain veneers. Note closure of interdental space.

need to alter the tooth slightly in the event you need greater composite opaquing. This can be done by slightly preparing a concave area on the tooth surface under the part of the veneer that requires greater masking.

Caution must be used during this phase of the try-in to avoid exposing the veneer and composite luting agent to the operating light, which may initiate the curing process. It also is important to completely remove the composite material used during the try-in period prior to the final process of luting. Be sure to remember that ceramic veneers are fragile and are subject to fracture prior to bonding.[91]

Final insertion

After spending considerable time preparing the teeth, taking impressions, and constructing and trying in the veneers, the most crucial step comes: that of final insertion with adhesive bonding. The reason why this step is potentially the most demanding of all is because the actual final placement, shade chosen for the cement, and the ability to achieve lasting adhesion to cementum, dentin, and enamel will ultimately determine how long the veneer remains esthetically and functionally viable.

There are also several phases to this process, which may best be done with a local anesthetic. (Figure 15.16A–Z4).

1. **Soft tissue control**. Gingival retraction cord should be placed to decrease the crevicular fluid flow, which would interfere with the adhesion and seal between the veneer and underlying enamel. It also allows for direct visibility of the gingival margin.

    Ideally, a rubber dam is the best way to secure overall moisture control. However, in many instances of subgingival margins it is either impossible or impractical to precisely seat the veneers with a rubber dam in place. Therefore, other methods of securing a dry field must be used. Using the retraction cord can help but if bleeding is present after retraction, due to inadequately healed tissue, the insertion should be postponed. Several rinses with saline (a teaspoonful of salt to a glass of water) may help to control the seepage. One thing is certain: unless bleeding and gingival seepage can be controlled, the life span of the veneers will be drastically shortened by reducing bond strength, especially in the gingival area, and increasing the chance for bacterial penetration and eventual unwanted stain beneath the veneer.

2. **Cleaning and etching**. In many cases the dental laboratory delivers veneer restorations with intaglio surfaces pre-etched with hydrofluoric acid (smoky white surface). This might make clinicians believe that the veneer is ready for adhesive bonding without further surface treatment, and silanation could be performed at the intaglio surfaces of the veneer immediately. Yet try-in procedures of veneers are necessary, which causes contamination of the bonding surface by saliva, blood, or the try-in glycerin paste (Figure 15.16A–C). Therefore, it is required to etch the intaglio surfaces once more with hydrofluoric acid for 20 s to 1 min, dependent on the composition of the silicate-based material used (Figure 15.16D). In case the ceramic surface was not pretreated by the laboratory, the veneer is cleaned with 99% isopropanol, and the inner surfaces are etched with 4.9% hydrofluoric acid for 60 s. The etched ceramic surface should be thoroughly sprayed with water for 60 s and dried with oil-free compressed air (Figure 15.16E).

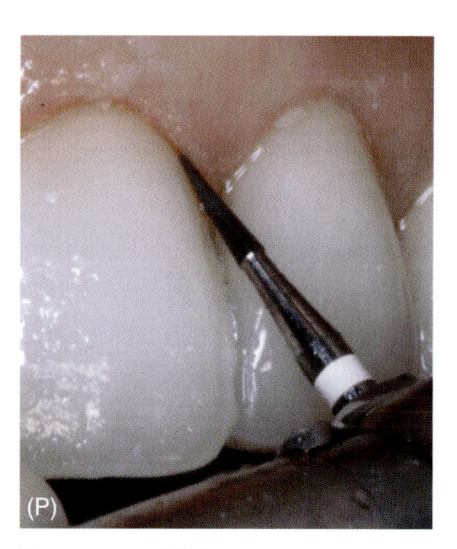

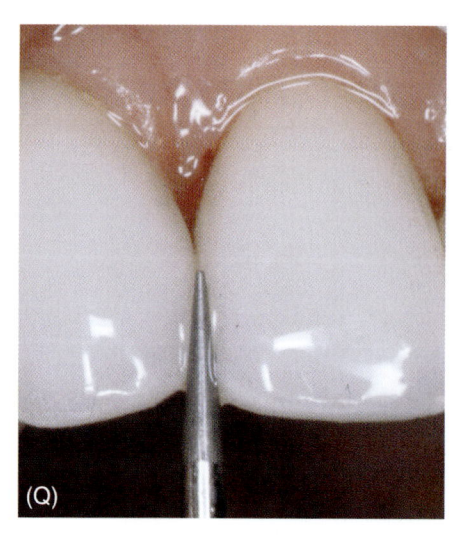

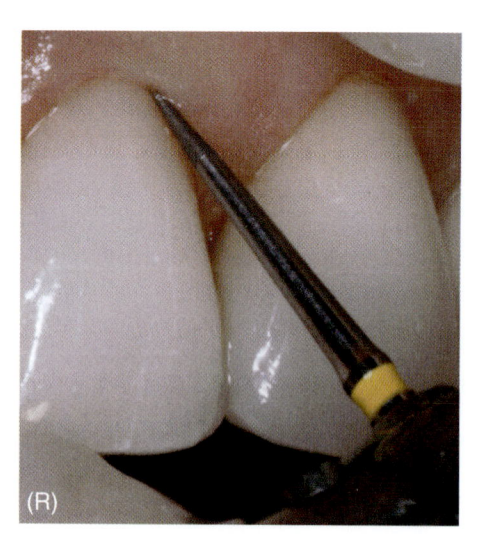

Figure 15.16 **(P)** The LVS-5 (Brasseler) is used to trim composite resin flash following polymerization. **(Q)** The LVS-6 is used to contour or reshape as necessary. **(R)** Gingival reduction shaping or contouring could also be easily managed with the LVS-7 15 μm diamond.

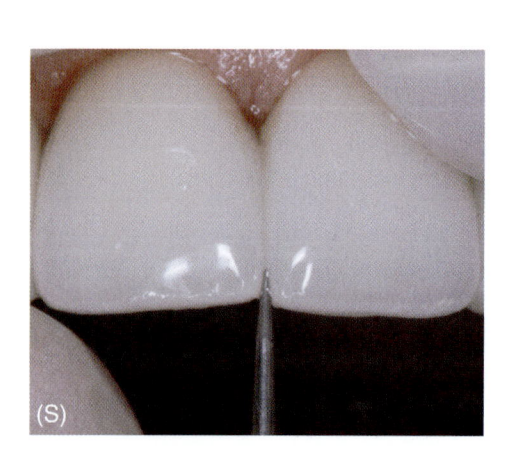

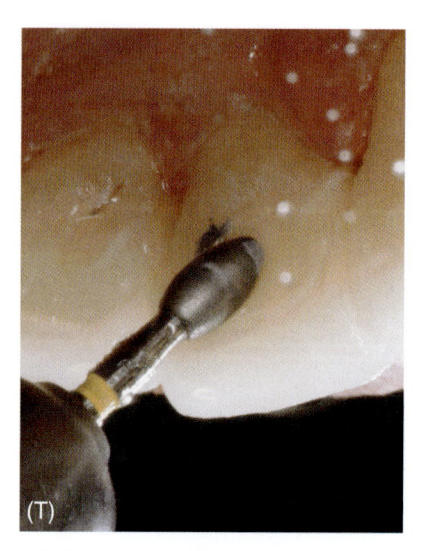

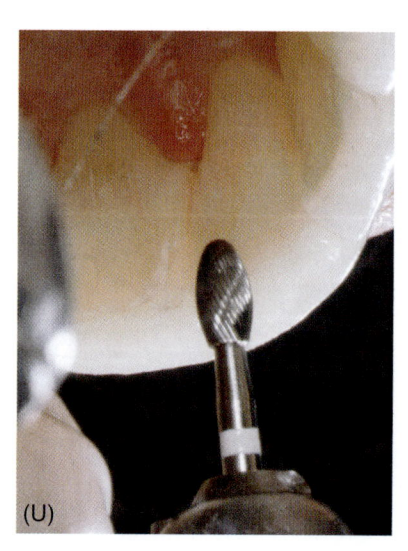

Figure 15.16 **(S)** The LVS-7 is also useful for contouring incisal embrasures. **(T)** The LVS-8 is helpful to establish appropriate occlusal anatomy and shape lingual surfaces. **(U)** Final porcelain finish should be done with the 30-bladed carbide (ETUF-OS1, Brasseler USA).

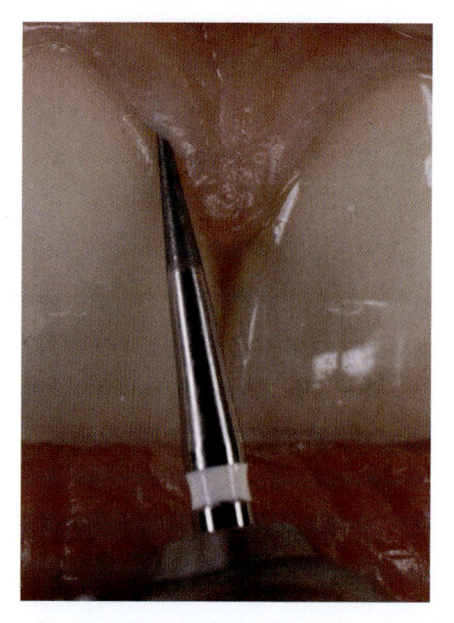

Figure 15.16 **(V)** Many clinicians prefer an 8 μm diamond (DET4UF) for final finishing of gingival margins.

3. **Silanation**. The bond of the porcelain veneer to the tooth is, in fact, a series of links: etched enamel to dental bonding agent to luting composite to hydrolyzing silane to etched porcelain. Common is the use of a one-component adhesive silane (e.g. Monobond-S, Ivoclar Vivadent or Etch 37, Bisco) (Figure 15.16 F). After a reaction time of 60 s the silanized ceramic surface can be dried with air (Figure 15.16G). Hereafter, the silanized intaglio surfaces of the veneer should not get in contact with water or other contaminants, or etching and silanization process needs to be repeated. Silane greatly enhances the adhesion between porcelain and resin and thus increases bond strength (Figure 15.16G).[92]

4. **Enamel etching**. Each prepared tooth is isolated, and then cleaned with a polishing brush and fluoride-free cleaning paste (e.g. Pell-ex Hawe Neos Dental, or Bisco). The prepared tooth structure is etched with 37% phosphoric acid (e.g. Total-Etch, Ivoclar Vivadent,), dentin for 15 s and enamel for 40 s (Figure 15.16H), sprayed with water for 15 s, and dried. 40 s etching time is sufficient if no dentin but only enamel is involved. (Figure 15.16I). The etchant must reach the entire periphery of the preparation where a tight seal is critical to the long-term success of the restoration. Gingival displacement is important to expose this margin and prevent contamination. If the patient rinses or in any way contaminates this etched enamel surface with saliva, the surface must be re-etched for 10 s, washed, and dried again (Figure 15.16I).

5. **Bonding**. Depending on the bonding system used, single or multiple steps are required to prepare the tooth surface. A classic and very durable three step bonding method is introduced here. A primer (e.g. Syntac Primer, Ivoclar Vivadent or All-Bond, Bisco) is applied to the etched surface with a brush for 15 s and blow-dried after a reaction time of 10 s. After conditioning of the surface with a primer, an adhesive (e.g. Syntac Adhesive, Ivoclar Vivadent or Porcelain Bonding Resin, Bisco) is applied for a reaction time of 10 s. Following, enamel and dentin are covered with an unfilled resin bonding liquid (e.g. Heliobond, Ivoclar Vivadent) blown to a thin layer. To avoid inaccuracies of fit, the unfilled resin bonding material should not be light-polymerized before restoration placement (Figure 15.16 J). The internal aspect of the veneer that has been silanated is now also coated with the unfilled resin bonding liquid, which is blown into a thin layer. The composite luting agent is now placed inside the veneer. Protect all these materials from strong light to prevent premature polymerization.

An alternate technique includes a universal self-etch material (All-Bond SE, Bisco), which combines etching, priming, and bonding in one step.

6. **Placement**. Generally, the distal-most veneers in the posterior should be seated and polymerized first, followed by the next mesial-most veneer until the canines. Next, seat central incisor veneers together, then the laterals, and finally, the canines. Be sure to refit your adjacent or next veneer before you attempt to cement it to place (Figure 15.16 K). Frequently, a small cement excess or slight placement variation in the previous veneer has caused the fit between them to vary. Use a 15 μm diamond ET6F, or LVS (Brasseler USA), to slightly shape the adjacent surface, and then refit the next veneer until the fit is again perfect before proceeding. If you need to remove the glazed surface of a seated veneer, you need to repolish the surface with a ceramic polishing system. The pivotal last veneer on each side may give you the most problems because there will be more sides to adjust if there is tightness in the fit. *Adjust the contacts of the already seated veneers until you again achieve a perfect fit.*

Handling a veneer full of cement is not as easy as positioning the cement-free veneer. Veneer carriers are available relying on glue tips or adhesive pads that can help to position the veneer correctly, although there is the distinct possibility that the glue bond might fail or the veneer might slide off, causing it to drop and become contaminated. When choosing to finger-hold the veneer you should avoid pushing the cement away from the edge of the veneer, leaving a bonding void. Also, make sure that well-fitting dental gloves are used.

The adjacent teeth should be separated with matrix strips during both acid etching and insertion so the cement does not

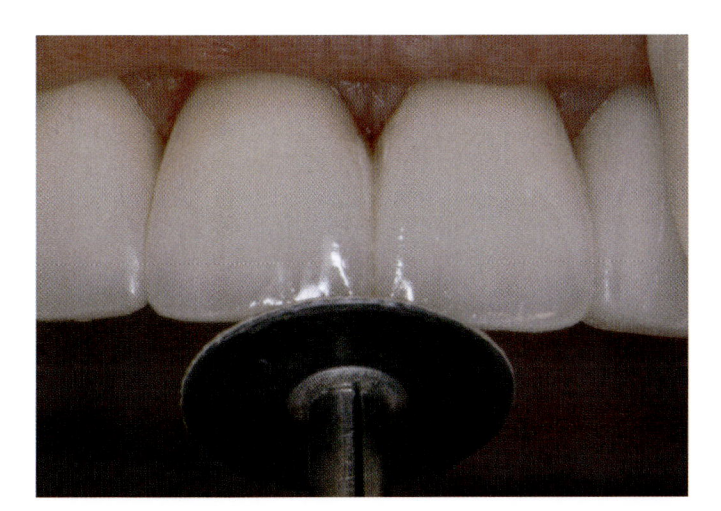

Figure 15.16 (**W**) The Soflex (3M) disk 1 s used to adjust the incisal length.

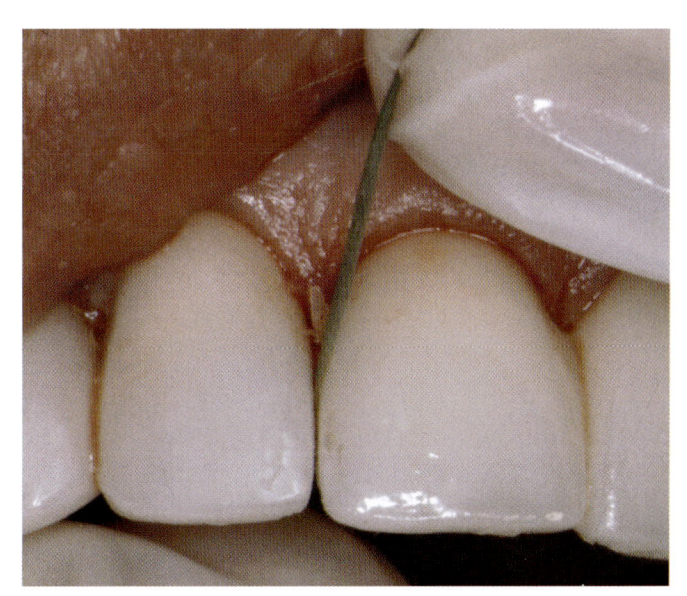

Figure 15.16 (**X**) Use waxed or unwaxed floss to test for any overhangs that might still need to be removed.

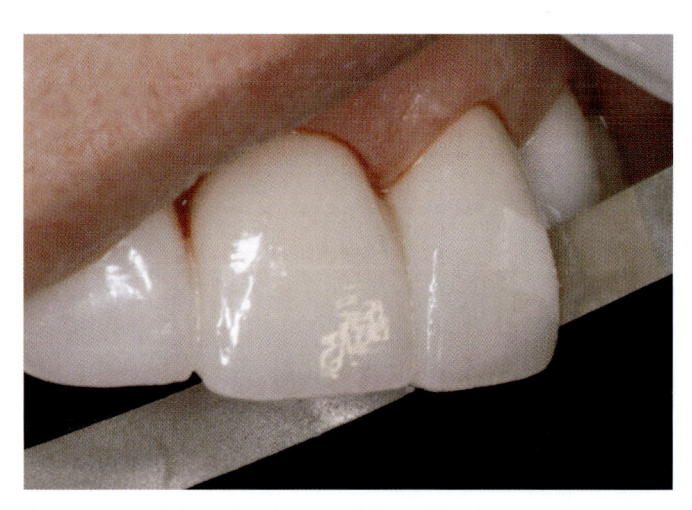

Figure 15.16 **(Y)** An ultrathin strip followed by abrasive strips, coarse to fine, will provide the best interproximal finish.

lock in or adhere to the adjacent tooth (Figure 15.16 L). Since most clear Dental Mylar strips are too thick, it is better to use the Artus occlusal registration strips or Variolink Esthetic LC System, which allow proper seating of veneers. Dual-polymerizing composite cement (e.g. Ivoclar Vivadent) is advised for adhesive fixation. Apply composite cement to the prepared tooth and inner restoration surfaces. Insert the veneers gently with increasing pressure ($\approx$5–10 N). Immediately remove excess cement in all marginal areas with foam pellets. Avoid cotton pellets, since cotton fibers will get stuck at the cementation composite. While placing the veneer, line up the incisal edge and the mesiolabial and distolabial line angles with the adjacent teeth. Use a sharp explorer to make certain the gingival margin is in place. Most of all, be careful not to torque the veneer, which could trap an air bubble underneath. Ten seconds of light polymerization at the incisal edge ensures stabilization of the veneer while other veneer surfaces should be covered with instruments or finger.[93] Remove residual interproximal cement gently with foam pellets, dental floss, and Superfloss (Oral-B) without dislocating the veneer. The most frustrating area for this to happen is at the gingival margin, since bacteria will usually penetrate, eventually causing a black stain to occur (see Figure 15.17). *In case the veneer moves or pulls away from the tooth in the gingival area*, it is highly advised to remove it, refill it with cement, and reseat it.

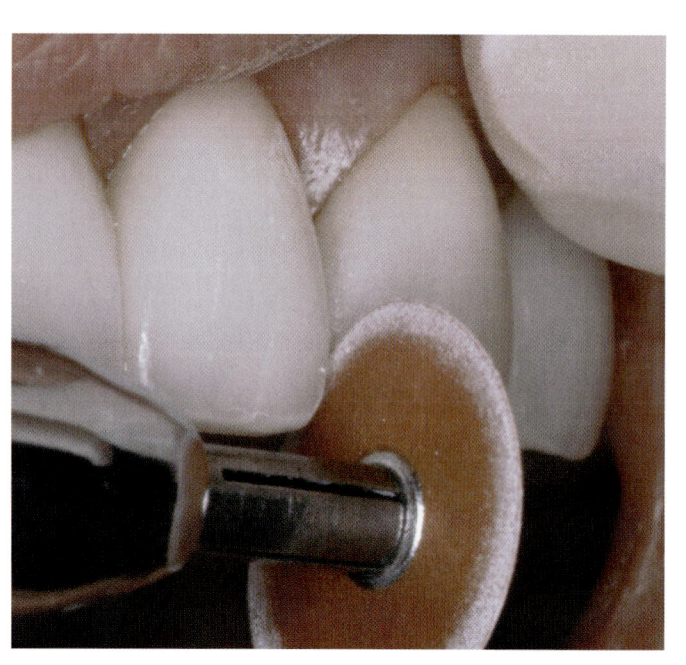

Figure 15.16 **(Z)** Ultrathin plastic pop-on discs could effectively reopen closed incisal embrasures.

7. **Polymerization**. A short polymerization period of about 5 s as you seat each veneer will be sufficient to allow you to remove the greatest bulk of marginal excess (Figure 15.16 M). Some flash or excess marginal cement is healthy to make certain that polymerization shrinkage does not cause a marginal void. Remove excess partially cured composite with a Novatech 12 (Hu-Friedy). This double-ended instrument is quite helpful because its chisel end can gently pry off excess labial and lingual composite cement, and the sickle end is extremely large but perfectly suited to remove interproximal excess composite cement. Glycerin gel application at all restoration margins (e.g. Liquid-Strip, Ivoclar Vivadent, Schaan, Liechtenstein) ensures oxygen inhibition during light polymerization. The polymerization process is completed by curing the various areas of the veneer for at least 60 s with light intensity of at least 650 mW/cm^2, or 10 s with an argon laser or xenon light (Figure 15.16 M–O). During this polymerization process it is essential to maintain complete stability of the relationship between the veneer and the underlying tooth. Although all flash should generally be removed; if you are inserting additional veneers, wait until the adjacent

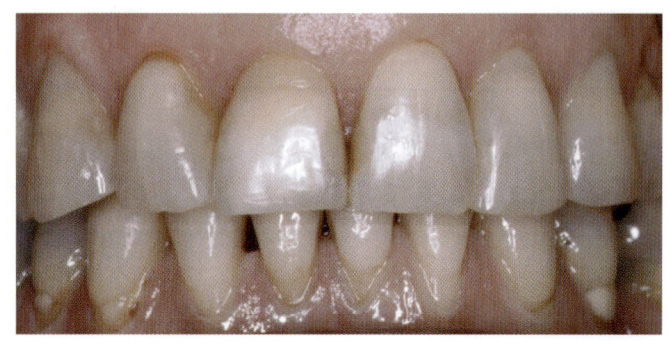

Figure 15.16 **(Z1)** This 49-year-old woman wanted a lighter and more prominent look to her teeth.

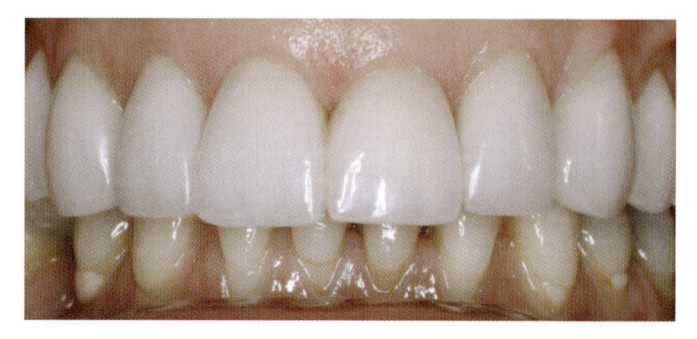

Figure 15.16 **(Z2)** Twelve porcelain veneers were placed to satisfy this patient's desire for perfection.

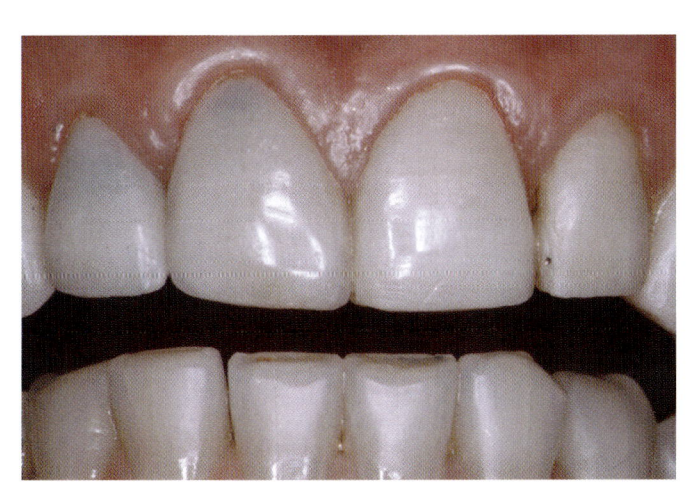

Figure 15.17 Torqueing or accidental moisture contamination during cementation can eventually cause marginal leakage. This can result in a black, gray, or blue stain appearing underneath a porcelain veneer. Although it can be repaired, the best solution to this problem is remaking the veneer.

veneer is seated before you do any subgingival trimming with the bur to avoid initiating bleeding or seepage.

8. **Finishing**. When polymerization is complete, excess composite should be chipped off manually with a finishing instrument (e.g. Novatech 12, Hu-Friedy). Further, residual excess composite cement can be removed with a 15c scalpel (#371716, Bard-Parker; Becton-Dickinson). This method is favorable for epi- or subgingivally positioned restoration margins. The scalpel allows for cement removal without alteration of the ceramic surface and gingival tissue trauma. A 30-bladed carbide finishing bur with a straight emergence profile (LVS-5) from the Veneer System (Brasseler USA) (Figure 15.16P) can be used to gently remove all remaining excess composite at the gingival margin. Use a copious water spray to avoid heat build-up.

If the veneer surface is not a smooth continuation of the subgingival enamel, then recontour the excess porcelain with a microfine diamond point (LVS-6) (Figure 15.16Q). A 15 μm grit polishing diamond (LVS-7) is then used to refine this interface of tooth/composite/porcelain (Figure 15.16R and S). Refine occlusion with microthin articulating film, 0.02 mm (AccuFilm II, Parkell), and adjust occlusion if necessary with a 15 μm diamond (LVS-8) (Figure 15.16T) and final finish with a 30-bladed carbide (ETUF-OS1) (Figure 15.16U). For final margin use an 8 μm diamond (DET 4, Brasseler USA) or a 30-bladed carbide ETUF 4 (Brasseler USA) of the same size (Figure 15.16V). The final polishing of the veneer is done with a series of ceramic polishing kits and diamond-dust-impregnated paste with non-webbed rubber cups. The edge of the rubber cup is brought to just beneath the free gingival margin to bring the junction between the veneer, composite, and tooth to a high luster, ensuring that this area does not become a repository for microbial plaque. This final polishing can take 5 min per tooth.

The lingual margin is finished with the LVS-8 to remove excess composite (Figure 15.16T). If the porcelain margin needs refining, use the 15 μm diamond (LVS-7). First, polishing is done with a series of flexible spirals (Dialite Feather Lite porcelain polishers, Brasseler USA) used in sequence. The final polishing is once again done with diamond impregnated polishing paste (Dialite intraoral porcelain polishing paste, Brasserler USA) on a disposable cotton polishing buff (Brasseler USA). Static and dynamic occlusion need to be checked. If necessary, adjust incisal length with flexible polishing discs (Brasseler or 3M ESPE) (Figure 15.16W).

A thorough study by Haywood and coworkers[94] compared various instruments and finishing and polishing sequences and found that the best results obtained were with a sequence consisting of diamond instruments with progressively smaller particle sizes at moderate speeds with water coolant, then a 30-blade carbide bur at high speed and dry, followed by a diamond polishing paste with a 2–5 μm particle size. In all polishing sequences, the best results were obtained with each individual instrument when diamond instruments were used at moderate speed, wet, and carbide instruments were used at high speed, dry.

Proximal contacts should be checked with dental floss (Figure 15.16X) and minor corrections can be made with a yellow-banded diamond finishing strip (VisionFlex Perforated diamond strips with Gateway, Brasseler USA). If the entire contact area needs thinning, then wider strips banded (Brasseler USA or Premier) (150 UF) can be used (Figure 15.16Y). In case the embrasure area needs to be reshaped, a 100 UF strip should be used. Incisal embrasures can be nicely thinned and polished with the ultrathin plastic discs (3M, Brasseler USA, or Premier) (Figure 15.16Z).

The patient should return at weekly intervals to be monitored for tissue response. In the event of inflammation, the veneers can be further refined with the LVS microfine diamonds for esthetic and functional harmony, making certain that no porcelain or composite impinges on the gingival tissue.

Post-treatment care and instructions

Once veneers are cemented and finished, it should be the goal to help the patient obtain the longest life expectancy for the veneers as possible. First and foremost, a night appliance should be constructed to protect the veneers from the possible damage due to abnormal chewing, grinding, or clenching during sleep. One of the easiest to make and most comfortable to wear is a flat upper occlusal plane made of hard acrylic, with a soft acrylic liner (Annalan Laboratory).

Office-based maintenance should consist of at least four professional cleanings per year. Be sure to train your hygienist to avoid ultrasonic scaling on any tooth with a porcelain veneer, and to avoid air-powered abrasive instruments, which can attack the porcelain surface.[95] When hand scaling, advise your hygienist to be careful not to scale against the veneer margin, which could produce chipping, fracture, or worse, debonding. Rather, scale either from the veneer onto the tooth or laterally parallel to the margins.

The highly esthetic outcome and longevity made traditional porcelain laminate veneers the treatment option of choice for restoring the anterior dentition.[16,48,96] Many authors state that fractures are the most frequent cause for clinical failure of ceramic veneer restorations,[96,97] yet the percentage of reported clinical unacceptable fractures is very low: Magne et al.[98] showed 0%, Peumans et al. 2%,[96] and Dumfahrt and Schaffer 3%.[70]

Calamia[99] reported a study of 115 etched porcelain veneers 2–3 years after placement and found a low fracture rate, low debond rate, no incidence of caries, and minimal negative periodontal response. Strassler recalled 196 porcelain veneers with up to 13 years of service and an average of 10 years. None had debonded and all were color-stable. Over the course of this long-term study, only seven veneers needed replacement due to porcelain chipping—a 96.4% success rate.[100] All-ceramic veneers involving the incisal edge, the approximal areas and larger parts of the palatal surface (full veneers[16]) should be considered more often as an alternative to full crowns[26,62,98] (Figures 15.18A–R and 15.19A–P). During a 5 year observation period, a study by Stappert showed promising survival rates of 97.6% and 100% for IPS Empress press-ceramic veneers with overlap- and full veneer preparation design, respectively.[21] The results remained the same for the 7 year follow-up.[47] Decrease in marginal adaptation and increase in marginal discoloration are the most common esthetic compromises for veneer restorations.[28] To prolong the survival rate of ceramic veneers, maintenance and care is highly advised:

1. Special care immediately following placement of veneers. During the 72–96 hours during which the bonding resin continues to cure, the patient should avoid hard foods, alcohol, some medicated mouthwashes, and extremes in temperature.

2. Eating and other habits must be altered indefinitely to avoid damaging, discoloring, or eroding the veneers. The patient should be instructed to avoid biting into hard foods, whether candy or meat with bones. Behaviors such as nail biting or pencil chewing endanger their new smile. Many dentists recommend that patients use a soft acrylic mouthguard when involved in sports or activities likely to result in impact to the mouth. Apart from concern with fracturing, the patient also should avoid large amounts of highly

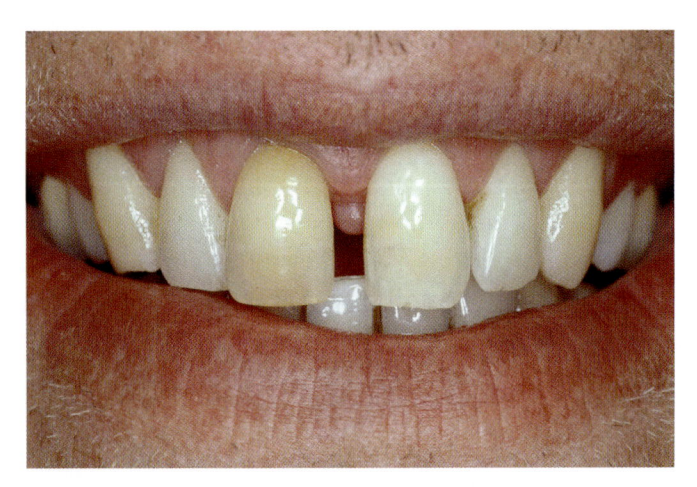

Figure 15.18 (A) This 30-year-old patient introduced himself for dental treatment of his upper diastema and color mismatched dentition.

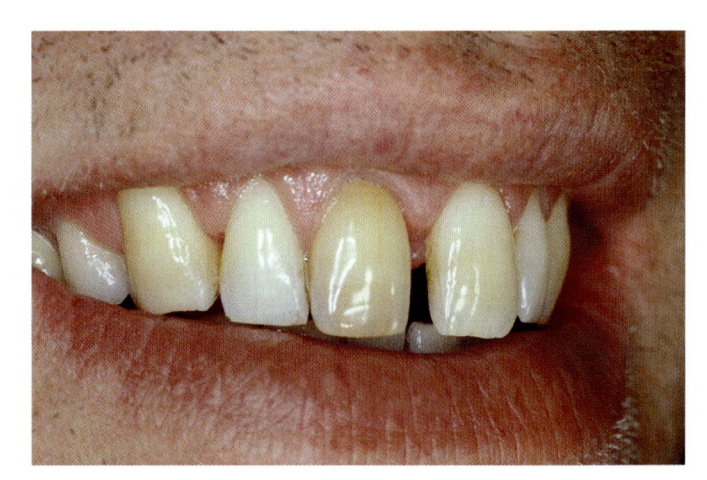

Figure 15.18 (B) The diastema between the two central incisors measured close to 3 mm. Also teeth #6, #8, and #11 were almost two shades darker than the adjacent teeth.

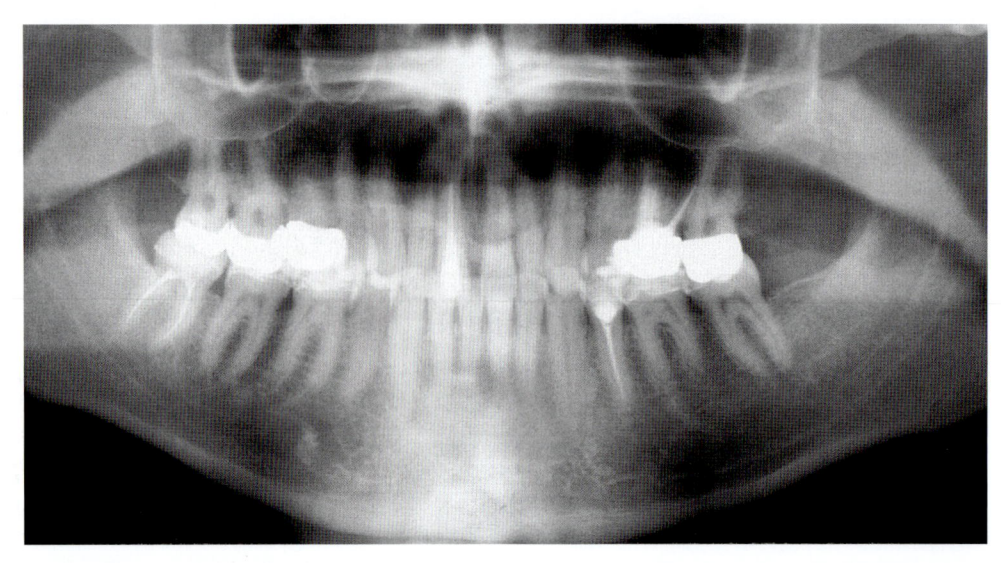

Figure 15.18 (C) Orthopantomogram demonstrates multiple posterior restorations, including a number of endodontic treatments, especially also for tooth #8.

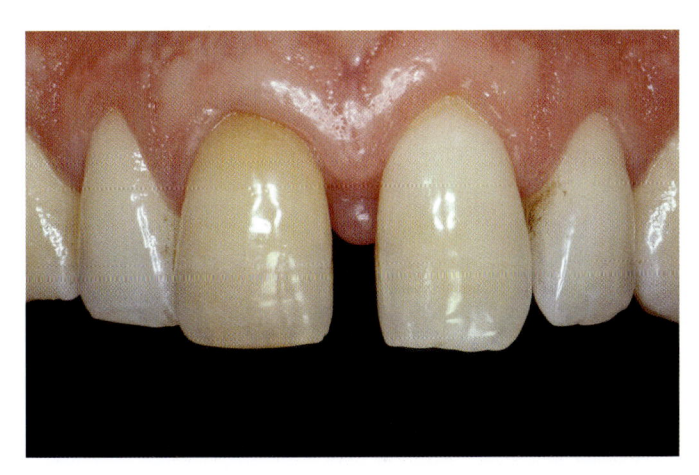

Chapter 15   Ceramic Veneers and Partial-Coverage Restorations

Figure 15.18 **(D)** Close-up view of the facial display of teeth #6–#11. Tooth #9 showed off-axis labial disposition, yet gingival conditions were stable.

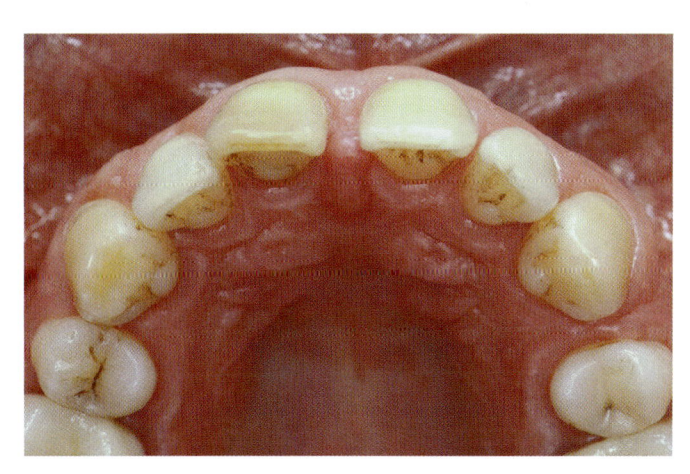

Figure 15.18 **(E)** Occlusal overview of the anterior dentition.

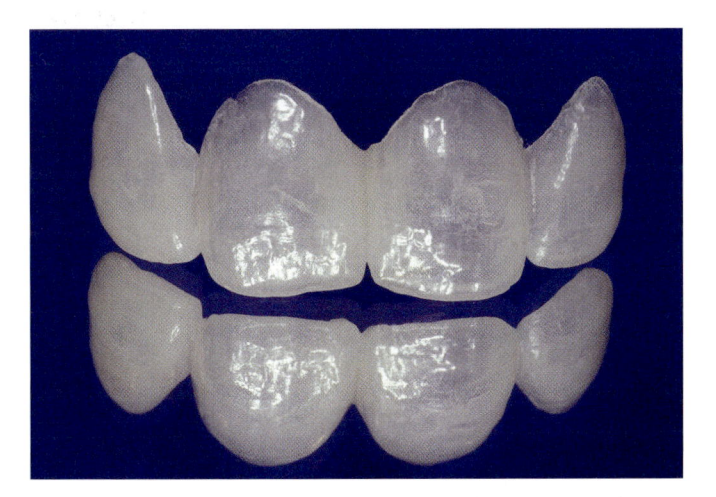

Figure 15.18 **(F)** Pre-fabricated shell provisional to restore teeth #7–#10 temporarily after extended veneer preparation.

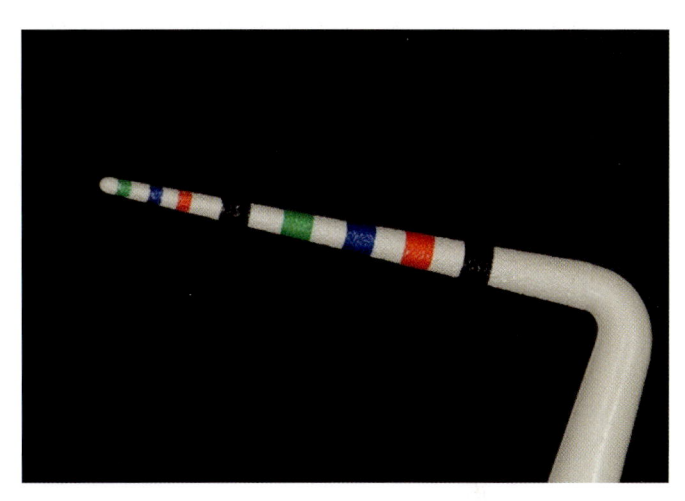

Figure 15.18 **(G)** The Goldstein multicolored ColorVue Probe (Hu-Friedy) is a useful device for measuring proper depth when preparing teeth for porcelain veneers since the tip of the probe to the red mark is in 0.5 mm increments and 1 mm increments afterwards.

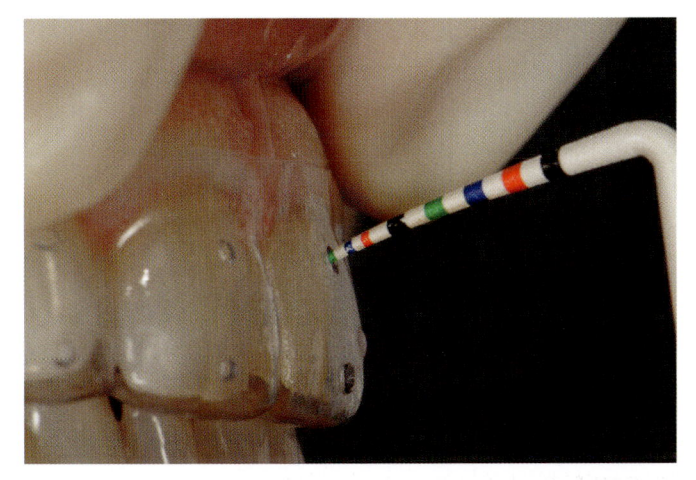

Figure 15.18 **(H)** A vacuform matrix with small holes for both gingival and incisal reduction combined with the bright colors of the probe assure sufficient uniform reduction for proper porcelain thickness.

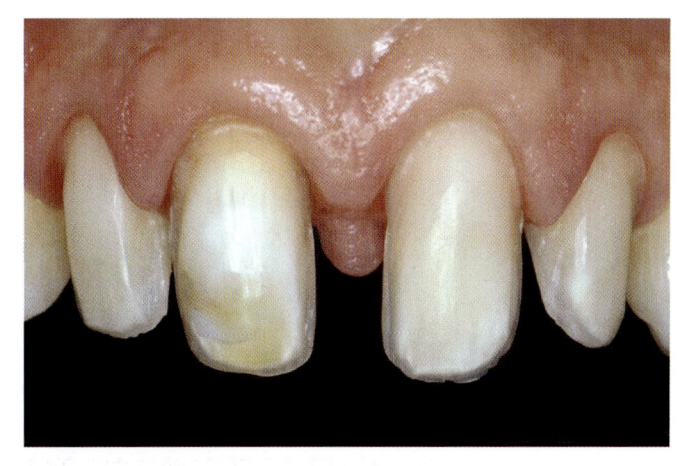

Figure 15.18 **(I)** Following a wax-up and model analysis, a butt joint veneer preparation was performed for teeth #7–#10 to allow for better distribution of spaces between the teeth. It was panned to extend the incisal width of the lateral incisors to balance wider central incisors to close the diastema space. The patient was not interested in orthodontic treatment.

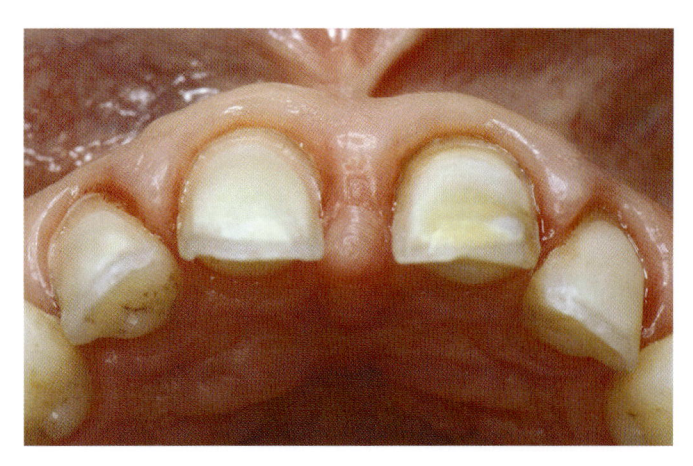

Figure 15.18 **(J)** Occlusal view of the anterior veneer preparations, following the arch form.

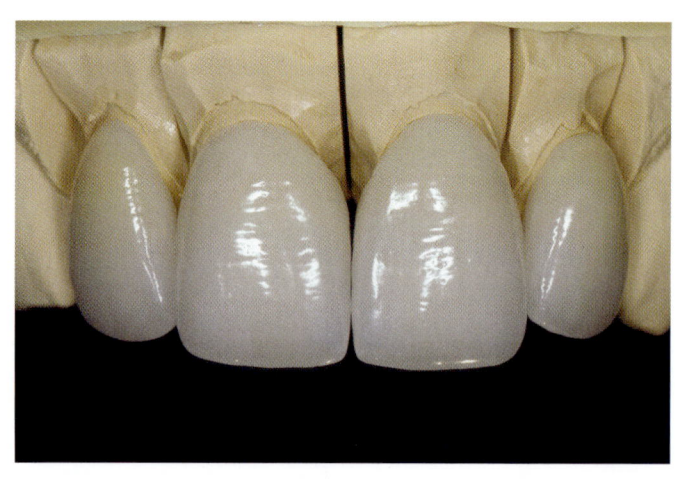

Figure 15.18 **(K)** Master cast of the final lithium-disilicate e.max Press restorations, utilizing the cut-back technique.

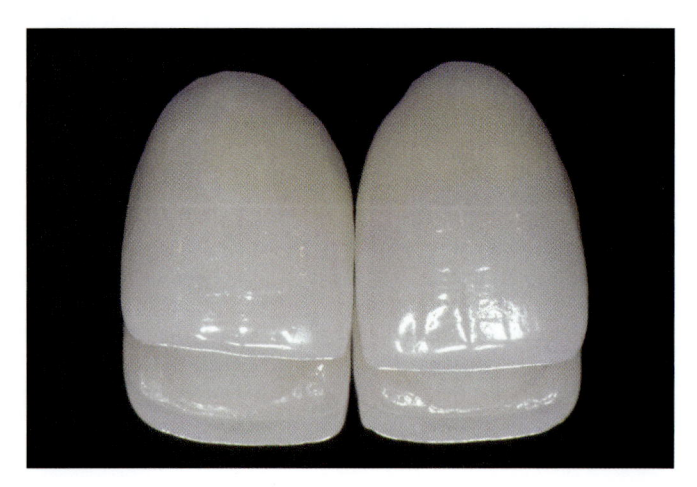

Figure 15.18 **(L)** Close-up of the two central incisor ceramic restorations to close the diastema.

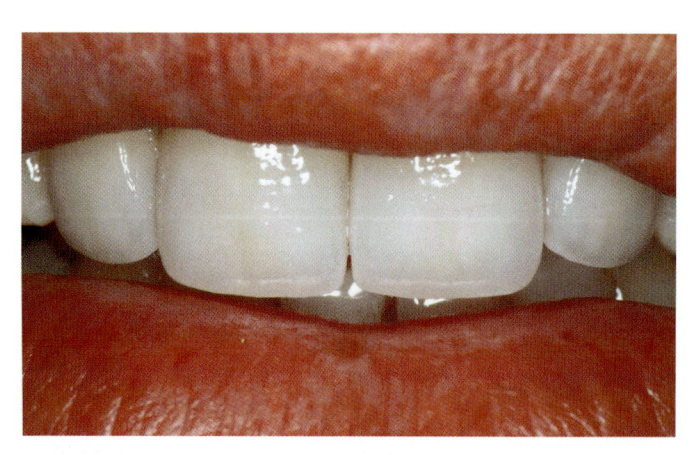

Figure 15.18 **(M)** Relaxed lip position under a light smile, displaying the upper anterior restorations after adhesive bonding under dry conditions.

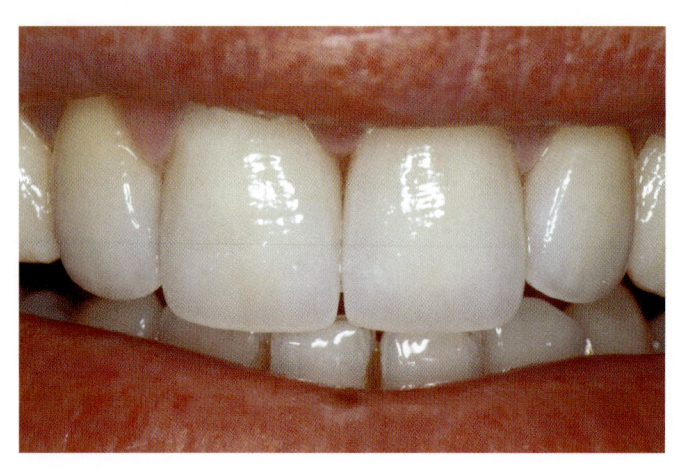

Figure 15.18 **(N)** Post-op facial view of the patients smile, four weeks after insertion.

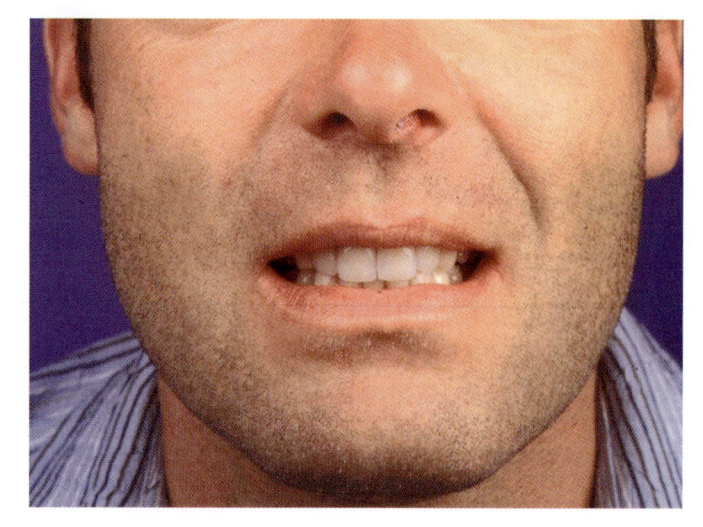

Figure 15.18 **(O)** Post-op: the patient's facial appearance and smile changed significantly. A week after the treatment, the patient showed improved self-confidence.

colored foods, tea, and coffee. And finally, the teeth can erode. Intrinsic erosion occurs primarily in anorexia nervosa or bulimia when gastric juices wash over the teeth during induced vomiting. But extrinsic erosion can also occur due to excessive consumption of acidic fruits and juices, which your patient should consume only at mealtimes or shortly before brushing.[101]

3. Home dental maintenance also takes on a slightly different nature. Instruct the patient to use a soft toothbrush with rounded bristles and to floss as with unrestored teeth. Maintenance of plaque-free teeth is essential to the longevity of the veneers as well as the health of the teeth and supportive tissues. Frequently the enamel has been lost and the softer dentin or cementum tends to decay much faster if not properly maintained. Mechanical plaque removal devices may be useful. In order to properly maintain cervical areas, especially when there is interdental tissue loss, a rotary cleaning device (Rotadent, DenMat) contains pointed brush tips that can easily clean these areas. The patient also should avoid acidulated phosphorus fluoride gels[102] or acidulated fluoridated mouthrinses, which can damage the surface finish of veneers. Nonacidic fluoride preparations (e.g. Prevident 1.1 % sodium fluoride; Prevident by Colgate Oral Pharmaceuticals or Clinpro 5000 by 3M ESPE) are effective in reducing caries and should be considered for patients with extensive porcelain or composite restorations.[103] Chlorhexidine antiplaque mouthrinses may stain veneers, although the stain can be removed by a hygienist.[68]

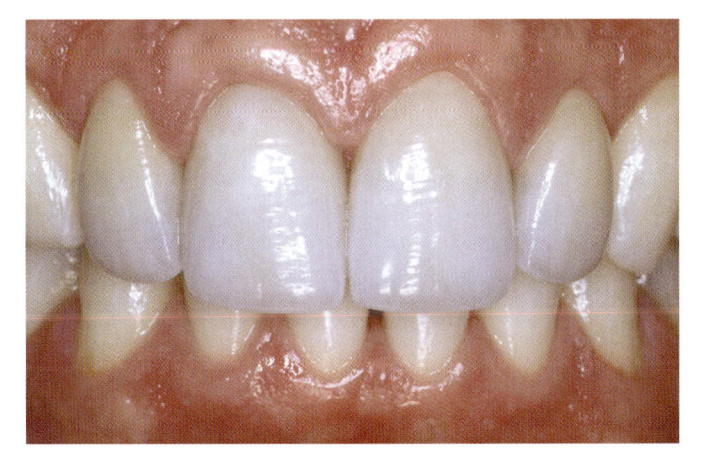

Figure 15.18 **(P)** Facial view of the intermaxillary anterior upper and lower dentition with extended ceramic restorations after 4 weeks.

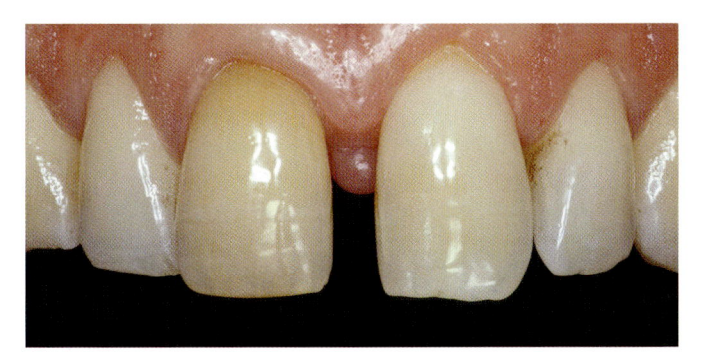

Figure 15.18 **(Q)** Facial view of the intermaxillary anterior upper dentition *before* extended ceramic restorations.

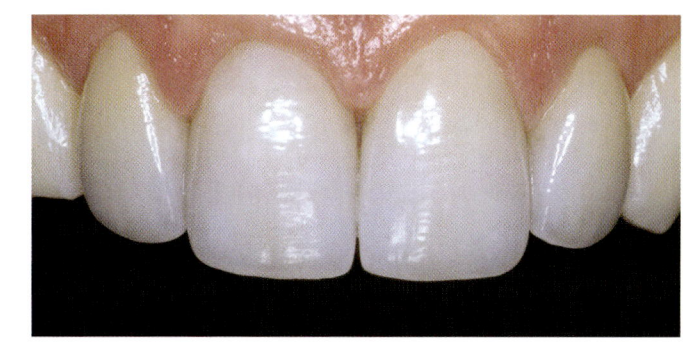

Figure 15.18 **(R)** Facial view of the intermaxillary anterior upper dentition *after* extended ceramic restorations.

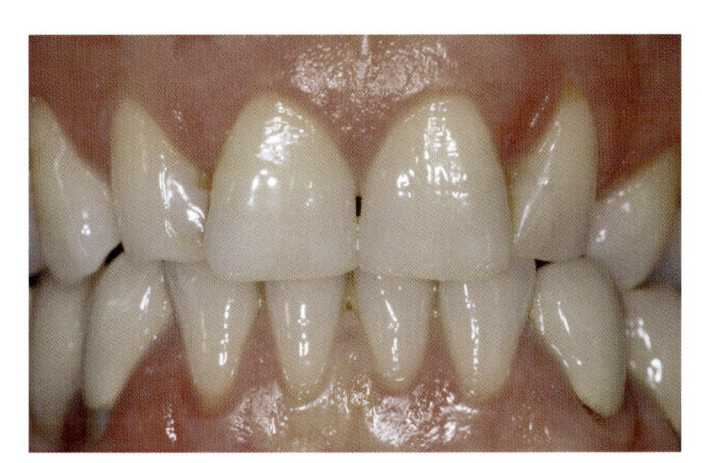

Figure 15.19 **(A)** A 44-year-old female patient presented with anterior crowding and bilateral reduction of the buccal corridor. Tooth #11 was missing and the first bicuspid had been moved orthodontically into the canine position, causing a crossbite occlusion on the left side. The patient refused additional orthodontic treatment.

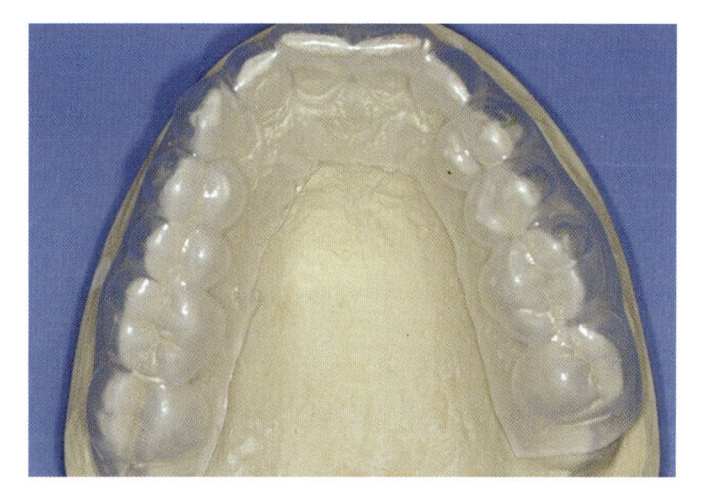

Figure 15.19 **(B)** Due to discoloration, multiple composite fillings, and tooth position, the patient mainly disliked her upper anterior dentition. Following dental hygiene treatment, home bleaching trays were fabricated.

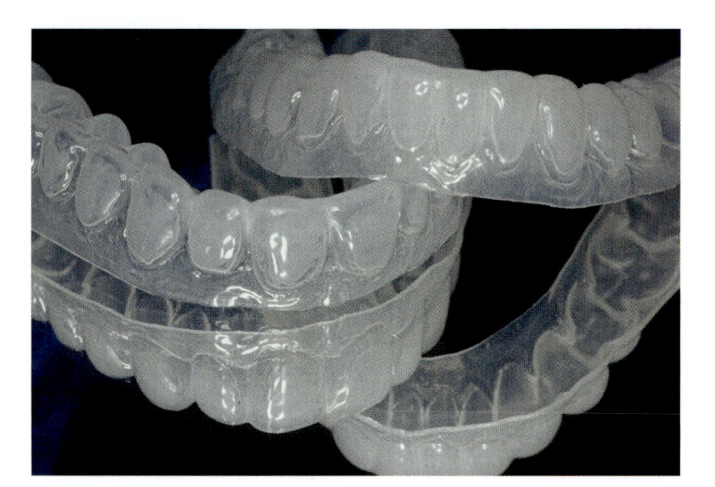

Figure 15.19 **(C)** Patient was instructed to perform six overnight sessions of home bleaching with 15% carbamide peroxide gel in the upper and lower jaw. The patient refused treatment on the lower crowns #22 and #27.

Posterior ceramic partial coverage restorations

Directly placed composite resins have made a tremendous impact on the field of esthetic restorations. But the current limitations of direct composites are most evident when you are working with posterior teeth.[104] The development of long-term wear-resistant, direct composite restorations that could stand up to the stresses of posterior occlusion and mastication has proven difficult.[105] Problems include fracture, post-insertion sensitivity, microleakage, loss of surface integrity, occlusal and proximal surface wear, and difficulty securing and maintaining interproximal contact.[106,107] Posterior composite placement and finishing techniques are markedly more difficult than for anterior teeth. When porcelain was introduced to restore the posterior dentition, Wiley[108] reviewed concerns of the potentially destructive nature of porcelain on the occluding surface. He concluded that the type of opposing occlusion should be the

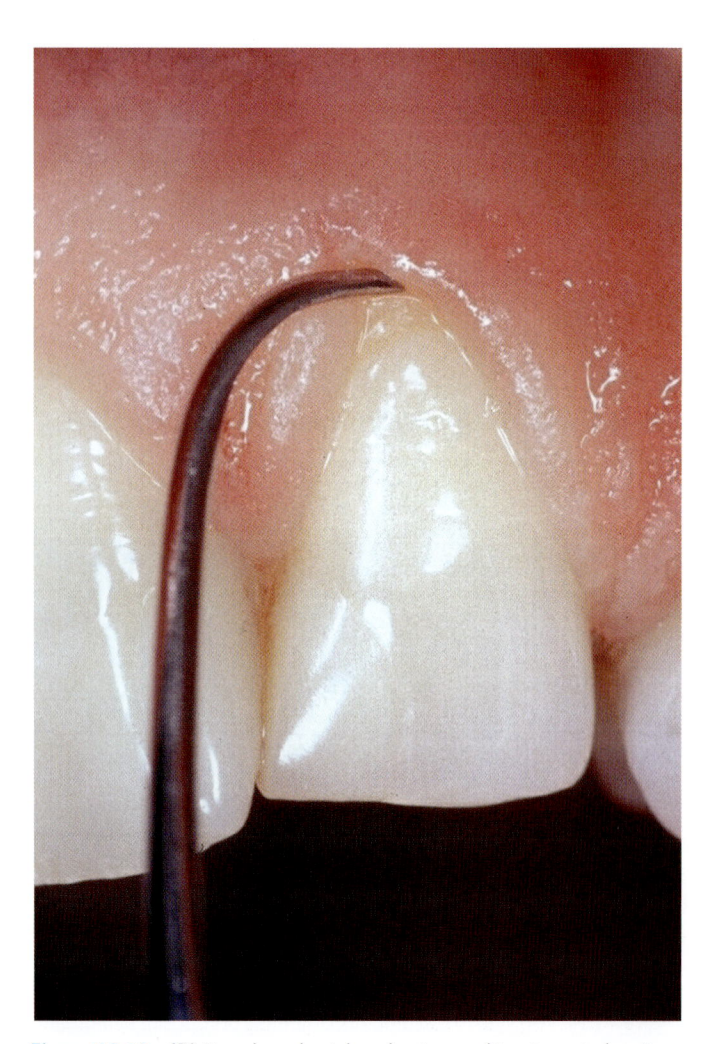

Figure 15.19 **(D)** Based on dental evaluation and treatment planning, a wax-up indicated a significant change with five partial coverage and full veneers. Soft tissue evaluation indicated the need for recession coverage of tooth #10.

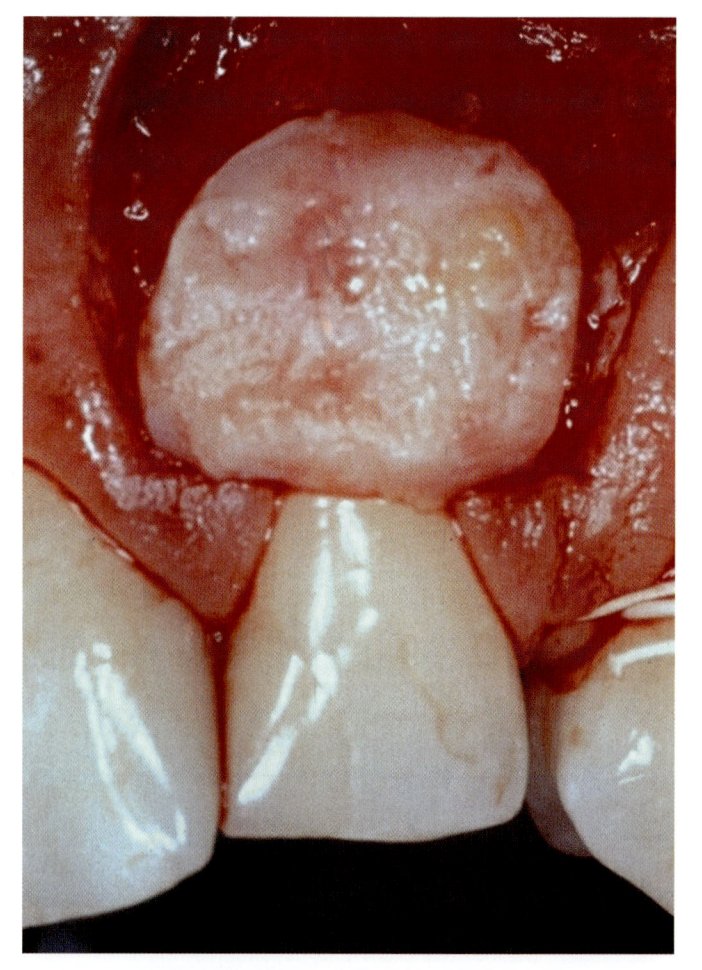

Figure 15.19 **(E)** Recession coverage with a connective tissue graft was performed on tooth #10.

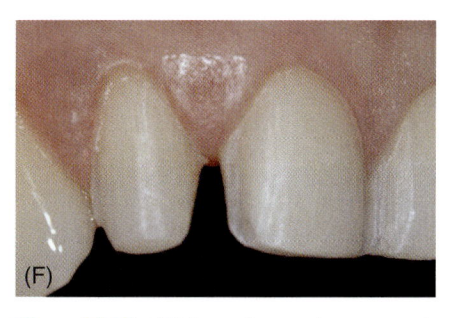

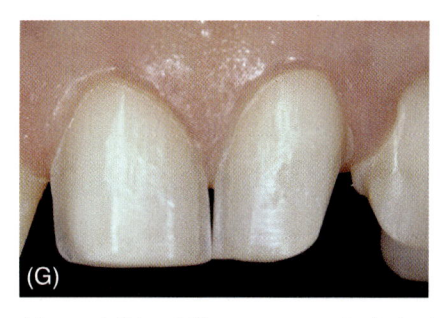

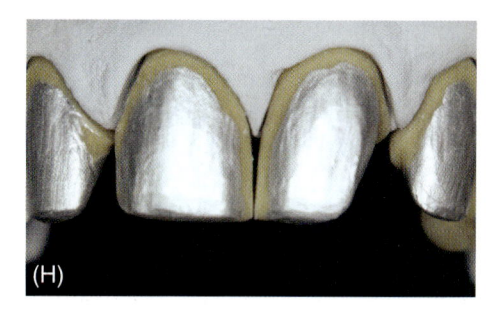

Figure 15.19 **(F)** According to the preparation guide, teeth #7 and #8 were prepared subgingival, including all the areas of former composite restorations. Tooth #7 required a full veneer preparation (360° veneer) and tooth #8 a facial incisal overlap preparation with a butt joint. **(G)** Due to a distal defect, tooth #9 required a combination of an incisal overlap and distal partial coverage veneer preparation. A full veneer preparation was performed at tooth #10. **(H)** A master model was fabricated to generate ceramic IPS Empress pressed veneers. Thin spacer was applied to the prepared surfaces, sparing the preparation margins.

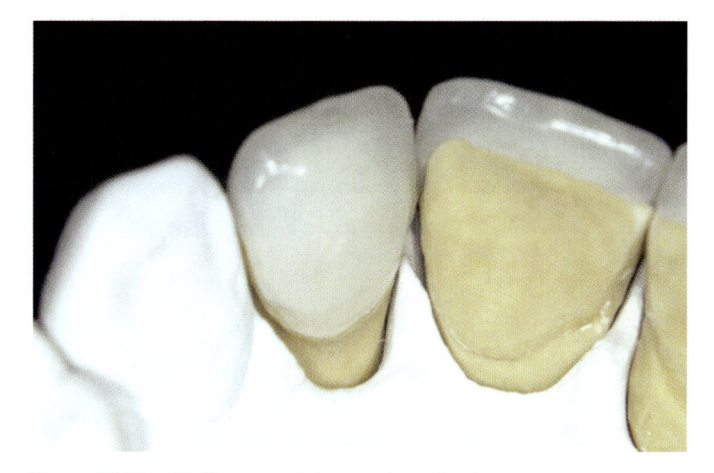

Figure 15.19 **(I)** When possible, anterior palatal tooth contact positions in centric should remain on natural tooth structure.[26] Defect size or tooth anatomy might require palatal tooth structure coverage shown at teeth #7 and #10.

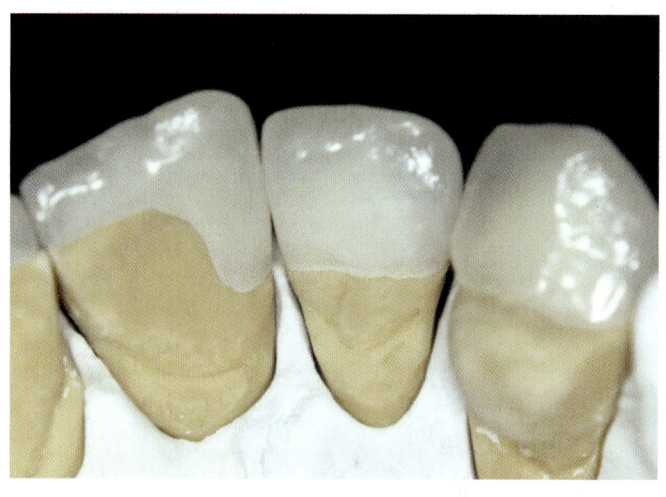

Figure 15.19 **(J)** The preparation on tooth #12 was adapted to create the illusion of an existing canine #11. The preparation extended from the occlusal surfaces to the lingual cervical side.

major consideration. Porcelain occluding against porcelain works best, with the least amount of opposing wear. The next best solutions would be porcelain against composite, then porcelain against enamel, and the worst is porcelain against gold, which can produce severe wear of the gold surface. Many researchers and clinical dentists recommend that composite resins be restricted to smaller posterior restorations not subject to strong occlusal forces.[109]

Although new developments continually improve the composite resins used for indirect inlays and onlays, ceramic has numerous advantages as described previously throughout this chapter.[110] Porcelain is most like enamel in appearance and most closely approximates its physical and chemical properties. Etched porcelain bonds successfully to etched enamel, with excellent marginal qualities, when a composite resin-based cement is used.[111] This bond to the tooth preparation is what gives porcelain, which by itself has a highly breakable nature, its strength as a dental restoration.[112] New glass-ceramic materials with improved mechanical properties and higher inert fracture strength, plus the progress in adhesive bonding techniques including dentin-enamel conditioning, and further developments of luting composites,[113] replaced porcelain for the application of posterior all-ceramic partial coverage restorations.

In general, the longevity of ceramic inlays, onlays and partial coverage restorations depends on many factors.[47,98,114–116] The processing- and operator-related factors include experience of the operator, correct indication, cavity preparation (size, type, finishing), impression technique, correct choice of the ceramic material and experience with the material, handling and application, cementation material and process, correct occlusion, and recall schedule. The patient-related factors include oral hygiene, preventive measures, compliance in recall, oral environment (for instance, quality of tooth structure, saliva), size, shape, location of the lesion and tooth (number of surfaces, vital versus nonvital tooth, premolar versus molar), cooperation during treatment, bruxism, habits (high sugar intake, smoking, frequent chewing of hard foods), and participation in contact sports. Long-term clinical studies with observation periods of up to 12 years showed that the survival rates of ceramic inlays, onlays, and partial coverage restorations might range between 74 and 100%.[47,114]

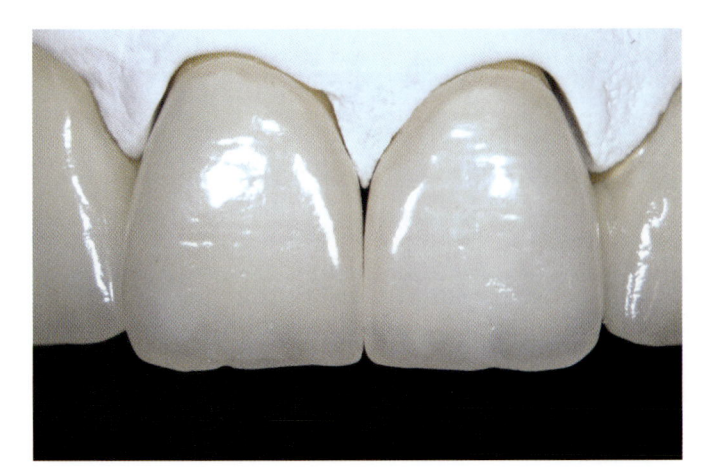

Figure 15.19 **(K)** Finalized ceramic IPS Empress pressed veneers, using the cut-back technique at the facial surfaces in combination with coloring and glazed finishing.

Indications

Etched ceramic partial coverage restorations are suitable for any clinical situation for which porcelain's superior esthetics, ability to restore strength to compromised teeth, and conservative treatment are indicated. The list of indications presented by Garber[50] remains current:

1. Small to moderate carious lesions for which the patient requests a highly esthetic restoration.
2. Large amalgam or composite restorations involving the mesio- or distolingual surface of a cuspid showing unacceptable discoloration or compromised contacts.
3. Large carious or traumatic lesions with undermined enamel to the extent that a cast metal restoration or a full crown would otherwise be necessary. In these situations the crosslinked resin-bonded ceramic restoration will bond to the remaining tooth structure, binding it together into what is, in effect, a homogeneous mass.
4. The endodontically compromised tooth where the access cavity has compromised the strength and prognosis of the tooth. An etched ceramic restoration can be a conservative alternative to a post-and-core and full-coverage crown.
5. Heavily undermined occlusal edge or proximal surface on a tooth requiring support to keep an otherwise pleasing intact tooth from fracturing.
6. Class IV restorations replacing missing occlusal and/or proximal aspects of the tooth.
7. Teeth opposed by existing porcelain restorations, which otherwise would tend to wear extensively.

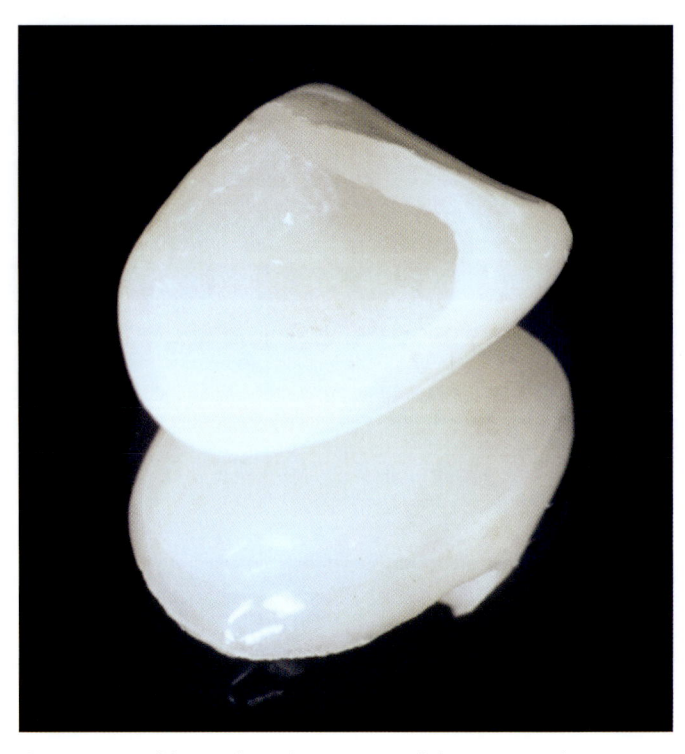

Figure 15.19 **(L)** Incisal overlap veneer with butt joint ending demonstrates the advantage of a metal free restoration.

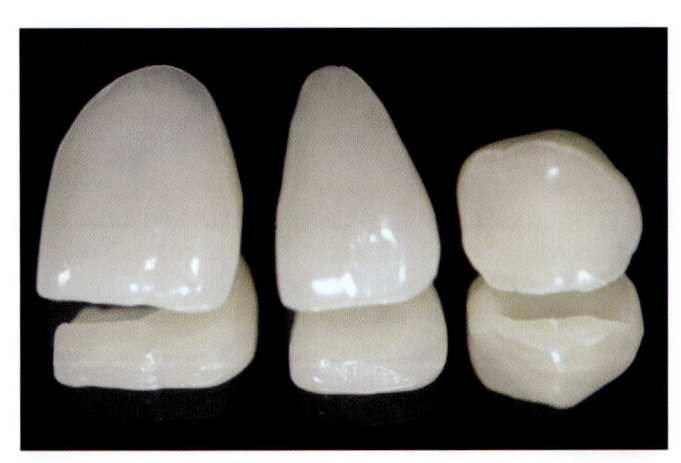

Figure 15.19 **(M)** Three pressed ceramic partial coverage and full veneers to restore teeth #10–#12. Restoration #12 demonstrates canine contour facially and occlusally.

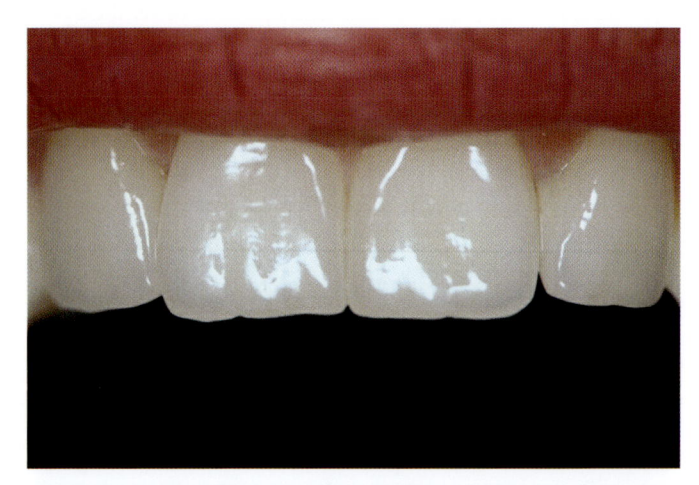

Figure 15.19 **(N)** Follow-up 15 month after insertion of the anterior veneer restorations. Tooth proportion and position of central and lateral incisors had been corrected.

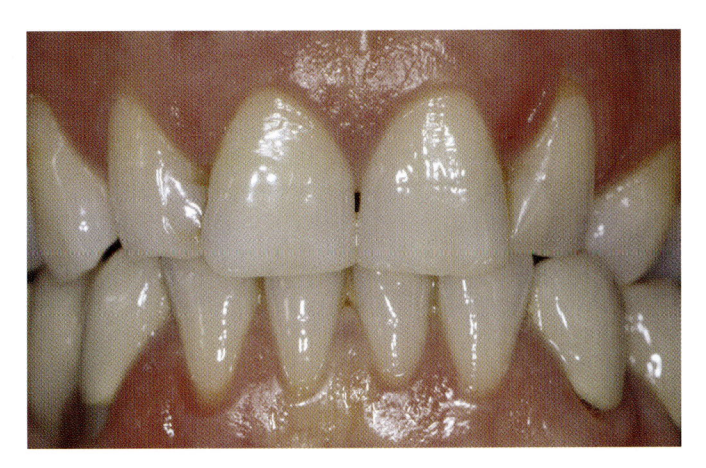

Figure 15.19 **(O)** Before the treatment with ceramic veneers, the patient was dissatisfied with function and esthetic appearance of her anterior teeth.

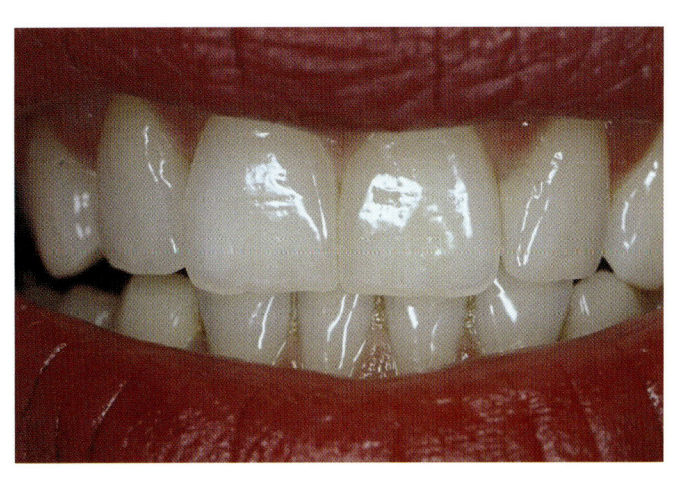

Figure 15.19 **(P)** After treatment: The patient liked the new appearance of her anterior dentition. Especially the changes on the left side, correcting the cross bite and reshaping a canine, had a significant impact on the symmetry of her smile. The restorations were inserted in 1999 and are still in place.

8. Teeth where it is difficult to develop retention form. The bonded restoration's adhesive nature may be more effective than other means of developing retention such as pins, periodontal crown lengthening, or a post and core after elective endodontic therapy.
9. Patients for whom allergy to metal is proven or suspected.

Contraindications

1. Patients who will continue excessive parafunctional habits that can damage the ceramic restoration.
2. Patients who exhibit aggressive wear.
3. Patients who have gold restorations in opposing teeth.
4. Ceramic posterior partial coverage restorations are not simple, and this factor needs to be considered against all the numerous advantages and the situations in which they are an excellent solution to a restorative problem. The problems of maintaining a dry field, obtaining precisely fabricated restorations, and the necessary high degree of attention to detail during placement have been called by Garber a "contraindication in itself" for many dentists.[50]

Many advantages can be gained by preserving as much of the healthy tooth structure as possible. This can be achieved best by using a defect-oriented tooth preparation. The general benefits of using partial coverage preparations are as follows:

1. Preserving healthy tooth structure.[47]
2. Facilitating superior periodontal health.[28,47,98]
3. Facilitating cementation without hydrolytic behavior.[22,117,118]
4. Preserving the pulp's health.[47,48,98]
5. Preserving the tooth's anatomical shape.[17,47]
6. Facilitating visual margin control.[47,97,114]
7. Facilitating easier performance of oral hygiene for the patient.[73,74,97]
8. Improving the reliability of tooth vitality testing.[21,98,114,119]

Technique: preparation

Laboratory requirements for fabrication of ceramic restorations, as compared to cast gold restorations, require certain preparation modification. Cavity preparation is somewhat simpler than for gold.[120] All line and point angles should be rounded to facilitate fabrication and decrease the potential for propagation of fractures. The cavosurface angle need not be beveled, and a hollow-ground chamfer confined to the marginal enamel will aid in developing a more effective seal.[50,121]

The basic premise of the preparation is to preserve all that remains; unlike some other restorations, only those aspects of the tooth already compromised by caries or trauma should be reshaped. This should be done before deciding on the definitive form of the preparation and final restoration.

To achieve the rounded angles needed for porcelain, the preparation is performed with a two-grit diamond in the shape of a tapered cylinder having a flat end and a rounded "corner" when the flat end and shank meet. It is favorable to produce a flat pulpal floor with calculated divergent axial walls and a rounded line angle between the two highly retentive axial walls, which increases the surface area for bonding and develops mechanical retention. Finally, a well-defined cavosurface margin at the occlusal surface is necessary to develop the hollow-ground chamfer at the margin.[50]

When using strength enhanced glass-ceramic materials, Stappert et al.[23] concluded that a defect-oriented tooth preparation in the posterior region for the restoration of a compromised tooth with a partial-coverage ceramic restoration is justifiable. All-ceramic partial coverage restorations for molars made of IPS e.max Press are fracture-resistant, showing results comparable with those of natural unprepared teeth. The preparation designs in this study include standard mesio-occlusal-distal (MOD) inlay, MOD with reduction of mesiopalatal cusp, MOD with reduction of both palatal cusps, MOD with reduction of both palatal and distobuccal cusps, and MOD with reduction of all cusps. Ceramic coverage of compromised cusps did not demonstrate an increase in fracture resistance after fatigue when compared to less invasive partial coverage restorations.[122]

Stappert et al.[116] also showed that maxillary molars restored with IPS e.max Press and ProCad restorations survived loads within the range of physiological mastication forces.

Veneer onlay

There are times when you may wish to veneer the buccal surface of a posterior tooth but encounter a defective one-, two-, or three-surface posterior restoration.[123] The question is: should you further reduce the buccal wall and have only a strong lingual wall to help retention, or would it be better to save the buccal enamel? You could save the buccal wall by laminating the buccal surface and extending that veneer into the mesio-occlusodistal preparation, making it a "veneer onlay" (Figure 15.20E). Goldstein introduced the concept of a "laminate onlay" in 1998.[124] In 2005, Stappert called this a "veneer onlay," modified as "full veneer," for the treatment of premolars with cervical and occlusal/proximal defects or existing fillings for press ceramic materials in 2005.[27] Pressable e.max Press ceramic (first published as Experimental Press Ceramic, or EPC) was scientifically investigated for this application for the first time. Full veneers made of e.max Press ceramic reached fracture strength values corresponding to those of natural unprepared premolars. All-ceramic full veneers for premolars offer an excellent esthetic solution for premolars with multiple defects and proved to be highly fracture-resistant restorations[27] (Figure 15.20A–G). Therefore, this form of treatment should be considered as a less invasive and esthetic alternative to full crowns. In 2015, McLaren, Figueira, and Goldstein used the term "vonlay" to further describe the technique. The technique used feldspathic porcelain and, according to Goldstein, it never caught on mainly because of fear of fracture in the posterior with the then available materials and bonding techniques.[125]

Impression

Impressions for posterior etched porcelain are best taken digitally or with PVS. Since the gingival margin ends in a rounded shoulder, tissue displacement with retraction cord should be sufficient to obtain an excellent, easy-to-read impression of this area.

Insertion

Insertion for the etched porcelain restorations involves try-ins, one at a time, then in groups if necessary. The occlusion should not be evaluated until all of the restorations are initially seated.

Cementation of posterior ceramic inlays, onlays, and partial coverage restorations is similar to anterior veneers with certain differences. Foremost is the consideration that the inlay, onlay, or partial coverage restoration is much thicker than the anterior veneer, requiring more emphasis on a dual cement, or self-curing cement, to bond properly.[126]

Usually, once the shade was taken properly and the ceramic ingot chosen accordingly, the ceramic restoration matches or blends sufficiently to the residual tooth structure. Due to the increased thickness of a partial coverage restoration when compared to a veneer, the influence of the luting composite has less impact on enhancing the color of the final restoration. However, there are times when it takes a significant amount of opacifier or stain to influence the shade of the cement sufficiently to blend the color of a ceramic posterior restoration that is too light for the tooth.

Finishing

A major consideration in cementation of posterior restorations is the attention that must be paid to removing excess cement in the interproximal areas. The LVS-5 should remove all excess resin cement. A Mylar strip through the intact areas during polymerization should only be used if it is approximately 0.002 mm thick or less (matrix strips made of Dupont Mylar 0.002 gauge, 10 cm × 1 cm; Henry Schein). The danger in using

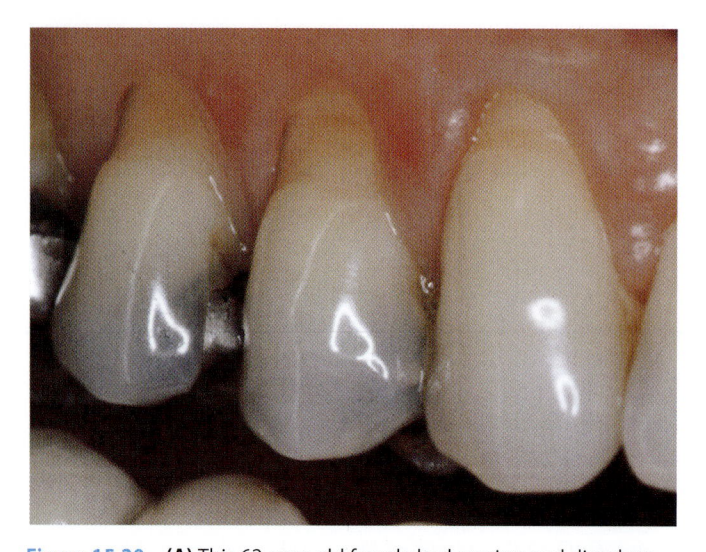

Figure 15.20 **(A)** This 62-year-old female had erosion and discoloration of her maxillary teeth. She was particularly concerned about the defective amalgam restorations showing through the maxillary right bicuspids and first molar.

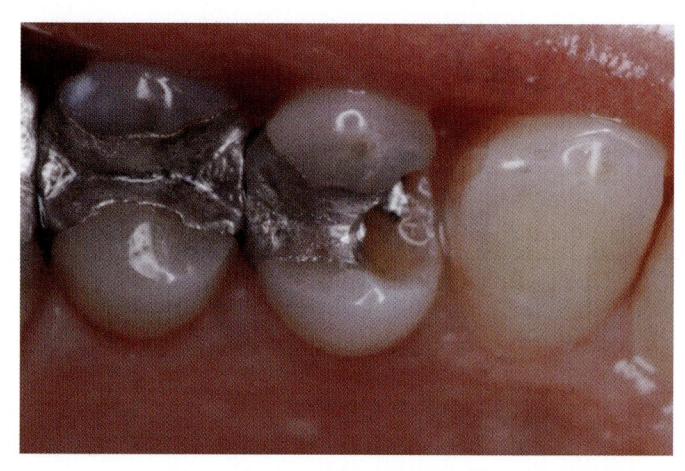

Figure 15.20 **(B)** The occlusal view shows how closely involved the posterior amalgams were to the buccal surface. Choices for treating this problem were posterior composites, posterior ceramic inlays/onlays, or full crowns. The compromise solution was the veneer onlay.

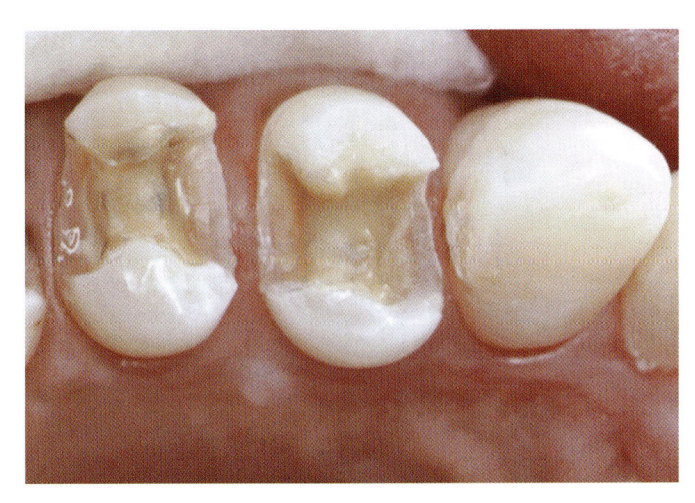

Figure 15.20 **(C)** CIP-I (Brasseler USA) diamond was used to prepare the occlusal portion, removing all defective amalgam, and then glass ionomer liners were placed as build-ups for the dentin defects.

anything thicker than this is in the increased possibility of not fully seating the restoration. It is wiser to insert the ceramic restoration and carefully observe the cementation set, using a 5–8 s polymerization time, and then removing the interproximal excess cement before final polymerization. Make sure that floss will clear the contact area. If the floss does not go through, an ET3 or end-cutting ET may be successful in removing the excess. Another quick way to break through the contact is to use a interproximal finishing and contouring strip (Brasseler ET Flex or Qwik Strip, Kerr). However, if some of these thin pieces remain, they may eventually be dislodged through normal occlusal function. Therefore, have the patient go home with a well-balanced occlusion, and check within 1 week to attempt clearing the contact area if excess cement still remains. Occlusal adjustment is accomplished by using the OS1 in a 30-or 15 µm grit. If necessary, the OS2 then places or corrects initial grooves, followed by the OS3 for final groove finishing plus smoothing of any pits or fissures. The final finishing is done with either a 30-bladed carbide or 8-mm diamond (DETUF series). Final polishing can be accomplished with impregnated points then porcelain polishers such as Dialite Feather Lite spiral porcelain polishers in sequence (Brasseler USA).

Patient instructions

Instructions to patients with new partial coverage restorations are similar to those for porcelain veneers, with emphasis on good homecare and plaque removal.

Alternative techniques

The production of ceramic restorations using the lost-wax press technique has been addressed already; yet modern CAD/CAM technology also allows fabricating veneers, inlays, onlays, and partial coverage restorations with similar precision and significant less laboratory procedures. Two representative CAD/CAM systems will be introduced, the CEREC and the Carestream systems.

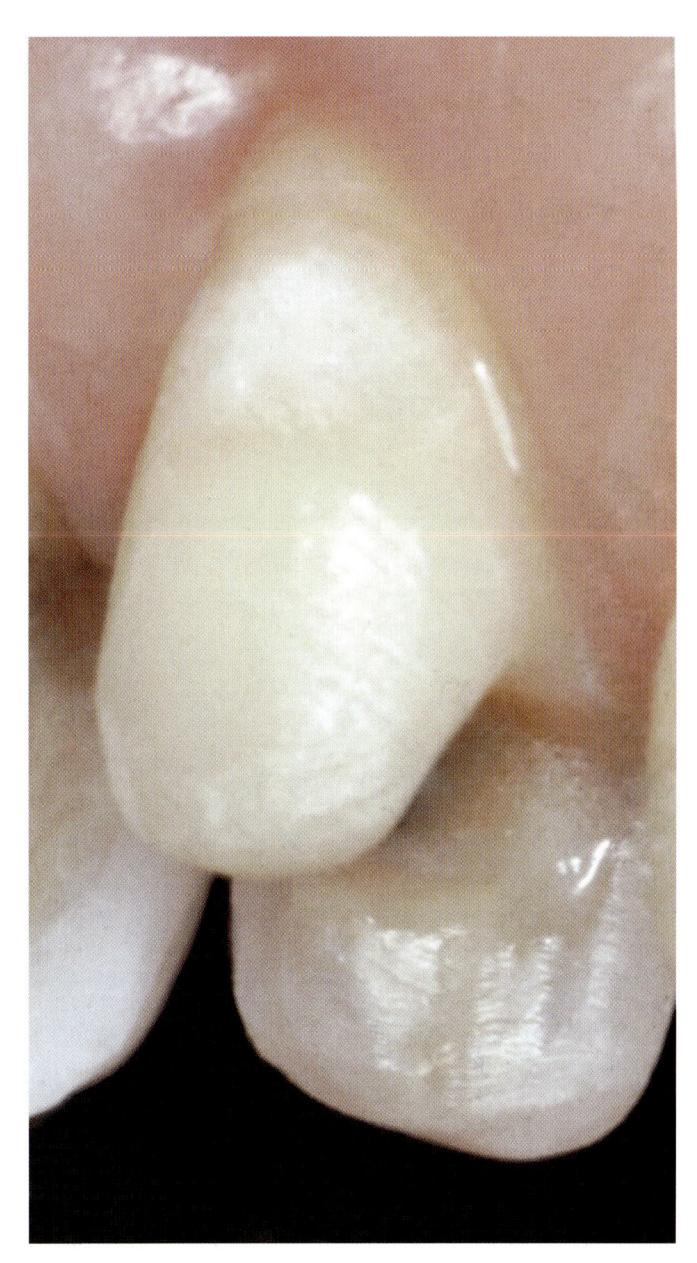

Figure 15.20 **(D)** The buccal view shows that the bucco-occlusal wall is reduced sufficiently so that the porcelain can lap over to the occlusal surface and have sufficient thickness and strength to resist breakage.

The CEREC system

The field of dentistry has witnessed a remarkable transformation in many areas, especially when considering digital impression technology for manufacturing indirect restorations. Ever since the development of CEREC, an acronym for *ce*ramic *re*construction, by W. Mörmann and M. Brandestini, the profession has taken advantage of providing same-day dentistry while maintaining quality in a best-practices approach. This CAD/CAM technology has evolved for the better part of 30 years; however, despite its longevity in the field, CEREC has made significant advances in recent years, not just on the technology frontier, but also as an increased treatment modality for the general practitioner. CEREC (Sirona) integrates computer technology with CAD/CAM and infrared optical imaging cameras,

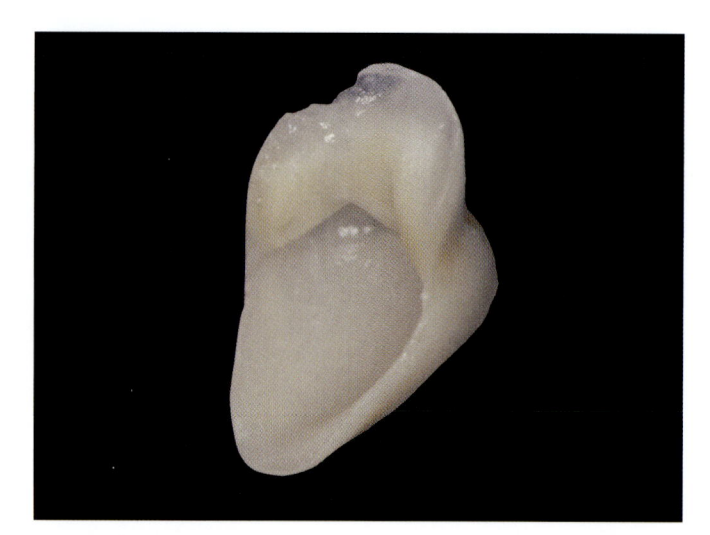

Figure 15.20 **(E)** This view of the veneer onlay shows the buccal portion and how it is connected to the posterior inlay portion.

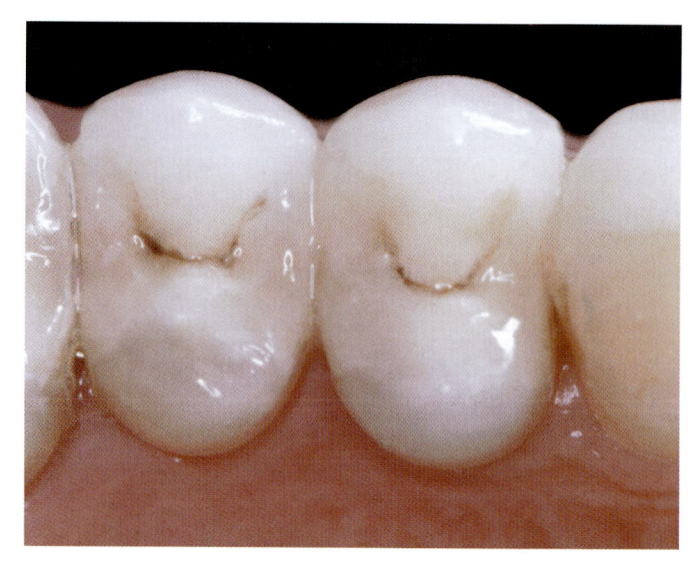

Figure 15.20 **(F)** This occlusal view shows the veneers cemented in place. Occlusion is correctly supported and there have been no fractures in the 20 year postoperative history.

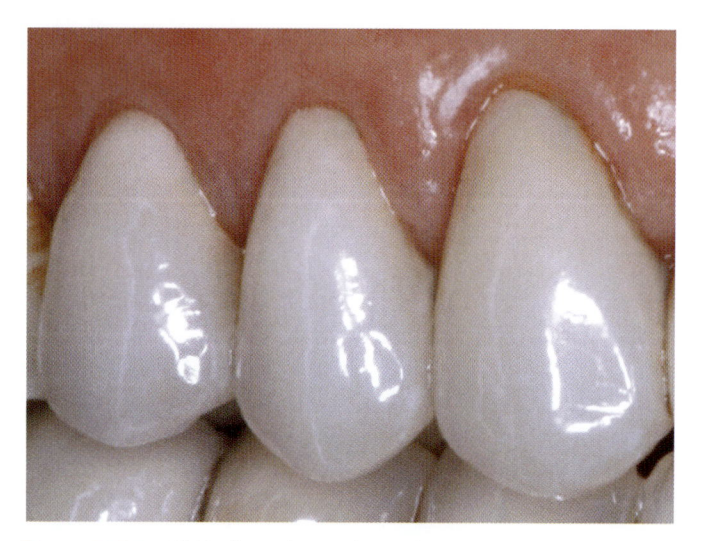

Figure 15.20 **(G)** The buccal view shows that the veneer onlays blend in as if they were full crowns. This means that on normal viewing the restoration looks more like a natural tooth, even more so than a simple veneer, which may not overlap onto the occlusal surface.

which then allows the design and milling of these porcelain/ceramic materials.

The system's chief appeal is its immediacy: restorations can be milled, fitted, seated, and finished in a single appointment. Another advantage of computer-generated restorations is that they provide a more economical restoration than the traditional, laboratory-produced ones. CEREC saves time and costs for both patient and dentist since it eliminates the impression, temporary restoration, and laboratory. Limitations of the early CEREC systems included their inability to do internal staining and the presence of greater marginal gaps than with conventional, indirect laboratory methods. The later generation, CEREC 3 was introduced based on 3D technology, while the first three models were based on 2D technology. 3D software was introduced in 2003, and allowed dentists to construct restorations based on virtual 3D models using the computer. Since 2006 software versions have included the options of automatic adjustment of a selected digital full-crown anatomy to the individual preparation, the proximal contacts, and the occlusion.[127] The latest software (CEREC software version 4.5.1) simplified the user interface that allows dentists to work on several restorations with a single process.

The CEREC Omnicam, launched in 2012, has many advantages over its predecessors. The main benefit is its ability to continuously acquire data, generating a 3D model in a powder-free manner. The length of the camera sleeve is 108 mm, the height and width of the tip are 18 mm, and it weighs 313 g. The size and weight allows the digital impression to be quickly taken, which is beneficial to the dentist and most importantly the patient.

In addition to the inlays and onlays produced by the original systems, the later generations are much more diverse, allowing the practitioner to manufacture veneers and crowns with the basic milling operating system.[74] The different ceramic materials even with the basic milling hardware include feldspar ceramic, glass-ceramic, lithium disilicate, translucent zirconium oxide (TZI), and hybrid and mono-sized polymer blocks. There is also a multitude of packages for the hardware and software if the practitioner is interested in complete autonomy from a dental laboratory. If the practitioner has an in-office laboratory, the possibilities allow access to the complete CAD/CAM spectrum including four-unit bridges, zirconium oxide and lithium disilicate abutments, and implant surgical guides. The practitioner can also digitally impress a field to be restored and send the digital information to a chosen laboratory via Sirona Connect, aiding in optimal dental esthetics. Another advantage of the CEREC system is utilizing integrated implantology for the surgical and prosthetic planning of implant placement.

There are now a multitude of ceramic blocks that can be selected depending on the type of indirect restoration. So, dentists can choose from an array of Sirona, Vita, 3M, or Ivoclar Vivadent blocks. Some of the commercially available ceramic blocks include feldspathic porcelain-based Vita Mark II, leucite glass-ceramic IPS Empress CAD, and lithium disilicate glass-ceramic IPS e.max CAD blocks.[128] Each block has advantages and disadvantages;

therefore, the dentist's knowledge of each available material is important.[115] Many factors need to be considered before choosing which material to use, but the most important factor to consider is the size of the preparation. The superior esthetics required for anterior restorations can easily be achieved through various forms of custom shade modification including external staining and in-office firing in a small porcelain furnace.[75]

CEREC uses a smaller diamond grain size to increase the marginal integrity of the restorations. There are different milling bur options, but as far as the orientation of the milling instruments, the left milling bur is a step bur designed to mill the intaglio surface of the restoration while the right milling bur is a cylinder pointed bur responsible for milling the occlusal surface of the restoration. These burs allow the restorations to be fabricated with significantly improved accuracy of ±25 μm.

Shade selection

Selecting the shade of the CEREC ceramic block requires visualizing the size, shape, and location of your intended restoration. Ideally, the dentist should determine the block shade at the outset before the tooth has had a chance to dry out and change color (Figure 15.21A–C). If color characterization is desired, you can make adjustments using stains or shaded bonding materials at the time of cementation. Conveniently, if the patient is dissatisfied with the crown after milling, a closer shade can be selected, finer detail can be adjusted to the restoration, and a new block can be milled if necessary.

Preparation

Clearly defined, smooth cavosurface and cervical preparation margins are recommended (Figure 15.21D–F). Important considerations for the practitioner are to avoid undercuts and "lips" or "spikes" specifically on the margin. Finally, finish the preparation with a fine or superfine bur to smooth all sharp angulations and artifacts. The reasoning behind this is the milling burs will not sacrifice material for the sharp artifact resulting in an inaccurate fit. It is important that the practitioner knows the minimal thickness requirements for each restorative material selected.

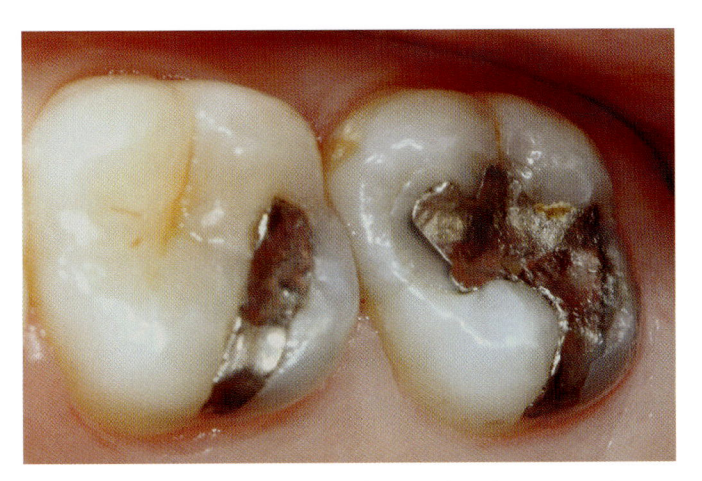

Figure 15.21 **(A)** Pre-op picture with secondary decay at teeth #14 and #15.

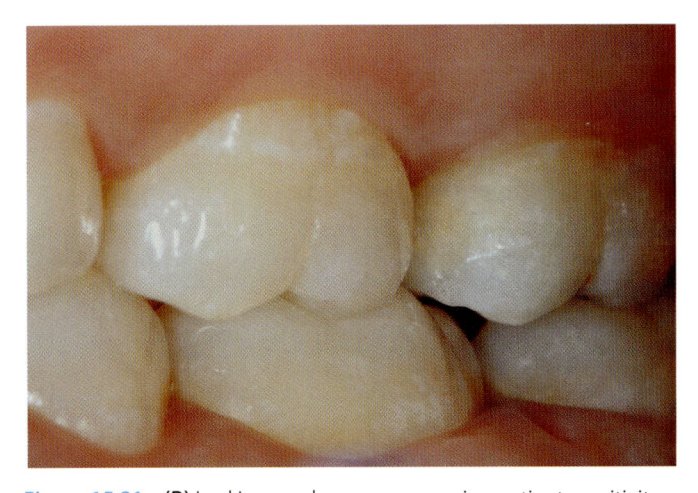

Figure 15.21 **(B)** Leaking amalgams were causing patient sensitivity.

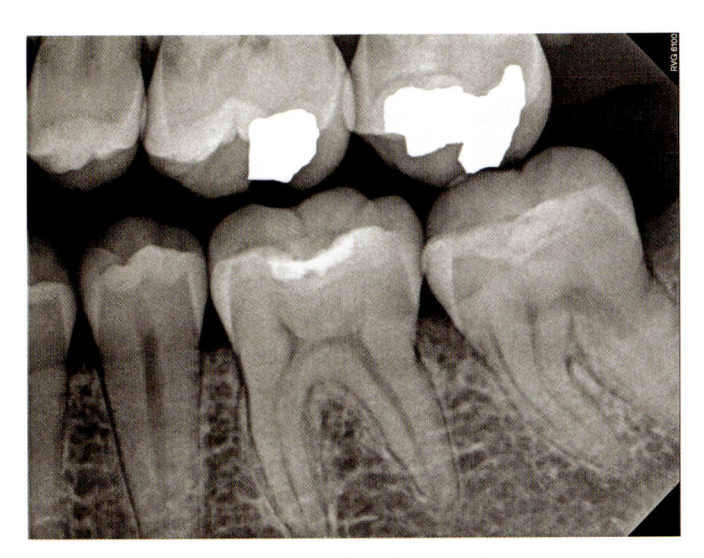

Figure 15.21 **(C)** Bitewing X-ray of teeth #14 and #15.

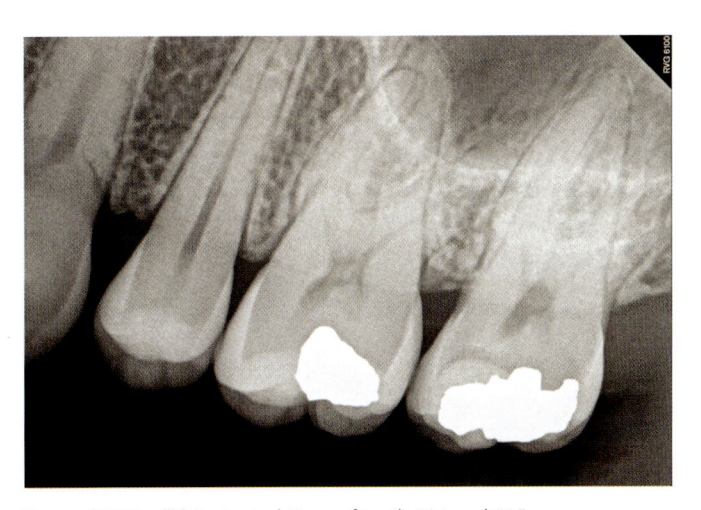

Figure 15.21 **(D)** Periapical X-ray of teeth #14 and #15.

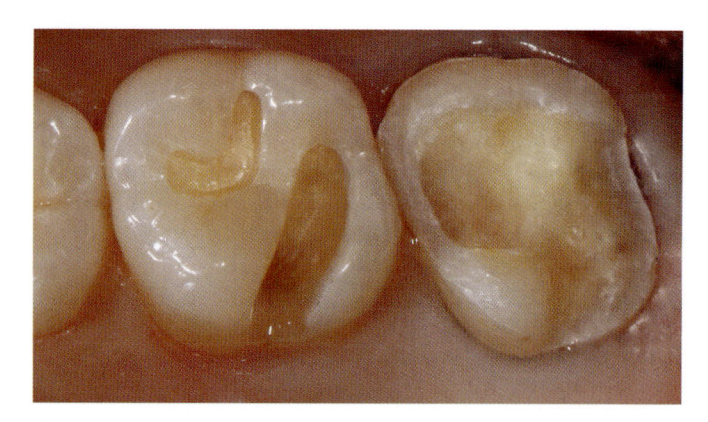

Figure 15.21 **(E)** Removal of amalgam restorations showed visible decay at teeth #14 and #15. Distal and lingual crack noted for tooth #15.

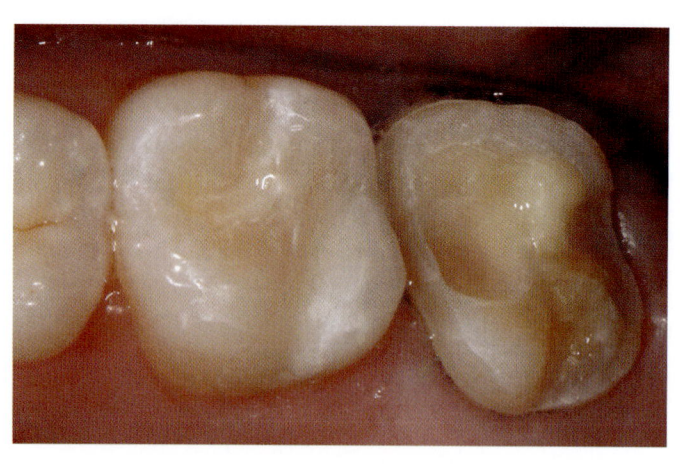

Figure 15.21 **(F)** Final result of tooth #14 with direct two-surface (occlusal, lingual) composite restoration. Restoration was finalized under rubber dam. Final preparation for an indirect CEREC onlay restoration was performed for tooth #15.

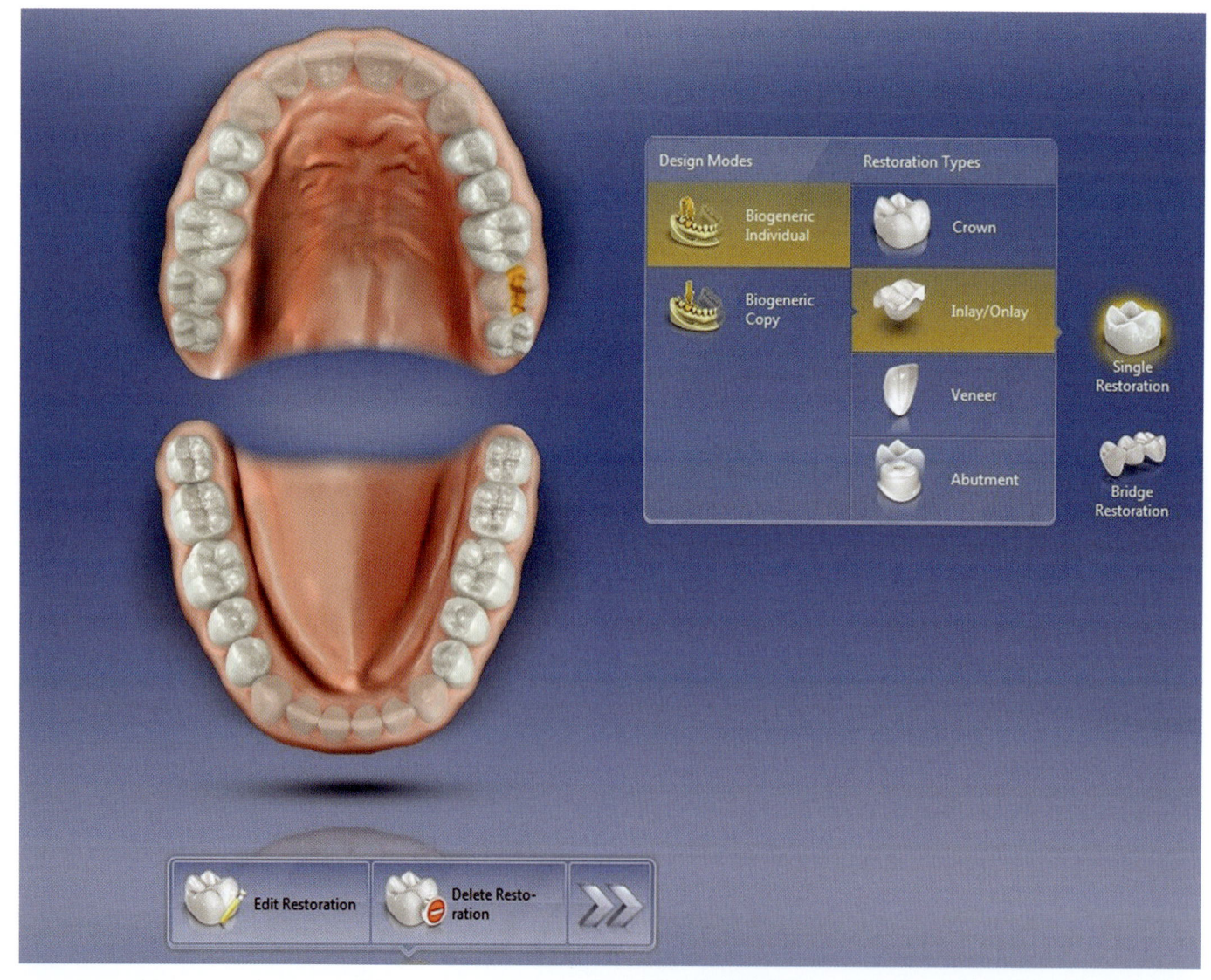

Figure 15.21 **(G)** Initiation of intraoral CEREC Omnicam scan for onlay restoration at tooth #15.

Digital impression

With the advances in technology with the Omnicam there is no need for powder when creating the digital impression, making it much easier for the practitioner and more convenient for the patient. The camera is moved 0–15 mm away from the tooth surface, capturing precise 3D images in natural color. The continuous capture of the tooth is simultaneously displayed on the monitor enabling the practitioner to efficiently move the camera over the field. The digital impression reduces chair time and improves the level of comfort and treatment acceptance for patients.[122,129,130] Another advantage of the digital impression is removing the need for impression trays, impression guns, and adhesives[130] (Figure 15.21G and H).

Design and milling procedures

During the design phase the practitioner has the ability to design the restoration with precision and efficiency, and there is a convenient tool to capture the original tooth anatomy (Figure 15.21I–J). The computer can then use this data to fabricate a final restoration that closely resembles the tooth prior to preparation. The practitioner also has the option to fabricate a customized restoration for each individual patient (Figure 15.21 K). After the restoration is designed, the computer analyzes the data and provides instructions to the milling machine. The milling of a single-tooth restoration can take upwards of 11 min and it is possible to digitally impress and design the restoration in 2–4 min (Figure 15.21 L). Once the practitioner becomes familiar with the software, it is possible to have the final crown milled approximately 15 min after the tooth is prepared (Figure 15.21 M and N).

Placement

The digital impression and milling processes reduce inaccuracies that can result from the laboratory fabrication process and the CEREC technology is able to manufacture a restoration that fits within the 50–75 μm range.[131,132] After the fit is assessed and approved, the restoration can be cemented in place using dual-cure microfilled composite resin cement (Figure 15.21O and P). Research has shown that the microfilled particle composite wears two to three times better than a hybrid composite.

The CEREC is a CAD/CAM system that produces full ceramic restorations of various kinds in a single step, by means of a fully automated grinding process, within a short period of time.[133] Computer-generated restorations can offer a lower-cost tooth-colored restoration for the patient and with the advances of technology and materials it is now possible to esthetically please the most demanding of patients even when considering a single anterior restoration. Therefore, for the great majority of patients, the advantage of a one-appointment ceramic restoration outweighs this slight esthetic deficit and makes it an ideal solution.

Research

In 2003, a study by Posselt and Kerschbaum evaluated 2328 ceramic inlays and onlays in 794 patients and reported a survival rate of 95.5% at 9 years.[134] A 10-year study completed by

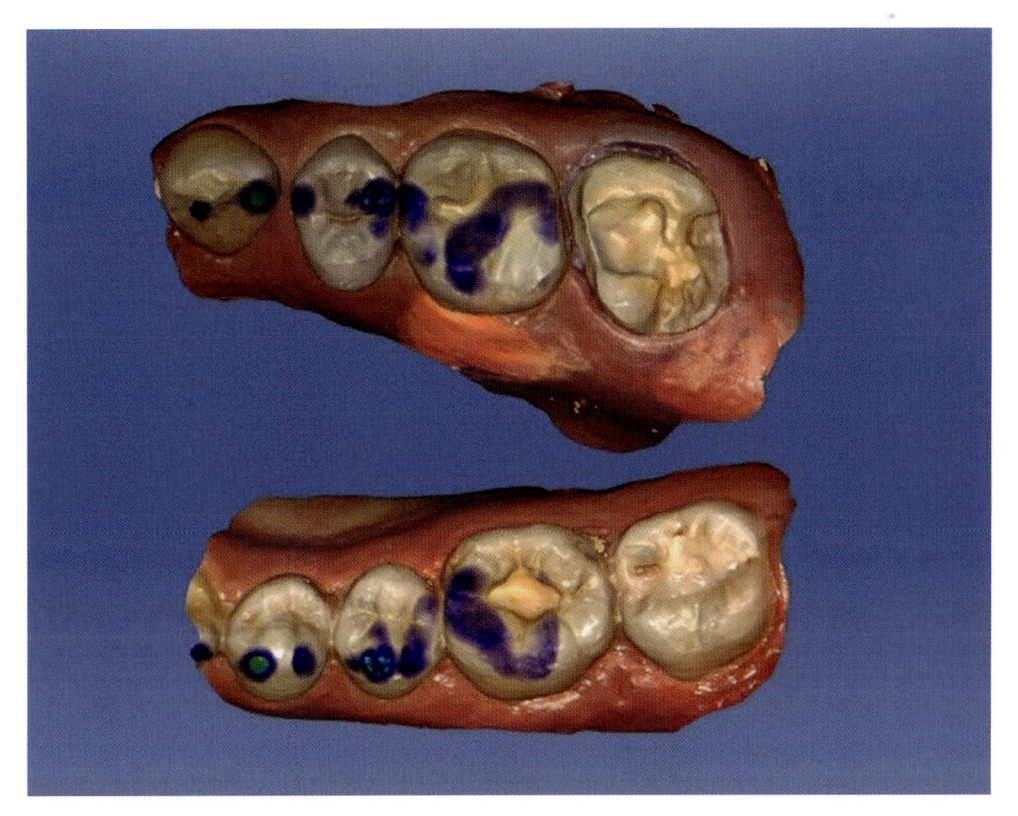

Figure 15.21 (H) Pictures of Omnicam digital impressions and restoration design.

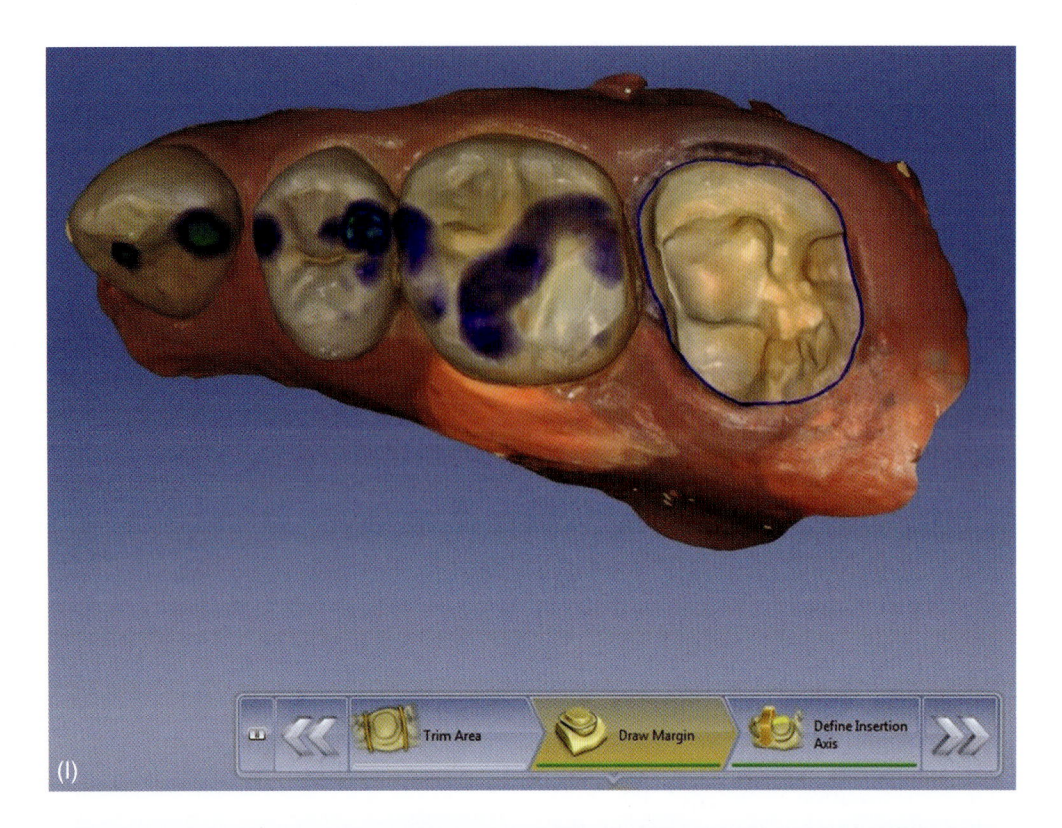

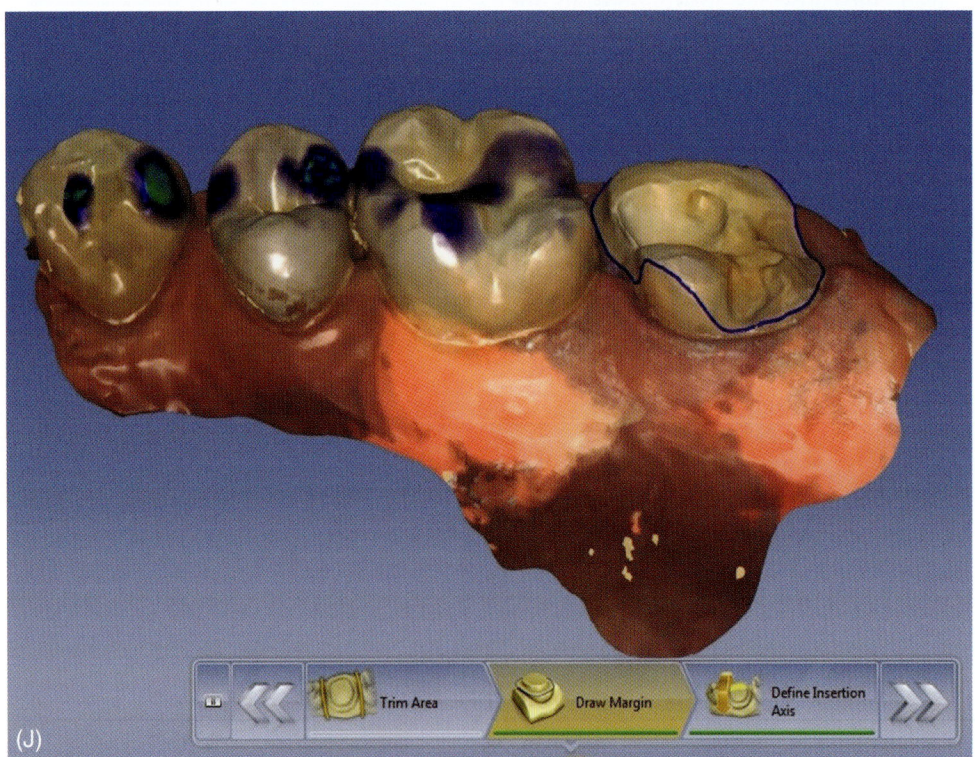

Figure 15.21 **(I and J)** Preparation margins are defined by drawing the borders of the onlay restoration: occlusal and lateral views.

Zimmer et al. assessed the longevity of the CEREC restorations placed in Class I and Class II preparations.[135] The study demonstrated a 94.7% survival rate after 5 years and an 85.7% survival rate after 10 years. They concluded that the CAD/CAM restorations are durable alternatives to direct and laboratory-fabricated restorations. In another 10 year study Sjögren et al. evaluated the performance of Class II CEREC inlay restorations with two different types of cement.[126]

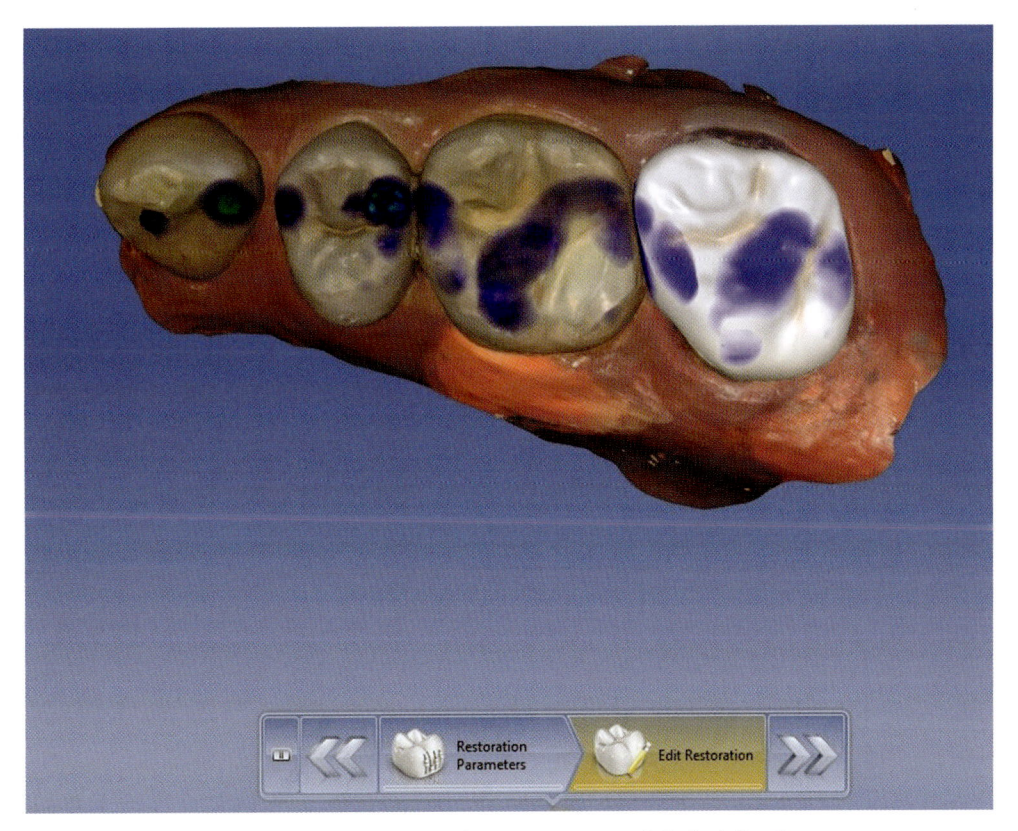

Figure 15.21 **(K)** Restoration parameters, restoration extension, and contact areas are digitally defined.

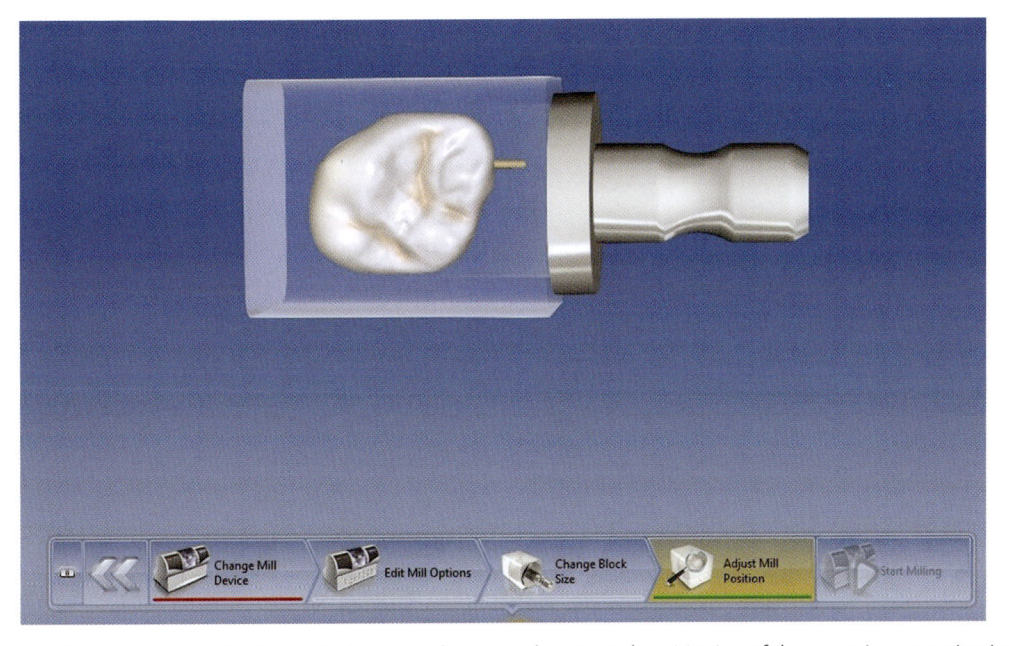

Figure 15.21 **(L)** The final workpiece gets finalized; block type and size are chosen, and positioning of the ceramic restoration in the milling block defined.

They showed an 89% survival rate after a 10 year reevaluation and demonstrated a statistically significant difference when comparing the survival of inlays cemented with dual-cured resin composite-luted inlays (77%) and chemically cured resin composite-luted inlays (100%). Furthermore, they state that "patient satisfaction with and acceptance of the CEREC inlays were high, and the performance after 10 years of clinical service was acceptable, especially regarding the inlays luted with

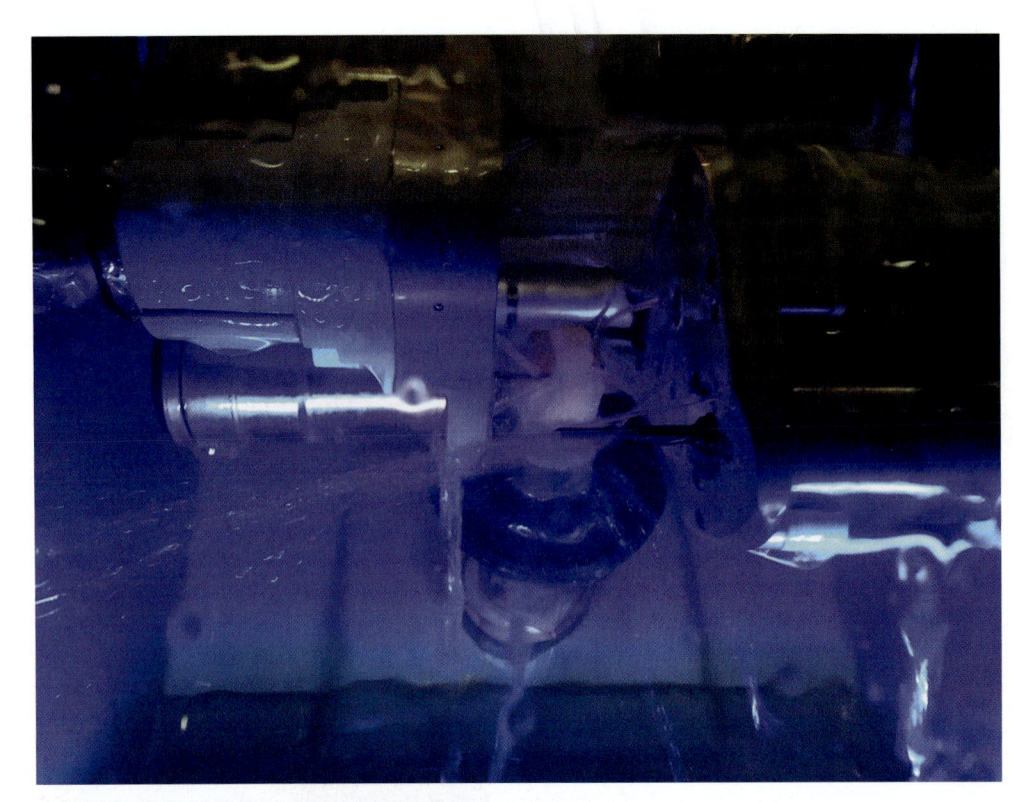

Figure 15.21 **(M)** CEREC milling of the CEREC e.max CAD restoration in process.

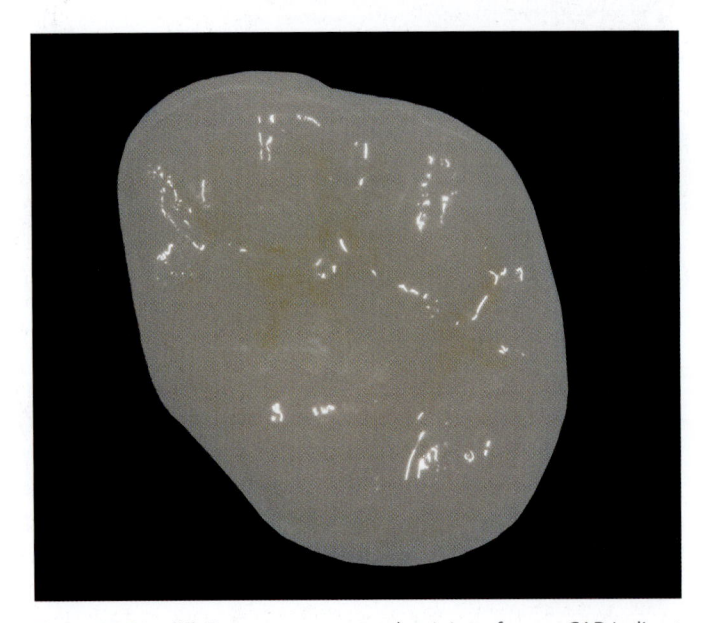

Figure 15.21 **(N)** Custom anatomy and staining of e.max CAD indirect restoration.

the chemically cured resin composite." Fasbinder concludes that CEREC restorations have reportedly approached a 97% survival probability for 5 years and a 90% survival probability for 10 years.[136] He states "the low rate of restoration fracture and long-term clinical survivability document the effectiveness of the CEREC system as a dependable, esthetic restorative option for patients."

Researchers measured margins of approximately 50 µm, suggesting that the marginal fit of CAD/CAM-generated restorations is clinically acceptable.[137,138] Denissen et al. reported average marginal accuracy of 85 µm for onlay restorations manufactured by CEREC 3, which was similar to laboratory-fabricated onlay restorations[139] (Figure 15.22A–D).

The Carestream system

CS Solutions from Carestream offers the ability to scan, design, and mill and place restorations in one appointment. It consists of an intraoral scanner, cone beam computed tomography (CBCT) impression scanning system, restoration design software, and a relatively small milling machine that can be easily placed in the dental office. As with other similar scanning systems, if the dentist does not want to mill in the office there is a web-based platform which can share and manage restoration cases between dentists and laboratories.

There is minimal training required via a light guidance system during image capture, easy but fast impression scanning, intuitive restoration design, and simple milling instructions. The entire milling process takes about 15 min.

Using the CS 3500 intraoral scanner images can be acquired in true color, and 2D and 3D digital impressions. It offers high-angulation scanning of up to 45° and goes to a depth from −2 mm to +13 mm. There is no powder required to obtain quite clear images. Its internal heater prevents mirror fogging during the scanning procedure. Once the scanning is complete, the CS Restore CAD software helps design the restoration, featuring advanced algorithms to help create contours and anatomy of the restoration (Figure 15.23A–C). However, there are also controls

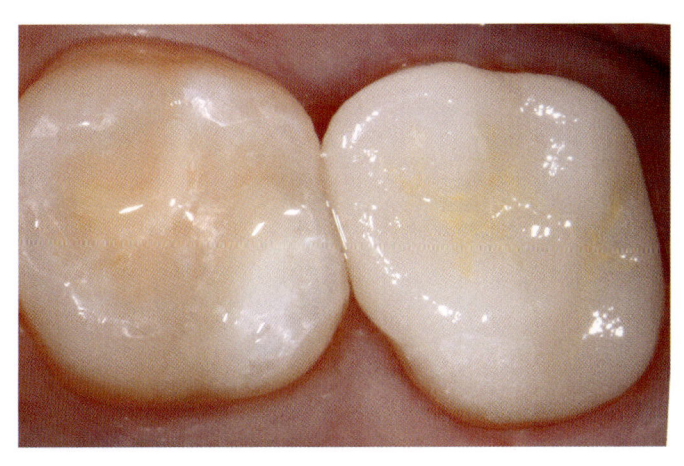

Chapter 15 Ceramic Veneers and Partial-Coverage Restorations

Figure 15.21 (**O**) Final adhesive bonded CEREC restoration at tooth #15, and final direct restoration at tooth #14, occlusal view.

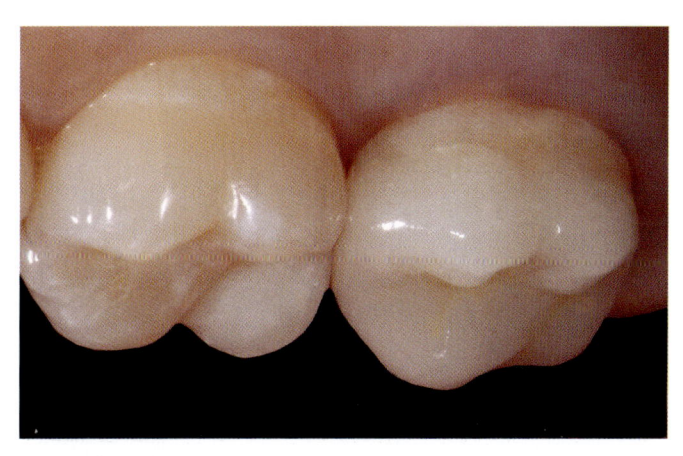

Figure 15.21 (**P**) Lateral view of restored teeth #15 and #14. Case courtesy of Jacob Truan DMD.

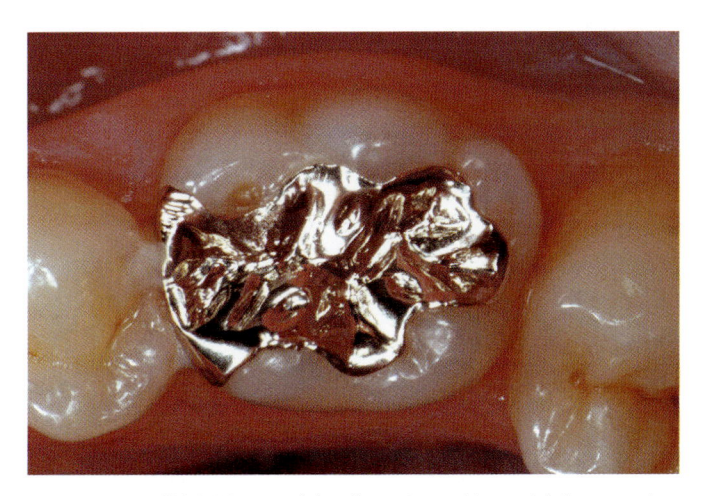

Figure 15.22 (**A**) A 28-year-old male patient with mesial decay under a gold restoration on tooth #30.

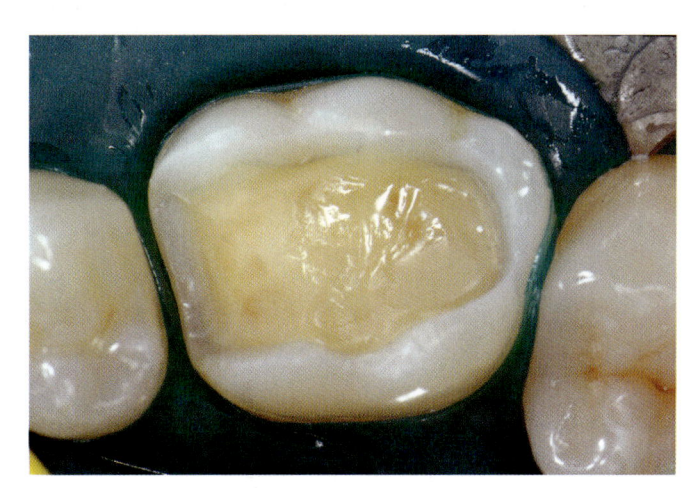

Figure 15.22 (**B**) The gold restoration was removed and decay eliminated. A preparation for a CEREC e.max CAD ceramic restoration was performed followed by an intraoral scan.

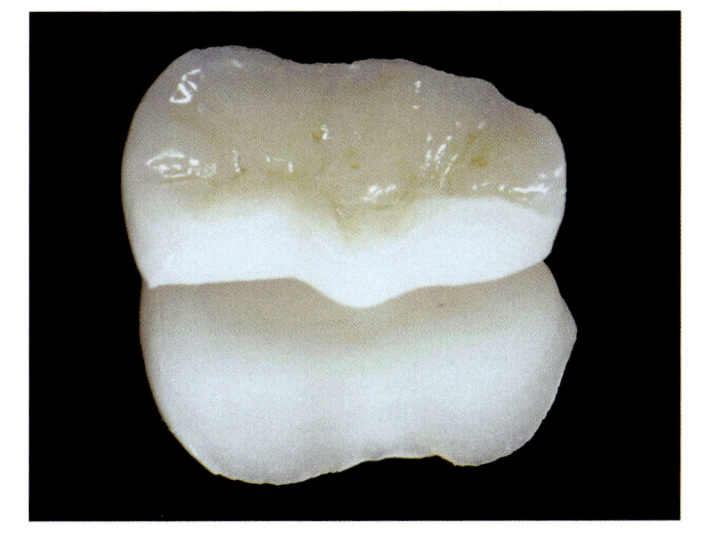

Figure 15.22 (**C**) Final CEREC CAD/CAM inlay restoration, with occlusal surfaces customized by coloring and glazing technique, was prepared with hydrofluoric acid and Monobond-S (silane) for adhesive cementation.

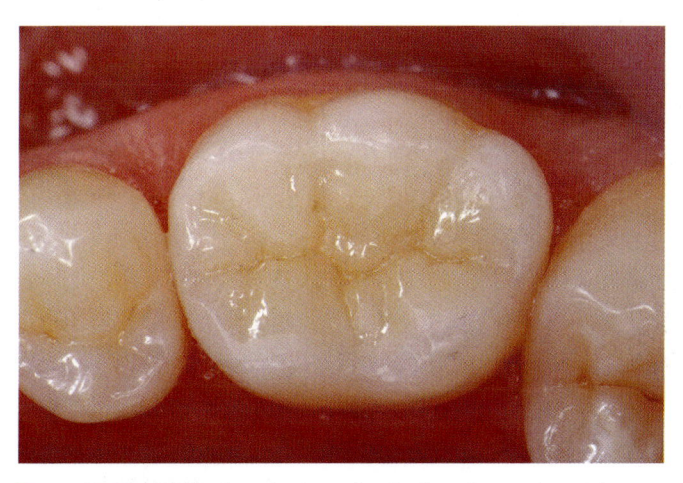

Figure 15.22 (**D**) Final result after adhesive bonding under rubber dam of the CEREC inlay restoration. Color match and marginal adaptation were achieved.

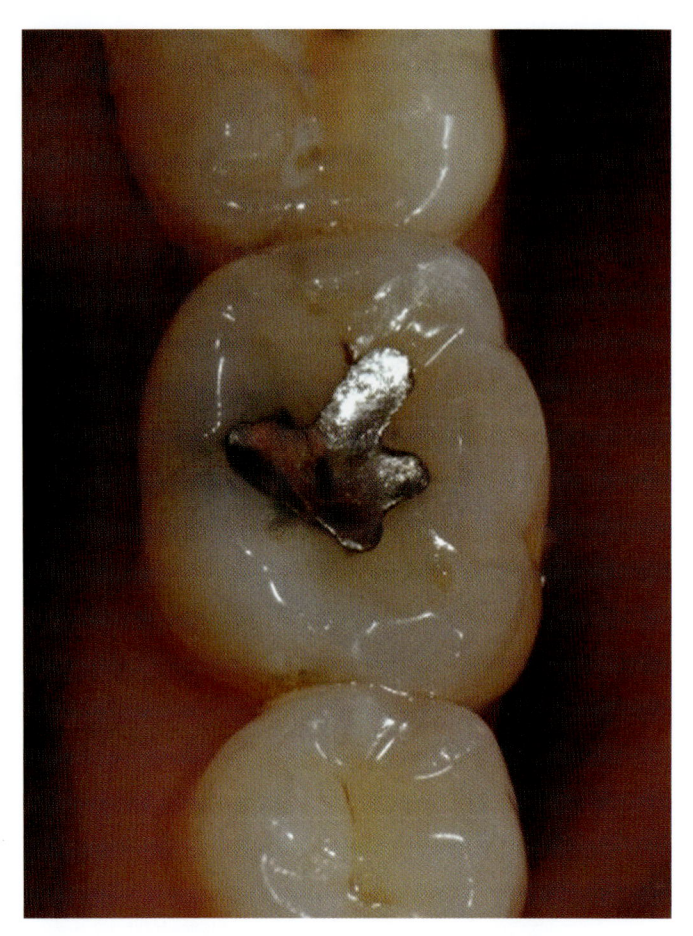

Figure 15.23 **(A)** This patient had caries under her old amalgam restoration plus occlusal-lingual and occlusal-buccal micro cracks.

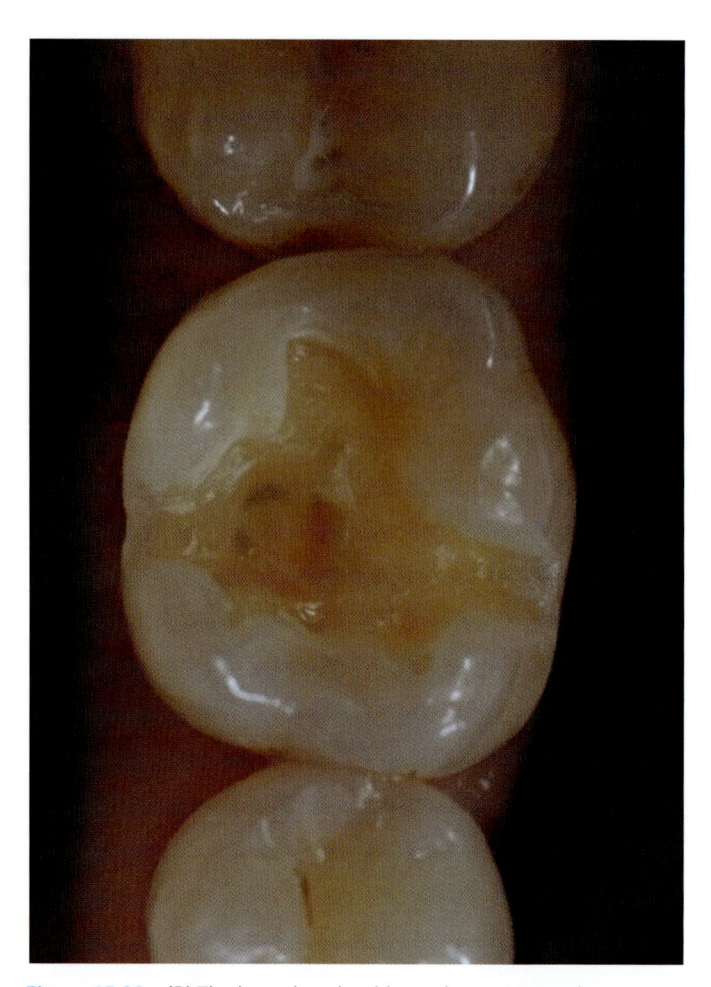

Figure 15.23 **(B)** The buccal-occlusal-lingual preparation shows caries removed in the central groove area.

to be able to individually customize the restoration by enlarging, taking away, and building up the occlusion or walls if desired (Figure 15.23D). One tip is to magnify the marginal lines to make sure they are precisely where you want them to be. If in doubt, extend the margin so it will not be necessary to redo the scan and repeat the design since it is much easier to just trim back any overextended margin.

The CS 3000 milling machine is a CAM unit that features a four-axis brushless motor that produces restorations with ±25 μm accuracy. It is relatively quiet and can even be rolled into the treatment room if desired (Figure 15.23E). Certainly one of the most important advantages of the entire system is that a trained dental assistant can perform much of the required procedures once the preparations are completed by the dentist (Figure 15.23 F–I).

Conclusion

The original purpose of offering reversible bonded restorations was to take advantage of future technology. That seems to have been a worthwhile approach. Many patients, who 10, 15, or even 20 years ago trusted us to give them restorations with what was then a new procedure called bonding, still have their composite resin posterior restorations and veneers in place. Some return to take advantage of the increasingly better materials and replace their composite restorations with porcelain restorations. The future of esthetic restorative dentistry will no doubt see considerable improvement in longer-lasting cementing materials, ease of construction, and the porcelain materials themselves. Finally, future advancements in CAD/CAM capability will no doubt have a positive effect on all aspects of both anterior and posterior restorations.

Acknowledgment

The authors are grateful to Pinhas Adar, MDT, Oral Design Center, Atlanta, GA, for his contribution to the CAD/CAM part of this chapter and Jacob Truan, DMD, Goldstein Center for Aesthetic and Implant Dentistry, Atlanta, GA, for his contribution to the CEREC part of this chapter.

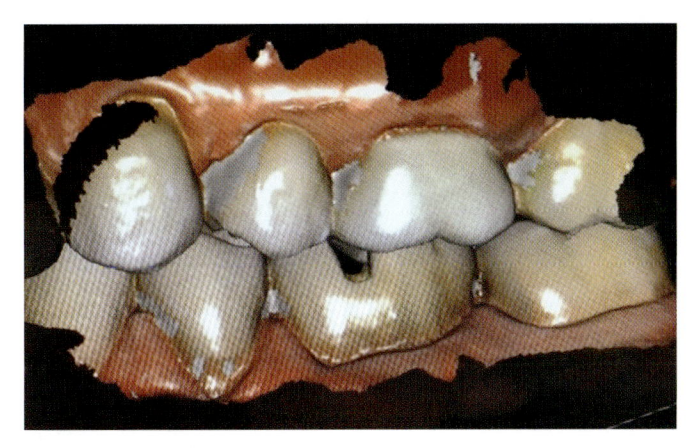

Chapter 15 Ceramic Veneers and Partial-Coverage Restorations 493

Figure 15.23 **(C)** The Carestream CS Solutions scanner was used to capture the restoration and occlusal bite registration.

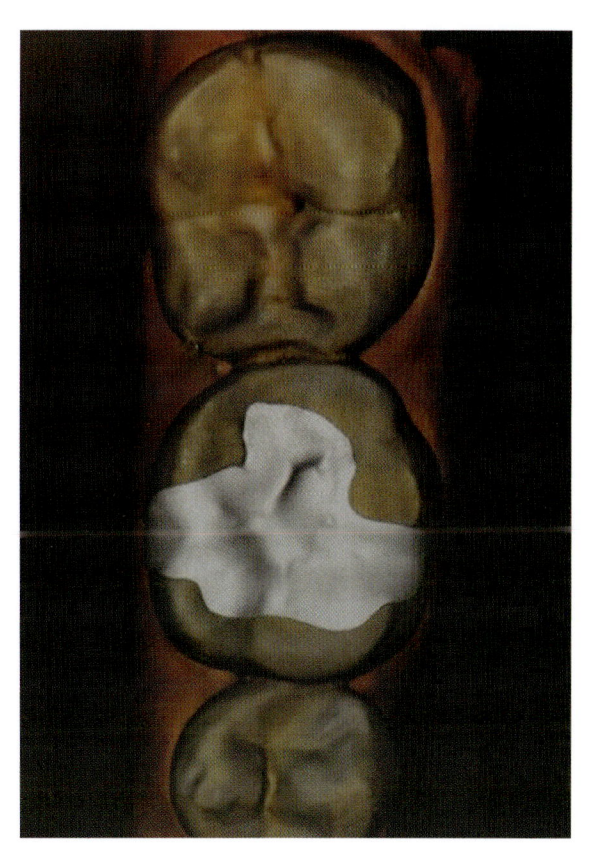

Figure 15.23 **(D)** The proposed restoration was easily designed for marginal fit and occlusal contact on the computer.

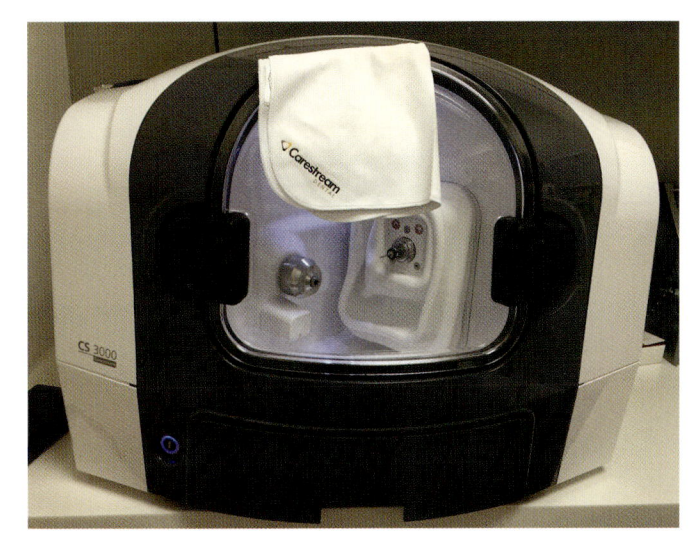

Figure 15.23 **(E)** The restoration was milled in 15 min on the Carestream CS 3000 milling unit.

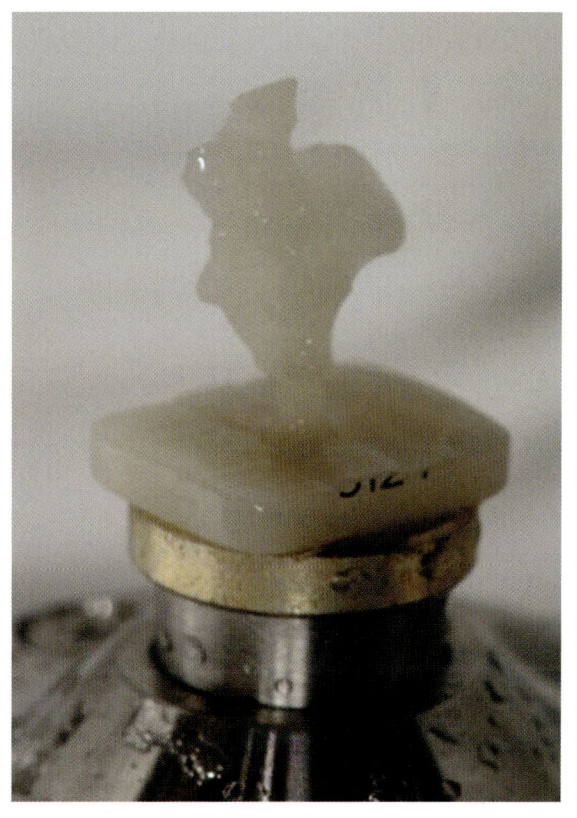

Figure 15.23 **(F)** Inlay restoration captured, still connected by the sprue pin to the CAD/CAM ceramic ingot.

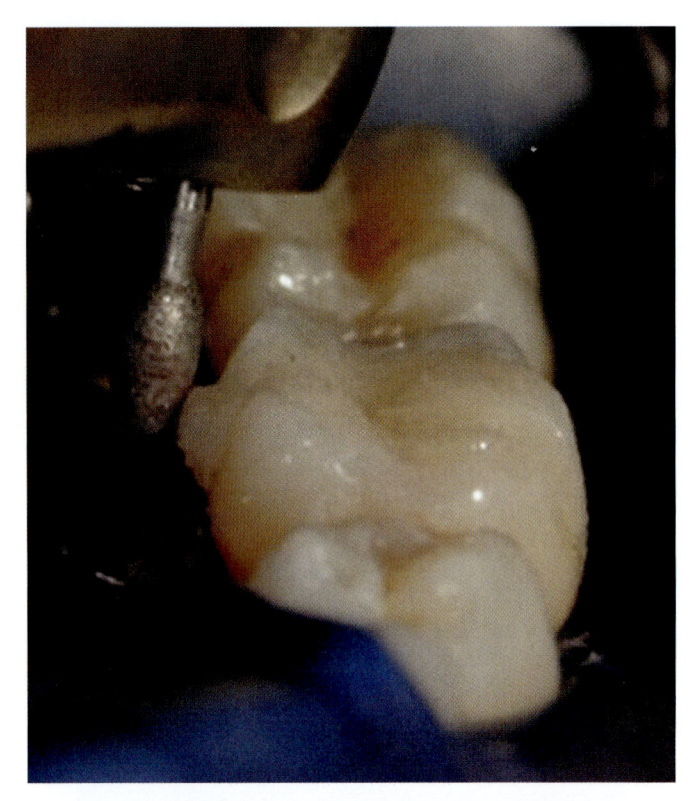

Figure 15.23 **(G)** Rubber dam is applied and the restoration cemented with a resin luting cement (Duo-Link Universal, Bisco). Then the sprue pin residue is cut off and contoured.

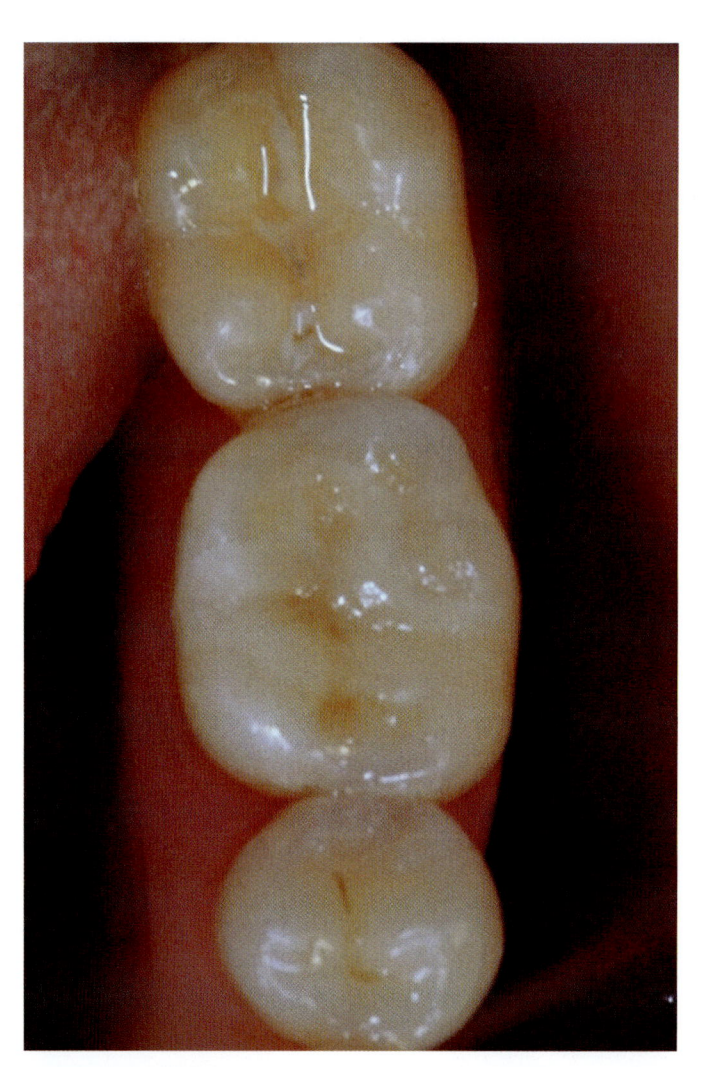

Figure 15.23 **(I)** The final ceramic restoration was placed to complete a 1 h appointment.

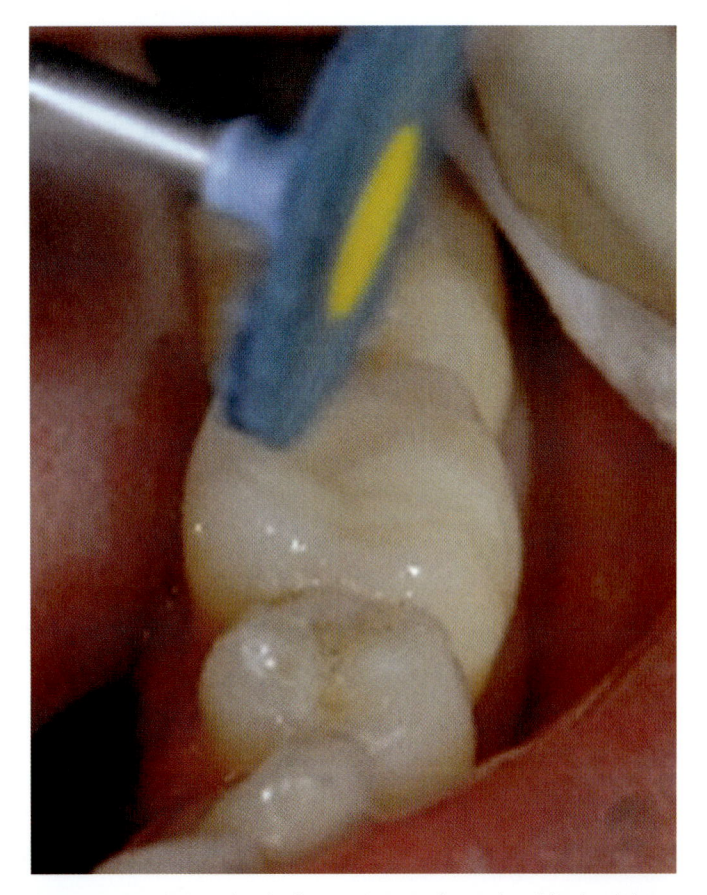

Figure 15.23 **(H)** Occlusal adjustment is performed and final polishing is accomplished using Dialite Feather Lite flexible spirals (Brasseler USA).

References

1. Pincus CR. Building mouth personality. *J Calif Stud Dent Assoc* 1938;14:125–129.
2. Buonocore MG. A simple method of increasing the adhesion of acrylic filling materials to enamel surfaces. *J Dent Res* 1955;34: 849–853.
3. Bowen RL. Properties of a silica-reinforced polymer for dental restorations. *J Am Dent Assoc* 1963;66:57–64.
4. Bowen RL (1958) *Development of a Silica-Resin Direct Filling Material*. Washington: National Bureau of Standards
5. Bowen RL, Paffenbarger GC, Sweeney WT. Bonding porcelain teeth to an acrylic resin denture base. *Dent Assoc* 1967;44:1018–1023.
6. McLaughlin G. Porcelain fused to tooth–a new esthetic and reconstructive modality. *Compend Contin Educ Dent* 1984;5:430–435.
7. Faunce FR. Tooth restoration with preformed laminate veneers. *Dent Surv* 1977;53:30–32.
8. Faunce FR, Myers DR. Laminate veneer restoration of permanent incisors. *J Am Dent Assoc* 1976;93:790–792.
9. Heymann HO. In: Garber DA, Goldstein RE, Feinman RAs, eds. *Proceedings of the Porcelain Laminate Veneers*. Chicago, IL: Quintessence; 1988: 126–132.

10. Kern M, Strub JR, Lu XY. Wear of composite resin veneering materials in a dual-axis chewing simulator. *J Oral Rehabil* 1999;26:372–378.
11. Rochette AL. A ceramic restoration bonded by etched enamel and resin for fractured incisors. *J Prosthet Dent* 1975;33:287–293.
12. Boksman L, Jordan RE, Suzuki M, et al. Etched porcelain labial veneers. *Ontario Dent* 1985;62:11, 13, 15–19.
13. Boksman L, Jordan RE. Posterior composite restorative technique. *Restor Dent* 1985;1:120, 122, 124–126.
14. Calamia JR. Etched porcelain veneers: the current state of the art. *Quintessence Int* 1985;16:5–12.
15. Calamia JR. Materials and technique for etched porcelain facial veneers. *Alpha Omegan* 1988;81:48–51.
16. Calamia JR, Calamia CS. Porcelain laminate veneers: reasons for 25 years of success. *Dent Clin North Am* 2007;51:399–417.
17. Frankenberger R, Tay FR. Self-etch vs etch-and-rinse adhesives: effect of thermo-mechanical fatigue loading on marginal quality of bonded resin composite restorations. *Dent Mater* 2005;21:397–412.
18. Magne P, Douglas WH. Porcelain veneers: dentin bonding optimization and biomimetic recovery of the crown. *Int J Prosthodont* 1999;12:111–121.
19. Magne P, Perroud R, Hodges JS, Belser UC. Clinical performance of novel-design porcelain veneers for the recovery of coronal volume and length. *Int J Periodont Restor Dent* 2000;20:440–457.
20. Stappert CF, Ozden U, Gerds T, Strub JR. Longevity and failure load of ceramic veneers with different preparation designs after exposure to masticatory simulation. *J Prosthet Dent* 2005;94:132–139.
21. Guess PC, Stappert CF. Midterm results of a 5-year prospective clinical investigation of extended ceramic veneers. *Dent Mater* 2008;24(6):804–813.
22. Cattell MJ, Chadwick TC, Knowles JC, et al. Flexural strength optimisation of a leucite reinforced glass ceramic. *Dent Mater* 2001;17:21–33.
23. Kelly JR, Benetti P. Ceramic materials in dentistry: historical evolution and current practice. *Aust Dent J* 2011;56(Suppl 1):84–96.
24. Kelly JR. Perspectives on strength. *Dent Mater* 1995;11:103–110.
25. Stappert CF, Ozden U, Att W, et al. Marginal accuracy of press-ceramic veneers influenced by preparation design and fatigue. *Am J Dent* 2007;20:380–384.
26. Stappert CF, Stathopoulou N, Gerds T, Strub JR. Survival rate and fracture strength of maxillary incisors, restored with different kinds of full veneers. *J Oral Rehabil* 2005;32:266–272.
27. Stappert CF, Guess PC, Gerds T, Strub JR. All-ceramic partial coverage premolar restorations. Cavity preparation design, reliability and fracture resistance after fatigue. *Am J Dent* 2005;18:275–280.
28. Stappert CF. Tooth structure preservation by extended veneer restorations. *Pract Proced Aesthet Dent* 2007;19:300–301.
29. Edelhoff D, Sorensen JA. Tooth structure removal associated with various preparation designs for anterior teeth. *J Prosthet Dent* 2002;87:503–509.
30. Rekow ED, Silva NR, Coelho PG, et al. Performance of dental ceramics: challenges for improvements. *J Dent Res* 2011;90:937–952.
31. Albakry M, Guazzato M, Swain MV. Fracture toughness and hardness evaluation of three pressable all-ceramic dental materials. *J Dent* 2003;31:181–188.
32. Guazzato M, Albakry M, Ringer SP, Swain MV. Strength, fracture toughness and microstructure of a selection of all-ceramic materials. Part I. Pressable and alumina glass-infiltrated ceramics. *Dent Mater* 2004;20:441–448.
33. Gorman CM, McDevitt WE, Hill RG. Comparison of two heat-pressed all-ceramic dental materials. *Dent Mater* 2000;16:389–395.
34. Bailey JH. Porcelain-to-composite bond strengths using four organosilane materials. *J Prosthet Dent* 1989;61:174–177.
35. Ferrari M, Patroni S, Balleri P. Measurement of enamel thickness in relation to reduction for etched laminate veneers. *Int J Periodont Restor Dent* 1992;12:407–413.
36. Tjan AH, Dunn JR, Sanderson IR. Microleakage patterns of porcelain and castable ceramic laminate veneers. *J Prosthet Dent* 1989;61:276–282.
37. Chu FC, Frankel N, Smales RJ. Surface roughness and flexural strength of self-glazed, polished, and reglazed In-Ceram/Vitadur Alpha porcelain laminates. *Int J Prosthodont* 2000;13:66–71.
38. Della Bona A, van Noort R. Shear vs. tensile bond strength of resin composite bonded to ceramic. *J Dent Res* 1995;74:1591–1596.
39. Calamia JR, Simonsen RJ. Effect of coupling agents on bond strength of etched porcelain. *J Dent Res* 1984;1:179 (Abstract 79).
40. Belser UC, Magne P, Magne M. Ceramic laminate veneers: continuous evolution of indications. *J Esthet Dent* 1997;9:197–207.
41. Chang JC, Nguyen T, Duong JH, Ladd GD. Tensile bond strengths of dual-cured cements between a glass-ceramic and enamel. *J Prosthet Dent* 1998;79:503–507.
42. Hooshmand T, van Noort R, Keshvad A. Bond durability of the resin-bonded and silane treated ceramic surface. *Dent Mater* 2002;18:179–188.
43. Frankenberger R, Krämer N, Sindel J. Repair strength of etched vs silica-coated metal-ceramic and all-ceramic restorations. *Oper Dent* 2000;25:209–215.
44. Kimmich M, Stappert CF. Intraoral treatment of veneering porcelain chipping of fixed dental restorations: a review and clinical application. *J Am Dent Assoc* 2013;144:31–44.
45. Kreulen CM, Creugers NH, Meijering AC. Meta-analysis of anterior veneer restorations in clinical studies. *J Dent* 1998;26:345–353.
46. Wakiaga J, Brunton P, Silikas N, Glenny AM. Direct versus indirect veneer restorations for intrinsic dental stains. *Cochrane Database Syst Rev* 2004:CD004347.
47. Aristidis GA, Dimitra B. Five-year clinical performance of porcelain laminate veneers. *Quintessence Int* 2002;33:185–189.
48. Fradeani M, Redemagni M, Corrado M. Porcelain laminate veneers: 6- to 12-year clinical evaluation--a retrospective study. *Int J Periodont Restor Dent* 2005;25:9–17.
49. Sheth JJ, Jensen ME. Luting interfaces and materials for etched porcelain restorations. A status report for the American Journal of Dentistry. *Am J Dent* 1988;1:225–235.
50. Garber DA. Direct composite veneers versus etched porcelain laminate veneers. *Dent Clin North Am* 1989;33:301–304.
51. Silva NR, de Souza GM, Coelho PG, et al. Effect of water storage time and composite cement thickness on fatigue of a glass-ceramic trilayer system. *J Biomed Mater Res B Appl Biomater* 2008;84:117–123.
52. Nixon R. *The Chairside Manual for Porcelain Bonding*. Wilmington, DE: B.A. Videographics.
53. Soares PV, Spini PH, Carvalho VF, et al. Esthetic rehabilitation with laminated ceramic veneers reinforced by lithium disilicate. *Quintessence Int* 2014;45:129–133.
54. Schmitter M, Seydler BB. Minimally invasive lithium disilicate ceramic veneers fabricated using chairside CAD/CAM: a clinical report. *J Prosthet Dent* 2012;107:71–74.

55. Webber B, McDonald A, Knowles J. An in vitro study of the compressive load at fracture of Procera AllCeram crowns with varying thickness of veneer porcelain. *J Prosthet Dent* 2003;89:154–160.
56. Chu FC, Sham AS, Luk HW, et al. Threshold contrast ratio and masking ability of porcelain veneers with high-density alumina cores. *Int J Prosthodont* 2004;17:24–28.
57. Zarone F, Apicella D, Sorrentino R, et al. Influence of tooth preparation design on the stress distribution in maxillary central incisors restored by means of alumina porcelain veneers: a 3D-finite element analysis. *Dent Mater* 2005;21:1178–1188.
58. Alghazzawi TF, Lemons J, Liu PR, et al. The failure load of CAD/CAM generated zirconia and glass-ceramic laminate veneers with different preparation designs. *J Prosthet Dent* 2012;108:386–393.
59. Alghazzawi TF, Lemons J, Liu PR, et al. Evaluation of the optical properties of CAD-CAM generated yttria-stabilized zirconia and glass-ceramic laminate veneers. *J Prosthet Dent* 2012;107:300–308.
60. Walls AW, Steele JG, Wassell RW. Crowns and other extra-coronal restorations: porcelain laminate veneers. *Br Dent J* 2002;193:73–76, 79–82.
61. Calamia JR. Etched porcelain facial veneers: a new treatment modality based on scientific and clinical evidence. *NY J Dent* 1983;53:255–259.
62. Crispin BJ. Expanding the application of facial ceramic veneers. *J Calif Dent Assoc* 1993;21:43–46, 48–49, 52–44.
63. el-Sherif M, Jacobi R. The ceramic reverse three-quarter crown for anterior teeth: preparation design. *J Prosthet Dent* 1989;61:4–6.
64. Brunton PA, Wilson NH. Preparations for porcelain laminate veneers in general dental practice. *Br Dent J* 1998;184:553–556.
65. McLean JW. Long-term esthetic dentistry. *Quintessence Int* 1989;20:701–708.
66. Shaini FJ, Shortall AC, Marquis PM. Clinical performance of porcelain laminate veneers. A retrospective evaluation over a period of 6.5 years. *J Oral Rehabil* 1997;24:553–559.
67. Rouse JS. Full veneer versus traditional veneer preparation: a discussion of interproximal extension. *J Prosthet Dent* 1997;78:545–549.
68. Garber DA, Goldstein RE, Feinman RA. *Porcelain Laminate Veneers*. Chicago, IL: Quintessence.
69. Gurel G. Porcelain laminate veneers: minimal tooth preparation by design. *Dent Clin North Am* 2007;51:419–431.
70. Dumfahrt H, Schaffer H. Porcelain laminate veneers. A retrospective evaluation after 1 to 10 years of service: Part II--Clinical results. *Int J Prosthodont* 2000;13:9–18.
71. Frankenberger R, Kern M. Dentin adhesives create a positive bond to dental hard tissue. *Int J Comput Dent* 2003;6:187–192.
72. Reid JS. Tooth color modification and porcelain veneers. *Quintessence Int* 1988;19:477–481.
73. Guess PC, Selz CF, Voulgarakis A, Stampf S, Stappert CF. Prospective clinical study of press-ceramic overlap and full veneer restorations: 7-year results. *Int J Prosthodont* 2014;27:355–358.
74. Glavina D, Skrinjaric I, Mahovic S, Majstorovic M. Surface quality of Cerec CAD/CAM ceramic veneers treated with four different polishing systems. *Eur J Paediatr Dent* 2004;5:30–34.
75. Wiedhahn K, Kerschbaum T, Fasbinder DF. Clinical long-term results with 617 Cerec veneers: a nine-year report. *Int J Comput Dent* 2005;8:233–246.
76. Williams PT, Jackson DG, Bergman W. An evaluation of the time-dependent dimensional stability of eleven elastomeric impression materials. *J Prosthet Dent* 1984;52:120–125.
77. Shen C. Impression materials In: Anusavice KJs, ed. *Proceedings of the Philips' Science of Dental Materials*. Saunders, 2003: 210–230.
78. Derrien G, Le Menn G. Evaluation of detail reproduction for three die materials by using scanning electron microscopy and two-dimensional profilometry. *J Prosthet Dent* 1995;74:1–7.
79. Giordano R, 2nd. Impression materials: basic properties. *Gen Dent* 2000;48:510–512, 514, 516.
80. Ciesco JN, Malone WF, Sandrik JL, Mazur B. Comparison of elastomeric impression materials used in fixed prosthodontics. *J Prosthet Dent* 1981;45:89–94.
81. Craig RG. Restorative Dental Materials. Elsevier St. Louis
82. Balkenhol M, Haunschild S, Lochnit G, Wostmann B. Surfactant release from hydrophilized vinylpolysiloxanes. *J Dent Res* 2009;88:668–672.
83. Donovan TE, Chee WW. A review of contemporary impression materials and techniques. *Dent Clin North Am* 2004; 48: vi-vii, 445–470.
84. Anusavice KJ. *Phillips' Science of Dental Materials*. Philadelphia, PA: Saunders.
85. Rubel BS. Impression materials: a comparative review of impression materials most commonly used in restorative dentistry. *Dent Clin North Am* 2007;51:629–642, vi.
86. Lacy AM, Fukui H, Bellman T, Jendresen MD. Time-dependent accuracy of elastomer impression materials. Part II: Polyether, polysulfides, and polyvinylsiloxane. *J Prosthet Dent* 1981;45: 329–333.
87. Garber DA. Porcelain laminate veneers: Ten years later. Part I: Tooth preparation. *J Esthet Dent* 1993;5:57–61.
88. Giordano R, 2nd. A comparison of all-ceramic restorative systems, Part 1. *Gen Dent* 1999;47:566–570.
89. Studer S, Lehner C, Schärer P. Seven-year results of leucite-reinforced glass-ceramic inlays and onlays. *Acta Med Dent Helv* 1998;3:137–146.
90. Studer S, Lehener C, Brodbeck U. Six-year results of leucite-reinforced glass ceramic crowns. *Acta Med Dent Helv* 1998;3:218–225.
91. Oliva RA. Handling and bonding of porcelain veneers–clinical evaluation of a new veneer handling instrument. *Quintessence Int* 1988;19:593–597.
92. Rucker LM, Richter W, MacEntee M, Richardson A. Porcelain and resin veneers clinically evaluated: 2-year results. *J Am Dent Assoc* 1990;121:594–596.
93. Stappert CF, Derks J, Gerds T, Strub JR. [Marginal accuracy of press-ceramic full veneers with different preparation before and after mouth motion fatigue]. *Schweiz Monatsschr Zahnmed* 2007;117:474–482.
94. Haywood VB, Heymann HO, Scurria MS. Effects of water, speed, and experimental instrumentation on finishing and polishing porcelain intra-orally. *Dent Mater* 1989;5:185–188.
95. Cooley RL, Lubow RM, Brown FH. Effect of air-powder abrasive instrument on porcelain. *J Prosthet Dent* 1988;60:440–443.
96. Peumans M, De Munck J, Fieuws S, et al. A prospective ten-year clinical trial of porcelain veneers. *J Adhes Dent* 2004;6:65–76.
97. Friedman MJ. A 15-year review of porcelain veneer failure-a clinician's observations. *Compend Contin Educ Dent* 1998;19:625–628, 630, 632.
98. Blatz MB. Long-term clinical success of all-ceramic posterior restorations. *Quintessence Int* 2002;33:415–426.
99. Calamia JR. Clinical evaluation of etched porcelain veneers. *Am J Dent* 1989;2:9–15.

100. Strassler HE, Nathanson D. Clinical evaluation of etched porcelain veneers over a period of 18 to 42 months. *J Esthet Dent* 1989;1:21–28.

101. Bassiouny MA, Pollack RL. Esthetic management of perimolysis with porcclain laminate veneers. *J Am Dent Assoc* 1987;115:412–417.

102. Jones DA. Effects of topical fluoride preparations on glazed porcelain surfaces. *J Prosthet Dent* 1985;53:483–484.

103. Goldstein RE. Status report: dentistry in the 1980's. *J Am Dent Assoc* 1988;116:617–624.

104. Kournetas N, Chakmakchi M, Kakaboura A, et al. Marginal and internal adaptation of Class II ormocer and hybrid resin composite restorations before and after load cycling. *Clin Oral Investig* 2004;8:123–129.

105. Krämer N, Garcia-Godoy F, Frankenberger R. Evaluation of resin composite materials. Part II: in vivo investigations. *Am J Dent* 2005;18:75–81.

106. Nasedkin JN. Porcelain posterior resin-bonded restorations: current perspectives on esthetic restorative dentistry: Part II. *J Can Dent Assoc* 1988;54:499–506.

107. Manhart J. Direct composite restorations in posterior region: a case history using a nanohybrid composite. *Dent Today* 2004;23:66, 68–70.

108. Wiley MG. Effects of porcelain on occluding surfaces of restored teeth. *J Prosthet Dent* 1989;61:133–137.

109. Jackson RD, Ferguson RW. An esthetic, bonded inlay/onlay technique for posterior teeth. *Quintessence Int* 1990;21:7–12.

110. Thordrup M, Isidor F, Horsted-Bindslev P. A prospective clinical study of indirect and direct composite and ceramic inlays: ten-year results. *Quintessence Int* 2006;37:139–144.

111. Mormann WH, Brandestini M, Lutz F, Barbakow F. Chairside computer-aided direct ceramic inlays. *Quintessence Int* 1989;20:329–339.

112. Dietschi D, Maeder M, Meyer JM, Holz J. In vitro resistance to fracture of porcelain inlays bonded to tooth. *Quintessence Int* 1990;21:823–831.

113. Krämer N, Lohbauer U, Frankenberger R. Adhesive luting of indirect restorations. *Am J Dent* 2000;13:60D-76D.

114. Hickel R, Manhart J. Longevity of restorations in posterior teeth and reasons for failure. *J Adhes Dent* 2001;3:45–64.

115. Kelly JR. Developing meaningful systematic review of CAD/CAM reconstructions and fiber-reinforced composites. *Clin Oral Implants Res* 2007;18 (suppl 3):205–217.

116. Stappert CF, Guess PC, Chitmongkolsuk S, et al. All-ceramic partial coverage restorations on natural molars. Masticatory fatigue loading and fracture resistance. *Am J Dent* 2007;20:21–26.

117. Burke FJ. The effect of variations in bonding procedure on fracture resistance of dentin-bonded all-ceramic crowns. *Quintessence Int* 1995;26:293–300.

118. Eidenbenz S, Lehner CR, Scharer P. Copy milling ceramic inlays from resin analogs: a practicable approach with the CELAY system. *Int J Prosthodont* 1994;7:134–142.

119. Kawai K, Hayashi M, Torii M, Tsuchitani Y. Marginal adaptability and fit of ceramic milled inlays. *J Am Dent Assoc* 1995;126:1414–1419.

120. Sadowsky SJ. An overview of treatment considerations for esthetic restorations: a review of the literature. *J Prosthet Dent* 2006;96:433–442.

121. McDonald A. Preparation guidelines for full and partial coverage ceramic restorations. *Dent Update* 2001;28:84–90.

122. Patzelt SB, Emmanouilidi A, Stampf S, et al. Accuracy of full-arch scans using intraoral scanners. *Clin Oral Invest* 2014;18:1687–1694.

123. Lin CL, Chang YH, Chang WJ, Cheng MH. Evaluation of a reinforced slot design for Cerec system to restore extensively compromised premolars. *J Dent* 2006;34:221–229.

124. Goldstein, R. *Esthetics in Dentistry*, 2nd edn. Hamilton, Ontario: B.C. Decker; 1998.

125. Mclaren, E, Figueira, J, Goldstein,R. Vonlays: A conservative esthetic alternative to full-coverage crowns. *Compendium* 2015;36: 282–289.

126. Sjögren G, Molin M, van Dijken JW. A 10-year prospective evaluation of CAD/CAM-manufactured (Cerec) ceramic inlays cemented with a chemically cured or dual-cured resin composite. *Int J Prosthodont* 2004;17:241–246.

127. Mormann WH. The evolution of the CEREC system. *J Am Dent Assoc* 2006; 137 (suppl):7S–13S.

128. Santos Jr GC, Santos Jr MJ, Rizkalla AS, et al. Overview of CEREC CAD/CAM chairside system. *Gen Dent* 2013;61:36–40.

129. Yuzbasioglu E, Kurt H, Turunc R, Bilir H. Comparison of digital and conventional impression techniques: evaluation of patients' perception, treatment comfort, effectiveness and clinical outcomes. *BMC Oral Health* 2014;14:10.

130. Patzelt SB, Lamprinos C, Stampf S, Att W. The time efficiency of intraoral scanners: an in vitro comparative study. *J Am Dent Assoc* 2014;145:542–551.

131. Nakamura T, Dei N, Kojima T, Wakabayashi K. Marginal and internal fit of Cerec 3 CAD/CAM all-ceramic crowns. *Int J Prosthodont* 2003;16:244–248.

132. Stappert CF, Chitmongkolsuk S, Silva NR, et al. Effect of mouth-motion fatigue and thermal cycling on the marginal accuracy of partial coverage restorations made of various dental materials. *Dent Mater* 2008;24:1248–1257.

133. Reiss B, Walther W. Clinical long-term reults and 10 year Kaplan Meier analysis of Cerec restorations. *Int J Comput Dent* 2000;3:9–23.

134. Posselt A, Kerschbaum T. Longevity of 2328 chairside Cerec inlays and onlays. *Int J Comput Dent* 2003;6:231–248.

135. Zimmer S, Gohlich O, Ruttermann S, et al. Long-term survival of Cerec restorations: a 10-year study. *Oper Dent* 2008;33:484–487.

136. Fasbinder DJ. Clinical performance of chairside CAD/CAM restorations. *J Am Dent Assoc* 2006;137 (suppl):22S–31S.

137. Estafan D, Dussetschleger F, Agosta C, Reich S. Scanning electron microscope evaluation of CEREC II and CEREC III inlays. *Gen Dent* 2003;51:450–454.

138. Reich S, Wichmann M, Nkenke E, Proeschel P. Clinical fit of all-ceramic three-unit fixed partial dentures, generated with three different CAD/CAM systems. *Eur J Oral Sci* 2005;113:174–179.

139. Denissen H, Dozic A, van der Zel J, van Waas M. Marginal fit and short-term clinical performance of porcelain-veneered CICERO, CEREC, and Procera onlays. *J Prosthet Dent* 2000;84:506–513.

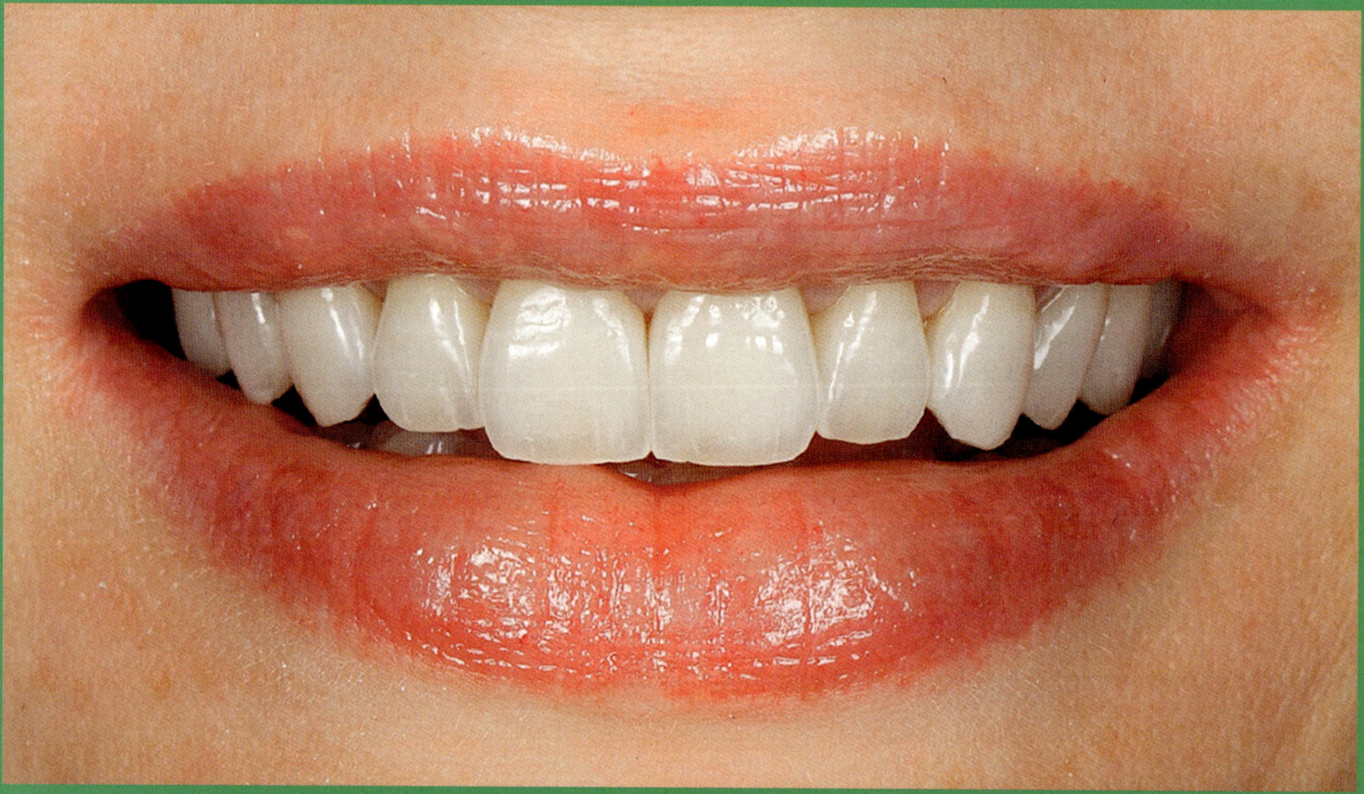

Chapter 16 Crown Restorations

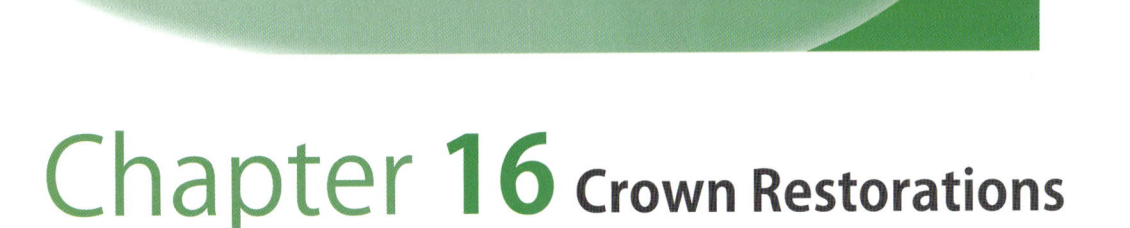

Kenneth A. Malament, DDS, MScD, Ronald E. Goldstein, DDS, Christian F.J. Stappert, MS, DDS, PhD, Mo Taheri, DMD, and Thomas Sing, MDT

Chapter Outline

Indications for a complete coverage crown	499
Diagnosis	500
Technical considerations	500
Choice of materials with associated technique considerations	502
IPS *Empress*	510
IPS *e.max*	512
Metal–ceramic restorations	514
Porcelain fused to metal	514
Adjunctive procedures	515
Esthetic considerations	516
Technical considerations	516
Tooth preparation	518
How to choose the right crown for esthetics	523
Specific problem: the discolored pulpless tooth	523
Opaquing	524
Principles for esthetic restorations	525
Lip line	525
Arch irregularity	526
Inclination of teeth	526
Tooth contour and shape	529
Final esthetic try-in	529
Tooth size	530
Correct occlusal registration	531
Tooth arrangement	531
Tooth color	532
Texture	532
Light	532
What to record	533
Review of tips for shade matching	535
Patient maintenance	536

A dental crown restoration can offer a remarkable service for a dental patient. The objectives of a crown are to restore function and esthetics for a treated tooth. This process may involve caries removal, endodontic therapy, periodontal therapy, and treatment of multiple teeth. A careful evaluation of the patient's occlusion provides the opportunity to establish ideal function. Meticulously observing tooth shape, shade, and texture ensures a pleasing result in the appearance of the new crown. When carefully crafted, the dental crown restoration has excellent long-term survival.

Indications for a complete coverage crown

The following are indications for a complete coverage crown:

- teeth with extensive caries
- teeth weakened by extensive restorations
- teeth with excessive wear
- teeth severely weakened or prone to fracture as a result of endodontic treatment

- teeth fractured or compromised with extensive microcracks
- restoration of the plane of occlusion as in the case of extruded teeth or teeth below plane of occlusion
- malformed teeth
- abutments for fixed partial dentures
- teeth with excessive interdental spaces
- teeth with excessive recession where soft tissue grafting is not appropriate
- restorations on implant abutments.

A patient should be informed of the ways that a full coverage crown can benefit them; however, the patient must also be informed of the potential complications of treatment. In some situations, detection of caries or cracks under existing restorations may require additional dental treatment, such as endodontic or periodontal therapy.

A crown can potentially remain functionally sound for the life of the tooth, but there are several factors that can affect the lifespan of a crown. After insertion of a restoration, the dentist should emphasize the importance of good home care and compliance with hygiene recall appointments, as a natural tooth is still susceptible to caries underneath the margins of a crown. Crown material fracture is a risk with all ceramics and porcelain. Changes in soft tissue and bone and changes in shade of adjacent natural teeth may also require remake of the crown at some point in the future.

Diagnosis

Some crown failures result entirely due to the lack of proper diagnosis and treatment planning from the onset. Major considerations that confront the dentist are patient expectations, existing disease, and esthetic and functional diagnosis. Treatment technique, material choice, and communication with the dental laboratory technologist are critical to successful patient care.

Adjacent teeth and the opposing ones need to be examined and evaluated for esthetics and function. An opposing tooth or neighboring tooth may need to be reshaped or restored to create a correct plane of occlusion or to give the desired esthetic result of a patient's smile (Figures 16.1A–B and 16.2A–F).

Photographs

Digital photographic records should be used as part of diagnosis. Photographs allow the dentist and the patient to see the issues from the same perspective and serves as a discussion point for esthetic and functional goals. Pretreatment photographs can help predict how complex the esthetic correction will be (Figures 16.1A and B). It should become evident to the patient that the range of problems present and the relative difficulty of the treatment can affect treatment time and case fee. *It is preferable to subtly introduce the relationship between difficulty and fees at this early stage rather than later.* Photographs also open a dialogue with the dental laboratory technician about the challenges they will encounter with the patient's treatment.

An effective photographic technique has been developed by Kuwata.[1] In this quick and easy-to-use system, photos can be made and stored in computer photographic software such as Apple's Aperture or Adobe's Lightroom™. The photographs can be downloaded to the storage program and minor adjustments made so that they are presentable to the patient and the images can be easily e-mailed to the technician or printed. The dentist can also place some images into presentation software such as Apple's Keynote or Microsoft's PowerPoint™ and draw lines defining symmetry and occlusal or esthetic planes. An extraoral digital video camera can also be very effective to determine the display of teeth during speaking, laughing, and with the smile analysis.

Technical considerations

An understanding of dental laboratory procedures is important because the quality and accuracy of the restorations may impact why esthetic restorations fail. Often, failure arises from poor planning and neglect of details by the dentist or the technician, so the dentist must give the technician a clearly defined and detailed laboratory prescription.

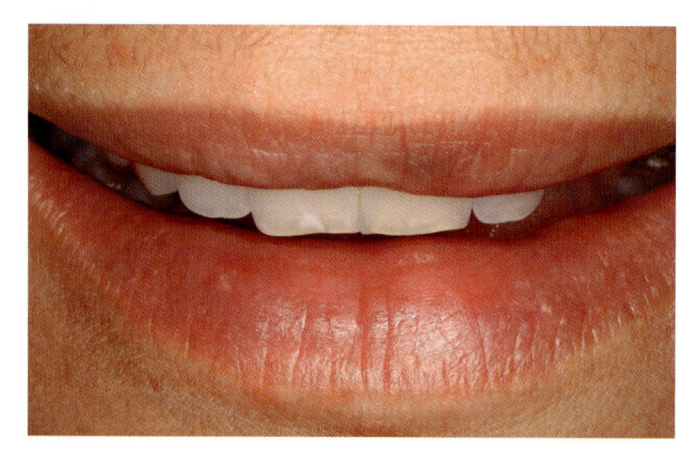

Figure 16.1 **(A)** This patient presented with esthetic and functional concerns. Due to a loss of vertical dimension and loss of canine guidance, the anterior incisors tooth length was significantly reduced. Additionally, a crossbite on the upper left side made her upper left teeth almost invisible.

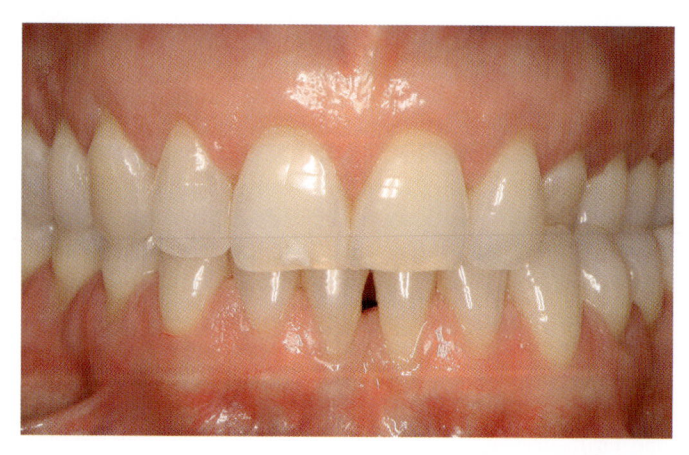

Figure 16.1 **(B)** Clinical thorough evaluation, planning models, wax-up simulation and photo documentation led to an comprehensive treatment planning to restore periodontal, functional and esthetic concerns of the patient (Figures 16-2A–F).

Chapter 16 Crown Restorations

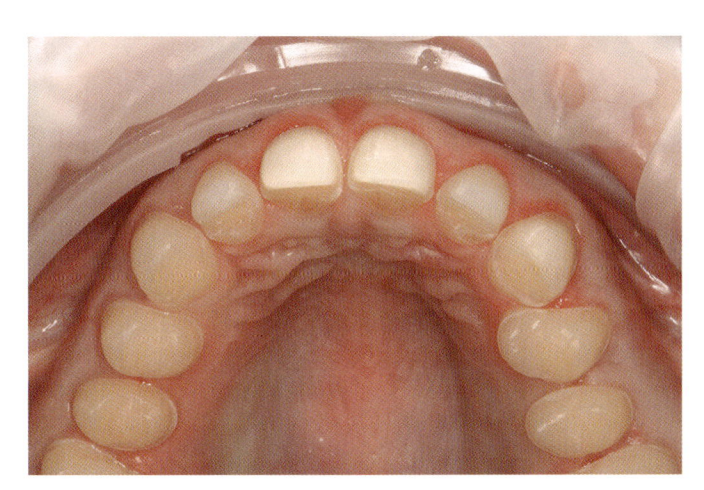

Figure 16.2 **(A)** After periodontal treatment, a mock-up of the new inter-maxillary dimension was used to minimize tooth structure reduction. The anterior dentition was prepared for butt-joint veneers, and the posterior dentition received thin lithium-disilicate 360° crown-veneers.

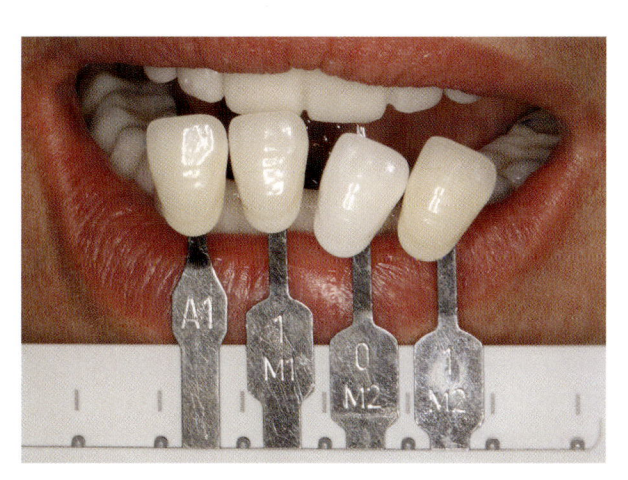

Figure 16.2 **(B)** The patient has high esthetic demands, and expectations. A request for 'very white teeth' should be addressed in a reasonable range of brightness, since too white teeth often lack recognizable surface texture and transparency.

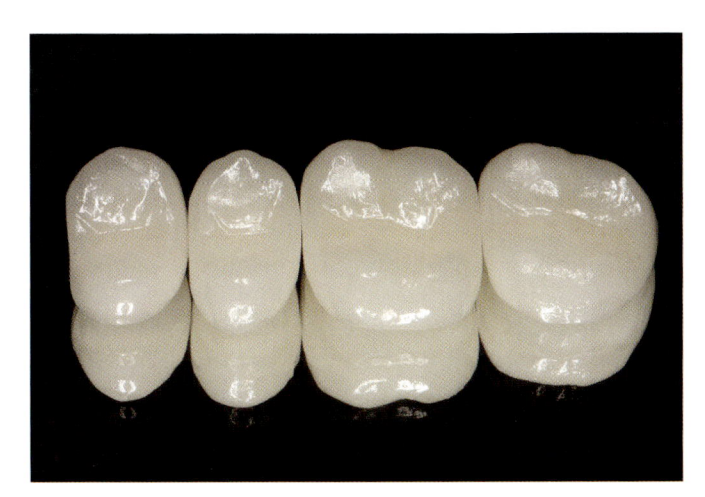

Figure 16.2 **(C)** To restore the dental display at the left buccal corridor, and adjust the vertical inter-maxillary dimension, IPS e.max Press 360° monolithic crowns and veneers were fabricated. Average ceramic thickness ranges from 0.3 to 1.2 mm.

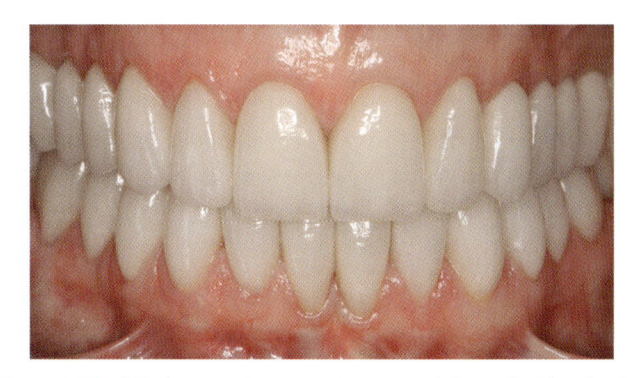

Figure 16.2 **(D)** The ceramic restorations were delivered with adhesive bonded resin cement under Rubberdam. Note the improvement in character, color, and shape. The new incisal position allowed for a steeper anterior guidance and provided adequate posterior separation.

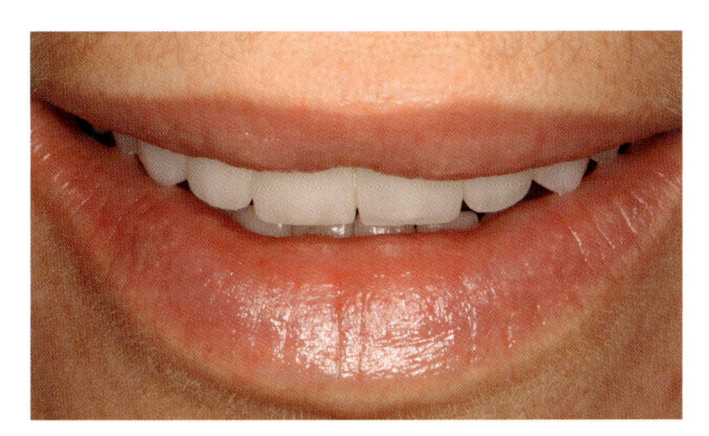

Figure 16.2 **(E)** Anterior central incisor and canine veneers follow the lower lip-line, barley touching the lower lip. Visibility of the upper and lower teeth during a light smile, creates a youthful impression.

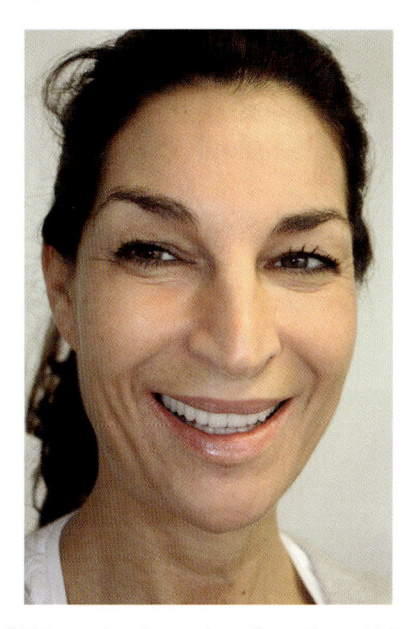

Figure 16.2 **(F)** The patient is seen happily smiling with her new ceramic restorations. The buccal corridor displays beautiful teeth on both sides evenly. The lower facial third becomes more recognizable, guiding the observer's view in a triangle between the patient's eyes and smile. Courtesy of Insititute of Advanced Dental Education GmbH, Zurich.

Successful esthetic and functional results primarily depend on adherence to sound principles of form, correct occlusion, articulation, and contacts. This is emphasized in a retrospective study of 320 crowns by Gropp et al.[2] Regardless of the materials used, abnormalities of occlusion and articulation were found in 14% of all crowns. Missing interproximal contacts were present in 19%, which caused noticeable inflammation in 9.5%, pocket formation in 5.5%, and radiographic abnormalities of the marginal periodontium in 6% of the cases. The cervical portion of the tooth was denuded in 31% of the cases, resulting in a 12% incidence of cervical caries. Esthetics will also be compromised when functional breakdown occurs.

Choice of materials with associated technique considerations

The choice of an appropriate restoration material depends on the functional and esthetic demands that will be placed upon it. Gropp et al.[2] also indicated that, functionally, the all-cast crown was the most successful, especially when precision casting techniques were used. This was followed in clinical acceptance by porcelain-fused-to-metal crowns, full ceramic crowns, and then full acrylic crowns. Whereas previously the standard of care for esthetic ceramic materials was porcelain fused to gold or all-ceramic materials, the standard for quality individual restorations today is principally a monolithic all-ceramic. The all-ceramic materials have developed from Dicor, In-Ceram, Ivoclar Porcelain System (IPS Empress), to bilayer zirconia–feldspathic porcelain combinations to monolithic IPS e.max Press or CAD and all-zirconia restorations.

Gold

The full gold crown has always been considered by dentists to be the most functionally sound, longest lasting restoration of its type. Its excellent marginal adaptation can be seen in Figure 16.3. It is a conservative restoration requiring much less reduction of tooth structure than an all-ceramic or porcelain-fused-to-metal crown, and its wear rate approximates that of natural enamel. If patients cannot see a gold restoration or they have little objection to it or the increasing cost, a yellow gold restoration is an excellent dental material to be used with partial or full coverage single tooth restorations. However, there are still some patients who prefer the longevity of full gold restorations (Figure 16.4A–C).

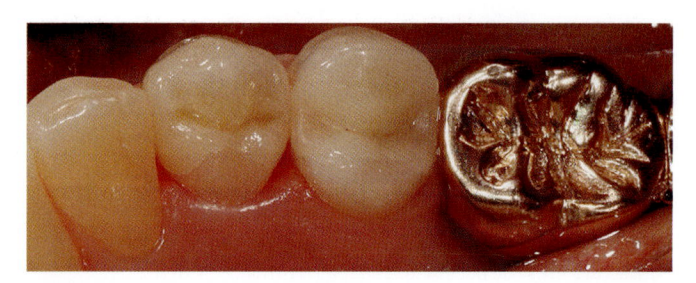

Figure 16.3 The gold crown exhibits excellent long-term stability and marginal integrity. The first bicuspid is restored with an e.max inlay, and the second bicuspid with an Empress crown.

Plus, a micro-etcher or air-abrasive device can dull or antique the gold sheen of the crown (Figures 16.5A–C and 16.6A and B).

Resins

Resin technology has developed significantly but does not have the physical strength characteristics necessary for use as final restorations with the expectation of long-term survival. Resin technology has been one of the most notable advancements in esthetic dentistry; therefore, it is important to understand a modern historic perspective of the different materials.

Acrylic resin or composite resins have been used to construct anterior full crowns (Figure 16.7A and B). Translucency, reasonable color stability, ease of construction and color matching, and economics have enhanced its popularity as a provisional restoration. It is relatively easy to obtain a good fit, and the material is biologically acceptable for short periods. Wear at the contact areas does not appreciably affect arch length or embrasure form. However, the material will abrade along the incisal edge. Because it also absorbs bacterial biofilms, leading to staining, it may be poorly tolerated by tissue and is too elastic.[3] An acrylic crown should be used as a long-term provisional fixed bridge or individual crown only in those instances where it is specifically indicated by circumstances or lifestyle, or when it may take the patient several years before they will be in a financial position to undergo correction in metal or ceramics, or a combination of the two. To reduce wear and staining, acrylic veneers or crowns can be hardened by heat processing[4] and curing under pressure.[5]

A later generation of veneering materials is light-polymerized composite resin (Dentacolor, Jelenko/Kulzer, Inc., Isosit-N, Ivoclar; and Visio-Gem, ESPE GmbH). Designed for indirect veneering in the laboratory, these composite resins had definite advantages over acrylic resins.[6] Composite resins may also be valuable in the repair of metal–ceramic restorations from which the porcelain has chipped off or fractured. If the restoration is otherwise serviceable, then the porcelain may be repaired by first creating micromechanical retention with an air abrasive, then acid etching, using silane coupling agents, and bonding with composite resin.

The two most significant problems with resins or composite resins are microleakage and occlusal wear. For example, Gallegos and Nicholls found that when opposing porcelain over a period of time, Isosit-N lost approximately 70% of its matrix filler, which was greater than that of Visio-Gem, but significantly less than the loss of porcelain under the same simulated functional forces.[7]

Composite resins often chip away from the restoration (Figure 16.8). Greenberg and Rafetto, studying Visio-Gem (ESPE), caution that it must be at least 1.5 mm thick and should not be used on masticatory surfaces because of its potential to chip.[8]

Feldspathic porcelain

Full-feldspathic porcelain crowns manufactured on platinum foils were one of the first attempts to create durable all-ceramic restorations. Today, glass-ceramic materials with enhanced fracture strength are predominantly used for all ceramic crown restorations, but all-feldspathic porcelain material is commonly used for esthetic porcelain veneers.

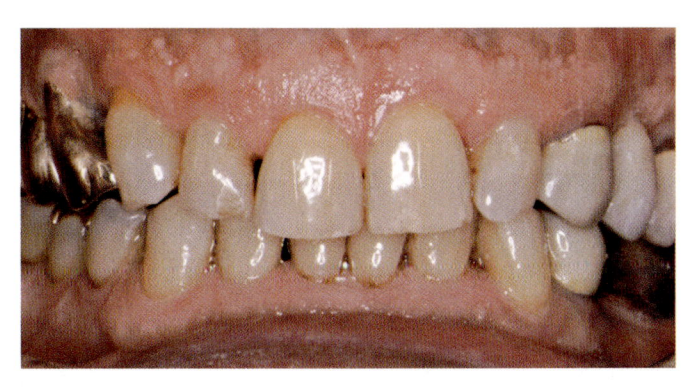

Figure 16.4 **(A)** This 69-year-old man had previously been functionally and esthetically satisfied with his all-gold crowns. However, when it came time for replacement, another dentist encouraged the patient to choose metal–ceramic, which shortly thereafter began to chip.

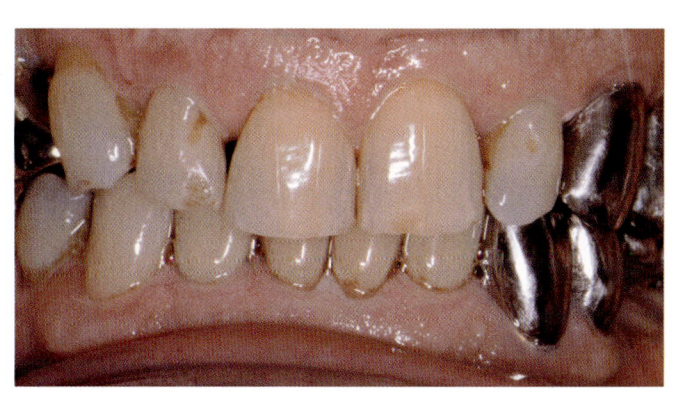

Figure 16.4 **(B)** The patient returned and had the restorations replaced with all-gold crowns.

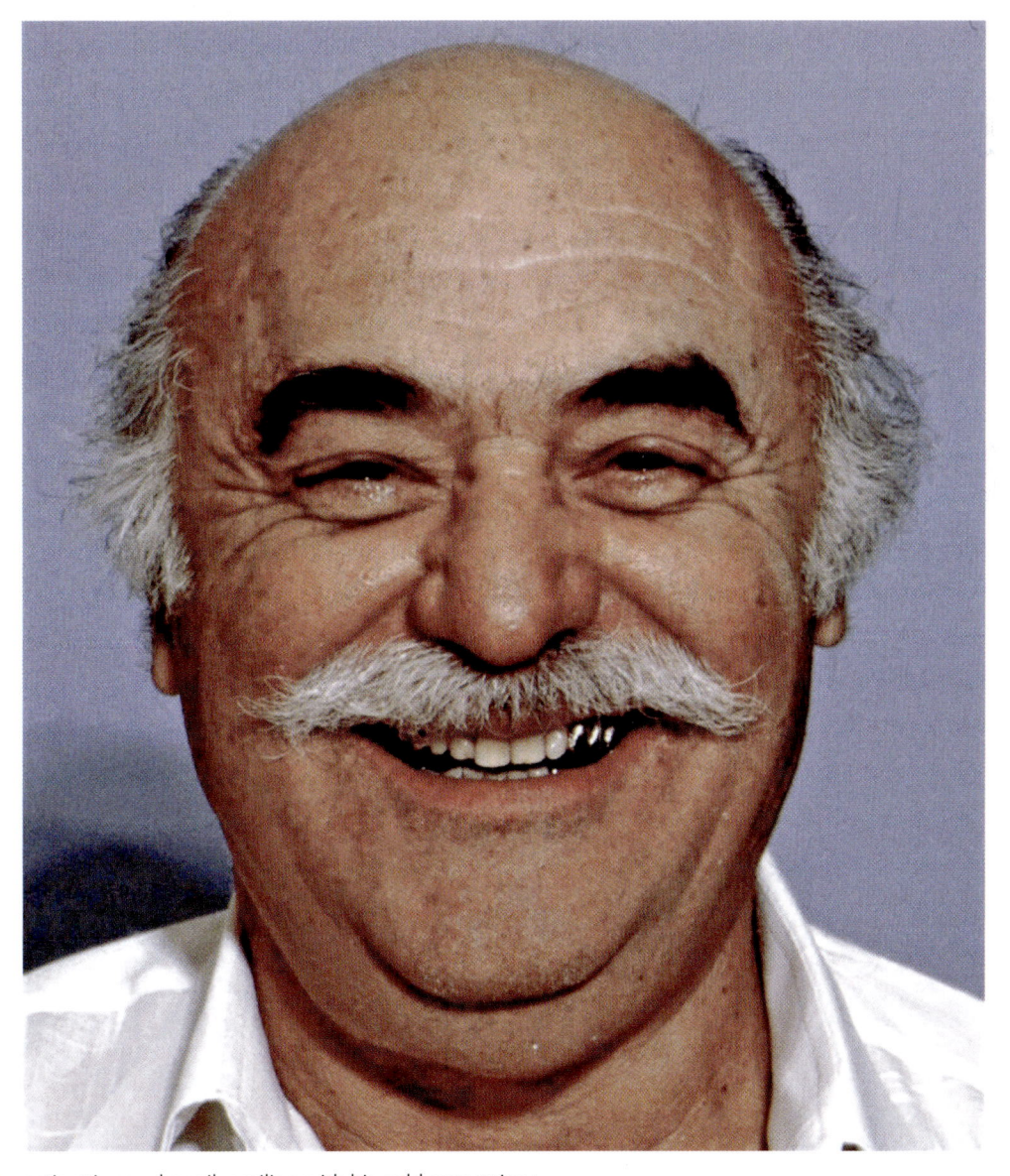

Figure 16.4 **(C)** The patient is seen happily smiling with his gold restorations.

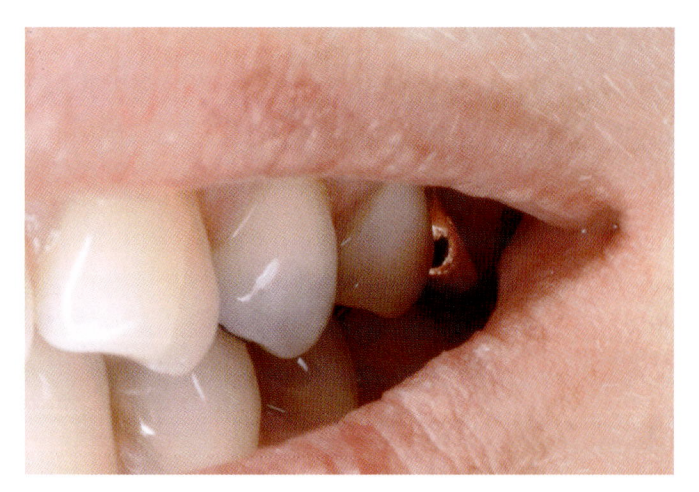

Figure 16.5 **(A)** This three-quarter gold crown on the maxillary first molar shows during smiling.

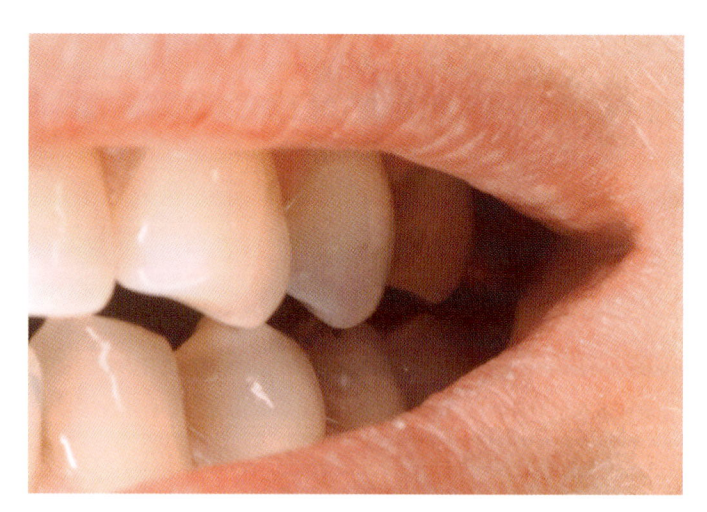

Figure 16.5 **(B)** Note the esthetic improvement when the patient smiles.

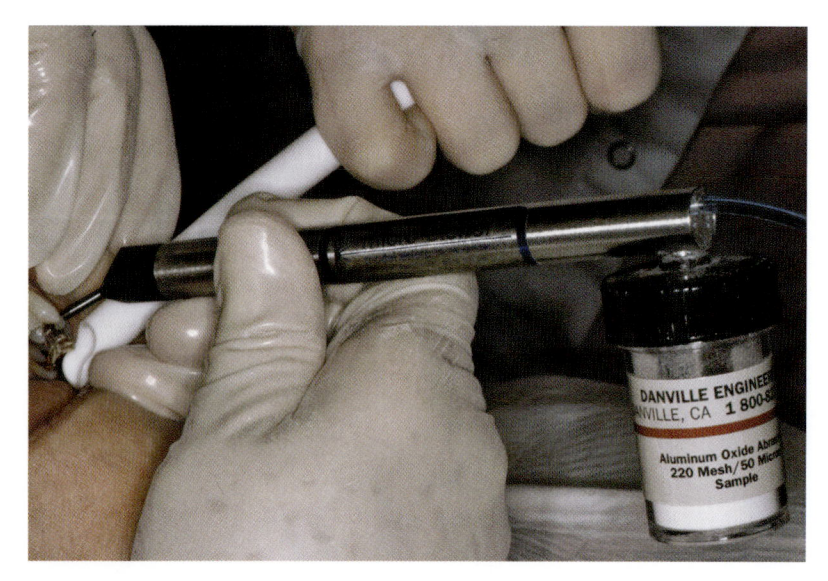

Figure 16.5 **(C)** A simple application with a micro-etcher (Paasche) or air-abrasive device dulls or antiques the gold sheen of the crown.

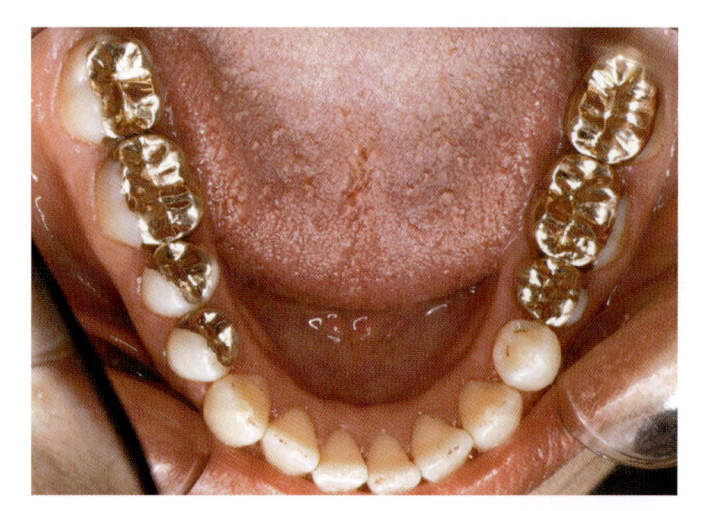

Figure 16.6 **(A)** This 35-year-old female wanted the longest lasting restorations available. Although she did not want gold showing, esthetics were a secondary consideration.

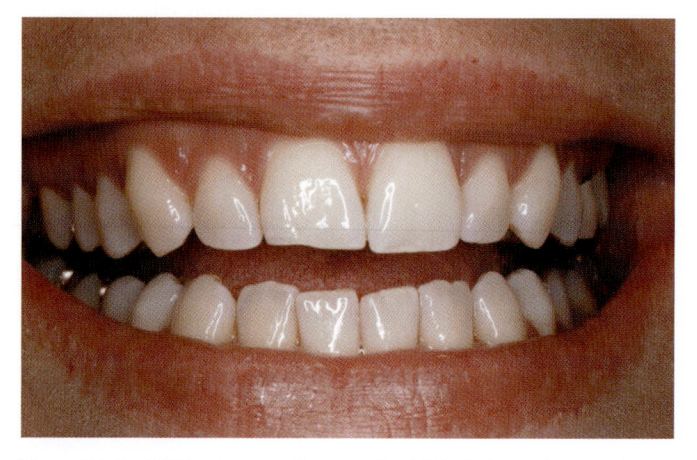

Figure 16.6 **(B)** The two small areas of gold that showed when she smiled did not concern this patient.

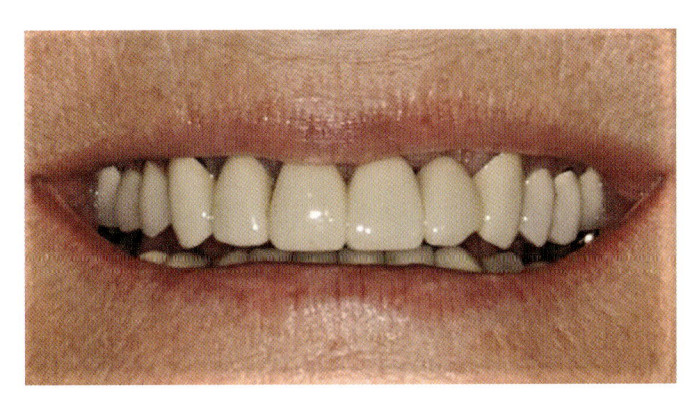

Figure 16.7 **(A)** This patient presented with a fractured fixed-partial denture spanning the maxillary anteriors. Beneath the fixed-partial denture, one of the abutments had fractured and soft tissue recession had occurred.

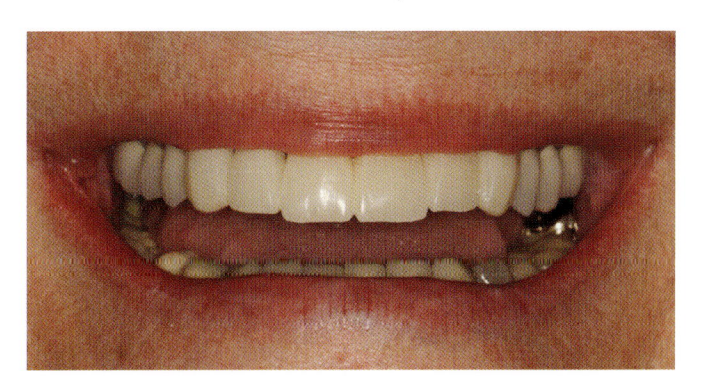

Figure 16.7 **(B)** Long-term poly(methyl methacrylate) provisionals were provided to allow for an esthetic interim restoration during grafting and endodontic procedures.

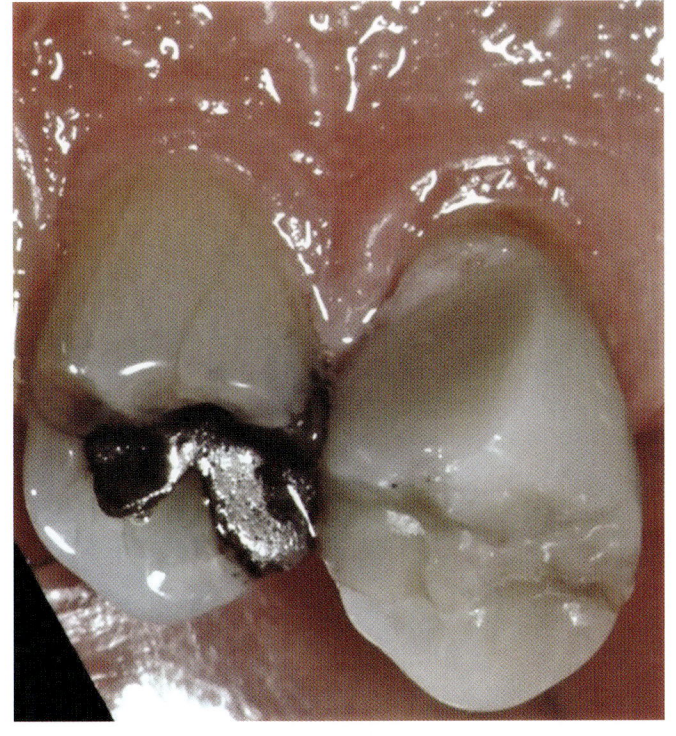

Figure 16.8 This indirect, composite resin crown fractured after only short-term use. *Source:* Photograph courtesy of Dr Joseph Greenberg, Philadelphia, PA.

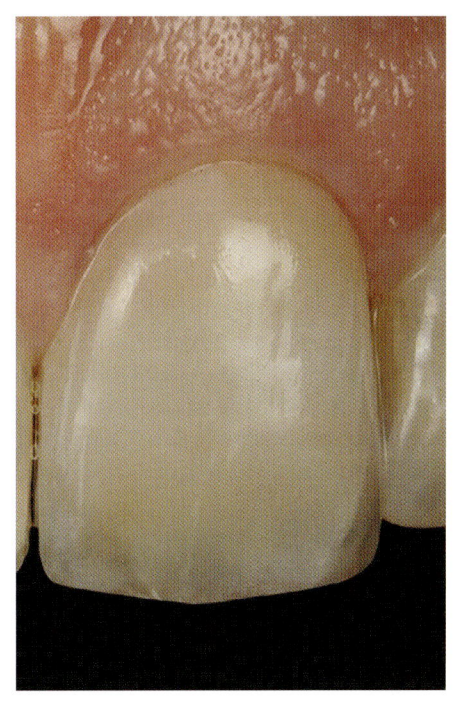

Figure 16.9 An excellent tissue response is typical of this well-fitting, all-porcelain crown.

Advantages

All-porcelain ceramic veneers are considered by many dentists to be state of the art, esthetically pleasing, and minimally invasive restorations. They have the potential to be translucent, color stable, brilliant, and lifelike. If they are acid etched and cemented principally to etched enamel, they have a long life expectancy in most patients. A properly fabricated and artistically produced porcelain veneer is often almost impossible to detect visually. The advent of vacuum firing has reduced bubbles, producing a fine-textured restoration with improved translucency, and increased impact strength. Porcelain is biologically acceptable and well tolerated by the soft tissues (Figures 16.9 and 16.10A and B).

Disadvantages

Feldspathic, IPS Empress, or IPS e.max ceramic veneers must be bonded and cemented preferable to etched enamel. If ceramic veneers are cemented to dentin, the moisture in dentin could hydrolyses the dentin bonding agent and in time could decrease the effectiveness of the bond strength of the adhesive cement.

Contraindications for traditional ceramic veneer use

1. When the tooth has limited enamel present or has interproximal composite resin restorations, where there is extensive dentin exposure.
2. When existing tooth color is so dark or low value that the veneer would not be likely to correct the unesthetic color. (For further information on ceramic veneers please see Chapter 15).

All-ceramic restorations

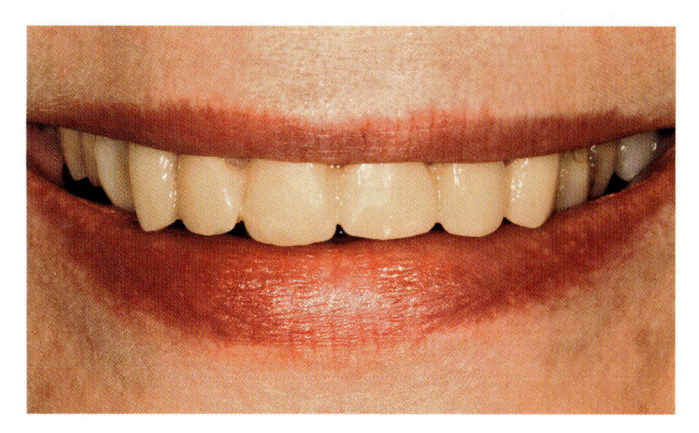

Figure 16.10 **(A)** This patient was displeased with her smile and requested full porcelain crowns for the longest restorative life expectancy.

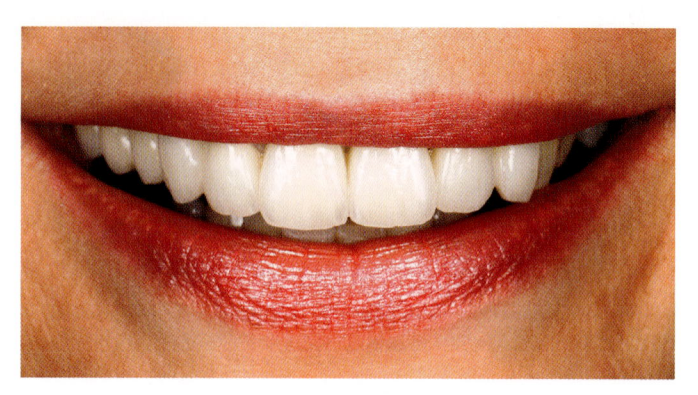

Figure 16.10 **(B)** A high degree of naturalness was obtained in these anterior all-porcelain crowns. Proper texture, shade variation, incisal translucency, contours, and embrasures contribute to the esthetic result.

Dicor

Dicor glass-ceramic material (Denstply International, York, PA) was developed by Peter Adair of Boston University Graduate School of Dentistry and David Grossman at Corning Glass Works[9,10] in 1978. After working out details for clinical applications,[11] the material was released to the dental community in 1982. Dicor was a fluorine-containing tetrasilicic glass-ceramic in the Pyroceram family of glass-ceramics. Restorations were made using the lost-wax technique. The casting had to be cerammed to develop internal mica-based crystals to create glass-ceramic form. Dicor was a well-researched dental material that could be used as a monolithic ceramic with surface metallic oxide colorants or used as a bilayer ceramic where it was used as a core with feldspathic ceramic applied as a veneering material. Dicor was first developed to be luted to teeth with zinc phosphate or glass ionomer luting agents. Grossman created a 10% ammonium bifluoride etchant[12] to both clean and etch the surface to allow composite resin luting. Clinical investigations have examined the many variables that might affect the long-term survival of Dicor complete coverage restorations.[13–15] Improved physical and clinical performance was described when Dicor was acid etched.[13] Other studies examined the effect of breaking strength of Dicor related to gender,[13] tooth position,[13] thickness,[14] margin design,[14] and the type of luting agent.[15] Studies have related the fracture resistance of Dicor crowns to crown length and the effect of varying the elastic moduli of the underlying supporting structure.[15,16] The effects that flaws in Dicor or luting agent spaces had on fracture potential and tensile strength were tested, as well as the effects of physiologic aging, abrasiveness, wear, and surface roughness.[4,17–30] The cast-glass preparation required a shoulder with rounded gingivoaxial line angles, or a deep (120°) chamfer. The axial surfaces should be reduced by 1.3–1.5 mm and the incisal or occlusal surface by 1.5–2.0 mm (Figure 16.11A–D) and free of undercuts. Impressions, casts, and dies are obtained in the usual manner. The crown was waxed to full contour, sprued, and invested in a phosphate-bonded investment. Once the crown was cast, it was then heated (cerammed) to grow the proper and mature crystalline form and increase strength. It was then shaded with surface metallic oxides and feldspathic colorants to match the shade and create translucency. Geller and coworkers[20,21] described another application for castable glass. This application involves using the cast glass as a substructure core, upon which porcelain Vitadur N or Vitadur Alpha can be baked (Willis glass). The advantages of using cast glass in this manner include precise marginal fit, margins that do not distort from multiple firings during the porcelain build-up process, favorable reaction of periodontal tissue to the glazed material, and improved esthetics.[22] The combination of a more translucent core, over which internally stained colors and effects are built in, can provide a highly esthetic result. Dicor was researched extensively, and many lessons were learned from its use. It has not been on the market for many years. Table 16.1 covers the most frequent problems concerning all-ceramic crowns.

In-Ceram

In-Ceram glass-ceramic material (Vita, Bad Sackingen, Germany) was developed by Michael Sadoun[7] and originally described as a slip-cast aluminum oxide ceramic. It initially consists of a densely packed slurry (80–82 wt%) of pure aluminum oxide, which is then fired at 1120 °C for 3 h on a refractory die. A lanthanum glass is infiltrated into the porous coping and fired again to 1100 °C for 4 h, producing a coping without shrinkage yet having high mechanical strength (In-Ceram alumina is similar in mechanical properties to 99.9% pure aluminum oxide). The infiltrated In-Ceram coping is dense, homogeneous, and of high strength. This opaque coping is veneered with feldspathic porcelain, creating a bilayer ceramic restoration (Figure 16.12A–L). To minimize surface cracks and to maintain its physical strength, the In-Ceram restoration cannot be acid etched and, like all all-ceramic materials, must never be sandblasted.[23] This ceramic can be luted with either conventional (reinforced glass ionomer) or composite resin luting agents. Clinical investigations have examined the long-term survival in function.[20,24] Because of its purported strength, posterior crowns were made, but the frequency of fracture and long-term survival did not meet expectations.

Chapter 16 Crown Restorations

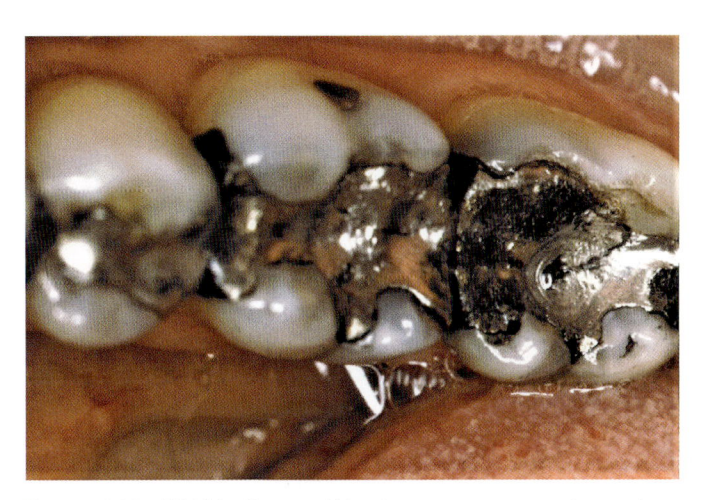

Figure 16.11 **(A)** This 51-year-old business woman wanted to replace her defective amalgam restorations with esthetic crowns that did not contain metal. Two cast-glass (Dicor, Dentsply) crowns were constructed for the first and second molars while more conservative porcelain onlays were made for the bicuspids.

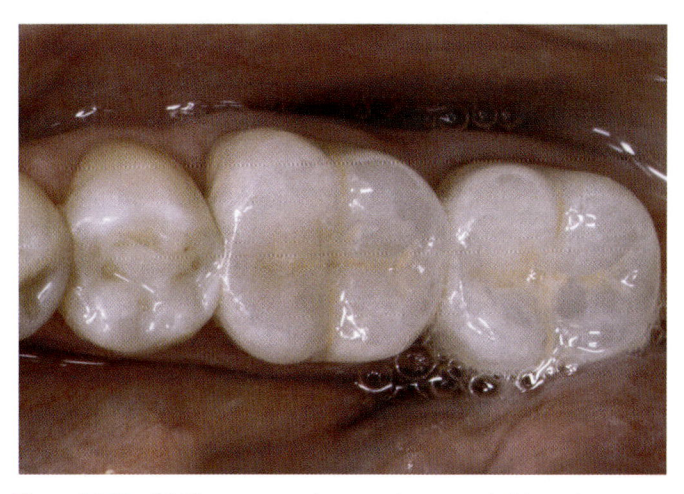

Figure 16.11 **(B)** The cerammed restorations are tried-in and cemented to place. Since the two cast-glass crowns were placed over amalgam-stained dentin, a colored opaque cement was used to help mask the discoloration.

Table 16.1 Troubleshooting Esthetics Guide for All-Porcelain Crowns

Problem	Solution
Tooth preparation is visible through porcelain	Add porcelain to labial aspect
	Reprepare the tooth to allow porcelain to be thicker
Teeth are unnaturally even	Provide for variation in tooth length and enhance illusion of spacing by shading and shape
	Open incisal embrasures
Glaze is too high	Break up light being reflected by texturing the porcelain
Crown is too opaque	Use more incisal shading or surface stains
Shade varies excessively	Select shade using color-corrected artificial light and outside light
	Laboratory must use same lighting
	Stain by using sectional shade chart (see Figure 16.2A)
Crown shade is dull	May be due to use of opaque-type cement
	Use a cement with more translucency, such as silicophosphate, composite, or glass ionomer
Porcelain is fractured	Correct to minimal occlusion in anterior teeth
	Provide greater thickness of porcelain
	Reduce stress factors by removing sharp edges or corners in tooth preparation
	Avoid inadequate length of preparation
	Change to aluminous porcelain or metal–ceramic

Alumina– or zirconia–feldspathic bilayers

Procera, Lava, Cercon, and Katana uses CAD/CAM technology to fabricate an all-ceramic crown incorporating a densely sintered zirconia or high-purity aluminum oxide coping. A computer-controlled design system in the dental office or laboratory collects tooth preparation and coping design data that is transmitted via modem to the manufacturing site. After fabrication, the coping is delivered to the dental laboratory where the ceramist completes the restoration with the addition of veneering porcelain. This system produces a crown that is color stable, translucent without being transparent, and biocompatible with the opposing dentition.[25]

Sadan and Hegenbarth[26] report that because the high-purity aluminum oxide copings are fabricated in an industrial process, the risk of introducing microcracks and flaws into the completed restoration is minimized. Furthermore, the high strength and accuracy of fit of the copings permit the utilization of these crowns in any segment of the dental arch. Labor-intensive, time-consuming, and technique-sensitive procedures for coping fabrication are eliminated while achieving an esthetic, strong, and durable restoration in a practical and simplified manner. This bilayer application can be used for the single crown and with the addition of zirconia for multiple unit all-ceramic anterior and posterior fixed bridges. The significant issue and reservation with the zirconia–feldspathic bilayer is severe and unpredictable chipping of the feldspathic veneering porcelain.[31] This has limited the use of this material, but with time improvements will be developed. It has been reported that slowing down the cooling rate after firing improves the reliability against chipping.[27]

The use of monolithic zirconia is increasing in popularity and has great potential in prosthetic dentistry. The ability to infiltrate colorants into the presintered zirconia that are improving the color properties of the restorations led to a breakthrough in dental acceptance. It would appear that monolithic zirconia will survive a very long time due to fracture strength exceeding more than 1500 MPa, without creating problems, and since it is

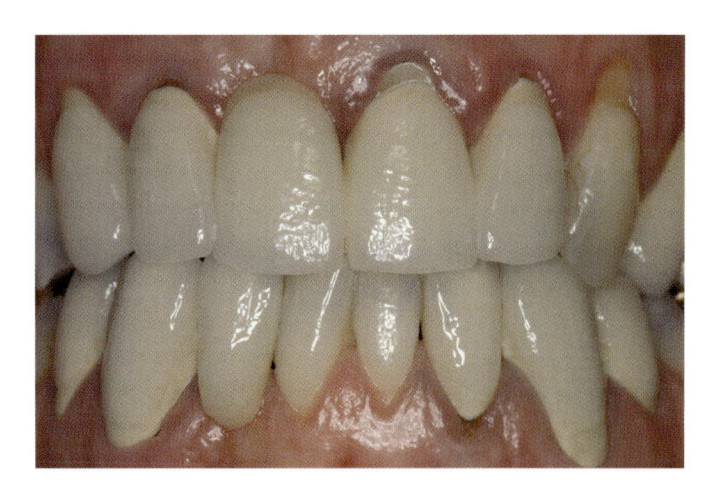

Figure 16.12 **(A)** This 39-year old patient had received multiple dental treatments - tooth loss, multiple endodontic treatments and many porcelain-fused-to-metal restorations (PFM). Being treated by various dentists over time, he was dissatisfied with his dental function and esthetics.

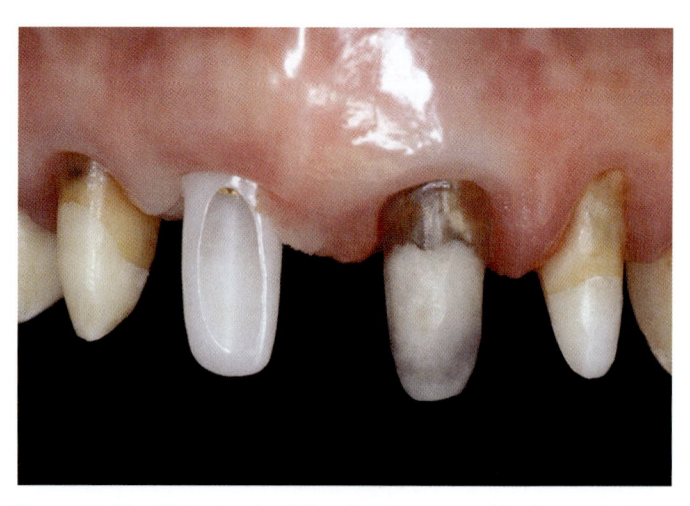

Figure 16.12 **(B)** Under the failing fixed crown and bridge work, the remaining teeth required core built-ups and endodontic revisions. Dental implants were placed. The restorable dental cores and the implant ceramic abutment (CerAdapt, Nobel Biocare) show a high variation in color.

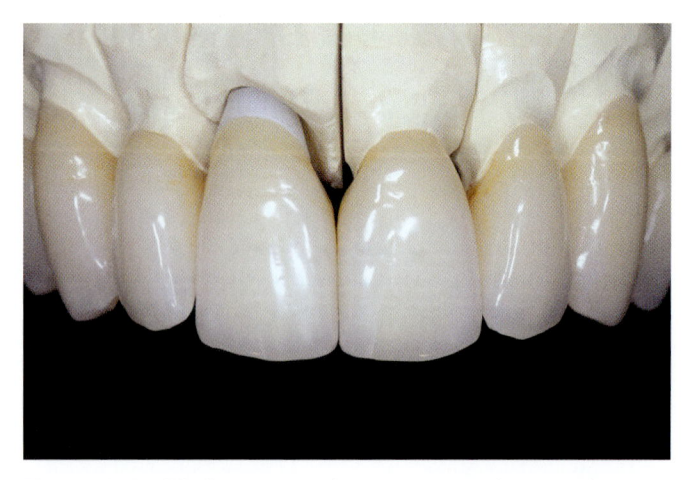

Figure 16.12 **(C)** Aluminum-oxide crown copings (Procera Alumina, Nobel Biocare) were manufactured and veneered with matching feldspathic veneering porcelain (Alumina Rondo, Nobel Biocare).

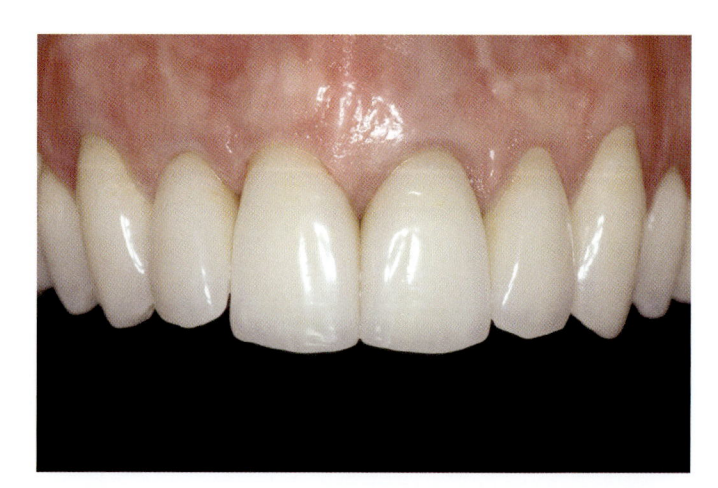

Figure 16.12 **(D)** The clinical outcome demonstrates the esthetic potential of alumina-oxide crown restorations. The opacity is sufficient to cover discoloration of the underlying tooth structure. Chipping rates were very low and clinical survival rates match PFM crown restorations.

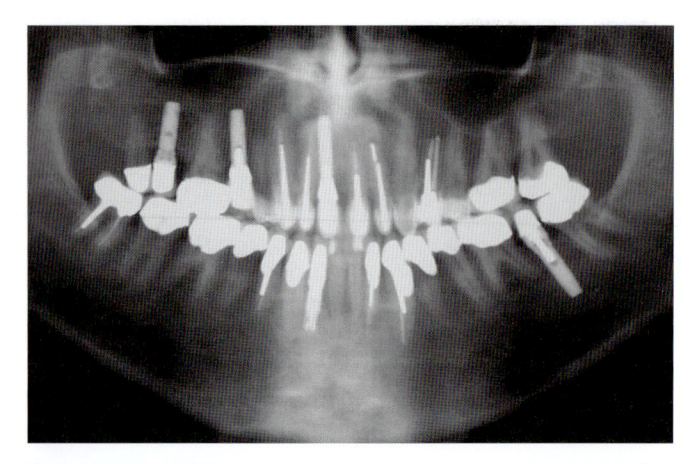

Figure 16.12 **(E)** The panoramic x-ray demonstrates the amount of dental procedures performed. The anterior dentition was treated with Alumina crowns (teeth # 4 to #13), posterior upper and lower teeth were conventionally treated with PFM restorations.

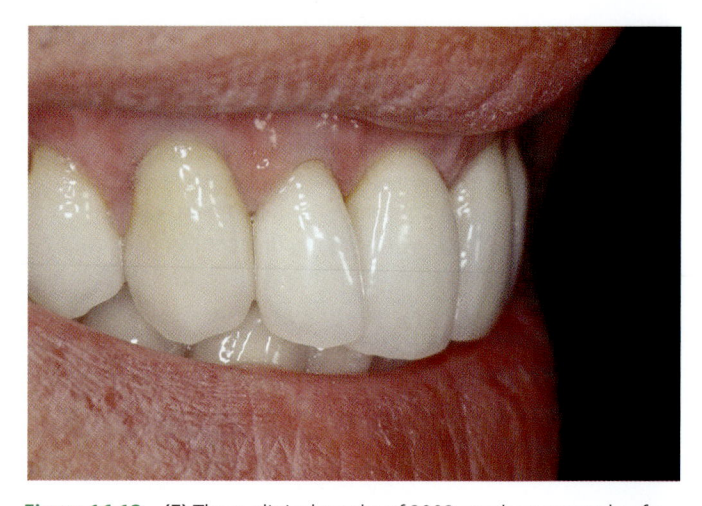

Figure 16.12 **(F)** These clinical results of 2002, mark an example of a coming change from metal-ceramic restorations to all-ceramic crown and bridge oral rehabilitations. Today, it is common to restore posterior teeth also with all-ceramic restorations.

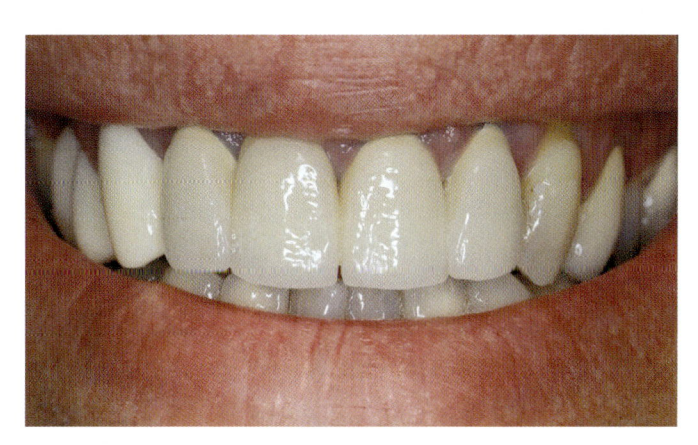

Figure 16.12 **(G) Before:** This image shows the initial metal-ceramic anterior bridge restoration and esthetic limitations. The biological response of the periodontal tissues was compromised.

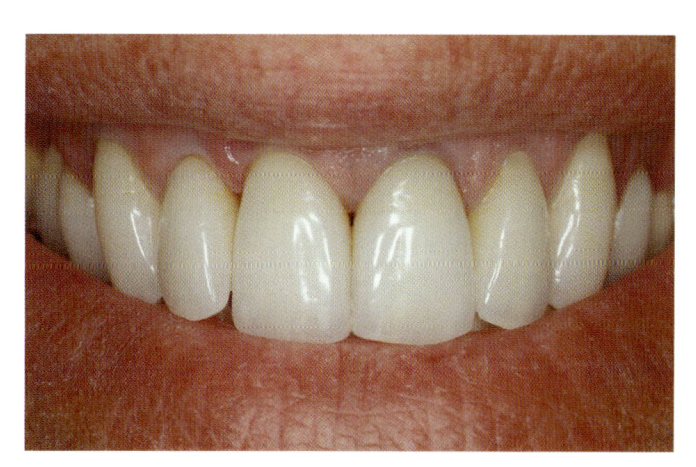

Figure 16.12 **(H) After:** The anterior Alumina rehabilitation, created a natural and transparent dentition, and proofed to be more bioinert to the soft tissue. Presently, the full rehabilitation is 16 years in-situ. Courtesy of Clinical Research Group, University of Freiburg, 2002.

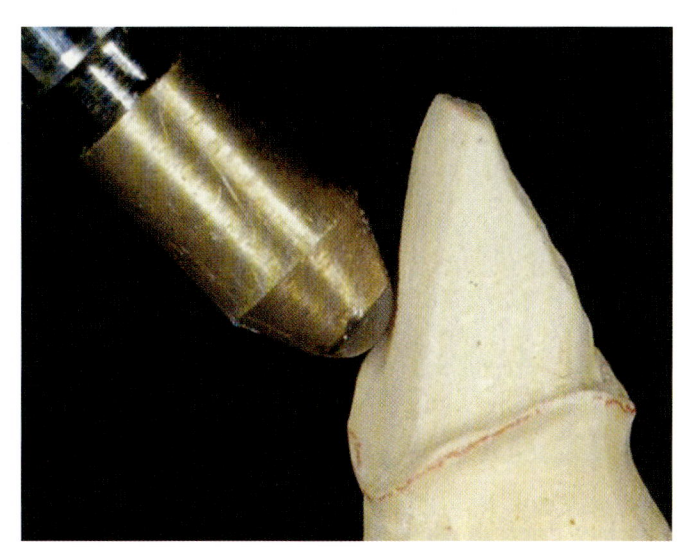

Figure 16.12 **(I)** The scanning probe reads every part of the tooth surface and inputs the measurements into the computer. Next the finish line and thickness of ceramic coping is established.

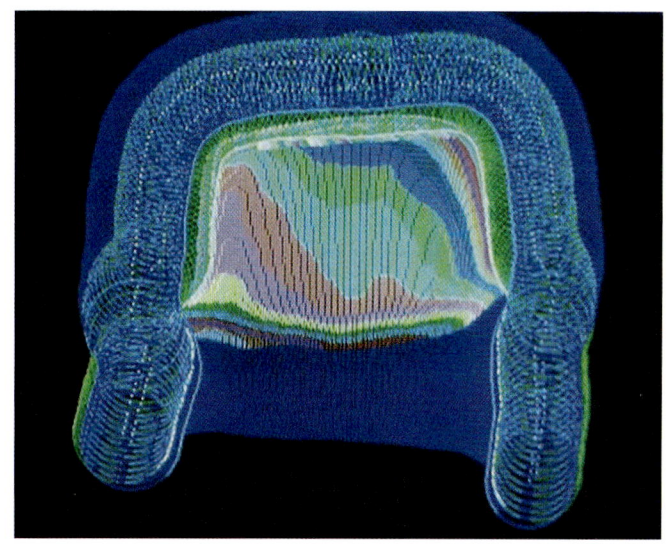

Figure 16.12 **(J)** This three-dimensional computer image is an example of the type of complete design for a molar all-ceramic core. The information is sent to Sweden.

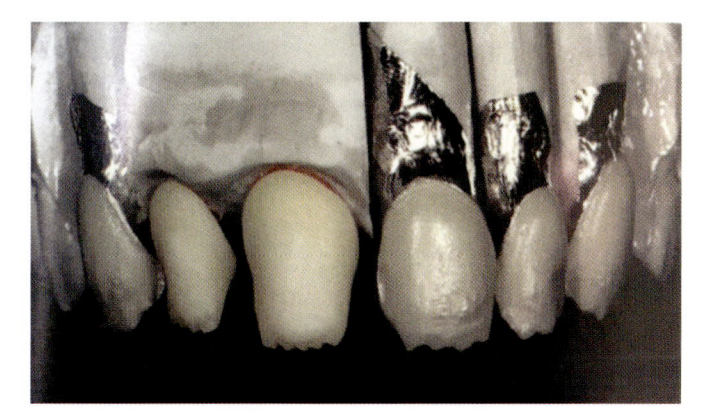

Figure 16.12 **(K)** Procera cores are fabricated in Sweden and sent to the dental office or laboratory in 4 days. Porcelain veneer preparations are prepared on foil and opacious dentin applied and then baked. Next, full-body and incisal affects will complete the veneer and full-crown buildups simultaneously.

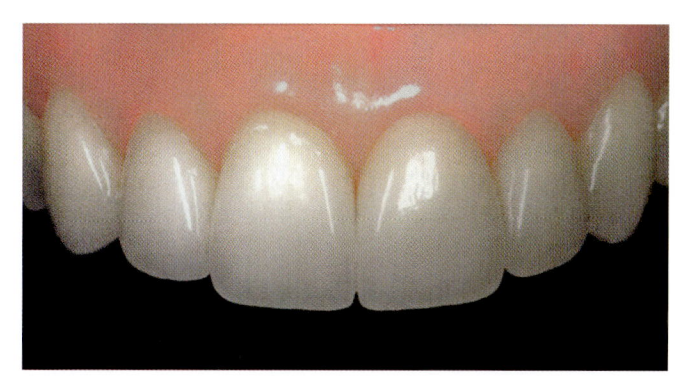

Figure 16.12 **(L)** The final veneers are bonded with Choice (Bisco) translucent dual cure resin cement, and the crowns are final cemented with Panavia (Kuraray). Note the harmonious blend of color and internal characterization.

such a dense, smooth surface, bacteria will not grow into it, and it will be clean. Significant improvements in this technology are occurring monthly. Concerns about wear are less today, and materials are being created to polish and adjust areas that have required alterations. Further details on full-zirconia restorations will be adressed at the end of this chapter.

IPS *Empress*

The IPS Empress all-ceramic material (Ivoclar Vivadent, Inc.,) was developed in association with Arnold Wohlwend and Peter Scharer[21] of the University of Zurich. A leucite-reinforced glass-ceramic, IPS Empress is manufactured through the controlled crystallization of minute leucite crystals found in the glassy matrix through the use of nucleation agents (Figure 16.13). As a monolithic ceramic, this material can be pressed to full or partial contour and colored appropriately; it can also be layered with a corresponding IPS Empress veneering ceramic powder, which is then sintered for an optimal color match. In this respect, it handles to some appreciable extent as feldspathic porcelain. IPS Empress as a silicate-based ceramic is amenable to acid etching and can then be luted to teeth with a composite resin cement system. Numerous authors have described the esthetic potential of this material, and various researchers have attested to its physical properties and long-term survival.[2,28] A major advantage of the all-ceramic crown over posterior metal–ceramic restorations is less occlusal reduction as possible in order to create a uniform thickness of the porcelain (Figure 16.14).

Because the ceramic can be somewhat translucent, the color of the underlying tooth structure may be transmitted through it. To account for this effect, a stump die resin material is available in seven different dentin shades to reproduce the shade of the dentin of the prepared tooth. A specially formulated shade guide, the stump or "dentin" shade guide, is used after tooth preparation to select the shade to be used. The shaded die materials contribute to the highly esthetic outcome of these restorations, as well as the material's inherent natural fluorescence.

The completion of the restoration can then be achieved in two ways: surface colorants or a layering technique. Surface colorants involve using glycerin on the internal surface of the restoration to transmit the color of the dentin-shaded die through to the final shaded restoration. The final intrinsically characterized restoration may require between two and four firings.

The layering technique of IPS Empress is a method recommended for developing ideal esthetics in the anterior region. An anatomic coping is fabricated from a colored ingot, and a cutback is done to provide the space required for the enamel and

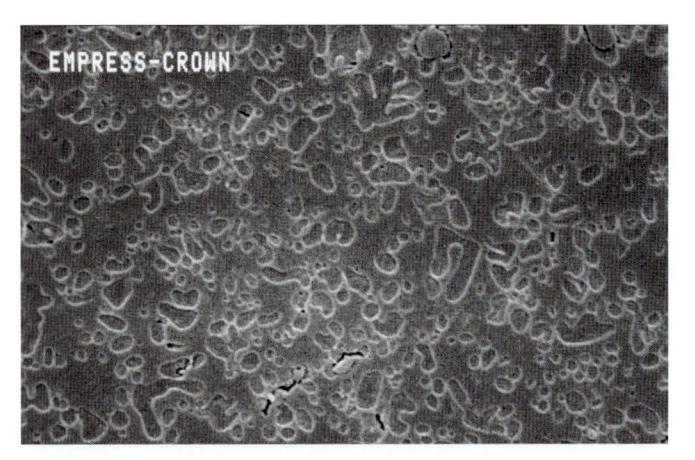

Figure 16.13 Empress is a ceramic that is made up of leucite-reinforced glass-ceramic within its crystalline form.

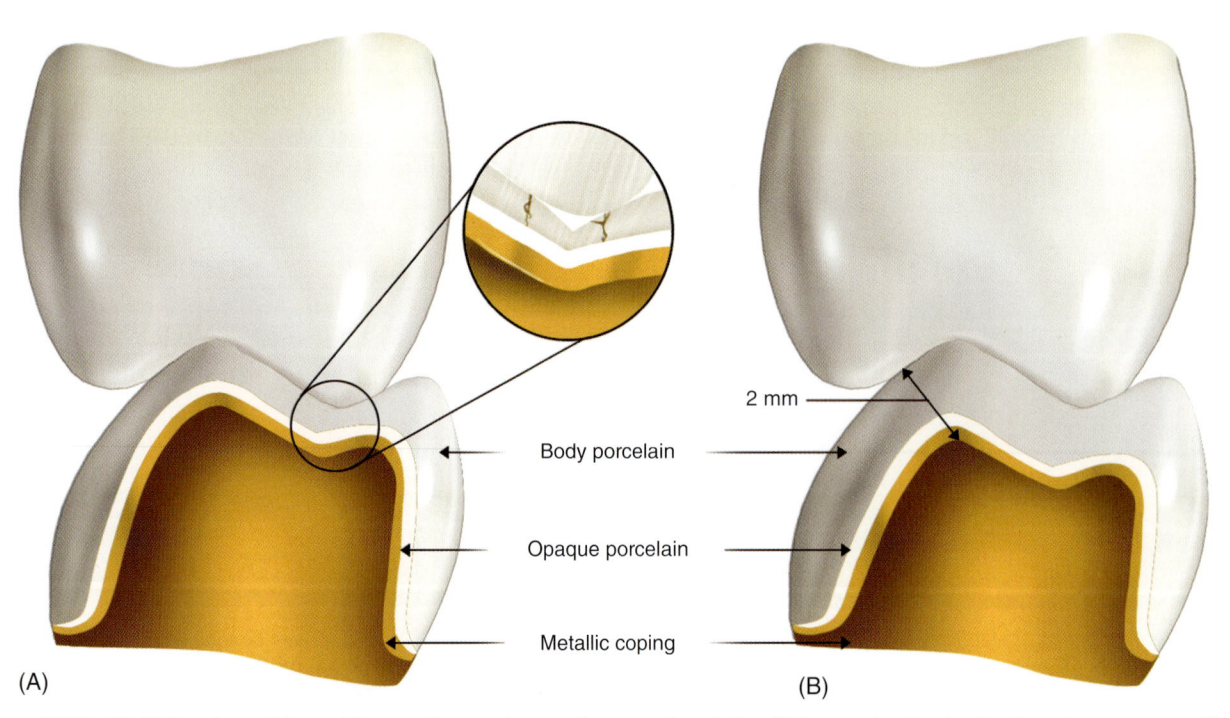

Figure 16.14 **(A, B)** A major problem with posterior metal–ceramic restorations is insufficient occlusal reduction in order to create uniform thickness of the porcelain. The failure to do this is one of the most frequent causes of fracture.

incisal layers. Body and incisal veneering ceramic (crushed Empress) and modifiers are applied when necessary to further customize internal structure, and the tooth form is fully developed and shaped (see Figure 16.15A–E).[24]

From an esthetic standpoint, surface characterization seems to be less crucial for IPS Empress, which is less opaque than conventional aluminous core restorations but less translucent than Dicor. IPS Empress has multiple ingots that provide different levels of translucency. To match more complex tooth shades, a body build-up (simulating dentin) is created, which is then covered with veneering porcelain up to 0.3 mm thick.[29] Lehner and Scharer found that several coats of a heavily pigmented colorant followed by a glaze (to total 50–60 μm in thickness) will enhance fracture resistance to external compressive forces.[29]

Advantages of the Empress system include simple processing, accurate reproduction of the wax pattern and margins, high flexural and tensile strength (which increases with each firing), and good esthetics. This new line of ceramic materials has a high degree of stability during the subsequent shading or layering technique. The IPS Empress ceramic has one of the best long-term survival rates[30] of any all-ceramic material previously tested but has been replaced in the market by the stronger and more durable IPS e.max lithium disilicate.

Lehner and Scharer point out that long-lasting esthetic results may be better achieved by using materials that allow internal colorants and shades rather than relying only on thin surface stains.[29] Also, external surface characterization is subject to surface loss due to the prescription acid-based stannous fluoride

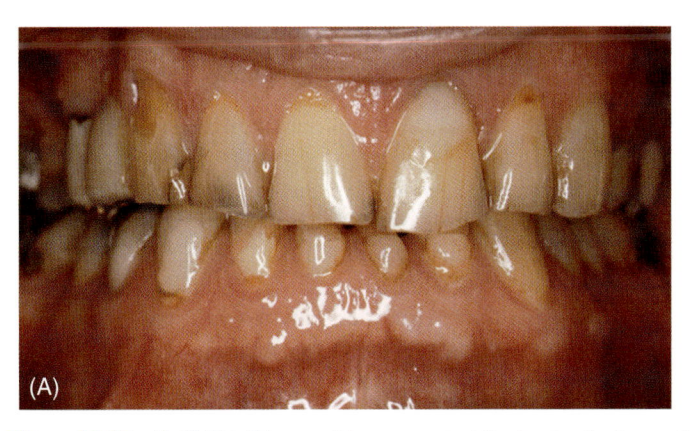

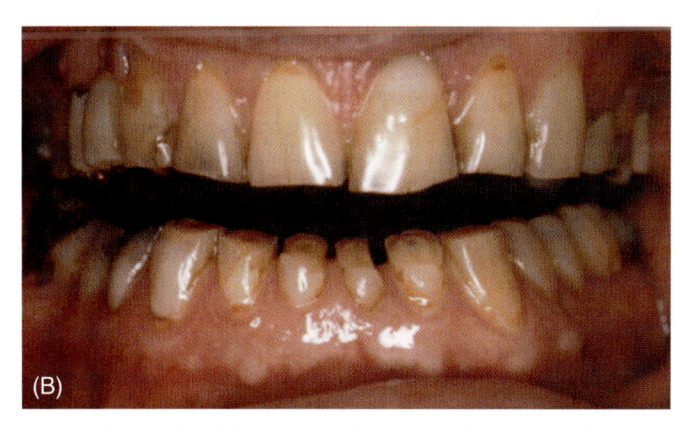

Figure 16.15 **(A, B)** This 71-year-old man wanted the best esthetic result without using metal on his lower anterior crowns. By cosmetically contouring the lingual surfaces of the maxillary anterior teeth, it was possible to create a favorable occlusion for cast-glass crowns.

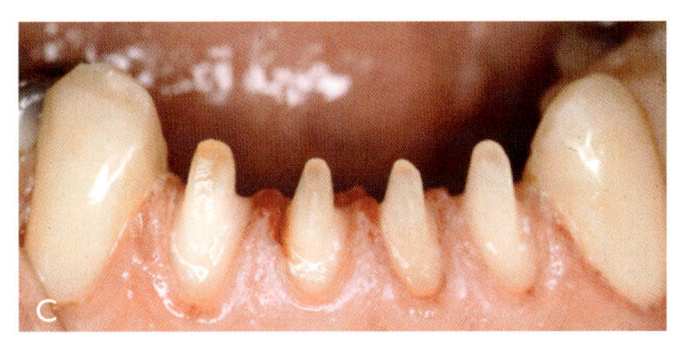

Figure 16.15 **(C)** The four incisors are prepared and ready for the impression.

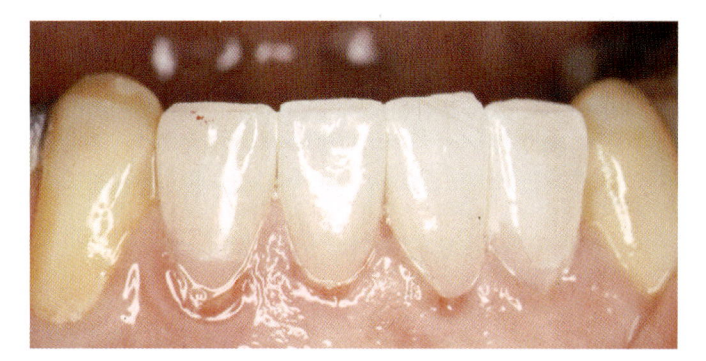

Figure 16.15 **(D)** It is essential that the occlusion be carefully and completely adjusted during the try-in.

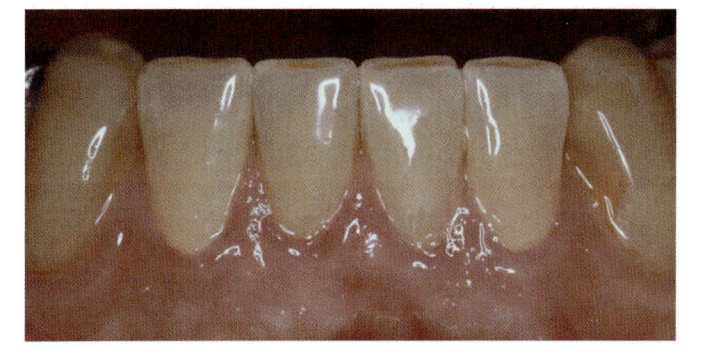

Figure 16.15 **(E)** The final shade is slightly lighter than, but in the same range as, the cuspids.

gels. Neutral fluorides must be prescribed for these patients. A long-term deficiency often seen when surface colorants are used to color or shade porcelain restorations is that, after years, there may be a loss of color as a result of functional demands and abrasion.[29] Surface roughness appears,[29] and there is clinical evidence that these materials generally abrade the enamel of the opposing teeth.[32] The color of an IPS Empress restoration, when fabricated from a colored ingot, is less affected by surface abrasion and occlusal attrition.

Marginal adaptation and occlusal harmony are dependent on the skill of the ceramist, who often has personal preferences. One needs to choose a ceramist (or ceramists) based on the unique needs of the practice and the results they can consistently deliver. Regardless of which ceramic system one may choose for a particular patient, the versatility of most ceramics should allow an acceptable esthetic result. Most systems have an esthetic range that will allow them to be used for most restorations. Only in cases of extreme opacity or translucency will it make a difference. This is one reason why the metal–ceramic restoration has remained so popular throughout the dental world.

IPS e.max

Lithium disilicate was developed by Ivoclar Vivadent and is principally a monolithic ceramic that can be utilized as a pressed (lost wax) or CAD/CAM ceramic. It is a highly esthetic, high-strength material that can be conventionally cemented or adhesively bonded. The pressable lithium disilicate material is indicated for inlays, onlays, veneers, partial crowns, anterior and posterior crowns, three-unit anterior bridges, three-unit premolar bridges, telescope primary crowns, and implant superstructures. In some cases, minimal tooth preparation is desired (e.g., thin veneers), and IPS e.max lithium disilicate enables laboratories to press the restorations as thin as 0.3 mm while still ensuring strength of 400 MPa. If sufficient space is available (e.g., a retruded tooth), no preparation is required. For laboratory ceramists, the versatility and performance of lithium disilicate enables them to optimize their productivity when fabricating restorations using this material, since either lost-wax pressing or CAD/CAM milling fabrication techniques can be used (see Figure 16.16A and B).

Glass-ceramics are categorized according to their chemical composition and/or application. Lithium disilicate is among the best-known and most widely used type of glass-ceramic. The IPS e.max lithium disilicate, for example, is composed of quartz, lithium dioxide, phosphor oxide, and other components. Overall, this composition yields a highly thermal shock-resistant glass-ceramic due to the thermal expansion that results when it is processed. This type of resistant glass-ceramic can be processed using either well-known lost-wax hot pressing techniques or state-of-the-art CAD/CAM milling procedures.

The pressable lithium disilicate (IPS e.max Press) is produced according to a unique bulk casting production process in order to create the ingots. This involves a continuous manufacturing process based on glass technology (melting, cooling, simultaneous nucleation of two different crystals, and growth of crystals) that is continuously optimized in order to prevent the formation of defects (e.g., pores, pigments). The microstructure of the pressable lithium disilicate material consists of approximately 70% needle-like lithium disilicate crystals that are embedded in a glassy matrix. These crystals measure approximately 3–6 µm in length (see Figure 16.17A). Polyvalent ions that are dissolved in the glass are utilized to provide the desired color to the lithium disilicate material. These color-releasing ions are homogeneously distributed in the single-phase material, thereby eliminating color pigment imperfections in the microstructure. Machineable lithium disilicate blocks are manufactured according to a similar process, but only partial crystallization is achieved in order to ensure that the blocks can be milled fast in a crystalline intermediate phase (blue, translucent state). The partial crystallization process leads to the formation of lithium metasilicate crystals, which are responsible for the material's processing properties, relatively high strength, and good edge stability. It is after the milling procedure and the restorations are fired that they reach their fully crystallized state and their desired strength. The microstructure of partially crystallized IPS e.max CAD lithium disilicate consists of 40% platelet-shaped lithium metasilicate crystals embedded in a glassy phase. These crystals range in length from 0.2 to 1.0 µm. The postcrystallization microstructure of IPS e.max CAD lithium disilicate materials consists of 70% fine-grain lithium disilicate crystals embedded in a glassy matrix (see Figure 16.17B). Similar to the pressable lithium disilicate, the millable IPS e.max CAD blocks are colored using coloring ions. However, the coloring elements demonstrate a different oxidation state during the crystalline intermediate phase

Figure 16.16 (A) Tooth #9 has a resin veneer that has aged and discolored. The patient wanted a more permanent esthetic solution.

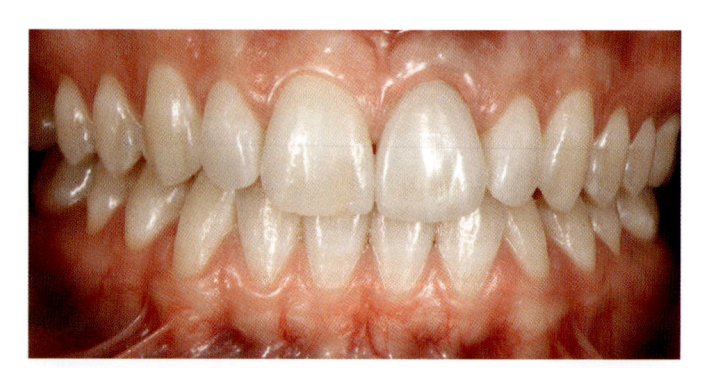

Figure 16.16 (B) A lithium disilicate e.max press crown was fabricated. The facial-incisal third was layered with fluorapatite to better match to the adjacent central incisor.

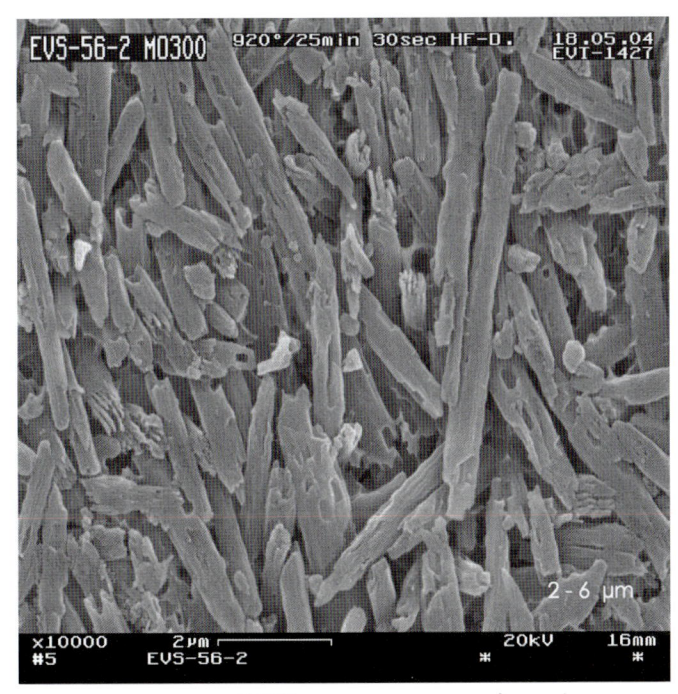

app. 70% coarser grained
lithium disilicate crystals

Figure 16.17 **(A)** The electron microscopic view of the e.max press crystalline structure shows highly compacted and coarse lithium disilicate crystals compared with the e.max CAD.

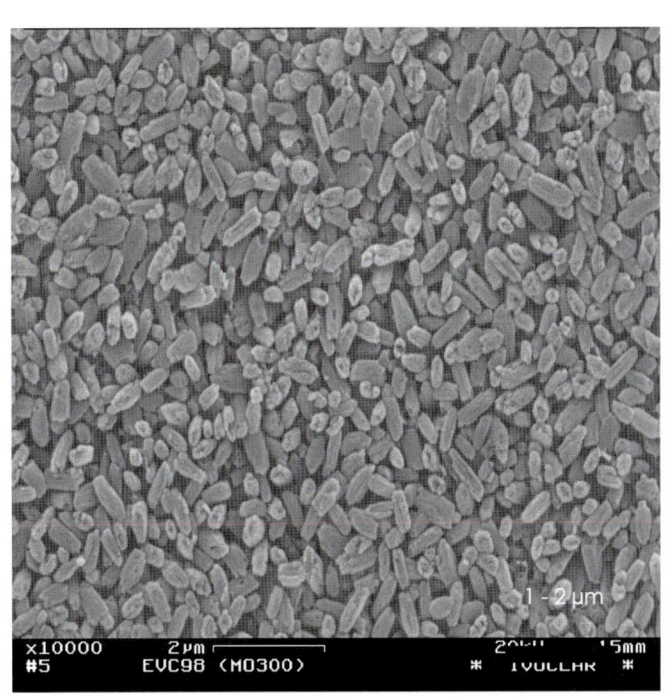

app. 70% fine grained
lithium disilicate crystals

Figure 16.17 **(B)** The crystalline structure of e.max CAD has finer lithium disilicate crystals.

Table 16.2 Clinical Gross Database of All-Ceramic Units to October 22, 2012

Ceramic	Dicor	In-Ceram	Empress	e.max	Totals
Start	Mar 1983	Feb 1990	Jun 1992	Dec 2008	Mar 1983
Months	356	273	245	47	356
Patients	414	137	692	391	1534
Gross nos.	1501	331	2130	1354	5316
Failures	239	49	97	0	385
Gross failure (%)	15.92	14.80	4.55	0	7.24
Chipping	4	13	30	3	50
Replaced	227	48	142	45	462

than in the fully crystallized state. As a result, the blocks exhibit a blue color. The material achieves its desired tooth color and opacity when the lithium metasilicate is transformed into lithium disilicate (during the postmilling firing process).

The lithium disilicate material (IPS e.max Press and IPS e.max CAD) has been in clinical trials for the past 4 years with adhesive and self-adhesive/conventional cementation, and the results have been extremely positive with minimal fracture, chipping, or need for replacement. In one study, over 1200 different-style restorations were completed with no failures and minimal chipping observed (Malament Clinical Database—see Table 16.2). Other physical tests have included mechanical testing of strength using static load with a universal testing machine, subcritical eccentric loading using a chewing simulator (Willytec), and a long-time cyclic loading with a chewing simulator (eGa). The results of these tests demonstrate that:

- To ensure maximum success using the lithium disilicate material, it is important to consider the minimum thickness of the lithium disilicate frame.
- The inside of the crown should *not* be sandblasted.
- Regardless of whether the in vitro test is performed, in comparison with various restorative dental material for crowns (e.g., leucite glass-ceramic, metal–feldspathic ceramic, zirconia–feldspathic ceramic), the lithium disilicate material demonstrates superior results.[33–35]

This is because the strength of the ceramic material in contact with opposing teeth, to fulfill masticatory functions, is about 100 MPa for veneering material and about 160 MPa for leucite glass-ceramic. However, for the pressed lithium disilicate (IPS e.max Press LT and HT), the strength is in the region of 400 MPa in its final anatomical-shaped crown form.

Indications for the machineable lithium disilicate material are inlays, onlays, veneers, partial crowns, telescope primary crowns, and implant superstructures. For a posterior crown fabricated to full contour using CAD methods, lithium disilicate offers 360 MPa of strength through the entire restoration. As a result, restorations demonstrate a "monolithic" strength unlike any other metal-free restoration. Overall, these materials demonstrate specific advantages to dentists and patients, including higher edge strength versus traditional glass-ceramic materials (i.e., can be finished thinner without chipping), low viscosity of heated ingot enabling pressing to very thin dimension (i.e., enabling minimal prep or no prep veneers), and chameleon effect due to higher translucency.

Metal–ceramic restorations

Porcelain fused to metal

History

The metal–ceramic restoration has been the standard of care in esthetic dentistry for more than 30 years. According to Kuwata,[1] in his book *Creating Harmony in Dental Ceramics*, Katz and Katz were the earliest pioneers in fusing feldspathic porcelain to metal, in the late 1940s, and first perfected this technology for dentistry. Later, with major investment backing from the Weinstein brothers, the first patent was granted to fuse porcelain to metal. Over time many people have played important roles in the early development, but Kuwata's contributions were significant, particularly in the areas of particle size and color pigment selection, as well as for his research on the coefficient of thermal expansion of both metal and porcelain to allow a long-term fusion. From an esthetic viewpoint, porcelain is a material capable of maintaining its surface texture and color for extended periods without losing its naturalness. However, because of excessive fragility, porcelain alone has its limitations. This limitation is overcome by the use of porcelain-fused-to-metal alloys.

Precious/nonprecious

The American Dental Association has developed a classification system for casting alloys. The classification is:

- high noble—≥60% gold, platinum, and palladium, and gold ≥40%;
- noble—≥25% gold, platinum, and palladium; and
- base—<25%.

(Noble metals are gold, platinum, palladium, and other platinum-group metals.) In the early 1970s, increased fluctuation in the cost of gold increased interest in alternative metals for casting, so base metals were developed. These metals are based on nickel and chromium. Other nonprecious ingredients are added to base metals to modify their properties, casting accuracy, and porcelain-to-metal compatibility.

Gettlemen defines noble metals differently. He states that noble metals are alloys of gold, palladium, and silver (not a noble metal), with smaller amounts of iridium, ruthenium, and platinum. They are primarily used as a substructure for ceramic application, with the rest used as inlays, onlays, and unveneered crowns. Base metal alloys, principally made of nickel, chromium, and beryllium, are used widely in the United States, owing to their lower cost and higher mechanical properties.[36] Most of the alternative base-metal casting alloys, he states, have superior mechanical strength, porcelain bond strength, high-temperature sag resistance, and corrosion resistance. The principle deficiencies of base metals are the potential for allergic reaction in patients who are hypersensitive to nickel, chromium, or beryllium.

When selecting an alloy the decision should be based on the type of restoration involved. The porcelain to be used is an important factor, in that only certain porcelains are compatible with specific metals. When a tooth is to be restored with a porcelain-fused-to-metal restoration, the alloy should be <5% silver due to the adverse effect silver has on porcelain color.[37] Different alloys offer different degrees of hardness; the differences are a result of the minor constituents added. For example, copper is added as a hardener. A long-span bridge would require a harder alloy than a single unit or a short-span bridge.[38] Nickel chromium base alloys also result in color changes, which are detectable by trained dental observers under ideal viewing conditions. However, it may be well within an acceptable range under normal viewing conditions.[37]

Indications for metal–ceramic restorations

1. For anterior crowns with complex color requirements.
2. Where there is need for multiple splinting of crowns together.
3. For fixed partial dentures with any number of pontics or short cantilevers.
4. With complex implant prosthodontics requiring gingival ceramics.

Contraindications for metal–ceramic restorations

1. Adequate tooth structure cannot be removed to allow ample space for both metal and porcelain.
2. The clinical crown is too short. Since an incisal or occlusal reduction of 2 mm is essential to allow space for metal and porcelain coverage, retention and stability of the crown may be inadequate.
3. Use in extensive long-span bridges or splints is not routinely recommended.

Technical problems

1. Pulp exposure can occur if required tooth structure is removed to allow for thickness of materials and to achieve sufficient parallelism for crown retention after insertion.
2. Breakage can be minimized by careful attention to tooth preparation, coping, or frame design.

3. Potential esthetic deficiency where single crowns, crowns splinted together, or fixed partial dentures using porcelain fused to metal suffer a loss of separateness that detracts from the appearance. As Bronstein points out, ideal deep interproximal carving is greatly limited by the proximity of the metal truss arms, which join the crowns. This is not as much of a problem in posterior segments of the mouth, where shadows and oblique angles make them less visible.[39]

Advantages

1. Porcelain fused to metal can be used to crown the abutment teeth of removable clasp-type partial dentures, since it resists abrasion by the clasp arms; and if necessary, rest seats can be made in the metal framework.
2. Porcelain may be contoured to provide desirable retentive undercuts and guiding planes for removable partial dentures.
3. They can be used for the placement of internal attachments for removable partial dentures. The cast metal can contain the female portion of the attachment.
4. Metal permits a good marginal seal and adds strength.[40]

Disadvantages

Aside from teeth that are heavily discolored, Zena and Abbott[41] propose that cervical shadowing or "black line" is caused by "disruption of the light harmony between the root and crown" of the prepared tooth and the overlying soft tissues. That is, the dentin and root structure of a tooth refract less ambient light, leaving a darkened, shadowed appearance of the root surface, as do metal substructures such as metal posts and cores (see Figure 16.18A–C). To avoid this esthetic problem, one may wish to place the facial margin subgingivally, but no more than halfway between the gingival crest and the depth of the sulcus. A soft tissue model can be used to ensure ideal facial emergence from the gingiva.

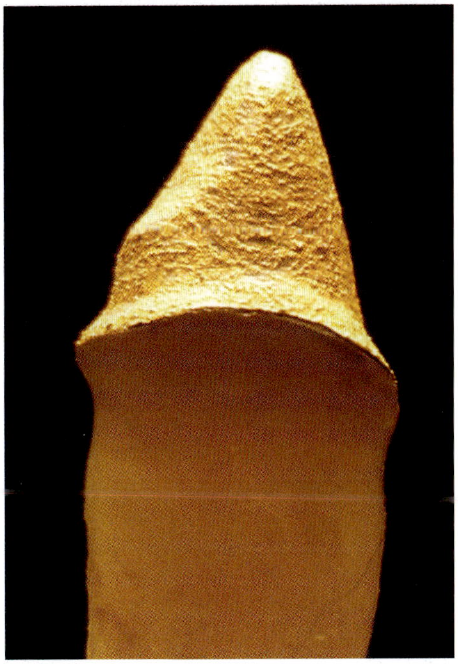

Figure 16.18 (B) Once a cast coping is placed over the prep, light stops being transmitted into the root and leaves a darkened cervical third, and even a shadow in the gingiva.

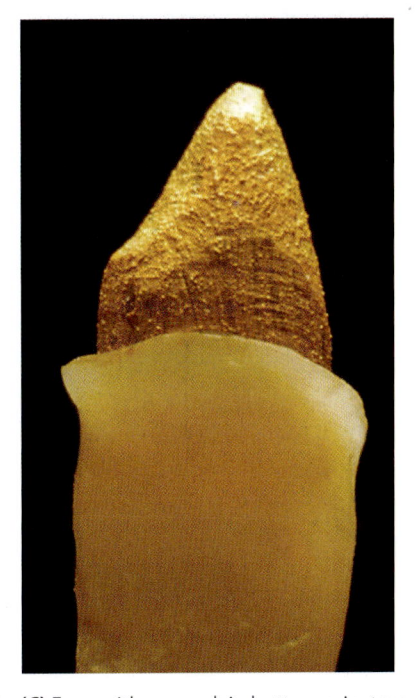

Figure 16.18 (C) Even with a porcelain butt margin, transmission of light into the root is impaired and can still yield a darkened cervical third.

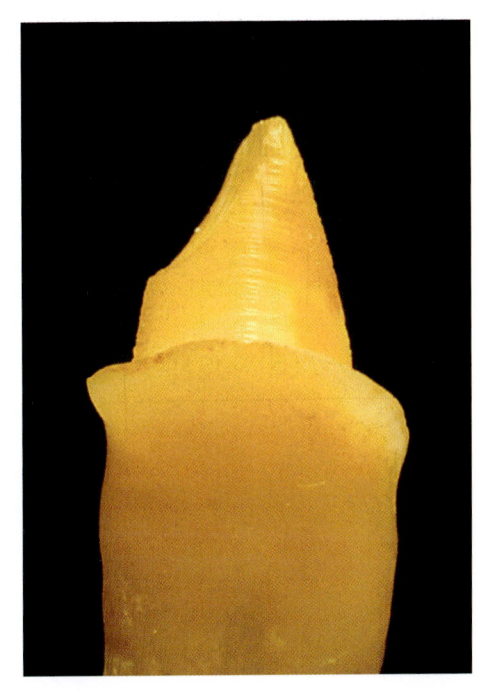

Figure 16.18 (A) One of the myriad of reasons for the use of all-ceramic crowns is their relative translucency. When light is passed through a prepared tooth (or natural tooth), it illuminates the root as well.

Adjunctive procedures

As noted by Pameijer,[42] the fabrication of a soft tissue cast has been strongly advocated to provide the laboratory technician essential information concerning the morphology of the gingival tissues surrounding the metal casting. An accurate replication of the height and contour of the marginal gingiva and of the interdental papilla is very helpful in establishing the emergence profile and cervical contour and helps the technician control the length of the metal collar for subgingival margins.

When writing the laboratory prescription, include as much information as possible in order to aid the technician in creating appropriately shaped teeth. Final shaping and contouring to reflect personality, age, and sex should also be done at this time.[28]

Esthetic considerations

With fixed partial dentures or splinted crowns, the loss of individuality in the anterior segment can be significantly improved by the design of the restorations where one may overlap crown forms to hide the opaqued or exposed connectors or by specific coloration technique for the interproximal porcelain. Eliminating the metal collar with a buccal butt porcelain margin improves esthetics. There should be subtle variation in the body and incisal porcelain to break up light and thus help create the illusion of naturalness.[42] The success of a buccal butt porcelain shoulder restoration is improved by proper tooth preparation.[43] Frame design is altered by finishing the labiogingival portion of the metal back to the gingivopulpal line angle, leaving metal substructure against the axial wall (which is 0.3–0.5 mm thick). This allows for an opaque porcelain layer from 0.2 to 0.3 mm thick and 0.7 to 1.0 mm of shoulder porcelain (see Figure 16.19).

The advantage of a porcelain shoulder in a porcelain-fused-to-metal crown, according to Harrison et al., is that the finish line can be kept supragingival or just slightly apical to the free gingival margin. Its major disadvantage is that the loss of metal along the facial margin may give less than an optimal margin closure, and it is possible that fracture of the facial porcelain caused by a lack of metal support may be increased. For this reason one must be careful if using a direct lift-off margination technique to avoid displacement or breaking of the porcelain shoulder build-up and deformation during firing.[43] However, the use of a bonded resin cement to either etched enamel or dentin helps to seal the margin and at the same time provides additional marginal support.

When both esthetics and strength are essential, consider the metal–ceramic butt joint (refer to Figure 16.20). This type of crown provides almost all the esthetics necessary, and yet the metal core adds great strength. Further discussion of esthetic considerations may be found later in this chapter.

New approaches to the metal–ceramic system compensate for the inherent esthetic problems with the advent of opalescent ceramic systems—Creation Porcelain (Jensen), Vintage Opal Porcelain (Shofu), and Omega Ceramic (Vita Co.).

These systems are based on the concept of opalescence, a naturally occurring phenomenon in the semiprecious opal stone. An opal's surface resembles that of enamel in opacity and translucency, so by mimicking enamel with a specially filled ceramic, which maintains its opalescence during firing, the metal–ceramic restoration appears more natural. An additional advantage is that laboratory construction is simplified, using only a two-layer build-up, versus the three needed for conventional porcelain restorations.[24]

Technical considerations

Substructure design

After diagnosis, treatment planning, and tooth preparation, the design of the metal substructure is of the greatest importance. As Dresden[40] states, poor design of the substructure is probably the primary reason for failure of the metal–ceramic restoration. Because of the strong influence of the opaque masking the metal framework on the final shade, uniform thickness of the body porcelain is paramount. Specific case design is usually determined by the nature of the preparation in relation to the esthetic and functional requirements. There are several major considerations in creating the metal substructure. The metal should be constructed to provide a uniform thickness of porcelain. Since labial surfaces may be particularly weak at the incisal and gingival areas, there should be incisal and gingival thickness to support the porcelain required for a full shoulder margin. A metal-reinforced margin, such as a chamfer or beveled

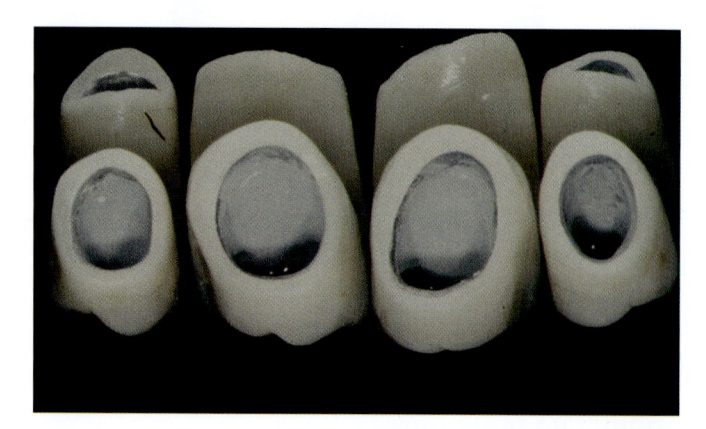

Figure 16.19 Porcelain butt margins on four anterior crowns. The metal does not extend onto the shoulder.

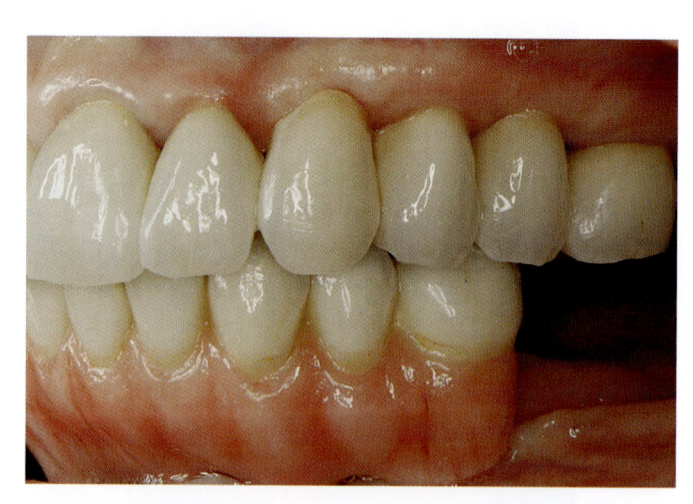

Figure 16.20 The maxillary arch is restored with individual porcelain-fused-to-metal restorations all with porcelain butt margins. The esthetic integration between the ceramic and the gingiva is heightened when the porcelain butt margins are used.

shoulder, can increase the strength. These may be designed in several ways for maximum function and esthetics. Figure 16.21A illustrates the beveled shoulder labially and lingually with porcelain fused to metal. The porcelain gingival margin is extended below the gingival crest. An alternative to this is porcelain coverage with the occluding surface in metal (Figure 16.21B).

Alternatives to the beveled shoulder margin are the porcelain butt joint (Figure 16.21C) and the chamfer margin (Figure 16.21D). The surfaces of the metal to which the porcelain is to be bonded must be well rounded with no sharp angles in concavities and convexities (Figure 16.22A and D). Especially sharp inner angles must be avoided, because porcelain shrinks

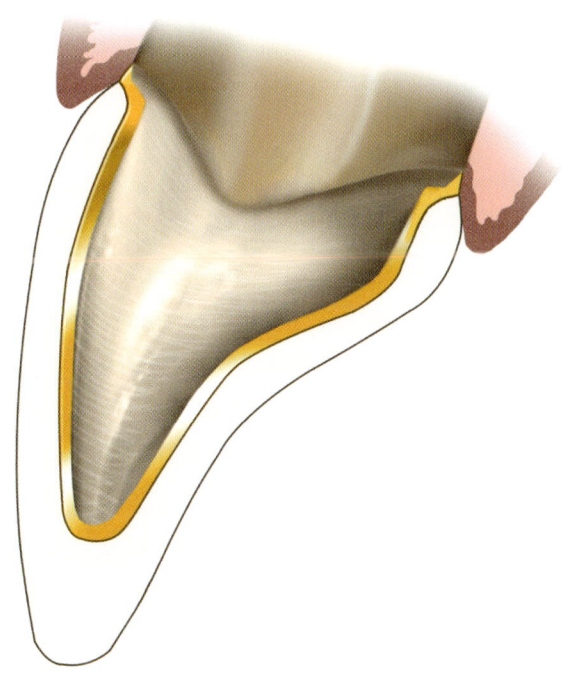

Figure 16.21 (A) The beveled shoulder margin can work well both labially and lingually when the patient has a low lip line or thick fibrous gingival tissue that diminishes the chance of tissue recession.

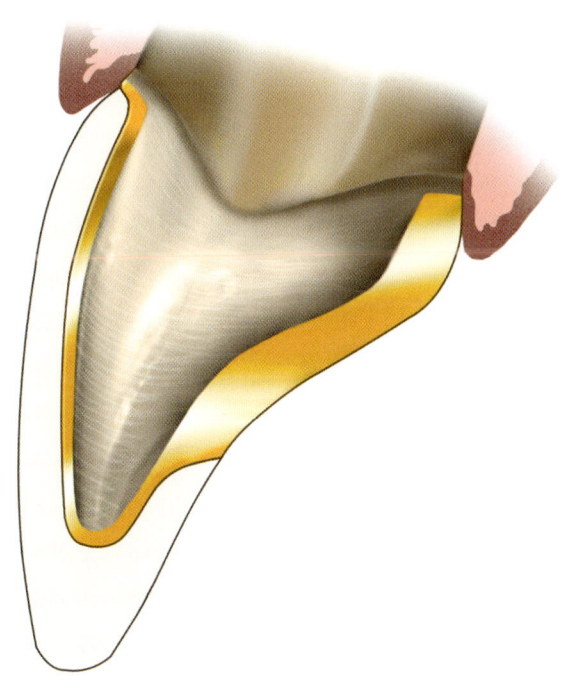

Figure 16.21 (B) An alternative to the porcelain lingual surface is to place the occluding lingual surface in metal.

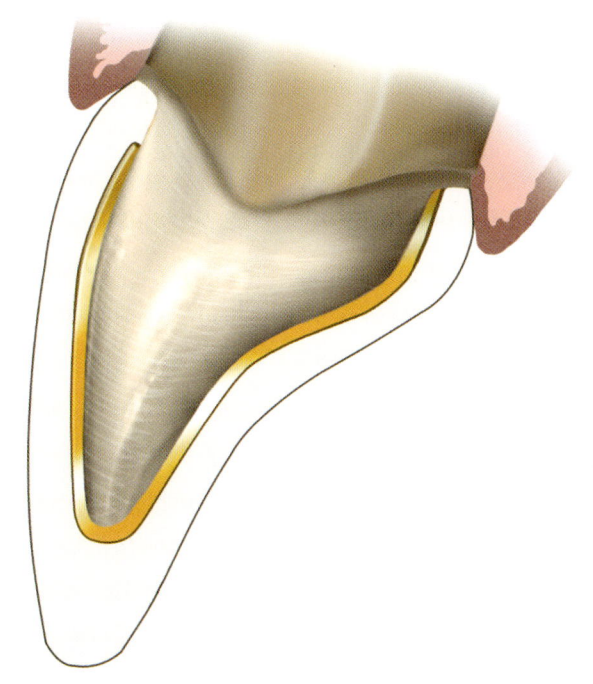

Figure 16.21 (C) For most situations the best esthetic margin is the porcelain butt joint.

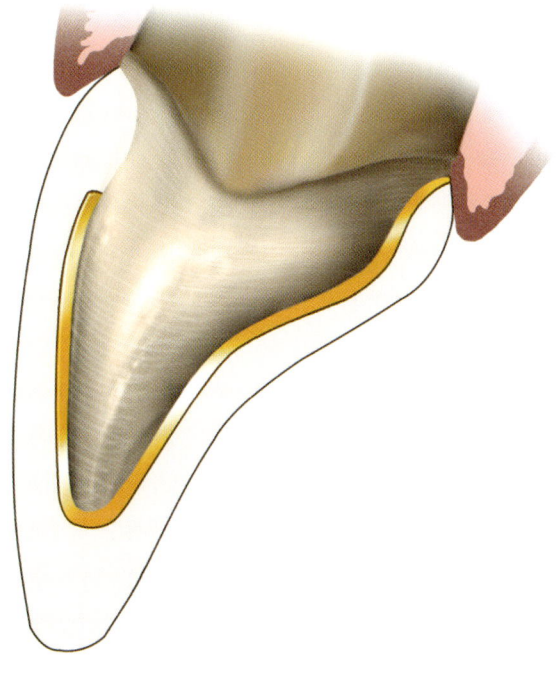

Figure 16.21 (D) There are situations where the chamfer margin is a good replacement for the beveled shoulder.

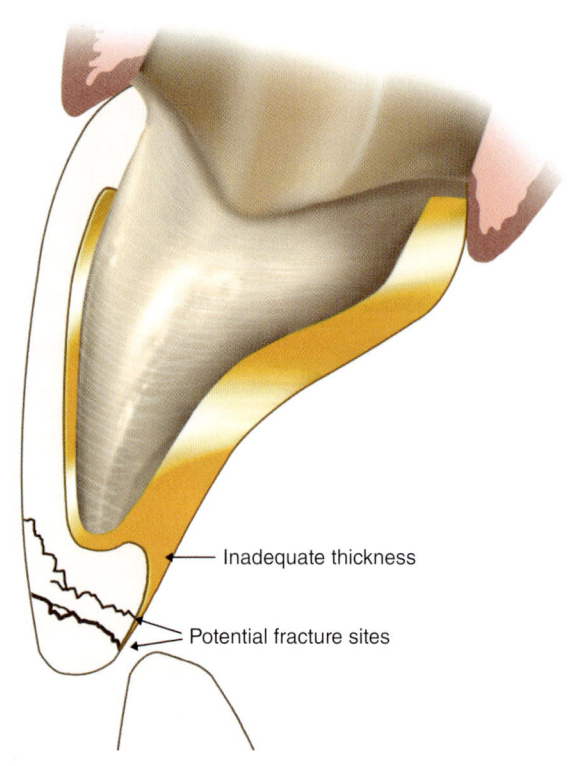

Figure 16.21 **(E)** An inadequate thickness of incisal metal can potentiate fracture, especially if the metal–ceramic junction occurs in an occluding area.

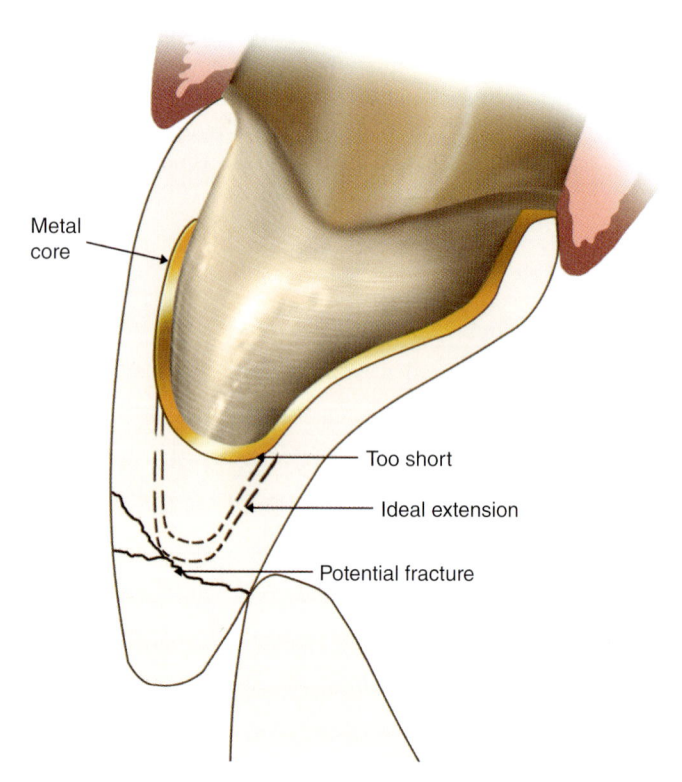

Figure 16.21 **(F)** The metal should always be constructed to provide for uniform porcelain thickness. If the substructure is too short it may require too much porcelain incisally, which could significantly weaken the restoration, causing fracture.

15–20% upon firing, and a layer of metal oxide develops to create a bond between metal and porcelain. Potential points of cleavage, which may occur if there is stress on the porcelain, will also be avoided by smoothing off any sharp angles.[44,45] Also, if the metal is too thin (less than 0.4 mm), porcelain shrinkage during firing can distort the fit of the metal substructure.

Metal fracture can also occur if the coping is poorly designed with an inadequate thickness of incisal metal (Figure 16.21E). This may result from deformation of the metal under masticatory stresses or when seating the preparation in the mouth. According to MacGibbon, failures may be due to the great difference between the elasticity of the porcelain and that of the metal employed.[46] Be certain, therefore, that the incisal metal coverage is thick and broad, not thin toward the lingual surface. If the substructure is too short, it may require too much porcelain incisally, and that could significantly weaken the restoration (Figure 16.21 F). The coping should be built up to allow for uniform porcelain thickness.[21] This principle also applies to full coverage, porcelain-fused-to-metal posterior restorations. Uniform material thickness is illustrated in Figure 16.23A. Note that the metal may be designed to go higher in the linguogingival area, unless the patient objects to the slight display of metal.

The type of labiogingival junction of porcelain and metal also depends on esthetic demands. If the patient has a high lip line when smiling, the porcelain should end beneath the crest of the gingiva. For upper posterior teeth, never place the visible porcelain–metal junction at the bucco-occlusal line angle in an occluding area, as this is a potential site of fracture. Instead, finish the porcelain on the lingual surface or halfway between the tip of the buccal cusp and the central fossa (Figure 16.23B).

Tooth preparation

Preparation

Successful esthetic and functional results obtained with all-feldspathic porcelain crowns cannot be credited solely to the quality of the particular material used. The method of preparation also has a significant influence on the final result. Control over the esthetics in the anterior porcelain crown is determined by the fit of the crown and its proper termination within the gingival sulcus. Strict observance of the rules of tooth preparation, soft tissue management, and techniques of impression is essential. Failure in any of these steps may result in poor crown adaptation, gingival irritation or destruction, and the resulting changes in tissue appearance. An adequately reduced (1.5 mm), clearly defined shoulder is necessary to achieve good margins and provide strength.[47] The strength of a porcelain restoration is highly dependent on proper crown preparation. Advocating careful preparation, Berger states that the shoulder should be carefully developed and brought to its final finishing line in the sulcus late in the process of preparing the tooth rather than establishing its location early in the procedure.[16]

Every effort should be made to minimize injury to the gingival tissues. The margin preparation must never exceed the depth of the sulcus. In a healthy mouth this distance may only be 1–3 mm. Therefore, the margin of the crown should be ideally placed in

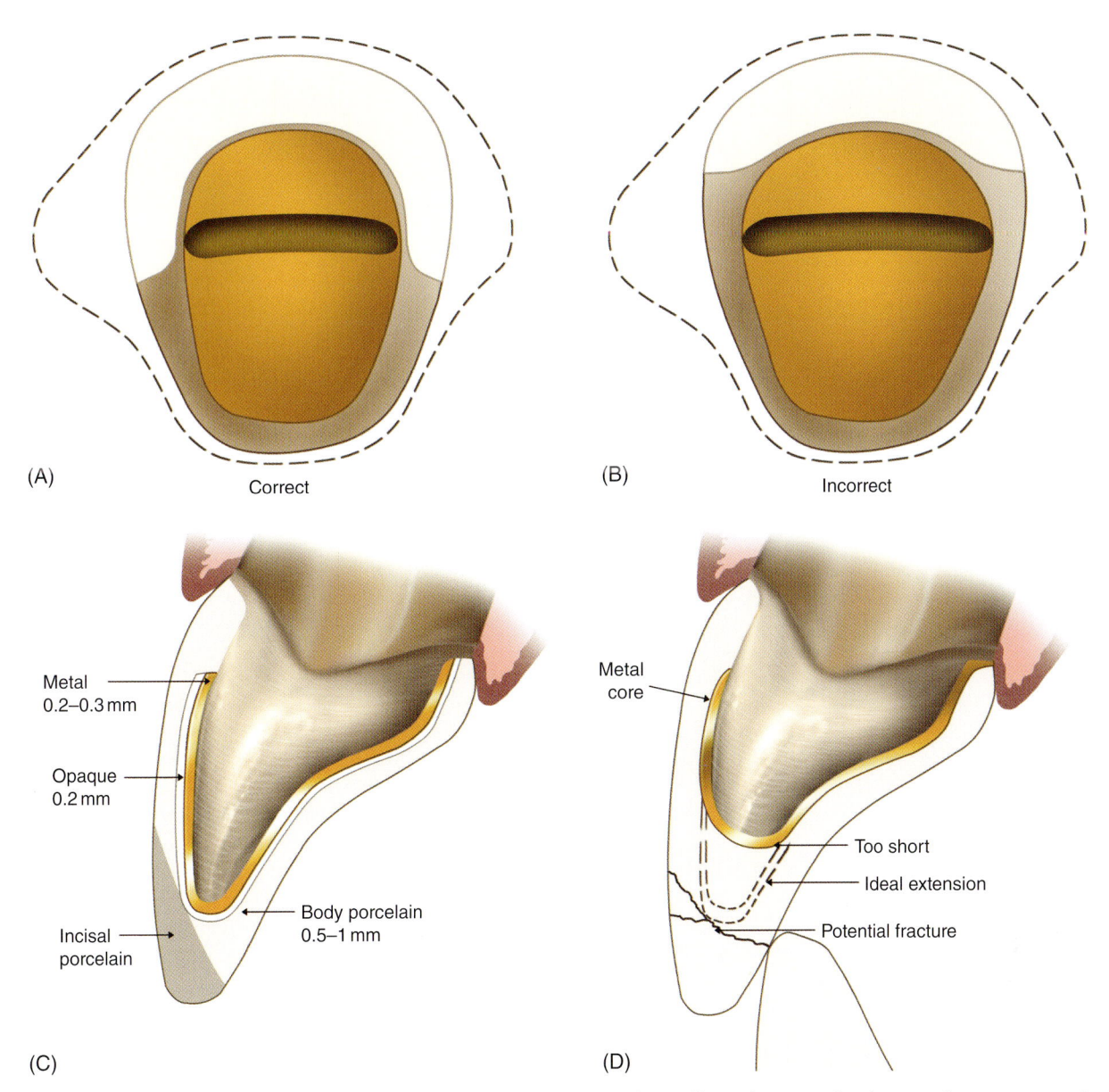

Figure 16.22 (A–D) These illustrations show the method of extending the porcelain well into the gingival embrasures for maximum esthetics. They also help to point out the use of rounded inner line angles to avoid potential points of cleavage, which may occur if there is stress on the porcelain. Figure 16.22C illustrates the correct thicknesses of each material layer of an anterior porcelain fused to metal crown and incisal edge design.

the sulcus 0.5 mm below the gingival crest.[38,48] Placing the margin of the shoulder as deep as possible into the sulcus can be a grave error. If the biologic width is compromised, there is a potential for changes in the underlying osseous structure with possible gingival recession and/or pocket formation. If recession can be avoided, then a major problem in esthetics is eliminated.[48]

Tooth structure apical to the margin is important also to ensure maintenance of the integrity of the gingival attachment apparatus. Extension of the crown too far apically can damage the attachment apparatus during try-in. Also, if the finish line is in an area that is inaccessible for cement removal, plaque can accumulate, and inflammation will result.[48] Kaiser and Newell state that margins should not be placed over 1.0 mm subgingivally to the retracted level of the free gingival margin to ensure that the margin is hidden under the healthy tissue.[49] They further emphasize that the potential for tissue recession is greatly dependent on its health before preparation; at cementation they endorse the use of a nonmedicated retraction cord of a size that does not require excessive pressure for its placement into the sulcus.

The problem of tissue recession may occur regardless of the care taken not to irritate the gingival fibers during preparation. The best way to avoid irritation is to extend the gingival margin into the sulcus after cord retraction so that clear vision is possible (Figure 16.24A and B). Deflection during gingival retraction and impression techniques can also produce enough irritation to the tissue to cause shrinkage and to eventually expose a margin;[50] therefore, use extreme care to avoid unnecessary deflection, in both duration and force, when inserting the cord. Interproximal

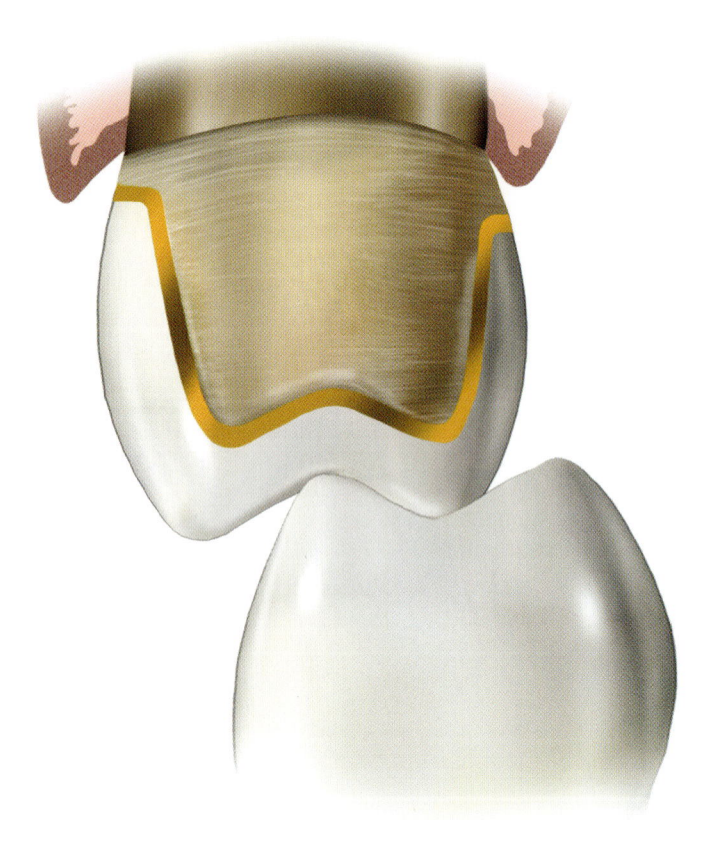

Figure 16.23 **(A)** The strongest metal–ceramic restoration is one that features wraparound, uniform porcelain thickness.

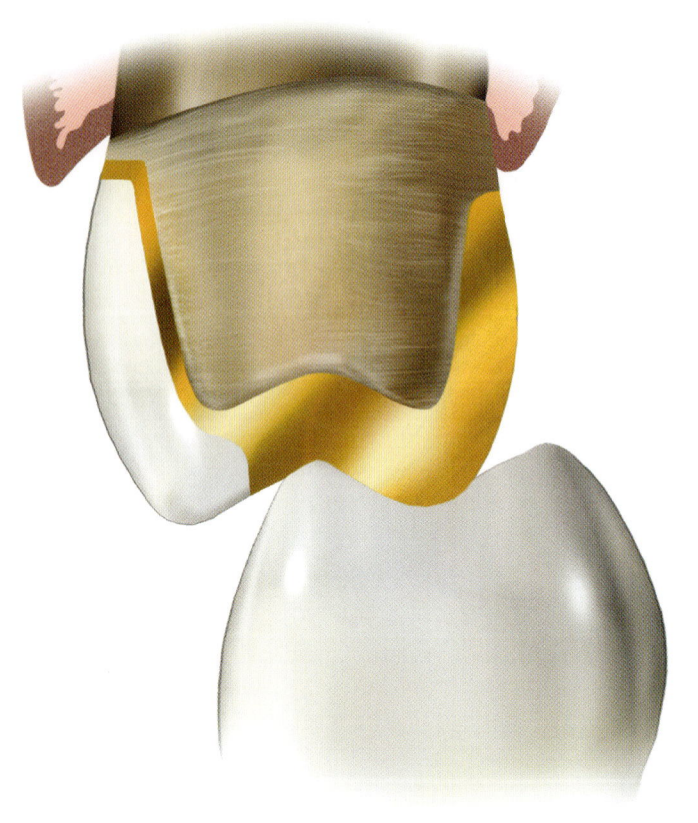

Figure 16.23 **(B)** Place metal–ceramic junctions in low- or no-stress areas.

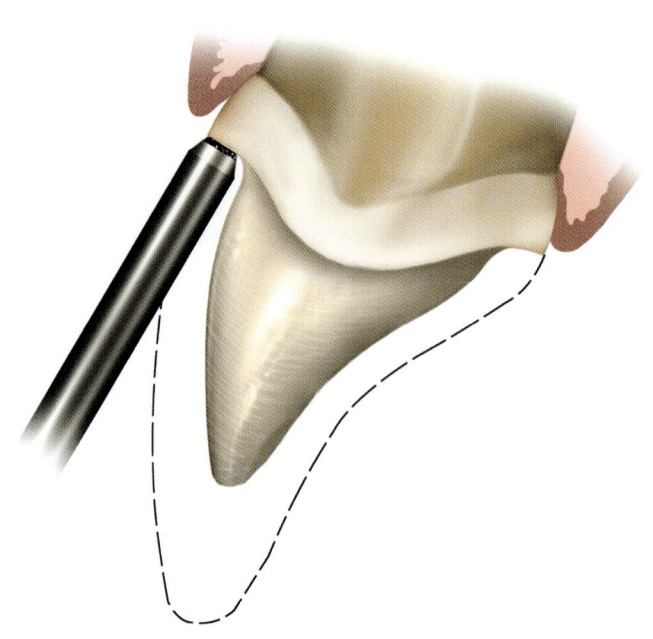

Figure 16.24 **(A)** This beveled end-cutting diamond (TPE-Shofu or TGE-Premier Dental Products) helps protect the gingival tissue as it extends the shoulder margin subgingivally.

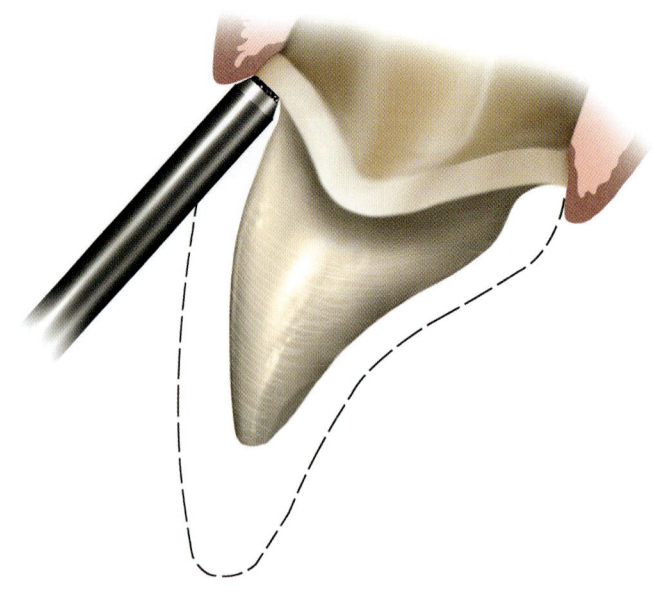

Figure 16.24 **(B)** As the diamond cuts the shoulder deeper into the gingival sulcus, the bevel protects the gingival epithelium by pushing it out of the way.

contacts between full crown restorations or with the natural dentition also play a role in maintaining gingival health. Southard et al. presented a study in which they conclude "posterior dental contact tightness, generally regarded by dentists as a static feature of occlusion, varies significantly as a function of posture."[51] The recumbent patient showed a mean decrease in posterior contact tightness, which increased after a return to an upright position. Aside from gingival health, as proposed by Sturdevant, excessive pressure between restored teeth may ultimately result in undesirable tooth movement.[51] From an esthetic standpoint, such shifting of the teeth may compromise the optimal restorative results one worked so hard to achieve.

Following the construction of the crown, check the shoulder fit and contour of the crown. Remove rough or excess porcelain, as it will increase plaque retention and cause gingival irritation. A poor marginal fit may eventually produce granulation tissue or gingival recession, which, in turn, may cause the gingival tissues to appear bluish or become puffy and reddened. Blame may be erroneously placed on the restoration rather than on poor planning or technique.[16] Some nonpathologic tissue changes occur with time. Under these circumstances, replacement for purely esthetic reasons is a matter for the patient to decide. Friedman and Jordan suggest that composite luting or bonding of the porcelain crown may reduce the incidence of fracture,[52] and they cite research that concludes that bonded porcelain crowns strengthen the remaining tooth structure to a degree comparable to the strength of a fully intact normal tooth.[53] In addition, the use of composite luting materials instead of traditional cements provides more control over the color of the restored tooth, because the composite functions like a core stain.[52]

Certain factors must be considered in preparation for metal–ceramic restorations. First, there must be adequate space for porcelain, opaque, and metal coverage (Figures 16.22C and 16.26). For anterior teeth this means reduction of 1.5 mm axially and 2 mm incisally (Figure 16.22C). Coughlin says the labioincisal reduction of the anterior teeth or the buccal cusp in posterior teeth should not be less than 2.0 mm and should roughly duplicate the contours of the original surface in order to gain uniformly adequate space for a metal coping, opaque porcelain, and body porcelain into which can be built occlusal anatomy.[54] The lingual cusp and marginal ridge should have a clearance of at least 1.0–1.5 mm in all lateral excursions. If this is sacrificed, shade control suffers, because all porcelains need depth to maintain shade. The porcelain must not be less than 0.5 mm thick anywhere. Otherwise, the shade is progressively lightened. Good porcelain coverage in the anterior restoration is illustrated in Figure 16.25A–E. Correct porcelain coverage design for the posterior restoration is illustrated in Figure 16.26. After impressions, casts and dies are made and a treatment wax-up that can be placed intraorally, which can help the dentist and technician

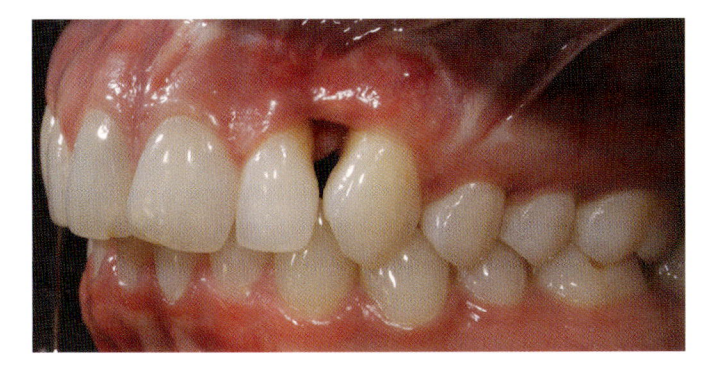

Figure 16.25 **(A)** The patient had a recurrent squamous odontogenic cyst excised from the papillary area between #6 and #7 and wanted a way to mask the defect.

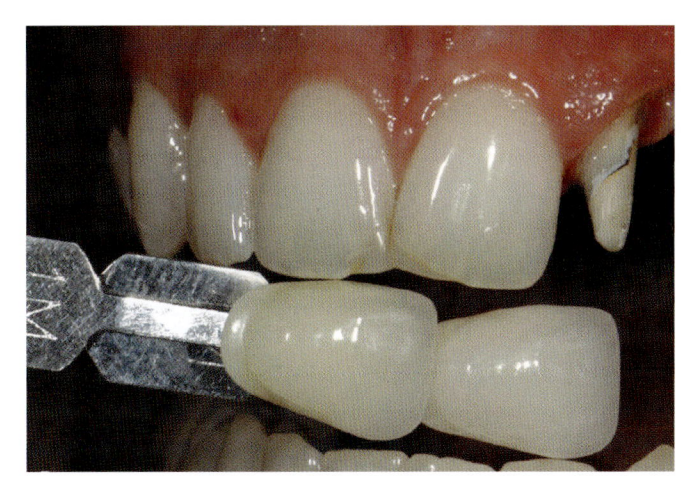

Figure 16.25 **(B)** To facilitate communication with the technician, a shade tab photograph is taken (or multiple). It is generally better to use the necks of the shade tabs, rather than the incisal edges.

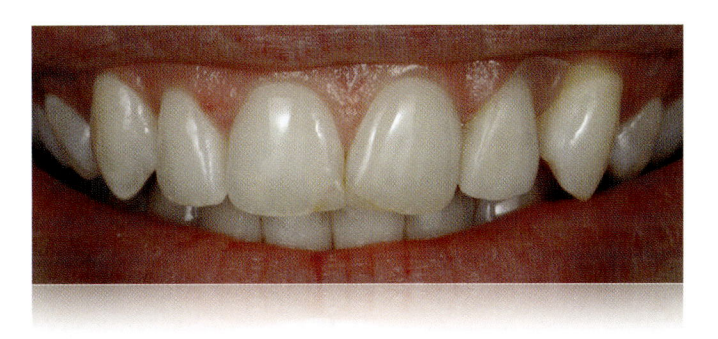

Figure 16.25 **(C)** A treatment wax was placed in the mouth before fabricating the final restoration to allow the patient to visualise the end result of the prosthesis.

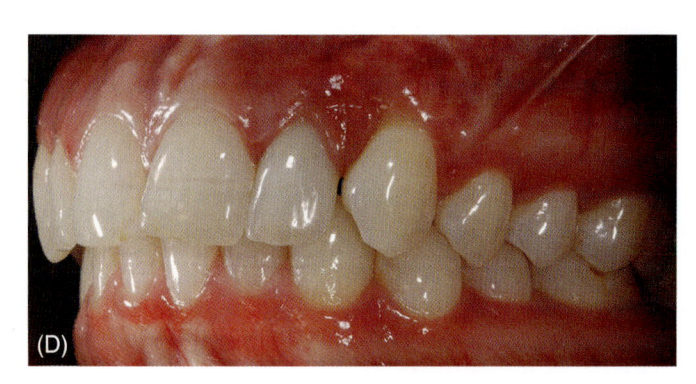

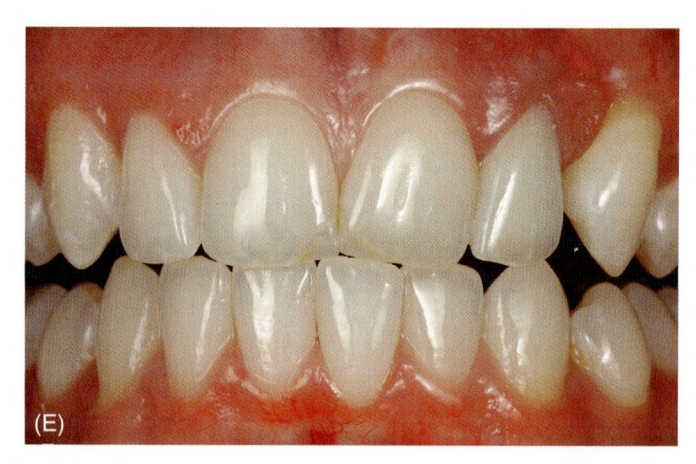

Figure 16.25 (D, E) The final restoration in place. The crown was fabricated with metal–ceramic in order to create the pink replacement papilla.

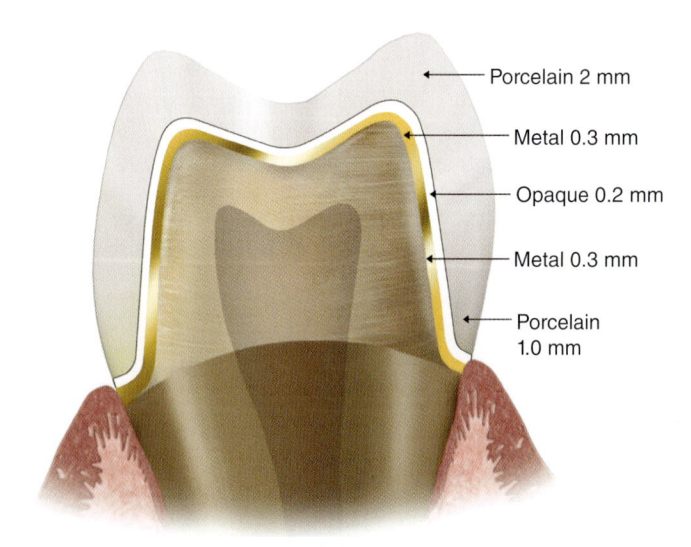

Figure 16.26 This diagram illustrates the correct thickness of a posterior metal–ceramic restoration using a bevel shoulder margin on the lingual and a porcelain butt joint on the labial.

Labels in Figure 16.26:
- Porcelain 2 mm
- Metal 0.3 mm
- Opaque 0.2 mm
- Metal 0.3 mm
- Porcelain 1.0 mm

visualize the potential esthetic results. With the patient's input, the treatment wax-up serves as a blueprint for both the metal–ceramic frame and the final ceramic restorations (see Figure 16.25C).

Choice of margin

Deciding what type of margin is obtainable is a prerequisite to crown selection. The best functional margin is gold supragingivally. However, when esthetics are of concern, the procedures of masking or covering the metal become essential.

The mere presence of metal in the mouth is enough to bother some patients. In this case, an all-ceramic crown or a porcelain-fused-to-metal crown with a porcelain butt joint should be used (see Figures 16.21C and 16.22C).

If periodontal disease is present, control of the depth of the sulcus is feasible if there is prior discussion of the esthetic goals among patient, dentist, and specialist. According to Kramer, periodontal treatment can be successful and still leave a manageable 2 mm deep sulcus to hide the metal margin.[55]

A number of finish line shapes have been discussed, including the labial shoulder chamfer and beveled shoulder. Any one of these provides adequate reduction in the labiocervical area, providing for good functional and esthetic results. This becomes particularly important where the maxillary anteriors or bicuspids are involved. Consideration must be given to how the finish line will ultimately relate to the marginal adaptation of the crown in the labial or buccal areas.

The possible labial margin designs using the previously mentioned finish lines include (1) a labiogingival porcelain–metal chamfer margin, (2) a labiogingival metal collar, and (3) a porcelain butt joint (Figures 16.21A–D). Almost always this can be hidden under the gingival sulcus, especially in maxillary anteriors and premolars. When the tissue is either thin and transparent or at zero sulcus depth, a porcelain butt joint is preferred. In designing the substructure, labial metal is carried to the shoulder but not on to it (Figure 16.26).

The labiogingival metal collar margin has an esthetic disadvantage in anterior restorations in cases where the metal collar is located incisal to the free marginal gingiva, thereby allowing for an unsightly display of metal. If the free gingival tissue on the labial is thin, the metal collar may create a dark bluish gray at the margin. Therefore, the metal collar seems most useful in the cervical areas of maxillary molars and in all mandibular teeth where the cervical areas are not visible, even if the patient smiles broadly.

Currently, according to Lanzano and Hill,[56] there are three main techniques being advocated for the fabrication of the metal collarless crown, but the finish line for all three techniques is identical. The facial finishing line should be a 90° shoulder of 1.5 mm in depth. This provides enough depth for adequate esthetic characteristics and sufficient bulk to provide strength. The lingual finishing line can be whatever the dentist would like to use with a traditional metal–ceramic restoration.[56]

The coping designs, as detailed by Anusavice and Hojjate, may terminate at the axiogingival junction or with the extension of the coping along the gingival floor but short of the facial margin. The most esthetic option is associated with the metal coping restricted to the axial wall and not extending into the shoulder area of the porcelain–butt joint margin.[10] A precise margin is difficult to obtain in porcelain, but methods have been developed to improve the fit in this critical area.

How to choose the right crown for esthetics

There is no one ideal crown for all situations. Each case is different, with varying factors that influence the choice of crowns. Patients have different esthetic demands that may or may not compromise function. The decision that one restoration is more esthetic than another is essentially based on visual interpretation. In certain mouths, anything will do (uniform tooth color, no distinguishing marks, etc.). In others, different identifying marks have to be matched, and a decision must be made as to whether to use gold, nonprecious metal, acrylic, or porcelain.

One should balance esthetics and function for each patient, and that balance will be different for each patient. To make the decision therefore, there must be an understanding of certain principles. Assuming the lithium disilicate or gold crown to be the most functional, it is the restoration of choice when esthetic needs are not compromised. For posterior teeth, if the patient agrees, full or partial coverage in lithium disilicate or gold should be used. Clearly, the advantages of the lithium disilicate restoration are that bacterial plaque does not form readily on its surface and that it is less thermally sensitive than gold. A disadvantage might be difficulty in maintaining adequate isolation for the bonding process.

The choice is ultimately based on a consideration of many factors.

1. **Lip line.** Does the gingival margin show when the patient speaks, smiles, or laughs? If so, one should select a crown system with an all-ceramic margin. Is the tooth to be crowned visible when smiling? Figure 16.29A shows a wide smile line of a female.
2. **Length of esthetic life expected by both patient and dentist.** This is a function of several factors:
   a. **Wear patterns.** Acrylic or composite resin restorations will not last as long as lithium disilicate or porcelain.
   b. **Acid content of the saliva.** Acid level and the amount of stain accumulated by natural and restored teeth are indicators of the life expectancy of acrylic, composite resin, and even cementing materials.
   c. Although still in its infancy, the known survival data of different ceramic materials today favor the lithium disilicate ceramic.
3. **Space limitations in tooth preparation.** For example, will the pulp preclude sufficient reduction for metal plus opaque plus porcelain? Evaluate the alveolar support.
4. **Occlusion.** Is the occlusion favorable for a full porcelain occlusal surface? It is always best to have porcelain functioning against porcelain. If the opposing occlusal surface is gold, the chances are the porcelain occlusal surface will wear the gold considerably faster. Even enamel can wear quickly against a porcelain occlusal surface. The lithium disilicate restorations wear very similarly to enamel.[57]
5. **The gingival sulcus.** Can one predict the long-term health of the sulcus? Even the most perfect gingival sulcus can become diseased and deformed within days, so one can never really be certain of long-term gingival margin coverage. How regularly is a patient receiving dental prophylaxis, and if previous disease was treated, is the patient maintained with periodontal care?
6. **Tissue type.** Is the tissue thin and transparent, thick and fibrous, or alveolar mucosa or keratinized attached gingiva? The thin, transparent type will be the most likely to recede or to show a metal margin. On the contrary, if a patient possesses thick fibrous tissue, one may choose a metal margin and be esthetically protected.
7. **Appearance of surrounding teeth.** How much translucency or opacity exists in adjacent or opposing teeth? Do they need to be recontoured before beginning treatment?
8. **Financial considerations.** Is the patient willing to pay for use of a high-quality laboratory or master ceramist, including specialized characterization procedures, or do they want the most economical treatment? Certainly, one of the more difficult decisions will be to match a fee to the level of difficulty presented by the patient. This difficulty may be expressed by the esthetic requirements of the patient, or even by the patient's attitude.

The patient and dentist should attempt to answer all these questions before a final decision to commence treatment is made. Many times, this choice cannot be made until the teeth are actually prepared, in order to determine how much space is available for the restoration.

The mouth must also be as disease-free as possible. The type of restoration should never be decided at the first or second appointment if there is periodontal disease or advanced caries or posterior bite collapse. Because the condition of the mouth can change, any decision would be premature. Since esthetic correction is accomplished in the provisional crowns or splinted fixed prosthesis, final decisions can be postponed and the options reevaluated later. When esthetics is a primary concern in both anterior and posterior teeth and there is not the need to splint restorations together, the all-ceramic restoration would be the primary choice for a long functional life and excellent esthetics.

Specific problem: the discolored pulpless tooth

Crowning one central incisor to match an adjacent tooth is one of the most difficult tasks in esthetic dentistry (see Figure 16.27A–D). When the compromised tooth happens to be nonvital and discolored, the procedure can become even more complex. The goal is to decide what type of restoration can best solve a patient's problems. The decision depends on what type of discoloration is present and whether or not a post and core will be needed that also could complicate the use of an all-ceramic crown. Recently,

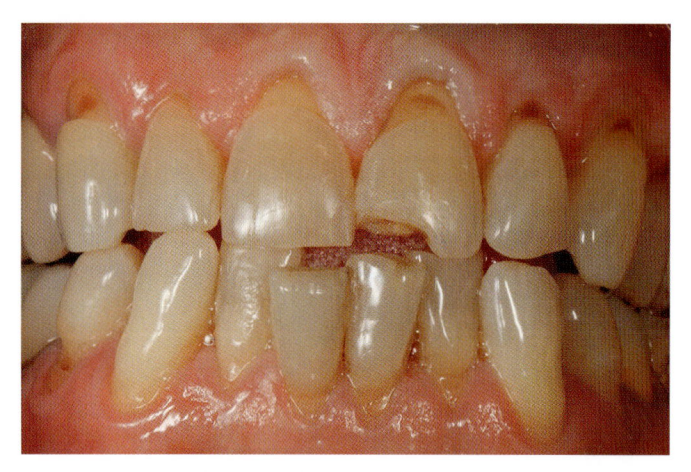

Figure 16.27 **(A)** The patient had a composite resin restoration that debonded and presented for a more permanent restoration. Because of the significant recession and the root caries, a crown was chosen as the restoration and lithium disilicate e.max as the material.

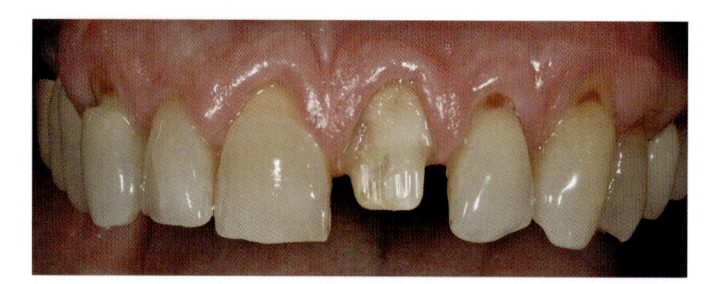

Figure 16.27 **(B)** With adequate reduction, matching the shape, hue, chroma, and value becomes less of a challenge.

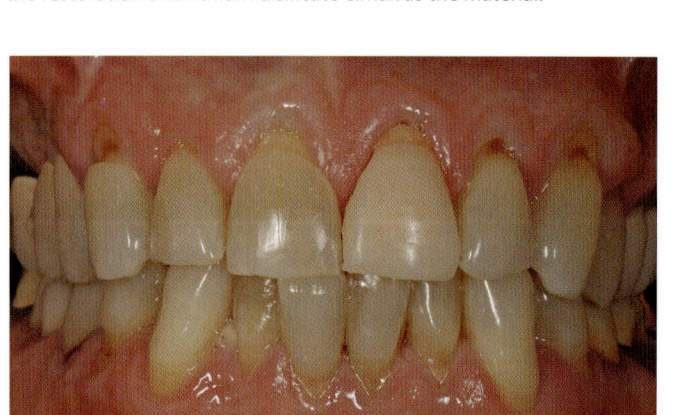

Figure 16.27 **(C)** A treatment wax is tried in, and the patient approves the esthetic direction chosen by the restorative dentist and the laboratory technician.

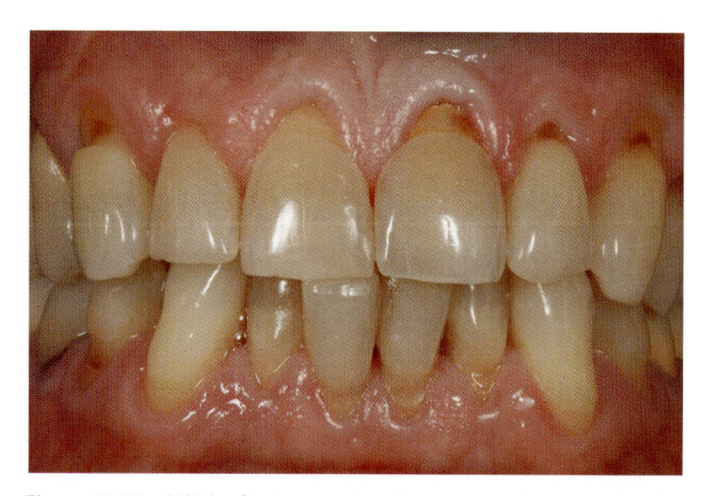

Figure 16.27 **(D)** The final restoration shows a very close match with the adjacent tooth. With adequate photography and shade communication, excellent matches can be achieved. Even radicular discoloration can be closely matched. Later the carious class V lesions will be restored with composite resin.

it has been possible to press lithium disilicate to a metal post and cover potentially more of the axial wall as an extended ferrule (see Figure 16.28). This can be very effective in masking the underlying discolored tooth.

If discoloration is the only problem, one may choose to use a porcelain veneer. However, this approach may make it more difficult to obtain a perfect match. One cannot remove extra tooth structure because porcelain veneers need to be bonded primarily to enamel. The problem of obtaining an optimal result can be made more difficult due to the effect of the underlying composite resin cement on the shade of the porcelain veneer. The tooth shade can also vary somewhat after seating the veneer because of a color shift in the polymerized composite resin cement. In fact, it may take several days to a week for the final color to be apparent, and by that time, one will obviously have no ability to change the color. Therefore, a crown may be the preferable choice, especially if the patient is a perfectionist. A crown's color and depth of stratification can be altered a few times as necessary to obtain the proper color.

Opaquing

Although an opaque can be applied to the tooth to mask the core and could conceivably help if the restoration is either a porcelain veneer or an all-ceramic crown, it may still be insufficient to mask the darkened tooth. The most predictable way is to have the laboratory incorporate the correct amount of opaquer in the ceramic material itself. Although this may sound like a simple solution, it is not. Until one actually seats the crown with cement one will not be assured the choice of material and opaquer is the correct one.

The most effective solution to this problem is to use a metal–ceramic crown with a metal substructure that is fully opaqued, masking out even the darkest of teeth or metal post and core. Masking of the opaque layer is also an esthetic necessity. It can be accomplished either by thickening the body porcelain layer or by tinting the opaque. To optimize esthetics, a porcelain shoulder that wraps around the entire preparation is quite

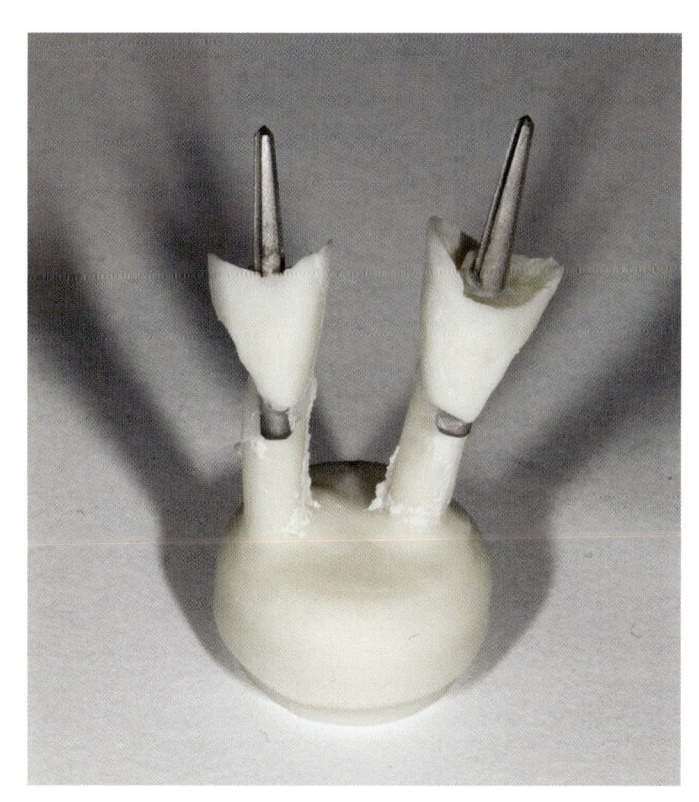

Figure 16.28 Lithium disilicate can be pressed onto a prefabricated gold–palladium post (Cendres Metaux) and used as a very rigid substrate to support an all-ceramic restoration.

effective, using metal along the axial walls only and not encroaching upon the visible marginal areas (see Figure 16.26). A problem can still exist if the root itself is discolored. In this condition, the margin area and gingival tissue may not be the correct color.

Principles for esthetic restorations

There is no substitute for the beautiful, healthy appearance of tooth enamel. This is precisely why it is so important to apply every conceivable esthetic principle in construction of a ceramic restoration. Using these principles is the best means of achieving the goal of a truly esthetic restoration. The concerned dentist must continually study the subject of esthetics, not only by attending courses and reading the literature, but also by being a keen observer of the natural smile and the use of diagnostic casts and digital photography. Shapes of teeth and their arrangement in the arch are crucial to obtain an esthetic result in artificial restorations, as the objective is to make the artificial restoration look believably natural. The following discusses some of these principles and solutions to the most common esthetic problems.

Lip line

The type of lip line almost always determines the number of teeth to restore. Observe not only the number of teeth exposed when the patient is smiling naturally, but also every tooth that is visible when the patient smiles widely. This is necessary to properly analyze the esthetic component (the teeth visible during smiling) in order to communicate to the patient exactly how the smile will look after restorative treatment. Often, the patient will seek to restore only the six anterior teeth, failing to realize that the improved shade or character of the restorations may call attention to the adjacent untreated teeth, which will no longer match. Thorough explanation of the smile analysis is necessary so that the patient can understand the results of the restoration before treatment begins. In addition, the use of lateral close-up and full-face views with computer imaging is essential in this instance. Few patients can visualize their smile past the six front teeth. To determine whether the lip line is high, medium, or low, observe the tooth length exposed when the patient smiles.[58]

High lip line

A high lip line is one in which all supragingival tooth structure and some gingival tissue are visible upon smiling (see Figure 16.29A).[58] The patient with the high lip line may not be the best candidate for a full crown because tissue tends to recede in time and a previously concealed margin may become visible. If the restoration is metal–ceramic, even a small metal collar may become exposed. Thin, transparent gingival tissue is more apt to recede. Even if the margin is not exposed upon insertion of the crown, such exposure may occur at a later time and make the patient extremely unhappy. It may be preferable to suggest a compromise treatment plan using ceramic veneers.

When the patient has a high lip line and a full crown becomes a necessary restorative choice, one should ideally use an all-ceramic restoration or with a metal–ceramic restoration the use of a full shoulder preparation on the labial surface with a porcelain butt joint as the margin. This will assist in maintaining an acceptable esthetic appearance if the tissue does recede in the future.

In the event that the tissue recedes after the impression appointment but before cementation, an immediate repair can be made to a porcelain butt margin. Even at the try-in appointment the labial shoulder margin can be extended into the gingival sulcus. Refit the crown with softened low-fusing compound attached to the labial margin. Make certain the new shoulder margin is recorded in the compound and pour a new die. After adapting foil to the die, the compound is removed and the porcelain added to establish the margin. An alternative impression compound would be polyether (Impregum, ESPE), since it has sufficient body hardness and is tenacious enough to record the new margin if one can achieve adequate tissue displacement.

Medium lip line

A medium lip line is one that shows up to, but does not include, the cervical margin of the anterior teeth (see Figure 16.29B).[58] A small portion of the interproximal gingival papilla also shows in a wide smile. The medium lip line presents only moderate difficulty in crown restoration, because the gingival margin is only seen in the widest of smiles. For normal speaking or slight smiling, there is no exposure of this area, thus a slight hint of a metal collar should present no unusual difficulty for most patients. However, for those patients who are extremely critical of any metal showing, the all-ceramic restoration should be used or the porcelain butt joint with a metal–ceramic crown.

Low lip line

In a low lip line the gingival margin is never revealed;[58] therefore, no problem exists with exposed margins except, possibly, in the patient's mind (see Figure 16.29C). Ideally, if the restoration can be a single unit, the all-ceramic crown is the state of the art. A metal–ceramic restoration with a metal collar is an ideal restoration when posterior teeth need to be splinted together or with fixed partial dentures only. If anterior teeth are splinted together the use of the buccal butt technique is required. The esthetic requirements may be less critical for a patient with a low lip line because with time the metal–ceramic restoration may display color deficiencies but they cannot be seen unless the patient retracts the lip with their fingers to look at the gingival margin; it becomes important to communicate this fact and allow the patient to participate in the final decision about treatment. It is necessary to explain to the patient exactly why their lip line will allow one to create the best possible biocompatible restoration. However, some patients, even those with low lip lines, may have emotional reservations about the presence of any exposed metal in their mouths; therefore, this must be dealt with on a psychological as well as a functional basis.

Arch irregularity

An arch irregularity generally exposes more coronal area on one side of the mouth than the other upon smiling (Figure 16.30). It is essential that the patient is made aware of this problem during the diagnostic stage. A patient needs to know that the crowns may not be bilaterally symmetrical in the final restoration. Take both full-face and close-up prerestorative photographs to preserve a good record of the patient's original intraoral condition in both smiling and lip-retracted positions. Computer imaging is also helpful to point out to the patient the irregularity and what one can do, if anything, to correct it.

Inclination of teeth

The inclination of teeth is an important consideration with all restorations. In the metal–ceramic restoration, because of the inherent qualities that exist in a crown with metal, opaque, and porcelain layers, this may be even more important. Proper color must be built into the restoration rather than relying on the use

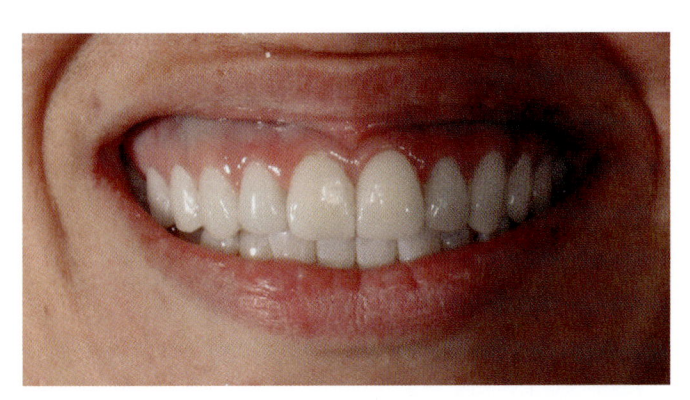

Figure 16.29 (A) A patient with a high lip line shows a continuous band of gingiva across the entire smile. These cases are considerably more challenging due to overwhelming exposure of the teeth and the supporting tissues.

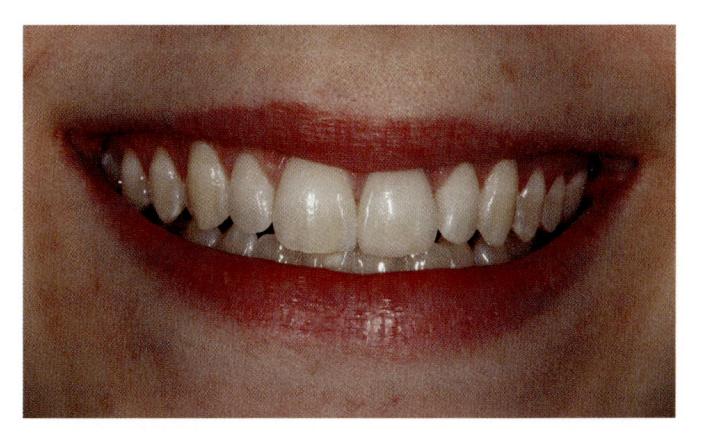

Figure 16.29 (B) A patient with a moderate lip line generally shows only the papilla. These cases can still be challenging, in particular with implant prosthodontics.

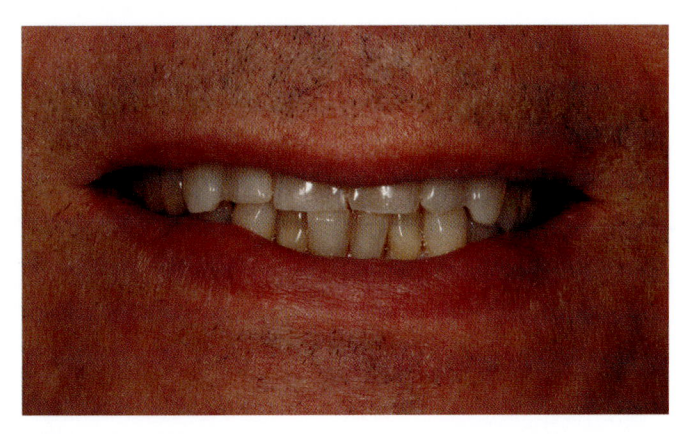

Figure 16.29 (C) A patient with a low lip line will show no tissue and, furthermore, only show a limited amount of tooth structure. This is widely considered to be the least difficult due to the limited amount of visibility.

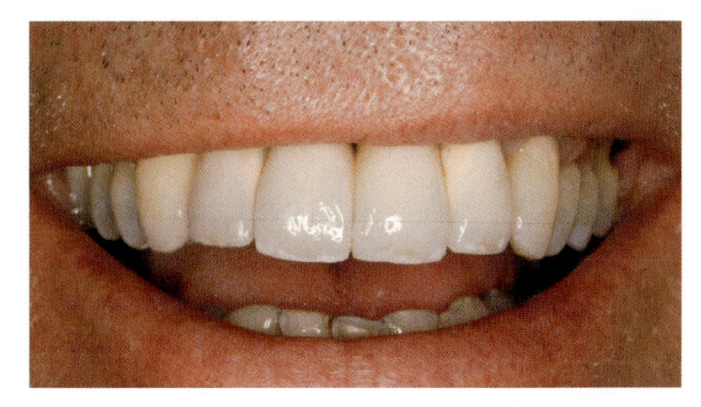

Figure 16.30 An arch and lip irregularity in the patient's smile causes more teeth to show on the patient's left side.

of surface stains. This will prevent lingually inclined upper anteriors from appearing to have different and darker shades in low lighting conditions. This may also apply in the case of extreme labially tipped upper incisors. Under certain conditions, when the head is tilted back exposing more of the lingual surface, the same situation may occur. Lingually inclined maxillary posterior teeth may need to be built out labially to achieve the most attractive overall smile.

If the crowns are satisfactory in their form and shade reproduction, the next concern is that they appear natural in their surroundings. Three factors that most often influence this are interincisal distance, and incisal and gingival embrasures.

Interincisal distance

The interincisal distance refers to the difference in incisal lengths of the maxillary central and lateral incisors. Generally, the central incisors should be slightly longer than the lateral incisors. The greater the distance, the younger the smile appears (Figure 16.31). As teeth wear, the incisal length of the centrals becomes reduced, making the four maxillary anterior teeth more equal in length. If an older look is desired, less interincisal distance is used. If a younger look is the objective, a greater interincisal distance is incorporated. This must be coordinated with incisal guidance, the incisal table of the mandibular incisors, and the cusp tips of the posterior teeth. Some patients can tolerate longer central incisors, whereas others may complain that their lips cannot accept the added length. Even speech can be a problem for them. One should observe the patient in saying "F," "V," and "S" sounds to understand the proper position of the anterior incisors. Whenever planning a greater interincisal distance, the patient should observe this in a treatment wax or a direct mock-up. The corrections may be created in the provisional restorations and ideally left to function for several weeks to determine the suitability of the altered incisal length.

When a high lip line exposes all the upper teeth in almost every facial expression, it is usually advantageous to vary the interincisal distance. Even altering the length of the central incisors by making one slightly longer than the other can create a more natural appearance, since this is frequently found in the natural dentition.

Incisal embrasure

The incisal embrasure refers to the space between the incisal tables of adjacent teeth. Lack of proper incisal embrasures usually results in an artificial-appearing restoration (Figure 16.32A and C). In each patient, it is usually best to duplicate the adjacent, natural incisal embrasures. Study photographs of the patient's smile as well as other people's smiles to appreciate the variation of incisal embrasures that exist in different individuals. An entire personality or cosmetic change can result from increasing or decreasing embrasure length and width.

Gingival embrasure

The esthetic restoration requires an adequate zone of attached gingiva and a proper embrasure that permits interdental tissue to exist without impingement (Figures 16.32B and D). One cause of

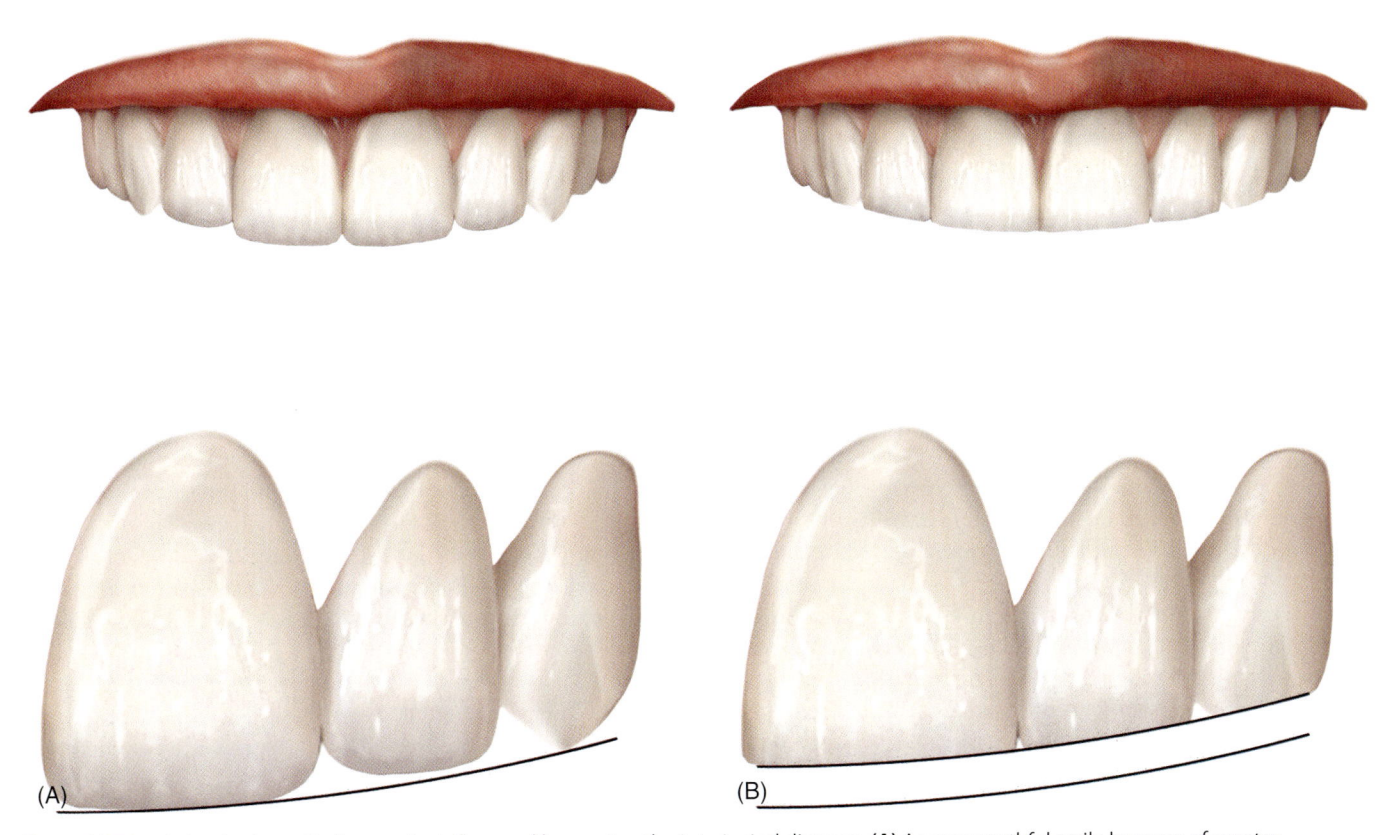

Figure 16.31 Aging in the smile line can be influenced by varying the interincisal distance. **(A)** A more youthful smile because of greater interincisal distance; **(B)** depicts increased wear, and thereby an older smile.

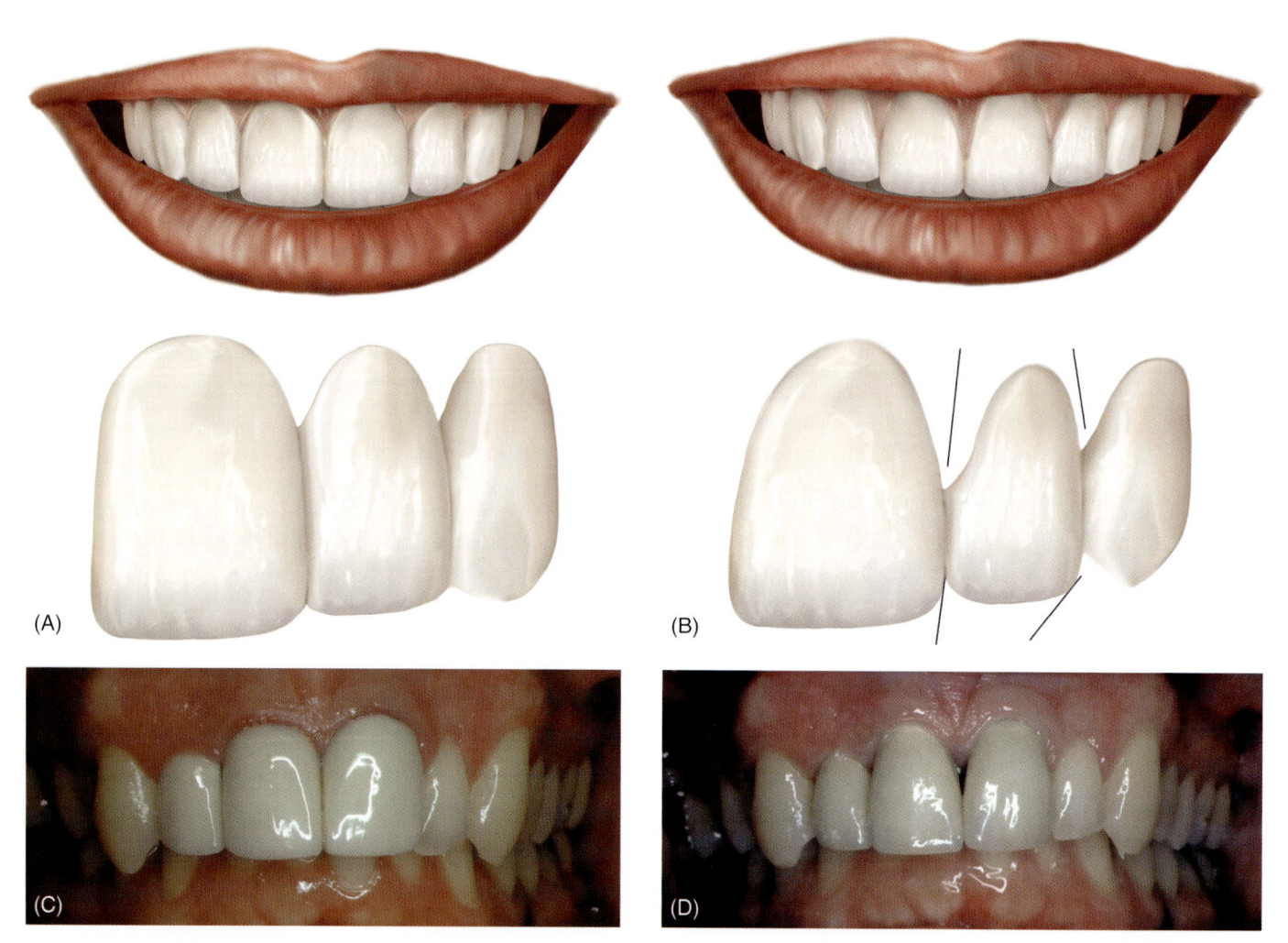

Figure 16.32 **(A–D)** Properly formed incisal and gingival embrasures are necessary for an esthetic restoration. (A, C) "Chicklet" appearance of a typical restoration lacking well-formed incisal and gingival embrasures. Absence of the gingival embrasures produces gingival impingement resulting in inflammatory response, which is unesthetic and functionally unacceptable. (B, D) Esthetic improvement is shown when both gingival and incisal embrasures have been included.

an unesthetic restoration is inflamed tissue due to overbuilding porcelain in the gingival area. The best prevention is, at the try-in, to mark the porcelain with a sharp pencil and open the area between adjacent teeth to encourage healthy tissue. An alternative method of creating proper gingival embrasures is to make a duplicate model showing exactly where the tissue is. Because tissue must be adequately supported, undercontouring porcelain may also cause a problem. A correct emergence profile is essential for both functional maintenance and an esthetic appearance. A gingival papilla will be present or absent in part by the amount of inter-root space that exists.[59] When roots or roots to implant are close, a gingival col anatomy will be present and generally the papilla will close the gingival embrasure. When the roots are far apart, the gingival anatomy becomes keratinized, and the gingival col flattens down and becomes convex. In this condition the papilla is lost.

The stage at which most problems should be resolved is before the impression, at the time one makes the provisional restoration. There are several reasons why all intended corrections should be incorporated in the provisional restorations. First, it allows the patient to wear the new look and to adjust to any esthetic and functional changes. Many esthetic changes may not be readily accepted by one's peers. This type of criticism is better to be received and evaluated during the temporary phase.

Second, it allows evaluation of the preparation before taking final impressions. After the intended shape and contour of the temporary restoration is completed, examine the thickness in every portion to be sure there will be sufficient room for metal, opaque, and body and incisal porcelains. If there are thin spots due to the labial convexities that are necessary to achieve an esthetic result, then alter the preparation to gain extra space for the final restoration. When presence of pulp tissue makes it impossible to remove additional tooth structure without potential damage, inform the patient that a vital pulp extirpation might be necessary to achieve the desired esthetic correction. It is important that the patient be a part of this decision, especially if the esthetic result would be compromised by an inadequate tooth preparation.

Another reason for making the provisional restoration before the impression is to examine the occlusion and make any alterations on the opposing arch that will improve the result.

These types of changes can only be made during tooth preparation. If one waits until the esthetic try-in, the final restoration may be a compromise rather than the esthetic result it can and should be. Always try to anticipate decisions of this sort so that the patient will be prepared and not become defensive when one realizes too late that one must reduce the opposing arch.

Tooth contour and shape

After the restorative material has been chosen, the next important factor is the shape and contour of the restoration. Natural teeth have rounded contours, rather than the square that may often be found in unnatural-appearing restorations. This is seen especially in the anterior teeth, where many ceramists tend to flatten the labial surfaces rather than place the proper contour and line angles in the mesial and distal aspects of that surface. Another common fault is lack of critical viewing from the incisal or occlusal aspect.

The ceramist is usually confronted with the problem of matching the contours of adjacent teeth. However, the esthetic appearance of the restoration can usually be improved by first altering the form of the adjacent teeth through cosmetic contouring or interproximal bonded ceramic veneers.

Yuodelis et al. found that correct morphological contours, although a vital part of any esthetic restoration, are of paramount importance during dental procedures that involve full-coverage restorations.[60] It has been suggested that the facial and lingual enamel bulges of human teeth protect the free gingival margin from the trauma of occlusion by deflecting food over the gingival crevice and onto the keratinized gingival tissue. Kramer, however, questions the effect of the curve and the evidence that indicates that crown contours protect tissue.[55]

Since microbial plaque is the principal cause of both caries and periodontal disease, its retention by tooth surfaces is to be avoided. Clinically, plaque retention is greatest in inaccessible areas, particularly the interproximal and the facial and lingual cervical areas of the teeth. To keep these areas plaque free, the relationship of morphology of crown contour and degree of accessibility must be understood. Overcontouring can encourage debris accumulation that may lead to functional and esthetic breakdown of supporting tissues.

In an experiment conducted by Perel that supports these findings, the effect of crown contours on gingiva was clearly demonstrated.[61] The mandibular teeth of mongrel dogs were remodeled by removing tooth structure from the labial, buccal, or lingual surfaces in different parts of the mouth. The labial surfaces of some teeth were overcontoured using self-curing resin. Results showed that supragingival undercontouring caused no apparent gingival pathology, whereas overcontouring caused inflammation and then collection of debris, hyperplasia, and engorgement of the marginal gingiva, scant keratinization, and deterioration of the fibers of the gingival collar.[61]

Thus, it may be seen that this so-called protective function of convex crown contour may in reality trap food and prevent vital stimulation of the gingival margin. In addition, particularly after periodontal therapy that involves osseous resection, a longer-than-normal clinical crown may be left. These lengthened clinical crowns are more difficult to keep plaque free due to the exposed furcations and different root shapes, especially proximal convexities that are much harder to clean.[60] In such cases, for an esthetic long-term result, the final restoration should not follow the original anatomic contour; instead, it should recreate at least the gingival contours of the root portion. This makes the gingival third of the furcation areas more accessible for cleaning. The crown contour debate has been active for years and clearly is real when studying teeth and their gingival relationships. In implant dentistry, where a tighter marginal seal is always present, this debate is of less importance.

While crown contour must establish an esthetic result, it must not compromise the patient's oral health. Although this responsibility lies solely in the hands of the dentist, too many practitioners try to pass it off onto the technician. Tooth preparation is extremely important to guarantee that the laboratory technician has sufficient room to create a well-shaped and contoured restoration. Although the laboratory procedure begins with the technician, it certainly ends with the dentist at chairside. No matter how well the technician has created a crown, some improvement and personalized changes can usually be performed by the dentist at chairside during the try-in appointment. Naturally, the better the technician, the less adjustment is necessary by the dentist. A faithful duplication of the matching tooth in the patient's natural dentition usually gives the best esthetic result, although occasionally an increase or diminution in overall size may be necessary due to tooth movement. The basic curves, angles, heights or contours, contact areas, and general outline form should be duplicated as closely as possible. Areas that need special attention are the mesial and distal incisal angles, the areas of contact, the concavities and convexities at the labial line angles in the gingival third of the crown, and the thickness of the incisal edge labiolingually.

A patient's appearance can be considerably altered depending on the shape of the crowns (Figure 16.33A). Notice in Figure 16.33B how different the smile can look when rounder, softer contours are used.

Another important factor to consider in the contour of the restoration is the shape of the pulp. If the pulp is unusually wide, this may be a contraindication for crowning. When some type of correction is imperative, a wide pulp requires a shallow preparation and a temporary crown for 6 months to 1 year to induce pulp recession through the formation of secondary dentin. The smaller the pulp in height and width, the greater the amount of tooth correction that can be made when necessary.[62]

Final esthetic try-in

The last chance to make corrections is at the esthetic try-in. Staining, final shaping, and contouring to influence personality, age, and sex, and any other improvements, should be done or planned at this time. The ceramist then has to add the necessary final touches to make an attractive and natural-appearing restoration, usually without seeing the patient. These changes must be determined at the chair. When writing the laboratory prescription, include as much information as possible in order to aid the technician.

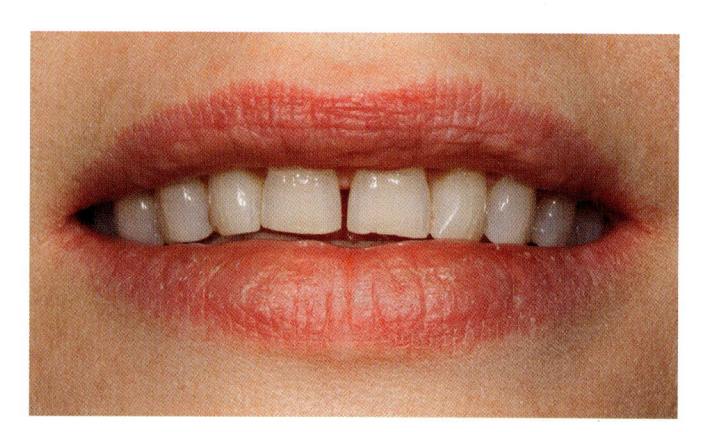

Figure 16.33 **(A)** This patient presented with a severely worn dentition. She felt that her teeth made her look masculine and wanted softer contours.

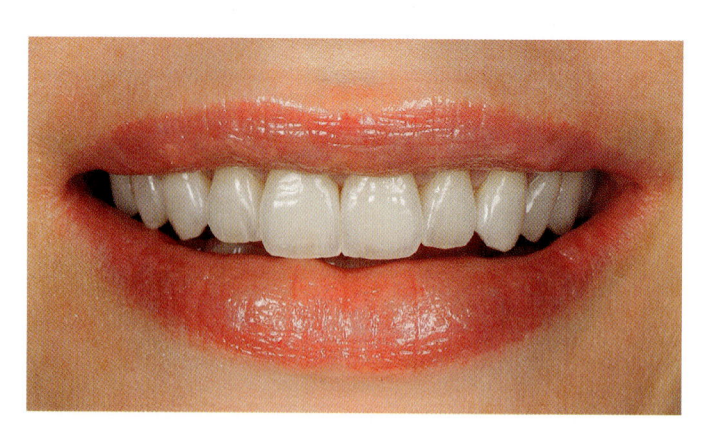

Figure 16.33 **(B)** The final delivery shows, in contrast to the originals, that the softer corners and open incisal embrasure can give a youthful appearance.

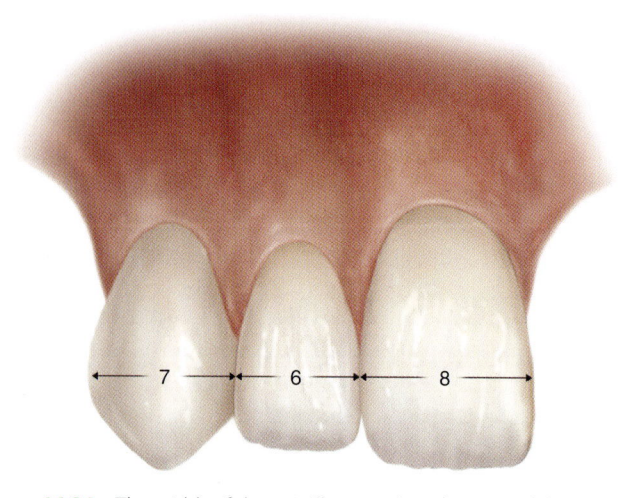

Figure 16.34 The width of the maxillary teeth in the natural dentition has a definite size variance. These dimensions can be used as a guide to the approximate proportion of anterior tooth width.

Tooth size

Computer imaging can help one in correctly proportioning the teeth. The principles of divine proportion should be built into a software program to give one a better idea of proper relative tooth size for a patient. Beaudreau suggests that the teeth can be proportioned in a general sense.[63] He proposes that when the central incisors are 8 mm wide the cuspids should be approximately 7 mm wide and the laterals should be 6 mm wide (Figure 16.34). Therefore, the lateral should be approximately 25% smaller in width than the central incisor, and the cuspid is approximately 13% narrower than the central incisor.

Long teeth

There are generally two causes of an extra-long tooth. The most common reasons for a long tooth are often caused by a skeletal malocclusion or periodontal disease that caused the teeth to be supraerupted. This problem is especially troublesome in the patient with a high lip line, where tooth symmetry, or lack of it, is all too apparent upon smiling. Periodontal treatment that includes grafting should be instituted before restorative treatment. If the existing restoration is still too long, then the replacement can incorporate gingival ceramic or a shorter root form that may improve the appearance.

Long teeth may be a result of periodontal surgery. A major consideration in crown preparation in these patients is the difficulty in preparing a modified chamfer on the root. Consequently, the resulting thin chamfer or knife-edge preparation does not allow for sufficient marginal depth to accommodate porcelain to conceal the metal or opaque color. In the final analysis, the patient's lip line can make the difference. If the patient has a medium or low lip line, there should be no problem.

When patients have extensive loss of interproximal tissue due to periodontal surgery, there are two solutions that can generally be applied to crown restorations: the addition of pink porcelain to the restoration to simulate interproximal tissue, or, if all else fails, a removable interproximal silicone tissue insert.

The use of gingival ceramics involves raising the gingival contact in porcelain and adding additional material lingually to close the space. One of the problems with this technique is the difficulty in matching the pink tone of the individual patient's gingiva. Request the laboratory to make several shade tabs of different combinations of pink porcelains to provide a range for matching the patient's gingival color, and ideally have the laboratory technician make the color analysis. An alternative to one of the prosthetic solutions to loss of interdental space is the possibility of orthodontic extrusion; this can sometimes work well when there are limited numbers of teeth involved.

Short teeth

If the tooth appears too short, first explore the possibility of lengthening the tooth by periodontal surgery to either apically reposition the tissue or, when there is excesses tissue, by a gingivectomy procedure. If not feasible, then resort to illusions in the crown to give an appearance of greater length. Eliminate horizontal lines and emphasize vertical characterizations and texture. Flatten the gingivoincisal dimension to help emphasize length. Rounding the proximal surfaces will make the tooth appear longer. Use stains to emphasize the length by darkening the interproximal porcelain and lightening the vertical dimension of the crown. Try to create vertical highlights by creating vertical, parallel lines on the labial surface that will reflect light in a vertical dimension.

Correct occlusal registration

An accurate interocclusal registration and the use of an articulator are essential in obtaining a successful esthetic result. As previously discussed, after master impressions and articulation, a dental technician should complete a treatment wax that can be placed in a patient's mouth to determine the correct tooth length, midline position, tooth cant, and the planes of occlusion (see Figure 16.35A–D). It may assist the technician if impressions are made of the provisional crowns to help determine the length of the restorations. Failure to do this may result in the crowns being too long at the try-in appointment. If this is not determined with the patient for their approval, alterations of the porcelain to correct the contour and occlusion may remove or affect ceramic stratification and occlusal or incisal translucency built into the ceramic color. Photographic or computer imaging may aid in this process.

Tooth arrangement

When the arch length to be restored is too small for normally sized crowns, it is sometimes better to overlap the lateral or central incisor crowns, when the patient permits, rather than simply reproducing smaller teeth. Another option is use of slightly larger crowns and elimination of one tooth in the restored arch. The solution should always depend on the patient's facial features, expressions, overall personality, and personal preferences. The intended correction should be made first on study casts and with computer imaging so that both the dentists and their patients can visualize and approve. Then, it is done on the

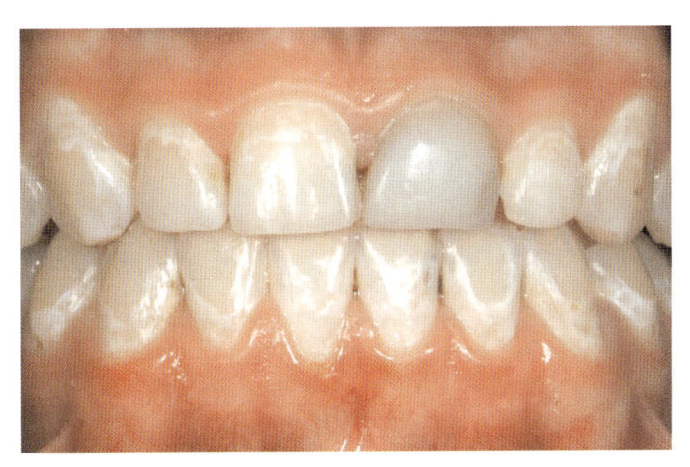

Figure 16.35 **(A)** This patient had seen an orthodontist for several years. Once the patient was debanded, his teeth exhibited substantial enamel hypoplasia and incipient caries. The anterior maxillary and mandibular six were the most severely affected. Couple that with a virtually nonexistent anterior guidance, so full crowns were indicated.

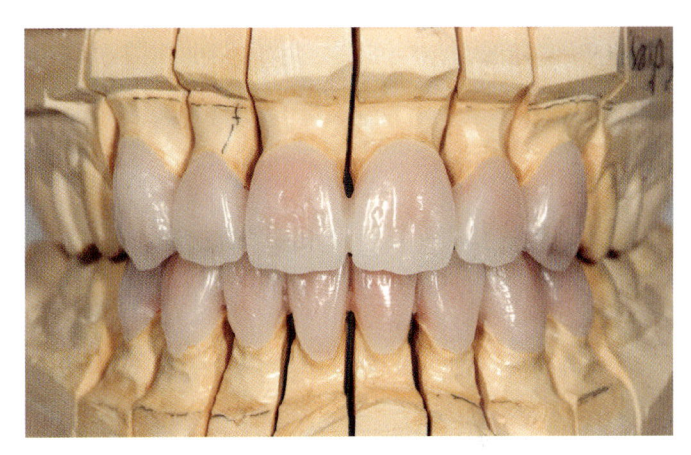

Figure 16.35 **(B)** The treatment wax is fabricated on the master cast and then transferred to the patient's mouth.

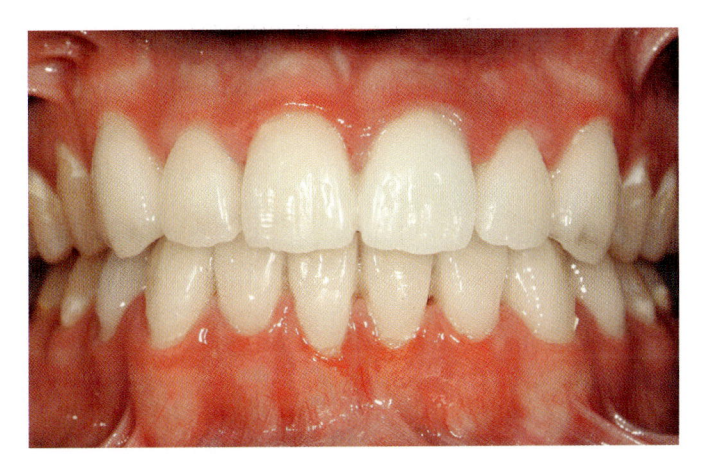

Figure 16.35 **(C)** In the mouth, the treatment wax can be used to allow the patient to freely communicate their esthetic desires. It also allows the technician to align their vision of the case with that of the patient and the restorative dentist.

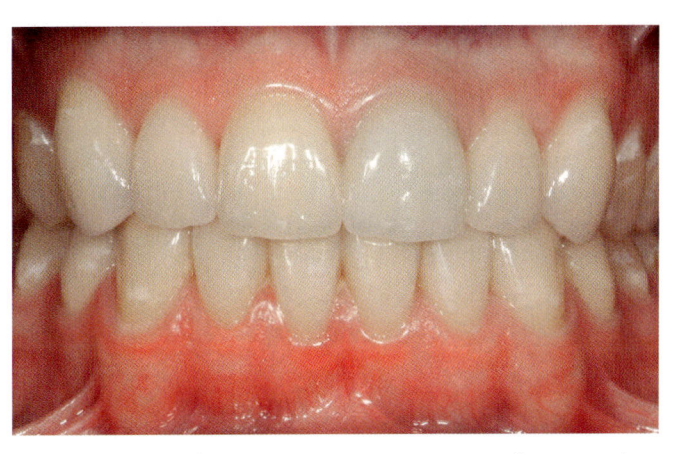

Figure 16.35 **(D)** After trying in the treatment wax and receiving the patient's approval, the technician can use it as a blueprint and fabricate the final restorations.

Tooth color

To deal with the perplexing problems of matching teeth, a thorough understanding of color is mandatory. With this increased knowledge and by applying some of the principles outlined in this chapter, more successful shade matching can be attained.

Culpepper[39] and others have described that one of the weakest links in shade making, regardless of shade guide or system used, is the eyes of the individual dentist. Although there have been many experiments in shade matching, few, if any, could be considered successful. What they did show was not only the tremendous variability in the way different dentists see color, but also the inconsistency in a given dentist's evaluation and judgment of color when tested at different times. Eyesight changes with age, and it also varies day to day, hour to hour, and appointment to appointment. This explains how a dentist or technician can select a shade, then look at this shade several days, or even minutes, later and see a different color. It also helps to explain how, regardless of how much care is taken, shades will sometimes be missed. Also, shade guides are just that: guides. They are rarely made of dental ceramics or the materials that will be used in the restoration. The matching of tooth color must be individualized for each patient.

Texture

After shape and shade selection, surface texture and characterization are important adjuncts to a natural esthetic appearance. An attempt should be made to copy the surface texture of adjacent teeth. Study natural teeth to note how small facets create natural shadows. Figure 16.36A and B shows examples of highly textured and nontextured teeth. Duplicating existing irregularities and heights of contour of adjacent teeth produces realism. Maximum highlights are reflected from the heights of contour, but realize that overprominent ridges and grooves on the labial surface are often associated with false teeth and add little to the esthetics of the restoration. A smooth, unbroken surface gives the impression of a long tooth, whereas texture can give the impression of a smaller tooth. At the try-in appointment, the moistened surface should be compared with adjacent teeth. This is most important when a single crown is to be placed next to a natural tooth.

An alternative method is to use a good color-balanced digital camera that can produce video. These digital images are an excellent method to convey to a technician an actual color representation of the condition of the patient's adjacent teeth, including shade variations.

Light

The light used to take a shade is critical. Since the eyes of the dentist and the laboratory technician are different, using different kinds of light sources can compound an error in color and judgment. For this reason, it is best for both the technician and dentist to use the same color-corrected light source.

The best light source for color selection is the light through a window with a northern exposure. If this is not available, take the patient outside, preferably with an assistant and laboratory technician. Be sure to include a full-face mirror for the patients so that they can participate in the selection procedure. An overcast sky is preferable, since a bright sky has a blue component that enhances the green color of the tooth. Early morning and late afternoon sunlight has a yellow component that enhances the yellow hue in the tooth. Inside, see how the shade may differ in incandescent light and in the lighting of the treatment room.

Even if outside light is available, one should use color-corrected fluorescent bulbs in the treatment rooms. In fact, one

Figure 16.36 **(A)** The amount of surface texture will affect the perception of color. A tooth with minimal surface texture will exhibit a flat, more opaque color.

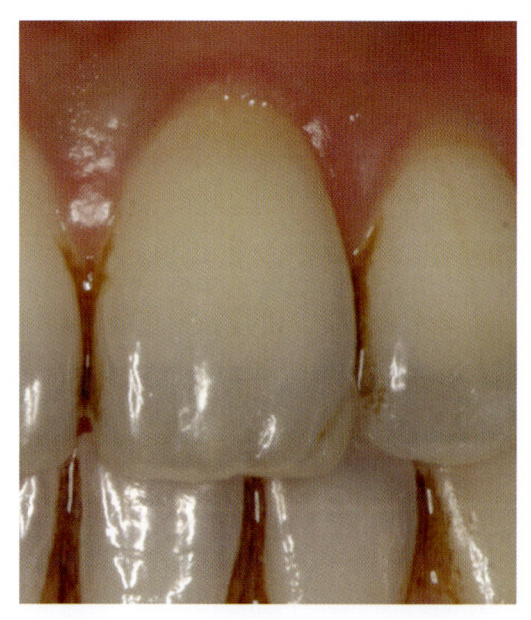

Figure 16.36 **(B)** In comparison, a tooth with greater surface texture will appear more translucent and have a more vital appearance.

of the best light sources available today is the color-corrected natural daylight fluorescent bulb. Used by major industries concerned with color control, it closely reproduces natural daylight and allows the truest relationship to exist between the shade guide and tooth. Request that the laboratory use them, because they can help achieve the best esthetic color result.

As an alternative, there are several hand-held light sources that one can use to help take a shade (Spectroshade, Vident, or Olympus). Ultimately, one will be using three light sources:

- fluorescent light
- outside light
- incandescent light.

In the event the shade appears different in the various light sources, make sure the patient is aware of this difference. Then ask in which light source he or she will be seen most of the time or in which light condition he or she wants the restoration to best match. *Although the entire dental team may participate in shade selection, the ultimate decision must rest with the patient.* Be sure to have them sign off on this final color selection. Otherwise, the patient may blame you if they become dissatisfied with the color of the final crowns.[64]

A patient's lipstick should be removed before they consider shades. When choosing the gingival shade, the lips of the patient should be raised and the incisal portion of the teeth covered. For selection of the incisal shade, the patient's lips should be in a speaking position to give one a better concept of shade and to eliminate any influence from the gingival third of the tooth. If using lip retractors, avoid drying out the teeth. Keep them wet during the entire process or the existing teeth may dry out sufficiently to change color. When selecting the shade, the patient's head should be erect and at your eye level. The dentist should stand between the patient and the light source. If there is no outside light, and only color-corrected light from overhead fixtures is being used, it may be necessary to tilt the patient back so that the light hits the tooth directly.

What to record

To construct a complete and accurate shade chart of a tooth, it is necessary to be able to see different colors in different sections of the tooth. Although dramatic differences may usually be seen in the broad gingival, body, and incisal portions of the tooth, there are often more subtle variations that occur in smaller areas of the tooth, varying with the angle at which one views the tooth. For example, a translucency may occur at either the mesial or distal line angle. It is rarely straight across or consistent, but often a broken line along the incisal one-third or one-fourth of the tooth and takes different shapes and forms in each tooth.

This should all be recorded on a shade chart that divides the teeth into sections to give the ceramist an understanding of where the colors are located. In this respect, a complete set of felt-tip colored pens is helpful (see Figure 16.37A and B). The different colors in the tooth can be diagrammed easily to give the technician a better understanding. To be as precise as possible, it may be necessary to give the technician several different shade tabs, with only portions of each marked, to correspond with specific sections of the tooth where that specific color is located. This way, the ceramist has a better idea of the hue, value, and chroma to be used. Another technique that can be used as an adjunct to digital photography is manipulation of the digital image. By maximizing the contrast and reducing the exposure of the image, the internal colors, and varying translucencies can be viewed. This technique, which can be seen in Figure 16.38A and B, works best when attempting to mimic an existing natural tooth (e.g., matching centrals). The shade will also depend on the position of the teeth. If central or lateral incisors are tilted lingually, the light is reflected differently than if they were in a marked labial inclination. If the patient is in a Class II or protrusive arrangement, choose a deeper or darker shade, since a lighter shade is more conspicuous and creates the appearance of false teeth. In a Class II patient with a high lip line, it is best to overdramatize the difference between the shades within the tooth. Accentuate the blues, greens, and oranges

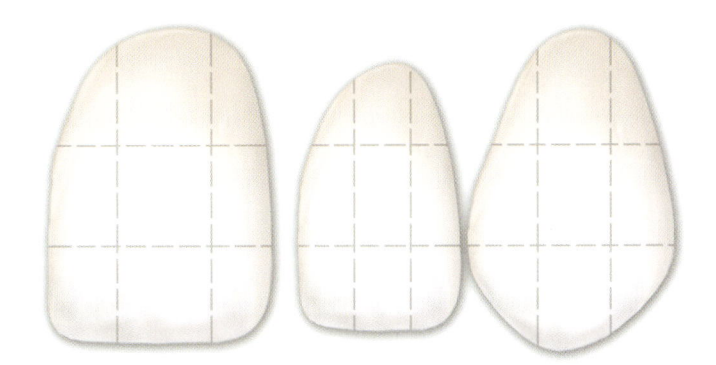

Figure 16.37 **(A)** This is an example how to divide the tooth surface to generate a functional shade chart. The teeth are divided into nine sections each for more exact shade mapping.

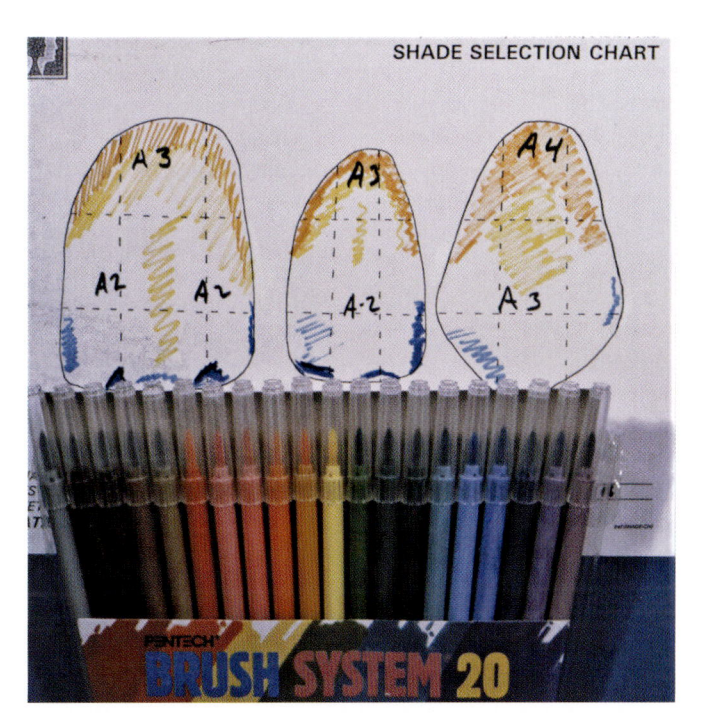

Figure 16.37 **(B)** Note how specifically the gingival intensity and incisal translucency can be designated with a complete set of felt-tip color pens.

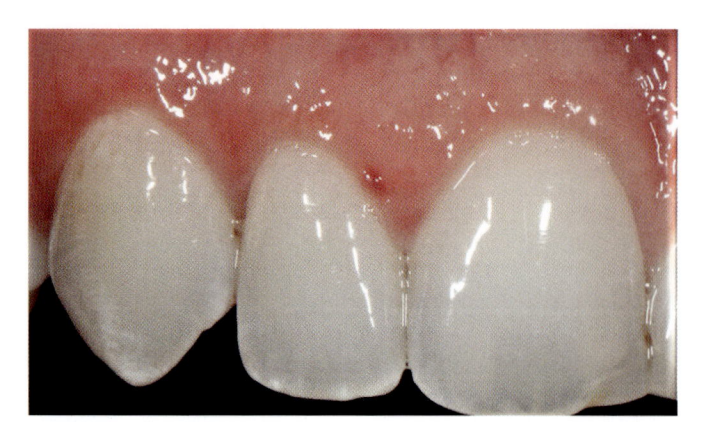

Figure 16.38 **(A)** When evaluating the internal coloring and defects in the tooth, a very useful technique is to increase the contrast and decrease the brightness. This will highlight incisal effects that may be difficult to see.

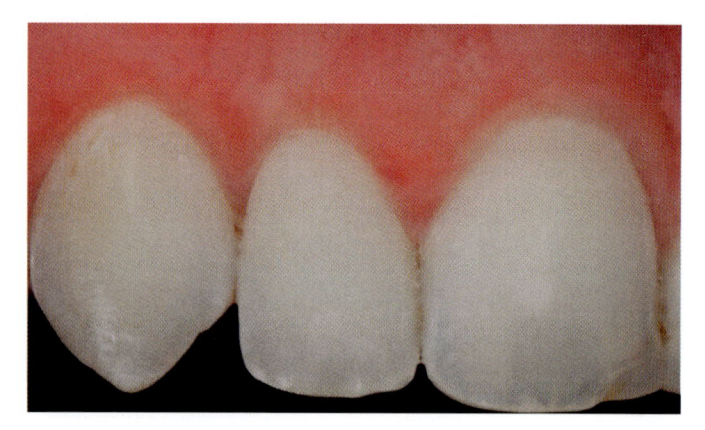

Figure 16.38 **(B)** After modifying the photograph, the technician can clearly see the incisal translucency and halo effect, as well as areas of hypercalcification and cracks.

and include any imperfections that simulate naturalness. Light reflection from a protruding tooth is much greater than from a tooth that is positioned lingually and thus shielded by the lips during smiling or speaking.

Conversely, beware of a dark tooth that is well concealed by the lips. To match this tooth, it is best to do so by choosing the appropriate shade of the basic dental ceramic. Frequently, to match the darker tooth, a mistake is made by using light-colored porcelain with surface stains to darken it. This may result in metamerism, or a tooth that will look different in different kinds of light. In changing light conditions, reflections will make the tooth look darker than it really is. It is critical to take sufficient time to choose the best possible shade and to view it under different forms of light before a final decision is made.

Shade selection should be as accurate as possible because, as shown by Mulla and Weiner, the appearance of the restoration that has been extrinsically stained cannot be precisely predicted. The changes for a particular type of stain, however, appear consistent, and it may be possible to judge the amount of stain to be applied on the basis of prior experience.[65]

McLean notes that custom staining should not be used for alteration of incorrect colors, except in marginal cases, but rather that custom staining be confined only to creating surface defects or colors that are present on the natural tooth surface. If one can narrow the choice of the basic shade to two, the one higher in value should be chosen, because a value can be lowered by staining, but a low value cannot be made lighter.[66–69]

However, there is no doubt that the most esthetic and esthetically long-lasting ceramic crown is one that has been constructed with color incorporated into the porcelain (stratification) internally, rather than by staining the surface. The internal color can come from layers of different shades of porcelain, from inlaid stains, or from special effects included into the building process. Good examples of natural-appearing, internally shaded, all-ceramic crowns are shown in Figure 16.39B.

Areas of stain, hypocalcification, translucency, crack lines, or other artifacts that one wants in the crown should be carefully placed on the shade chart to record their exact position on the tooth. The more accurate the rendition, the better the final result.

For anterior crowns, if there are no adjacent, opposing, or nearby natural anterior teeth to match, evaluate the shape, texture, and shade of the uncrowned, posterior teeth. Note the presence or absence of multiple colors, translucencies, or artifacts. The posterior teeth can serve as a relative guide for the missing anterior teeth. One can also ask the patient to provide photographs that clearly show the anterior teeth when they were unrestored. If there are no photographs or unmarked or undamaged teeth in the mouth, one is free to choose any acceptable shade. Since all these must be done before one begins any treatment on the tooth, a preliminary shade chart should be completed at the first appointment. The tooth should be checked again at the next appointment to confirm or make any necessary changes. Also take color digital photographs of the patient during one of these visits to obtain an accurate guide that may be given to the laboratory technician when the preparations are completed and impressions are made. Make certain that the photograph is an accurate representation of the actual tooth shade. The technician must be able to see the color and any shade differences and to grasp a visual concept of the shape and characterization of the tooth.

There is a definite advantage to having one's own laboratory technician or having an outside technician present at a shade-taking visit. The technician can see the shade as one takes it. Frequently, the technician will suggest certain shades based on their knowledge and experience with porcelain in the laboratory.

Shade guides

It is obvious that whatever manufacturer's product is being used, the corresponding shade guide should also be used. But be careful, because even the shade tabs of one shade number may differ from one supposedly identical shade guide to another. One may also find that there are many times when the only way to arrive at a proper representation of the colors involved is to use different manufacturers' shade guides. One may even use three different manufacturers' shade tabs to delineate separate cervical, body, and incisal parts of a patient's tooth.

Many dentists like to develop their own shade guides. Usually, dentists who have their own laboratory technicians do this. However, an outside laboratory can also do it, if the dentist

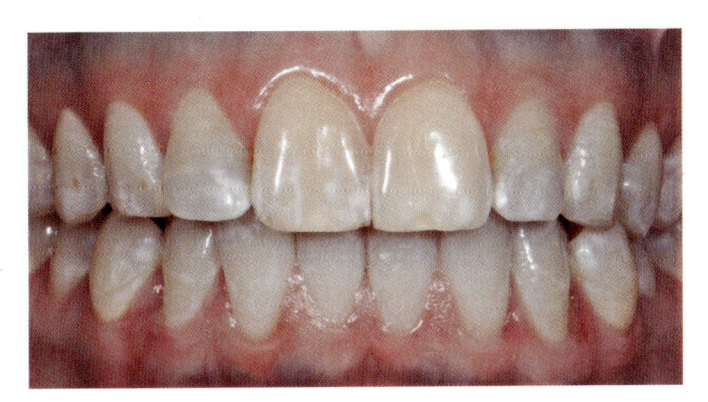

Figure 16.39 **(A)** With a large amount of resin composites exhibiting microleakage and recurrent caries, crowns were the best option to provide the patient with an esthetic result.

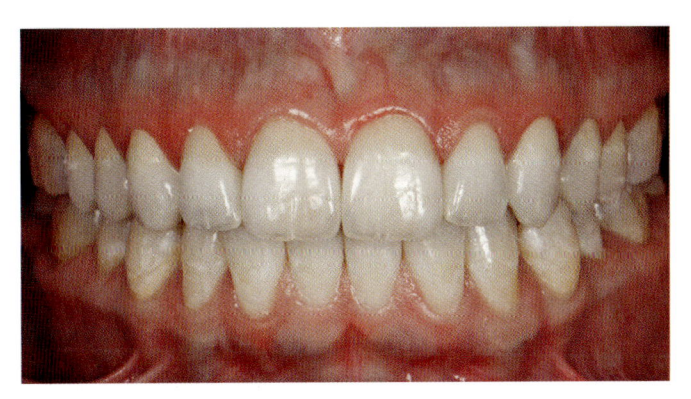

Figure 16.39 **(B)** With a highly skilled technician, internal colorants, translucency, and surface texture can be employed to create ceramic crowns with a highly natural and esthetic appearance.

requests it. Because of the multiplicity of shade guides (Figure 16.40) and the variety of shades made by individual manufacturers, the exact shade button (or buttons) that was chosen should be sent to the laboratory. If the choice of restoration is metal–ceramics, the metal backing must be the same as routinely employed for the individual dentist's everyday application, including the usual opaque and porcelain thickness.

Probably the most difficult task after the shade has been taken is communicating this to the laboratory so that a reasonably accurate crown comes back for the try-in. Naturally, some correction can be done with staining (provided the required value is higher and the chroma is lower), but the closer the original match, the easier and better the final esthetic result will be. Along with the photographs, which should be sent digitally (including images of the selected shade tabs adjacent to the prepared tooth), send the shade chart, notes on texture and characterization, casts, and anything else that can help. Remember, unless one has an in-office laboratory, the ceramist will most likely never have seen the patient, and they will have to rely totally on the information to create the crown. Again, the more accurate the information, the better the result.

Convey also to the laboratory technician the intensity of the different hues. For instance, in the incisal coloration or translucency, how gray or how blue is a "grayish" or "bluish" tint (Figure 16.41)? Unless some type of shade guide with approximating color can be given to the ceramist, it is mere guesswork as to what shade is being requested.

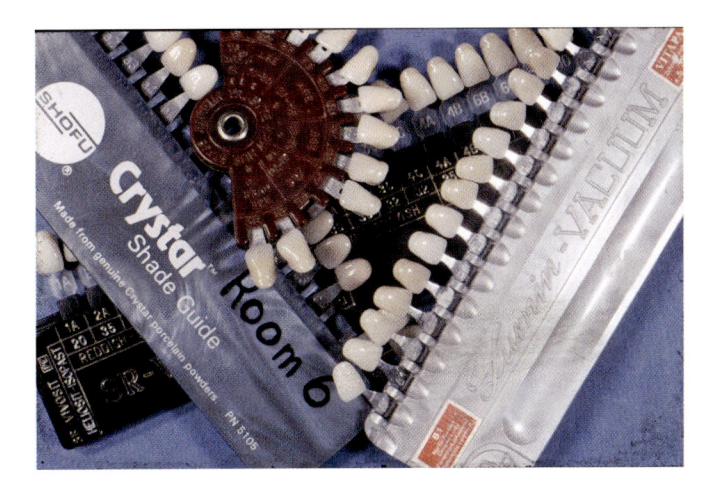

Figure 16.40 It is ideal to use the same manufacturer's shade guide as the porcelain selected. However, if one goal is to match an existing tooth, find a shade tab that comes as close as possible to the tooth to be matched (regardless of the manufacturer) and send that to the laboratory.

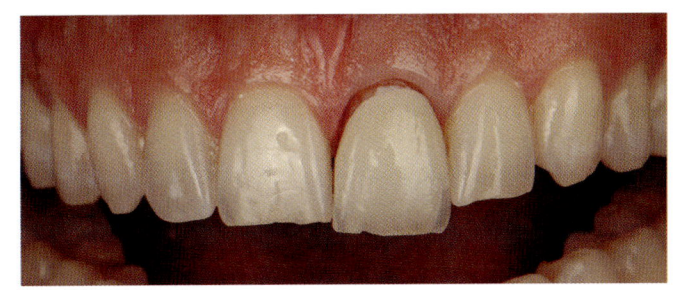

Figure 16.41 Without a photograph it would be extremely difficult to communicate the color, translucency, and degree of surface texture to the technician. Without this information, fabricating a crown to match this tooth would be highly improbable.

Review of tips for shade matching

1. Determine the correct hue; different shades within the hue can then be selected (chroma value).
2. Do not look too long at any particular shade, but compare several different ones with the patient in different positions. In addition to observing the tooth directly, try looking slightly away from the tooth so that just a color difference can be seen out of the corner of the eye. The shade that blends most closely with the tooth will usually be the correct one.
3. Make sure the patient is not wearing any brightly colored makeup or clothing. If so, drape the patient in a neutral-colored apron.
4. Do not be limited by one shade guide. Use shades from different guides to let the ceramist know exactly what color occurs in different parts of the tooth.
5. Use three different light sources: fluorescent, natural, and incandescent. When using outside lighting, avoid direct sunlight. Choose a shaded area that is bright enough to permit visualization of the important differences between teeth. To determine the proper value level, it is best to squint.

To achieve a highly esthetic result in a single crown, meticulous attention must be given to each of the various esthetic considerations. If care is applied to each step, everyone can enjoy the result: an esthetic, harmonious appearance of the mouth and face.

Patient maintenance

Much of the longevity and esthetic success of the crown restoration relies on both maintenance and prevention routines adopted by the patient. However, one can provide them with the best chance for longevity by making sure that one has created the most maintainable restoration possible. This means that one has provided for:

- marginal integrity during the impression, construction, and finishing stages of the crown;
- strong interproximal contact areas;
- restoration contours and materials that resist the retention of plaque and food debris; and
- the complete removal of excess cements and calculus.

Next, it is incumbent upon one to have a strong, comprehensive, and flexible patient maintenance program that focuses on inspiring participation by patients. Promote positive programs with careful professional monitoring. These programs should be tailored to each patient's existing oral condition, as well as to their lifestyle. It is especially important not to overwhelm a patient with too many tasks and devices, particularly with the mobile lifestyle of today's society. As an example, fewer tasks for the patient coupled with more frequent prevention visits to the office may be a better solution. The frequency of these in-office visits with a hygienist can vary from three to six times yearly, or even more in certain situations.

Motivation differs among patients, and not everyone will respond equally. Many patients will follow the esthetic maintenance and soft tissue management instructions to the letter. Others will continue with or fall back on old habits and ignore the prescribed instructions. One can advise that the breakdown and failure of the restoration may cause the patient to need even more drastic restorative treatment, which may include pain, and additional money and time. For these recalcitrant patients, and perhaps for all patients, and quite possibly for one's own protection, it is best to put patient maintenance and prevention instructions in writing, and have the patient sign two copies. Keep one in the patient chart as part of the official record and send the other copy home with the patient. Regardless of the prevention agenda one creates for their patients, the basics in oral hygiene care need to be reinforced:

- thorough brushing on a daily basis, preferably with an electric cleaning device (Oral B Smart Series, Pro Dentec, Rotadent, Sonicare);
- daily flossing regardless of the brushing method used; and
- plaque-reducing rinses.

It is important for the dental hygienist to make a critical evaluation of home care during a prevention appointment for both the patient and dentist. It is equally important for the hygienist to adjust the hygiene procedures for patients with esthetic restorations. Of significant importance in assuring ideal service and longevity of a porcelain restoration is its treatment during routine dental prophylaxis. Jones,[70] Sposetti et al.,[71] and Wunderlich and Yaman,[72] as well as many others, have demonstrated the ability of acidulated fluoride gel to etch a porcelain surface. Therefore, a neutral pH product should be substituted for patients with ceramic restorations. Additionally, never use ultrasonic scalers or air-abrasive polishing systems as they may damage the surface of the restoration.

As a part of follow-up and recall, special attention should be paid to the patient's caries index, and a risk assessment should be made. A risk level of low, moderate, high, and extreme can be assigned based on the following parameters: visible caries or radiographic penetration of caries into dentin, radiographic approximal enamel lesions, enamel decalcification on smooth surfaces, and restorations placed within the past 3 years.[73] Risk factors and protective factors for each patient also need to be assessed and monitored throughout the patient's recall schedule. *Streptococcus mutans* bacterial tests and salivary quantity and quality tests also aid in the risk determination. High-risk patients and extreme-risk patients must be very carefully monitored, and adherence to the established guidelines should be maintained. Jenson et al. have proposed guidelines to recall based on the patient's risk level. Patients who present with one or more carious lesions are assigned to the high-risk category.[74] High-risk patients should have bitewing radiographs every 6–18 months, caries recall examinations every 3–4 months, salivary flow and bacterial test every recall appointment to assess the patient's cooperation, chlorhexidine gluconate 0.12% rinse for 1 week every month, and 1.1% NaF toothpaste instead of regular fluoride paste.[74] Patients who present with one or more carious lesions and hyposalivation are assigned to the extreme-risk category. Extreme-risk patients should have bitewing radiographs every 6 months, caries recall exams should be done every 3 months, salivary flow and bacterial test every recall appointment, chlorhexidine (as per the high-risk patient) and xylitol (6–10 g daily) in gum or candies, 1.1% NaF toothpaste and NaF varnish at the 3-month recalls, acid-neutralizing mouth rinses, and calcium phosphate paste application daily.[74,75] Appropriate caries risk identification and treatment can be vital to the long-term survival of any complex restorative case.

Finally, always attempt to encourage a patient to be part of the "oral care team" that is dedicated to maximizing the investment in their mouth.

Appendix - Zirconium-oxide restorations

Indirect ceramic materials have been developed to higher levels of strength and esthetics, resulting in materials like lithium-disilicate glass-ceramics, aluminum-oxide and Yttrium-stabilized zirconium-oxide. Glass-ceramic materials serve mainly for single unit dental restorations, like crowns, inlays, onlays or veneers. To fabricate all-ceramic framework structures for extended tooth and implant supported fixed-dental-prostheses, monolithic zirconia was utilized to allow for increased mechanical stability and translucency, replacing traditional metal frameworks.[76] Initially introduced zirconia structures were known for their too opaque white appearance. Veneering porcelain needed to be applied to achieve acceptable esthetic results.[77] Multiple international scientific investigations were performed, to understand the early failures of this new material in dentistry, causing high clinical veneering porcelain chipping rates between 20-45%.[78–81] Framework design, veneering porcelain composition,[82] porcelain veneering thickness, coefficient of thermal expansion matching of veneer and core, correct furnace cooling rates and controlling the three-dimensional shrinkage process from the green stage to the final framework of a fixed-dental-prosthesis had to be investigated.[77,82–84] Research of the last 15 years helped to minimize the risk of porcelain chipping of zirconia dental restorations. Yet, based on the practitioners fear of clinical porcelain chipping,[85] and the time and cost consuming process of ceramic veneering dental frameworks, the focus shifted to monolithic pure zirconia dental restorations.[77] Digital workflow in the dental office, interlinked with computer-aided design/computer-assisted manufacture (CAD/CAM) procedures, allow to simulate oral rehabilitation, simplify the production process, and design restorations from single units to full arch frameworks out of zirconia ceramics. To allow for esthetic monolithic zirconia fixed-dental-prostheses, the introduction of dyeing color liquids of different shades was substantial (Prettau Zirconia, ZirkonZahn). The color liquids get applied and absorbed by the green stage monolithic framework under a drying lamp before the final sintering process. The final color becomes indelible through the sintering process.

The progressive development of currently introduced next-generation zirconias, drive toward greater translucency while preserving adequate strength and toughness of monolithic zirconia materials.[86,87] Four examples of current high-translucency monolithic zirconia materials are BruxZir Shaded 16, BruxZir HT, BruxZir, Lava Plus, 3 M, and inCoris TZI C, Dentsply Sirona. It should be mentioned that the enhanced translucency properties are achieved by using different dopants in the starting zirconia powders, for instance 0.2 mol% La_2O_2 into 3Y-TZP, which diminishes mechanical properties of the high-translucency monolithic zirconias, compared to the original Y-TZP frameworks.[86,88] Yet, the residual fracture strength is still considered sufficient to allow for full arch restorations.[77,86]

Current monolithic high-transparent zirconia restorations can generate exceptional esthetic results (Figures 16.42A and B), which have been esthetically matched with lithium-disilicate ceramics in the literature. The initial concern of excessive wear of the opposing dentition through the hardness of monolithic dental restorations was not confirmed, yet the degree of surface roughness should be minimized by surface polishing after occlusal adjustments. Full-contour monoliths are less susceptible to occlusal surface or cementation interface fracture damage. Based on state of the art treatment planning, x-ray and intermaxillary occlusal relation analysis, high-transparent zirconia restorations post an excellent alternative to conventional crown- and bridgework rehabilitations (Figures 16.43A and B).

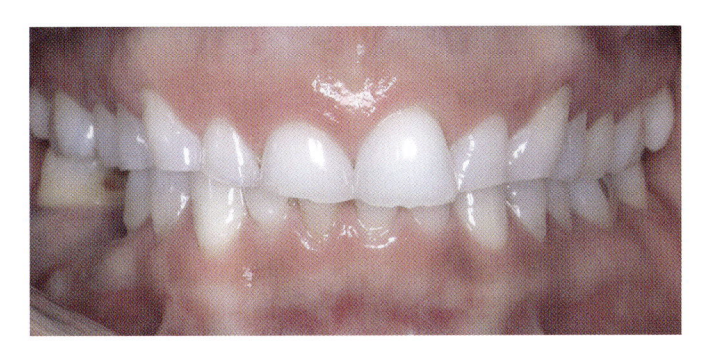

Figure 16.42 (A) This patient presented with chief complaint, "My teeth are worn down, what can be done?".

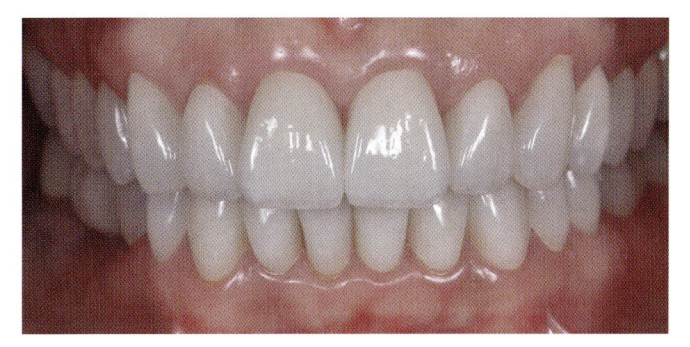

Figure 16.42 (B) After orthodontics, the patient received crown lengthening, and restoration of vertical dimension with monolithic zirconia crowns (Noritake Katana STML) (Courtesy of J. Londono, G. Chiche, M. Tadros, and S. Bin Im).

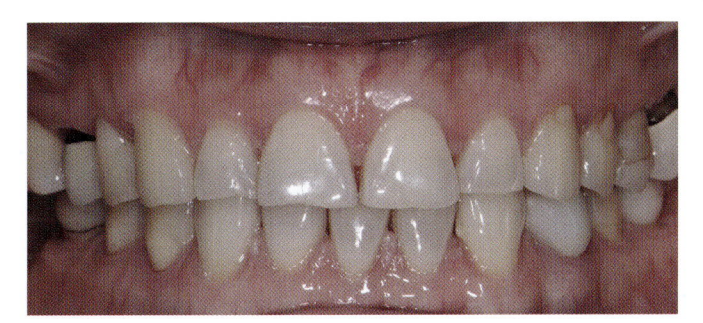

Figure 16.43 (A) Before: This patient had severe headaches, TMJ dysfunction, jaw pain and difficulty in eating and speaking due to her worn teeth due to bruxism.

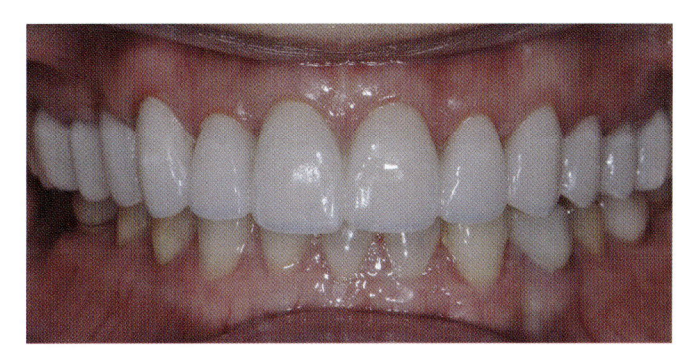

Figure 16.43 (B) After: Vertical dimension was restored with 12 medium translucency Zirconia full crowns on her maxillary teeth which eliminated all previous symptoms, plus cosmetic contouring and bleaching on the mandibular arch.

Conclusion

Although unique problems occur in the construction of a crown, if properly fabricated this restoration can be as esthetically pleasing as any other type of restoration. Knowing its limitations and providing for and adhering to the basic esthetic principles outlined in this chapter will help ensure successful results. The dentist interested in obtaining predictable results with esthetic restorations is urged to continually study natural and artificial dentitions (Table 16.3).

Table 16.3 Advantages and Disadvantages of Bonding Veneering and Crowning

Procedure	Advantages	Disadvantages
Bonding	No anesthesia required	Can chip or stain
	Little or no tooth reduction necessary	Limited esthetic life
	Immediate esthetic results	May not work if insufficient tooth structure
	Color change possible	Limited ability to realign teeth
	Less expensive than crowning or laminating	Teeth may appear somewhat thicker without enamel reduction
	Can usually be a reversible process	
Veneering	Little tooth reduction required	Can chip or fracture; repairs may be difficult or impossible
	Highly esthetic	More costly than bonding
	Does not stain	Requires two appointments
	Can mask dark color	Irreversible procedure if tooth form altered
	Longer esthetic life than bonding	Limited ability to realign teeth
	Easier to obtain good tooth form and proportion	Teeth may appear thicker unless sufficient enamel reduction is performed
	Less wear than bonding	
	May not require anesthesia	
Crowning	Teeth can be lightened to any shade	Can fracture
	Some realignment of teeth is possible	Requires anesthesia
	Can serve as abutment for fixed or removable restorations	Original tooth form altered
	Longer esthetic life than bonding or veneering	More costly than bonding
	Offers greatest latitude in improving tooth form and proportion	Requires two or more appointments
	Most "natural" results	An irreversible procedure

References

1. Kuwata M. *Creating Harmony in Dental Ceramics (Form, Color, and Illusion)*. Tokyo: Ishiyaku; 1998.
2. Gropp HP, Schwindling R, Eichner K, Voss R. Statistical studies on faulty crown formation with results on tooth, periodontium and gingiva. The crown edge. Discussion using a retouched tape recording and shortened to the main trains of thought. *Dtsch Zahnarztl Z* 1971;26:734–757 (in German).
3. Sousa RP, Zanin IC, Lima JP, et al. In situ effects of restorative materials on dental biofilm and enamel demineralisation. *J Dent* 2009;37:44–51.
4. Binkley CJ, Irvin PT. Reinforced heat-processed acrylic resin provisional restorations. *J Prosthet Dent* 1987;57:689–691.
5. Solnit SG. The effect of methylmethacrylate reinforcement with silane-treated and untreated glass fibers. *J Prosthet Dent* 1991;66:310–314.
6. Rehany A, Hirschfield Z. Veneering serviceable restorations. *Quintessence Int* 1988;19:787–792.
7. Gallegos LI, Nicholls JI. In vitro two-body wear of three veneering resins. *J Prosthet Dent* 1988;60:172–177.
8. Greenberg JR, Rafetto Jr RF. Laboratory light-cured composite resins: a clinical study. Part I. *Compend Contin Educ Dent* 1985;6:402, 404, 406.
9. Anusavice KJ, Hojjatie B. Effect of thermal tempering on strength and crack propagation behavior of feldspathic porcelains. *J Dent Res* 1991;70:1009–1013.
10. Anusavice KJ, Hojjate B. Stress distribution in metal-ceramic crowns with a facial porcelain margin. *J Dent Res* 1987;66:1493–1498.
11. Anusavice KJ, Dehoff PH, Gray A, Lee RB. Delayed crack development in porcelain due to incompatibility stress. *J Dent Res* 1988;67:1086–1097.
12. Bailey LF, Bennett RJ. DICOR surface treatments for enhanced bonding. *J Dent Res* 1988;67:925–931.
13. Malament KA, Socransky SS. Survival of Dicor glass-ceramic dental restorations over 14 years: part I. Survival of Dicor complete coverage restorations and effect of internal surface acid etching, tooth position, gender, and age. *J Prosthet Dent* 1999;81:23–32.
14. Malament KA, Socransky SS. Survival of Dicor glass-ceramic dental restorations over 14 years. Part II: effect of thickness of Dicor material and design of tooth preparation. *J Prosthet Dent* 1999;81:662–667.
15. Malament KA, Socransky SS. Survival of Dicor glass-ceramic dental restorations over 16 years. Part III: effect of luting agent and tooth or tooth-substitute core structure. *J Prosthet Dent* 2001;86:511–519.
16. Berger CC. Control of esthetics for anterior crowns. *Dent Surv* 1965;41:54–57.
17. Bertolotti RL. Removal of "black-line" margins and improving esthetics of porcelain-fused-to metal crowns: update in technique. *Quintessence Int* 1990;21:643–646.

18. Boghosian AA. Sunrise: a new and versatile ceramic system. *Pract Periodontic Aesthet* 1990;2(3):21–24.
19. Braggi A. Esthetic crowns on vital teeth. *Odont Pract* 1970;5:197.
20. Geller W, Kwaitkowski SJ. The Willi's glass crown: a new solution in the dark and shadowed zones of esthetic porcelain restorations. *Quintessence Dent Technol* 1987;11:233–242.
21. Geller W, Kwiatkowski SJ. Willis Glass: Glaskeramische Synthese zur Vermeidung der Dunkel- und Schattenzonen im Gingivalbereich [Willis glass: a glass-ceramic synthesis to avoid dark and shadow zones on gingiva]. *Quintessenz Zahntech* 1987;13:39–57.
22. Savitt ED, Malament KA, Socransky SS, et al. Effects of colonization of oral microbiota by a cast glass-ceramic restoration. *Int J Periodontics Restorative Dent* 1987;7:22–35.
23. Tysowsky G. Ceramic or ceramist? Category 1—the ceramic restoration. *Compend Contin Educ Dent* 1992;XIII(4):257–266.
24. Garber DA. Esthetics and the ceramo-metal restoration. *Compendium*, 1992.
25. Razzoog ME, Lang BR. Research evaluations of a new all-ceramic system. *Pract Periodontics Aesthet* 1998;1(10):1–3.
26. Sadan A, Hegenbarth EA. A simplified and practical method for optimizing aesthetic results utilizing a new high-strength all-ceramic system. *Pract Periodontics Aesthet* 1998;1(10):4–9.
27. Tan JP, Sederstrom D, Polansky JR, et al. The use of slow heating and slow cooling regimens to strengthen porcelain fused to zirconia. *J Prosthet Dent* 2012;107:163–169.
28. Goldstein RE, Feinman RA, Garber DA. Esthetic considerations in the selection and use of restorative materials. *Dent Clin North Am* 1983;27:723–730.
29. Lehner CR, Scharer P. All-ceramic crowns. *Curr Opin Dent Prosthodont Endod* 1992;2:45–52.
30. Heintze SD, Rousson V. Fracture rates of IPS Empress all-ceramic crowns—a systematic review. *Int J Prosthodont* 2010;23:129–133.
31. Stawarczyk B, Ozcan M, Roos M, et al. Load-bearing capacity and failure types of anterior zirconia crowns veneered with overpressing and layering techniques. *Dent Mater* 2011;27:1045–1053.
32. Lehman MI. Stability and durability of porcelain jacket crowns. *Br Dent J* 1967;23:419.
33. Silva NR, Thompson VP, Valverde GB, et al. Comparative reliability analyses of zirconium oxide and lithium disilicate restorations in vitro and in vivo. *J Am Dent Assoc* 2011;142(suppl 2):4S–9S.
34. Guess PC, Zavanelli Ra, Silva NR, et al. Monolithic CAD/CAM lithium disilicate versus veneered Y-TZP crowns: comparison of failure modes and reliability after fatigue. *Int J Prosthodont* 2010;23:434–442.
35. Borges GA, Caldas D, Taskonak B, et al. Fracture loads of all-ceramic crowns under wet and dry fatigue conditions. *J Prosthodont* 2009;18:649–655.
36. Gettleman L. Noble alloys in dentistry. *Curr Opin Dent* 1991;2:218–221.
37. Crispin BJ, Seghi RR, Globe H. Effect of different metal ceramic alloys on the color of opaque and dentin porcelain. *J Prosthet Dent* 1991;65:351–356.
38. Crispin BJ, Watson JF. Esthetic considerations for the placement of anterior crown margins. *J Prosthet Dent* 1980;44:290.
39. Culpepper WD. A comparative study of shade matching procedures. *J Prosthet Dent* 1970;24:166–173.
40. Dresden JD. Porcelain-fused-to-metal restorations. *Northwest J Dent* 1970;49:123.
41. Zena RB, Abbott LJ. Light harmony of crowns and roots: understanding and managing the black line phenomenon. *Pract Periodontics Aesthet* 1991;3(4):27–31.
42. Pameijer JHN. Soft tissue master cast for esthetic control in crown and bridge procedures. *J Esthet Dent* 1989;1:47–50.
43. Harrison L, Huggman T, Goldfogel M. All-porcelain labial margin for ceramo-metal crowns. *J Esthet Dent* 1992;4:154–158.
44. Davis DR. Comparison of fit of the two types of all-ceramic crowns. *J Prosthet Dent* 1988;59(1):12–16.
45. Shelby DS. Esthetics and fixed restorations. *Dent Clin North Am* 1967;(Mar):57–70.
46. MacGibbon DJ. The failure of a porcelain-fused-to-metal crown. *Dent Digest* 1971;77:520.
47. Mahalick JA, Knapf J, Weiter EJ. Occlusal wear in prosthodontics. *J Am Dent Assoc* 1971;82:154–159.
48. Nevins M, Skurow H. The intracervicular restorative margin, the biologic width and the maintenance of the gingival margin. *Int J Periodontics Restorative Dent* 1984;3:31–49.
49. Kaiser DA, Newell DH. Technique to disguise the metal margin of the metal/ceramic crown. *Am J Dent* 1988;1:217–221.
50. Ruel J, Schuessler PJ, Malament K, Mori D. Effect of retraction procedures on the periodontium in humans. *J Prosthet Dent* 1980;44:508–515.
51. Southard TE, Southard KA, Tolley EA. Variation of approximal tooth contact tightness with postural change. *J Dent Res* 1990;69:1776–1779.
52. Freidman M, Jordan RE. Bonded porcelain crowns. *J Esthet Dent* 1989;1:120–125.
53. Probster L. Compressive strength of the two modern all-ceramic crowns. *Int J Prosthodont* 1992;5:409–414.
54. Coughlin JW. Variabilities in the bonded porcelain veneer crown. *J Acad Gen Dent* 1970;18:30.
55. Kramer GM. Dental failures associated with periodontal surgery. *Dent Clin North Am* 1972;16:13–31.
56. Lanzano JA, Hill TJ. The fabrication and clinical utilization of the collarless veneer crown. In: Renner RP, ed., *QDT Yearbook*. Lambert, IL: Quintessence; 1988:75–81.
57. Rosentritt M, Preis V, Behr M, et al. Two-body wear of dental porcelain and substructure oxide ceramics. *Clin Oral Investig* 2012;16:935–943.
58. Tjan AHL, Miller ED, The JGP. Some esthetic factors in a smile. *J Prosthet Dent* 1984;51:24–29.
59. Martegani P, Silvestri M, Mascarello F, et al. Morphometric study of the interproximal unit in the esthetic region to correlate anatomic variables affecting the aspect of soft tissue embrasure space. *J Periodontol* 2007;78:2260–2265.
60. Yuodelis RA, Weaver JD, Sapkos S. Facial and lingual contours of artificial complete crown restorations and their effect on the periodontum. *J Prosthet Dent* 1973;29:61–66.
61. Perel ML. Axial crown contours. *J Prosthet Dent* 1971;25:642–649.
62. Pincus CL. Cosmetics—the psychologic fourth dimension in full mouth rehabilitation. *Dent Clin North Am* 1967:71–88.
63. Beaudreau DE. *Atlas of Fixed Partial Prosthesis*. Springfield, IL: Charles C. Thomas; 1975.
64. Preston JD, Bergen SF. *Color Science and Dental Art*. St. Louis, MO: CV Mosby; 1980.
65. Mulla FA, Weiner S. Effects of temperature on color stability of porcelain stains. *J Prosthet Dent* 1991;65:507–512.
66. McLean JW. Ceramics in clinical dentistry. *Br Dent J* 1988;164(6):187–194.

67. McLean JW, ed. *Dental Ceramics: Proceedings of the First International Symposium on Ceramics*. Chicago, IL: Quintessence; 1983.
68. McLean JW. The alumina reinforced porcelain jacket crown. *J Am Dent Assoc* 1967;75:621–628.
69. McLean JW, Hughes TH. The reinforcement of dental porcelain with ceramic oxides. *Br Dent J* 1965;119:251–267.
70. Jones DA. Effects of topical fluoride preparations on glazed porcelain surfaces. *J Prosthet Dent* 1985;53:483–484.
71. Sposetti VJ, Shen C, Levin AC. The effect of topical fluoride application on porcelain restorations. *J Prosthet Dent* 1986;55:677–682.
72. Wunderlich RC, Yaman P. In vitro effect of fluoride on dental porcelain. *J Prosthet Dent* 1986;55:385–388.
73. Featherstone JD, Domejean-Orliaguet S, Jenson L, et al. Caries risk assessment in practice for age 6 through adult. *J Calif Dent Assoc* 2007;35:703–707, 710–713.
74. Jenson L, Budenz AW, Featherstone JD, et al. Clinical protocols for caries management by risk assessment. *J Calif Dent Assoc* 2007;35:714–723.
75. Featherstone JD, Singh S, Curtis DA. Caries risk assessment and management for the prosthodontic patient. *J Prosthodont* 2011;20:2–9.
76. Denry I, Kelly JR. State of the art zirconia for dental applications. *Dent Mater* 2008;24(3):299–307.
77. Zhang Y, Kelly JR. Dental ceramics for restoration and metal veneering. *Dent Clin North Am* 2017;61(4):797–819.
78. Sax C, Hämmerle CH, Sailer I. 10-year clinical outcomes of fixed dental prostheses with zirconia frameworks. *Int J Comput Dent* 2011;14(3):183–202.
79. Kimmich M, Stappert CF. Intraoral treatment of veneering porcelain chipping of fixed dental restorations: a review and clinical application. *J Am Dent Assoc* 2013;144(1):31–44.
80. Swain MV. Unstable cracking (chipping) of veneering porcelain on all-ceramic dental crowns and fixed partial dentures. *Acta Biomater* 2009;5(5):1668–77.
81. Molin MK, Karlsson SL. Five-year clinical prospective evaluation of zirconia-based Denzir 3-unit FPDs. *Int J Prosthodont* 2008;21(3):223–7.
82. Stawarczyk B, Ozcan M, Roos M, Trottmann A, Sailer I, Hämmerle CH. Load-bearing capacity and failure types of anterior zirconia crowns veneered with overpressing and layering techniques. *Dent Mater* 2011;27:1045–53.
83. Baldassarri M, Zhang Y, Thompson VP, Rekow ED, Stappert CF. Reliability and failure modes of implant-supported zirconium-oxide fixed dental prostheses related to veneering techniques. *J Dent* 2011;39(7):489–98.
84. Rues S, Kroeger E, Mueller D, Schmitter M. Effect of firing protocols on cohesive failure of all-ceramic crowns. *J Dent* 2010;38(12):987–94.
85. Groten M, Huttig F. The performance of zirconium dioxide crowns: a clinical follow-up. *Int J Prosthodont* 2010;23(5):429–31.
86. Zhang Y, Lawn BR. Novel zirconia materials in dentistry. *J Dent Res* 2018;97(2):140–147.
87. Koutayas SO, Vagkopoulou T, Pelekanos S, Koidis P, Strub JR. Zirconia in dentistry: part 2. Evidence-based clinical breakthrough. *Eur J Esthet Dent* 2009;4(4):348–80.
88. Kim JW, Covel NS, Guess PC, Rekow ED, Zhang Y. Concerns of hydrothermal degradation in CAD/CAM zirconia. *J Dent Res*. 2010 Jan;89(1):91–5.

PART 3
ESTHETIC CHALLENGES OF MISSING TEETH

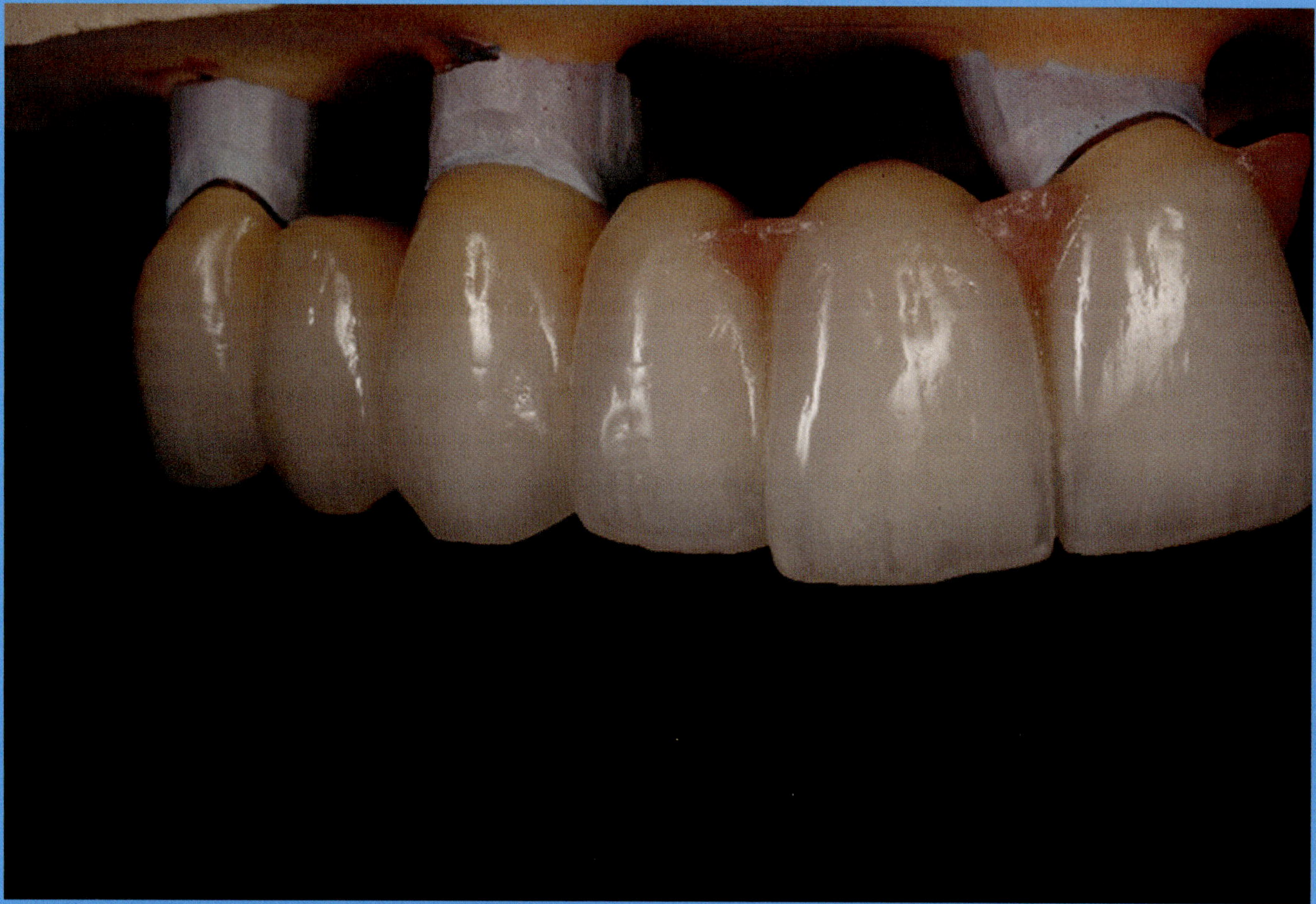

Chapter 17: Replacing Missing Teeth with Fixed Partial Dentures

Jacinthe M. Paquette, DDS, Jean C. Wu, DDS,
Cherilyn G. Sheets, DDS, and Devin L. Stewart, DDS

Chapter Outline

Diagnosis	543
Intraoral examination	544
Extraoral examination	544
Radiographic examination	544
Diagnostic study casts	545
The diagnostic wax-up	545
Esthetic considerations	545
Functional considerations	546
Interdisciplinary consultations	547
Retainers	547
Partial-coverage retainers	549
Complete-coverage retainers	550
Margin location	551
Margin materials	552
Porcelain–metal junction	553
Anterior restorations involving one missing tooth	555
Splinting	555
Use of telescoping crowns as abutments	555
Evolving technologies	562
Use of precision attachments	564
Pontics	565
Pontic design	565
Preparation of tissue	566
Pontic materials	570

Although fixed prosthodontics has been greatly enhanced by implant dentistry, there will continue to be situations that require fixed prostheses for the replacement of missing teeth. A fixed partial denture has been described in the "Glossary of prosthodontics terms" as any fixed dental prosthesis that is luted, screwed, or mechanically attached or otherwise securely retained to natural teeth, tooth roots, and/or dental implant abutments that furnish the primary support for the dental prosthesis. This may include replacement of 1 to 16 teeth in each dental arch. If a metallic or ceramic component is included within the fixed dental prosthesis, that component is termed the framework.[1(p.38)] When choosing a fixed partial denture as the restoration of choice for a given edentulous area, a systematic sequence of diagnosis and treatment planning must be followed to achieve a successful esthetic and functional outcome.[2-4]

Diagnosis

In order to establish a positive working relationship and a successful treatment outcome for a patient, there are two critical psychological factors that need to be recognized by a dentist: the patient's attitude toward the dental treatment and prior dental experiences. The patient's chief complaint should be ascertained;

specific esthetic desires, expectations, and needs should also be assessed. Any esthetic shortcomings with previous prostheses and esthetic challenges with the presenting condition should be noted and communicated with the patient. Once all of these elements have been established and a good working relationship exists between the dentist and the patient, the mutually agreed treatment for that patient can be pursued.

Intraoral examination

Whether the patient's presenting condition appears simple or complex in nature, it is recommended that a comprehensive intraoral examination be performed for all patients. The recording of preexisting restorations and any existing pathoses should be a routine procedure. All diagnoses, such as missing teeth, periodontal status, pulpal pathosis, caries, fractures, wear, unesthetic restorations, muscle and temporomandibular joint pathosis, and oral cancer screening, should be documented. A comprehensive evaluation of the patient is necessary to ensure a thorough treatment plan, rather than only addressing the specific edentulous area and adjacent tooth structure. It is of paramount importance that a comprehensive treatment plan be developed to provide appropriate oral health objectives. A complete diagnosis and treatment plan will ensure a successful and sound prosthodontic treatment outcome.[5]

Additionally, the use of an intraoral camera (see figure 2-7A–C in *Esthetics in Dentistry*, Volume 1, 2nd edition)[6,7] or surgical microscope (Figure 17.1) can further assist in the documentation and planning of the presenting condition of the patient.[8] Revelations such as hidden microcracks, defective restorative margins, and other tooth and/or tissue defects can determine if single or multiple retainers are indicated when weakened teeth, thought to be in good condition, are exposed. Each tooth should be individually evaluated and its condition recorded in the patient record for diagnostic and legal purposes.

Extraoral examination

An extraoral evaluation is always important in a comprehensive patient evaluation, and is critical when treating esthetically motivated patients. This evaluation should include assessment of the patient's facial symmetry, muscle hypertrophy, and possible loss of vertical dimension of occlusion. Additionally, a smile analysis that determines the amount of tooth display, smile line, lip line, arch form, and the balance of the hard and soft tissues should be considered.

Radiographic examination

A full-mouth series of radiographs and/or a panoramic radiograph with selected periapical radiographs of the proposed abutment teeth are necessary in the evaluation for treatment with a fixed partial denture. The primary purpose of radiographs

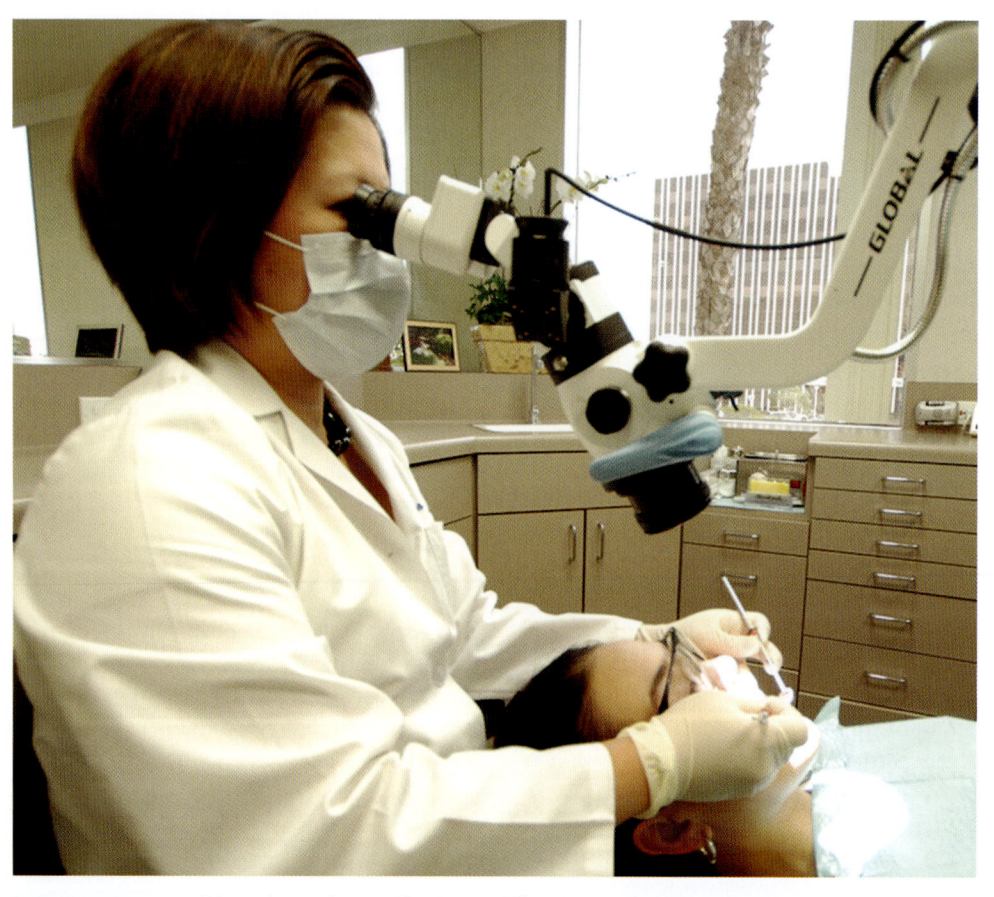

Figure 17.1 The clinical microscope provides enhanced magnification and illumination for better visualization and diagnosis.

is to disclose hidden areas and structures, such as the root morphology, crown/root ratios, pulpal health, periodontal ligament spaces, and existing caries.[9] In some situations, preexisting full-coverage restorations are present that mask the integrity of the underlying coronal tooth structure radiographically. In these instances, an accurate assessment of adequate tooth structure may not be possible without the removal of the existing restorations.

Computerized digital radiographs[10,11] are also an effective way to communicate the observations made to the patient. The ability to colorize the radiographic findings combined with the ability to isolate and enlarge segments of the root or crown in question provides an avenue to enhance the patient–doctor relationship and improve communication.[12,13]

Diagnostic study casts

Diagnostic study casts are imperative during the diagnostic and treatment planning phases. The casts serve as an educational aid for the patient while also providing the dentist with a record of the preexisting condition. Casts mounted on a suitable articulator, at the treatment position, will enable the restoring dentist to evaluate the condition of the patient's mouth. Clinical crown lengths, tipped or rotated teeth, ridge form, and the span of the edentulous area can all be evaluated, thereby helping the dentist in the decision-making process. The interarch space and the occlusal plane can also be evaluated on the diagnostic casts. This may lead to the diagnosis of lost interocclusal space or supraeruption of a segment of the dentition. If these compromised conditions are noted, other interdisciplinary efforts may be required to create a more solid or idealized foundation for the future restorative goals. These treatments may involve crown lengthening, ridge reduction/augmentation, endodontic therapy, orthodontic repositioning of teeth, segmental osteotomy, and/or surgical extraction. Properly mounted, accurate diagnostic casts serve an extremely important role in the comprehensive diagnosis and treatment planning for a fixed partial denture.

The diagnostic wax-up

A diagnostic wax-up of the proposed fixed partial denture can be invaluable in determining the esthetic requirements of a treatment plan. It provides the opportunity to observe the abutment tooth–pontic relationship and the pontic–ridge relationship. The diagnostic wax-up also allows the dentist to evaluate and work within the confines of the edentulous space. The edentulous area itself may be resorbed or reduced in the mesio-distal dimension and require surgical correction with bone grafting, soft tissue, or both. Often, other treatment issues or necessary modifications are more readily visible at this point in the planning process.[14] Frequently, orthodontic treatment is the best solution for limited space, rotated, tipped, and/or malposed teeth. This may be done in place of or prior to fabrication of a fixed partial denture. In some situations, the diagnostic wax-up will indicate the need for endodontic treatment when the required tooth preparations may involve the pulp of slightly malposed or tipped teeth at the time of preparation (Figure 17.2A–D).

Esthetic considerations

A significant part of the complete diagnosis is ascertaining the extent of the patient's esthetic requirements. Understanding the patient's esthetic desires may dictate the type of retainer margin, margin placement in relation to the gingiva, and the type of dental materials to be considered. The dentist should know what the patient's esthetic expectations are before treatment begins, to avoid dissatisfaction and costly retreatment. Although the maxillary anterior region is usually the most demanding area to treat owing to its obvious visibility, certain patients will place just as much esthetic demand in the posterior region of the mouth.

The arch in which the prosthesis is to be placed, the restoration's position in that arch, the amount of display of the prosthesis, and the patient's esthetic desires all have to be considered when designing the elements of an esthetic fixed partial denture. These elements include tooth shape, symmetry, shade, retainer selection, material, amount of tooth coverage, margin location, ceramic–metal junction location on

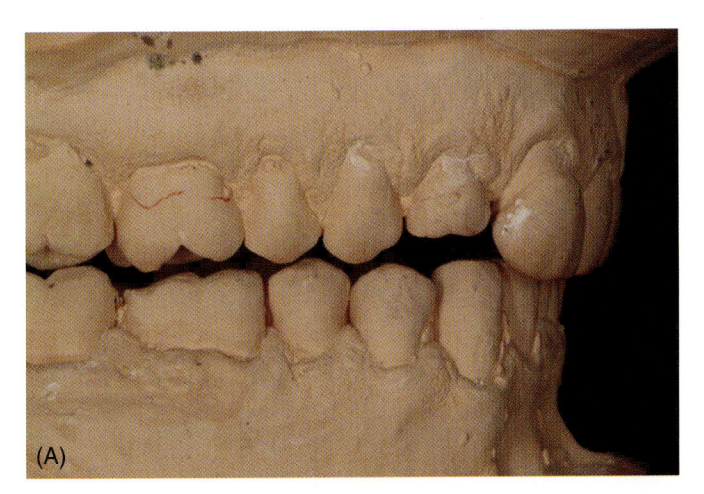

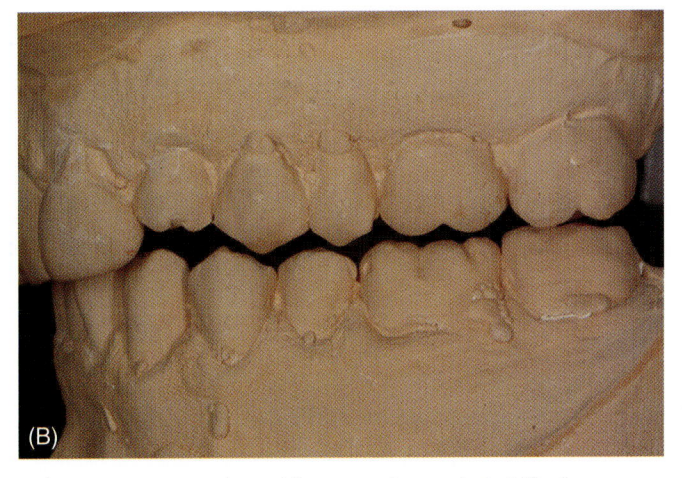

Figure 17.2 **(A)** Right and **(B)** left lateral views of the study casts of a patient who was treatment planned for a complete oral rehabilitation. Clinically, it appeared that an increase in the vertical dimension of occlusion would be necessary to create space for the restorations planned.

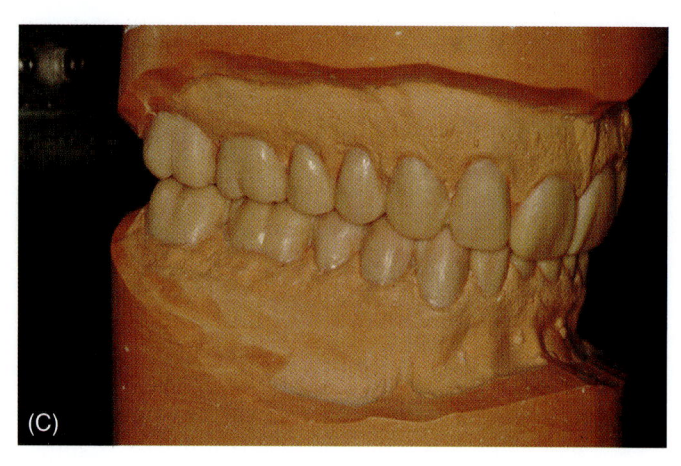

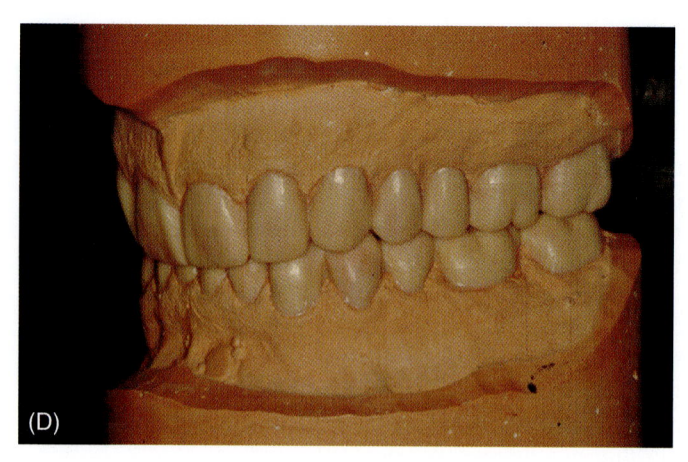

Figure 17.2 **(C)** Right and **(D)** left lateral views of the completed diagnostic wax-up of the proposed treatment at the planned vertical dimension of occlusion.

metal–ceramic crowns, and pontic design. All of these esthetic considerations must be coupled with biologic and functional considerations (such as span length, need for splinting, periodontal support, soft-tissue management, and the use of provisional restorations) and the need for adjunctive care (such as orthodontics, endodontics, periodontics, and oral and maxillofacial surgery).

The anterior fixed prosthesis can often present the most difficult of esthetic challenges, and artistic skill and know-how are important to obtain a pleasing result. Correct functional occlusal schemes and loading characteristics must also be integrated into the final restorations.

Ideally, a pleasing esthetic result can best be achieved when the restorations blend inconspicuously with the patient's remaining natural dentition. An exception to this rule is when the entire dentition is changed. Esthetic templates created from a preliminary diagnostic wax-up can assist the patient to visualize the possibilities of the treatment being recommended (Figure 17.3A–D). Also, thin resin shells of the proposed treatment (Hollywood templates) can be used to help the patient see the proposed results. The form of the lip line will often help to determine the treatment choice. When a tissue disharmony exists, such as excessive or insufficient gingival volume, periodontal plastic surgery may be required to create the ideal environment for an implant or fixed partial denture.

Computer-generated analyses and imaging can also serve as an effective diagnostic adjunct when considering esthetic goals.[15,16] One of the greatest advantages of this technique is the ability to evaluate proposed tooth sizes and shapes before the final restoration is constructed. Although digital imaging can assist in demonstrating the esthetic appearance of the proposed final result, the esthetic elements can be too difficult to clearly visualize on the computer screen. More exacting esthetic analyses before the commencement of treatment provide valuable information for the fabrication of the provisional restorations and subsequently the final restorative design.

Functional considerations

Functional considerations, by their nature, are an integral part of the esthetic evaluation. The type and number of abutments (retainers) utilized for the future fixed prosthesis require

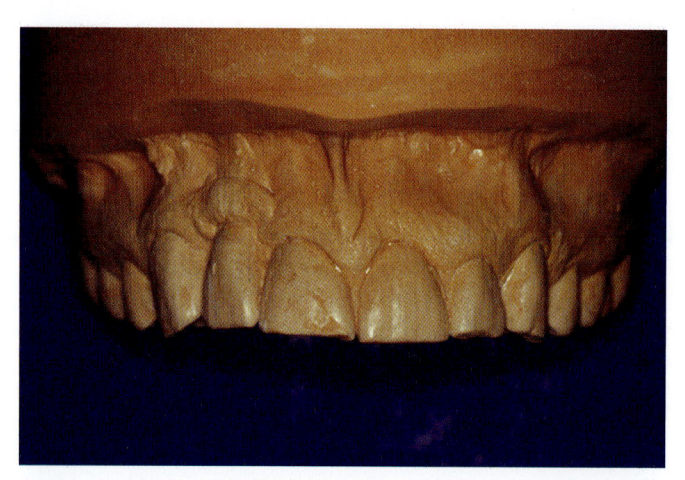

Figure 17.3 **(A)** A study model of patient with advanced wear of her maxillary incisors. The right lateral incisor presented with significant tissue abnormalities after implant placement and a free gingival grafting.

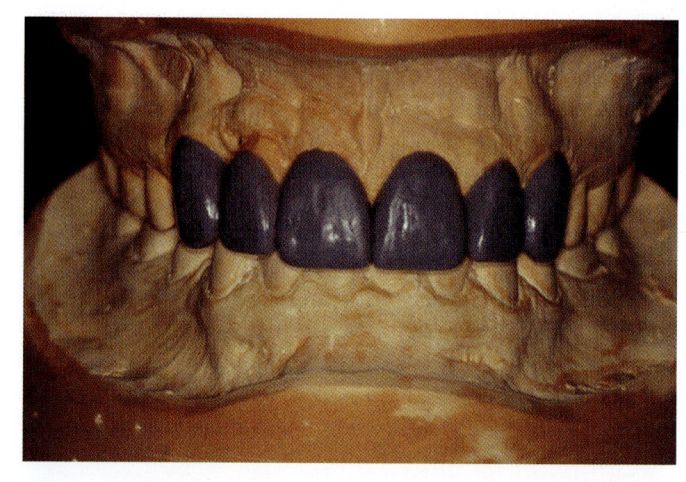

Figure 17.3 **(B)** A diagnostic wax-up was completed to illustrate the treatment objectives with porcelain veneers and connective tissue refinement around the implant at the lateral incisor position.

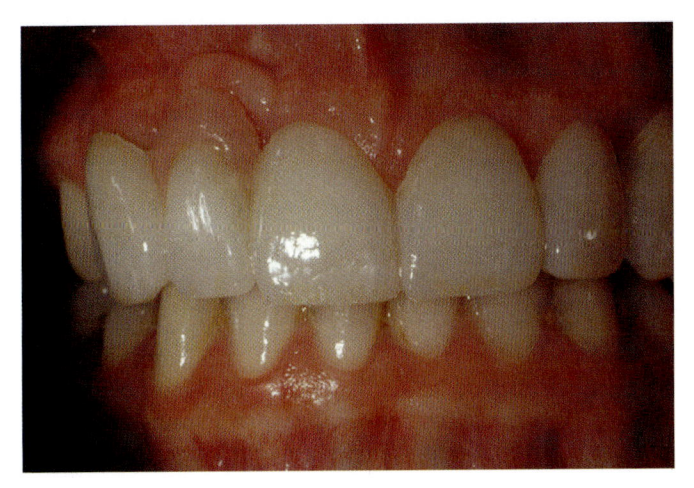

Figure 17.3 (C) The completed diagnostic wax-up was replicated in resin to create a "Hollywood template" or "esthetic template."

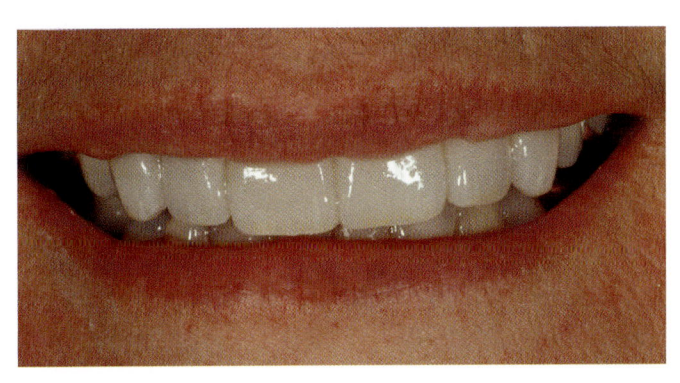

Figure 17.3 (D) The esthetic template allowed the patient to better visualize the esthetic outcome possible with the proposed treatment.

functional considerations, which in many instances can affect the esthetic result. The use of intracoronal or extracoronal retainers depends on the length of the space to be restored, the functional stresses that will be placed on the prosthesis, and the age of the patient. If extracoronal retainers are chosen, the same considerations apply to the choice of either complete- or partial-coverage crowns that apply to intracoronal retainers.

Patients with deep vertical overlap or those with a history of bruxism or clenching can be at risk for restoration fracture, especially in the anterior region. In these instances, whenever possible, orthodontic intervention should be incorporated to improve the interocclusal relationships and a better occlusal functional scheme.

Interdisciplinary consultations

Interdisciplinary consultations and treatment referrals are important when providing comprehensive care. Multiple treatment modalities and treatment options for the patient should be investigated and presented during the treatment planning phase.[17]

Once the diagnostic process has been completed, treatment options may be selected from the following choices:

I. Retainers
   A. Partial coverage
      1. Cemented
      2. Resin bonded
      3. Porcelain veneers
   B. Complete coverage
      1. All metal
      2. All ceramic
      3. Metal–ceramic
         a. Margins
            - Location
            - Material
            - Metal collar margin
            - Disappearing metal margin
            - Porcelain margin
         b. Porcelain–metal junction
   C. Other considerations
      1. Cantilever fixed partial denture
      2. Implants
      3. Splinting
      4. Use of telescoping crowns as abutments
II. Pontics
   A. Design
   B. Edentulous ridge form
   C. Material.

Retainers

The history of the patient's condition plays a vital role in the treatment planning process. When selecting appropriate retainers for a fixed partial denture, esthetics is only one of three important factors to be considered. The other two are biologic considerations and functional/mechanical considerations. Some biologic and mechanical considerations are the size of the abutment tooth, the amount of remaining tooth structure, the size and type of restoration for the tooth, the status of the pulp, the clinical crown length, the location of the tooth in the mouth, the type of occlusal load, the interocclusal space, the opposing dentition or prostheses, the edentulous span length, and consideration of the insertion path. A patient who presents with a pre-existing fixed partial denture, which has served the patient well for many years, may serve as an indicator of the prognosis if this treatment option is being considered again. This may be an indication that potentially the functional objectives and underlying retainers will provide suitable support for the future fixed prosthesis (Figure 17.4A–F).

Fixed partial denture retainers can be separated broadly into two categories: partial- and complete-coverage retainers. Usually, the most esthetic material the restoring dentist can choose to match the patient's existing dentition is natural tooth structure. This display of natural tooth structure in the esthetic zone is

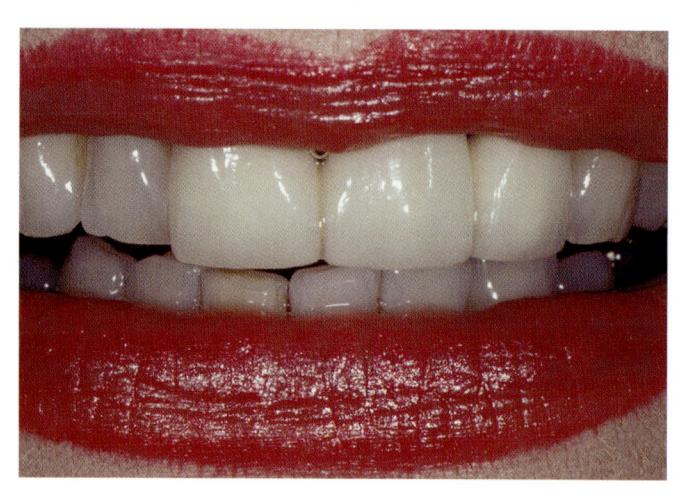

Figure 17.4 **(A)** This patient presented with an unesthetic fixed partial denture.

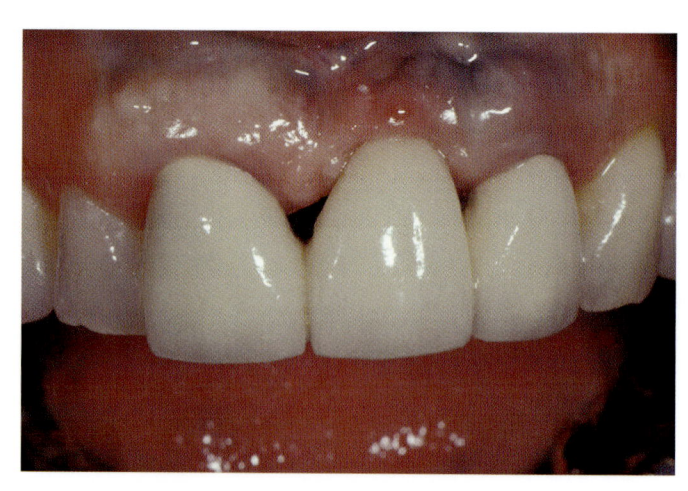

Figure 17.4 **(B)** She had become dissatisfied with the appearance of her smile due to the significant wear of the adjacent incisors, ill-matching shades, and black triangles from recession.

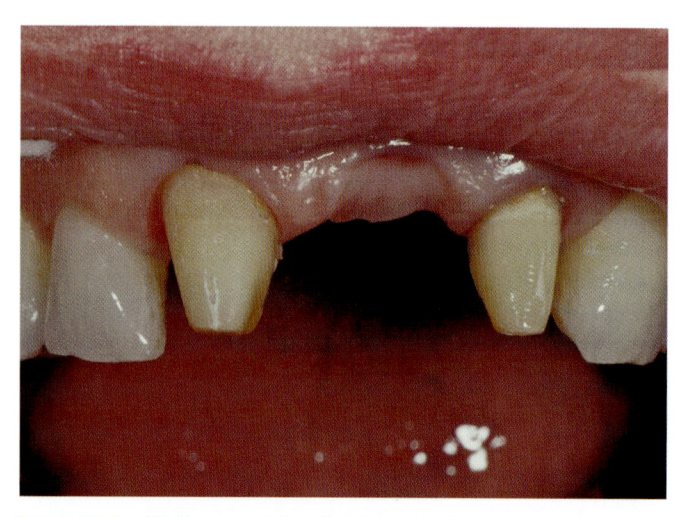

Figure 17.4 **(C)** The preexisting fixed prosthesis demonstrates insufficient tooth reductions at the gingival margin that did not allow sufficient room for the restorative materials.

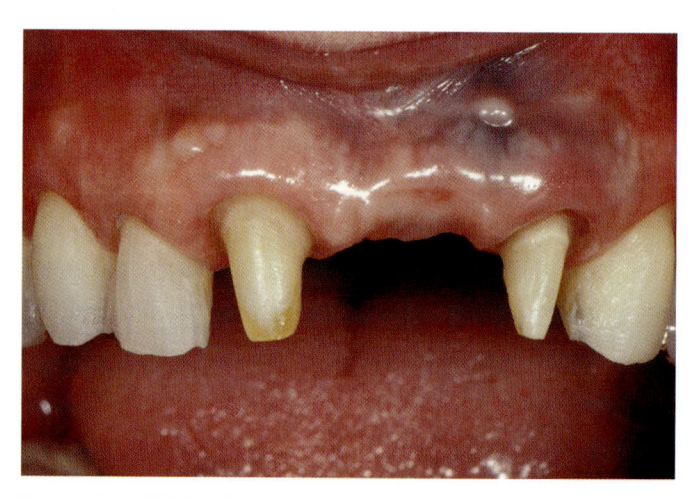

Figure 17.4 **(D)** The abutment teeth were reprepared to allow space for a more natural emergence profile, contour, and enhanced color optics.

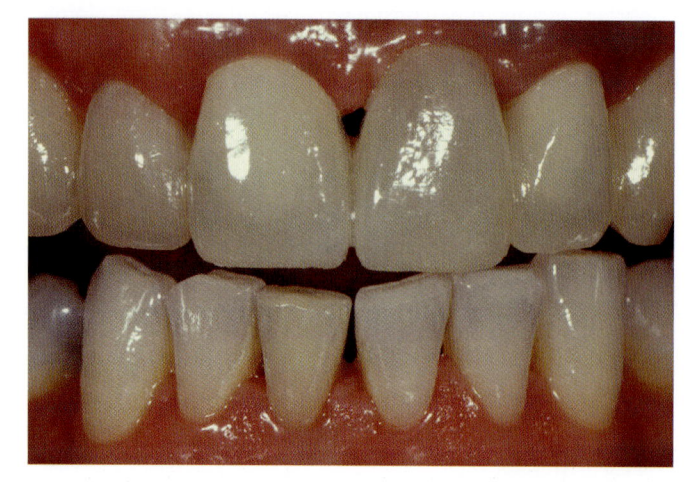

Figure 17.4 **(E)** Tissue grafting had been considered and discussed with the patient to correct the black triangles. Owing to sufficient closure of the spaces noted at the time of provisionalization, the doctor and patient decided that an acceptable esthetic outcome could be achieved without tissue augmentation.

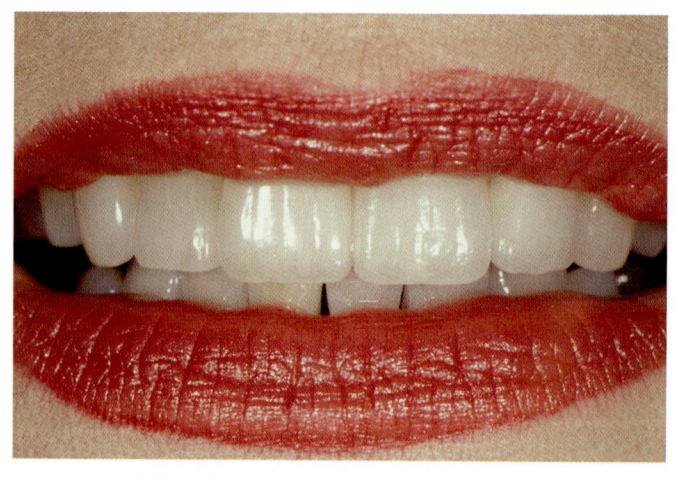

Figure 17.4 **(F)** The final esthetic treatment outcome achieved with porcelain veneers and the replacement of a fixed dental prosthesis.

accomplished by way of partial-veneer restorations. As retainers, these are the most conservative and can be the most esthetic treatment option.[18]

Partial-coverage retainers

The most traditional of the partial-coverage retainer designs is the metal inlay, onlay, or three-quarter crown. These are usually made of a gold alloy and cemented with traditional, mechanically retentive cements. Owing to the retention and resistance form necessary to make these retainers successful, it is virtually impossible to avoid some display of metal at the proximal, incisal, and/or occlusal line angles. This show of metal often makes this retainer design unacceptable in the anterior region of the mouth for the esthetically conscious patient. It can be acceptable in less esthetically critical areas of the mouth. The best application is on large and relatively unrestored second premolars and first molars in the maxillary arch.

Currently, the most widely used partial-coverage retainer is the resin-bonded retainer. In its original form, it was described as the "prepless bridge."[19-21] The preparation design is conservative, without resistance form, and relies almost entirely on the resin bond to enamel for retention. This design is especially useful for short-term provisional restorations prior to future implant treatment. The documented success rates for these early restorations varied widely. As a long-term restorative option, the preparation design for resin-bonded retainers has evolved to the classic three-quarter crown preparation. Additionally, parallel grooves can be incorporated to improve resistance and retention form, and can be further augmented with pins or ledges.[22-26] The only modification for esthetics is the lack of the incisal offset and proximal metal display seen in the classic three-quarter crown preparation. This is compensated for by the use of base metal alloys that are relatively rigid in thin sections and the micromechanical retention potential between the cement and metal and between the cement and tooth enamel.[27] These preparation specifics can be challenging to create. For this reason, properly constructed long-term resin-bonded fixed partial dentures have fallen from favor just as traditional partial-coverage retainers.

Resin-bonded partial-veneer fixed partial dentures would be the restoration of choice, particularly in the anterior part of the mouth, if the following conditions are present: the abutment teeth are esthetically acceptable to the patient in their present size, form, and color; the teeth are free of restorations or have only minimal restoration that does not involve the crown margins; and the abutment teeth are of adequate length to afford preparation resistance and retention and of adequate thickness of tooth structure to prevent metal shadowing from the lingual surface. For the best results, the resin-bonded partial-veneer retained prosthesis should only replace one tooth. The teeth should have minimal mobility, as failure rates rise rapidly with increased numbers of pontics and with mobile abutment teeth. The pontic space must be ideal in width, as little widening or narrowing of the edentulous space can be accomplished with partial-veneer retainers. One of the most frequently seen esthetic challenges with this type of retainer is the difficulty of shade matching. If the adjacent retainers are metal, light translucency of the abutment teeth is diminished, resulting in possible shade variance.

A third type of partial-coverage restoration made from traditional crown materials and cemented or bonded to tooth structure is the porcelain veneer. It is one of the most esthetic of all partial-coverage restorations but has limited long-term clinical studies. The connector dimensions are often limited by anatomic configurations, material properties, and esthetic expectations. A connector dimension of at least 3 mm × 3 mm has favorable fracture resistance, based on several in-vitro studies.[28,29] The clinical performance of cantilevered resin-bonded fixed partial dentures has been shown to be superior to the two-retainer designs.[30,31] A 2.5-year follow-up study on zirconia-based resin-bonded fixed partial dentures showed satisfactory functional and esthetic results.[32] In Figure 17.5A, the 17-year-old patient was unable to proceed with implant-supported crowns to replace the congenitally missing upper lateral incisors, and she was seeking an improvement in the esthetics of her resin-bonded bridges. Owing to the thin dimensions of her central incisors, all-ceramic (zirconia) resin-bonded bridges were preferred to avoid the gray show-through of a metal framework (Figure 17.5B). On removal of the pontics, the thin incisal edges were evident (Figure 17.5C).

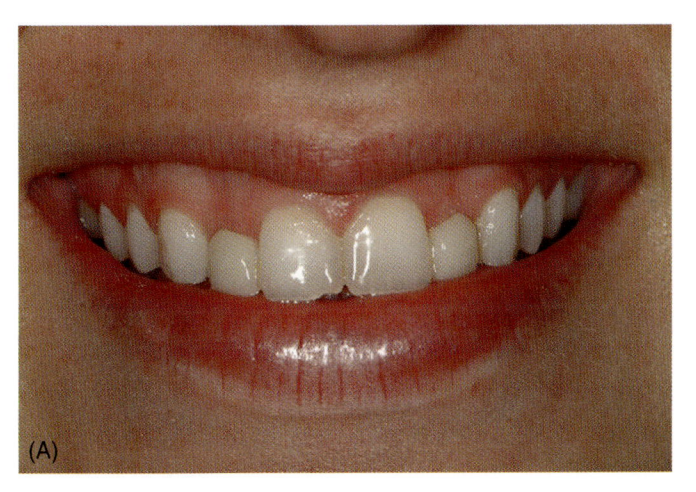

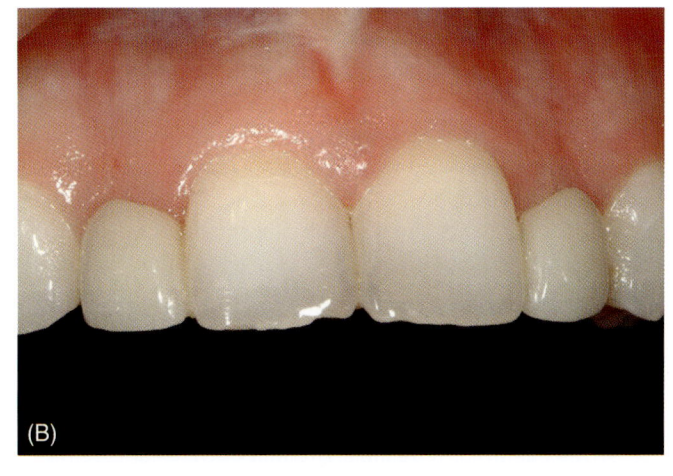

Figure 17.5 (A, B) A 17-year-old girl presented seeking esthetic replacement of the congenitally missing lateral incisors.

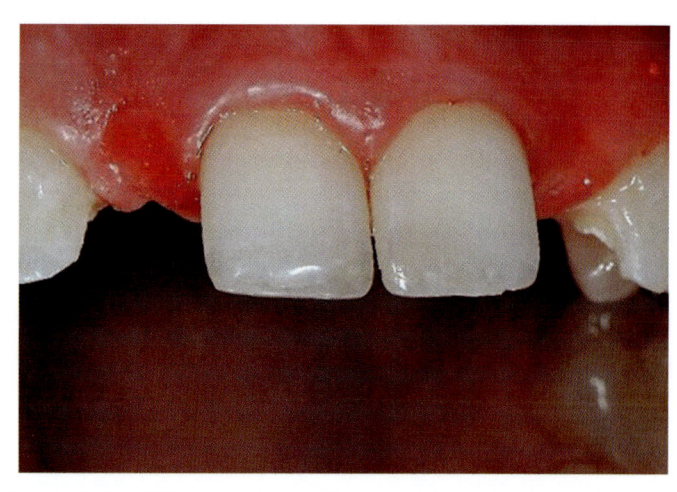

Figure 17.5 **(C)** Retracted view after removal of resin pontics showing thin, translucent incisal edges that would allow show-through of a metal framework. The phase I treatment included fabrication of partial-coverage adhesive zirconia bridges to replace the maxillary lateral incisors. Phase II treatment would be augmentation of the edentulous ridges and implant crowns to replace both lateral incisors.

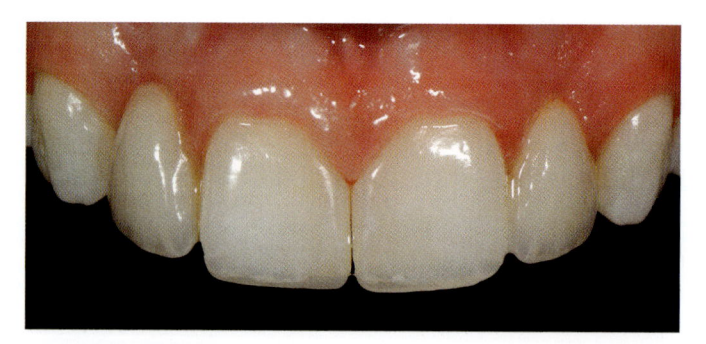

Figure 17.5 **(D)** Bonded zirconia framework adhesive bridges with improved pontic contours and more harmonious proportions. The patient was very satisfied with the stronger framework and improved esthetics, providing a more stable restoration while waiting for phase II.

The retracted view of her preexisting bridges shows the unsatisfactory proportions of the pontics. The final bonded zirconia bridges provided improved pontic contours, and more harmonious proportions (Figures 17.5D). A reduction in the framework thickness from 0.5 to 0.3 mm for single crowns on bridge frameworks can reduce the fracture resistance by 35%.[33]

Complete-coverage retainers

Full-veneer retainers are the most popular of all retainers for fixed partial dentures. They generally fall into three categories: all-metal, all-ceramic, and metal–ceramic retainers.

All-metal crowns are not particularly esthetic and therefore should be used only in patients who have low esthetic demands and in esthetically less demanding regions of the mouth. Typically, they are placed in areas of the mouth that virtually cannot be viewed by observers or the patient. They are ideal for maxillary and mandibular second and third molar abutments and for the occasional maxillary first molar in patients with low smile lines that do not expose this tooth. It is fortunate that these areas of the mouth lend themselves to all-metal crowns since it is rare to find second or third molars, particularly mandibular molars, that have sufficient gingivo-occlusal height to allow sufficient reduction for porcelain occlusal coverage. The major advantages of all-metal retainers are less tooth reduction compared with the metal–ceramic or all-ceramic crown preparation, strength, and lack of wear of the opposing dentition. The chief disadvantages are the lack of esthetics and high thermal conductivity.

All-ceramic systems are an esthetic alternative to metal–ceramic systems for fixed partial dentures. Zirconium dioxide ceramics have superior mechanical properties, high flexural strength, and fracture toughness compared with the conventional feldspathic porcelains or leucite or lithium disilicate reinforced ceramics. The majority of zirconia frameworks have been made with yttria-stabilized, tetragonal zirconia polycrystal ceramics[22] which undergo "transformation toughening." Zirconia blocks can be milled at three different stages: green, presintered, and fully sintered. Frameworks milled from the green-stage and presintered zirconia blocks are enlarged to compensate for future material shrinkage (20–25%).[34] Fully sintered zirconia blocks are more difficult and time consuming to mill, but are not subject to the dimensional changes that occur with the green-stage and presintered zirconia materials. Computer-aided design and computer-aided manufacturing (CAD/CAM) technology is used to fabricate most zirconia-based restorations. Precise tooth preparation with rounded shoulder/chamfer margins is recommended to facilitate laser scanning. Sharp axiogingival line angles are difficult to scan, and consequently may result in compromised internal and marginal fit[2,24,35] (Figure 17.6A–G).

The marginal fit of zirconia-based fixed partial dentures can be equal or superior to metal–ceramics, and serve as a viable alternative to metal–ceramic systems.[19] High survival rates (over 95%) has been reported in 5-year clinical studies of zirconia-based posterior fixed partial dentures.[36–38] The most commonly reported complication is chipping of the veneering porcelain. This is often attributed to inappropriate support of the veneering porcelain, although temperature control and ceramic compatibility may play a role as well. A full contour wax-up should be utilized for the zirconia coping design to ensure adequate support for the veneering porcelain[25] (Figure 17.7). The zirconia coping thickness should follow the outback of the wax-up to allow a uniform thickness of veneering porcelain. Future fabrication methods involving pressing to the zirconia coping may improve the clinical outcomes currently seen with traditional layering techniques.[39]

Recent improvements in second-generation lithium disilicate ceramic materials have resulted in smaller and more homogeneous crystals providing improved physical properties such as flexural strength and fracture toughness. Studies indicate that monolithic lithium disilicate ceramic can be used to fabricate three-unit fixed partial dentures to replace anterior teeth and premolars[8,40] When used to replace molars, there were catastrophic failures.[41] The 10-year survival rates ranged from 87.0 to 89.2%, with a rate of ceramic chipping of only 6.1% (similar to that of metal–ceramic fixed partial dentures).[4,42]

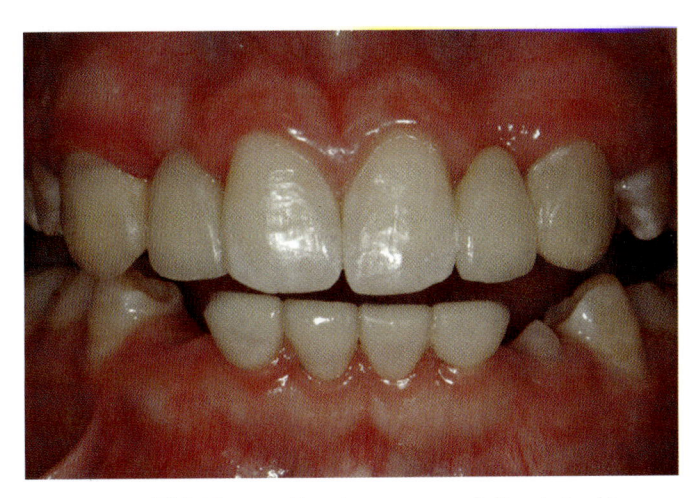

Figure 17.6 **(A)** A 15-year-old male was congenitally missing his laterals. He was evaluated as too young for dental implants and the needed ridge augmentation procedure. There was a tooth size discrepancy evident within the maxillary incisors.

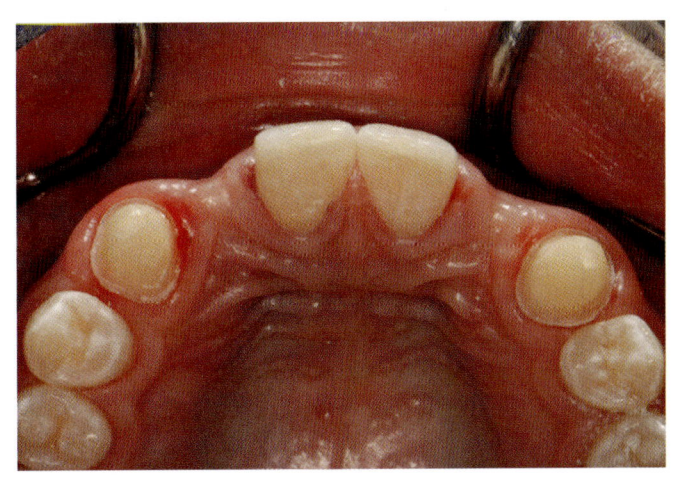

Figure 17.6 **(B)** To be conservative, provide stability, allow for growth, and correct esthetic proportions, the two cuspids were prepared for porcelain-fused-to-zirconia cantilever bridges. To correct the size discrepancy, no-prep porcelain veneer pieces were created for the distal of the two centrals, and no-prep porcelain onlays were created for the right and left first bicuspids.

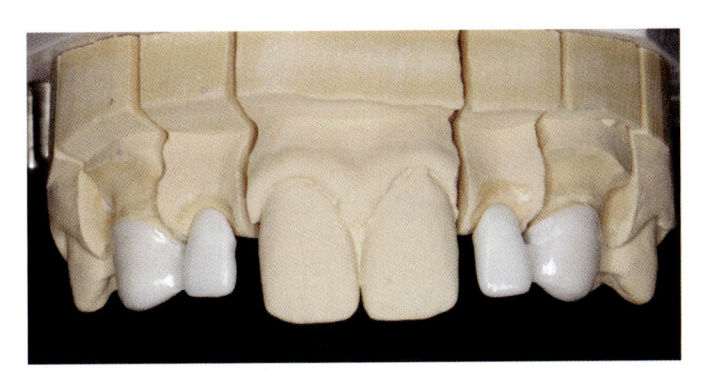

Figure 17.6 **(C)** Right and left CAD/CAM zirconia frameworks seated on the master cast. Note the space created for the partial porcelain veneer that will be used to widen the central incisors.

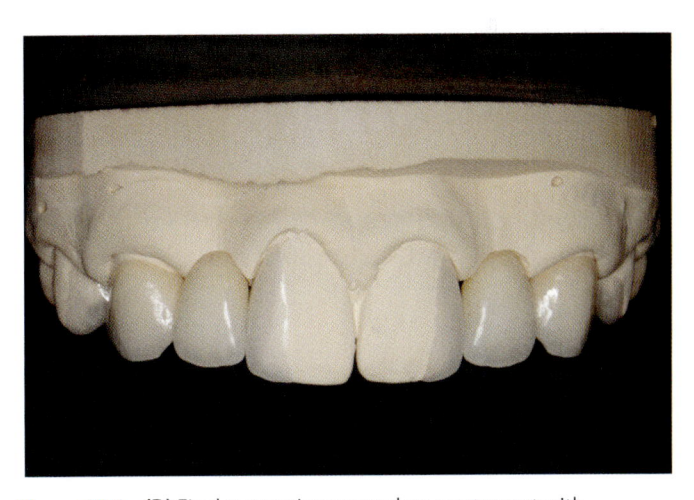

Figure 17.6 **(D)** Final restorations seated on master cast with corrected tooth contours. Note that conservative restorative choices were provided to allow for growth and additional options in the future.

By far the most commonly used retainer for fixed partial dentures has been the metal–ceramic crown. During the last 30–40 years, this restoration has proven to be very satisfactory. Some of the variables that should be considered with metal–ceramic retainers are the location of the margins in relation to the gingiva, the materials utilized, and the location of the porcelain-metal junction on the occlusal surface.[18]

Margin location

Numerous studies have shown that the biologic acceptance of an artificial crown by the gingival apparatus is generally healthier and more favorable when the artificial material remains supragingival.[43] Supragingival margins are also easier to prepare, impress, and evaluate for accuracy of fit. Although it has been shown that soft-tissue health can be maintained in the presence of subgingival margins,[44] the general consensus is that margins should only be placed into the gingival sulcus when necessary for esthetics, wall height for resistance and retention, or extension beyond preexisting caries or restorations.[30] In one study, it was shown that less than 50% of the population evaluated revealed the gingival third of any of their mandibular teeth during facial expression (without manually retracting their lower lips).[45] A smaller percentage in the same study did not reveal their maxillary gingival margins during facial expression. It was the author's observations that many patients do not show the gingival margin of maxillary molars at all. In general, subgingival metal–ceramic margins should be limited to a patient's visible esthetic zone. In the esthetically critical areas, the equigingival porcelain shoulder butt margin can be utilized to any desired extent of the tooth circumference up to a 360° porcelain margin (see also figure 15–11 in the second edition). For any margin location selected, the restorative objective is to create precise, well-fitting margins that will ensure longevity of the restorations and idealized periodontal health (Figure 17.8A and B).[46]

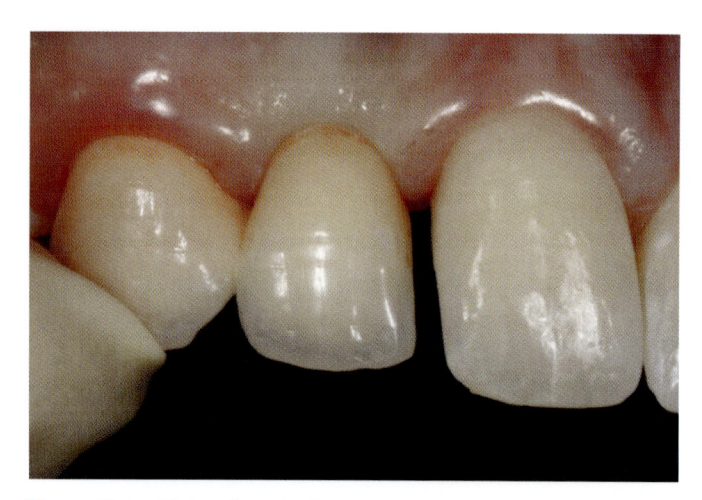

Figure 17.6 **(E)** Cantilever bridge in place showing size discrepancy for central incisors.

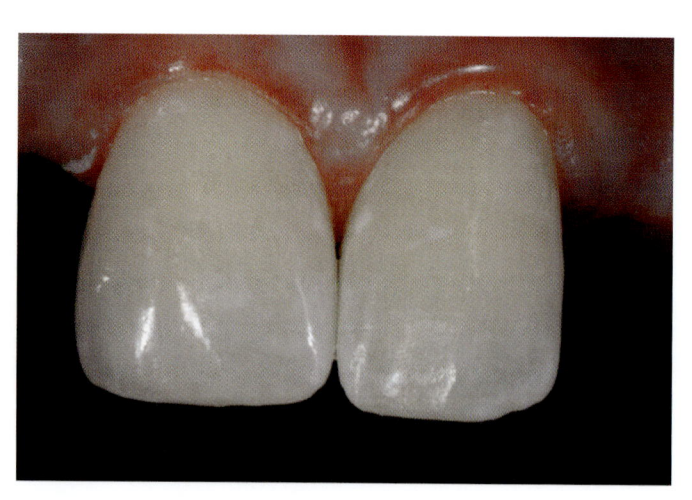

Figure 17.6 **(F)** Right central incisor porcelain veneer (no-prep) expanding width of central incisor to normal proportions. Compare with the unrestored, undersized left central incisor.

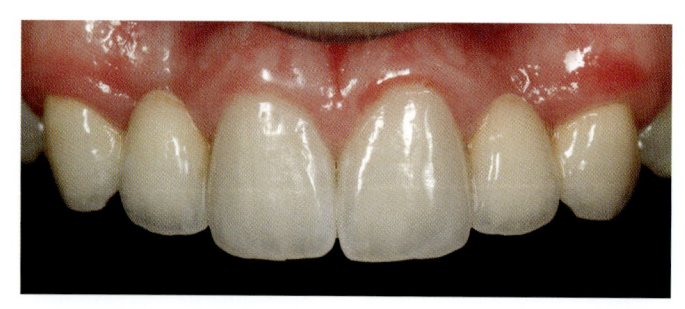

Figure 17.6 **(G)** A retracted view of the final esthetic outcome.

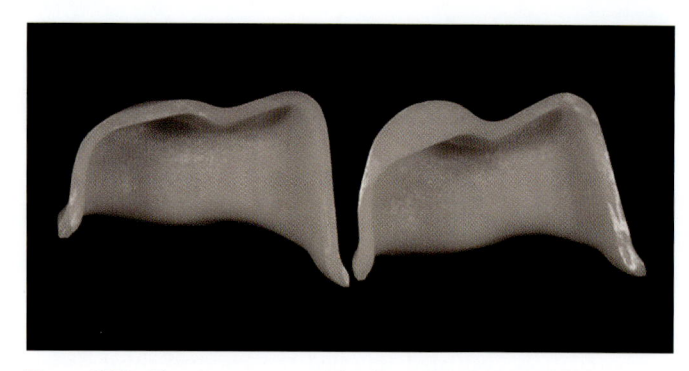

Figure 17.7 The zirconia coping thickness should follow a full contour wax-up to allow a uniform thickness of veneering porcelain and provide adequate support and prevent porcelain fracture. The right coping was modified from a typical uniform coping thickness (as seen in the left coping).

Margin materials

Not all subgingival margins result in an esthetic outcome. For patients with a delicate, thin biotype, a metal margin can sometimes show through the thin gingival sulcus. There are three different approaches to a metal–ceramic crown margin. The first is the classic metal collar, in which a small band of metal creates the terminus for the crown with no overlaying porcelain.

Historically, the metal collar margin was the technique for all early metal–ceramic crowns and is currently used for posterior restorations or areas with heavy occlusal forces.

The unpredictability of consistently hiding the metal collar subgingivally led to the second approach to metal–ceramic crown margins. This is a compromise variously named the metal–porcelain margin, the covered metal margin, or the disappearing metal margin. This technique involves a thin metal collar with an overlay of porcelain to hide the metal margin. This margin design is contraindicated because the metal is often extremely thin and can often distort during porcelain firing.[38] Second, owing to the thinness of the porcelain overlying this metal, it is almost all opaque porcelain. This opaque porcelain is virtually unglazable and unpolishable, resulting in a rough, plaque-retentive marginal surface that is often overcontoured. Therefore, this marginal design can only produce limited esthetic benefit with potential compromises to the biologic health of the surrounding gingiva.

The third approach to achieving an esthetic metal–ceramic crown margin is the porcelain margin. This is accomplished by cutting back the metal supportive coping to the internal line angle of the shoulder of the preparation as far proximally as is required for esthetics and for the creation of a porcelain shoulder. Some techniques also reduce the metal coping to some distance up the facial surface to further maximize the esthetics of

Figure 17.8 **(A)** A radiographic view of ill-fitting restorations and extruded cement. Incomplete marginal closure leads to compromised periodontal health and risk of recurrent caries.

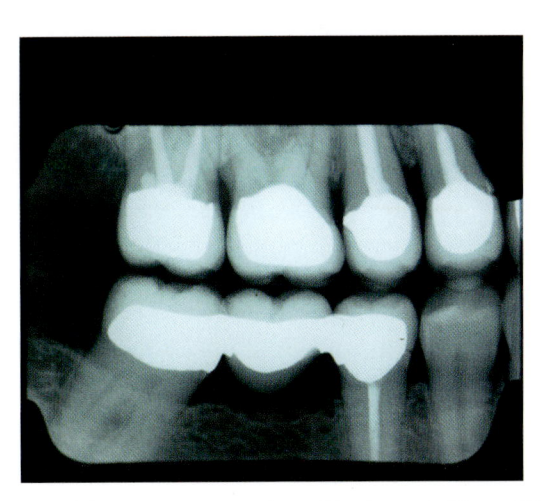

Figure 17.8 **(B)** A posttreatment view of the image in Figure 17.8A illustrating new restorations with well-sealed margins, ideal for the long-term maintenance of periodontal health.

the porcelain and the light-reflective properties of the metal coping.[47] It was originally thought that this technique would not yield sufficiently accurate marginal adaptation to be clinically acceptable. Yet, several studies have shown that margins of equal clinical acceptability as metal margins can be created with this design and by many different porcelain application techniques.[48–50] Historically, ceramic margins were not expected to be strong enough to withstand clinical loads. However, research has indicated that, once cemented on the abutment teeth, all-ceramic margins have equal or possibly greater strength than metal collar margins.[51]

Our recommendation for margin selection for metal–ceramic retainers is to use metal collar margins in esthetically noncritical areas. Porcelain margins should be used in the patient's esthetic zone or for patients with higher esthetic demands, and the combination metal–porcelain margin should be avoided whenever possible (Figure 17.9A–F).

Porcelain–metal junction

The final aspect to consider in the esthetics of the metal–ceramic crown is the location of the porcelain–metal junction. Often, the most esthetic choice is to cover the entire metal coping with porcelain in all areas of the mouth where the abutment retainer is visible. This design is effective as long as the underlying metal coping is of sufficient thickness to provide sufficient rigidity to support the overlying porcelain.[52] Yet, the clinician must make certain there is adequate occlusal reduction for the restorative materials being placed. Otherwise, compromised esthetics or a vulnerability to porcelain fracture can result.[53]

The mandibular arch is also an esthetically demanding area, and complete-porcelain coverage of the mandibular premolars and first molar is often desired. The occlusal and lingual surfaces of these teeth are readily visible when the mouth is open. In some patients, even the mandibular second molar is visible. For many

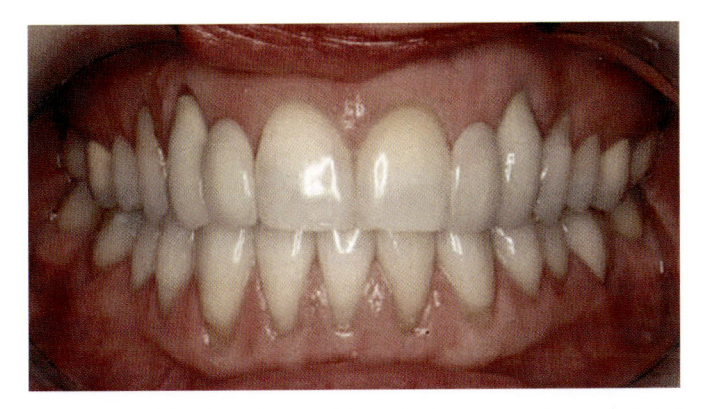

Figure 17.9 **(A)** A frontal view of the esthetic compromises associated with generalized recession, a constricted maxillary arch, and narrow spaces for congenitally missing maxillary lateral incisors. After an extensive review of interdisciplinary treatment options, periodontal tissue grafting and a comprehensive restorative treatment plan were coordinated to correct the patient's esthetic problems.

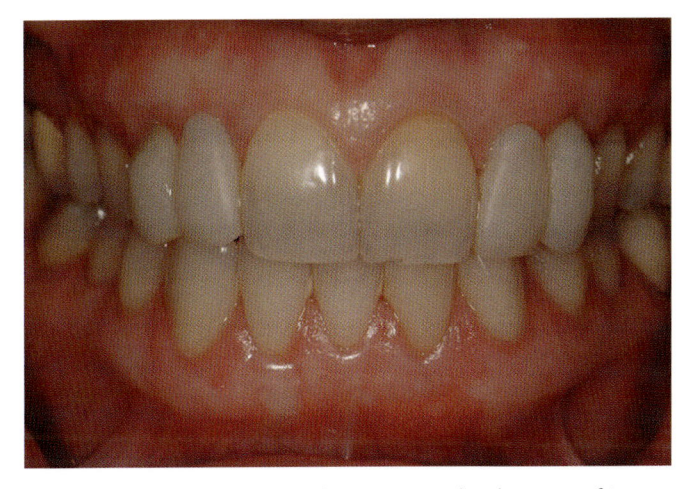

Figure 17.9 **(B)** The patient underwent generalized tissue grafting to restore the gingival harmony and balance throughout her dentition. This anterior view with provisional restoration at the cuspid and cantilevered lateral incisor illustrates the graft results.

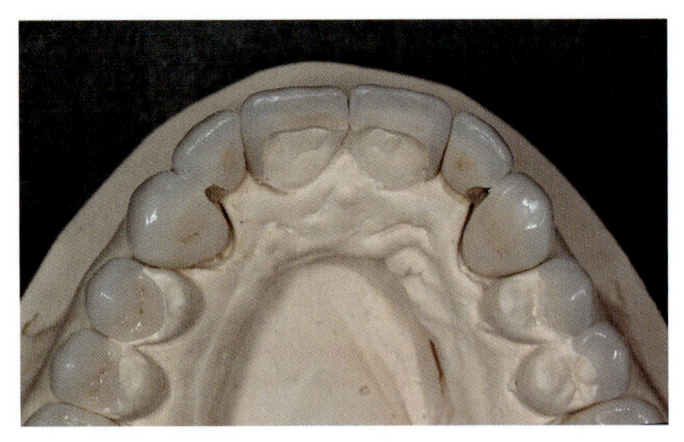

Figure 17.9 **(C)** A broadened arch form was achieved through the use of a combination of porcelain-bonded restorations, full crowns, and cantilevered fixed partial prosthesis for the replacement of the congenitally missing lateral incisors.

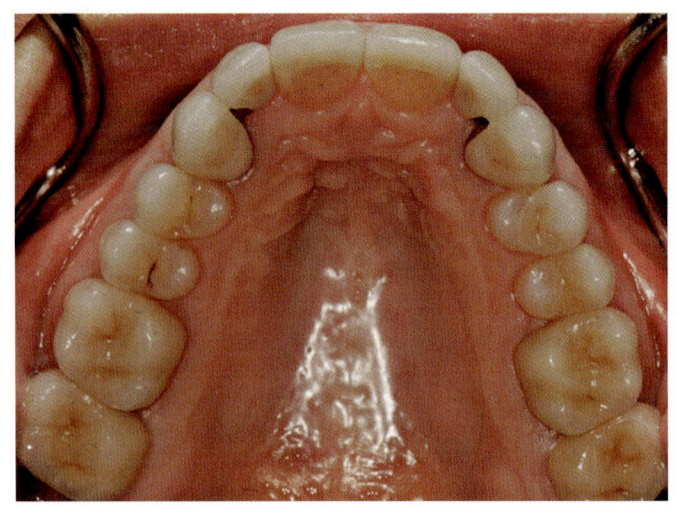

Figure 17.9 **(D)** A maxillary occlusal view of the completed treatment.

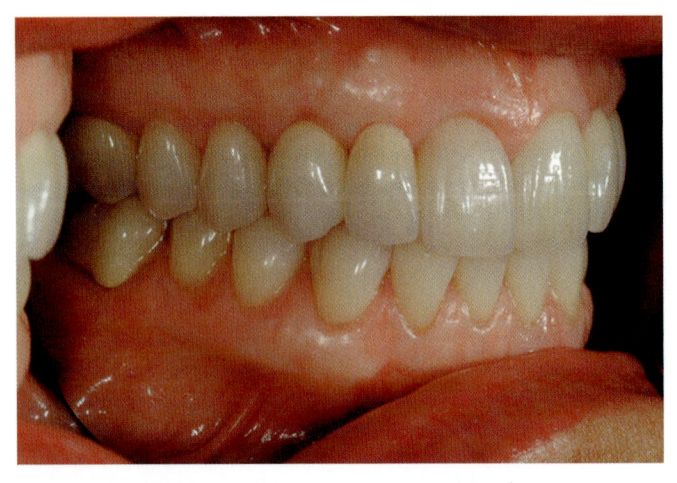

Figure 17.9 **(E)** A right lateral view of the completed treatment. The esthetic restorative objectives could be achieved once the preexisting tissue recession issues were corrected with connective tissue grafting procedures.

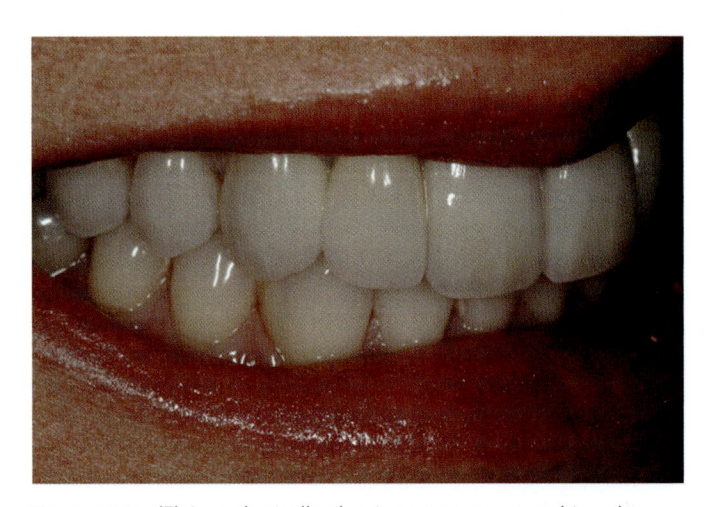

Figure 17.9 **(F)** An esthetically pleasing outcome was achieved through comprehensive treatment and clear communication on esthetic goals.

patients, the porcelain–metal junction location on mandibular anterior restorations is rarely of importance esthetically or functionally. Biologically, owing to the small size of mandibular anterior teeth, overcontouring of the lingual surface of the restorations is best avoided by locating the junction as far incisively as esthetics will allow.

The delicate balance of porcelain occlusal coverage for esthetics and prevention of wear of the opposing dentition may be compensated for in the posterior occlusion if the patient possesses a mutually protected occlusion in lateral and protrusive excursive movements. Without an anterior disclusive occlusal scheme, porcelain wear of the opposing dentition may need to be addressed with a protective occlusal splint. A well-constructed protective occlusal splint is recommended following any extensive esthetic rehabilitation to ensure protection of the restorations created and longevity of the results. Occlusal splint protection is especially important for patients with nocturnal and daytime parafunctional habits (Figure 17.10).

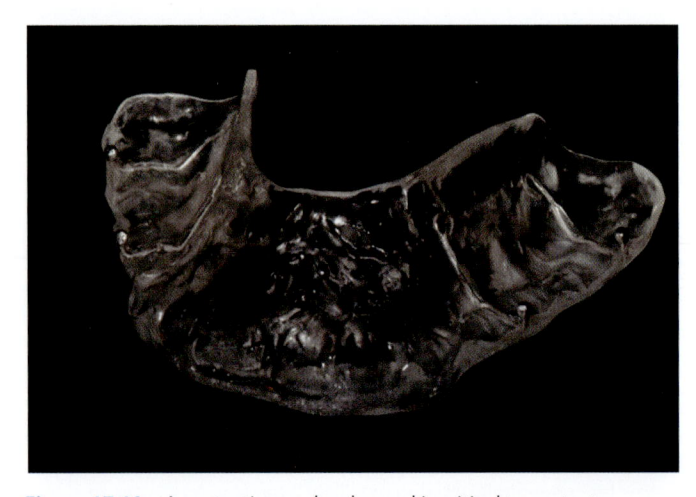

Figure 17.10 A protective occlusal guard is critical to protect porcelain restorations due to parafunctional activity.

Anterior restorations involving one missing tooth

The ideal choice for the replacement of a single missing tooth is the single-tooth implant. Dental implants have become the standard of care, and it is important to evaluate each patient possessing an edentulous space for the possibility of replacing that space with an implant. The patient has a right to know the potential functional and esthetic success associated with the placement of an implant instead of a fixed or removable prosthesis.

However, there are times when an implant may not be possible or practical. In these instances, a conservative alternative is the cantilever fixed partial denture involving one or more abutment teeth. A cantilever in a mesial location to the abutment tooth is the most favorable functionally as it causes less stress to the abutment tooth. The cantilevered restoration is highly desirable esthetically (especially in areas adjacent to unrestored teeth). This conservative treatment can be an excellent treatment choice for a young patient, where implant surgery is contraindicated until complete growth is achieved. Additionally, for the more mature patient, cantilever bridges can offer an esthetic and conservative treatment where implants are not possible and one of the abutments is not requiring restoration (Figure 17.11A–E).

The question of whether to select an implant prosthesis rather than a tooth-borne fixed partial denture is generally decided by the dentist and the patient after a thorough analysis of the advantages and disadvantages of each treatment modality (Figure 17.12A–I). A thorough discussion of the treatment alternatives must include a conscientious and thorough analysis of the longevity, costs, and esthetic appearance of each proposed treatment.[54]

Splinting

Esthetically, it is much better not to splint the incisors when possible to maintain the individuality of teeth. Either separation or the appearance of separation helps to make a missing tooth replacement appear natural. In addition, the lack of splinting will promote easier maintenance and good oral hygiene. The decision to splint is determined by the mobility patterns of the abutment teeth, support and integrity of the abutment teeth, and potential esthetic challenges that might result when functional requirements indicate splinting.

To achieve a pleasing natural appearance, restorations should appear to have some bilateral symmetry and the maintenance of natural tooth proportions. This may sometimes require the incorporation of some minor crowding of the pontics within the edentulous space. There should also be harmony in the gingival contour and incisal levels to idealize the esthetic appeal of the visible smile.

Use of telescoping crowns as abutments

Advantages

In situations that would often be considered dentally hopeless, the use of telescoping restorations can offer treatment options that will provide an esthetic, functionally stable, and long-lasting result. Numerous benefits exist with this technique. One of the greatest benefits is the ability to ensure complete marginal closure around each of the abutments as they are cemented independently of the splinting suprastructure. This advantage is significant in long-span splinting, especially with periodontally involved abutments. The technique also assures long-term protection of each abutment in case of the intrusion of weak abutments in parafunctionally active patients. Intrusion of a telescoped abutment tooth results in cement failure between the coping and the suprastructure, rather than the abutment and the fixed prosthesis, thereby preventing recurrent decay, potential abutment loss, and the need for a new prosthesis.

Additional advantages focus on the tooth preparation criteria and overall biomechanical advantages for the restorative materials. Telescoping crown preparations do not need to conform to a strict common path of insertion.[55] Only the functional surfaces of the created copings require drawing to a common path. Telescoping restorations also provide the ability to strategically link different segments of fixed partial dentures to limit the length of each segment for better biomechanics, strength, and precision in marginal adaptation. This is particularly useful

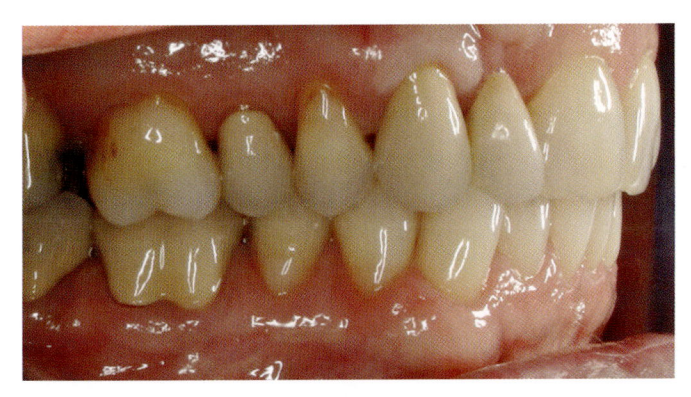

Figure 17.11 **(A)** Note deficient tissue in maxillary right lateral incisor pontic site resulting in a food trap and unesthetic appearance.

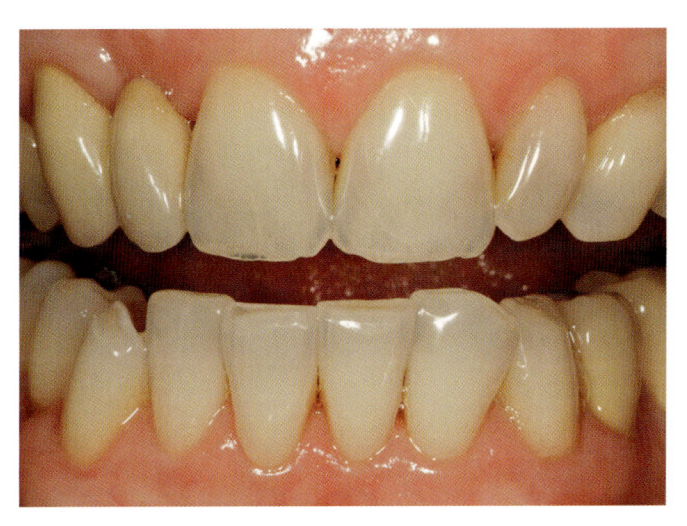

Figure 17.11 **(B)** A frontal view of the same patient illustrates the thin, chipped, and worn edges of her maxillary centrals.

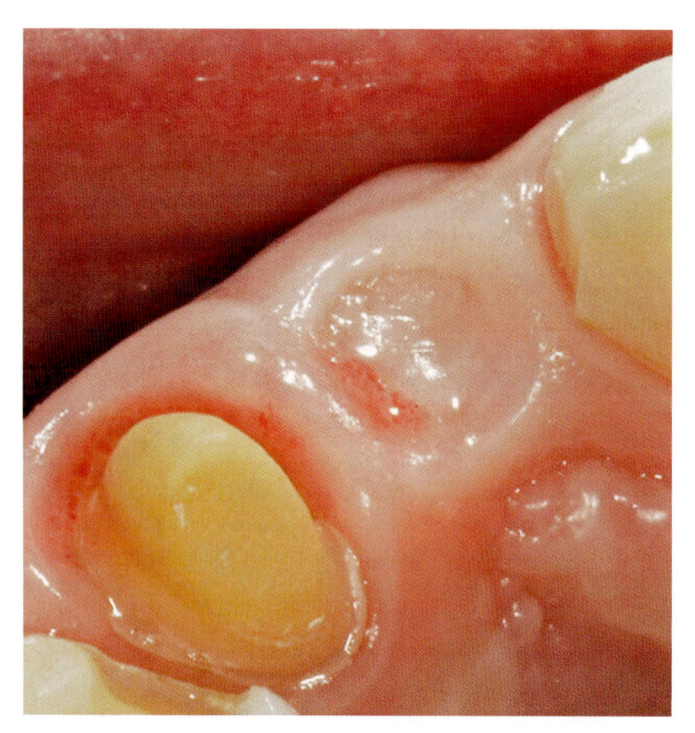

Figure 17.11 **(C)** Occlusal view postperiodontal surgery with a connective tissue graft to create contours for an ovate pontic.

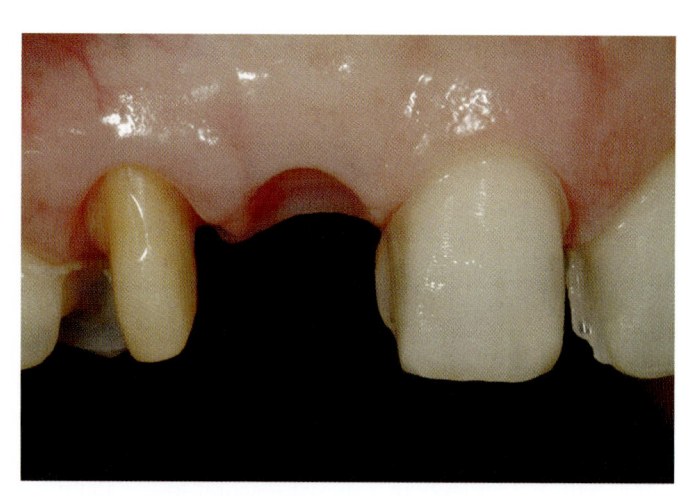

Figure 17.11 **(D)** A frontal view of the tooth preparations for the cantilevered fixed partial denture and porcelain-bonded restorations. Note the labial view of the ovate pontic site.

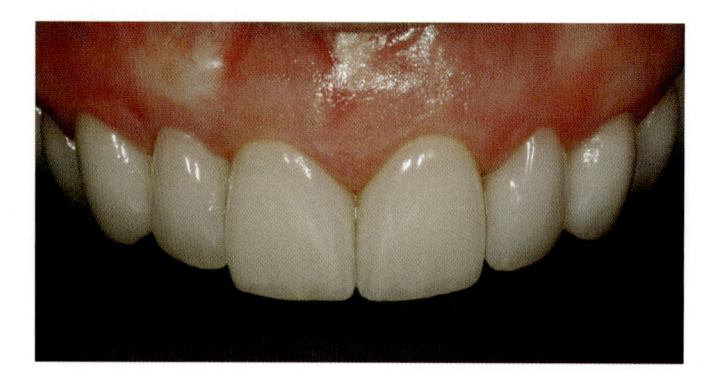

Figure 17.11 **(E)** Postoperative view showing the cantilevered fixed partial denture blending with the surrounding dentition and newly created harmonious tissue contours.

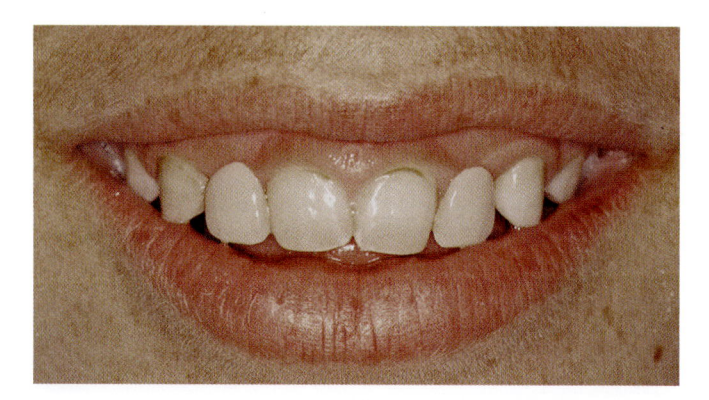

Figure 17.12 **(A)** Patient presented postorthodontic treatment, with an upper removable appliance replacing her congenitally missing lateral incisors.

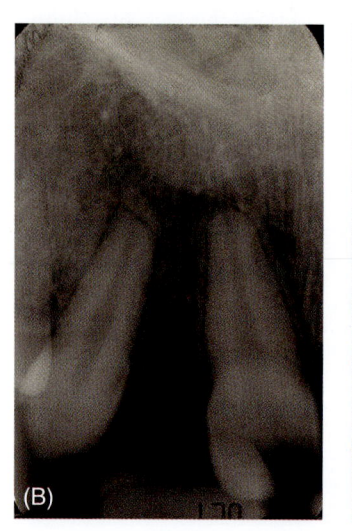

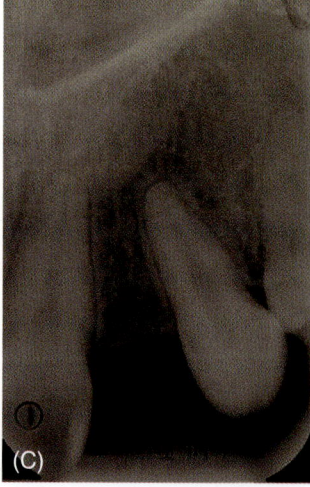

Figure 17.12 **(B, C)** Radiographs of the future implant sites illustrate the limited space for the future implants due to converging roots.

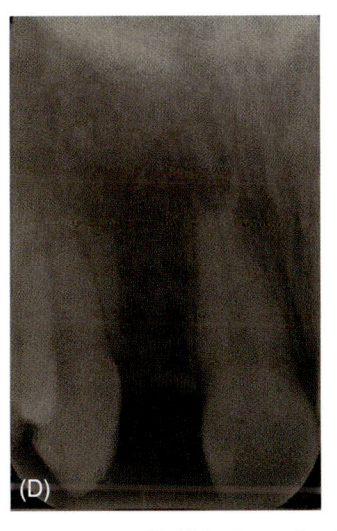

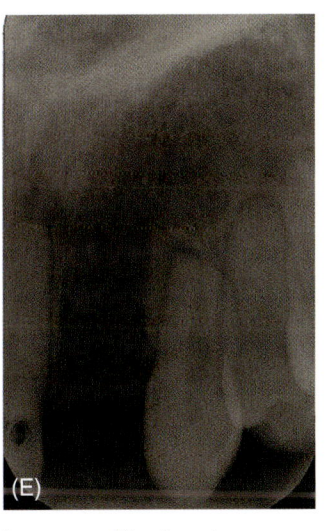

Figure 17.12 (D, E) Radiographs of the corrected implant sites following orthodontic retreatment.

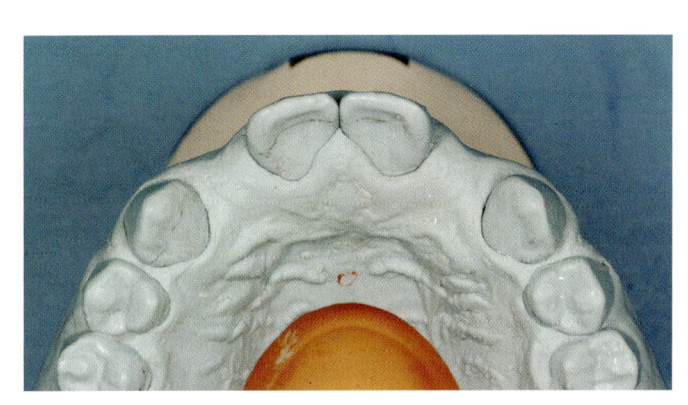

Figure 17.12 (F) Master cast prior to tissue augmentation. Note lack of volume in future implant sites due to underdeveloped alveolar ridges.

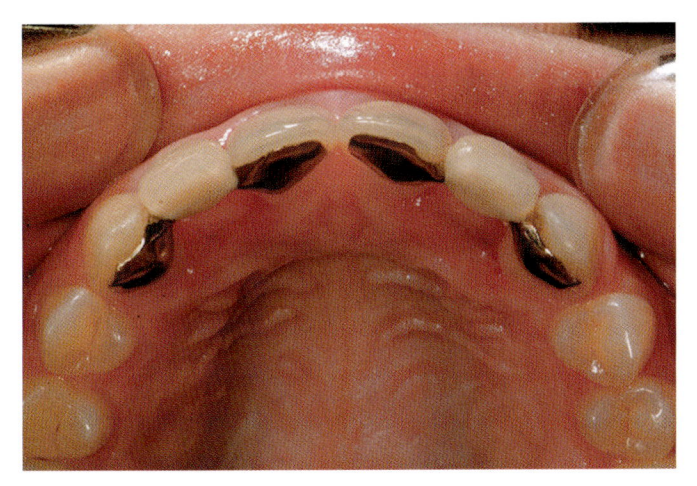

Figure 17.12 (G) Provisional no-prep adhesive bridges, after tissue augmentation and implant site preparation.

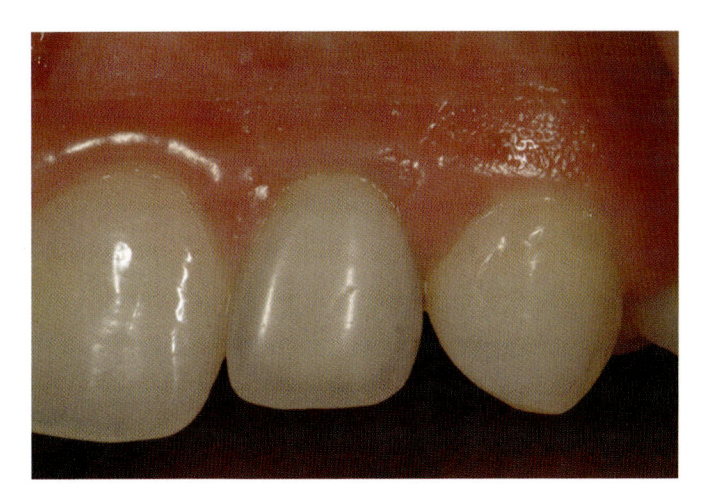

Figure 17.12 (H) Final results with implants, custom gold abutments, and porcelain-fused-to-gold implant restorations. All of the surrounding teeth are unrestored.

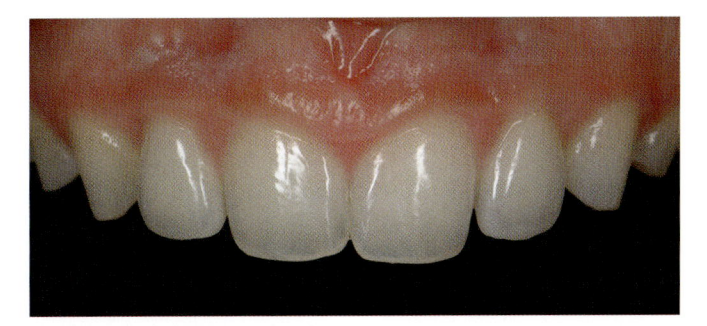

Figure 17.12 (I) A 5-year posttreatment view.

when using a metal–ceramic or all-ceramic prosthesis where a long span may produce excessive flexure and, subsequently, increase the possibility of fracture. Smaller spans are less vulnerable to flexure and can be more easily removed for repairs or potential future endodontic procedures.[56]

Telescoped superstructures are delivered with temporary cement providing the benefit of retrievability when future alterations in design are required. For example, in the event of the loss of a posterior abutment, the superstructure may be removed and modified by filling the former abutment retainer with composite resin, turning it into a pontic. This option provides an immediate cost-effective solution, preserves the integrity of the prosthesis, and protects the investment made by the patient. With thoughtful design and engineering of the suprastructure, flexible solutions for future complications can be pre-engineered into the prosthesis.

Owing to the success of endosseous implants, strictly tooth-borne prostheses are limited to the medically compromised patients where implant surgery may be contraindicated.[43,57] Since teeth and implants have different attachment mechanisms to bone, it is not recommended to attach teeth and implants. Otherwise, problems such as natural tooth intrusion can result.[58–60] In complex restorative care, implants and teeth can be combined in the overall treatment plan, but restored in different segments through the use of telescoping abutments, copings, and suprastructures.

An example of this more complex form of treatment is illustrated in Figure 17.13A–H. A male patient referred by his periodontist for restorative retreatment had only seven salvageable teeth in the maxillary arch. The maxillary right first bicuspid to the left cuspid were to be retained, and his posterior teeth would be replaced with implant-supported fixed partial dentures. Owing to the severe periodontal breakdown and structural damage of the anterior teeth, it was determined that periodontal splinting of the remaining natural dentition was indicated. Individual, gold-milled copings and a suprastructure were chosen as the treatment of choice to provide stabilization of the natural teeth, separation of the tooth- and implant-borne segments, and retrievability for potential abutment loss in the future. Figure 17.13B shows the master cast of the milled copings for the anterior teeth and the milled implant abutments for the posterior segments. An intraoral view of the cemented anterior copings is seen in Figure 17.13C. The importance of dividing the tooth-borne and implant-borne suprastructures has been emphasized throughout the literature. Figure 17.13D illustrates the importance of well-designed and contoured connections between the individual segments providing an esthetic natural appearance with seamless transitions of hard and soft tissues while providing

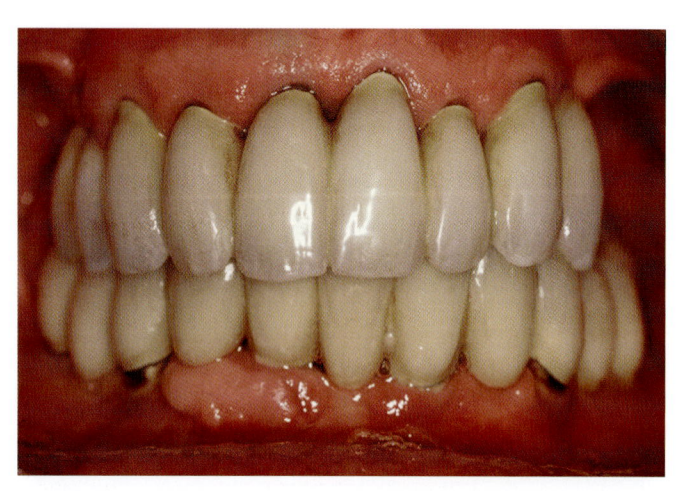

Figure 17.13 (A) Preliminary photo of patient's maxillary arch. Only his maxillary right first bicuspid to the left cuspid were restorable. All posterior teeth needed replacement with implant-supported fixed partial dentures.

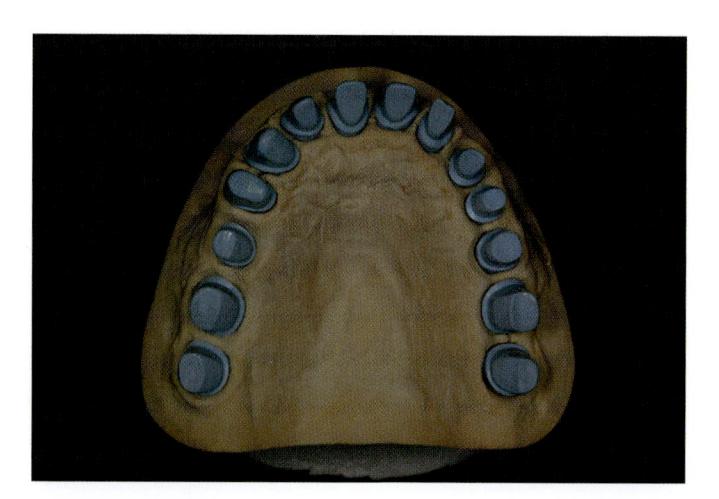

Figure 17.13 (B) Occlusal view of the maxillary master cast showing the milled implant abutments and natural tooth copings. The final prosthesis will be segmented into three separate tooth supported and implant supported fixed partial dentures.

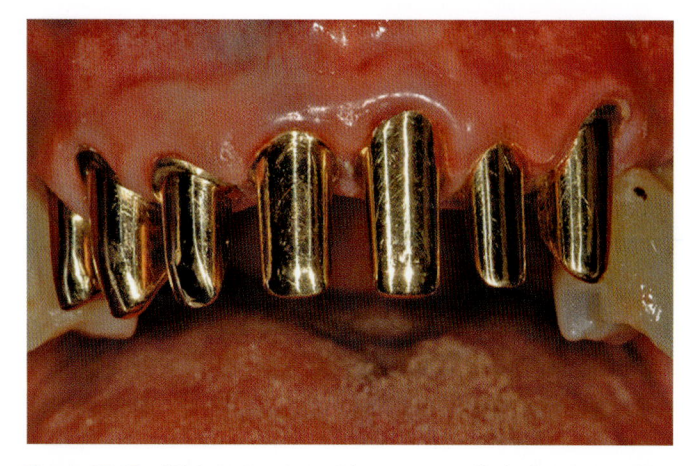

Figure 17.13 (C) Anterior view of the custom milled telescopic gold copings for the seven remaining natural teeth. The implant-supported fixed partial dentures are seated in the posterior segments.

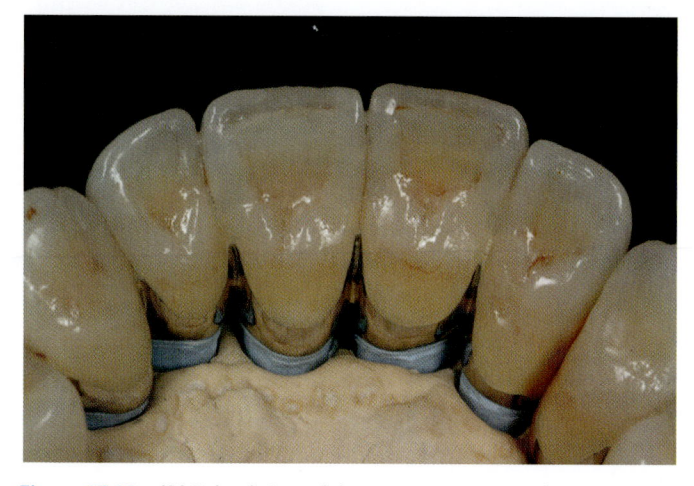

Figure 17.13 (D) Palatal view of the superstructure on the master cast illustrates the creation of natural-appearing contours. Attention must be paid to create interproximal contours that are easily accessible for adequate hygiene and long-term gingival health.

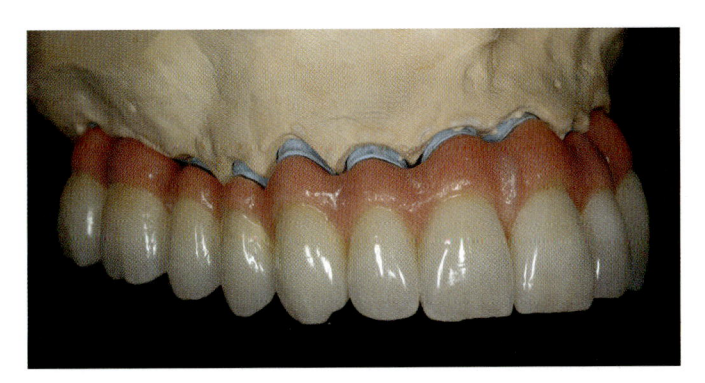

Figure 17.13 **(E)** All three superstructures seated on the master cast showing the hard- and soft-tissue replacements created in porcelain-fused-to-gold restorations.

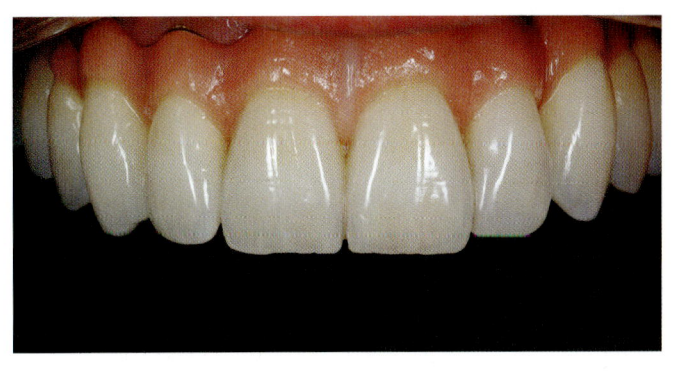

Figure 17.13 **(F)** Retracted anterior view of all copings, abutments and superstructures at the clinical try-in appointment.

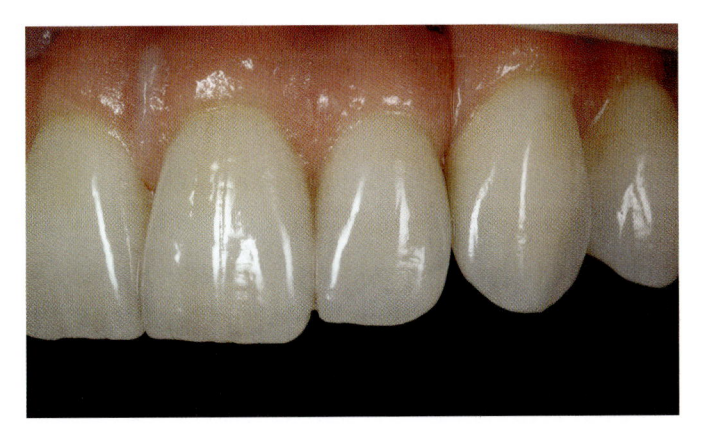

Figure 17.13 **(G)** Magnified view of the separation between the anterior tooth-borne superstructure and the maxillary left implant-borne superstructure.

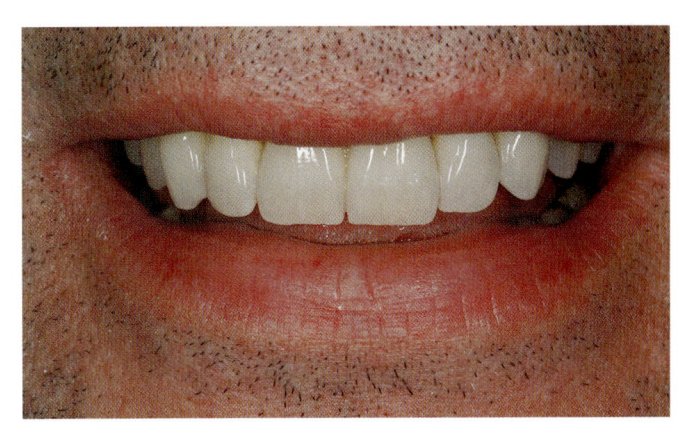

Figure 17.13 **(H)** Patient smile with the new restorations in place. Esthetic, mechanical, biologic, and psychologic goals have been accomplished.

easy cleansability. For the patient, correcting hard- and soft-tissue defects through dental bioengineering can help create better self-esteem and a more relaxed smile (Figure 17.13H).

The telescopic copings were cemented with a definitive cement for maximum longevity and stability. Suprastructures were cemented with a provisional cement for retrievability. For this patient, this advantage was realized when a tooth abutment was lost many years later. His superstructure was removed, the failing tooth was extracted, the superstructure was modified with composite resin to create a pontic, and the prosthesis was recemented during the same appointment. The patient was pleased with the minimal expense, preserved esthetics, additional longevity of his prosthesis, and minimal interruption of his daily life. The superstructures need to be designed with exposed metal at the connector site to prevent damage or fracture of the porcelain if a reverse hammer is used to tap off the superstructure.

Disadvantages

The main disadvantage associated with telescopic restorations is increased expense and the three-dimensional (3D) space requirement necessary to accommodate two full-coverage restorations. Even though the expense can sometimes be justified for the many advantages to this procedure, it is still significant.

The biomechanical needs of telescoping require careful preoperative planning between the dentist and the dental technician to achieve success. If sufficient interproximal space is lacking, strategic extractions may be required to create more space. Even when the overall spacing will allow for the increased restorative bulk of materials, it is critical that individual tooth preparations be designed to allow for the additional layer of metal, associated cement space, and fuller interproximal contours. Therefore, using telescoping crowns in small, flat teeth should be avoided owing to mechanical limitations.

Another potential esthetic disadvantage with the coping and telescope procedure is the need for a more prominent gold collar at the junction of the coping and the superstructure. Potential treatment solutions for this problem include minimizing the collar heights or the creation of an anterior coping design modification that does not cover the gingival half of the tooth, allowing cross-linkage without the compromise in esthetics.[41,61]

With stronger all-ceramic materials, another possible solution is the use of zirconia copings combined with zirconia superstructures, eliminating the esthetic concerns associated with metal materials. As previously mentioned, recognizing the success of osseointegrated implants today, if contraindications or concerns with salvaging compromised teeth become significant, implants should be considered as an alternative.

Copings are well suited in the patient with a low lip line to mask the esthetic compromises. However, patients' esthetic tolerances vary greatly and it is important that the patient is fully informed of the design and is able to pre-approve the esthetic appearance in a provisional restoration. During provisionalization, the patient can personally experience that the gingival portion of the tooth will not be seen during normal conversation, laughing, or smiling, and may become more accepting of this treatment alternative.

The example in Figure 17.14A–G shows the pretreatment photographs of a female patient who was suffering from severe periodontal disease and was dissatisfied with the appearance of her smile. The patient reported that she wanted to retain her teeth as long as possible. She declined a removable treatment option and was receptive to orthodontic treatment as an adjunct to her restorative treatment. The bone loss in the right and left bicuspid areas would have created severe esthetic and technological challenges. The full mouth series of radiographs shows the severity of the destruction. It was determined that the extrusion of the maxillary right and left bicuspids and the left cuspid would provide esthetic and mechanical advantages for the future implant sites.[9,61] Molar implants were placed and then ultimately used as orthodontic anchorage to extrude the periodontally compromised teeth, bringing the bone and tissue to develop the implant sites. Upon extraction and bone grafting, a full-arch maxillary provisional was placed as an interim restoration to restore esthetics and function. Subsequently, dental implants were placed in the healed extraction sites, and the implants and teeth were restored with gold milled abutments, gold milled tooth copings, and three separate suprastructures. The final results were mechanically stable, functionally ideal, and esthetically improved.

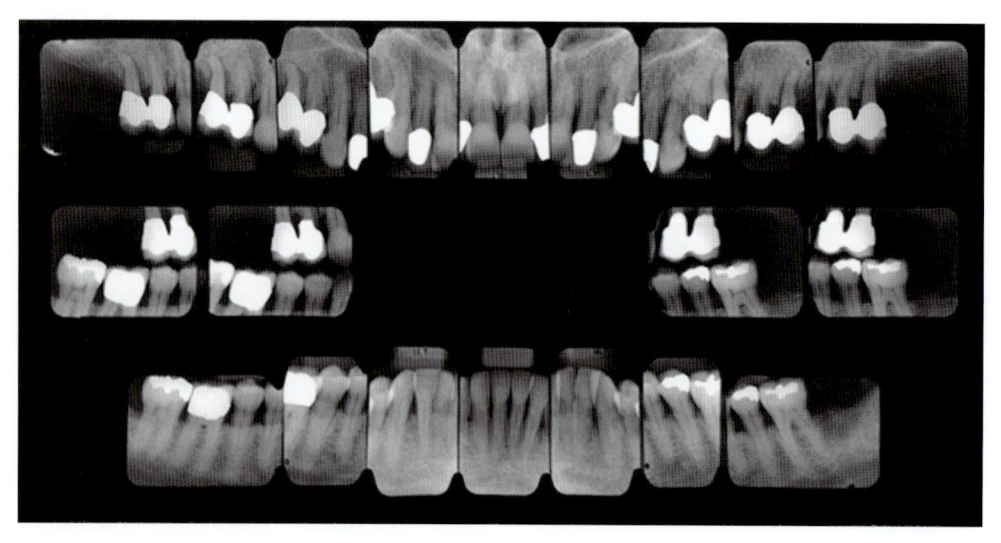

Figure 17.14 (A) Radiographs of a patient with severe periodontal disease and terminal posterior teeth and significant horizontal bone loss and mobility.

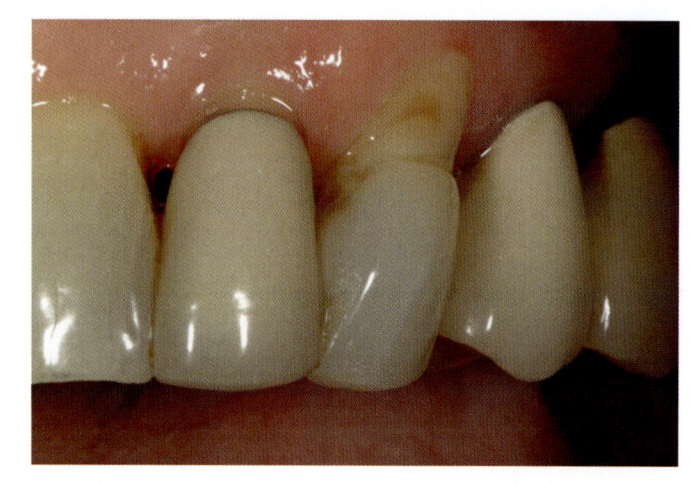

Figure 17.14 (B) To prepare the posterior maxillary bone for implants, the left cuspid and premolars were treatment planned for orthodontic extrusion to bring the tissue and bone levels occlusally. Implant placement was staged so that molar implants were used for leverage to assist in tooth extrusion.

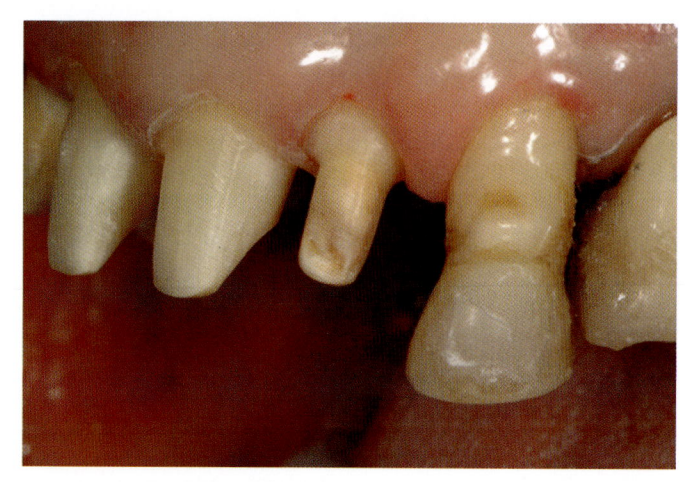

Figure 17.14 (C) Postorthodontic extrusion and provisional preparations on remaining maxillary incisors. Note tissue level correction from prior image in Figure 17.14B.

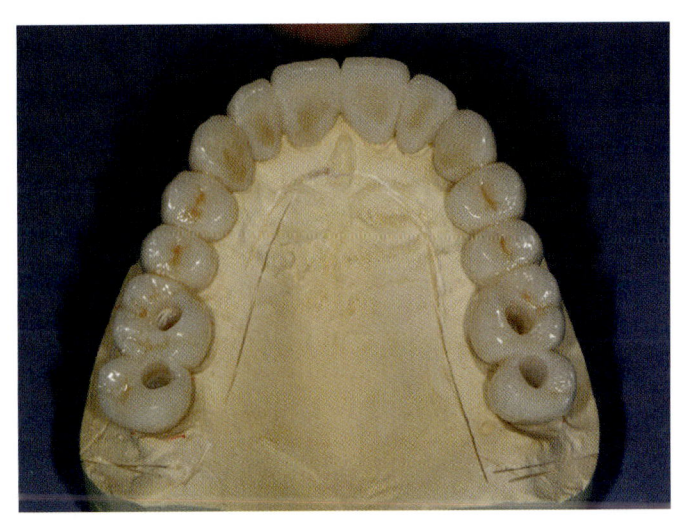

Chapter 17 Replacing Missing Teeth with Fixed Partial Dentures

Figure 17.14 (D) Maxillary occlusal view of the provisionals on the master cast of the provisional restoration for the maxilla.

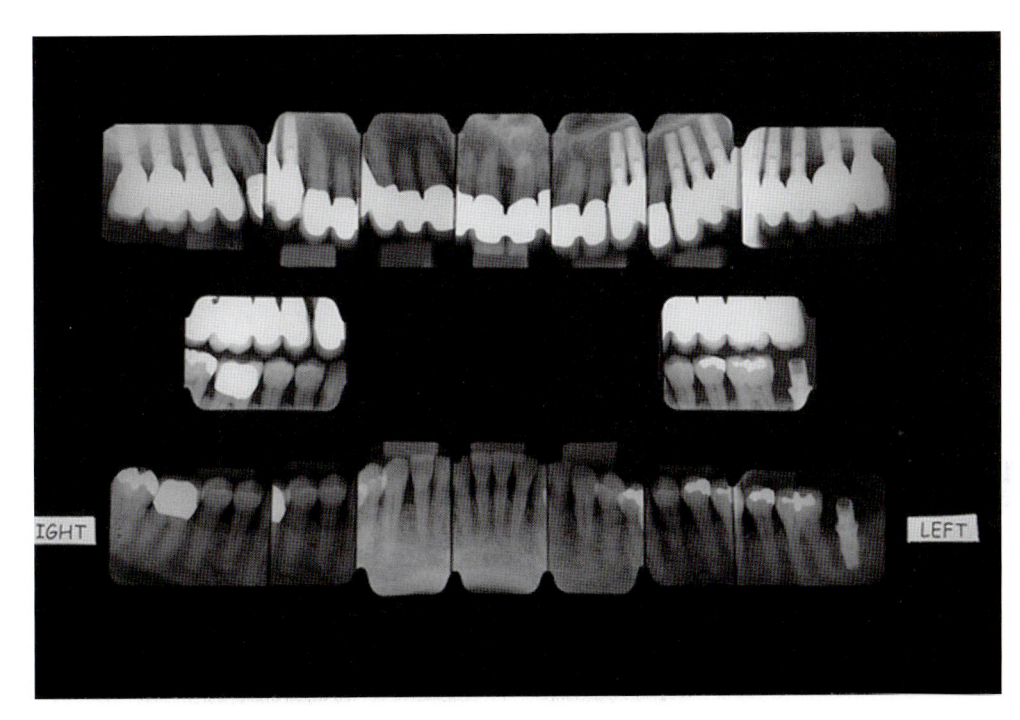

Figure 17.14 (E) Final radiographs.

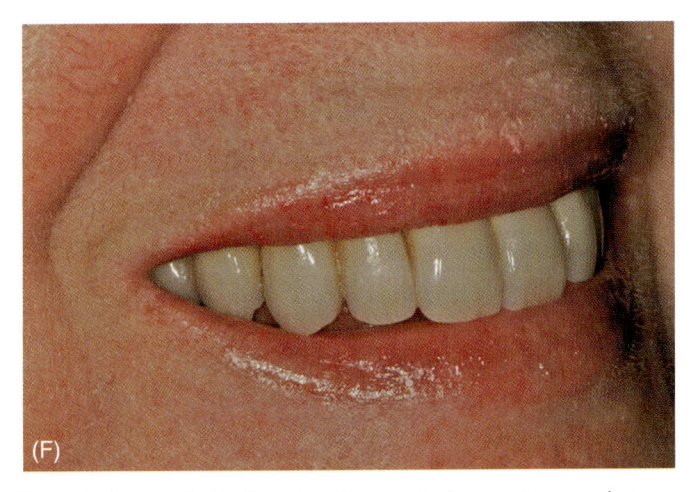

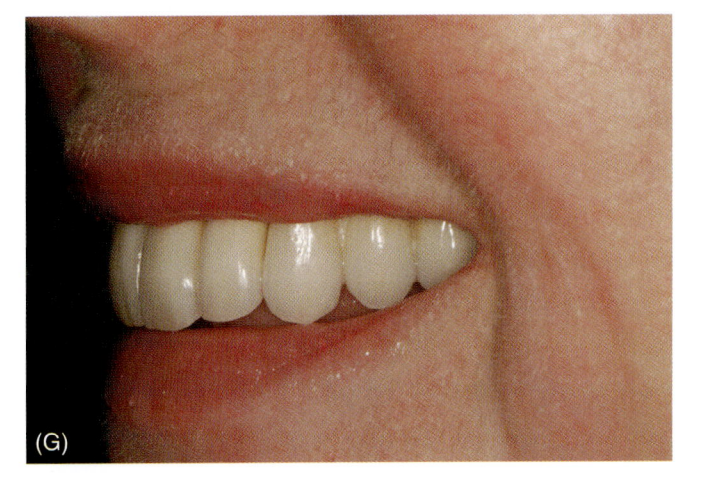

Figure 17.14 (F, G) Final photos of completed restorations in place.

An alternative in the posterior region, where vertical height is often restricted, is the open-telescopic technique. The occlusal surface of the restoration is wholly or partially a part of the inner coping, and the outer crown fits around the inner coping. Provision must be made for occlusal seating by incorporating a shoulder in the coping.

It is of paramount importance that the patient be educated on the advantages and limitations of the telescoping and superstructure technique prior to the commencement of treatment.

Evolving technologies

Today's evolving technologies are providing us with exciting new treatment options for the diagnosis and treatment of missing teeth. These new diagnostic and technological breakthroughs have provided the clinician with improved data for the 3D diagnosis of pathology, virtual 3D treatment planning capabilities, including placement of dental implants, virtual diagnostic wax-up, and design of abutment support and superstructure frameworks, and the final actual CAD/CAM prosthesis ready for the technologist's final esthetic customization. The new materials available, if utilized properly, are stronger, have potentially more accurate marginal fit than traditional techniques, and can provide excellent esthetic results.

The patient in Figure 17.15A–H reported esthetic dissatisfaction with her severely worn 18-year-old implant-supported hybrid denture. She was 88 years old and required disassembly of her prostheses every 3 months for hygiene maintenance as the implants were inaccessible for cleaning due to the large ridge lap design of the prosthesis. She routinely required chronic repairs to the maxillary prosthesis, and the bilateral zygomatic implants were failing, probing over 20 mm with suppuration. The previously placed pterygoid implants were unloaded owing to the patient's inability to keep them clean and were painful due to their position in the unattached buccal mucosa.

The treatment plan was to submerge the pterygoid implants, shorten and submerge the remaining zygomatic implants, use cone beam computed tomography to plan additional implants for

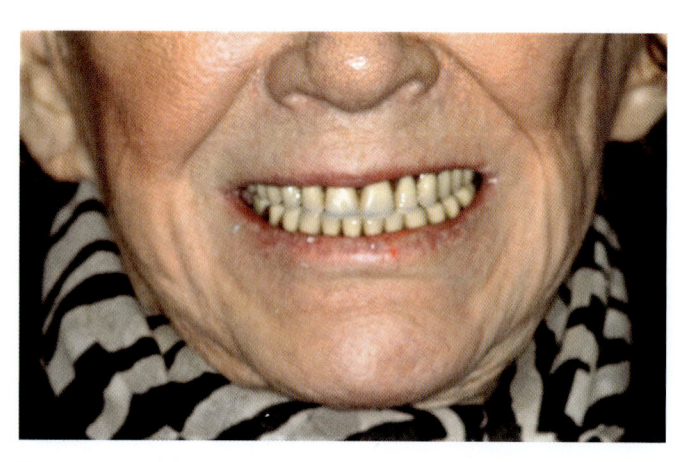

Figure 17.15 (A) A patient presented with a traditional, 20-year-old, maxillary hybrid prosthesis that was in chronic need of removal for repairs and proper hygienic access on recall visits.

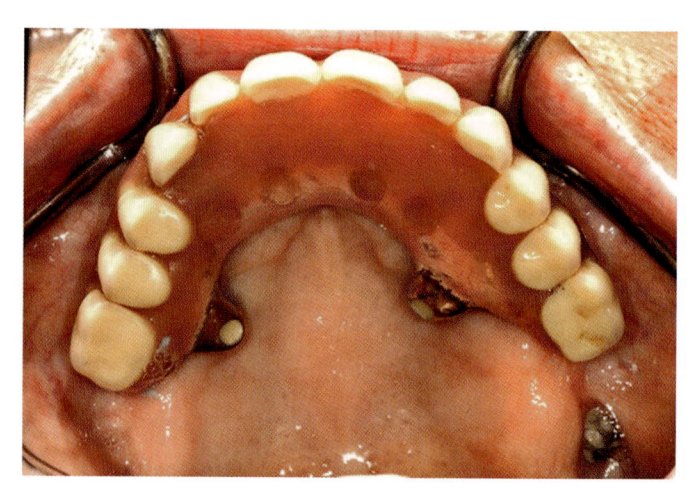

Figure 17.15 (B) An intraoral view of the prosthesis in place illustrates the challenging implant position that resulted in unhygienic contours and impingement into the patient's tongue space.

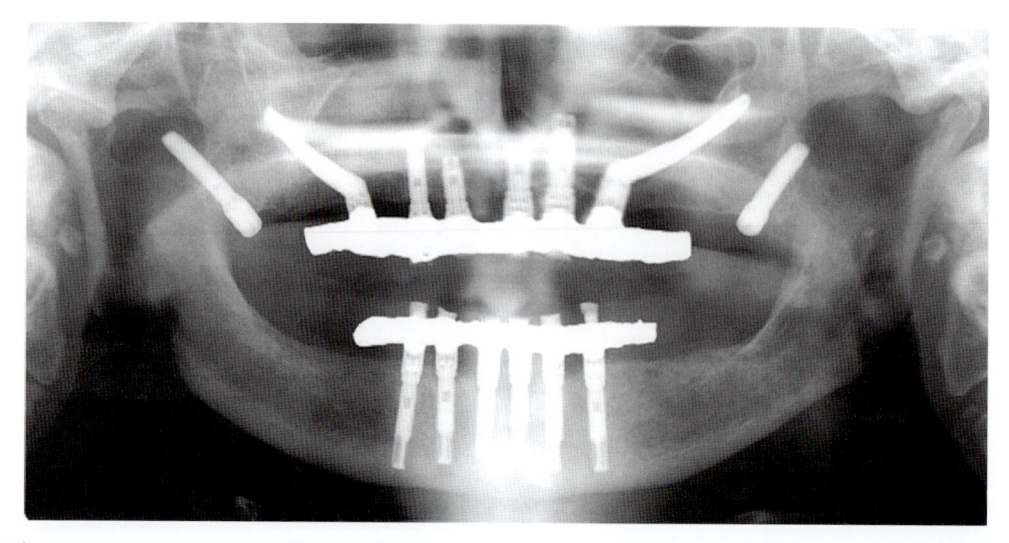

Figure 17.15 (C) Before treatment: panoramic radiograph demonstrates preexisting prosthesis with failing zygomatic implants.

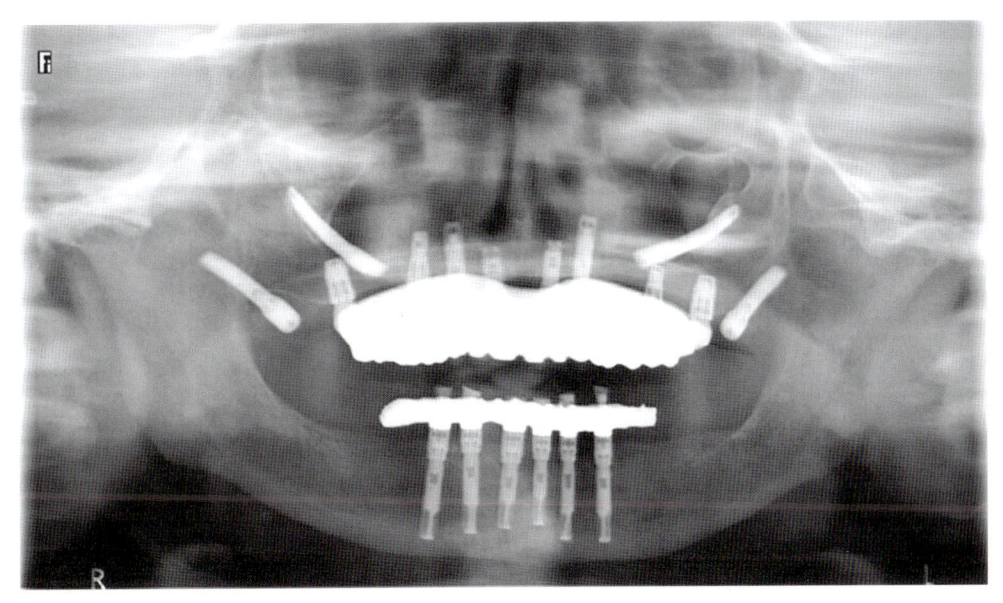

Figure 17.15 **(D)** After treatment: panoramic radiograph demonstrates new prosthesis in place with four new implants for fixed retention and unloading and submersion of the zygomatic implants.

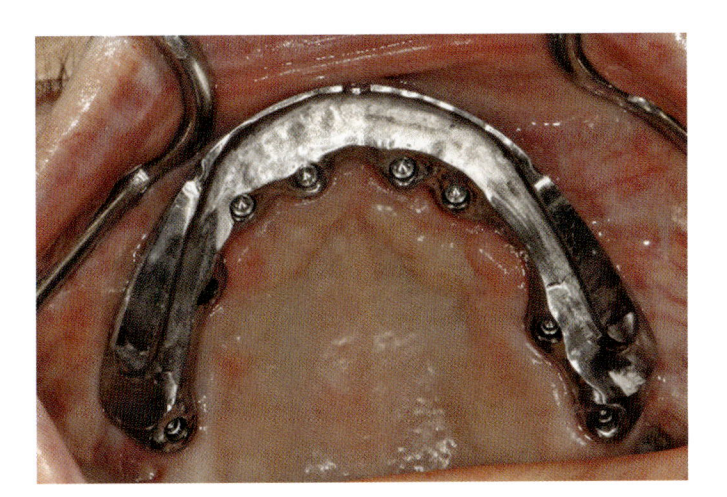

Figure 17.15 **(E)** Intraoral occlusion view of maxillary supportive (substructure) titanium bar in place.

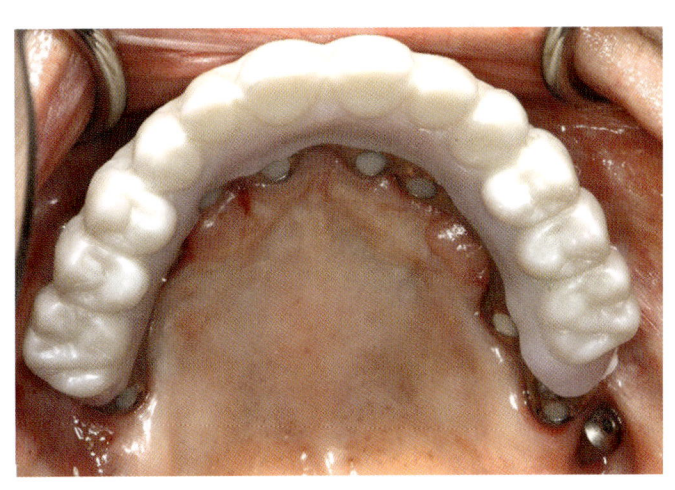

Figure 17.15 **(F)** Intraoral view of maxillary zirconia preliminary suprastructure in place for esthetic try-in.

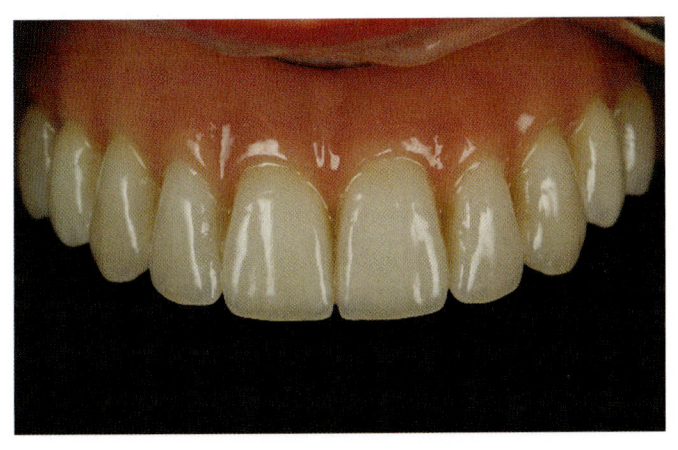

Figure 17.15 **(G)** Retracted view of final esthetic outcome. Note pleasant esthetic outcome achieved with zirconia prosthesis conservatively veneered with feldspathic porcelain for the six anteriors.

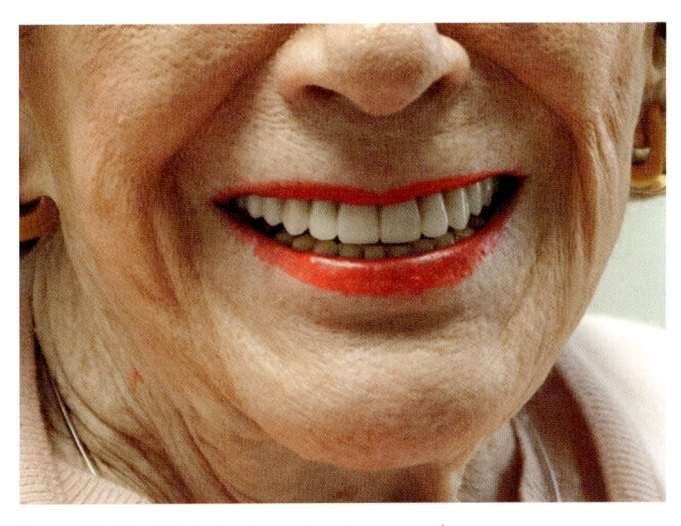

Figure 17.15 **(H)** Patient's posttreatment smile.

required support, and then design a new CAD/CAM maxillary prosthesis. Four new implants were planned and placed to augment the preexisting, still serviceable dental implants. The newly placed implants enabled a reconfiguration of the maxillary superstructure design with a reduced ridge lap for hygiene access.

The infection was eliminated by the debridement and submersion of the zygomatic and pterygoid implants. The patient had improved access for oral health maintenance, improved esthetics, and improved biomechanics. The patient was elderly and medically compromised, and the elimination of infection was of critical importance to her health. On completion of the restoration, the patient reported an improvement in her overall health and was very pleased with the improvement in esthetics.

Radiographic examination/cone beam computed tomography

Three-dimensional analyses and visualization are critical to accurately and safely perform the surgical plan and execution of treatment. This is especially critical when there is a deficiency of bone or critical anatomical structures. The ability to transfer the surgical plan into a surgical guide/stent and a preoperative model on which the restoration can be fabricated has increased the efficiency, cost, and accuracy of implant-supported prostheses. Historically, conventional two-dimensional radiographic analyses were challenging and supplemented by direct visualization at the time of surgery. Computerized tomography can assist the evaluation of regional anatomy but is costly and also exposes the patient to a higher dosage of radiation.

All-ceramic/zirconia fixed partial dentures

There is increasing use of zirconia (yttria-containing tetragonal zirconia polycrystal) not only for single crowns, but also for short-span fixed partial dentures and full-arch zirconia frameworks.[62,63] Zirconia's high flexural strength (900–1200 MPa) and high fracture toughness (9–10 MPa m$^{1/2}$) enable its use in full-arch restorations.[64] Milled, partially sintered zirconia is popular for the fabrication of fixed partial dentures owing to their consistent fit, reliability, and reduced labor and material costs.

The phenomenon of low-temperature degradation is when water penetrates a surface crack, resulting in propagation of the microfracture, grain pullout, and surface roughness.[65] Currently, there is no definitive relationship between low-temperature degradation and the clinical failure of zirconia fixed partial dentures.[66] There are very few studies on the clinical performance of implant-supported zirconia fixed partial dentures and single crowns, or long-term clinical trials.[67-70] Catastrophic fractures of fixed partial dentures through the zirconia core after 2–5 years were 1–8% and were 7% for single crowns after 2 years. Occlusal overloading in bruxers resulting in fractures through the zirconia core were also attributed to insufficient framework thickness <0.3 mm, especially through the connector in long-span fixed partial dentures.[71,72] Higher rates of fracturing of the veneering porcelain were reported for implant-supported single crowns (8%) than for tooth-supported single crowns, where there was a 2–9% failure of the veneering porcelain after 6 months–3 years. Implant fixed partial dentures had porcelain veneer fracture rates of 53% after 1 year compared with 3–30% for tooth-supported fixed partial dentures after 1–5 years.[62] To minimize failure of the veneering porcelain, a full-contour wax-up and cut-back is recommended to control the thickness of the zirconia coping and support the overlying porcelain. Careful adjustment of the zirconia is critical to minimize the formation of surface microfractures and roughness, and avoidance of postsintering modifications is recommended.[73,74]

Use of precision attachments

When it is not advisable or feasible to use a one-piece superstructure, interlocking suprastructure segments can assist in creating cross-arch stabilization in a segmented superstructure. Precision attachments that have an open rod and sleeve design can be preferable compared with the dictated sequence of removal required of the male/female attachments.

Semiprecision or precision internal attachments in fixed partial dentures may improve the quality of the prosthesis significantly. Precision attachments can eliminate parallelism problems, interlock smaller segments to avoid lengthy spans of porcelain-fused-to-metal restorations, and provide splinting of periodontally mobile segments. Additionally, they can provide a stress breaking protection in cases of cuspid abutments attached to posterior fixed partial dentures (Figure 17.16A–C).

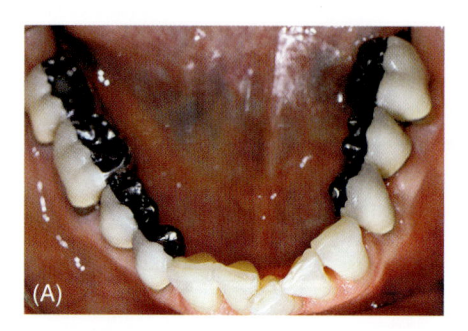

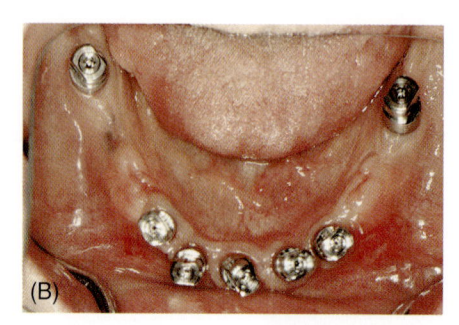

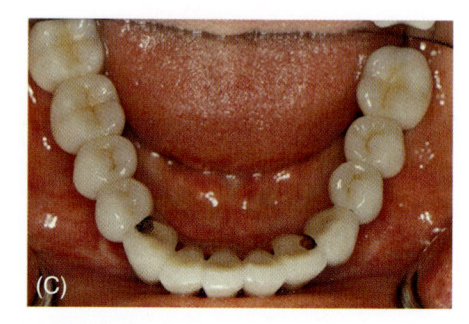

Figure 17.16 (A) Intraoral occlusal view of a hopeless mandibular natural dentition. All remaining teeth were planned for extraction and replacement with endosseous implants. (B) Impression copings in place for the final impression for the fabrication of an implant-retained complete mandibular rehabilitation. The superstructures were planned for solderless joint connections distal to the cuspids for retrievability and improved accuracy for fabrication. (C) Occlusal view of the completed implant-retained prosthesis in place. Note the solderless joints placed distal to the cuspid restorations.

Pontics

Pontic design

The overall objective in pontic design is to achieve esthetics, function, and cleansability. Additionally, the tooth substitute should be in harmony with the abutment teeth and the remaining dentition. Concealing the pontic as an artificial replacement is accomplished with attention to its outline form, size, alignment, embrasure form, contour, surface texture, and color. In addition, it must function with the opposing occlusion and provide comfort and support to the adjacent tissues (Figure 17.17A–F).

There are several pontic designs available for fixed partial dentures. The choices include ridge lap (saddle), modified ridge lap, conical or bullet, hygienic (sanitary), and the ovate pontic (Figure 17.18A–E). Esthetics, phonetics, edentulous ridge anatomy, and the patient's ability to maintain adequate hygiene must be considered during pontic design. Hygienic pontics are relegated to the posterior, nonesthetic zone and act to restore occlusal function while preventing the drifting of adjacent teeth. Conical or bullet-shaped pontics are indicated for thin mandibular ridges; however, they may have larger embrasure spaces, resulting in a tendency to collect debris. The ridge-lap pontic is the least favorable design owing to the patient's inability to maintain adequate oral hygiene and is not recommended.

To optimize esthetics and create a natural-appearing emergence profile, the modified ridge lap[75] and the ovate pontic[35,76] are the preferred pontic designs. Certain conditions are required to accomplish a favorable esthetic outcome. The pontic must have the proper incisogingival or occlusogingival length in relation to the abutment teeth. Excessively open interproximal embrasures or "black triangles" must be avoided in the anterior

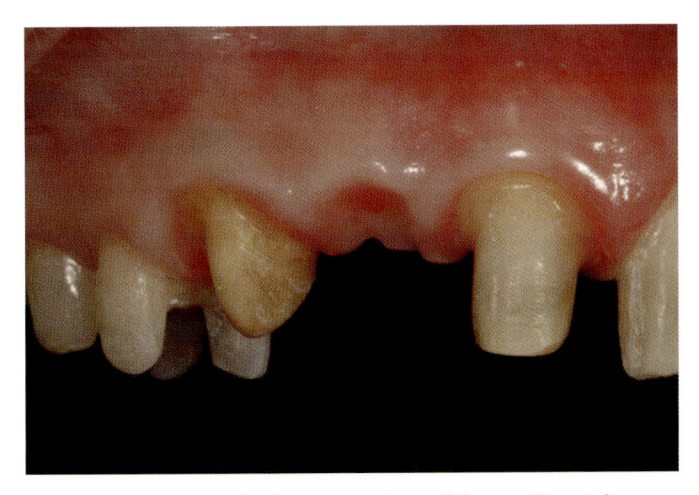

Figure 17.17 (A) Final bridge preparations of the maxillary right cuspid to central with ovate pontic site preparation utilizing connective tissue grafts for tissue augmentation.

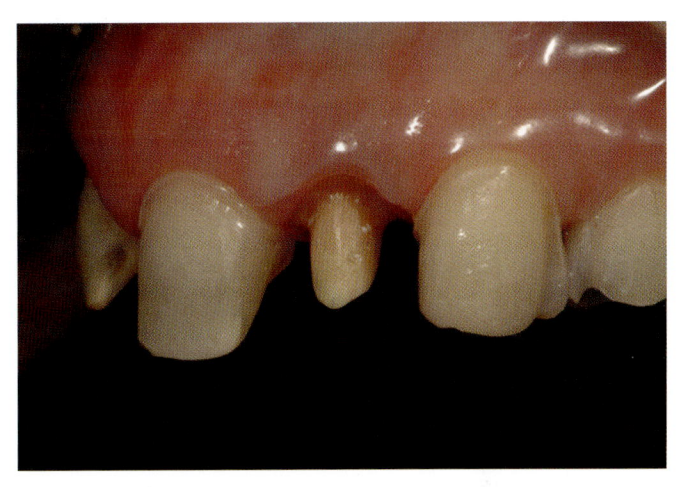

Figure 17.17 (B) Contralateral tooth preparations illustrating symmetry of natural contours with the grafted pontic site.

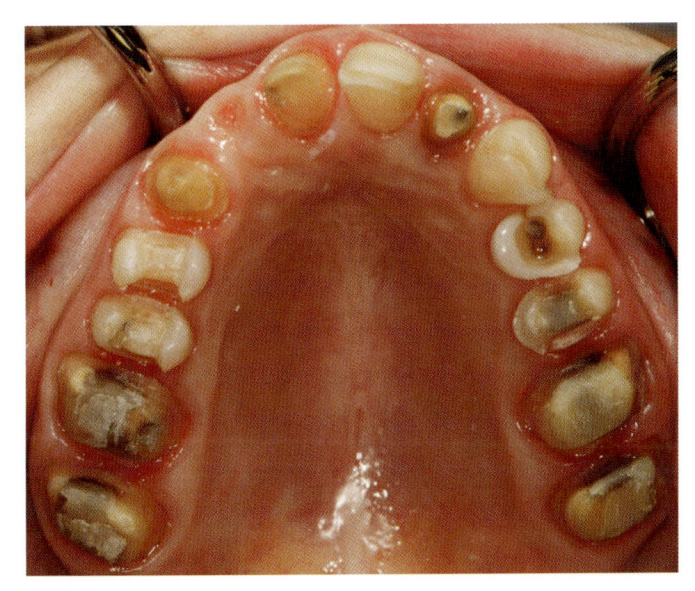

Figure 17.17 (C) Occlusal view of the maxillary arch demonstrating tooth-specific preparation designs ranging from porcelain veneers, inlays, veneer onlays, to full-coverage restorations.

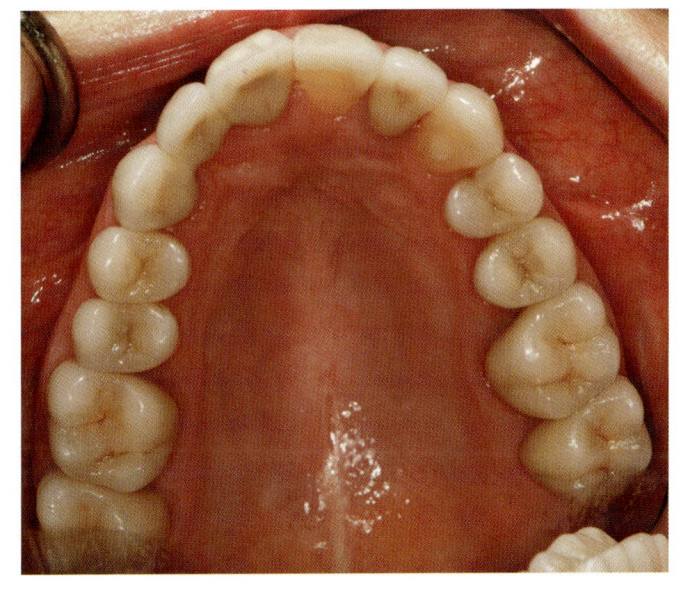

Figure 17.17 (D) Occlusal view of maxillary arch.

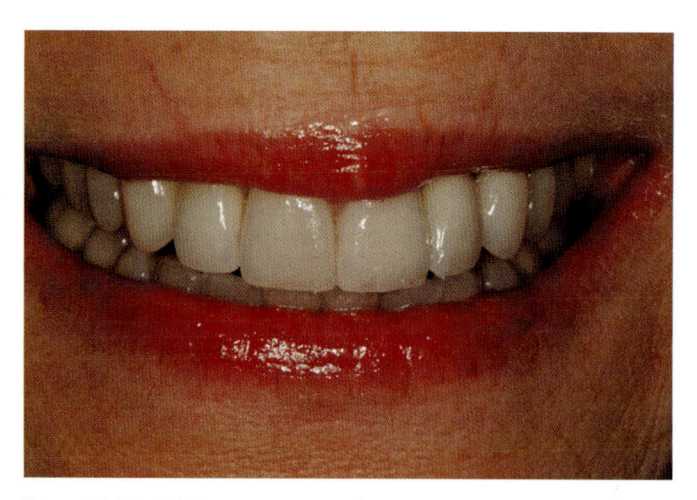

Figure 17.17 **(E)** Posttreatment smile.

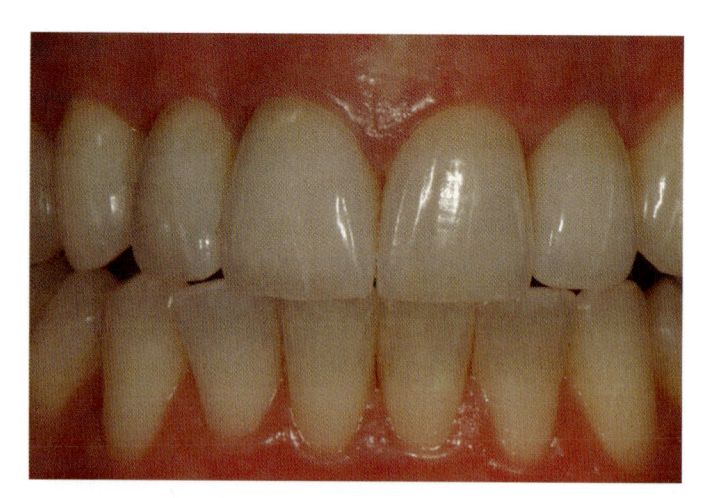

Figure 17.17 **(F)** Anterior view of final restorations.

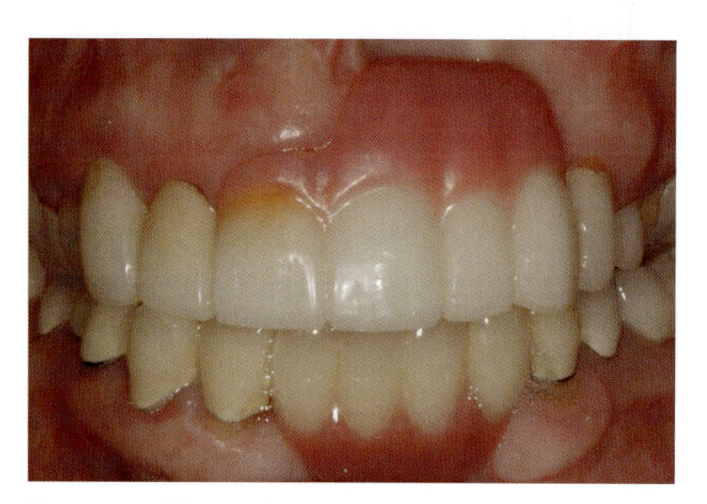

Figure 17.18 **(A)** Pontic design: total ridge lap.

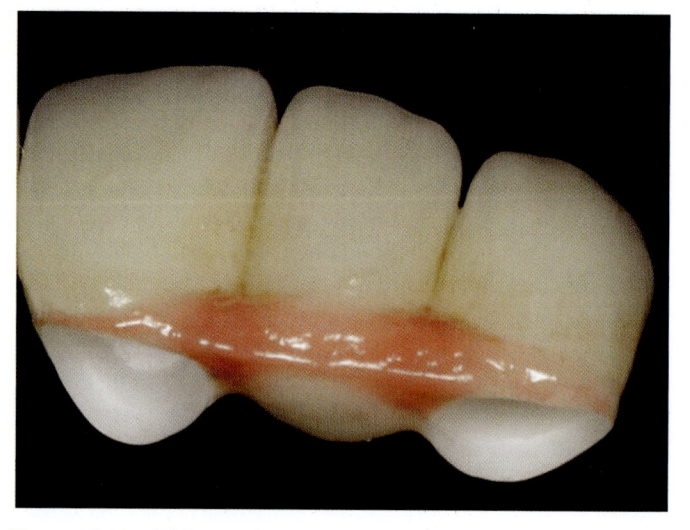

Figure 17.18 **(B)** Pontic design: intaglio surface of modified ridge-lap pontic.

region, and a proper labiolingual or buccolingual relationship with the abutment teeth should be obtained for a natural emergence profile. To accomplish these three requirements, ideal edentulous ridge form is imperative. Preprosthetic surgery is often required to enhance the edentulous ridge to achieve the desired esthetic goals.

Preparation of tissue

A diagnostic wax-up of the planned fixed partial denture will aid in assessing the pontic–ridge relationship to determine whether the three design requirements are met.

The edentulous ridge with ideal dimensions both buccolingually and occlusogingivally can be treated with a modified ridge-lap pontic design, meeting all three esthetic design requirements. Ridge contour for the modified ridge-lap pontic should be slightly convex in a labiolingual direction and gently concave mesiodistally.[77] Modified ridge-lap pontic contours should not extend lingually past the middle of the edentulous ridge. For the edentulous ridge that has excessive hard or soft tissue, surgical reduction can be performed. If the soft tissue is thick, scalloping of the tissue may create a favorable pontic site. If the hard tissue is excessive with a minimal soft-tissue covering, osseous recontouring or resection may be necessary.

Ovate pontic designs are generally used in two types of clinical situations: the healed edentulous ridge and new extraction sites. When a healed edentulous ridge exists, the recipient site requires a surgical procedure of hard tissue, soft tissue, or both to provide proper emergence from the tissue. In a new extraction site, the abutment teeth can be prepared and the fixed partial denture provisional fabricated. Then, the ovate pontic provisional can be placed so that it emerges from the immature extraction site. This type of procedure quite often leads to a highly acceptable esthetic effect, but requires an adequately wide labiolingual ridge dimension.[32]

Frequently, a deficient edentulous ridge involves adjunctive soft- and/or hard-tissue augmentation. Deficient pontic areas may occur as a result of trauma, periodontal disease, root or buccal plate fractures, periapical lesions, or developmental

Figure 17.18 **(C)** Pontic design: clinical view of modified ridge lap.

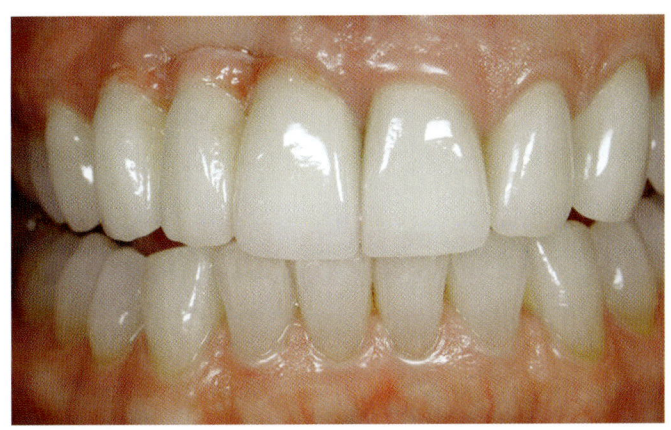

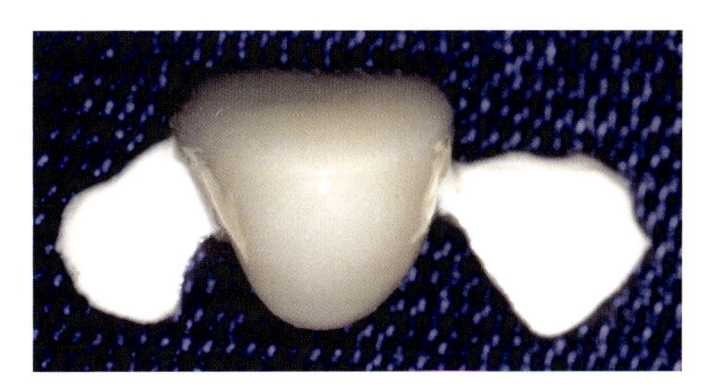

Figure 17.18 **(D)** Pontic design: intaglio surface of ovate pontic.

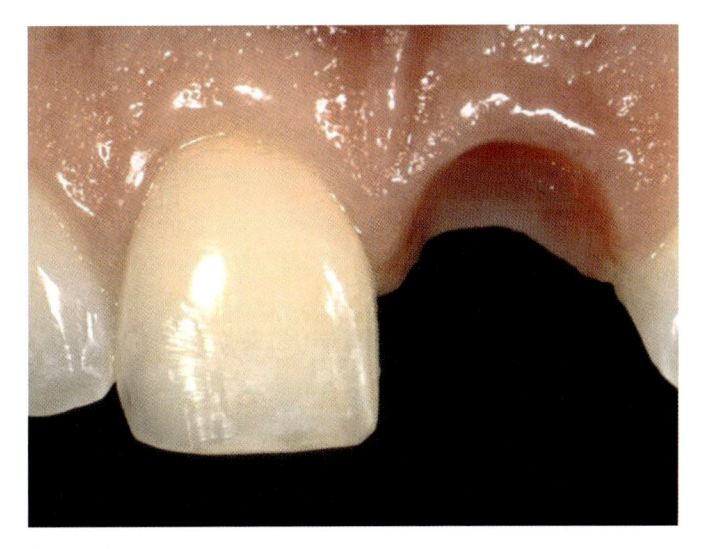

Figure 17.18 **(E)** Pontic design: clinical view of ovate pontic site.

defects. The edentulous area may be deficient in height, width, or both, depending on the individual situation. The classification system by Seibert describes: (1) buccolingual loss of tissue with normal ridge height (Class I), (2) apicocoronal loss of tissue with normal ridge width (Class II), or (3) combined loss of ridge contour in both the buccolingual and apicocoronal dimensions (Class III).[78] For the deficient ridge, adjunctive treatment involves surgical augmentation, which can be accomplished using an autogenous or allogenic bone graft, placement of subepithelial connective tissue grafts, rolling a pediculated flap buccally, an alloplastic graft, or a combination of these techniques depending on the amount of donor tissue needed to repair the defect of augmentation required.[38,76,77,79–81] The volume of donor tissue needed to repair the defect and the availability of such tissue will affect the selection of the graft material.[82] Larger augmentations quite often involve multiple surgeries to achieve optimal results. For sites that can be augmented with soft tissue alone, esthetic results can often be obtained with one surgical grafting procedure.[83] If the deficient site cannot be augmented, for reasons that may include cost, medical history, or too severe a defect, another modality such as a removable partial denture should be considered or tissue replacement with the use of a pink restorative material (Figure 17.19A–H).[84]

The goal of the pontic site tissue preparation procedure is to provide a ridge in which the pontic displays a natural emergence profile and is harmonious with the surrounding dentition. Although the hard tissue gives the augmented site the necessary structure and support, proper soft-tissue contours and thickness provide the illusion of a natural tooth emergence in an edentulous site. Tissue thickness over the edentulous ridge areas can vary depending on the location. In Stein's study of 50 anterior ridges and 50 posterior ridges, he found that, regardless of the degree of ridge atrophy, the mean tissue thickness of the posterior regions was 2.05 mm. The mandibular anterior region was similar to the posterior regions, whereas the maxillary anterior regions showed a mean tissue thickness of 4.13 mm.[85] This study and many others have shown that a certain thickness of tissue needs to be maintained, and encroachment on the tissue by the pontic may lead to an inflammatory process. If additional tissue thickness is generated over the ridge, soft-tissue modification can be performed.[75] Seibert Class I category defects can be treated with a soft-tissue augmentation procedure buccally to improve esthetics. This is a highly successful and fairly predictable procedure. Seibert Class II and Class III defects are much less predictable and quite often require multiple surgeries to increase the likelihood of a successful esthetic result.

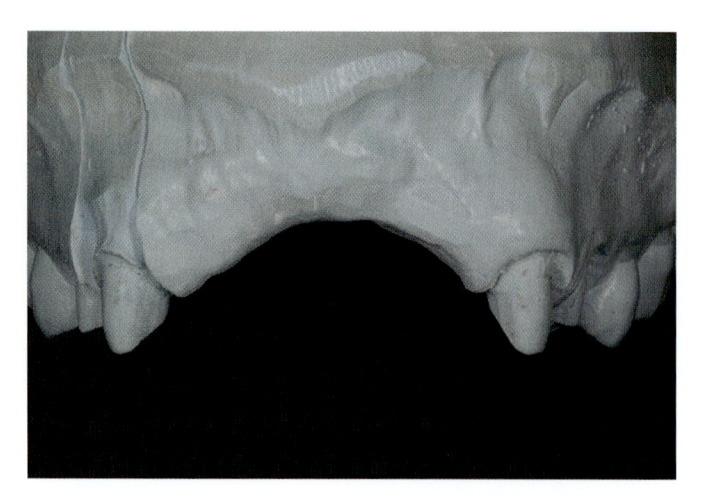

Figure 17.19 **(A)** A patient had experienced extensive bone loss in the anterior maxilla. After two failed attempts at dental implants and bone grafting, a conventional tooth-borne fixed prosthesis was determined to be the most suitable treatment option.

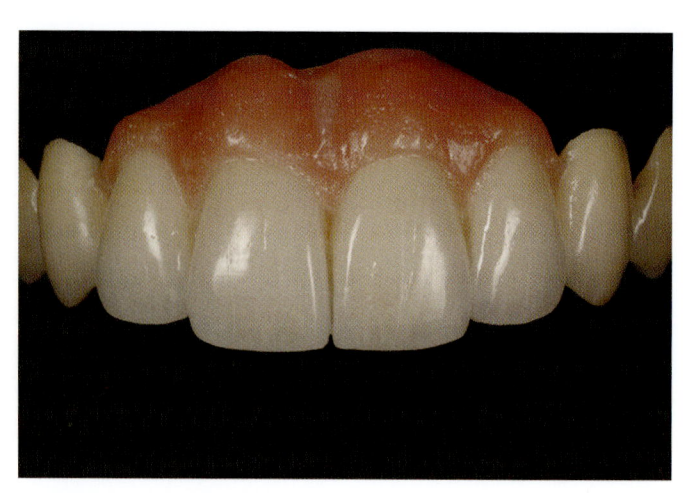

Figure 17.19 **(B)** The fixed prosthesis was created to simulate the replacement of both the teeth and the osseous and gingival tissues.

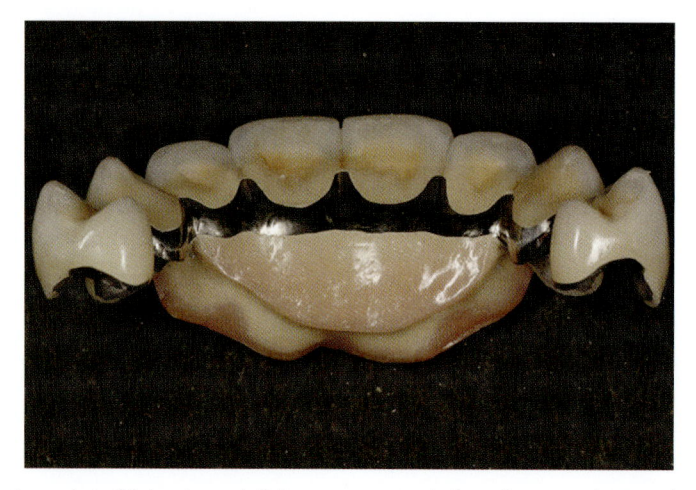

Figure 17.19 **(C)** The elaborate pontic made to fill the tissue deficiency was ovate in form for ease of proper hygiene and overall longevity of the restoration.

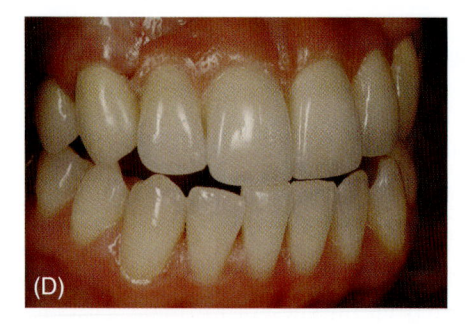

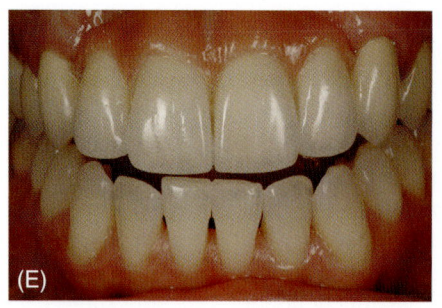

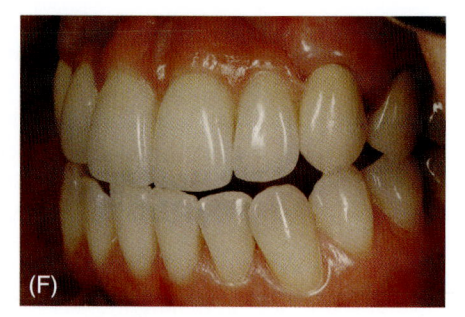

Figure 17.19 **(D–F)** Retracted views of the completed treatment with the fixed partial prosthesis cemented into place.

The future pontic site often has a nonrestorable tooth with deficient attachment apparatus, resulting in a soft-tissue defect. Orthodontic extrusion before extraction may be an alternative that can help modify the ridge and benefit pontic site design by bringing down the bone as the tooth erupts, thus eliminating or reducing any preexisting defects.[78]

Prosthodontic preparation prior to ridge augmentation is necessary in order to facilitate a successful esthetic outcome (Figure 17.20A–G). Prior to ridge augmentation, the abutments are prepared and a provisional acrylic resin fixed partial denture is fabricated. The proper form and function of the prosthesis are created in the provisional, and the pontic intaglio surface (the tissue-borne surface) is designed to simulate the position and contour desired in the final prostheses. At the surgical appointment, the provisional is removed and the ridge is augmented. The surgeon uses the intaglio surface of the pontic as a reference

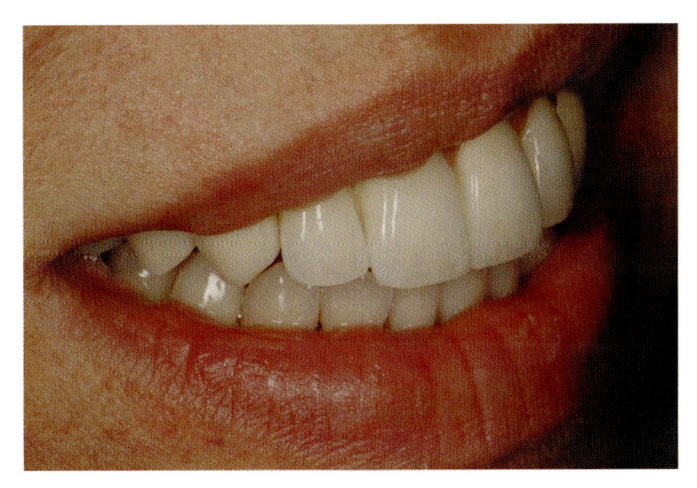

Chapter 17 Replacing Missing Teeth with Fixed Partial Dentures

Figure 17.19 **(G)** A lateral view of the patient's completed smile illustrates the efforts made to create natural tooth contours and alignment that complement the patient's facial profile and lip contours.

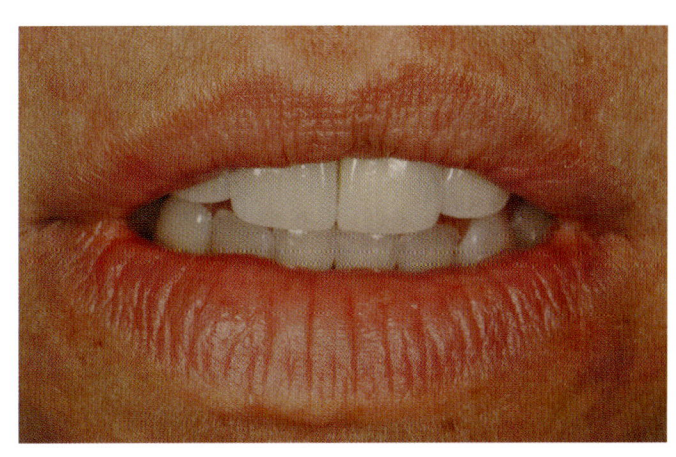

Figure 17.19 **(H)** An esthetic outcome was achieved in all facial expressions.

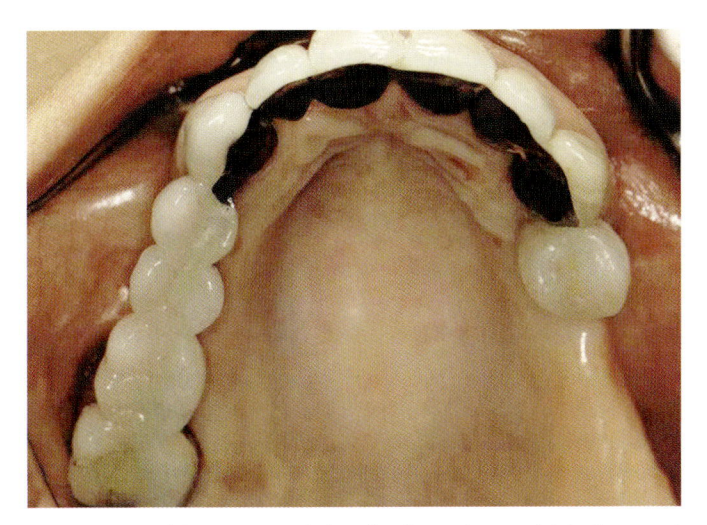

Figure 17.20 **(A)** Preexisting failing fixed prostheses with leakage and recurrent decay.

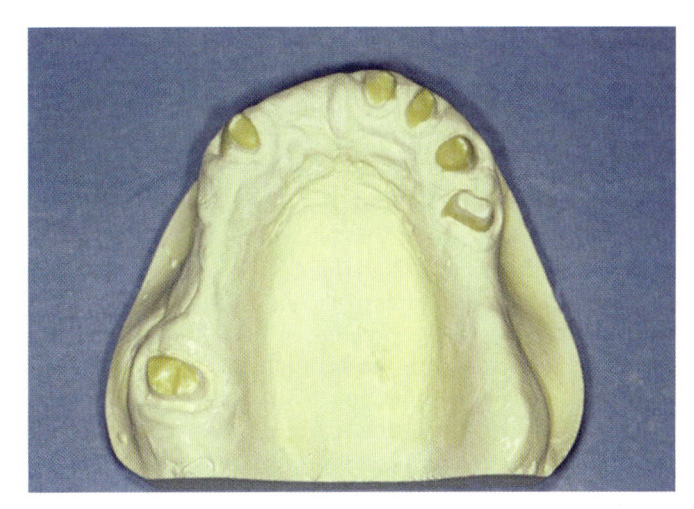

Figure 17.20 **(B)** The maxillary stone cast of the remaining abutments. Bone/ridge augmentations were required to allow implants to be placed in the posterior regions and improve tissue architecture in the anterior region where a tooth-borne fixed prosthesis was planned.

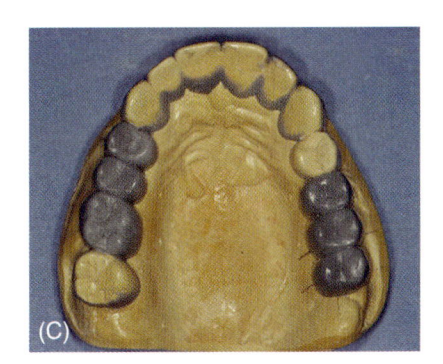

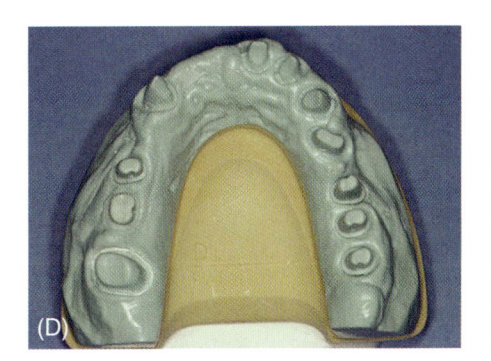

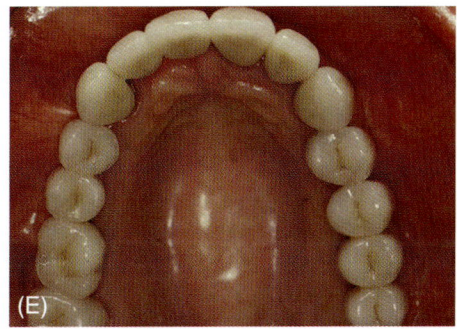

Figure 17.20 **(C)** A view of the maxillary arch wax-up following completion of the augmentation procedures. **(D)** An occlusal view of the maxillary arch illustrates the augmented ridges and implant placement compared with the prior configuration seen in Figure 17.20B, created for the support of the future restorations. **(E)** An occlusal view of the completed treatment. The tooth-borne and implant-borne prostheses are cemented independent of one another for biomechanical reasons.

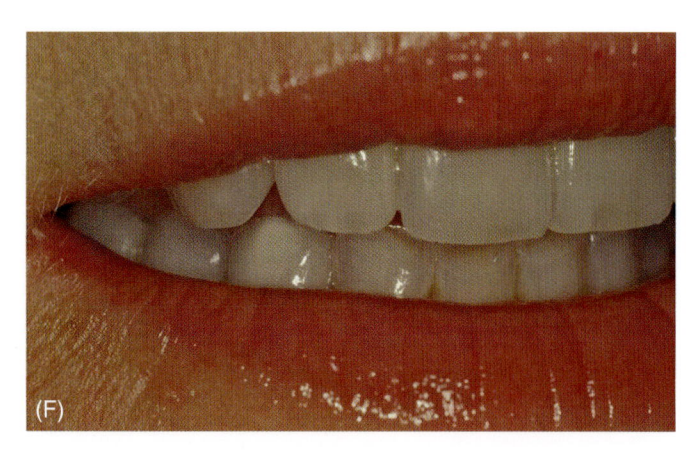

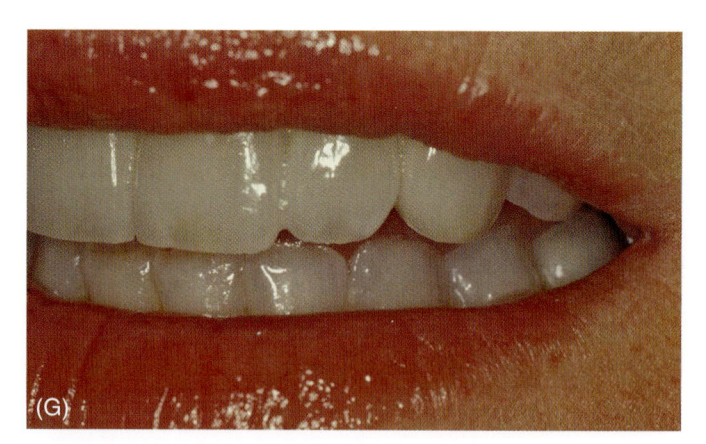

Figure 17.20 **(F, G)** The final esthetic outcome of the treatment combining both tooth-borne and implant-borne final prostheses for the rehabilitation of the maxillary arch.

point for the amount of augmentation, making sure to compensate for tissue shrinkage. The intaglio surface of the pontic is then modified prior to recementation, ensuring little to no tissue contact. The surgical site is allowed to heal for 6–8 weeks, depending on the location (longer period for anterior esthetic areas). Once adequate healing has occurred, the provisional fixed partial denture is removed and the pontic intaglio surface is modified by forming acrylic resin to the ideal shape. At this point of healing, the soft tissue is modified either by electrosurgery, a surgical blade, laser surgery, or rotary instrumentation to a contour adaptive to the provisional. The highly polished provisional is temporarily cemented and the area allowed to heal for an additional 6–8 weeks prior to making the final impression for the definitive prosthesis. "Scalloping" the soft-tissue site and adapting the fabricated provisional to the scalloped site affords the clinician the opportunity to shape the tissue, creating an esthetic prosthesis. The tissue scalloping allows the pontic to closely mimic the emergence of the abutment teeth. The pontic–ridge relationship will look natural, and the three requirements for an esthetic pontic/edentulous ridge will be met.[86]

If attempts at surgery are unsuccessful or even only moderately successful, resulting in small black triangles, then esthetic masking must take place in the fabrication of the prosthesis. This can take the form of either fixed or removable tissue inserts. The fixed tissue insert can be fabricated from tissue-colored ceramic or composite resin material. Great longevity should be expected if ceramics are used to replace the interdental tissue. Gingival porcelain replaces the lost hard and soft tissue and may prevent food impaction and allow for better phonetics by preventing percolation of saliva during speech.[35] Alternatively, some patients use a removable tissue insert fabricated from acrylic resin.

Pontic materials

The type of material utilized for the pontic depends on the esthetic result required and potentially the materials utilized for the adjacent areas. Pontic material types can be all metal, metal–ceramic, all ceramic, or metal with acrylic resin. Porcelain covering all exposed areas is the most esthetic. Metal with acrylic resin is occasionally used today in the posterior regions when retainer

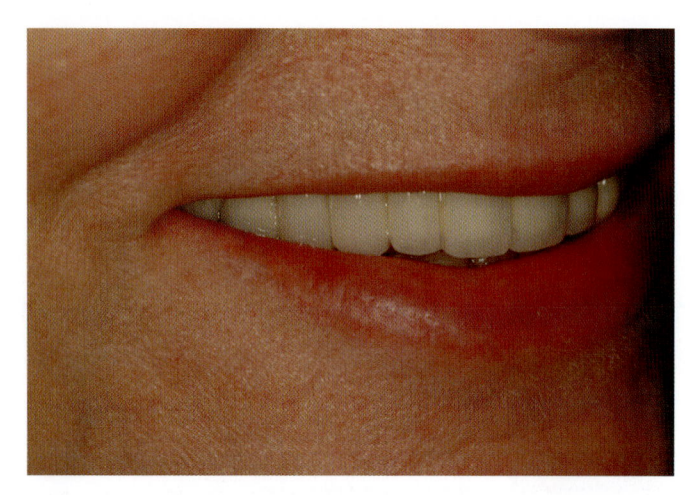

Figure 17.21 **(A)** A right lateral view of a patient's presenting condition. The patient was unhappy with the presenting fixed prosthesis and surrounding restorations. Limiting the tooth size to the contours of the limited edentulous space, often associated with tooth loss, creates and aged/"denture look" to the restorations.

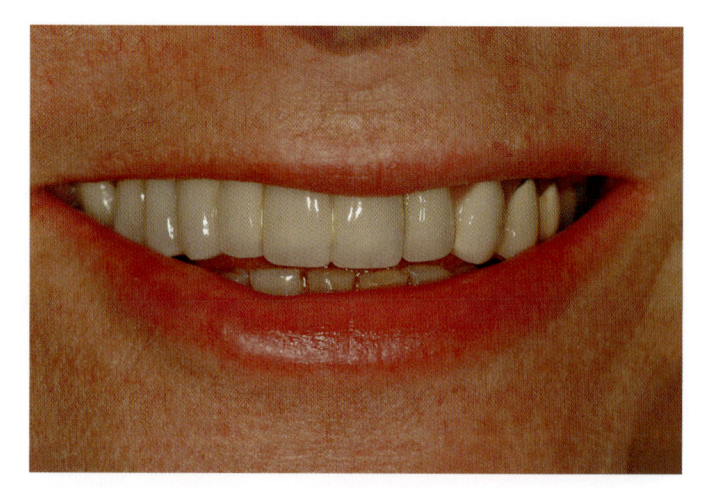

Figure 17.21 **(B)** A frontal view of the patient's smile illustrates the irregularities in the occlusal plane and the lack of symmetry and balance in relation to the patient's natural smile line.

design dictates type III gold. The length of span of a fixed partial denture can influence material choice. Many failures associated with the fixed partial denture can be related to the choice of materials.[87] For longer span fixed partial dentures, a more rigid (higher modulus of elasticity) predominantly base-metal alloy such as Rexillium III (Jeneric/Pentron, Wallingford, CT) may be the alloy of choice to minimize flexure.[88]

Proper pontic–tissue contours and surface finish are the key to healthy tissue response. Pontic design has been found to be the foremost factor in obtaining inflammatory-free pontic–ridge relationships.[85] Surface smoothness and polish are critical factors; there is no observable advantage with porcelain, acrylic resin, or gold. However, Stein also found that modification of the pontic outline form without attention to the surface smoothness did not prevent gingival inflammation.[85] Other studies have found that glazed porcelain and highly polished gold are the preferable materials for tissue contact[45,55] (Figure 17.21A–S).

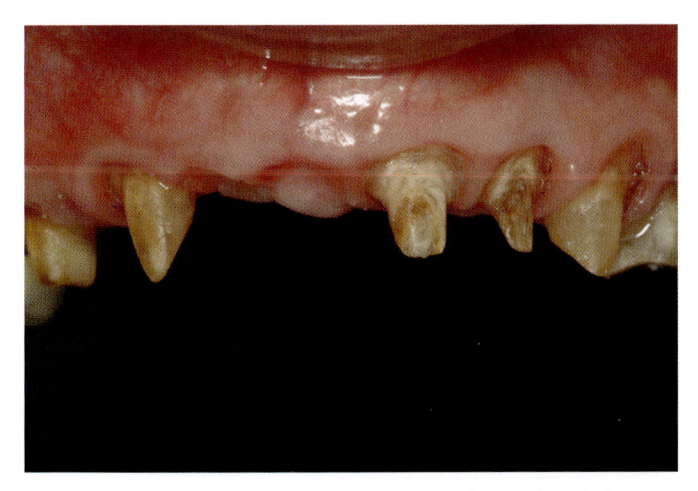

Figure 17.21 (C) The patient underwent several periodontal plastic surgeries, connective tissue grafts, crown lengthenings, and pontic site developments to idealize the overall tissue harmony.

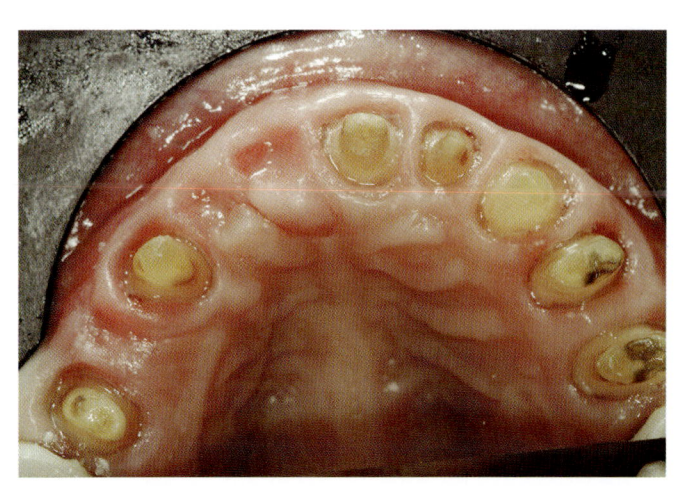

Figure 17.21 (D) An occlusal view of the final tissue harmony and the gingival symmetries established sites for the future fixed prosthesis.

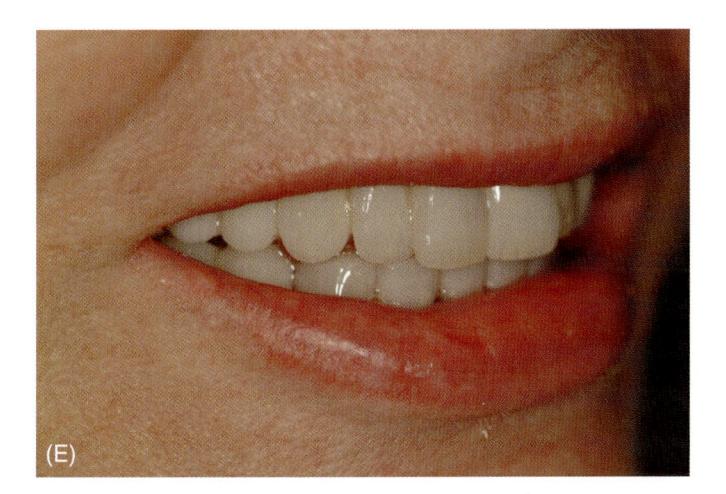

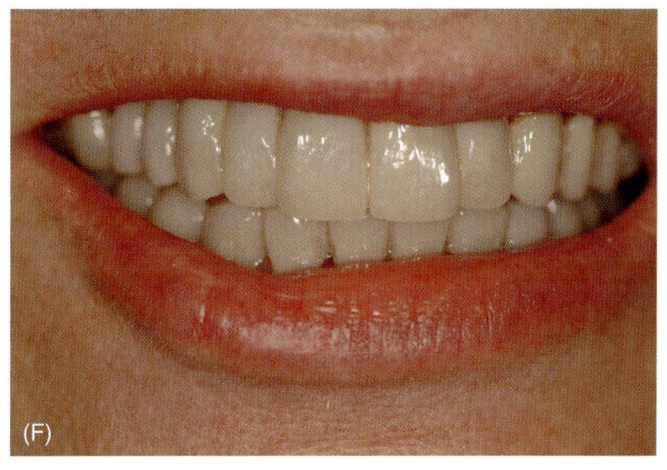

Figure 17.21 (E, F) The provisional restorations for this patient were adjusted over a few separate visits. The occlusal plane, vertical dimension of occlusion, and tooth esthetics were all refined to achieve an esthetic template for the final restorations.

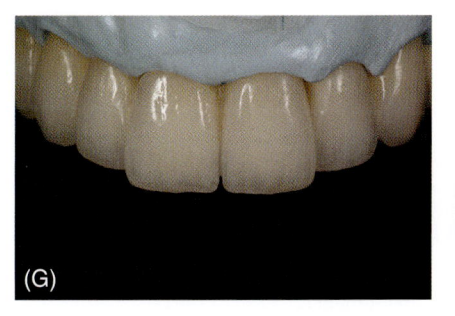

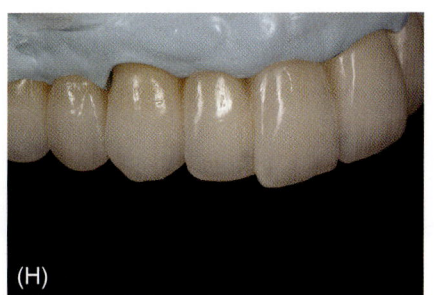

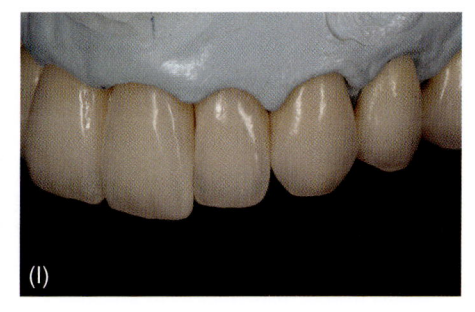

Figure 17.21 (G–I) The completed final prostheses on the master model.

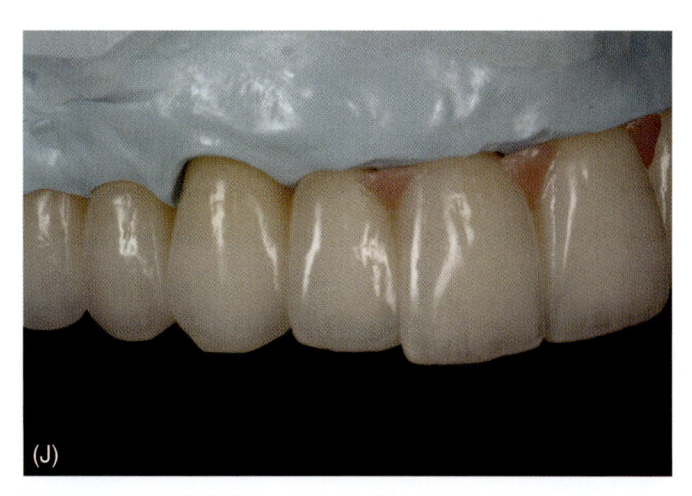

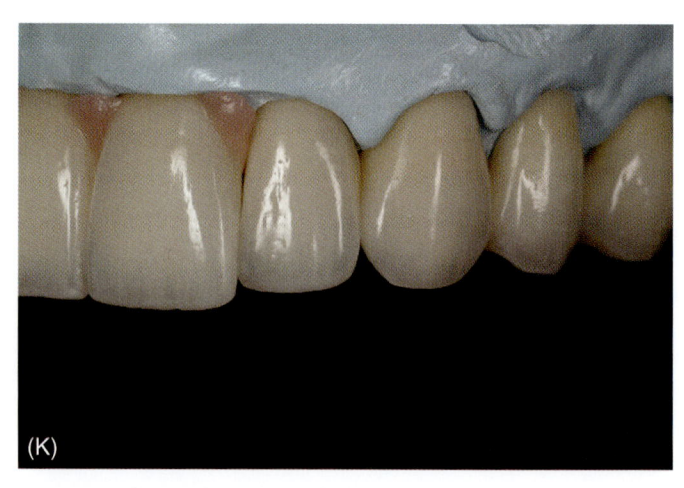

Figure 17.21 **(J, K)** Pink porcelain papilla added to the prosthesis created a more natural tissue harmony with sharp papilla interproximally. The addition of papilla was first tested in the provisional restoration to ensure patient approval and hygienic contours.

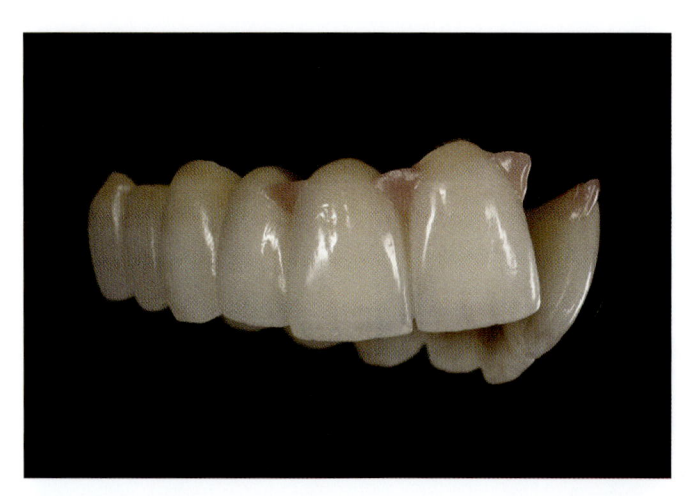

Figure 17.21 **(L)** A close-up view of the pink porcelain papilla added to the fixed partial prosthesis to maximize the esthetic outcome of the patient with a moderately high lip line.

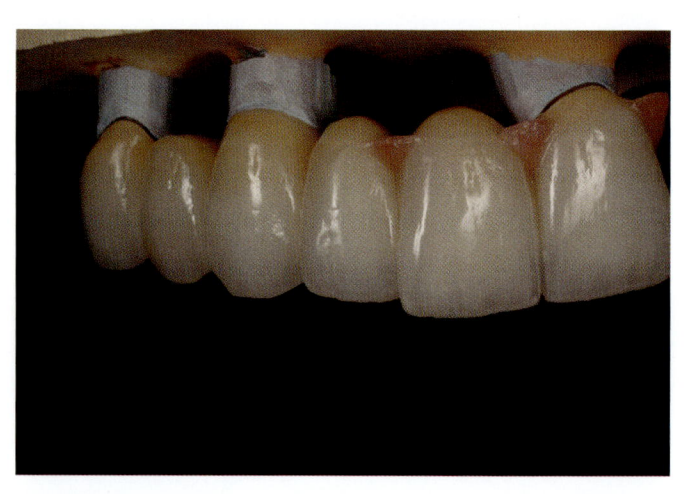

Figure 17.21 **(M)** Three tooth abutments (retainers) were utilized to retain this fixed prosthesis.

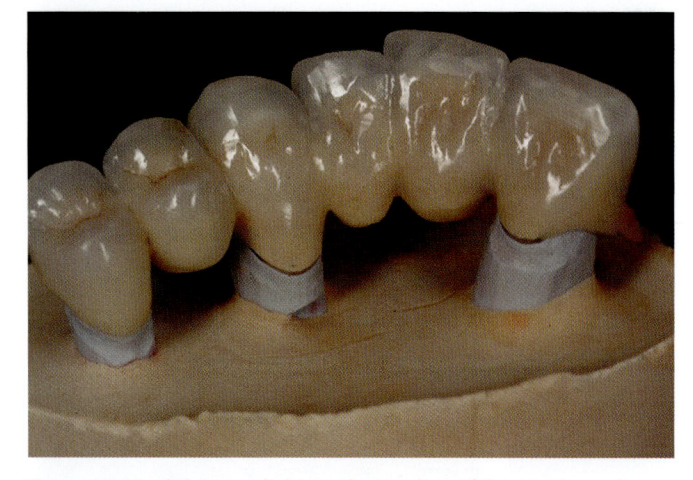

Figure 17.21 **(N)** Some slight tooth crowding of the pontics and abutment crowns creates natural tooth dimensions that will assist in creating a natural esthetic outcome.

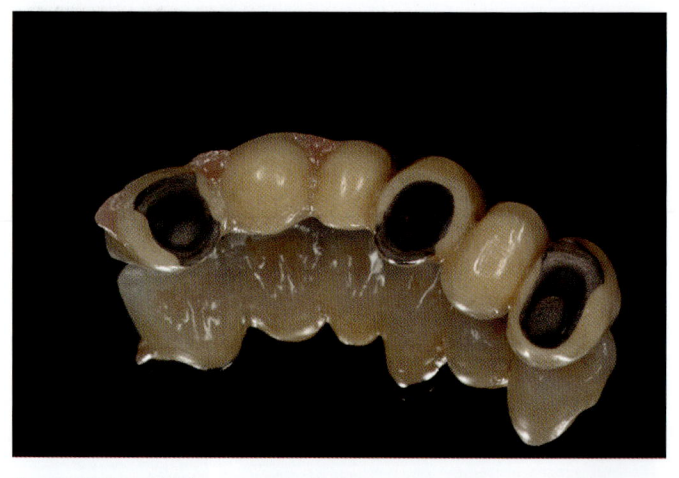

Figure 17.21 **(O)** Ovate pontic designs with contours created for good hygiene access and maintenance.

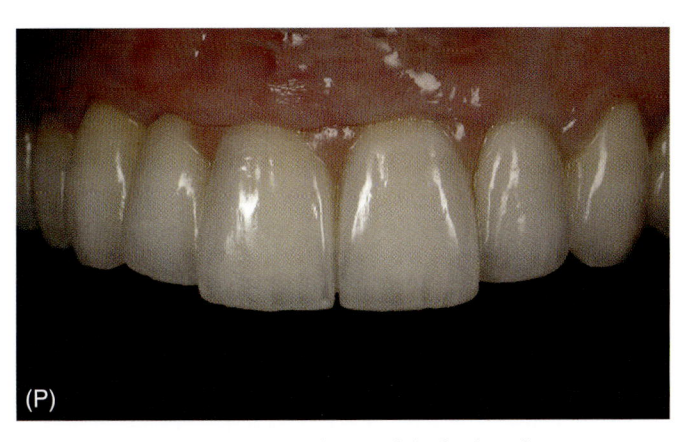

Figure 17.21 **(P, Q)** The retracted view of the final result.

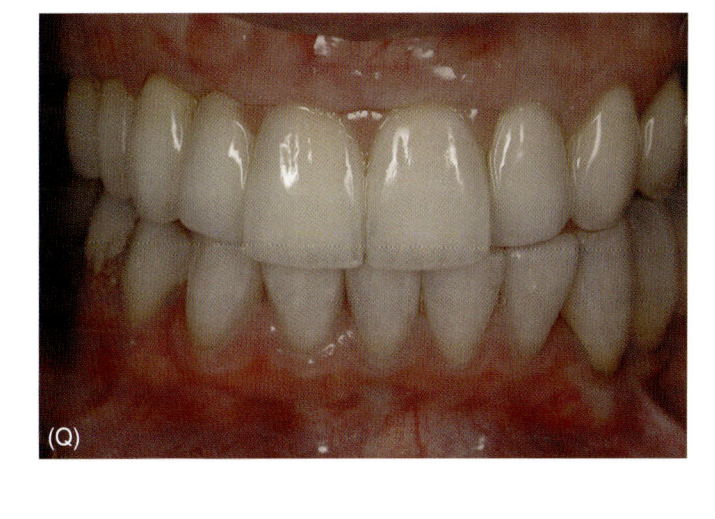

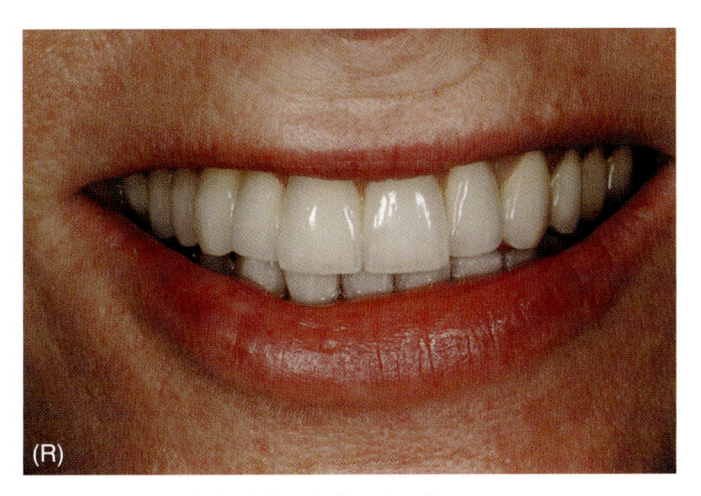

Figure 17.21 **(R, S)** The full and relaxed smile.

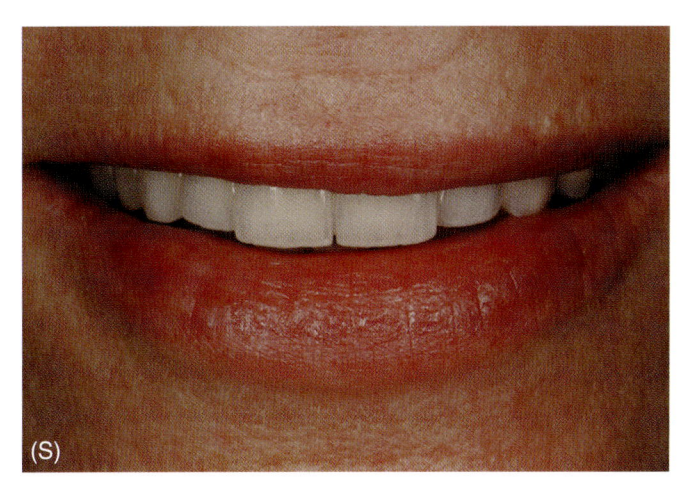

References

1. The Nomenclature Committee. Glossary of prosthodontic terms. *J Prosth Dent* 2005;94(1):10–92.
2. Bindl A, Mormann WH. Marginal and internal fit of all ceramic CAD/CAM crown copings on chamfer preparations. *J Oral Rehabil* 2005;32:441–447.
3. Boyle JJ, Jr, Naylor WP, Blackman RB. Marginal accuracy of metal ceramic restorations with porcelain facial margins. *J Prosthet Dent* 1993;69:19–27.
4. Heintze SD, Rousson V. Survival of zirconia-and metal-supported fixed partial dental prostheses: a systematic review. *Int J Prosthodont* 2010;23(6):493–502.
5. Johnson PF, Taybos GM, Grisius RJ. Prosthodontics; diagnostic, treatment planning, and prognostic considerations. *Dent Clin North Am* 1986;30:503–518.
6. Gardner FM, Tillman-McCombs KW, Gaston ML, Runyan DA. In-vitro failure load of metal-collar margins compared with porcelain facial margins of metal–ceramic crowns. *J Prosthet Dent* 1997;78:1–4.
7. Goldstein RE, Miller MC. High technology in esthetic dentistry. *Curr Opin Cosmet Dent* 1993;1:5–11.
8. Holand W, Schweiger M, Frank M, Rheinberger V. A comparison of the microstructure and properties of the IPS Empress 2 and IPS Empress glass-ceramics. *J Biomed Mater Res* 2000;53(4):297–303.
9. Korayem M, Flores-Mir C, Nassar U, Olfert K. Implant site development by orthodontic extrusion. A systematic review. *Angle Orthod* 2008;78(4):752–760.
10. Musikant BL, Cohen BI, Deutsch AS. The surgical microscope, not just for the specialist. *N Y State Dent J* 1996;62:33–35.
11. Preston JD. Rational approach to tooth preparation for ceramo-metal restorations. *Dent Clin North Am* 1977;21:683–698.
12. Shrout MK, Russell CM, Potter BJ, et al. Digital enhancement of radiographs: can it improve caries diagnosis? *J Am Dent Assoc* 1996;127:469–473.
13. Van der Stelt PF. Improved diagnosis with digital radiography. *Curr Opin Dent* 1992;2:1–6.
14. O'Boyle KH, Norling BK, Cagna DR, Phoenix RD. An investigation of new metal framework design for metal ceramic restorations. *J Prosthet Dent.* 1997;78:295–301.
15. Dewey KW, Zugsmith R. An experimental study of tissue reactions about porcelain roots. *J Dent Res* 1933;13:459–472.
16. El Salam Shakal MA, Pfeiffer P, Hilgers RD. Effect of tooth preparation on bond strengths of resin-bonded prostheses: a pilot study. *J Prosthet Dent* 1997;77:243–249.

17. Goldstein CE, Goldstein RE, Garber DA. Computer imaging: an aid to treatment planning. *J Calif Dent Assoc* 1991;19:47–51.
18. Silness J. Periodontal conditions in patients treated with dental bridges. 2. The influence of full and partial crowns on plaque accumulation, development of gingivitis and pocket formation. *J Periodont Res* 1970;5:219–224.
19. Gonzalo E, Suarez MJ, Serrano B, Lozano JF. A comparison of the marginal vertical discrepancies of zirconium and metal ceramic posterior fixed dental prostheses before and after cementation. *J Prosthet Dent* 2009;102:378–384.
20. Livaditis GJ. Cast metal resin-bonded retainers for posterior teeth. *J Am Dent Assoc* 1980;110:926–929.
21. Preiskel H. Telescopic prosthesis. *Israel J Dent* 1969;18:12–19.
22. Christel P, Meunier A, Heller M, et al. Mechanical properties and short-term in-vivo evaluation of yttrium-oxide-partially-stabilized zirconia. *J Biomed Mater Res* 1989;23:45–61.
23. Crispin B, Watson J. Margin placement of esthetic veneer crowns. Part 1: anterior tooth visibility. *J Prosthet Dent* 1981;45:278–282.
24. Kmine F, Iwai T, Kobayashi K, Matsumura H. Marginal and internal adaption of zirconium dioxide ceramic copings and crowns with different finish line designs. *Dent Mater J* 2007;26:659–664.
25. Marchack BW, Futatsuki Y, Marchack CB, White SN. Customization of milled zirconia copings for all-ceramic crowns: a clinical report. *J Prosthet Dent* 2008;99:169–173.
26. Saad AA, Claffey N, Byrne D, Hussey D. Effects of groove placement on retention/resistance of maxillary anterior resin-bonded retainers. *J Prosthet Dent* 1995;74:133–139.
27. Rochette AL. Attachment of a splint to enamel of lower anterior teeth. *J Prosthet Dent* 1973;30:418–423.
28. Sundh A, Molin M, Sjogren G. Fracture resistance of yttrium oxide partially-stabilized zirconia all-ceramic bridges after veneering and mechanical testing. *Dent Mater* 2005;21:476–482.
29. Vult von Steyern P. All-ceramic fixed partial denture. Studies on aluminum oxide- and zirconium dioxide-based ceramic systems. *Swed Dent J Suppl* 2005;(173):1–69.
30. Kern M. Clinical long-term survival of two-retainer and single retainer all ceramic resin-bonded fixed partial dentures. *Quintessence Int* 2205;36:141–147.
31. Ries S, Wolz J, Richter EJ. Effect of design of all ceramic resin-bonded fixed partial dentures on clinical survival rate. *Int J Periodontics Restorative Dent* 2006;26:143–149.
32. Komine F, Tomic M. A single-retainer zirconium ceramic resin-bonded fixed partial denture for single tooth replacement: a clinical report. *J Oral Sci* 2005;47:139–142.
33. Reich S, Petschelt A, Lohbauer U. The effect of finish line preparation and layer thickness on the failure load and fractography of ZrO_2 copings. *J Prosthet Dent* 2008;99:369–376.
34. Vagkopoulou T, Koutayas SO, Koidis P, Strub JR. Zirconia in dentistry: Part 1. Discovering the nature of an upcoming bioceramic. *Eur J Esthet Dent* 2009;4:130–151.
35. Comlekoglu M, Dundar M, Ozcan M, et al. Influence of cervical finish line type on the marginal adaptation of zirconia ceramic crowns. *Oper Dent* 2009;34:586–592.
36. Raigrodski AJ, Chiche GJ, Potiket N, et al. The efficacy of posterior three-unit zirconium-oxide-based ceramic fixed partial denture prostheses: a prospective clinical pilot study. *J Prosthet Dent* 2006;96:237–244.
37. Sailer I, Feher A, Filser F, et al. Five-year clinical results of zirconia frameworks for posterior fixed partial dentures. *Int J Prosthodont* 2007;20:383–388.
38. Molin MK, Karlsson SL. Five-year clinical prospective evaluation of zirconia-based Denzir 3-unit FPDs. *Int J Prosthodont* 2008;21:223–227.
39. Raigrodski AJ, Hillstead MB, Meng GK, Chung K-H. Survival and complications of zirconia-based fixed dental prostheses: a systematic review. *J Prosth Dent* 2012;107:170–177.
40. Marquaedt P, Strub JR. Survival rates of IPS Empress 2 all ceramic crowns and fixed partial dentures: results of a 5-year prospective clinical study. *Quintessence Int* 2006;37(4):253–259.
41. Kern M, Sasse M, Wolfart S. Ten-year outcome of three-unit fixed dental prostheses made from monolithic lithium disilicate ceramic. *JADA* 2012;143(3):234–240.
42. Sailer I, Pjetursson BE, Zwahlen M, Hammerle CHF. A systematic review of the survival and complications rate of all-ceramic and metal-ceramic reconstructions after an observation period of at least 3 years, part II: fixed dental prostheses. *Clin Oral Implants Res* 2007;18(Suppl 3):86–96.
43. Nevins M. Periodontal prosthesis reconsidered. *Int J Prosthodont* 1993;6(2):209–217.
44. Levin RP. Building your practice with an intraoral video camera. *Compendium* 1990;11:52, 54, 56.
45. Brehm TW. Diagnosis and treatment planning for fixed prosthodontics. *J Prosthet Dent* 1973;30:876–881.
46. Richter WA, Ueno H. Relationship of crown margin placement to gingival inflammation. *J Prosthet Dent.* 973;30:156–161.
47. Johnson GK, Leary JM. Pontic design and localized ridge augmentation in fixed partial denture design. *Dent Clin North Am* 1992;36:591–605.
48. Belser UC, MacEntee MI, Richter WA. Fit of three porcelain-fused-to-metal margin designs in vivo: a scanning electron microscope study. *J Prosthet Dent* 1985;53:24–29.
49. Bowley JF, Stockstill JW, Attanasio R. A preliminary diagnostic and treatment protocol. *Dent Clin North Am* 1992;36:551–568.
50. Prichard JF, Feder M. A modern adaptation of the telescopic principle in periodontal prosthesis. *J Periodont* 1962;33:360–364.
51. Del Castillo R, Ercoli C, Delgado JC, Alcaraz J. An alternative multiple pontic design for a fixed implant-supported prosthesis. *J Prosth Dent* 2011;105:198–203.
52. Shillingburg HT, Hobo S, Fisher DW. Preparation design and margin distortion in porcelain-fused-to-metal restorations. *J Prosthet Dent* 1973;29:276–284.
53. Wanserski DJ, Sobczak KP, Monaco JG, McGivney GP. An analysis of margin adaptation of all-porcelain facial margin ceramometal crowns. *J Prosthet Dent* 1986;56:289–297.
54. Reynolds MJ. Abutment selection for fixed prosthetics. *J Prosthet Dent* 1968;19:483–488.
55. Johnson LA. A systemic evaluation of intraoral cameras. *J Calif Dent Assoc* 1994;22:34–42, 44–47.
56. Walton JN, Gardner FM, Agar JR. A survey of crown and fixed partial denture failures: length of service and reasons for replacement. *J Prosthet Dent* 1986;56:416–421.
57. Salama H, Garber DA, Salama MA, et al. Fifty years of interdisciplinary site development: lessons and guidelines from periodontal prosthesis. *J Esthet Dent* 1998;10(3):149–156.
58. Sheets CG, Earthman JC. Tooth in implant-assisted prostheses. *J Prosthet Dent* 1997;77(4):39–45.
59. Sheets CG, Earthman JC. Natural tooth intrusion and reversal in implant-assisted prosthesis—evidence of and a hypothesis for the occurrence. *J Prosthet Dent* 1993;70(6):513–520.
60. Schlumberger TL, Bowley JF, Maze GI. Intrusion phenomenon in combination tooth–implant restorations: a review of the literature. *J Prosthet Dent* 1998;80:199–203.

61. Kim SH, Tramontina VA, Papalexiou V, Luczyszyn SM. Orthodontic extrusion and implant site development using an interocclusal appliance for a severe mucogingival deformity: a clinical report. *J Prosthet Dent* 2011;105(2):72–77.
62. Larsson C, Vult von Steyern P, Nilner K. A prospective study of implant-supported full-arch yttria-stabilized tetragonal zirconia polycrystal mandibular fixed dental prostheses: three-year results. *Int J Prosthodont* 2010;23(4):364–369.
63. Manicone PF, Rossi Iommetti P, Raffaelli L. An overview of zirconia ceramics: basic properties and clinical applications. *J Dent* 2007;35(11):819–826.
64. Christel P, Meunier A, Heller M, et al. Mechanical properties and short-term in-vivo evaluation of yttrium-oxide-partially-stabilized zirconia. *J Biomed Mater Res* 1989;23(1):45–61.
65. Tholey MJ, Berthold C, Swain MV, et al. XRD^2 micro-diffraction analysis of the interface between Y-TZP and veneering porcelain: role of application methods. *Dent Mater* 2010;26(6):545–552.
66. Chevalier J. What future for zirconia as a biomaterial? *Biomaterials* 2006;27(4):535–543.
67. Cehreli MC, Kokat AM, Akca K. CAD/CAM zirconia vs. slip-cast glass-infiltrated alumina/zirconia all-ceramic crowns: 2-year results of a randomized controlled clinical trial. *J Appl Oral Sci* 2009;17(1):49–55.
68. Sailer I, Feher A, Filser F, et al. Five-year clinical results of zirconia frameworks for posterior fixed partial dentures. *Int J Prosthodont* 2007;20(4):383–388.
69. Beuer F, Edelhoff D, Gernet W, et al. Three-year clinical prospective evaluation of zirconia-based posterior fixed dental prostheses (FDPs). *Clin Oral Investig* 2009;13(4):445–451.
70. Roediger M, Gersdorff N, Huels A. Prospective evaluation of zirconia posterior fixed partial dentures: four-year clinical results. *Int J Prosthodont* 2010;23(2):141–148.
71. Aboushelib MN, Feilzer AJ, Kleverlaan CJ. Bridging the gap between clinical failure and laboratory fracture strength tests using a fractographic approach. *Dent Mater* 2009;25(3):383–391.
72. Taskonak B, Yan J, Mecholsky JJ Jr, et al. Fractographic analyses of zirconia- based fixed partial dentures. *Dent Mater* 2008;24(8):1077–82.)
73. Marchack B, Futatsuki Y, Marchack C, et al. Customization of milled zirconia copings for all-ceramic crowns: a clinical report. *J Prosthet Dent* 2008;99(3):163–173.
74. Guess PC, Zhang Y, Kim JW, et al. Damage and reliability of Y-TZP after cementation surface treatment. *J Dent Res* 2010;89(6):592–596.
75. Podshadley AG. Gingival response to pontics. *J Prosthet Dent* 1968;19:51–57.
76. De Kanter RJ, Creugers NH, Verzijden CW, Van't Hof MA. A five-year multi-practice clinical study on posterior resin-bonded bridges. *J Dent Res* 1998;77:609–614.
77. Abrams L. Augmentation of the deformed residual edentulous ridge for fixed prosthetics. *Compend Contin Educ Dent* 1980;3:205–214.
78. McCracken WL. Differential diagnosis: fixed or removable partial dentures? *J Am Dent Assoc* 1961;63:767–775.
79. Reel DC. Establishing esthetic contours of the partially edentulous ridge. *Quintessence Int* 1988;19:301–310.
80. Salama H, Salama M. The role of orthodontic extrusive remodeling in the enhancement of soft and hard tissue profiles prior to implant placement: a systematic approach to the management of extraction site defects. *Int J Periodont Restor Dent* 1993;13:313–333.
81. Seibert JS. Reconstruction of deformed, partially edentulous ridges, using full thickness onlay grafts. Part I. Technique and wound healing. *Compend Contin Educ Dent* 1983;4:437–453.
82. Garber DA, Rosenberg ES. The edentulous ridge in fixed prosthodontics. *Compend Contin Educ Dent.* 981;2:212–223.
83. Schart DR, Tarnow DP. Modified roll technique for localized alveolar ridge augmentation. *Int J Periodontic Restorative Dent* 1992;2(5):415–425.
84. Silverman SI. Differential diagnosis. Fixed or removable prosthesis? *Dent Clin North Am* 1987;31:347–362.
85. Stein RS. Pontic–residual ridge relationship: a research report. *J Prosthet Dent* 1966;16:251–285.
86. Cavazos E, Jr. Tissue response to fixed partial denture pontics. *J Prosthet Dent* 1968;20:143–153.
87. Prichard JP. *Advanced Periodontal Diseases*, 2nd edn. Philadelphia, PA: WB Saunders; 1972.
88. Thompson VP, Del Castillo E, Livaditis GJ. Resin-bonded retainers. Part 1: resin bond to electrolytically etched non-precious alloys. *J Prosthet Dent* 1983;50:771–779.

Additional resources

Garber DA, Adar P, Goldstein RE, Salama H. The quest for the all-ceramic restoration. *Quint Dent Tech* 2000;23:27–37.

Goldstein RE. *Esthetics in Dentistry*. Philadelphia, PA: JB Lippincott; 1976.

Goldstein RE. Diagnostic dilemma: to bond, laminate, or crown? *Int J Periodont Restor Dent* 1987;87(5):9–30.

Goldstein RE. Esthetic principles for ceramo-metal restorations. *Dent Clin North Am* 1988;21:803–822.

Goldstein RE. *Change Your Smile*, 3rd edn. Carol Stream, IL: Quintessence; 1997.

Goldstein RE, Adar P. Special effects and internal characterization. *J Dent Technol* 1989;17:11.

Goldstein RE, Feinman RA, Garber DA. Esthetic considerations in the selection and use of restorative materials. *Dent Clin North Am* 1983;27:723–731.

Goldstein RE, Garber DA, Schwartz CG, Goldstein CE. Patient maintenance of esthetic restorations. *J Am Dent Assoc* 1992;123:61–66.

Goldstein RE, Garber DA, Goldstein CE, et al. The changing esthetic dental practice. *J Am Dent Assoc* 1994;125:1447–1457.

Gregory-Head B, Curtis DA. Erosion caused by gastroesophageal reflux: diagnostic considerations. *J Prosthodont* 1997;6:278–285.

Grippo JO. Abfractions: a new classification of hard tissue lesions of teeth. *J Esthet Dent* 1991;3:14–19.

Grippo JO. Noncarious cervical lesions: the decision to ignore or restore. *J Esthet Dent* 1992;4(Suppl):55–64.

Hacker CH, Wagner WC, Razzoog ME. An in vitro investigation of the wear of enamel on porcelain and gold in saliva. *J Prosthet Dent* 1996;75:14–17.

Harris EF, Butler ML. Patterns of incisor root resorption before and after orthodontic correction in cases with anterior open bites. *Am J Orthod Dentofac Orthop* 1992;101:112–119.

Hazelton LR, Faine MP. Diagnosis and dental management of eating disorder patients. *Int J Prosthodont* 1996;9:65–73.

Hertzberg J, Nakisbendi L, Needleman HL, Pober B. Williams syndrome—oral presentation of 45 cases. *Pediatr Dent* 1994;16:262–267.

Heymann HO, Sturdevant JR, Bayne S, et al. Examining tooth flexure effects on cervical restorations: a two year clinical study. *J Am Dent Assoc* 1991;122:41–47.

Hicks RA, Conti P. Nocturnal bruxism and self reports of stress-related symptoms. *Percept Mot Skills* 1991;72:1182.

Hicks RA, Lucero-Gorman K, Bautista J, Hicks GJ. Ethnicity and bruxism. *Percept Mot Skills* 1999;88:240–241.

Horsted-Bindslev P, Knudsen J, Baelum V. 3-year clinical evaluation of modified Gluma adhesive systems in cervical abrasion/erosion lesions. *Am J Dent* 1996;9:22–26.

Hsu LK. Epidemiology of the eating disorders. *Psychiatr Clin North Am* 1996;19:681–700.

Hudson JD, Goldstein GR, Georgescu M. Enamel wear caused by three different restorative materials. *J Prosthet Dent* 1995;74:647–654.

Hugoson A, Ekfeldt A, Koch G, Hallonsten AL. Incisal and occlusal tooth wear in children and adolescents in a Swedish population. *Acta Odontol Scand* 1996;54:263–270.

Ikeda T, Nishigawa K, Kondo K, et al. Criteria for the detection of sleep-associated bruxism in humans. *J Orofac Pain* 1996;10:270–282.

Imfeld T. Dental erosion. Definition, classification and links. *Eur J Oral Sci* 1996;104:151–154.

Imfeld T. Prevention of progression of dental erosion by professional and individual prophylactic measures. *Eur J Oral Sci* 1996;104:215–220.

Ingleby J, Mackie IC. Case report: an unusual cause of toothwear. *Dent Update* 1995;22:434–435.

Jagger DC, Harrison A. An in vitro investigation into the wear effects of selected restorative materials on enamel. *J Oral Rehabil* 1995;22:275–281.

Jagger DC, Harrison A. An in vitro investigation into the wear effects of selected restorative materials on dentine. *J Oral Rehabil* 1995;22:349–354.

Jarvinen VK, Rytomaa II, Heinonen OP. Risk factors in dental erosion. *J Dent Res* 1991;70:942–947.

Johansson A. A cross-cultural study of occlusal tooth wear. *Swed Dent J Suppl* 1992;86:1–59.

Josell SD. Habits affecting dental and maxillofacial growth and development. *Dent Clin North Am* 1995;39:851–860.

Josephson CA. Restoration of mandibular incisors with advanced wear. *J Dent Assoc S Afr* 1992;47:419–420.

Kaidonis JA, Richards LC, Townsend GC, Tansley GD. Wear of human enamel: a quantitative in vitro assessment. *J Dent Res* 1998;77:1983–1990.

Kampe T, Hannerz H, Strom P. Ten-year follow-up study of signs and symptoms of craniomandibular disorders in adults with intact and restored dentitions. *J Oral Rehabil* 1996;23:416–423.

Kelleher M, Bishop K. The aetiology and clinical appearance of tooth wear. *Eur J Prosthodont Restor Dent* 1997;5:157–160.

Khan F, Young WG, Daley TJ. Dental erosion and bruxism. A tooth wear analysis from south east Queensland. *Aust Dent J* 1998;43:117–127.

Kidd EA, Smith BG. Toothwear histories: a sensitive issue. *Dent Update* 1993;20:174–178.

Kiliaridis S, Johansson A, Haraldson T, et al. Craniofacial morphology, occlusal traits, and bite force in persons with advanced occlusal tooth wear. *Am J Orthodont Dentofac Orthop* 1995;107:286–292.

Kleinberg I. Bruxism: aetiology, clinical signs and symptoms. *Aust Prosthodont J* 1994;8:9–17.

Knight DJ, Leroux BG, Zhu C, et al. A longitudinal study of tooth wear in orthodontically treated patients. *Am J Orthod Dentofacial Orthop* 1997;112:194–202.

Kokich VG. Esthetics and vertical tooth position: orthodontic possibilities. *Compend Contin Educ Dent* 1997;18:1225–1231.

Lambrechts P, van Meerbeek B, Perdigao J, et al. Restorative therapy for erosive lesions. *Eur J Oral Sci* 1996;104:229–240.

Lavigne GL, Rompre PH, Montplaisir JY. Sleep bruxism: validity of clinical research diagnostic criteria in a controlled polysomnographic study. *J Dent Res* 1996;75:546–552.

Lee CL, Eakle WS. Possible role of tensile stress in the etiology of cervical erosive lesions of teeth. *J Prosthet Dent* 1984;52:374–380.

Lee CL, Eakle WS. Stress-induced cervical lesions: review of advances in the past 10 years. *J Prosthet Dent* 1996;75:487–494.

Leinfelder KF, Yarnell G. Occlusion and restorative materials. *Dent Clin North Am* 1995;39:355–361.

Leung AK, Robson WL. Thumb sucking. *Am Fam Physician* 1991;44:1724–1728.

Levine RS. Briefing paper: oral aspects of dummy and digit sucking. *Br Dent J* 1999;186:108.

Lussi A. Dental erosion clinical diagnosis and case history taking. *Eur J Oral Sci* 1996;104:191–198.

Lussi A, Portmann P, Burhop B. Erosion on abraded dental hard tissues by acid lozenges: an in situ study. *Clin Oral Investig* 1997;1:191–194.

Mair LH, Stolarski TA, Vowles RW, Lloyd CH. Wear: mechanisms, manifestations and measurement. Report of a workshop. *J Dent* 1996;24:141–148.

Marchesan IQ, Krakauer LR. The importance of respiratory activity in myofunctional therapy. *Int J Orofac Myol* 1996;22:23–27.

Maron FS. Enamel erosion resulting from hydrochloride acid tablets. *J Am Dent Assoc* 1996;127:781–784.

Matis BA, Cochran M, Carlson T. Longevity of glass-ionomer restorative materials: results of a 10-year evaluation. *Quintessence Int* 1996;27:373–382.

McCoy G. The etiology of gingival erosion. *J Oral Implantol* 1982;10:361–362.

McCoy G. On the longevity of teeth. *J Oral Implantol* 1983;11:248–267.

McIntyre JM. Erosion. *Aust Prosthodont J* 1992;6:17–25.

Mehler PS, Gray MC, Schulte M. Medical complications of anorexia nervosa. *J Womens Health* 1997;6:533–541.

Menapace SE, Rinchuse DJ, Zullo T, et al. The dentofacial morphology of bruxers versus non-bruxers. *Angle Orthod* 1994;64:43–52.

Mercado MD. The prevalence and aetiology of craniomandibular disorders among completely edentulous patients. *Aust Prosthodont J* 1993;7:27–29.

Mercado MD, Faulkner KD. The prevalence of craniomandibular disorders in completely edentulous denture-wearing subjects. *J Oral Rehabil* 1991;18:231–242.

Metaxas A. Oral habits and malocclusion. A case report. *Ont Dent* 1996;73:27.

Millward A, Shaw L, Smith AJ. Dental erosion in four-year-old children from differing socioeconomic backgrounds. *ASDC J Dent Child* 1994;61:263–366.

Millward A, Shaw L, Smith AJ, et al. The distribution and severity of tooth wear and the relationship between erosion and dietary constituents in a group of children. *Int J Paediatr Dent* 1994;4:151–157.

Milosevic A. Tooth wear: an aetiological and diagnostic problem. *Eur J Prosthodont Restor Dent* 1993;1:173–178.

Milosevic A, Dawson LJ. Salivary factors in vomiting bulimics with and without pathological tooth wear. *Caries Res* 1996;30:361–366.

Milosevic A, Brodie DA, Slade PD. Dental erosion, oral hygiene, and nutrition in eating disorders. *Int J Eat Disord* 1997;21:195–199.

Milosevic A, Lennon MA, Fear SC. Risk factors associated with tooth wear in teenagers: a case control study. *Community Dent Health* 1997;14:143–147.

Morley J. The esthetics of anterior tooth aging. *Curr Opin Cosmet Dent* 1997;4:35–39.

Moses AJ. Thumb sucking or thumb propping? *CDS Rev* 1987;80:40–42.

Moss RA, Lombardo TW, Villarosa GA, et al. Oral habits and TMJ dysfunction in facial pain and non-pain subjects. *J Oral Rehabil* 1995;22:79–81.

Murray CG, Sanson GD. Thegosis—a critical review. *Aust Dent J* 1998;43:192–198.

Nel JC, Bester SP, Snyman WD. Bruxism threshold: an explanation for successful treatment of multifactorial aetiology of bruxism. *Aust Prosthodont J* 1995;9:33–37.

Nel JC, Marais JT, van Vuuren PA. Various methods of achieving restoration of tooth structure loss due to bruxism. *J Esthet Dent* 1996;8:183–188.

Nemcovsky CE, Artzi Z. Erosion-abrasion lesions revisited. *Compend Contin Educ Dent* 1996;17:416–418.

Neo J, Chew CL. Direct tooth-colored materials for noncarious lesions: a 3-year clinical report. *Quintessence Int* 1995;27:183–188.

Neo J, Chew CL, Yap A, Sidhu S. Clinical evaluation of tooth-colored materials in cervical lesions. *Am J Dent* 1996;9:15–18.

Nunn J, Shaw L, Smith A. Tooth wear—dental erosion. *Br Dent J* 1996;180:349–352.

Nunn JH. Prevalence of dental erosion and the implications for oral health. *Eur J Oral Sci* 1996;104:156–161.

Nystrom M, Kononen M, Alaluusua S, et al. Development of horizontal tooth wear in maxillary anterior teeth from five to 18 years of age. *J Dent Res* 1990;69:1765–1770.

Okeson JP. Occlusion and functional disorders of the masticatory system. *Dent Clin North Am* 1995;39:285–300.

Osborne-Smith KL, Burke FJ, FarlaneTM, Wilson NH. Effect of restored and unrestored non-carious cervical lesions on the fracture resistance of previously restored maxillary premolar teeth. *J Dent* 1998;26:427–433.

O'Sullivan EA, Curzon ME, Roberts GJ, et al. Gastroesophageal reflux in children and its relationship to erosion of primary and permanent teeth. *Eur J Oral Sci* 1998;106:765–769.

Owens BM, Gallien GS. Noncarious dental "abfraction" lesions in an aging population. *Compend Contin Educ Dent* 1995;16:552–562.

Paterson AJ, Watson IB. Case report: prolonged match chewing: an unusual case of tooth wear. *Eur J Prosthodont Restor Dent* 1995;3:131–134.

Pavone BW. Bruxism and its effect on the natural teeth. *J Prosthet Dent* 1985;53:692–696.

Pierce CJ, Chrisman K, Bennett ME, Close JM. Stress, anticipatory stress, and psychologic measures related to sleep bruxism. *J Orofac Pain* 1995;9:51–56.

Pintado MR, Anderson GC, DeLong R, Douglas WH. Variation in tooth wear in young adults over a two-year period. *J Prosthet Dent* 1997;77:313–320.

Powell LV, Johnson GH, Gordon GE. Factors associated with clinical success of cervical abrasion/erosion restorations. *Oper Dent* 1995;20:7–13.

Priest G. An 11-year reevaluation of resin-bonded fixed partial dentures. *Int J Periodont Restor Dent* 1995;15:238–247.

Principato JJ. Upper airway obstruction and craniomandibular morphology. *Otolaryngol Head Neck Surg* 1991;104:881–890.

Ramp MH, Suzuki S, Cox CF, et al. Evaluation of wear: enamel opposing three ceramic materials and a gold alloy. *J Prosthet Dent* 1997;77:523–530.

Ribeiro RA, Romano AR, Birman EG, Mayer MP. Oral manifestations of Rett syndrome: a study of 17 cases. *Pediatr Dent* 1997;19:349–352.

Ritchard A, Welsh AH, Donnelly C. The association between occlusion and attrition. *Aust Orthod J* 1992;12:138–142.

Rivera-Morales WC, McCall WD, Jr. Reliability of a portable electromyographic unit to measure bruxism. *J Prosthet Dent* 1995;73:184–189.

Robb ND, Cruwys E, Smith BG. Regurgitation erosion as a possible cause of tooth wear in ancient British populations. *Arch Oral Biol* 1991;36:595–602.

Rogers GM, Poore MH, Ferko BL, et al. In vitro effects of an acidic by-product feed on bovine teeth. *Am J Vet Res* 1997;58:498–503.

Schmidt U, Treasure J. Eating disorders and the dental practitioner. *Eur J Prosthodont Restor Dent* 1997;5:161–167.

Schneider PE. Oral habits—harmful and helpful. *Update Pediatr Dent* 1991;4:1–4, 6–8.

Schwartz JH, Brauer J, Gordon-Larsen P. Brief communication: Tigaran (Point Hope, Alaska) tooth drilling. *Am J Phys Anthropol* 1995;97:77–82.

Seligman DA, Pullinger AG. The degree to which dental attrition in modern society is a function of age and of canine contact. *J Orofac Pain* 1995;9:266–275.

Seow WK. Clinical diagnosis of enamel defects: pitfalls and practical guidelines. *Int Dent J* 1997;47:173–182.

Sherfudin H, Abdullah A, Shaik H, Johansson A. Some aspects of dental health in young adult Indian vegetarians. A pilot study. *Acta Odontol Scand* 1996;54:44–48.

Silness J, Berge M, Johannessen G. A 2-year follow-up study of incisal tooth wear in dental students. *Acta Odontol Scand* 1995;53:331–333.

Silness J, Berge M, Johannessen G. Longitudinal study of incisal tooth wear in children and adolescents. *Eur J Oral Sci* 1995;103:90–94.

Silness J, Berge M, Johannessen G. Re-examination of incisal tooth wear in children and adolescents. *J Oral Rehabil* 1997;24:405–409.

Smith BG, Robb ND. The prevalence of toothwear in 1007 dental patients. *J Oral Rehabil* 1996;23:232–239.

Smith BG, Bartlett DW, Robb ND. The prevalence, etiology and management of tooth wear in the United Kingdom. *J Prosthet Dent* 1997;78:367–372.

Sognnaes RF, Wolcott RB, Xhonga FA. Dental erosion I. Erosion-like patterns occurring in association with other dental conditions. *J Am Dent Assoc* 1972;84:571–576.

Speer JA. Bulimia: full stomach, empty lives. *Dent Assist* 1991;60:28–30.

Spranger H. Investigation into the genesis of angular lesions at the cervical region of teeth. *Quintessence Int* 1995;26:183–188.

Steiner H, Lock J. Anorexia nervosa and bulimia nervosa in children and adolescents: a review of the past 10 years. *J Am Acad Child Adolesc Psychiatry* 1998;37:352–359.

Stewart B. Restoration of the severely worn dentition using a systematized approach for a predictable prognosis. *Int J Periodont Restor Dent* 1998;18:46–57.

Suzuki S, Suzuki SH, Cox CF. Evaluating the antagonistic wear of restorative materials when placed against human enamel. *J Am Dent Assoc* 1996;127:74–80.

Taylor G, Taylor S, Abrams R, Mueller W. Dental erosion associated with asymptomatic gastroesophageal reflux. *ASDC J Dent Child* 1992;59:182–185.

Teaford MF, Lytle JD. Brief communication: diet-induced changes in the rates of human tooth microwear: a case study involving stone-ground maize. *Am J Phys Anthropol* 1996;100:143–147.

Teo C, Young WG, Daley TJ, Sauer H. Prior fluoridation in childhood affects dental caries and tooth wear in a south east Queensland population. *Aust Dent J* 1997;42:92–102.

Thompson BA, Blount BW, Krumholz TS. Treatment approaches to bruxism. *Am Fam Physician* 1994;49:1617–1622.

Timms DJ, Trenouth MJ. A quantified comparison of craniofacial form with nasal respiratory function. *Am J Orthod Dentofac Orthop* 1988;94:216–221.

Touyz LZ. The acidity (pH) and buffering capacity of Canadian fruit juice and dental implications. *J Can Dent Assoc* 1994;60:448–454.

Turp JC, Gobetti JP. The cracked tooth syndrome: an elusive diagnosis. *J Am Dent Assoc* 1996;127:1502–1507.

Tyas MJ. The Class V lesion—aetilogy and restoration. *Aust Dent J* 1995;40:167–170.

Ung N, Koenig J, Shapiro PA, et al. A quantitative assessment of respiratory patterns and their effects on dentofacial development. *Am J Orthod Dentofac Orthop* 1990;98:523–532.

Villa G, Giacobini G. Subvertical grooves of interproximal facets in Neandertal posterior teeth. *Am J Phys Anthropol.* 1995;96:51–62.

Waterman ET, Koltai PJ, Downey JC, Cacace AT. Swallowing disorders in a population of children with cerebral palsy. *Int J Pediatr Otorhinolaryngol* 1992;24:63–71.

West NX, Maxwell A, Hughes JA, et al. A method to measure clinical erosion: the effect of orange juice consumption on erosion of enamel. *J Dent* 1998;26:329–335.

Westergaard J, Moe D, Pallesen U, Holmen L. Exaggerated abrasion/erosion of human dental enamel surfaces: a case report. *Scand J Dent Res* 1993;101:265–269.

Woodside DG, Linder-Aronson S, Lundstrom A, McWilliam J. Mandibular and maxillary growth after changed mode of breathing. *Am J Orthod Dentofac Orthop* 1991;100:1–18.

Yaacob HB, Park AW. Dental abrasion pattern in a selected group of Malaysians. *J Nihon Univ Sch Dent* 1990;32:175–180.

Yamaguchi H, Tanaka Y, Sueishi K, et al. Changes in oral functions and muscular behavior due to surgical orthodontic treatment. *Bull Tokyo Dent Coll* 1994;35:41–49.

Young DV, Rinchuse DJ, Pierce CJ, Zullo T. The craniofacial morphology of bruxers versus nonbruxers. *Angle Orthod* 1999;69:14–18.

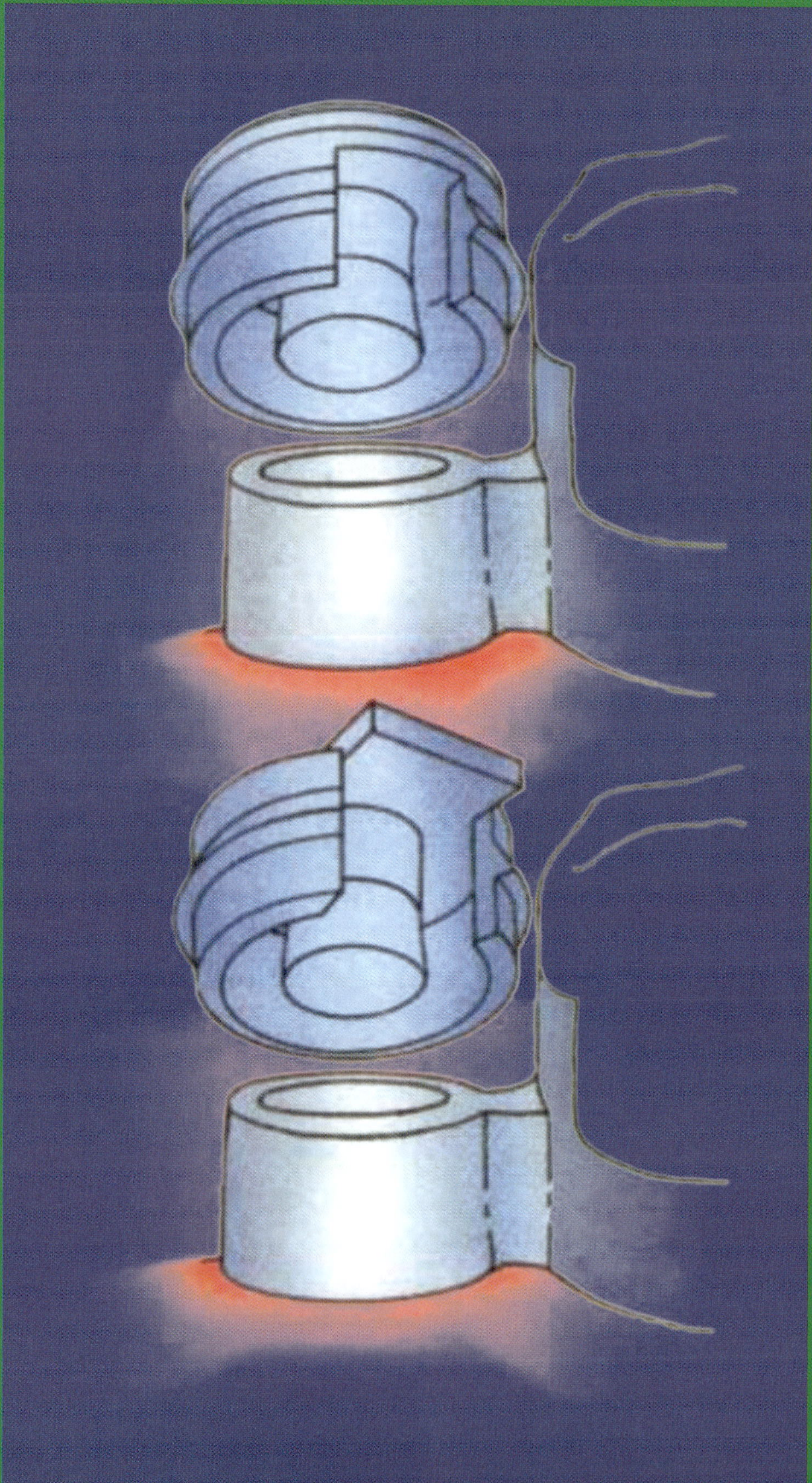

Chapter 18 Esthetic Removable Partial Dentures

Carol A. Lefebvre, DDS, MS, Roman M. Cibirka, DDS, MS, and Ronald E. Goldstein, DDS

Chapter Outline

Classification overview	582	Other esthetic considerations	589
Principles of design	582	Alternative treatment modalities	589
Use of a surveyor	583	Adjunctive mechanisms for minimizing metal display	590
Biomechanics	583	Rotational path removable partial dentures	590
Problem situations	584	Attachments for removable partial dentures	590
Specific clasp types and esthetic considerations	584	Diagnosis and treatment planning	590
Circumferential clasp	584	General considerations for attachments	591
I-, Y-, T-, or modified T-bar clasp	584	Biomechanics and support	594
Rest–proximal plate–I-bar clasp	585	Path of insertion	595
Mesial groove reciprocation clasp	585	Indirect retention	595
Ring clasp	585	Tooth preparation	595
Embrasure clasp	588	Attachment selection considerations	595
Combination clasp	588	Intracoronal attachments	597
Retention enhancement	588	Types of intracoronal attachments	597
Rest seats	588	Extracoronal attachments	599
Flange design	589	Types of extracoronal attachments	600
Replacement teeth	589	Special-use attachments	605

The patient who has lost a number of teeth has several treatment alternatives. The patient may remain partially edentulous until esthetics or function is compromised, or treatment in the form of a fixed partial denture (FPD), removable partial denture (RPD), or implant(s) may be pursued.

The highly esthetic demands of contemporary dental patients compel dentists to satisfy their requests. RPDs designed without prudence and skillfulness may result in functional or esthetic insufficiency. Esthetic deficiencies may be shrouded by functional criticisms. Patients may present with frequent functional complaints of unaccountable pain or inability to chew when, in fact, they are discontented with the appearance. Unesthetic RPDs can be avoided with appropriate diagnosis and design using conventional clasping or attachment-aided prostheses.

Classification overview

Universal classification systems for the partially edentulous arch have been devised to enhance communication and aid in design. Although numerous classification systems exist, the most widely accepted is that proposed by Kennedy[1] and further modified by Applegate.[2] There are four classes in the Kennedy classification system (Figure 18.1). The Kennedy Class I consists of bilateral edentulous areas located posterior to the remaining natural teeth and is the most common of the partially edentulous situations.[3] The Kennedy Class II has a unilateral edentulous area located posterior to the remaining natural teeth. The Kennedy Class III consists of a unilateral edentulous area with natural teeth remaining both anterior and posterior to it. The rarest class of the Kennedy classification is the Kennedy Class IV, which is a single, bilateral (crossing the midline), edentulous area located anterior to the remaining natural teeth. Edentulous areas other than those determining the classification are termed modification spaces.

Principles of design

The prudent treatment plan embraces a comprehensive analysis of the patient's dentition and supportive soft tissues. The health and distribution of the teeth will influence partial denture component selection and the anticipated esthetics. Likewise, the quality of the supportive soft tissues dictates the measure of force transferred to the abutments and guides the component selection for the tooth-tissue-supported RPD. The greater the tissue support required, the more likely it is that the forces imparted to the abutment teeth will increase. The most destructive force is that of torque in the distal extension design. Minimization of torque should be considered of paramount importance in the design of the RPD.

Therefore, RPD design should be based on the available support. Kennedy Class I, II, and large IV RPDs are considered tooth-tissue-supported. In general, flexible direct retainer assemblies, mesioocclusal rests on posterior distal extension abutments, and indirect retainers to limit rotation are indicated for tooth-tissue-supported RPDs.[4]

Kennedy Class III and small IV arches are considered tooth-supported RPDs. In these situations, no additional support from the tissue is generally needed. For these designs, clasp assemblies may be more rigid, and indirect retainers are usually not indicated.

Examination of the patient requires clinical and radiographic diagnosis of the teeth and soft tissues for judgment of the support available for the partial denture. Radiographic interpretation should include (1) periodontal status, (2) responses of the teeth to previous stress, (3) vitality of the remaining teeth, and (4) pathosis. The quantity or height and quality of bone support often predict the prognosis of an abutment tooth or may influence the design of an RPD component. Proper diagnosis necessitates high-quality radiographs, devoid of angulation errors. Vertical bone heights will provide a measure of clinical crown : root ratios. A clinical crown : root ratio greater than 1 : 1 should be considered an endangered abutment with a poor prognosis for RPD support. Stress-breaking direct retainers and contingency planning should be included in the design of RPDs to use an abutment with marginal support.

Bone indices have been described;[5] however, they may be difficult to discern on some radiographs. A 25% error in actual bone calcification levels may be found with normal radiographs. Optimum bone qualities are expressed as normal-sized interdental trabecular spaces that tend to decrease in size slightly near the coronal portion of the root. Normal bone responds favorably to stresses within clinical limits. Favorable reaction to stresses from an existing RPD may be considered indicative of a future reaction to stress. Teeth that have experienced previous heavy stress from RPD support or in conjunction with abnormal occlusal forces and demonstrate normal to slightly condensed trabeculation, a dense lamina dura, and a heavy cortical layer are designated as having a positive bone index or factor. Abnormal stresses will be evidenced as a reduction in the size of the trabeculae being most pronounced adjacent to the lamina dura. The reduced trabeculae size may be termed bone condensation and may be indicative of aberrant forces that could result in bone loss if the patient becomes less resistant. A compaction of trabecular spaces and significant alterations to the cortical layer or lamina dura may be considered a negative bone index or bone factor.

Lamina dura is considered a radiographic measure of abutment tooth health. The structure is hard cortical bone lining the tooth sockets with a primary function of withstanding mechanical strain. The lamina dura should be intact and cross interdental spaces to adjacent teeth as a fine, radiopaque white line.

The supportive elements will generally respond to build support where needed and predict the degree of future response. Mechanical insults from poorly designed RPDs may overload

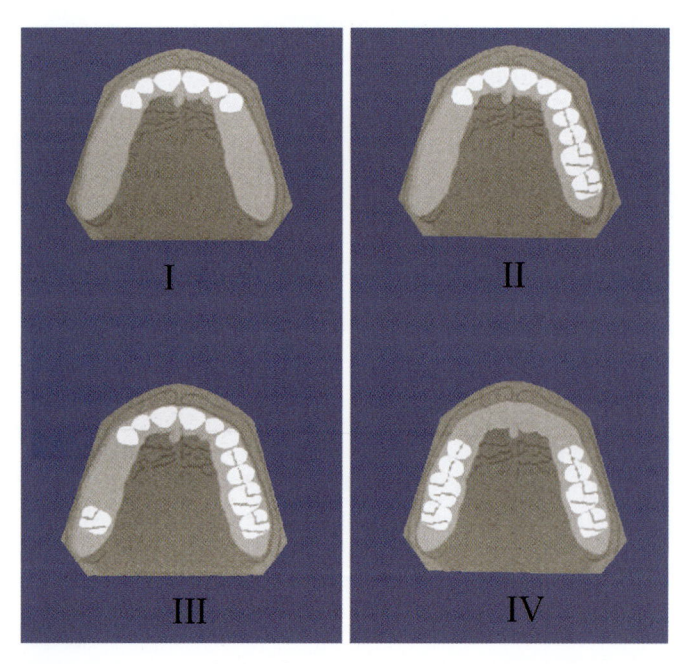

Figure 18.1 Kennedy classification: Class I, bilateral distal extension; Class II, unilateral distal extension; Class III, unilateral edentulous area bounded by natural teeth; and Class IV, single bilateral (crossing the midline) area located anterior to the remaining natural teeth.

the remodeling capacity of the body, resulting in tissue destruction. Bone is approximately 30% organic and stores little protein; therefore, any alterations in body health will be reflected in the ability to maintain support. Systemic diseases that alter the reparative capacity of the body should be strongly considered with RPD design. The patient's future health status and manifestations of aging should be considered in the selection of abutment teeth for loading.

Use of a surveyor

The dental surveyor is a fundamental instrument for RPD design and treatment planning. Additionally, the dental surveyor is indispensable for the dental laboratory technician to fabricate an RPD and fabricate supportive elements such as surveyed, telescopic, or attachment restorations.

The surveyor may be used for diagnostic cast analysis, contouring abutment tooth restorations, placement of attachment retainers, and milling internal rests and reciprocal elements. Survey objectives include: (1) determination of an acceptable path of insertion to eliminate interference with placement or removal of either hard or soft tissues; (2) identification of proximal tooth surfaces to be made parallel to act as guiding planes for placement and removal; (3) location and measurement areas of teeth for undercut and suitable esthetic clasp placement; (4) delineation of heights of contour; and (5) recording of cast position, or tripod, for future reference.[5,6]

An esthetic determinant of the survey is establishing one path of placement to minimize the retentive element and acrylic resin or denture base display. Retentive areas may influence the placement of retentive elements, so areas of retention should be selected to enhance the esthetic value of the RPD. When an anterior modification space is present, a path of placement should be selected to minimize excessive modification of adjacent abutment teeth and eliminate placement interferences. Anterior tissue undercuts may dictate a posteriorly directed path of placement to avoid excessive need for tissue blockout and inherent lip fullness from the overcontoured denture base flange. Restoration of highly esthetic anterior regions should be accomplished through fixed prosthodontics whenever possible or when the path of placement required for accomplishment of esthetics might limit the functional efficacy of the partial denture.

Biomechanics

The design of an RPD must value the mechanics and the biologic considerations. Maxwell stated that "Common observation clearly indicates that the ability of things to tolerate force is largely dependent upon the magnitude or intensity of the force."[5] The structures supporting a partial denture, teeth, and residual ridges are "living things" subjected to forces. The attributes, frequency, and magnitude of the force will foretell the success or failure of the RPD and remaining dentition.

Forces applied to an RPD are generally classified into three cranial planes: vertical, sagittal, and coronal. However, it should be recognized that functional forces are a summation of individual vector forces in the three cranial planes. Therefore, the actual force encountered by an abutment may be the result of two differing planar vector forces of varied intensity. Knowledge of the functional movements patients generate should be considered in the selection of abutment teeth, retainers, and partial denture design. Widely distributed abutment teeth with poor periodontal support in a patient with a parafunctional bruxism habit whose native diet includes nuts will obligate the dentist to develop a different design than for a patient with sound periodontal support and few other potentially damaging functional considerations.

A lever is a rigid rod supported somewhere between its two ends at a point, termed a fulcrum, which allows movement around that point.[5] The lever system allows magnification of force applied at one end of the rod proportional to the length of the rod from the fulcrum. Consequently, a small magnitude of force remote to the fulcrum will amplify to potentially destructive levels, depending on the design of the prosthesis. This is most apparent in distal extension designs, where the length of the lever arm predicts the degree of force applied to the abutment teeth. Likewise, the dissimilar characteristics of support from the teeth and soft tissues yield rotation in three cranial planes.

The tooth : tissue dissimilarity of support is a preeminent concern in distal extension and Class I, II, or large IV partial denture designs. Class I, II, or large IV partial dentures derive most of their support from the residual ridges and a limited amount from the abutment teeth. These types of RPDs generate the most potentially destructive lever forces. The fulcrum is generally established through a line connecting the most distal abutment teeth or the rests on those teeth. The Class III or small IV partial denture design is generally tooth supported with the fulcrum positioned between the abutment teeth bordering the edentulous space.

The residual ridge has a fibrous connective tissue covering the bone and underlying the mucosa. The thickness of subepithelial tissue defines the displaceability of the tissue overlying the residual bone. The displaceability and the amount of keratinized mucosa overlying the residual ridge will distinguish the amount of support anticipated from the edentulous regions. The periodontal ligament is composed of collagenous fibers, blood vessels, and interstitial fluid to act as a shock absorber for the dentition. This ligament or membrane may vary in composition or thickness depending on the amount of force applied to the tooth. However, the compressibility of the residual ridge tissues and tooth ligament is not comparable. In fact, a tissue : tooth ratio of approximately 13 : 1 exists in healthy tissues.[5] This phenomenon requires careful deliberation when designing and fabricating a distal extension RPD.

Occlusion is of primary interest in the distal extension prosthesis. Accentuated occlusal forces or aberrant, parafunctional occlusal forces on the most remote portion of the distal extension base will impart a greater degree of leverage force to the supportive elements. Formation of a precise occlusal scheme will ensure harmonious function and enhance the prognosis of the abutment teeth.

Tooth morphology should be considered when evaluating potential abutment teeth. Clinical crown contours and occlusion will often dictate direct retainer, major and minor connector selection, and rest seat placement.[7,8] Root anatomy is frequently overlooked as a critical component of the supportive element for a removable prosthesis. In general, single-rooted teeth are less favorable abutments than multirooted abutments. Divergent roots render more support than fused roots. Circular roots offer the least resistance to rotational forces than do oblong root contours. For this reason, premolars, particularly mandibular premolars, are poor choices to serve as solitary abutments for distal extension RPDs. Ideally, an FPD or implant should be provided from the second premolar to the canine to avoid using the second premolar as a solitary abutment. Periodontally weakened roots provide disproportionately less surface area for anchorage owing to their conical shape.

Problem situations

Perhaps the most difficult situation is the distal extension RPD. This is complicated when the missing teeth are located unilaterally, since functional requirements make it more difficult to esthetically mask the abutment attachments. However, if the entire arch is to be restored, then the situation becomes amenable to either an overdenture, precision attachment, or implant-retained prosthesis. If this is not the case, then the determination of the lower lip when smiling will help determine the type of attachment or clasp assembly to use.

Specific clasp types and esthetic considerations

The use of conventional clasping in esthetic regions of the mouth can present difficulties with patient acceptance. Proper surveying and mouth preparation may circumvent complications. Clasps may approach undercuts from a suprabulge or infrabulge region. Proper abutment tooth selection for clasps and placement of the clasps far enough into the infrabulge or distal region will maximize the esthetic benefit. Ideally, suprabulge clasps should be placed in the middle one-third of the tooth in the region of the proximal plate. The retentive tip should be located in the gingival one-third but not encroach on the free gingival margin (Figure 18.2). Placing the suprabulge clasp in this manner will improve the esthetic result and diminish the torquing forces applied to the tooth by the clasp. Infrabulge clasps will generally provide more enhanced esthetics, although they may have limitations to their use owing to anatomic considerations. The height of the vestibule, position of frena and soft tissue, or bony prominences may limit their application or necessitate preprosthetic surgery.

Circumferential clasp

Owing to its rigidity, this suprabulge clasp is generally reserved for tooth-supported abutments in posterior regions of the mouth. It is a cast clasp of either a round or half-round configuration, both of which provide little flexibility. When serving as a retentive element, the clasp should only engage a 0.25 mm undercut to avoid excessive torquing of the tooth. This clasp may also serve as a bracing or reciprocal element and is positioned above the height of contour. Owing to the relative size (thickness and diameter) of this clasp, use of the clasp above the height of contour for reciprocation should be limited in esthetic regions of the mouth. In situations where increased flexibility is necessary, but there is no place to remote solder a wrought wire clasp, such as the tooth-supported side of a Kennedy Class II arch, a cast round clasp may be used. A 20-gauge cast round clasp has been shown to have the same flexibility as a 19-gauge wrought wire clasp.[9]

I-, Y-, T-, or modified T-bar clasp

The infrabulge approach of this clasp optimizes esthetics for patients with reasonably high lip lines or in situations where clasping of maxillary first or second premolars is indicated (Figure 18.3). It is generally cast as part of the framework and

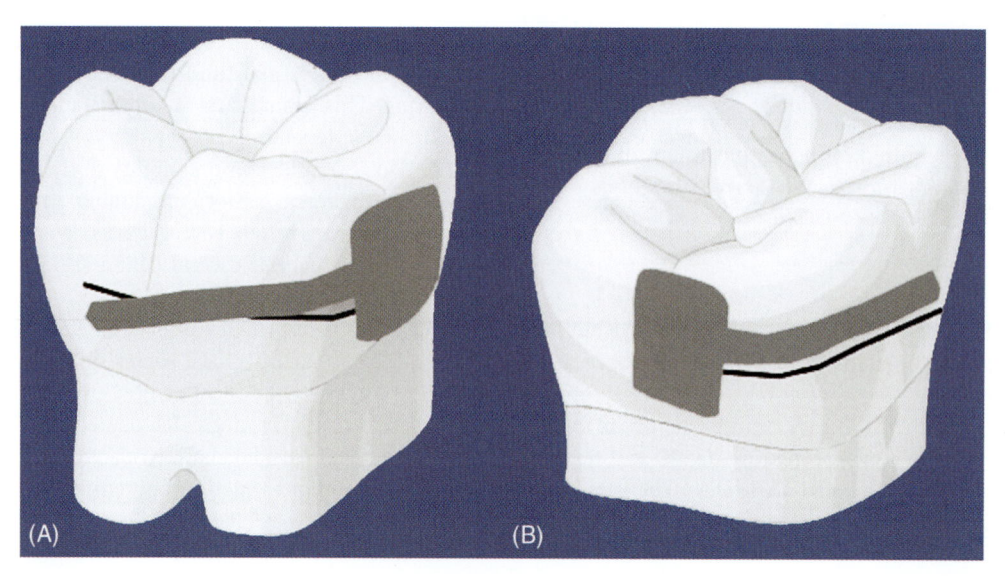

Figure 18.2 Proper placement of the retentive and reciprocal arms. **(A)** The retentive arm exits the abutment tooth in the middle one-third and terminates in the gingival one-third; only the retentive tip (terminal one-third) is placed below the height of contour. **(B)** The reciprocal arm exits the abutment tooth in the middle one-third and remains completely above the height of contour.

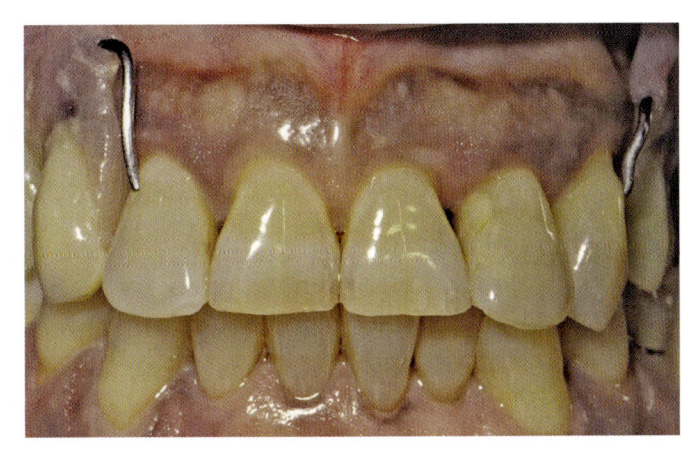

Figure 18.3 The use of the infrabulge bar (I-bar) clasp optimizes esthetics, particularly in the maxillary arch.

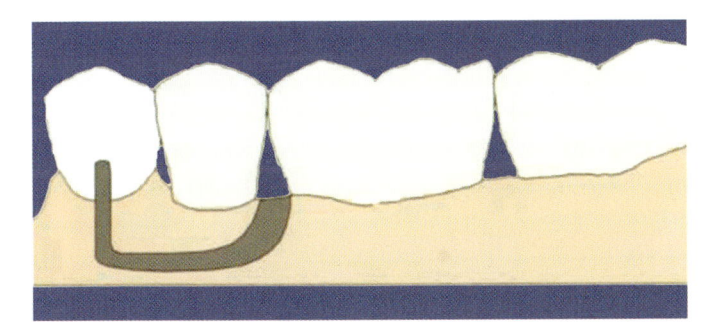

Figure 18.4 The approach arm of the I-bar is placed approximately one tooth distal to the abutment tooth. It exits the meshwork in the interdental area between the replacement teeth to minimize grinding of the replacement teeth.

should exit the meshwork approximately one tooth distal to the abutment tooth. This allows for optimal tooth positioning without excessive grinding of the replacement tooth, which would reduce the esthetic value of the denture tooth. In Figure 18.4, correct positioning of the approach arm of the I-bar allows the clasp to traverse from the framework through the interproximal embrasure region of the first and second replacement tooth. This minimizes the need to shorten the most anterior denture tooth to allow for the clasp to traverse from the framework more anteriorly.

The T- or Y-bar configuration achieves undercut engagement of 0.25 mm on either the mesial or distal surfaces of the tooth. A common error is to place both tips of the T- or Y-bar clasp into an undercut (Figure 18.5A and B). The esthetic value may be diminished if the anterior arm of the T- or Y-bar remains while using a distal undercut. Removal of the anterior arm should be considered, and a modified T-bar clasp should be selected (Figure 18.6A and B). A functional advantage of the modified T-bar is elimination of the mesial arm, limiting mesial undercut engagement of the clasp during a seating movement of the denture base toward the residual ridge. This will reduce the torque and distal tipping of the tooth. As a general rule, clasps should disengage during denture base movements toward the residual ridge and become active only on dislodging movements away from the residual ridge. If the height of contour is located in the incisal or occlusal one-third of the tooth, this clasp design should not be used because of the space created under the approach arm.

Rest–proximal plate–I-bar clasp

The rest–proximal plate–I-bar (RPI) clasp, described by Kratochvil[10,11] and later modified by Krol and coworkers,[12,13] consists of the following components: (1) mesioocclusal rest, (2) proximal plate, and (3) I-bar clasp. The retentive tip of the I-bar should engage a 0.25 mm midfacial undercut (Figure 18.7). As for the T- or Y-bar clasps, the approach arm should traverse from the meshwork approximately one tooth distal from the abutment tooth. Esthetically, the RPI clasp fulfills all requirements of a conventional clasp yet demonstrates minimal tooth coverage, relatively limited metal display, and an infrabulge approach. The mesioocclusal rest stabilizes the tooth and resists distal tipping. The design is indicated for distal extension situations and allows for disengagement of the clasp under occlusal force to the denture base. As with the T- or Y-bar, this infrabulge approach may not be desirable if adequate vestibular height is not present or anatomic structures, such as frena, are present. Infrabulge clasps may be more esthetically pleasing for patients with a low lip line.

Mesial groove reciprocation clasp

The mesial groove reciprocation (MGR) clasp, described by McCartney,[14] is indicated for maxillary distal extension RPDs when canines serve as the abutment teeth (see Figure 18.3). Facial bracing is important because, unlike premolars, the mesiolingual contour of the canine does not usually present enough surface to resist distal movement. Adequate bracing is necessary to resist distal movement that would disengage the retentive portion of a distally placed clasp from the surface of the canine and result in a loss of retention.[15]

When necessary, the labial surface should be prepared so that its height of contour is at the same occlusogingival level as that of the lingual surface. A distal guide plane is not prepared. A 1 mm depression is prepared in the center of the distal half of the labial surface, gingival to its height of contour (Figures 18.8, 18.9, and 18.10). Retention is attained with a 19-gauge cast or wrought wire I-bar engaging a 0.25 mm undercut on this surface. The MGR clasp incorporates a prepared mesial groove to provide reciprocation. A vertical mesial groove guiding plane 1–2 mm in length is prepared in the mesiolingual surface within the mesial marginal ridge enamel. To complete the abutment modification, the mesial reciprocation groove is extended over the mesial marginal ridge to terminate in a spoon-shaped mesial rest seat. Occasionally, a small amalgam restoration may be required when dentin is exposed while preparing sufficient depth for lateral force resistance.

Ring clasp

This clasp is used for inclined maxillary or mandibular molars with natural undercuts on the mesiobuccal or mesiolingual surface respectively. The ring clasp should never be used as an unsupported ring, known as a back-action clasp, as it cannot

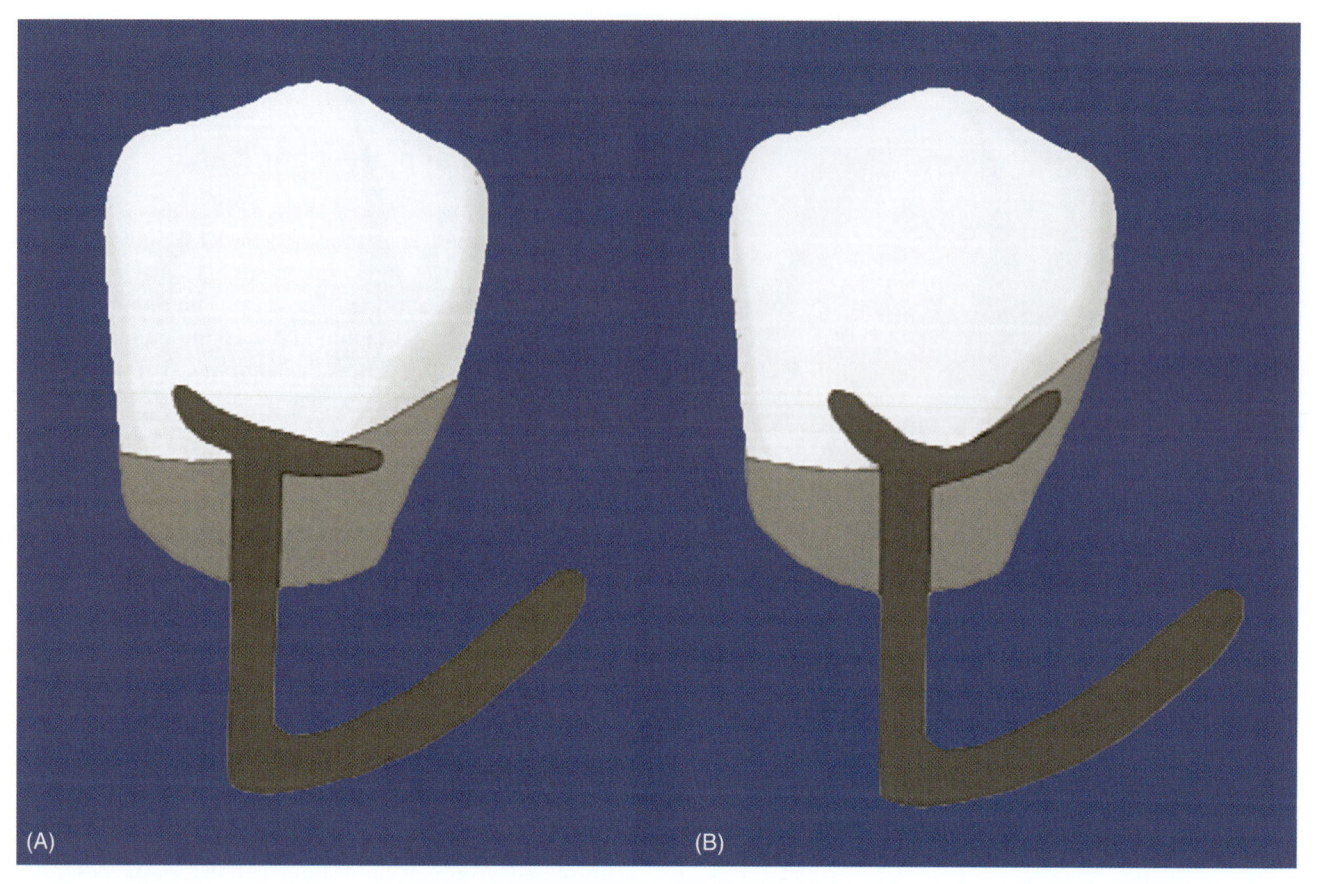

Figure 18.5 **(A, B)** Only one tip of the T- or Y-bar clasp should be placed in the retentive undercut. The other tip provides support only.

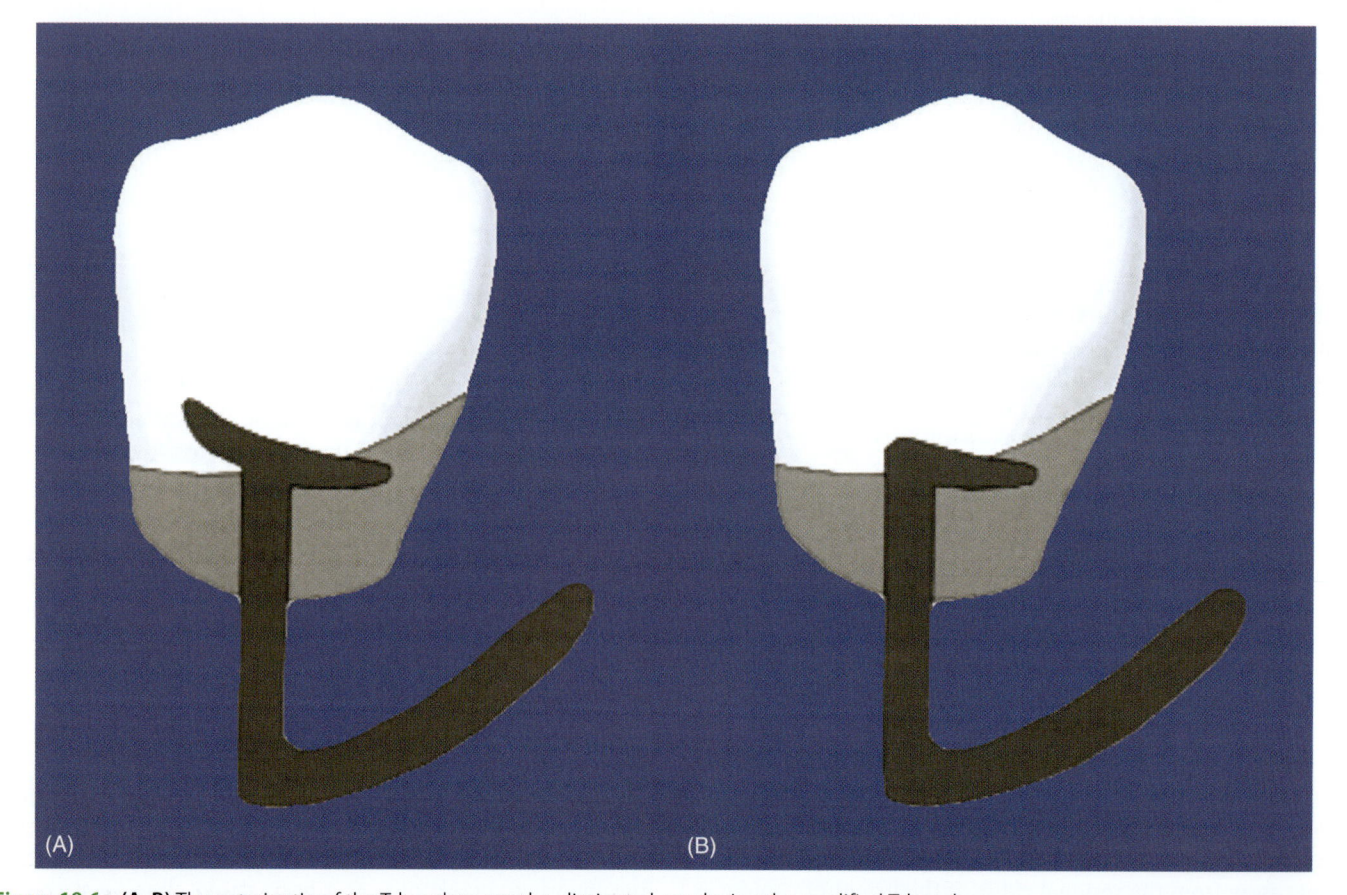

Figure 18.6 **(A, B)** The anterior tip of the T-bar clasp may be eliminated, producing the modified T-bar clasp.

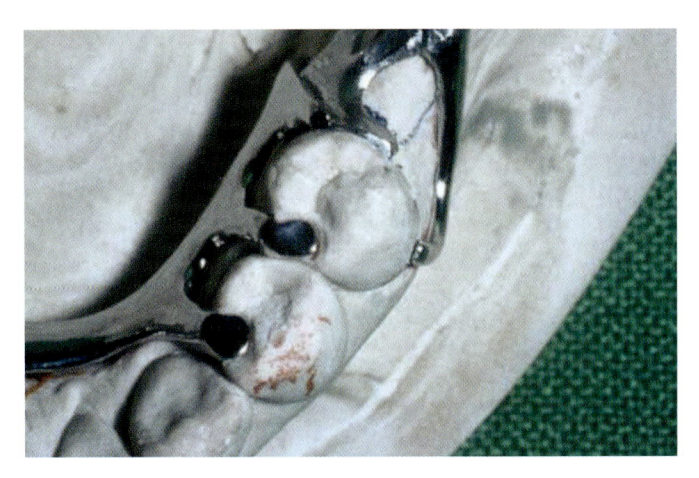

Figure 18.7 The RPI clasp design consists of a mesioocclusal rest, proximal plate, and midfacial I-bar clasp. *Source:* Courtesy of Dr John R. Ivanhoe.

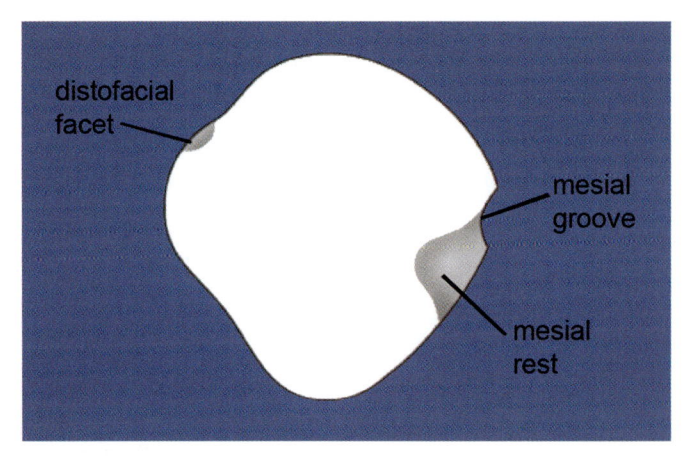

Figure 18.8 MGR clasp natural tooth preparation. A distal guide plane is not prepared. A 1 mm depression is prepared in the center of the distal half of the labial surface, gingival to the height of contour. A mesial groove that provides reciprocation extends over the mesial marginal ridge to a mesial rest seat.

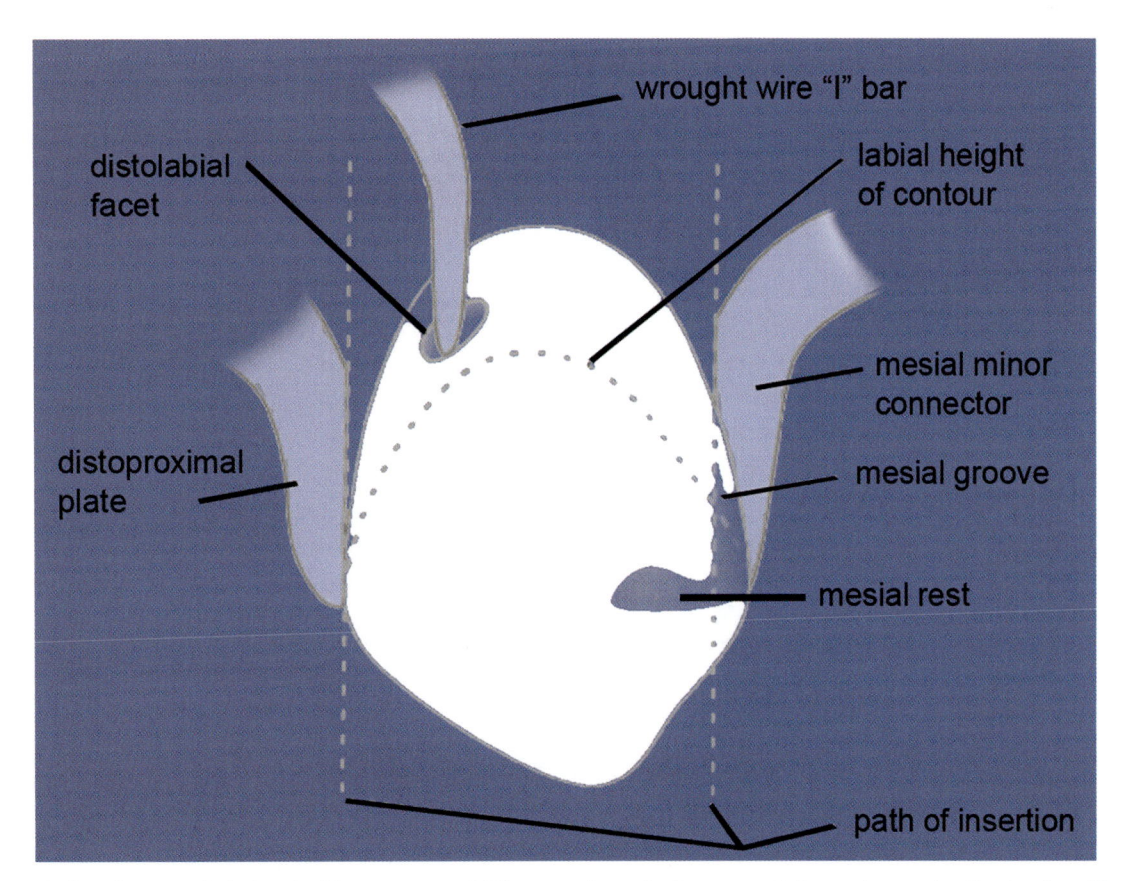

Figure 18.9 MGR clasp framework design. An I-bar engages a 0.25 mm undercut in the prepared depression on the distal surface. The mesial minor connector contacts the mesial groove and terminates in the mesial rest seat.

provide both reciprocation and stabilization.[5] It is usually designed with an additional bracing arm to prevent excessive flexing. An additional rest seat placed on the opposite side of the tooth enhances the rigidity of the clasp assembly and may aid in resisting further mesial migration of the tooth. The entire clasp assembly, except for the retentive tip, must lie above the height of contour. Consequently, it is not an esthetic clasp assembly and is reserved for molar abutments.

Embrasure clasp

This clasp will be used in posterior regions of the mouth in the quadrant without an edentulous space, as in Class II situations. This clasp avoids excessive distal extension of the major connector. The embrasure clasp is a suprabulge clasp that should have an adequate sluiceway prepared through the embrasure of the abutment teeth to allow for proximal rests and emergence of the suprabulge clasp arm elements near the height of contour (Figure 18.11A and B). Adequate sluiceway depth will also provide for proper metal thickness to ensure rigidity and avoid occlusal interference from the opposing dentition.

Combination clasp

The combination clasp consists of a wrought wire clasp arm and cast reciprocal arm (Figure 18.12).[16] It is most frequently used adjacent to a distal extension base to promote stress-breaking characteristics to the abutment tooth. The wrought wire, being more flexible (less brittle), may be used in smaller diameter with less danger of fracture. A 19-gauge wrought wire in a 0.5 mm mesial undercut is generally indicated for canine and premolar distal extension abutments. Remote soldering of the clasp to the framework provides increased flexibility.[17] Owing to its round form, light refraction is decreased, making the metal display less noticeable than with the broader surface of a cast clasp.

Retention enhancement

Traditionally, enamelplasty or a cast restoration has been indicated for an abutment tooth with an inadequate undercut. The improvements in composite resins have made them a conservative, cost-effective, and minimally invasive method for enhancing retention. However, variable results have been reported from the studies using composite resin to enhance retention. In-vitro studies have shown that cast I-bars produced wear of the composite resin,[18] whereas stainless steel round clasps did not cause a noticeable loss of retention.[19] The use of a partial-coverage porcelain laminate bonded to a tooth to enhance retention is a viable alternative.[20]

Rest seats

In general, mesioocclusal rest seats are indicated for posterior distal extension abutments when the occlusion permits.[10,21] For tooth-supported RPDs, rest seats are placed on either side of the

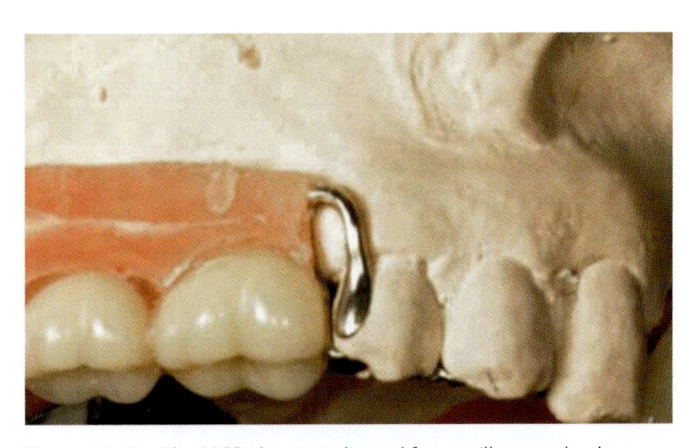

Figure 18.10 The MGR clasp is indicated for maxillary teeth where esthetics is a concern.

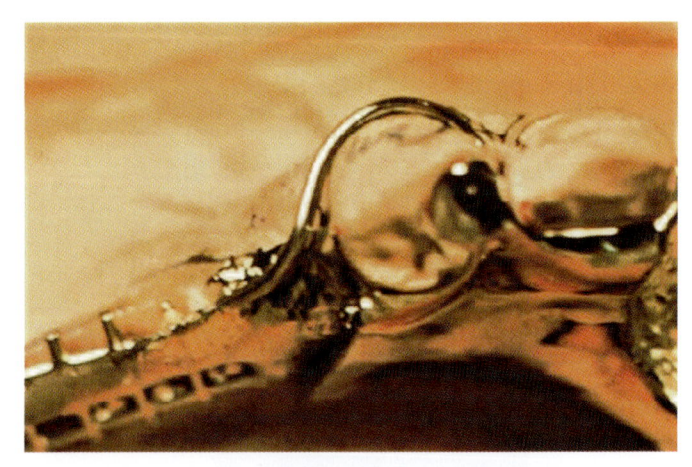

Figure 18.12 The combination clasp consists of a wrought wire retentive arm with a cast reciprocating arm or plated surface. *Source:* Courtesy of Dr John R. Ivanhoe.

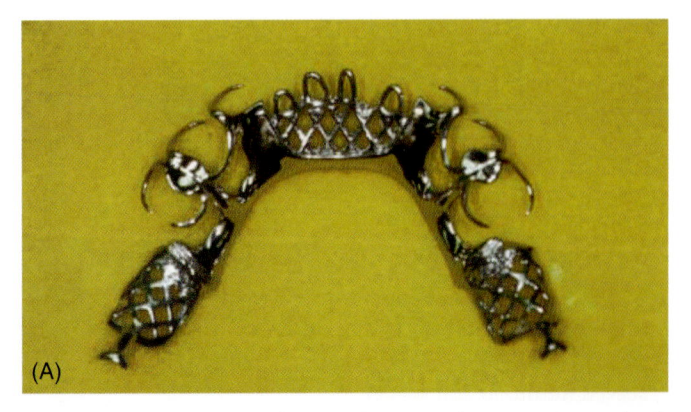

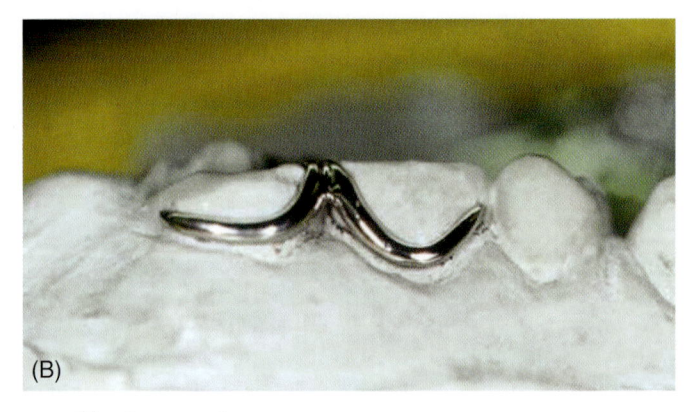

Figure 18.11 (A, B) The embrasure clasp is used on posterior teeth where no modification space is present.

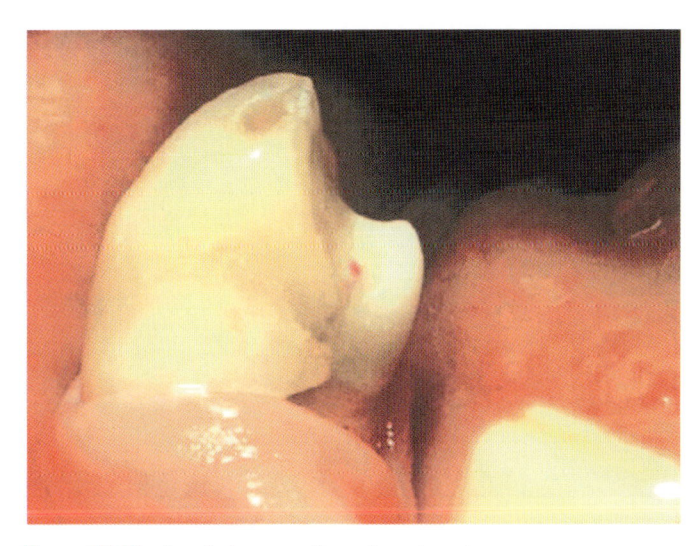

Figure 18.13 Bonded composite resin rest seat.

modification space to prevent tissueward movement of the RPD and for ease of fabrication. Cingulum rest seats are indicated for anterior teeth. However, the lack of adequate enamel often precludes placement of a positive cingulum rest seat on the mandibular anterior teeth. Traditionally, incisal rests have been advocated for mandibular anterior teeth. Unfortunately, they are unesthetic, may interfere with the occlusion, and may increase torquing forces on the teeth. Bonded composite resin or metal rest seats have been shown to provide a satisfactory and esthetic alternative to the incisal rest (Figure 18.13).[22,23]

Flange design

A labial flange in the anterior region is indicated when residual ridge resorption has occurred and additional lip support is needed. The flange should extend to the junction of the attached and unattached mucosa and should be contoured to blend in with the adjacent teeth. Also, the flange should not extend into an undercut apical to the adjacent teeth.[24] Occasionally, tinting of the denture base to match the pigmentation of the patient may be indicated.[25–27]

Replacement teeth

Teeth should be selected to match the size, shape, shade, and contour of the adjacent teeth. In some instances, it will be necessary to contour the tooth, and, occasionally, it may be necessary to stain the artificial tooth or place a restoration in the tooth to match adjacent teeth. A technique to modify the shade, contour, and occlusal contacting surfaces of denture teeth with light-polymerized composite resin has been described.[28] Microfilled resins for veneering facial surfaces are advocated because these are more easily polished and provide an improved esthetic appearance. These changes are most easily accomplished when the artificial tooth is fabricated from acrylic resin. The acrylic denture base resin should be contoured to match the size and contour of those of the adjacent teeth. The artificial teeth should be positioned to simulate the position of the natural teeth. If natural teeth remain, they may be used as a guide for placing the artificial teeth in a harmonious arrangement.

Other esthetic considerations

The patient should be assessed in totality rather than as an aggregate of singular entities. The potential consequence that one treatment has on another region of the mouth and the overall result requires careful appraisal. Although it is the intent of most clinicians to maximize the esthetic value of treatment for the patient, the esthetic awareness and desire of the patient merit consideration. The implementation of complex components that potentially increase the cost, maintenance, or difficulties with hygiene for a patient unconcerned with esthetics is not prudent. However, the assessment of patient awareness needs to be bona fide. The apathetic patient can create postinsertion obstacles if a genuine esthetic concern is not detected. This type of patient will frequently respond to queries of esthetics with "Do whatever you think would look good, doctor," or "I don't care about the appearance, as long as I can chew." Caution should be exercised when managing the prosthetic care of these patients.

Skeletal anomalies that may affect esthetics should be brought to the patient's attention prior to treatment. Any discussion following the completion of care may often be interpreted as an excuse. Particular examples would include patients who believe that the RPD will correct skeletal discrepancies, overt facial wrinkling, or other esthetic concerns normally requiring surgical intervention. A skeletal Class II patient or a patient with vertical maxillary excess will be particularly aware of a maxillary anterior modification space for the RPD. The excessive acrylic resin display or lip displacement justifies consultation prior to RPD fabrication, allowing the patient the opportunity to consider alternative treatment options to meet their esthetic needs.

Tooth morphology and anticipated placement require evaluation of presurgical diagnostic casts. Most patients will request replacement of the missing dentition to maintain their previous esthetic situation. This should be readily accomplished, although if a suitable replacement is not feasible the limitations should be discussed with the patient prior to commencing treatment. Encumbrances may be due to tooth size or shape limitations or positioning difficulties, which may detract from the function of the partial denture. Examples may include the patient with natural anterior teeth that were much larger than the commercially available artificial dentition or the request to maintain the anterior tooth display in a patient demonstrating an excessive vertical overlap of the maxillary incisors. Clearly, esthetic and functional concerns may create the need for investigation of alternative treatment options or acceptance of the limitations by compromising either the esthetics or functional design. Any of these situations should remain well documented and explained to the patient completely.

Alternative treatment modalities

In situations demanding maximal esthetics, alternatives to conventional RPD design must be in the clinician's armamentarium. Alternative treatment modalities will often produce a result in prudent design with function and esthetics. The use of dental attachments is discussed in this chapter; however, finances, as

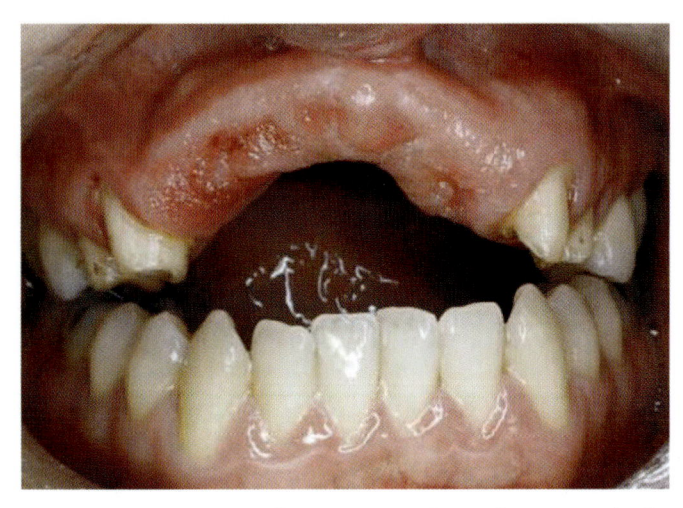

Figure 18.14 (A) The maxillary anterior teeth were lost as a result of a traumatic injury. The bone loss in the anterior maxilla is significant.

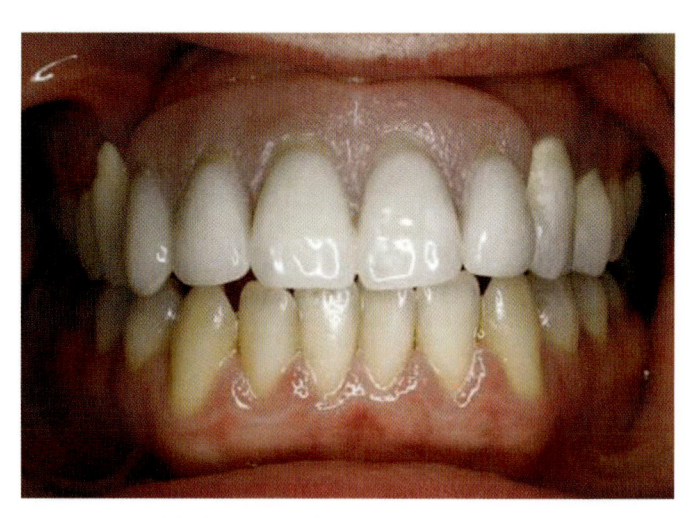

Figure 18.14 (B) The rotational path RPD allows the elimination of anterior clasp arms to improve esthetics.

well as dexterity or the ability to complete or maintain complex care, often dictate the need for conventional alternatives.

Adjunctive mechanisms for minimizing metal display

Camouflaging of RPD clasps, including the addition of acrylic or composite resin, has been reported in the literature.[29,30] The difficulty with the use of acrylic or composite resin to veneer to RPD metals lies in the differences between their abilities to flex and their coefficients of thermal expansion. Non-noble metals possess strength and resist significant flexure. However, resins are subjected to greater deformation from physical and thermal conditions. The composite resin matrix also tends to be brittle beyond its elastic limit. As a result, the abilities of the metals and resins to deform plastically are incompatible. Other concerns include the effect of the intraoral forces of mastication, the adjustability of veneered clasps, and the additional bulk of the clasp created by the addition of the veneering material. Excessive shortening and thinning of the clasp should be avoided to ensure rigidity and minimize the breakage potential of the clasp.[31]

Rotational path removable partial dentures

The rotational path RPD is a relatively uncomplicated method that eliminates the use of esthetically objectionable clasping in the anterior region of the mouth (Figure 18.14A and B).[32–35] It uses an anterior rigid portion of the framework and a conventional flexible posterior retentive clasp as the retentive components. The primary advantage of this design is the minimal use of clasps. The esthetic result is enhanced, and the tendency toward plaque accumulation is reduced. However, both the clinical and laboratory procedures required for the rotational path RPD are technique sensitive.

The rotational path RPD should be limited to tooth-supported situations to prevent torquing of abutment teeth. This design also requires that positive rest seats be used. Cingulum and extended occlusal rest seats are indicated for canine and premolar abutments respectively (Figures 18.15A and B and 18.16). For premolars, the rest seats should be extended to 1.5–2.0 mm deep occlusogingivally with nearly parallel facial and lingual walls. A restoration may be indicated to adequately contour the rest seat.

The cast is first surveyed at a 0° tilt to determine the adequacy of undercuts on the mesial surfaces of the anterior abutments and the distofacial surfaces of the posterior abutments (Figure 18.17). The amount of undercut needed for the anterior teeth is 0.25–0.5 mm. This position is registered using tripod marks. The cast is then tilted until the undercuts of the anterior abutments are eliminated. The analyzing rod is then used to determine whether access exists for the rests to be seated. There must be no interferences for the anterior segment to go to place (Figure 18.18). If it is satisfactory, the second cast tilt should be registered on the cast with a second set of tripod marks (Figure 18.19A and B). Major connectors with minimal palatal or lingual tooth contact are indicated to avoid interferences to seating of the framework. It is important that, during the framework trial insertion appointment, there is minimal adjustment of the anterior proximal plate; otherwise, the anterior retentive component may be lost. The rotational path RPD is not indicated for distal extension RPDs, arches with lingually inclined teeth, severely tapered arches, and arches with multiple edentulous areas.

Attachments for removable partial dentures

Diagnosis and treatment planning

The demands for highly esthetic dental restorations provide the catalyst for the attachment RPDs. The esthetic expectations of a patient should be the primary directive for attachment use. The psychological component of treatment planning of the RPD remains crucial to the success or failure of the rehabilitation. Meeting the patient's esthetic and functional expectations while not exceeding the biomechanical attributes of the supportive structures will result in successful therapy. The anticipated

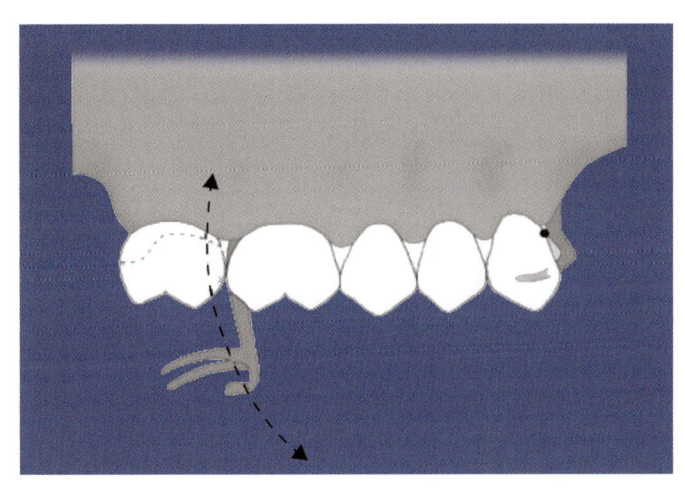

Figure 18.15 **(A)** The rotational path RPD uses an anterior rigid portion of the framework that engages an undercut and a conventional flexible posterior retentive clasp. After engaging the anterior undercut, the prosthesis is rotated into the fully seated position along an arc.

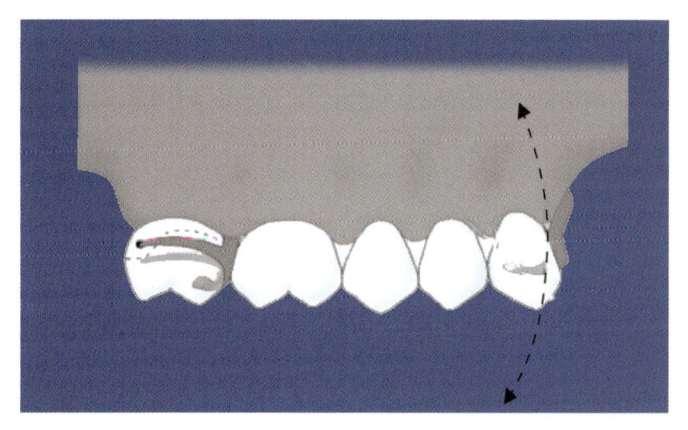

Figure 18.15 **(B)** This arc demonstrates the arc along which the anterior rigid retainer would have to move for the prosthesis to be dislodged.

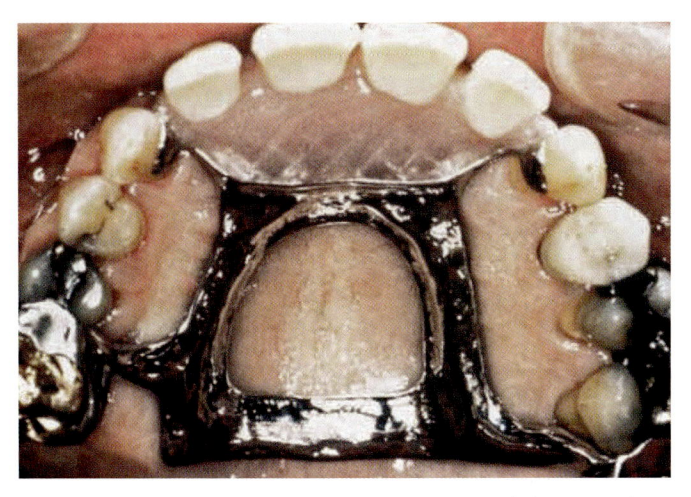

Figure 18.16 The rotational path design uses extended rests on the anterior abutments.

function of the prostheses by the patient must not exceed the physiologic capacity of the teeth and tissues.

Proper treatment planning of the attachment RPD encompasses similar concepts to the conventional RPD. Fundamental biologic tenets must be adhered to for successful treatment. The components of guiding planes, rigid major and minor connectors, and indirect retention remain important in the philosophy of design. Suitable tissue preparation, accurate border extension, and tissue coverage without impingement are important adjuncts. Correct prosthetic planning will reduce the possibility of tissue abuse and enhance the prognosis for success.

Definition

An attachment is a connector consisting of two or more parts.[36] One part is connected to a root, tooth, or implant and the other part to a prosthesis. Attachment RPDs have been empirically termed "precision attachments" for years. The terminology of precision attachment partial dentures is frequently misused. Attachment partial dentures should be classified by the nature of the attachment fabrication, location, and biomechanical properties. Attachments used in RPDs are most commonly classified as (1) precision, (2) semiprecision, (3) intracoronal (nonresilient and resilient), and (4) extracoronal (nonresilient and resilient).[36-38]

Attachments are subdivided into two general categories: precision and nonprecision.[36,39] Precision attachments consist of machined components of special alloys under precise tolerances within 0.01 mm. The metallurgic properties of the alloys are controlled to minimize the intra-attachment wear and are designed in a manner that affords most wear to occur on interchangeable elements. The intra-abutment portion of the attachment will generally evidence little to no wear, allowing accurate replacement while maintaining the specific tolerances designed. These systems allow ease of replacement interchangeability of the standard components.

Semiprecision attachments require the direct casting of plastic, wax, or refractory patterns. They are considered semiprecision because they are subject to inconsistent water : powder ratios, burnout temperatures, and other variables. The resulting components may dimensionally change and reduce the preciseness of their accuracy of fit. The primary advantages of the semiprecision attachments are economy, ease of fabrication, and ability to be cast in a wide variety of alloys without the problem of coefficiency differences between the casting alloy and the attachment alloy.[36,39]

General considerations for attachments

The variability in the circumstances for use of attachments and the variety of attachments available preclude the establishment of a standard model. Selection should be based on the functional and physiologic requirements of the restoration. Consideration of the laboratory expertise in using particular attachments must be contemplated. Selection of an attachment with specific biomechanical and functional attributes may be finalized by the dental laboratory technician's ability to use the attachment and fabricate the prosthesis.

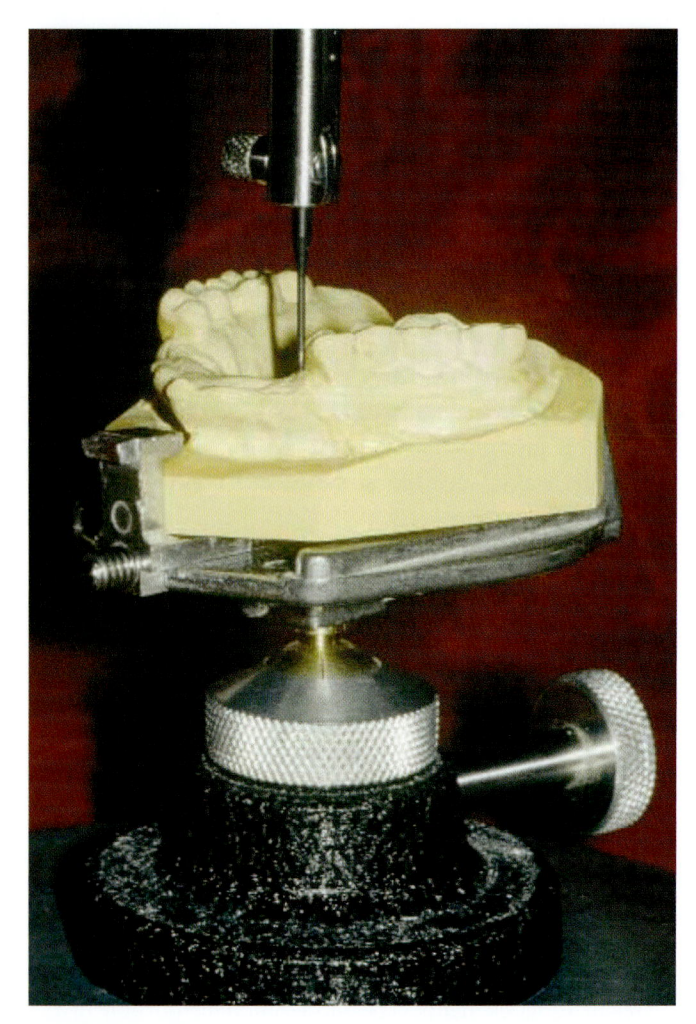

Figure 18.17 The cast is first surveyed with a 0° tilt to determine the adequacy of undercuts on the mesial surfaces of the anterior abutments and on the distal facial surfaces of the posterior abutments. This position is registered using tripod marks.

Attachment use

A significant consideration in the selection of an attachment should be the long-term maintenance. Retrievability should be regarded with equality to function in the design and selection of an attachment for the esthetic RPD. Repeated use of similar attachments increases the knowledge of the clinician and dental laboratory technician alike. This repetition will prove beneficial for efficacious delivery of care, management of difficult situations, and postoperative maintenance. The dental team should limit the application of dental attachments to a selection that meets the functional and esthetic requirements of the majority of patients and the level of expertise of the team. Other attachments may be considered periodically; however, use of other attachments may prove to be the rarity rather than the norm. This self-imposed limitation will ensure correct fabrication of the partial denture, untroubled delivery of care, and unrestricted maintenance of the prosthesis. Periodic planned or unplanned maintenance of the attachment prosthesis will be required. Consistent use of an attachment selection may safeguard adequate supply of replacement parts in the event of accidental breakage.[40]

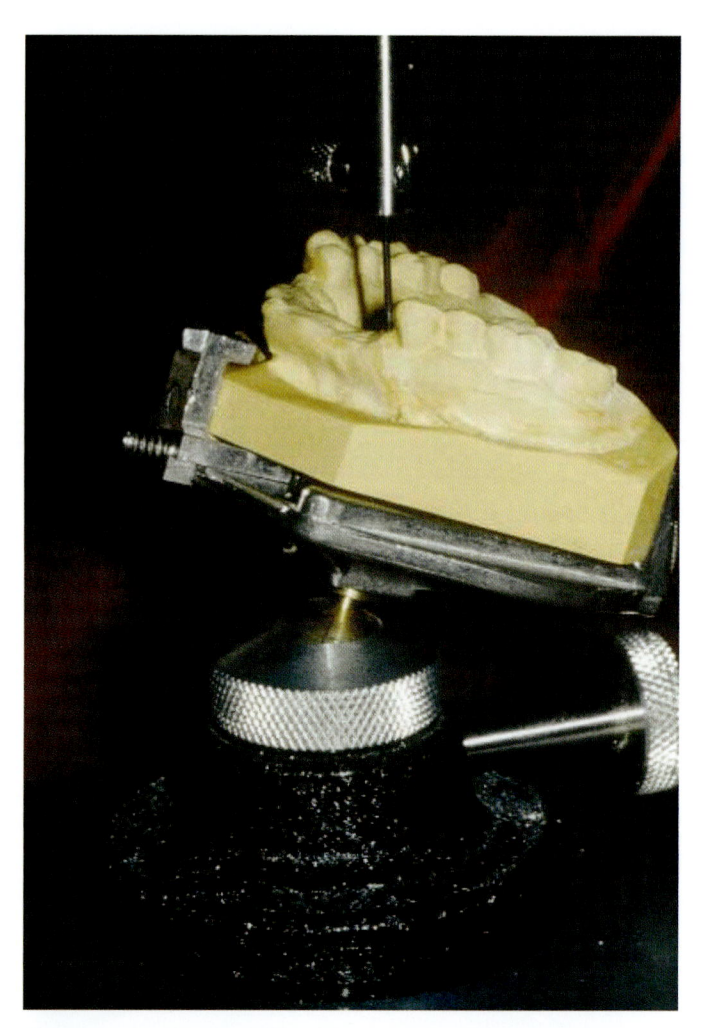

Figure 18.18 The cast is then tilted to eliminate the undercuts of the anterior abutments. This tilt is registered with a second set of tripod marks.

Indications and contraindications

The overwhelming indication for the attachment RPD is esthetics. Numerous skillfully designed conventional RPDs are not worn simply because the patient does not like the appearance. Elimination of the buccal or labial direct retainer or clasp arm is a key factor in establishing an esthetically acceptable design. Once the need for an attachment-assisted RPD is established, the selection of the attachment type should be based on the biomechanical, physiologic, and functional attributes of the patient or technical expertise of the dental team.[39,41]

The contraindications to the use of attachments in RPDs are numerous. One must consider anatomic, biomechanical, personal, and physiologic factors in determining the selection of attachments. The health and morphology of the abutment teeth remain a significant factor in the selection of an attachment. Short clinical crowns prove to be the foremost contraindication to the use of attachments in the fabrication of RPDs. The tooth must have adequate clinical crown height to house the attachment components and effectively offset the leverage forces exerted on the tooth and supporting apparatus. The leverage forces are most often observed in distal extension RPDs.

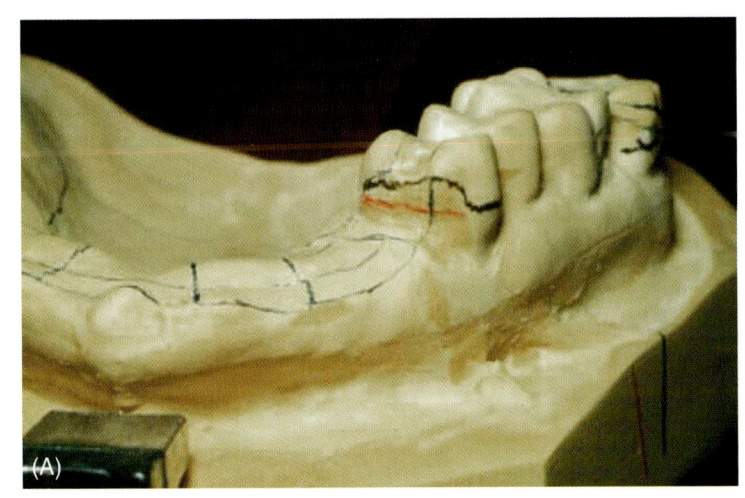

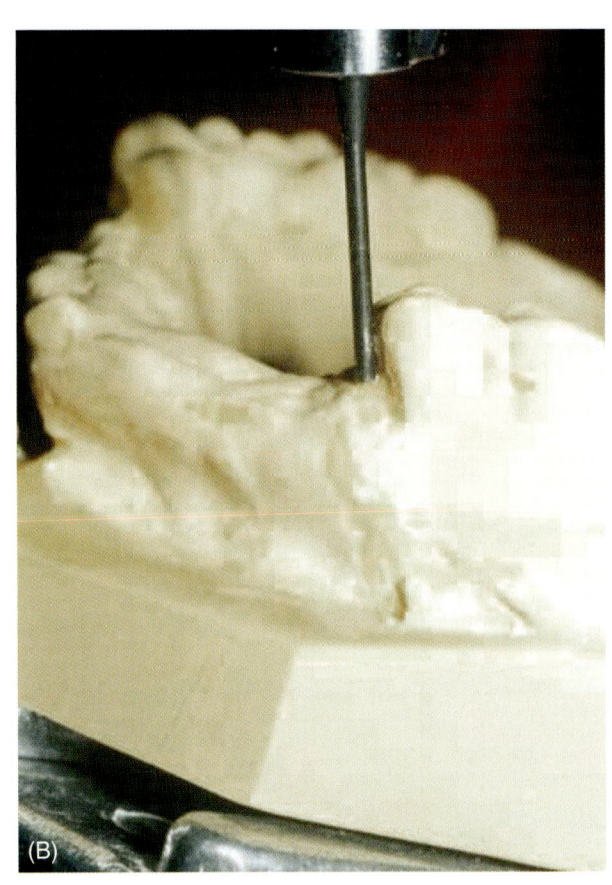

Figure 18.19 (A, B) The heights of contour made at the two paths of insertion. The superior height of contour is made at the 0° tilt. The inferior height of contour represents the path of insertion whereby the undercuts of the anterior abutments are eliminated. The area between the two lines represents the undercut into which the anterior rigid section of the framework is seated. Care must be taken during finishing and fitting of the framework in this area; otherwise, retention may be lost.

In addition, adequate height must be present for the corresponding attachment components to be housed within the RPD framework or supportive acrylic resin while allowing proper artificial tooth placement.[36–41] Too little vertical height will preclude the use of attachments or require modifications to the attachment thereby reducing its strength or functionality; this also may result in insufficient space for replacement teeth and resin on the RPD, resulting in reduced esthetics, reduced function, or unanticipated fractures in this area.

Adjunctive procedures

Gingivectomy, or crown-lengthening procedures, may overcome the clinical disadvantage of short clinical crown height. This pre-prosthetic procedure will generally improve fixed prosthesis retention and resistance form and may increase the effective undercut, thereby enhancing the retention for a conventional clasping mechanism. This may avoid the need for placement of a surveyed crown when attachments are not a feasible treatment modality. Gingival crown-lengthening procedures may be required to provide adequate occlusal cervical space for attachment positioning while maintaining the functional attributes of the selected attachment to be used.

Orthodontic therapy should be considered with the presence of tipped or malpositioned teeth. The orthodontic correction of malpositioned teeth will avoid excessive tooth preparation, enhance vertical loading, avert the need for endodontics, and provide easier development of a common path of placement for the attachment partial denture. A particular degree of parallelism is required of all attachments. Orthodontic correction of malpositioning will allow proper attachment orientation. A non-resilient precision attachment requires the higher degree of parallelism.

Teeth with large pulps will not allow for incorporation of an internal box within the crown preparation to accommodate certain attachments.[37,39,41] The result of improper preparation would be an excessively overcontoured tooth resulting in a periodontal compromise. Endodontic therapy may be required in certain instances for the use of attachments. Endodontics should also be considered when preparation of a tooth with a large core restoration might provide little resistance to fracture. The placement of an intraradicular core might offer enhanced resistance to fracture under the functional loading of an attachment RPD.

The placement of attachments in pontics is an option that can avoid possible violations of biologic principles during tooth preparation or the need for adjunctive procedures (Figure 18.20). The use of attachments lingually positioned in a traditional pontic or distally located in a cantilevered pontic has been described.[42]

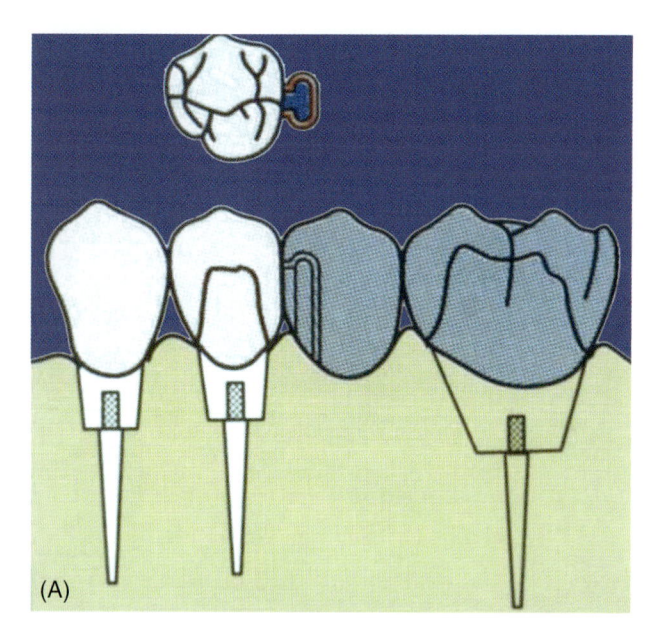

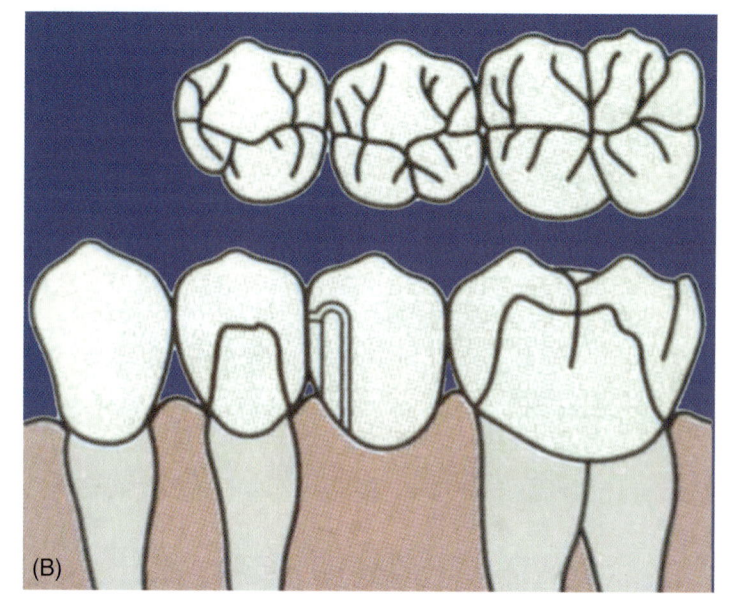

Figure 18.20 Intracoronal attachment types, such as the Score-BR, PDC, Omega-M, Beyeler, and others (Attachments International, San Mateo, CA). **(A)** The matrix is placed upside down and cast to the anterior abutment. The patrix is waxed over the matrix, and the waxing of the FPD is completed. **(B)** The FPD is invested, cast, and finished. *Source:* Reproduced with permission from Staubli.[36]

Dexterity

Poor patient dexterity remains a strong contraindication for the placement of an attachment RPD. Patients lacking adequate hand coordination may encounter significant difficulty manipulating the prosthesis intraorally. For some, it may be a virtual impossibility. While the average life expectancy increases, more patients become potential candidates for RPD treatment. Debilitating diseases affecting neuromuscular control and joint mobility are likely to correspondingly increase. Arthritis, Parkinson's disease, cerebrovascular accidents, and other situations that influence fine motor skills might preclude efficacious attachment partial denture use or, at least, direct the attachment selection. Consequently, dexterity should remain a strong diagnostic consideration with all potential attachment RPD patients. Patients demonstrating average dexterity will generally be able to manipulate placement and removal with relative ease over time. A resilient attachment will generally be more easily accommodated rather than a rigid intracoronal attachment with a precise path of placement.

Cost

The design and fabrication of the complex attachment RPD treatment are costly. Cost in terms of time, effort, and resource commitment can be anticipated. The economic factors may predict the feasibility of using attachments. The prudent clinician should anticipate an increased amount of diagnostic effort, laboratory expense, chair time, and maintenance in this form of therapy. These factors should be explained to the patient. The patient should anticipate charges for periodic attachment maintenance or replacement. Subsequently, these considerations support the use of a limited number of different attachments for efficacious delivery of care and reduced chair time.[40]

Oral hygiene maintenance

A final factor to be considered in the possible exclusion of attachment use for patients is the long-term maintenance of the prosthesis. It must be anticipated that periodic evaluation, adjustment, or replacement of attachment components will be required. The inability of patients to travel or return on a regular or periodic basis should be considered contraindications to the use of attachments. Oral hygiene may also be considered a parameter of attachment selection. Attachments will accumulate plaque and calculus, limiting the effectiveness or intended function of the attachment. Additionally, attachment use implicates the fabrication of full- or partial-coverage castings. Patients with high caries rates may experience a diminished prognosis with rehabilitations consisting of multiple fixed restorations.

Biomechanics and support

Once a decision has been made to restore a region with an attachment prosthesis, the manner in which the vertical and horizontal forces are to be supported requires consideration. A partial prosthesis may be tooth borne or tooth–tissue borne. The forces imparted to the prosthesis and its supportive elements should be as widely distributed as possible.

The periodontal health and support of the natural teeth should be considered in the selection of an attachment design. The forces should be equitably distributed over as many teeth as possible within the biologic and physiologic capacity of the supportive dentition. The denture bases should offer the broadest support possible for mucosal coverage.

Distal extension situations raise the dilemma of load distribution between the teeth and mucosa. The amount of soft-tissue compressibility over the distal extension residual ridge remains disproportionate to the abutment teeth. This phenomenon will create unharmonious movement of the partial denture, imparting leverage forces to the abutment teeth, possibly resulting in harm to the abutment teeth, mucosa, and residual ridge, if not considered in the selection of an attachment. Only teeth with suitable clinical crown height and periodontal stature should be considered for attachment use. The presence of excessive tissue compressibility or unsupported tissue might prescribe the need for preprosthetic surgical intervention.[37–39,41]

Path of insertion

With the aid of a surveyor, the anticipated path of insertion must be considered to develop appropriate guiding planes and attachment placement within the confines of the natural dentition. A less resilient attachment will generally dictate a smaller degree of tolerance or more parallelism relative to the path of insertion. Rigid and intracoronal attachments must closely accommodate nonsurgically correctable tissue/anatomic limitations or undercuts. For example, distal extension situations may require a distally inclined path of placement to accommodate extension into the retromylohyoid fossa, whereas an anterior modification space may require a labially inclined path of insertion and attachment orientation.[37,38]

Knowledge of the anticipated path of insertion may guide the attachment selection to a more resilient, universal design that can offer a greater tolerance to the path of placement. The path of insertion of the abutment crowns may be determined at this time and may indicate the need for preprosthetic endodontics or surgery.

Once a prosthesis has been placed along its path of insertion, anterior, posterior, and lateral forces alone or in combination influence the stability of the prosthesis. The tendency of the forces to dislodge the prosthesis must be counteracted through direct and indirect retainers. Direct retention may occur through friction of the attachment components, framework components with the teeth, or mucosal coverage of the denture bases. The forces of adhesion, cohesion, and surface tension between the base, saliva, and mucosa cause a pressure reduction on compression and further inhibit denture base movement.

Indirect retention

Resistance to lateral displacing forces must be provided through rigid bracing components and the vertical height of the residual ridges. Bilateral distal extension bases use the mucosa and teeth of both sides of the dental arches for resistance to lateral forces. A force on one side of the arch is resisted by the components or tissue/base integrity of the contralateral side. This supports the increased stability usually found in bilateral distal extension bases compared with unilateral designs. The design of certain attachments will provide indirect retention; however, the effectiveness of the indirect retention will vary. In attachment systems that offer little or no indirect retention, it must be incorporated in the framework design. In general, the more precise or rigid the attachment design is, the greater is the degree of indirect retention inherent in the design. Additionally, the more widely spaced the retainers are, the greater the support and stability are when compared with a design with retainers placed closely together.[36–41,43]

As attachment designs increase in the degree of indirect retention, a generally greater amount of force to the supportive elements will be generated. Because of this increase in leverage forces transferred to the abutment teeth by the prosthesis, many teeth treated with castings incorporating attachments must be splinted to adjacent teeth. This concept safeguards the functional and biomechanical overloading of the supportive elements.[44–47]

Tooth preparation

Preparation design should anticipate an increased degree of the forces to be applied to the teeth by the attachment mechanism. Avoidance of excessive taper, replacement of suspicious or weakened core restorations, and adequate axial wall height will reduce the risk of tooth fracture or decementation of the restoration. Therefore, most teeth will require full crown coverage for adequate retention and resistance form.

The preparations should consider the morphology of the tooth as related to the attachment selection. Adequate tooth structure must be present in all dimensions to allow incorporation of the attachment pattern yet retain the emergence profile and clinical crown contours of the tooth. Buccolingual, incisocervical, and mesiodistal space must be considered before a bur is placed to the tooth tissue. Alternative attachment selection or adjunctive procedures should be planned prior to preparation to allow for completion of the intended restoration and to enhance the functional and periodontal success of the restoration.

Attachment selection considerations

Proper attachment selection requires evaluation of five factors: location, function, retention, available space, and cost. Location can be subdivided into intracoronal, extracoronal, radicular, and bar types of attachments.[36]

Location

Intracoronal attachments are incorporated entirely within the contours of the cast crown for the tooth. It is imperative that adequate space exists in all three dimensions for both incorporation of the attachment and the maintenance of natural tooth contours to ensure proper use of the attachment and a positive prognosis of the restoration and the tooth. If it is not possible to place a box in the preparation to accommodate the matrix component of the attachment, an alternative attachment selection should be made. The advantage of the intracoronal attachment is that the forces exerted by the prosthesis are applied more closely to the long axis of the tooth. All intracoronal attachments are nonresilient and may require double abutting or splinting of the adjacent teeth. This form of attachment offers indirect retention and a more precise path of placement. Most wear will occur on placement and removal. In situations with diminished attachment length as a result of reduced interocclusal height, milled lingual bracing arms should be considered (Figure 18.21A–C). Careful consideration should be given to the amount of reduction in attachment length that will also allow for maintenance of the

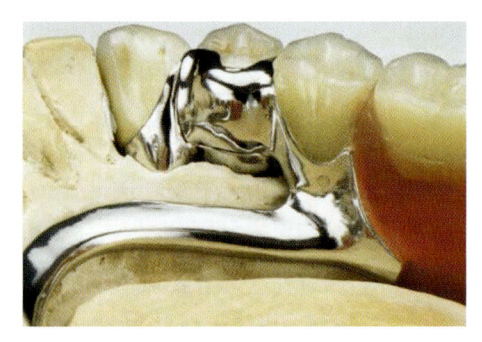

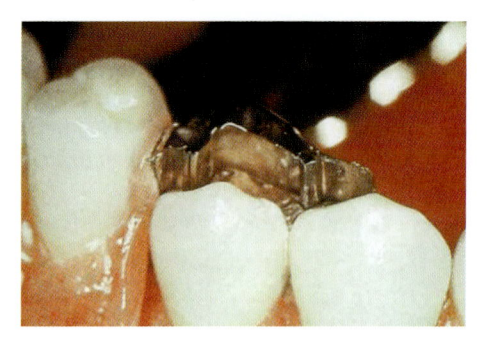

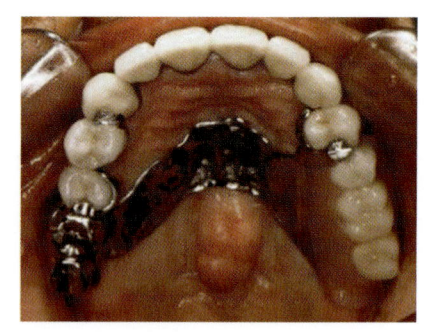

Figure 18.21 **(A)** Milled lingual bracing arm on an RPD framework. The design allows development of normal crown contours with placement of the RPD. **(B)** The Biloc and Plasta attachment (Attachments International) allows the bracing arm to be incorporated into the crown contours. **(C)** A traditional lingual bracing or reciprocal arm may create bulk or result in tongue irritation.

functional aspects of the attachment. Most manufacturers state the optimal and minimal lengths of the attachment.

Extracoronal attachments are situated external to the developed contours of the crown. Normal emergence profile and tooth contours may be maintained while minimizing the amount of tooth structure preparation. The more conservative preparation reduces the risk of or need for devitalization.

The majority of extracoronal attachments have resilient attributes. This will improve the ability of patients demonstrating dexterity problems when inserting the prosthesis. However, the extracoronal positioning will increase the likelihood of hygiene difficulties. Patients will require fastidious hygiene instruction using floss and adjunctive periodontal aids to prevent food entrapment and calculus accumulation. Inadequate hygiene will generally result in hyperplastic tissue inflammation subjacent to the attachment apparatus.

Function

The functional attributes of an attachment require differentiation between the intention of the prosthesis as being solid or resilient. Kennedy Class III and small to moderate-size (replacement of less than seven teeth) Class IV tooth-supported prostheses should be considered solid, whereas large Class IV and distal extension I or II prostheses are increasingly tissue supported and should be considered resilient.

Rigid attachment mechanisms may include locking pins. Locking and nonlocking attachments allow for virtually no movement between the prosthesis and the abutment tooth. Resilient attachments allow for a spectrum of movement ranging from limited uniplanar to universal. Staubli has categorized rigid and resilient attachments into six classifications, from rigid to universal resiliency.[36] The higher classification number correlates with a greater degree of resiliency and suggests less torque transfer to the root or implant abutment. The classifications are shown in Table 18.1.

Retention

Retention of the attachment components may be based on frictional, mechanical, frictional–mechanical, magnetic, and suction characteristics. Frictional retention is developed by the resistance to the relative motion of two or more surfaces in contact. Greater intimate surface contact will usually correlate with an increase in the amount of retention. Mechanical retention implies the resistance to relative motion by means of a physical undercut. The degree of undercut and the ability to adjust the physical component will predict retention. Frictional–mechanical retention combines parameters previously discussed and should be considered in situations necessitating increased retention with appropriate abutment support. Magnetic retention is created by attraction of certain materials to a surrounding field of force produced by the motion of electrons and atomic alignment. This type of retention is not largely used and may be diminished by corrosion of the elements. Suction is created by a negative pressure similar to the intaglio surface of a denture to the supportive residual ridge.

Space

Space is a principal consideration for the selection of an attachment. Vertical space is measured from free gingival margin to the marginal ridge of the abutment. Avoidance of tissue impingement and maintenance of a proper emergence profile is paramount at the cervical region. Cautious placement of the superior aspect of the attachment will circumvent occlusal interferences. The length of attachments that rely on frictional retention should be maximized to maintain resistance to dislodgment. Placement of the attachment should be as low on the tooth as possible to reduce the tipping or leverage forces applied. Buccolingual space is equally important to avoid overcontouring the crown. Additional bulk will be required buccal and lingual to the attachment for the casting alloy. Proper analysis of mesiodistal

Table 18.1 Classification of Attachments

Class 1a	Solid, rigid, nonresilient
Class 1b	Solid, rigid, lockable with U-pin or screw
Class 2	Vertical resilient
Class 3	Hinge resilient
Class 4	Vertical and hinge resilient
Class 5	Rotational and vertical resilient
Class 6	Universal, omniplanar

Source: Reprinted with permission from Staubli.[36(p.5)]

measurement ensures proper proximal contour and will provide an indication of a need for boxes in the development of the preparation. The largest attachment possible should be selected. This requires careful prepreparation analysis that includes the arrangement of denture teeth in a diagnostic waxing. This will help ensure the highest functional and esthetic value to the reconstruction.

Cost

Cost is related to the complexity of the attachment and the material components. In general, precision attachments are machined from noble alloys. The accuracy, manufacturing, and precious nature of the composition will demand a higher cost. Semiprecision attachments are made of plastic or other refractory materials subject to variables in the casting procedure possibly resulting in inaccuracies in the preciseness of fit; however, the materials and processes significantly reduce the cost of using these attachments.

Intracoronal attachments

Advantages

Intracoronal attachments, if used correctly, are incorporated entirely within the contours of the crown. This is advantageous for maintenance of tooth dimension and morphology. The positioning of the attachment near the long axis of the tooth allows force direction to be located along the long axis of the tooth. This creates a more advantageous biomechanical loading and force transfer to the tooth with a reduction in adverse leverage forces. Maintenance of natural tooth contours and the ability to properly place an adjacent replacement tooth without excessive recontouring or alteration for adaptation around an external attachment generally make intracoronal attachments more esthetic. Less possibility of food entrapment near the gingival tissues will enhance long-term prognosis and comfort.[36–39,41,43]

Disadvantages

A disadvantage of intracoronal attachments is the more excessive tooth reduction required for proper positioning of the attachment. Teeth with large pulps or young patients often contraindicate the use of intracoronal attachments or necessitate endodontic therapy for attachment use. The three-dimensional size of the tooth will predict the functional or biomechanical success with this attachment. Large clinical crowns (at least 4 mm) are usually required for intracoronal attachments. Decreasing the length by half reduces the retention by a factor of eight. This may be overcome by using a mechanical type of retentive element. The cost and precision of intracoronal attachments may be a limiting factor. Patient dexterity, maintenance, and repair are disadvantages or possible contraindications to the use of this type of attachment. Attachment alignment is critical owing to the limited resilience and finite path of placement possible. This creates a limited path of placement for the prosthesis.[36–39,41,43]

It is the authors' intention to present commonly used attachments that meet the considerations previously described. However, it is recognized that other attachments similar in design and meeting the functional and biomechanical criteria for use may be prescribed. The intracoronal attachment obligates a sound abutment tooth and demand for high esthetic value. A clinical crown of greater than 4 mm is generally required with a similar faciolingual width. The preparation depth of the internal box is approximately 2 mm. The frictional retention attachments must maximize clinical length to offer the greatest degree of retention. Generally, in situations where the clinical crown will be 3.5 mm or less, a mechanical retention attachment type should be considered.

Types of intracoronal attachments

The Stern G/A, Stern G/L, and Stern Type 7 are intracoronal precision attachments providing frictional retention and allowing for some degree of adjunctive mechanical retention.[43] The Stern G/A attachment may be considered for segmenting an FPD, which may require modification to an RPD in the future. The gold alloy patrix offers an expansion slot on the gingival edge for enhancement of frictional retention. The Stern Type 7 does not offer conversion from an FPD to an RPD, although it has similar adjustment of the frictional retention through the use of expansion slots. The Stern G/A expansion slot design (Figure 18.22) allows for the patrix faceplate to remain flat against the matrix wall, thereby reducing wear. The Stern G/L employs a gingival latch mechanism to provide mechanical retention in addition to the frictional retention of the similar Stern G/A and Type 7 (Figure 18.23). The Stern G/L patrix is produced in two designs: the flat-back and the "tail" on the back of the patrix (ESI), and in two faciolingual widths, 0.70 and 0.96 inches. The width characteristics are axiomatic, although the shape characteristics predict the method of attachment to the RPD framework. The flat-back design requires soldering to the framework or casting a retentive arm to the attachment for acrylic resin retention within the denture base. The ESI offers greater versatility, allowing soldering, electrosoldering, and acrylic resin attachment to the RPD framework (Figure 18.24). Owing to the presence of the mechanical gingival lock, this type of attachment allows one of the shortest clinical crown height requirements of 2.7 mm.

The Stern McCollum (Sterngold) attachment (Figures 18.25 and 18.26) offers an adjustment slot on the face of the patrix that allows access when the slot is situated lingually for cross-arch stabilization.[43]

The Biloc and Plasta attachments (Attachments International, San Mateo, CA) offer conversion possibilities from FPDs to RPDs.[36] The Biloc and Plasta attachment, an intracoronal semiprecision attachment, offers a machined patrix in two alloy possibilities and a castable plastic matrix. A lingual bracing arm is recommended and is indicated in fixed Kennedy Class I or II situations (Figure 18.27). The patrix portion of the attachment types described are either similar in metallurgic properties or possess characteristics allowing a greater degree of wear when compared with the matrix. Consequently, the frictional wear of the patrix reduces retention and supports the adjustment capacity of the components. When the amount of wear or loss of retention exceeds the adjustment capacity, replacement of the patrix component is necessary. This clarifies the advantage of a

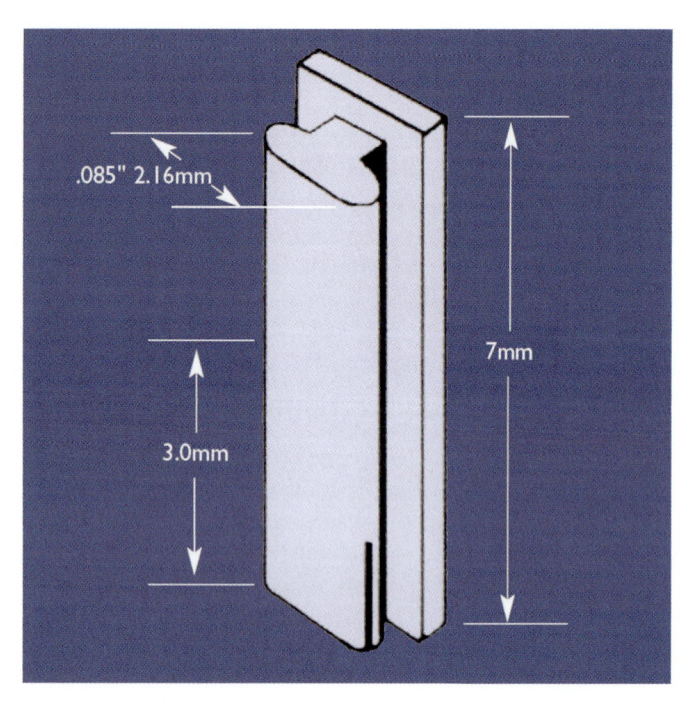

Figure 18.22 Stern G/A dimensions and illustration of expansion slot to allow for frictional retention adjustment. *Source:* Reproduced with permission from Sterngold, International.[43]

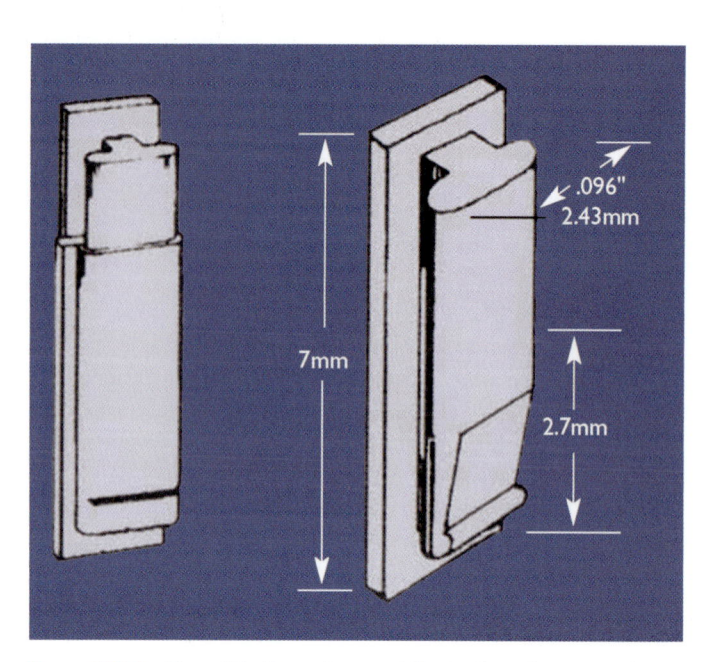

Figure 18.23 Stern G/L dimensions and illustration of an expansion slot to allow for frictional retention adjustment and gingival latch component. *Source:* Reproduced with permission from Sterngold, International.[43]

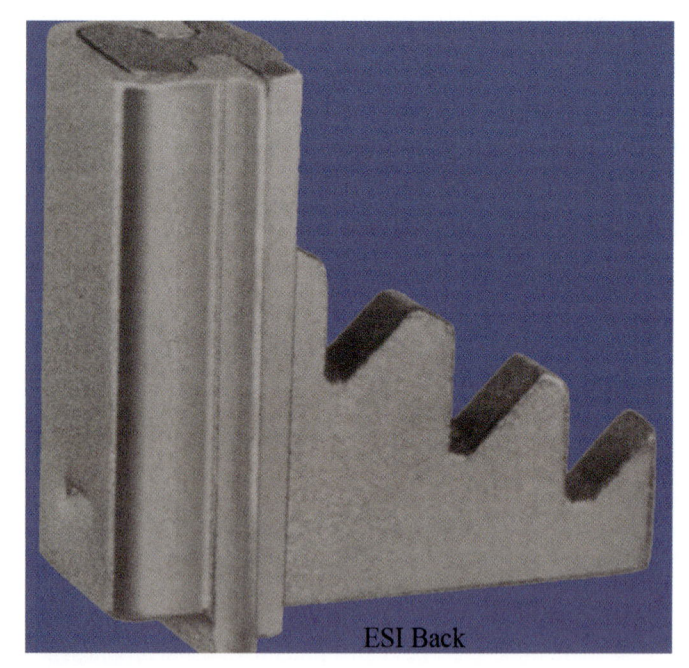

Figure 18.24 Stern G/L ESI back allows for acrylic resin retention to the RPD framework during attachment relation. Acrylic resin retention allows for retrievability of the attachment for ease of maintenance. *Source:* Reproduced with permission from Sterngold, International.[43]

precision-milled component. For replacement, a new patrix is purchased and replaced into the RPD without concern for casting inaccuracies or difficulties retrofitting the patrix portion to the abutment matrix, as might be experienced with semiprecision attachments.

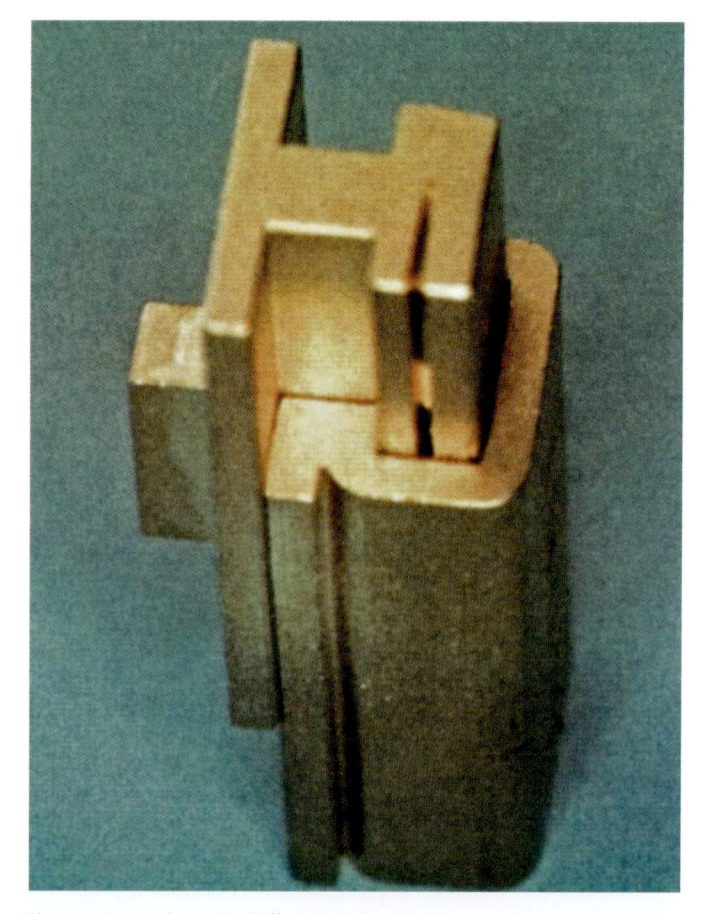

Figure 18.25 Stern McCollum attachment (Sterngold). Note that the expansion slot must be positioned to face buccally.

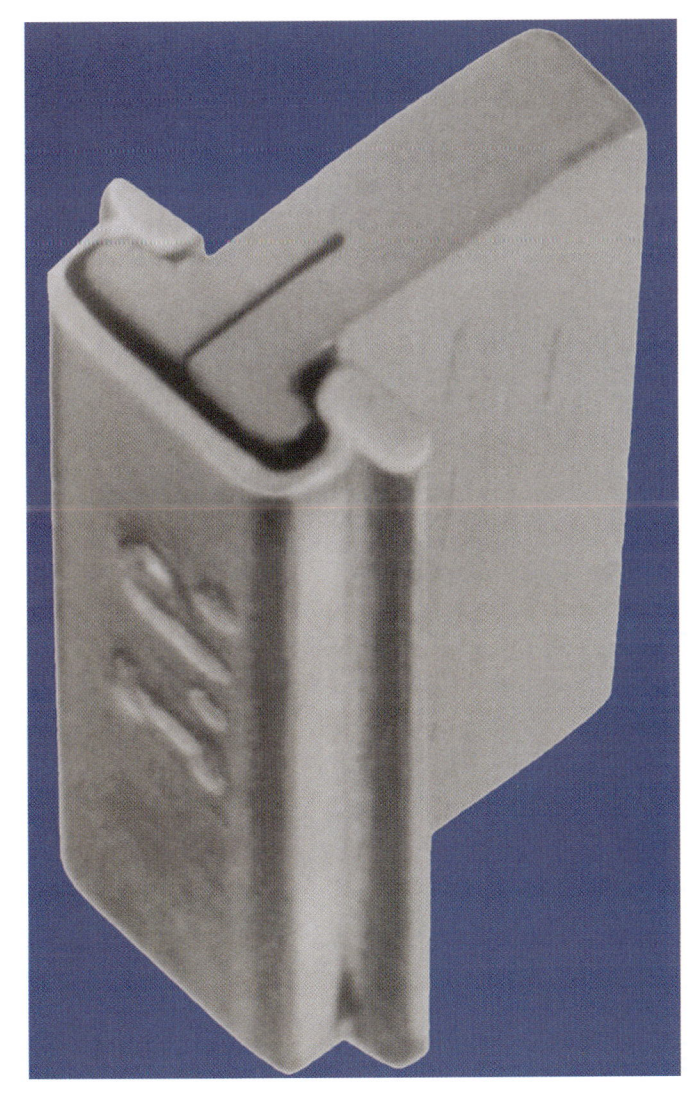

Figure 18.26 Stern McCollum (Sterngold) attachment. Note that the expansion slot is positioned on the face of the attachment oriented along the ridge crest. *Source:* Reproduced with permission from Sterngold, International.[43]

Attachment connection to the RPD may be accomplished in a variety of ways, as previously described. Soldering to the framework remains the most permanent and possibly the most common method. However, acrylic resin attachment of the patrix or patrix portion of the attachment to the RPD provides the highest degree of retrievability. In acrylic resin attachment patrices, the worn patrix component is retrieved from the RPD, and the new patrix is luted into place with autopolymerizing acrylic resin, often without disturbing the artificial teeth (Figure 18.28). The disadvantages of this technique are the discoloration and potential weakness of the acrylic resin. However, this technique remains more time and resource efficient than rebasing the RPD to retrieve a soldered-to attachment. A soldered technique requires artificial tooth removal and replacement owing to the excessive heat generated from the retrieval and resoldering of the patrix to the framework.

Extracoronal attachments

Advantages

The advantages of extracoronal attachments include resiliency in certain designs and less abutment tooth preparation. The conservative nature of the preparation required would suggest less harm to the pulp and reduced risk of potential endodontic intervention. The resiliency in design provides advantageous stress-breaking characteristics in distal extension situations (i.e., Class I or II arches). Attachment alignment is not as critical in highly resilient extracoronal attachments due to the omniplanar motion possible. This creates the advantage of multiple paths of placement for the prosthesis. Patients with biomechanical limitations not withstanding a rigid attachment apparatus or anatomic limitations precluding a finite path of placement are strong candidates for resilient attachments.[36–39,41,43]

Disadvantages

The adverse aspects of extracoronal classification include the potential for torque imparted by the attachment to the tooth and hygiene maintenance. Careful recall evaluation is necessary to

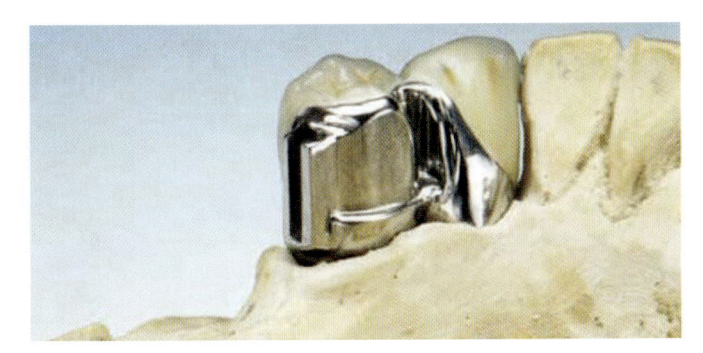

Figure 18.27 The Biloc and Plasta attachment (Attachments International) allows for fabrication of an intracoronal attachment with a milled bracing arm. This design offers incorporation of the RPD bracing arm into the proper clinical crown contours. The mesial portion of the bracing arm is similar in orientation and function to the intracoronal portion of the attachment on the distal of the crown.

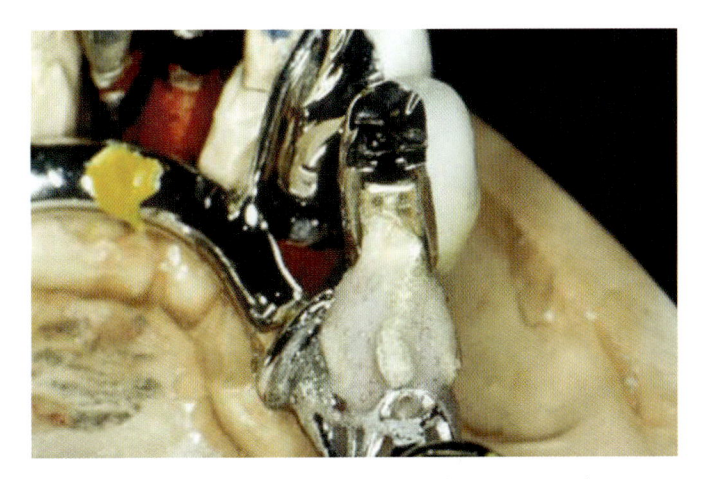

Figure 18.28 Patrix attachment with autopolymerizing acrylic resin to the RPD framework allows for easy retrievability and attachment replacement. This type of patrix placement increases the accuracy of the framework relation to the tissues and the abutment teeth.

ensure proper base–tissue relationships and fastidious oral hygiene. Tooth positioning around the attachment apparatus is often difficult and diminishes functional or esthetic value if adequate space is not available. Some resilient extracoronal attachments do not allow for "locking" to a rigid state. This may create difficulties with relining and rebasing procedures. Indirect retention and bracing are not incorporated into most extracoronal attachment designs and will necessitate the addition of components to provide these functions.[36–39,41,43] As with intracoronal attachments, it was our intention to present commonly used attachments, while understanding that other attachments similar in design and meeting the functional and biomechanical criteria for use may be prescribed.

Types of extracoronal attachments

Dalbo attachment system (Cendres & Métaux SA)

This attachment is one of the oldest and most successful extracoronal attachments and is classified as an adjustable, directed-hinge distal extension attachment.[36,43] This system features lateral stability, vertical resiliency, and hinge movement (Figure 18.29A–D). The advantages of the Dalbo system are the intrinsic direct retainer and excellent stability owing to the vertical beam. The attachment may be used in unilateral or bilateral applications (Figure 18.29E–J). The unilateral configuration provides a larger vertical bar for enhanced lateral stability. The attachment is offered in two sizes, although the mini version lacks vertical resiliency (see Figure 18.29D). The vertical resiliency is rendered through the presence of a spring and found only in the standard unilateral and bilateral designs. The difference between the standard and the mini is approximately 2 mm in clinical crown height requirement, 1.7–2.0 mm in preparation depth, and 1 mm in faciolingual width requirement. As in all extracoronal attachments, the amount of space required in the denture base is approximately 5.5–6.0 mm. This often creates difficulty with tooth placement and inadequate strength for the acrylic resin. The minimum amount of acrylic resin recommended should be strictly adhered to so as not to compromise the strength of the denture base in the region of the attachment.

This extracoronal retainer offers a mechanism to "lock" the attachment for reline procedures.

Octolink

The Octolink system (Attachments International), an extracoronal precision/semiprecision attachment, provides a large degree of movement and is classified as a universal hinge with vertical resiliency (Figure 18.30A–D).[43] The patrix button is adjustable and is screwed into a metal keeper, or retention nut, which is retained in the acrylic resin or may be spot-welded to the RPD framework. The matrix becomes incorporated into the crown through either a cast-to technique or a castable plastic technique (Figure 18.30E–I). A minimum of 4.0 mm of vertical abutment tooth height is necessary, although a minimum of 6.0 mm of space is mandatory for the retentive keeper and patrix component in the denture base.

Stern ERA-RV, ERA-RV offset and micro

The Stern ERA and Stern-RV (reduced vertical) (Sterngold) are commonly used semiprecision attachment providing universal hinge and vertical resiliency (Figure 18.31A–E).[43] Retention may be varied through use of four color-coded nylon patrices indicating four levels of retention (Figure 18.31F and G). An optional metal jacket serves as a keeper for the patrix retentive element, which may be alternatively retained within the acrylic resin (Figure 18.31H). However, this is more difficult to change once retention is diminished. Patrices may be easily changed without the use of acrylic resin. The Stern ERA requires a minimum of 4 mm of vertical height, whereas the Stern-RV requires 3.5 mm of vertical space (Figure 18.32). No additional preparation depth is required for matrix incorporation to the crown restoration. A large space of 6.5 mm is required within the denture base for the patrix component and an additional 0.3–0.5 mm for the optional ERA metal jacket. The manufacturer recommends an additional 1.0 mm of acrylic resin for patients demonstrating parafunction or "habitually strong occlusions." The patrix component is the variable between the Stern ERA and the Stern-RV. Both patrices fit with the selected matrix.[43,48]

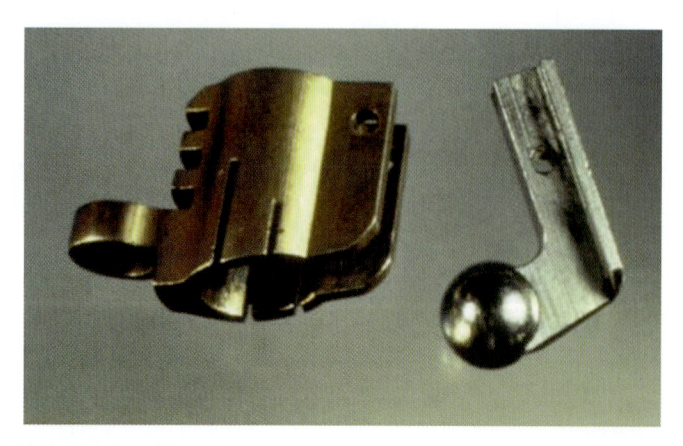

Figure 18.29 (A) Dalbo attachment (Cendres & Métaux).

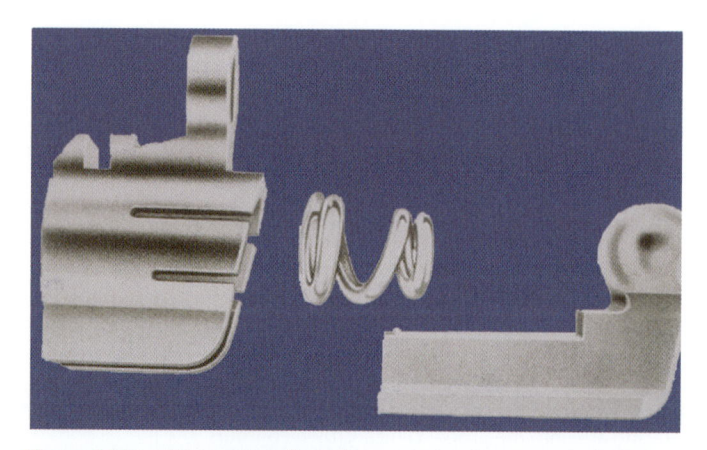

Figure 18.29 (B) A spring allows for vertical resiliency, and a ball allows for horizontal rotation.

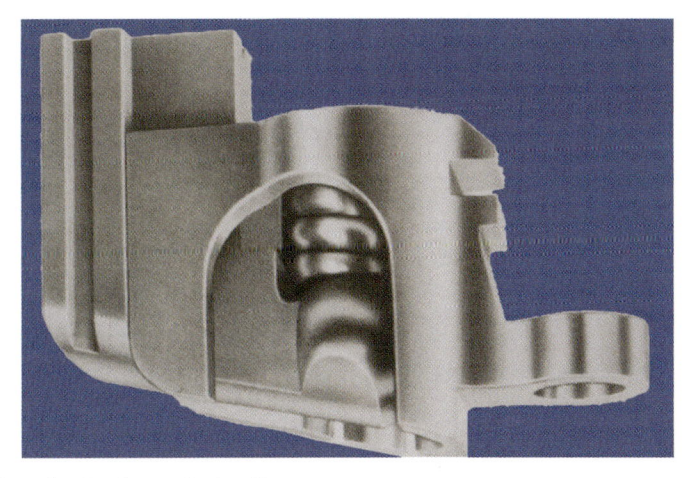

Figure 18.29 (C) A compressed spring allowing for vertical resiliency.

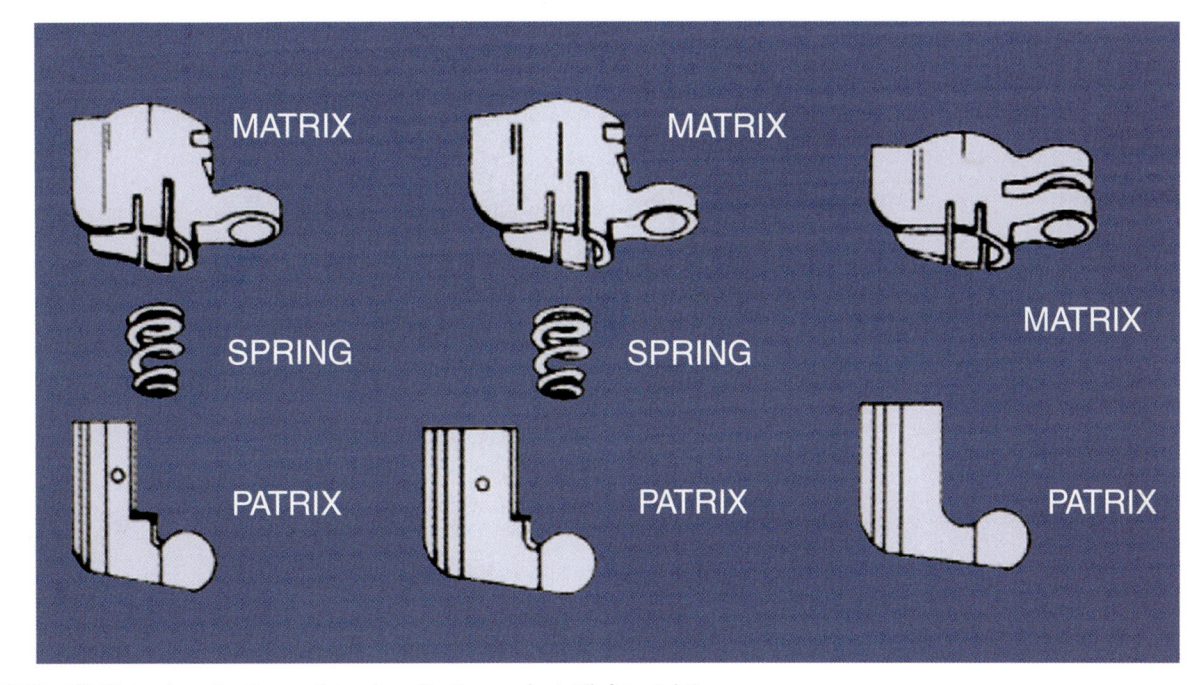

Figure 18.29 (D) Bilateral application, unilateral application, and mini (left to right).

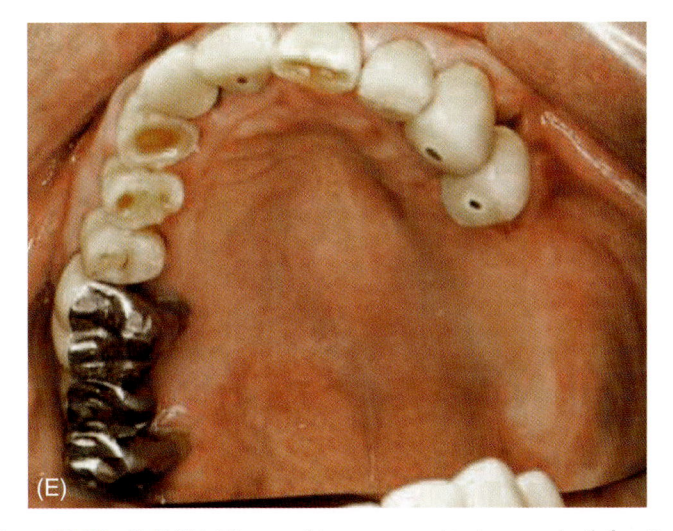

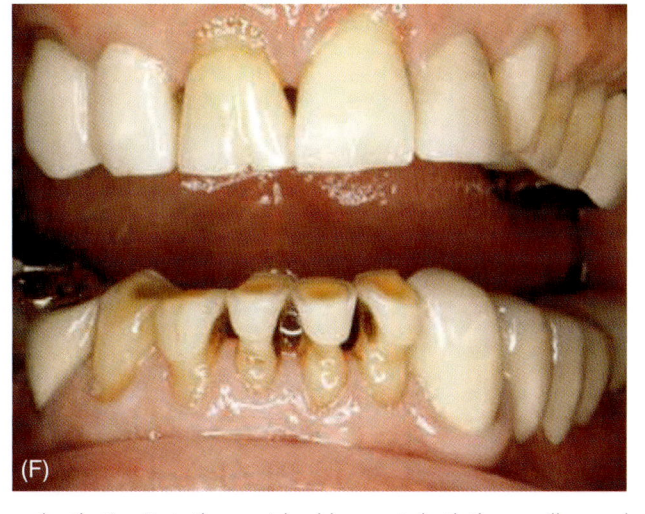

Figure 18.29 (E, F) This 75-year-old man wanted to improve both function and esthetics. Note the considerable wear in both the maxillary and mandibular dentitions.

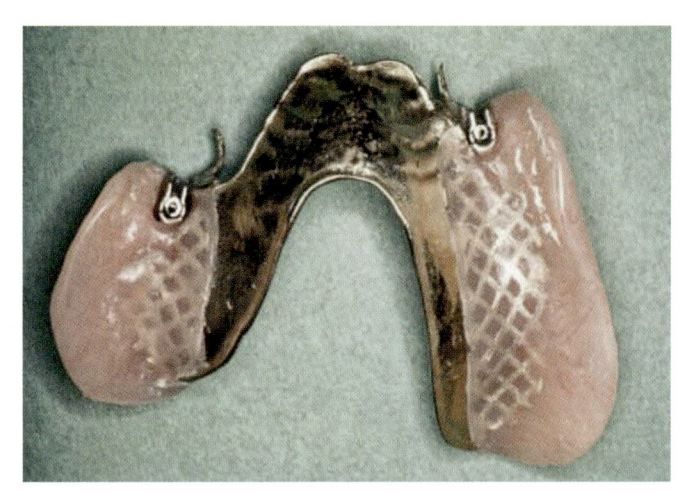

Figure 18.29 **(G)** A removable prosthesis with Dalbo attachments in place.

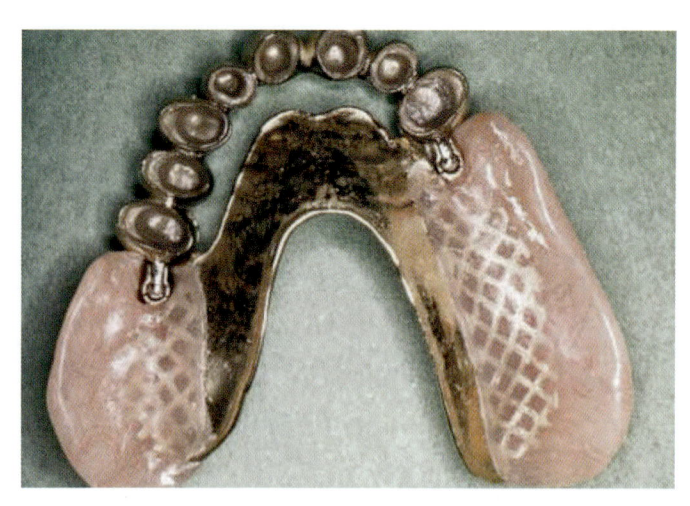

Figure 18.29 **(H)** The metal–ceramic framework is easily fixed to the Dalbo attachments.

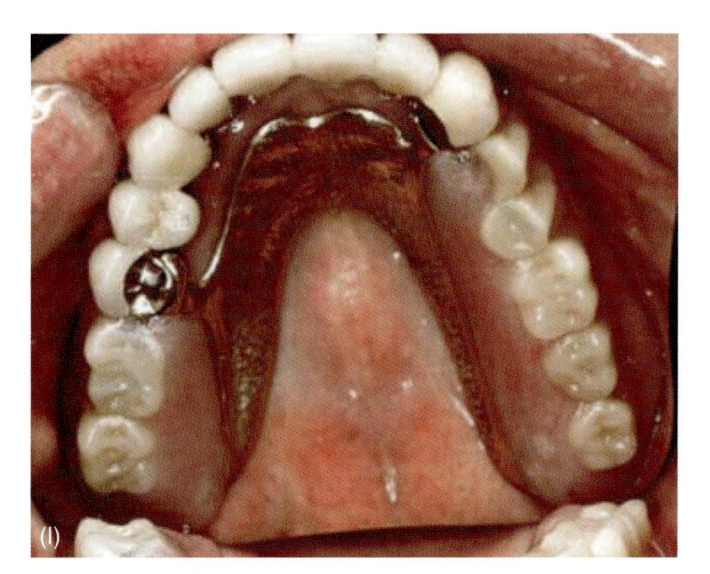

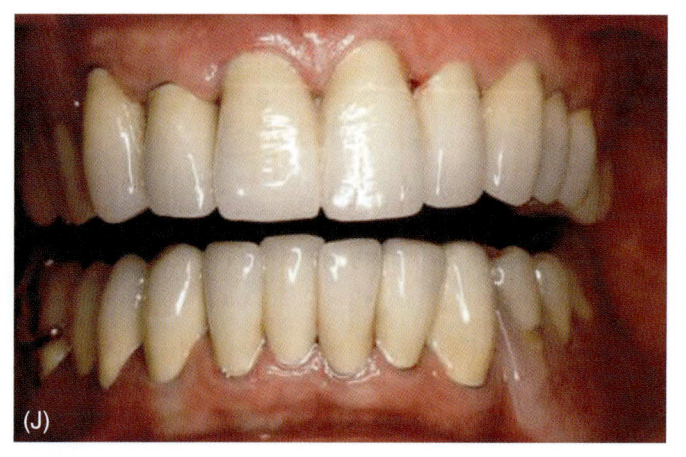

Figure 18.29 **(I, J)** Fixed metal–ceramic prostheses combined with Dalbo attachments provided maximum function and esthetics and were easy for this patient to insert and remove.

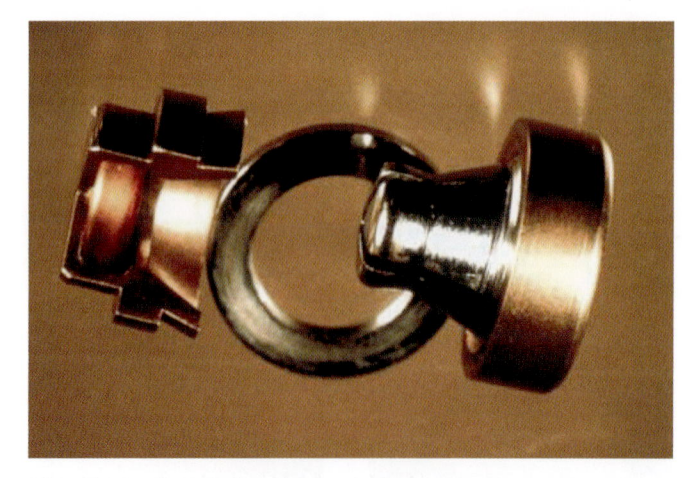

Figure 18.30 **(A)** Octolink attachment (Attachments International).

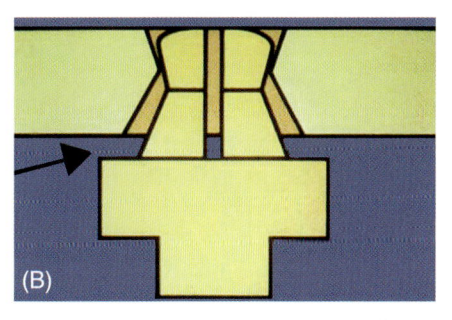

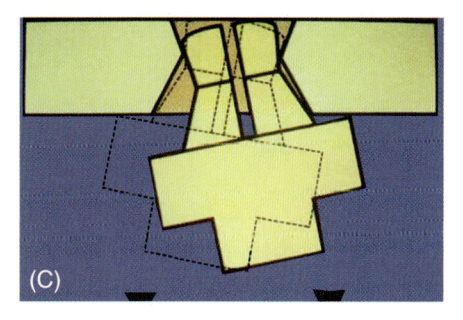

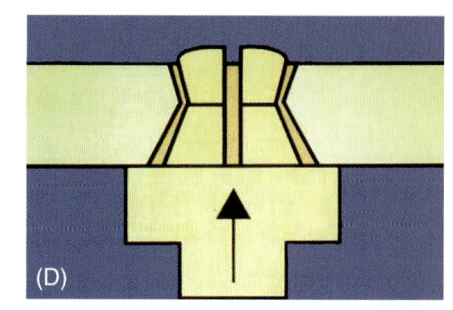

Figure 18.30 **(B)** Spacer used to allow for vertical resiliency. **(C, D)** Note the vertical and omniplanar resiliency of the attachment.

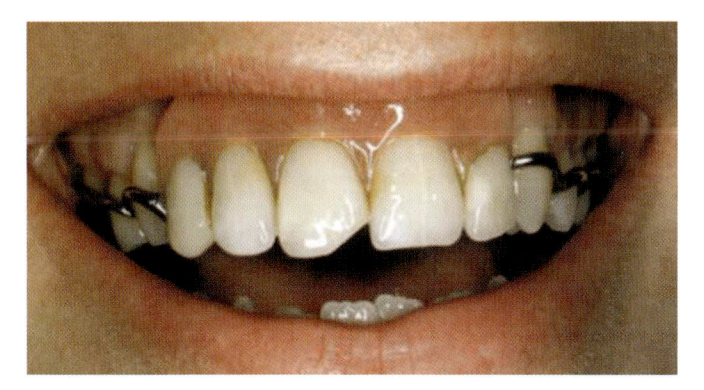

Figure 18.30 **(E)** This 30-year-old man was embarrassed because the clasps of his removable prosthesis showed when he smiled.

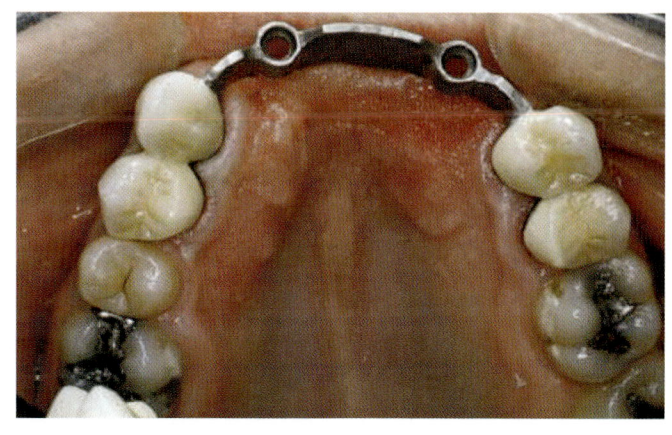

Figure 18.30 **(F)** A four-unit metal–ceramic splint combined with an Octolink (Attachments International) framework would better support the removable prosthesis.

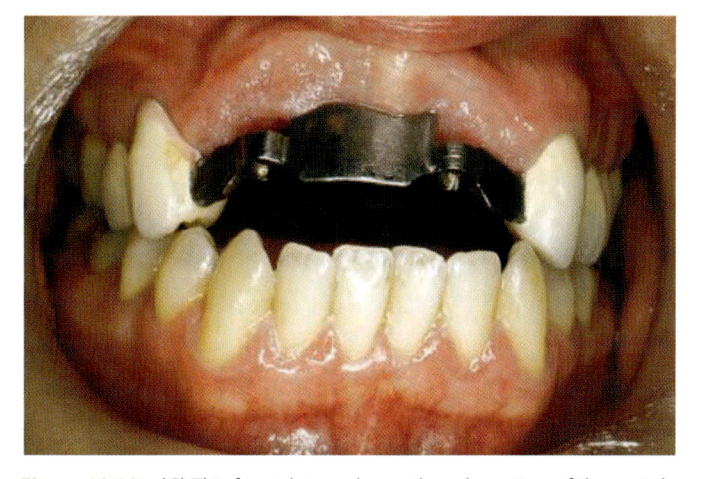

Figure 18.30 **(G)** This frontal view shows the adaptation of the metal framework to the alveolar ridge.

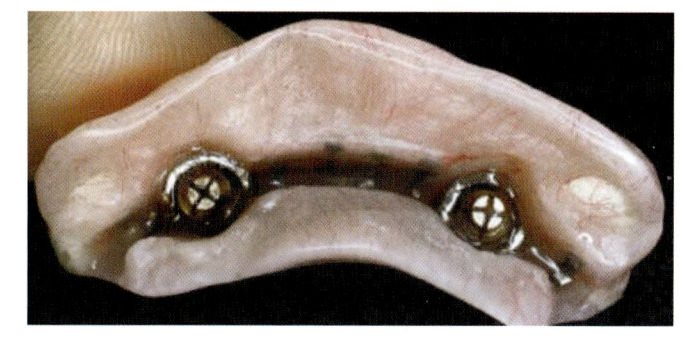

Figure 18.30 **(H)** This view shows how the Octolink (Attachments International) attachments will fit into the removable prosthesis.

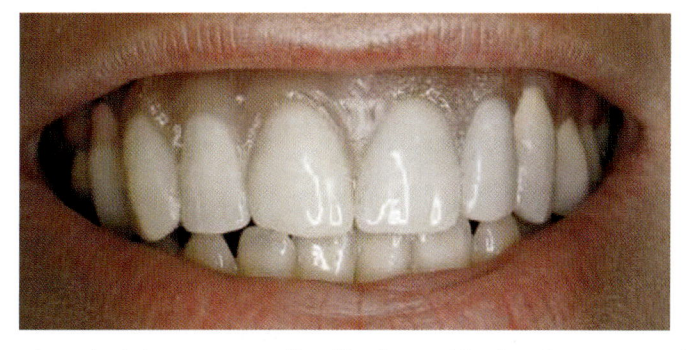

Figure 18.30 **(I)** The final smile shows the esthetic improvement offered by the combination of a secure attachment and a natural-looking acrylic flange.

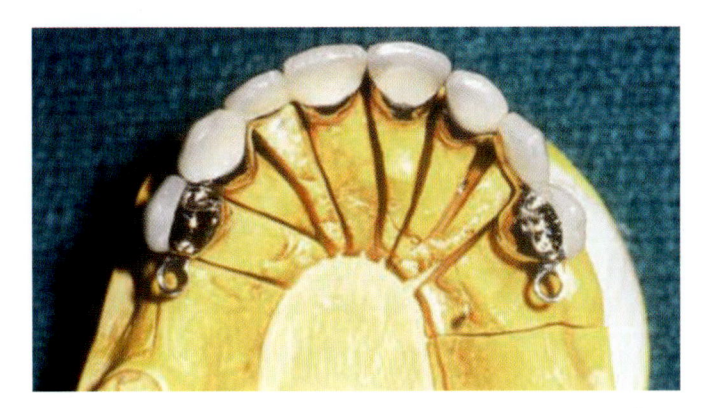

Figure 18.31 (A) Maxillary bilateral distal extension application of Stern ERA attachments.

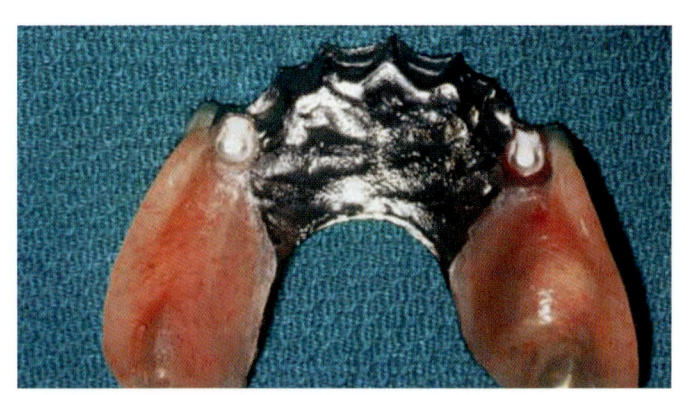

Figure 18.31 (B) Patrix placement within an RPD framework. *Source:* Courtesy of Dr Steven K. Nelson.

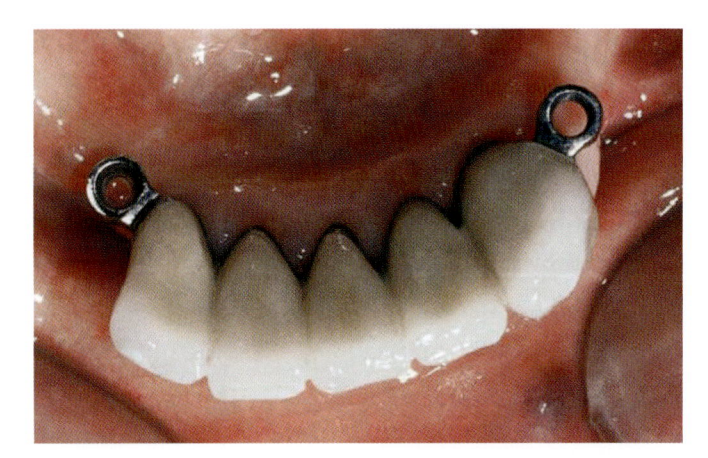

Figure 18.31 (C) The need for parallelism with each other in the sagittal plane is not required. Note the splinting of fewer than six remaining anterior teeth.

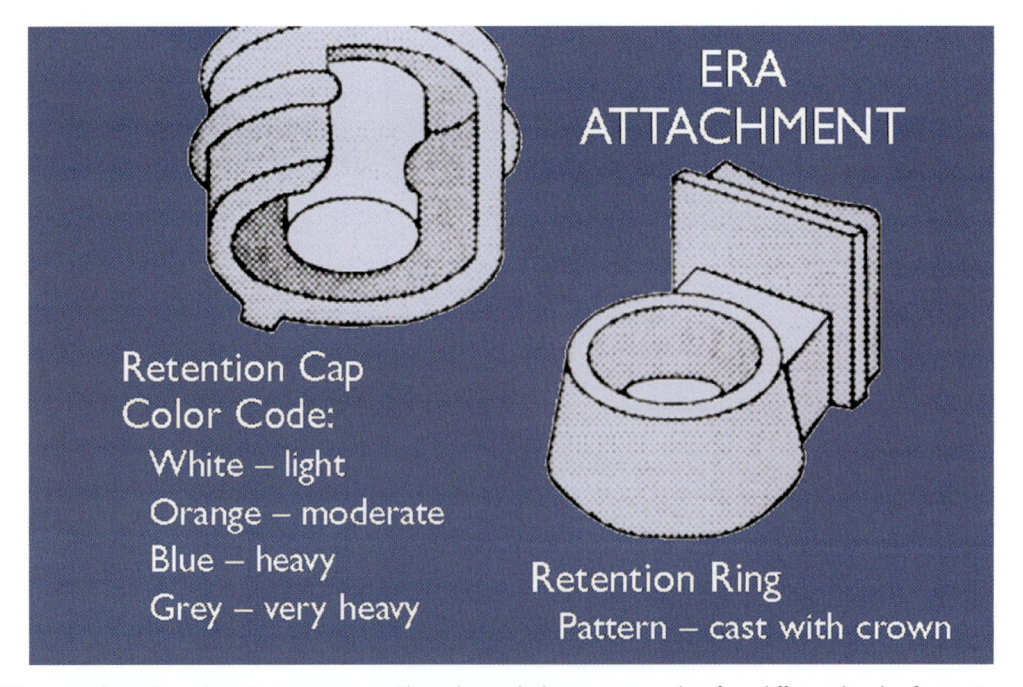

Figure 18.31 (D) Diagram of matrix and patrix components. The color-coded retentive cap has four different levels of retention. *Source:* Reproduced with permission from Sterngold, International.[43]

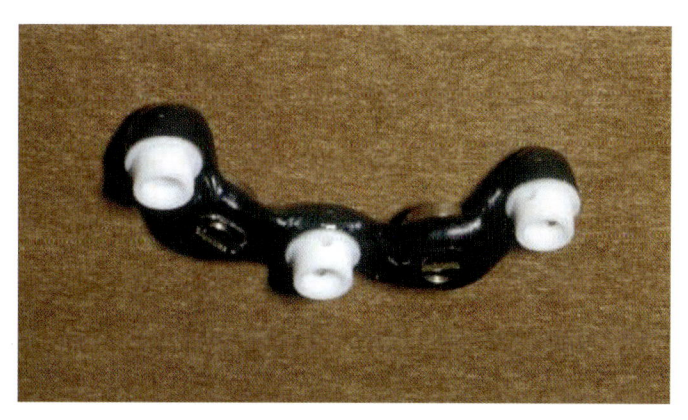

Figure 18.31 **(E)** An ERA attachment can be used with bar overdentures on implants or natural teeth.

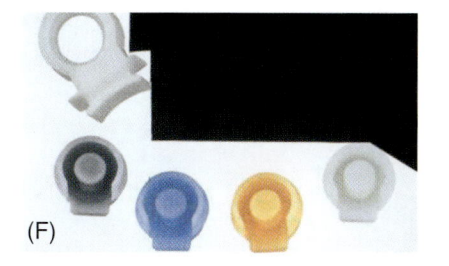

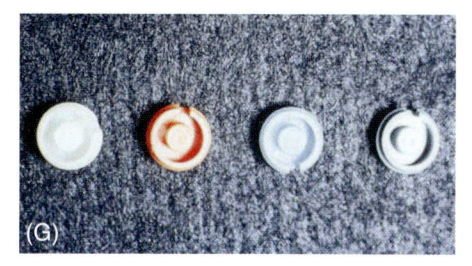

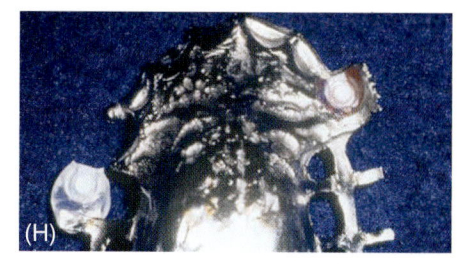

Figure 18.31 **(F)** Color-coded retentive caps and plastic pattern cast to abutment. *Source:* Reproduced with permission from Sterngold, International.[43(p.21)] **(G)** Color-coded retentive caps. **(H)** Retentive caps incorporated into the framework design and retained with autopolymerizing acrylic resin.

Hader vertical

This extracoronal semiprecision attachment (Attachments International) is compatible with conventional clasping on the contralateral side.[43] The resilience of the attachment allows slight hinging movement, although it will load abutment teeth more strongly than other resilient attachments. This attachment requires a 4.5 mm vertical tooth height without internal preparation limitations.

Special-use attachments

Special-use attachments should be considered for limited use based on the esthetic, functional, or anatomic needs of the patient. These types of attachments augment the armamentarium of the practitioner, although they may often increase the complexity and expense. Plunger-type or pawl attachments are an excellent adjunct for esthetic anterior teeth with required function as retentive abutments.[49] Classified as an intracoronal attachment, the spring-loaded plunger allows for a full range of motion, mimicking a universal-type extracoronal design. This attachment may be used with conventional or attachment partial dentures. A reciprocal lingual arm should encompass 180° and terminate in a rest seat. Matrix components or concavities are incorporated into the natural tooth or crown dependent on the situation or attachment, whereas patrix components are luted with acrylic to the framework and not soldered. Examples of plunger attachments are the Hannes anchor, the IC attachment, and the SwissTac/Tach E-Z (Attachments International) (Figure 18.33A–C).[36,43]

Splint bar designs incorporate Hader/EDS, Dolder, CM bar and rider or Ackermann clips, ABS, CBS, or PPM bar systems.[36,43] Selection is based on the degree of resilience, anatomic limitations, or convenience. The primary indication would be the splinting of abutment teeth while providing retention for the RPD. Careful consideration for the degree of resilience and interocclusal space for tooth arrangement must be provided (Figure 18.34A–F).

Dental implant placement offers a highly predictable treatment approach for overpartial dentures. Long tooth-bounded modification spaces requiring a significant amount of tissue support for the partial denture bases can benefit from application of overdenture abutment attachments supported by endosseous dental implants. Class I and II RPD classifications may have significant improvement in retention and stability by dental implant placement in the distal region of the edentulous residual ridge. The support offered by the overdenture concept using a dental implant would dramatically reduce the tipping and leverage forces imparted to the distal abutment teeth. This treatment modality may offer support comparable to the Class III RPD.

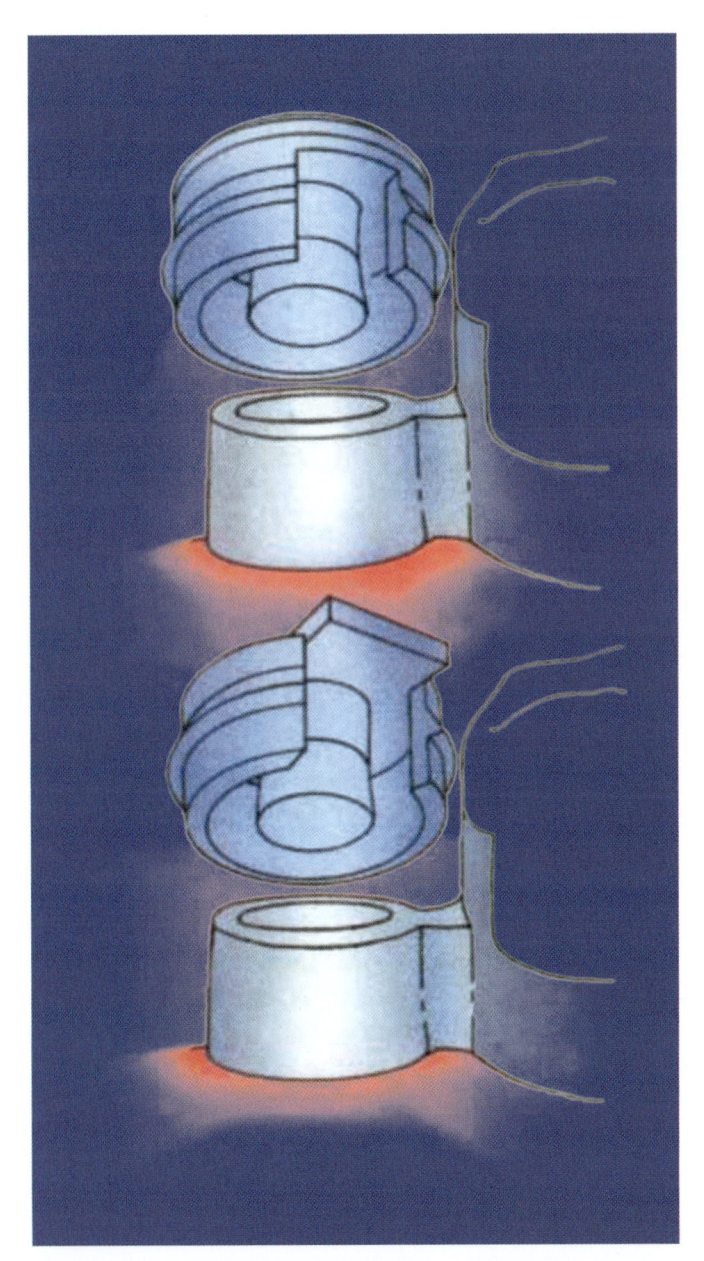

Figure 18.32 Comparison of the Stern ERA and the ERA-RV. The retentive cap varies in vertical height. *Source:* Reproduced with permission from Sterngold, International.[43]

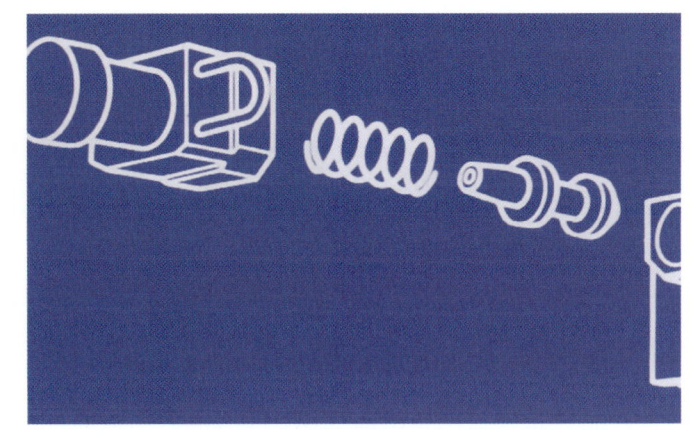

Figure 18.33 **(A)** Diagram of an IC plunger attachment.

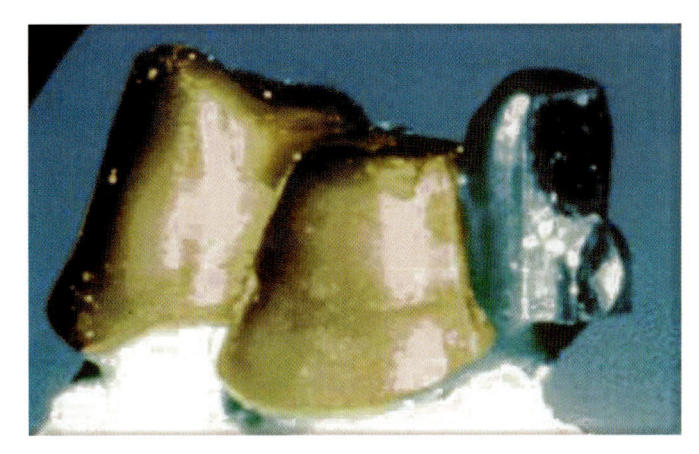

Figure 18.33 **(B)** Matrix cast into abutment restoration.

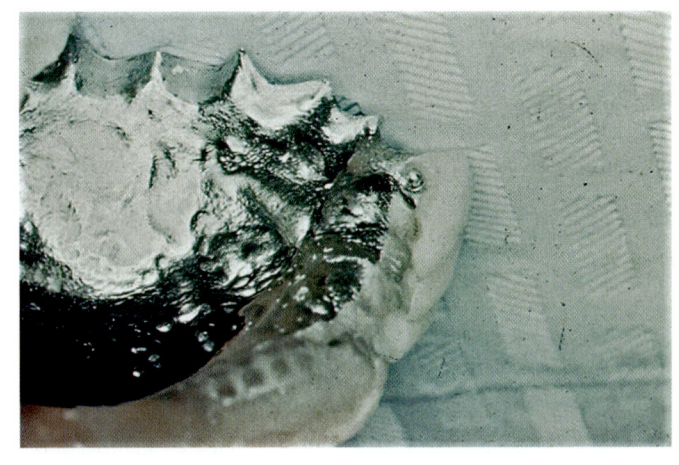

Figure 18.33 **(C)** Plunger and spring apparatus incorporated into acrylic resin or RPD.

Milled lingual ledges have been described as an adjunctive component that will accommodate placement of lingual bracing arms, generally providing compensation for short attachment length.[36,43] A technique of providing frictional retention of components through precision milling has been described. Spark erosion technology to create a precision milled fit has proved to be successful.[50] Adjunctive elastoclips may offer additional retention. The intimacy of fit developed with spark erosion or precision milling provides frictional retention, nearly eliminating any resilience. This type of attachment technology must be considered nonresilient and should be applied to the appropriate supportive elements. Additionally, the cost of this treatment approach may be prohibitive. A preprosthetic laboratory analysis of the anticipated cost may be useful in establishing the degree of remuneration required for the success of the rehabilitation.

Chapter 18 Esthetic Removable Partial Dentures

Figure 18.34 **(A)** A 60-year-old man complained about his appearance. Examination revealed posterior occlusal collapse, extreme breakdown of his remaining teeth, and periodontal disease.

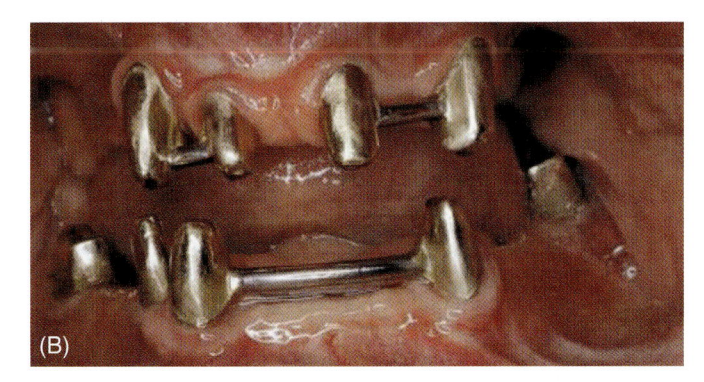

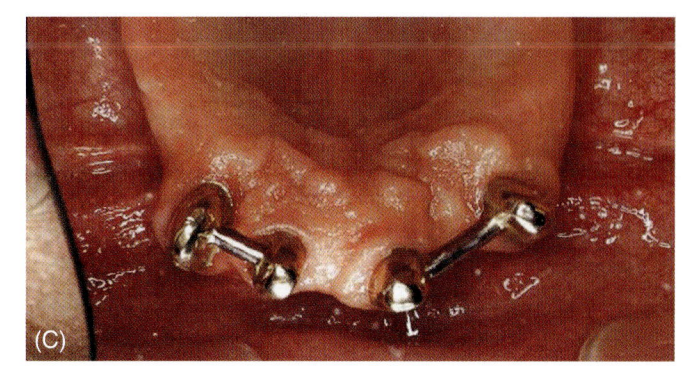

Figure 18.34 **(B, C)** Following periodontal surgery, maxillary and mandibular overdentures were constructed using Dolder bar attachments. Note the access that provides the patient with the ability for proper hygiene.

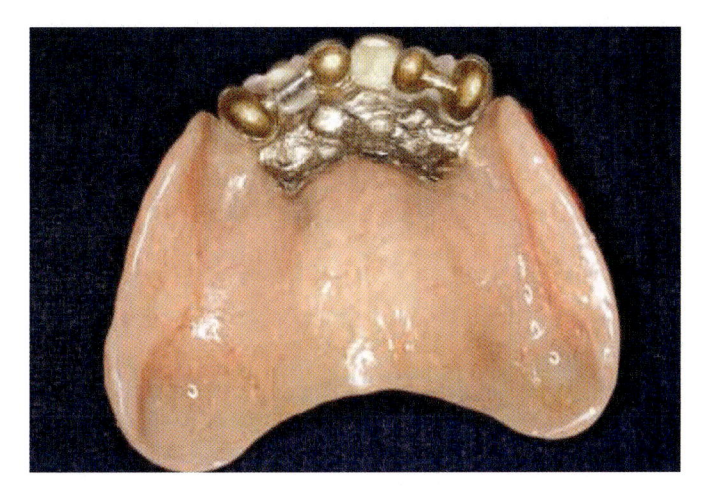

Figure 18.34 **(D)** This removable FPD provides excellent ridge adaptation plus Dolder bar secure retention for an ideal overdenture.

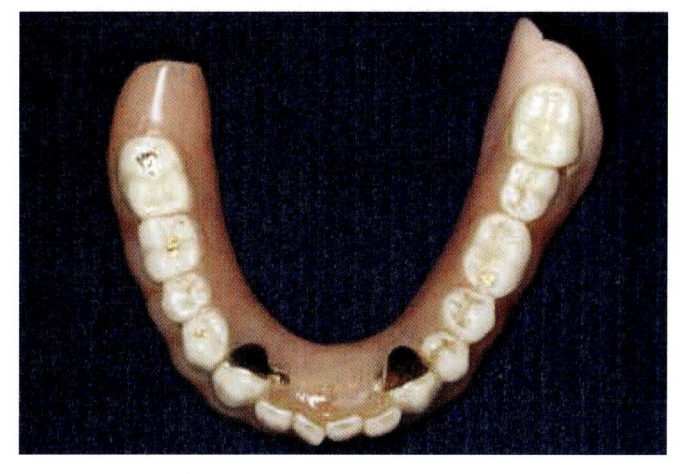

Figure 18.34 **(E)** The patient wanted some exposed gold and a somewhat crowded anterior tooth arrangement for what he considered a "natural look."

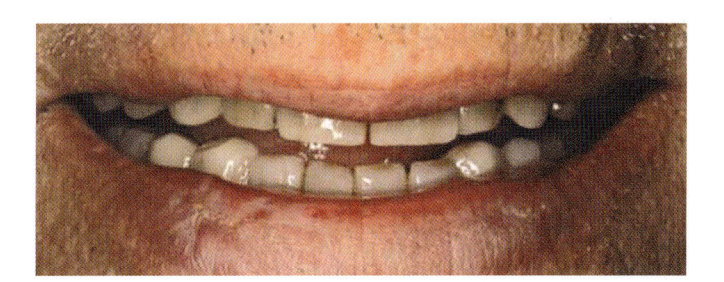

Figure 18.34 **(F)** A custom tooth staining and natural tooth arrangement gave the patient the appearance he thought appropriate.

References

1. Kennedy E. *Partial Denture Construction*. Brooklyn, NY: Dental Items of Interest Publishing Co.; 1928:3–8.
2. Applegate OC. The rationale of partial denture choice. *J Prosthet Dent* 1960;10:891–907.
3. Curtis DA, Curtis TA, Wagnild GW, Finzen FC. Incidence of various classes of removable partial dentures. *J Prosthet Dent* 1992;67:664–667.
4. Becker CM, Kaiser DA, Goldfogel MH. Evolution of removable partial denture design. *J Prosthodont* 1994;3:158–166.
5. McGivney GP, Castleberry DJ. *McCracken's Removable Partial Prosthodontics*, 9th edn. St. Louis, MO: Mosby; 1995.
6. Stewart KL, Rudd KD, Kuebker WA. *Clinical Removable Partial Prosthodontics*, 2nd edn. St. Louis, MO: Ishiyaku EuroAmerica; 1992.
7. Goodkind RJ. The effects of removable partial denture design on abutment tooth mobility: a clinical study. *J Prosthet Dent* 1973;30:139–146.
8. Myers RE, Pfeifer DL, Mitchell DL, Pelleu GB. A photoelastic study of rests on solitary abutments for distal-extension removable partial dentures. *J Prosthet Dent* 1986;56:702–707.
9. Frank RP, Brudvik JS, Nicholls JI. A comparison of the flexibility of wrought wire and cast circumferential clasps. *J Prosthet Dent* 1983;49:471–476.
10. Kratochvil FJ. Influence of occlusal rest position and clasp design on movement of abutment teeth. *J Prosthet Dent* 1963;13:114–124.
11. Kratochvil FJ. *Partial Removable Prosthodontics*. Philadelphia, PA: WB Saunders; 1988.
12. Krol AJ. Clasp design for extension base removable partial dentures. *J Prosthet Dent* 1973;29:408–415.
13. Krol AJ, Jacobson TE, Finzen FC. *Removable Partial Denture Design Outline Syllabus*, 4th edn. San Rafael, CA: Indent; 1990.
14. McCartney JW. The MGR clasp: an esthetic extra-coronal retainer for maxillary canines. *J Prosthet Dent* 1982;46:490–493.
15. Hansen CA, Iverson GW. An esthetic removable partial denture retainer for the maxillary canine. *J Prosthet Dent* 1986;56:199–203.
16. Kotowicz WE, Fisher RL, Reed RA, Jaslow C. The combination clasp and the distal extension removable partial denture. *Dent Clin North Am* 1973;17:651–660.
17. Brudvik JS, Wormley JH. Construction techniques for wrought wire retention arms as related to clasp flexibility. *J Prosthet Dent* 1973;30:769–774.
18. Tietge JD, Dixon DL, Breeding LC, et al. In vitro investigation of the wear of resin composite materials and cast direct retainers during removable partial denture placement and removal. *Int J Prosthodont* 1992;5:145–153.
19. Davenport JC, Hawamdeh K, Harrington E, Wilson HJ. Clasp retention and composites: an abrasion study. *J Dent* 1990;18:198–202.
20. Dixon DL, Breeding LC, Swift EJ Jr. Use of a partial-coverage porcelain laminate to enhance clasp retention. *J Prosthet Dent* 1990;63:55–58.
21. Zach GA. Advantages of mesial rests for removable partial dentures. *J Prosthet Dent* 1975;33:32–35.
22. Toth RW, Fiebiger GE, Mackert JR, Goldman BM. Shear strength of lingual rests prepared in bonded composite. *J Prosthet Dent* 1986;56:99–104.
23. Wong R, Nicholls JI, Smith DE. Evaluation of prefabricated lingual rest seats for removable partial dentures. *J Prosthet Dent* 1982;48:521–526.
24. Smith BJ. Esthetic factors in removable partial prosthodontics. *Dent Clin North Am* 1979;23:53–63.
25. Berte JJ, Hansen CA. Custom tinting denture bases by visible light cure lamination. *J Prosthodont* 1995;4:129–132.
26. Gerhard R, Sawyer N. Dentures to harmonize with heavily pigmented tissues. *J Am Dent Assoc* 1966;73:94–95.
27. Haeberle CB, Khan Z. Construction of a custom-shaded interim denture using visible-light-cured resin. *J Prosthodont* 1997;6:153–156.
28. Weiner S, Krause AS, Nicholas W. Esthetic modification of removable partial denture teeth with light-cured composites. *J Prosthet Dent* 1987;57:381–384.
29. Moreno de Delgado M, Garcia LT, Rudd KD. Camouflaging partial denture clasps. *J Prosthet Dent* 1986;55:656–660.
30. Snyder HA, Duncanson MG Jr, Johnson DL, Bloom J. Effects of clasp flexure on a 4-META adhered light polymerized composite resin. *Int J Prosthodont* 1991;4:364–370.
31. Morris HF, Brudvik JS. Influence on polishing of cast clasp properties. *J Prosthet Dent* 1986;55:75–77.
32. King GE, Barco MT, Olson RJ. Inconspicuous retention for removable partial dentures. *J Prosthet Dent* 1978;39:505–507.
33. Krol AJ, Finzen FC. Rotational path removable partial dentures: part 1. Replacement of posterior teeth. *Int J Prosthodont* 1988;1:17–27.
34. Krol AJ, Finzen FC. Rotational path removable partial dentures: part 2. Replacement of anterior teeth. *Int J Prosthodont* 1988;1:135–142.
35. Zarb GA, MacKay HF. Cosmetics and removable partial dentures—the Class IV partially edentulous patient. *J Prosthet Dent* 1981;46:360–368.
36. Staubli PE. *Attachments & Implants: Reference Manual*, 6th edn. San Mateo, CA: Attachments International; 1996.
37. Baker JL, Goodkind RJ. *Precision Attachment Removable Partial Dentures*. San Mateo, CA: Mosby; 1981.
38. Preiskel HW. *Precision Attachments in Dentistry*. St. Louis, MO: Mosby; 1968.
39. Burns DR, Ward JE. A review of attachments for removable partial denture design: part 1. *Classification and selection. Int J Prosthodont* 1990;3:98–102.
40. Schuyler CH. An analysis of the use and relative value of the precision attachment and the clasp in partial denture planning. *J Prosthet Dent* 1953;3:711–714.
41. Burns DR, Ward JE. A review of attachments for removable partial denture design: part 2. Treatment planning and attachment selection. *Int J Prosthodont* 1990;3:169–174.
42. Lepe X, Land MF. Use of an intra-pontic attachment as cosmetic support for a removable appliance. *Ill Dent J* 1990;59:280–283.
43. Sterngold-ImplaMed, Int. *Advanced Restorative Products Catalog*. Attleboro, MA: Sterngold-ImplaMed; 1998.
44. Berg T, Caputo A. Load transfer by a maxillary distal-extension removable partial denture with cap and ring extracoronal attachments. *J Prosthet Dent* 1992;68:784–789.
45. Berg T, Caputo A. Maxillary distal-extension removable partial denture abutments with reduced periodontal support. *J Prosthet Dent* 1993;70:245–250.
46. Chou TM, Eick JD, Moore DJ, Tira DE. Stereophotogrammetric analysis of abutment tooth movement in distal-extension removable partial dentures with intracoronal attachments and clasps. *J Prosthet Dent* 1991;66:343–349.
47. El Charkawi HG, El Wakad MT. Effect of splinting on load distribution of extracoronal attachment with distal extension prosthesis in vitro. *J Prosthet Dent* 1996;76:315–320.

48. Williamson RT. Removable partial denture fabrication using extracoronal attachments: a clinical report. *J Prosthet Dent* 1993;70:285–287.
49. Bagley D. Versatile uses for plunger attachments. *Trends Tech Contemp Dent Lab* 1993;10:33–35.
50. Weber H, Frank G. Spark erosion procedure: a method for extensive combined fixed and removable prosthodontic care. *J Prosthet Dent* 1993;69:222–227.

Additional resource

Goldstein RE. *Esthetics in Dentistry*, 1st edn. Philadelphia, PA: JB Lippincott; 1976:110–135.

⅙×

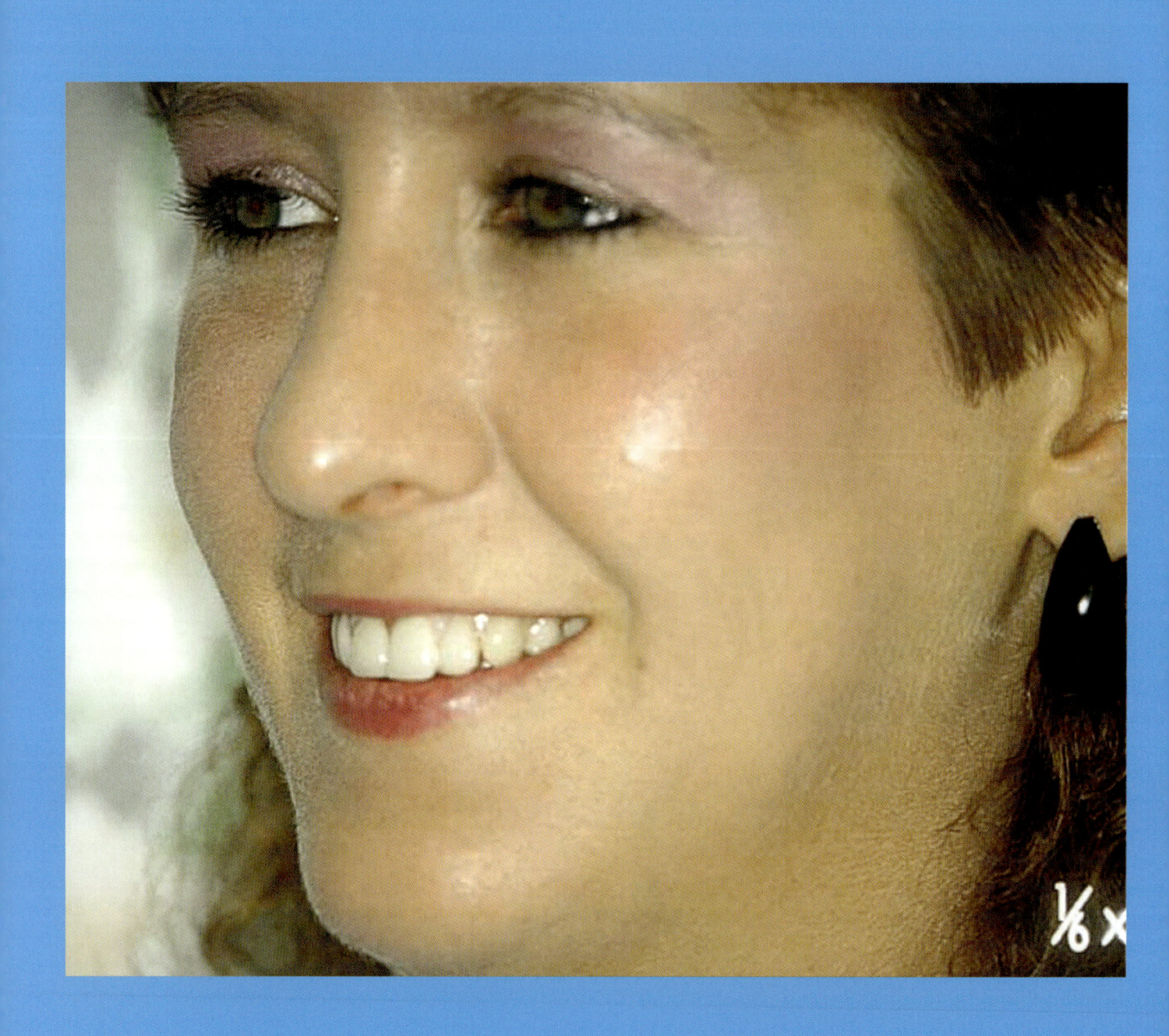

Chapter 19 The Complete Denture

Walter F. Turbyfill Jr, DMD

Chapter Outline

Occlusion: the complete denture	613	Tips on creating a natural-looking denture base	623
The art of creating esthetic dentures: four esthetic harmonies	614	Clinical examples of esthetic dentures	625
		Bone quantity and quality dictates every procedure	625
Tooth selection	614	Porcelain versus plastic	626
Tooth color	616	Dentures that oppose natural teeth	628
Tooth arrangement	616	Implants and complete dentures	629
Denture base	623		

Dental esthetics and beauty of the smile are of prime importance in today's society. The edentulous patient is no exception, yet creating a natural-appearing smile for this patient is very difficult to obtain. The edentulous patient will no longer accept the prosaic straight line over the ridge denture esthetics of the past (Figure 19.1A). Dentists, not patients, must be educated that it does not have to be this way. The dentist has an awesome responsibility to the edentulous patient to produce a prosthetic appliance that appears so natural that it defies detection as a prosthetic replacement (Figure 19.1B).[1–3] This chapter is primarily concerned with denture esthetics; however, comfort and function must be addressed. The failure of a complete denture treatment can be traced to three areas: comfort, function, and esthetics. A denture can be functional and comfortable. However, if it is ugly in the eyes of the patient, it is a total failure. On the other hand, a denture can be esthetically superior, but if it is not functional and comfortable it is still a failure. Complete denture prosthetics has been taught in schools the very same way since the turn of the 20th century.[4]

Materials are far superior (i.e., impression materials, teeth, acrylic, base tints, and precision processing equipment); however, the basic approach to satisfying the patient's needs has remained the same. Impressions are made, and bases and wax rims are constructed. The wax rims are adjusted in the mouth for tooth display, high lip line, and midline, and a jaw relation is determined. The teeth are set on the articulator by the technician or the dentist many times, with few guidelines. Then the wax-up is presented for patient approval. This is frustrating and may result in several resets to achieve patient acceptance. The denture is processed and delivered. In many cases, it is now when the patient begins to speak, eat, and observe the esthetics over a period of several days that the real problems arise. Unfortunately, many patients and dentists are far too familiar with the heart-breaking results using this unpredictable approach.

In the practice of fixed restorative dentistry, comfort, function, and patient acceptance of the esthetics are ensured prior to final prosthesis construction by first providing a provisional

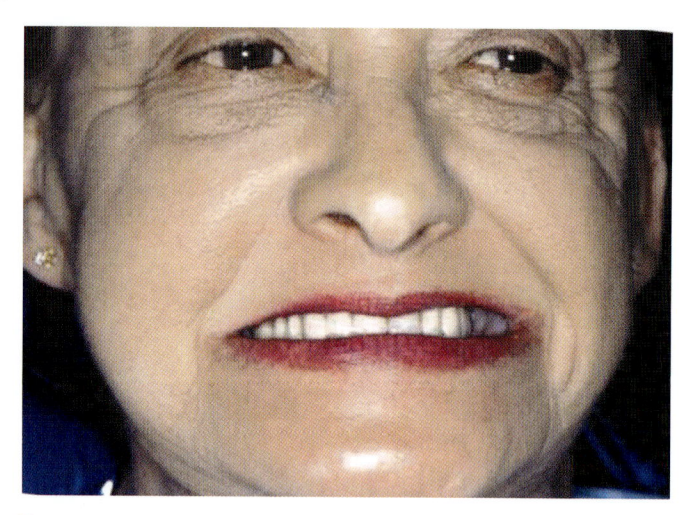

Figure 19.1 **(A)** Unesthetic denture.

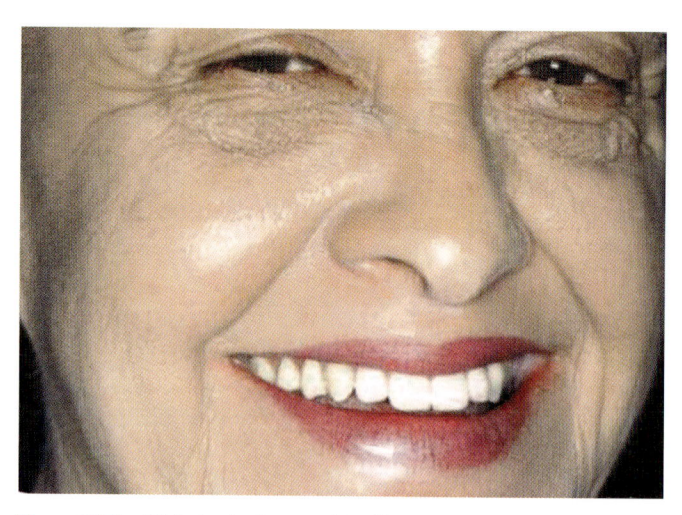

Figure 19.1 **(B)** Esthetic denture. Maxillary anterior teeth are in the proper position; therefore, the entire denture is esthetic. The proper positioning of the anterior teeth guide all the teeth in the denture.

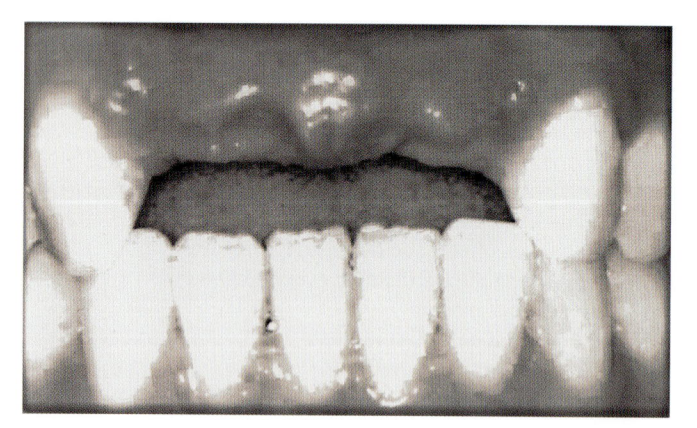

Figure 19.2 Maxillary anterior edentulous area to be treated with a fixed partial denture.

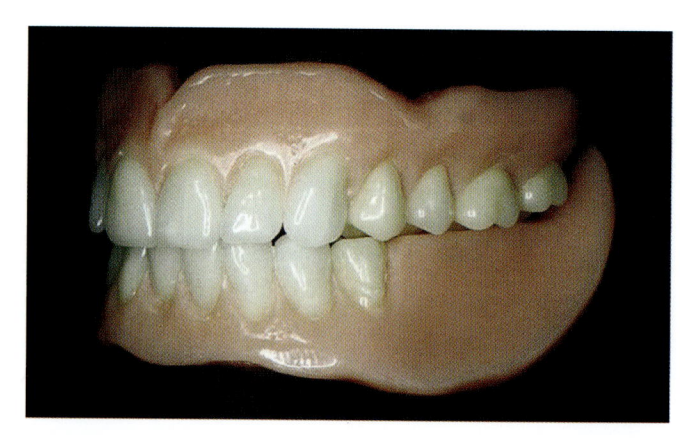

Figure 19.4 Maxillary and mandibular provisional training denture.

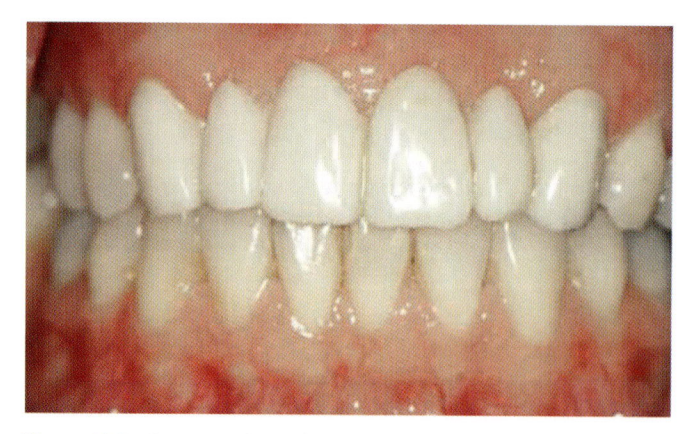

Figure 19.3 Provisional prosthesis placed to gain patient acceptance and to test esthetic and functional values.

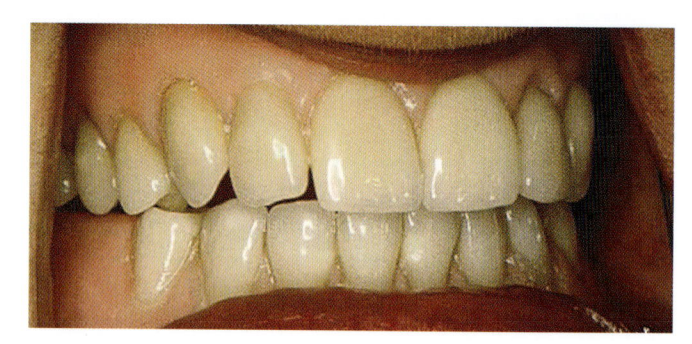

Figure 19.5 Provisional training denture placed to prove all aspects of denture function, esthetics, and comfort and to gain patient acceptance.

prosthesis (Figures 19.2 and 19.3). In the modern practice of complete denture prosthetics, the edentulous patient is first provided with a provisional denture.[5–9] This provisional denture will allow the dentist to refine all of the functional esthetic aspects of the denture to their and their patient's satisfaction (Figures 19.4 and 19.5). After complete acceptance by the dentist and patient, the provisional denture is used much like a blueprint to construct the final continuance denture. This approach leads to patient happiness without the frustrating surprises of the past. This technique makes the practice of denture prosthetics very predictable. While the patient wears the treatment denture, an added benefit is the creation of functional

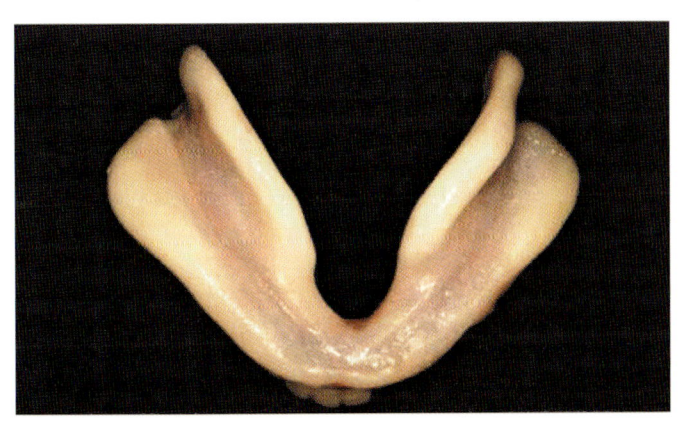

Figure 19.6 Mandibular functional impression is created as the patient wears the provisional denture.

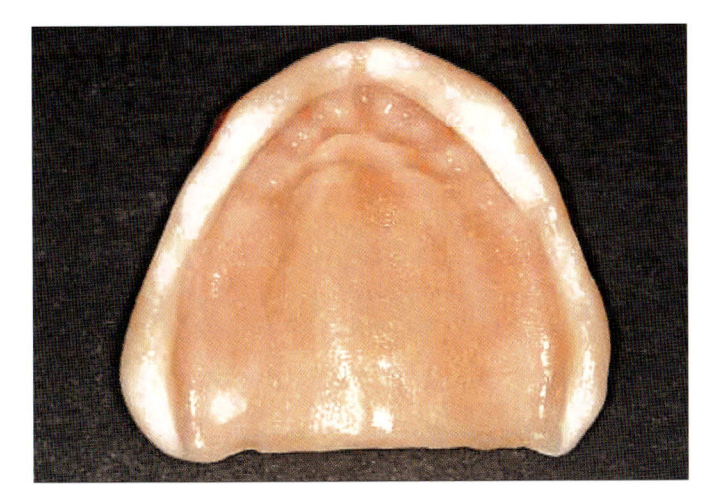

Figure 19.7 Maxillary functional impression is created as the patient wears the provisional denture.

impressions (Figures 19.6 and 19.7). It is my experience that, after final delivery of the denture, few, if any, postinsertion adjustments are necessary.

Occlusion: the complete denture

No discussion of complete dentures can be complete without addressing the occlusion. Of all the causes of denture failure, the lack of a balanced occlusion in centric relation accounts for 90% of all denture failures. The most difficult challenge in denture prosthetics is occlusion. All of the denture teeth must occlude evenly as the mandible opens and closes on the arc of closure (Figure 19.8). Personal experience tells the dentist that patients with natural teeth many times function for a lifetime in a maximum intercuspal position that is not coincidental with centric relation. This is not true with the edentulous patient. These patients have lost most of the occlusal awareness, and the occlusion must be built to the repeatable position of centric relation.

This is often a difficult task because the precise jaw relation must be registered on two movable bases. In the treatment denture in Figure 19.5, the mandibular posterior teeth are replaced with a noninterfering bite block. This bite or chewing block acts as a superior repositioning splint to help the dentist obtain the optimum position of centric relation. Registering and confirming the occlusal relation position is done with various waxers and central bearing recording devices. The occlusal scheme is referred to as a lingualized occlusion that is characterized with a single maxillary lingual cusp that functions into a mandibular fossa. This occlusion seems to be very efficient and stable for the denture patient (Figures 19.9 and 19.10).

Figure 19.9 shows the posterior esthetics of lingualized occlusion with the natural maxillary facial cusp.

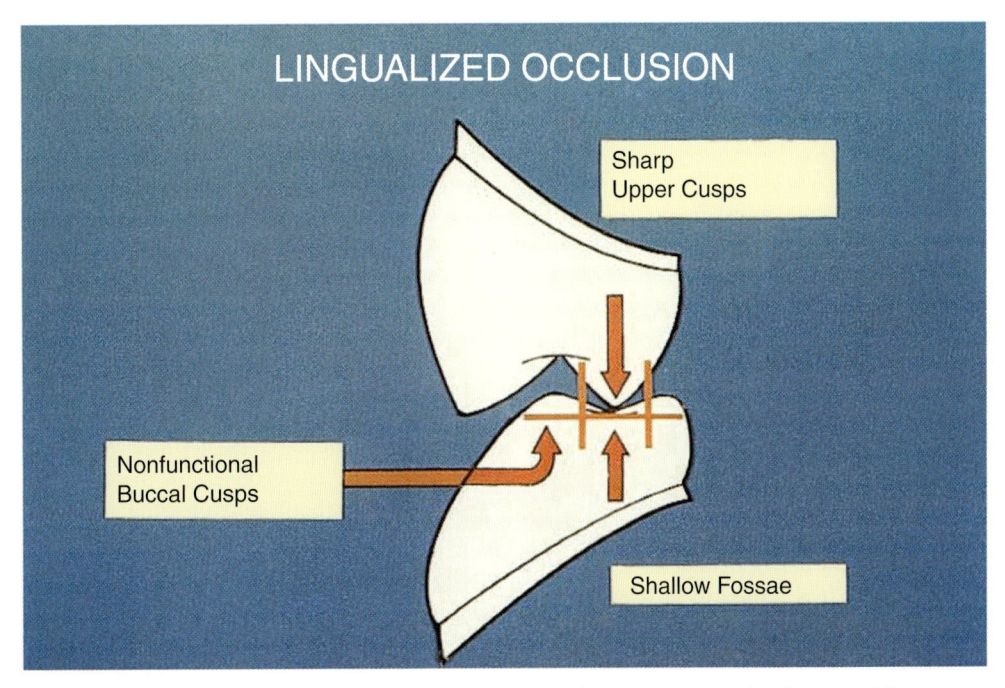

Figure 19.8 Schematic of lingual contact occlusion. Maxillary lingual cusp will function in a mandibular central fossa with no contact of the mandibular buccal cusp and the occlusal incline of the maxillary buccal cusp. *Source:* Reproduced with permission from Turbyfill.[10]

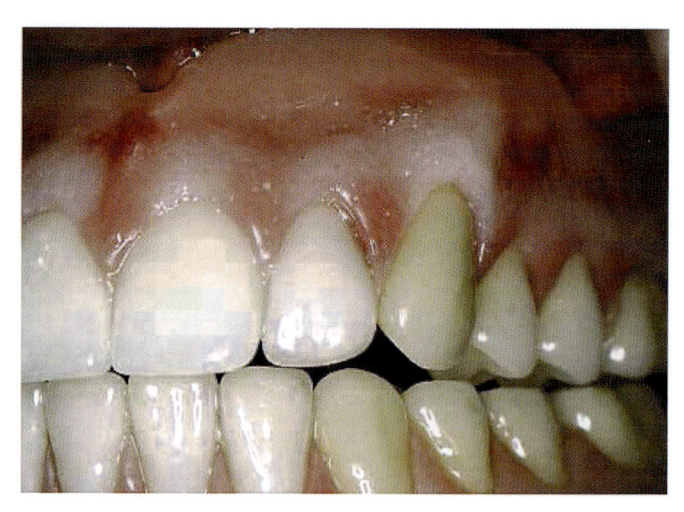

Figure 19.9 Lingualized occlusion in the completed denture.

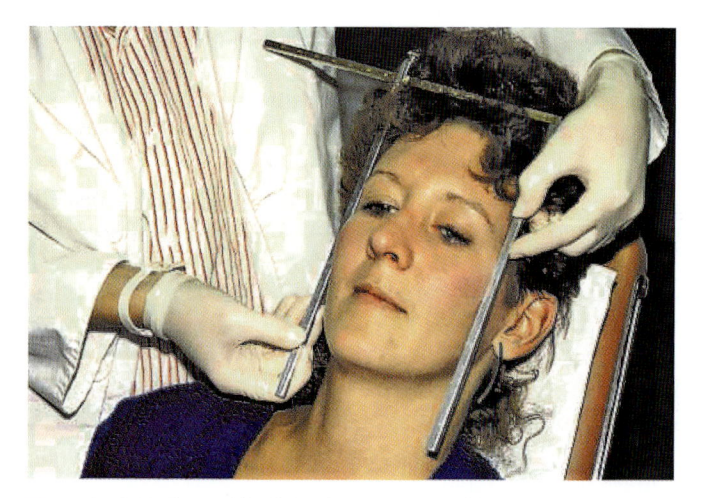

Figure 19.10 The width of the face is measured from 1 inch behind the outer canthus of the eye. *Source:* Reproduced with permission from Turbyfill.[11]

The art of creating esthetic dentures: four esthetic harmonies

There are four esthetic harmonies that must be considered to produce a denture that will satisfy the patient's esthetic demands. These esthetic harmonies are (1) tooth size and form, (2) tooth color, (3) tooth position, and (4) background. The background is the denture base, which should be formed and colored to look like human gingiva and tinted to blend with the patient's overall complexion.

Of the four harmonies, the most important are tooth position and size. If the teeth are placed into the position that the natural teeth once occupied and in a size that is in harmony with the face, most of the esthetic requirements will have been achieved. In the consideration of tooth position and arrangement, it must be understood that everything that is done in this area has an influence on the esthetics. These considerations include the proper midline, incisal plane, posterior occlusal plane, horizontal and vertical positions of the maxillary anterior teeth, and horizontal and vertical positions of the mandibular anterior teeth.

Tooth selection

Size and form

Tooth size and form are considered simultaneously. The selection of the maxillary incisors is the starting point in creating esthetic dentures. There are many suggested ways to select teeth, including (1) preextraction records, (2) patient photographs, (3) patient desires, and (4) facial measurements.

The four methods of tooth selection are used routinely in complete denture prosthetics. There have been several theories set forth. It must be understood that none of these ways are accurate in all cases.[12–16] However, the selection is made; it is a guide or a starting place. In 1887, the temperamental theory was proposed.[17] It was one of the earliest to propose that a person's personality might influence the morphology of the teeth. In 1914, Williams[18] rejected the temperamental theory as a fallacy, proposing what is known as the geometric theory, and concluded that the shape of the face and the shape of the central incisor are related. This approach is still being used by many dentists. In 1939, House and Loop[19] expanded on Williams's works to include not only pure typal forms (square, tapered, and ovoid) but also combinations of typal forms and the discovery of the relationship of the width of the face and the width of the central incisor. In a study of 555 subjects, House and Loop found that the majority of central incisors were not only in harmony with facial outlines but they were also one-sixteenth of the size of the face. A study by LaVere et al. has confirmed their findings.[20] I still use this method as a basic starting place for tooth selection when other data are not available.

In 1955, Frush and Fisher[21] brought forth the sex, personality, and age (SPA) theory of tooth selection. By 1959, five additional articles followed describing the methods of applying the SPA factors. They concluded that tooth size is related to the width of the nose. With the use of the alameter (Productivity Training Corporation, Morgan Hill, CA), it is determined whether the patient needs a small, medium, or large central incisor. Although the esthetics achieved using the SPA method is very good, one study shows that it may not be anatomically accurate.[22]

At the annual session of the American Academy of Esthetic Dentistry in 1981 in San Francisco, an interesting study was conducted by Abrams.[22] One hundred slides of human teeth were chosen, and the audience, consisting of several hundred dentists, was asked to choose whether each slide was a male or a female (lips were blocked out so that only the teeth were visible). After the results were tabulated, it was determined that (1) gender cannot be determined by tooth morphology or arrangement and (2) the older the patient, the more the audience thought that the patient was a male purely because wear denotes vigorousness to most dentists. Nevertheless, using this approach can produce many quite esthetic and pleasing results.[23] Although none of these methods is absolutely accurate,[12–15] it must be reiterated that there must be a starting point.

Clinical tooth selection

From a clinical standpoint, measurement of the face is the first step. House and Loop have shown that the width of the central

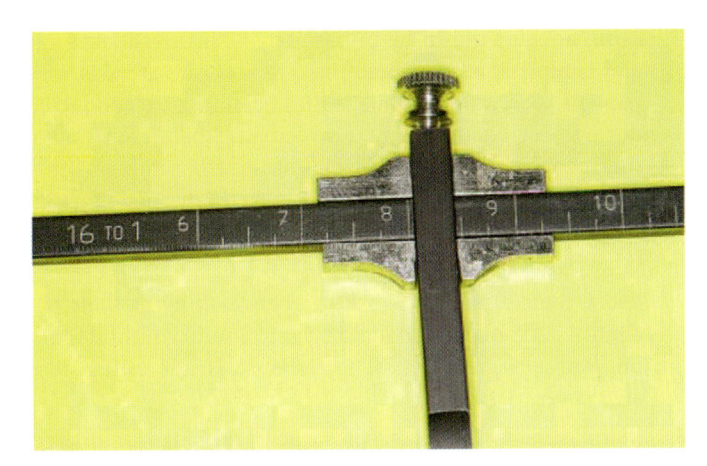

Figure 19.11 The measuring device reads the facial width in millimeters at a ratio of 1 to 16.

incisor is one-sixteenth of the width of the face as measured from 1 inch behind the outer canthus of the eye (see Figure 19.10). The length of the tooth is determined by measuring from the hairline to the lower border of the chin. If there is hair loss, then the top furor of the forehead is used. The measurement is made by using a device first described by House and Loop (Figure 19.11). The measurements have been interpolated to read in millimeters one-sixteenth of the width of the face.

Tooth form and mold

Most instruction on tooth selection suggests that tooth form be matched to the patient's facial form; that is, square, tapered, ovoid, or, in some manufacturers' teeth, combination form types. These combinations include square/tapered, square/ovoid, tapered/ovoid, and so forth. Some tooth manufacturers make only the basic square, tapered, and ovoid but do not make the combination forms. Other manufacturers make only different size teeth and no teeth designated for the different facial forms. However, these manufacturers do make molds that exhibit different amounts of incisal wear.

I rarely consider tooth mold in terms of square, tapered, or ovoid. Once the proper tooth size is selected, the mold is selected to fit the patient's maturity. Younger patients get more rounded molds with unworn tips on the cuspids. More mature patients will get teeth that show more incisal wear and cuspids where the incisal tip is worn flatter. I put tapered teeth in ovoid faces or square teeth in tapered faces and do not like ovoid teeth in most cases (see tip 2 in the "Tips on tooth selection" section).

After the upper anterior teeth are selected, the lower anterior teeth are selected as recommended by the manufacturer. For example, the 44E (DENTSPLY/Trubyte) maxillary anterior mold is opposed by mandibular mold F (DENTSPLY/Trubyte), and the Universal Lactona maxillary anterior mold M45 (Universal Lactona Dental) is opposed by mandibular mold M45 (Universal Lactona Dental). The combined width of the recommended six lower anterior teeth is generally 10 mm less than the combined width of the upper six anterior teeth (see tip 6 in the "Tips on tooth selection" section).

Tips on tooth selection

1. Facial width of one-sixteenth is determined to give the width of the central incisors. The laterals and cuspids in any mold are sized to be in harmony with this measurement. The facial length is never used because the length of the teeth is more determined by lip height and the size of the residual ridge. This maxillary central size is always in harmony with the size of the patient's face. Next, the shape or mold of the teeth must be selected. I use another method called "heart and imagination." This is hard to explain. Credit is to be given to Fillastre (Fillastre, personal communication, 1980). After the appropriate size is selected, the dentist pictures the patient in their mind's eye with the mold chart in front of them and imagines what mold would look good for the patient.

2. Facial types—square, tapered, or ovoid—have little to do with mold selection. The amount of incisal wear is a more appropriate guideline. The older the patient, the flatter the incisal edges. The younger patient will require more rounded edges that show less wear. Older patients tend to have flatter, more worn cuspids. There is basically no difference in molds for male or female.

3. Patients should be asked to bring pictures of them before they lost their natural teeth. This can show anterior tooth arrangement and situations such as diastemas. A trick to using a portrait-size picture is to measure tooth width on the photograph and also the interpupillary width on the photograph. Then the interpupillary width on the patient is measured. By using a simple mathematical proportion, the actual tooth size is determined.

4. Patients should bring pictures of people from magazines who have teeth that they think are attractive. This is done to point out that teeth are not set over the residual ridge[8] with small teeth hidden back in the mouth. Pretty teeth are prominent and support the lip. Most attractive people show all of their teeth when they smile, and many show some or all of their gingiva. This exercise allows the teeth to be placed more in the position that the natural teeth once occupied.

5. The molds are mixed. For example, the central and cuspids from one mold and the laterals from another are used. Also, the use of laterals from two different molds can create a nice effect. The patient must be educated to the fact that bilateral symmetry does not occur in nature and that this is not esthetic.

6. Manufacturers' suggestions for a mandibular anterior mold to use with a specific maxillary anterior mold are dictated by a combined upper and lower width that will allow the first bicuspids, maxillary and mandibular, to blend in harmony with the maxillary and mandibular cuspids and with the cuspids in a Class I relationship. To be esthetic, a denture must be in harmony with nature. It is good to remember that, in establishing natural denture esthetics, the teeth are to be set in harmony with original jaw relations, whether it is Class I, II, or III. In these cases, the mandibular anterior mold may have to be varied in size to produce a nice harmonic transition from the cuspids to the first bicuspids during setup.

7. In selecting posterior teeth, my preference is to use an anatomic maxillary posterior tooth (33° cuspid tooth) that occludes in a lingualized fashion into the central fossae of the lower.[8,24] The esthetics is far superior to flat plane and other lesser degree teeth. The beautiful maxillary buccal cusps look natural (see Figure 19.9). The purpose of the maxillary buccal cusp is esthetics, food manipulation, and overjet to prevent jaw biting.

8. Facial profiles can be important in denture tooth selection. For example, an individual with a flat profile might look better with a flat mold tooth, and the patient with a curved profile might look better with a more curved or rounded facial contour.

9. A choice is made between porcelain or acrylic teeth. Porcelain teeth keep their luster. They will not wear excessively, causing loss of vertical dimension, which leads to serious esthetic problems. There are times when, because of interarch space, acrylic teeth must be used. In these cases, metal occlusal surfaces should be used to prevent further loss of vertical dimension. The use of acrylic teeth does not reduce the pressure on the underlying bone. Rapid bone loss is caused by malocclusion. With plastic teeth, the malocclusion is soon worn in; with porcelain teeth, the malocclusion is there forever.

10. The newer composite resin teeth have certain advantages. Ro Youdalis (personal communication, 1985) pointed out that the hardness of these teeth will make many metal occlusal surfaces unnecessary because of their wear resistance.

Tooth color

The hues found in most natural teeth fall into the ranges of yellow, brown, and orange. The lightness and darkness of teeth are controlled by the value (degree of gray or white). Chroma (the saturation of hue) increases with advanced age, whereas the value decreases. Tooth color and gingival tissue seem to be related to tissue tones and the general overall complexion of the individual. The light-complexion, blue-eyed blond will usually display very light teeth, with little or no yellow. Contrasting this is the dark-complexion brunette and redhead whose teeth generally show more yellow, brown, and orange. As these individuals grow older, the yellow–brown of the brunette is intensified by a deeper color and lower value. As the blue-eyed blond advances in age, the greatest change is lower value. The teeth become more gray but still exhibit very little yellow–brown. There are always exceptions. It is not unusual at all to see a dark-complexion brunette with very white teeth with no yellow. There are exceptions to all of these rules.

Tips on tooth color

1. Consultation with the patient is the best way to establish rapport in the matter of tooth color.[25] No attempt should be made to convince a patient to accept any other shade than what they want.[26] All patients want nice white teeth, and the older denture patient is no exception. (A personal note on this subject is in order. In the early days, I tried to select teeth as my mentor did to be in harmony with the patient's age and complexion. It seemed that I was always at odds with patients who wanted white teeth.) Seminars are conducted during which dentures are provided for patients. Since all of the shades cannot be available during the seminars, only light shades are stocked. There is never a discussion about shades at the seminars. The fact that every patient gets young bright teeth is a key to success.

2. Every female patient is asked when looking at their old denture, "Wouldn't you like a brighter, more youthful tooth on your new denture?" The response is interesting: it is always yes.

3. Many patients love to see the artist in their dentist emerge. The dentist could try using central incisors of one shade and then change the shades of the laterals. The patient with the love of naturalness will respond.

4. Lower anteriors are one shade darker than the upper incisors.

Tooth arrangement

Once a proper tooth has been selected for the patient, the maxillary anterior teeth will be positioned on the base. The most important consideration in creating an esthetic denture is the position of the maxillary anterior teeth. This position will directly influence the position of every other tooth in the denture. Frank Lloyd Wright said, "Form and function are one." So it is with dentures: the closer the artificial teeth are placed to the position once occupied by the natural teeth, the better the function will be. Another advantage of natural tooth placement is that they will fall within the neutral zone, which is the neutral point of muscle balance between the lips and cheeks and the tongue. E. Pound (personal communication, 1975) said that, in the early days, when motion pictures became talking pictures, many actors lost their jobs because of poor dentistry and poor phonetics. He said that the sound people at the studios knew as little about speech as he did. Pound said that he strove to make dentures exquisitely esthetic and that the better they looked, the better they spoke. This is how his lifetime study of phonetics began. In the practice of complete denture prosthetics, if the dentist can position the artificial teeth in the position the natural teeth occupied, the better the esthetics and function will be.

Key to denture esthetics: proper placement of maxillary anterior teeth

The single most important thing that must be done to create an esthetic denture is proper placement of the maxillary anterior teeth. The key is the placement of the maxillary central incisors. If these two teeth are correct, they will directly influence the position of every other tooth in the denture. Correctly placed, the maxillary six incisors should be as close as possible to the exact position once occupied by the natural teeth. The notion that teeth should be set over the ridge to gain a mechanical advantage is simply outdated and untrue. If the teeth are set to anatomic harmony, then they will be in the neutral zone and vice versa.

Over the years, I have measured casts of natural maxillary anterior teeth to find a common position. A common average position of the maxillary anterior teeth to constant landmarks has been found by measuring hundreds of casts of natural healthy teeth. These measurements are (1) the distance of the incisal labial one-third of the maxillary central incisors from the center of the incisive papilla (Figure 19.12) and (2) the distance down the incisal edge from the general height of the maxillary anterior labial vestibule (Figure 19.13).

This position will not be appropriate for every patient. It will put the teeth in a reasonable position all of the time. Variations from this position require a judgment on the dentist's part. I have observed that when positioned in this manner, about 4 in 10 patients are close to ideal. The other 60% will need slight changes.

In Figure 19.14A, the patient has very unesthetic dentures. The ridges are healthy and well formed (Figure 19.14B). A stabilized base is constructed onto the cast of the maxillary edentulous ridge. A wax rim is placed onto the stabilized base. The wax rim is built 10 mm out from the center of the incisal papilla and 20 mm down from the general height of the labial vestibule. In addition, the wax rim is built level to the interpupillary line and parallel to Camper's line. Camper's line runs from the middle of the tragis of the ear to the base of the ala of the nose. The wax rim is tried into the edentulous mouth. The level of the incisal plane and Camper's line is verified. The facial midline is marked (Figure 19.14C–E).

The maxillary central incisors are set onto the wax rim (Figure 19.14 F) and confirmed in the mouth (Figure 19.14G and H).[27-29] Once the proper position of the central incisors is verified, then the remainder of the maxillary incisors is set (Figure 19.14I). At this point, the basic tooth position has been determined. Detailed esthetics, such as lapping of the lateral incisors and tipping of the cuspids, is done in the laboratory. Once the maxillary anterior basic tooth position has been verified, as a demonstration, a silicone matrix has been made onto the setup. In this case, the central incisors ended up 9 mm anterior to the center of the incisive papilla. The teeth follow the curvature of the edentulous ridge (Figure 19.14J). If the ridge should be more square or more "V" shaped, this would be reflected in the

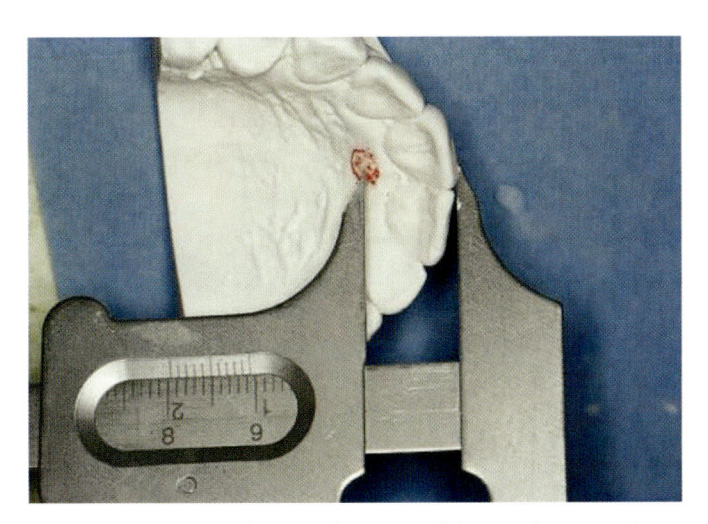

Figure 19.12 Average horizontal position of the maxillary central incisors is determined by measuring the distance from the center of the incisive papilla and the labial incisal one‑third of the central incisors.

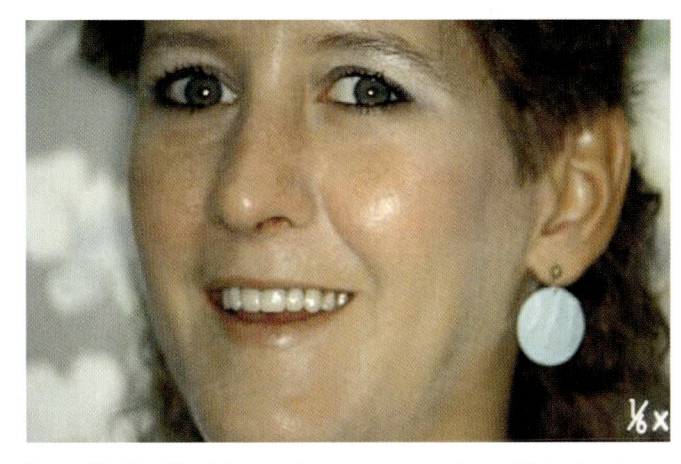

Figure 19.14 **(A)** A 32-year-old edentulous patient with teeth set over the ridge with a straight line setup resulting in the typical denture look.

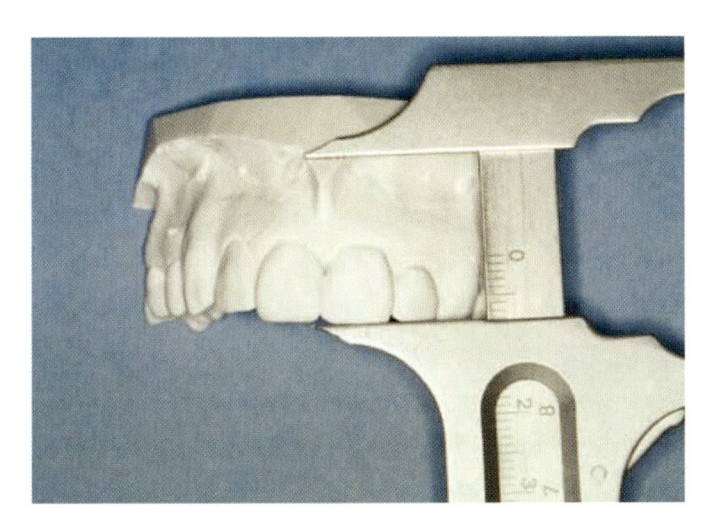

Figure 19.13 Average vertical position of the maxillary central incisors is measured from the general height of the anterior labial vestibule down to the incisal edge of the central incisors.

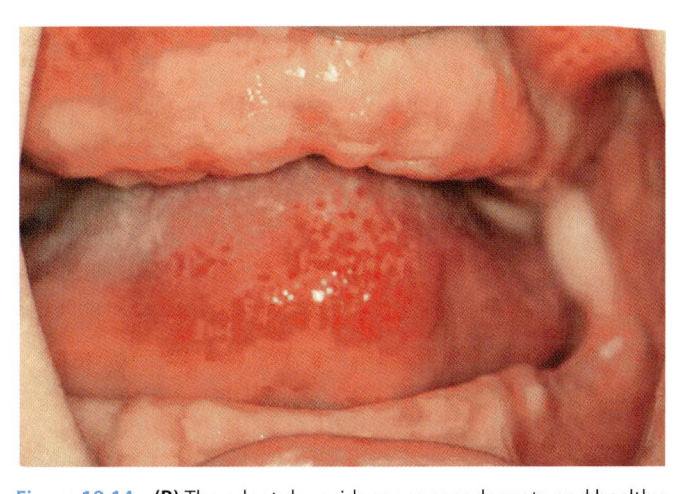

Figure 19.14 **(B)** The edentulous ridges appear adequate and healthy.

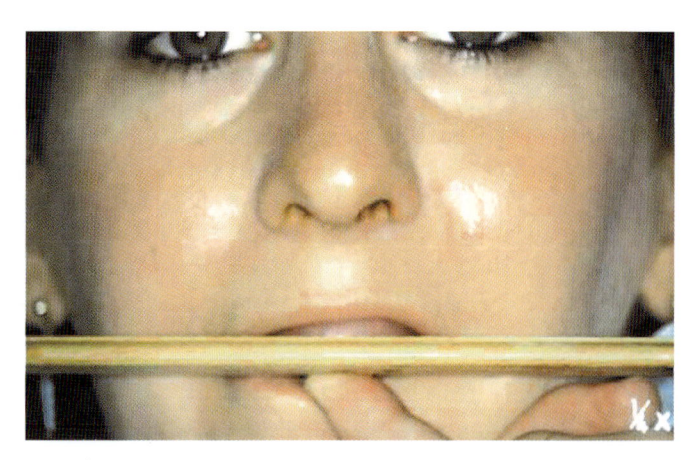

Figure 19.14 **(C)** The maxillary bite rim is built 10 mm anterior from the center of the incisive papilla horizontally and vertically 20 mm down from the general height of the labial vestibule. It is built level so that it is parallel to the interpupillary line. *Source:* Reproduced with permission from Turbyfill.[11]

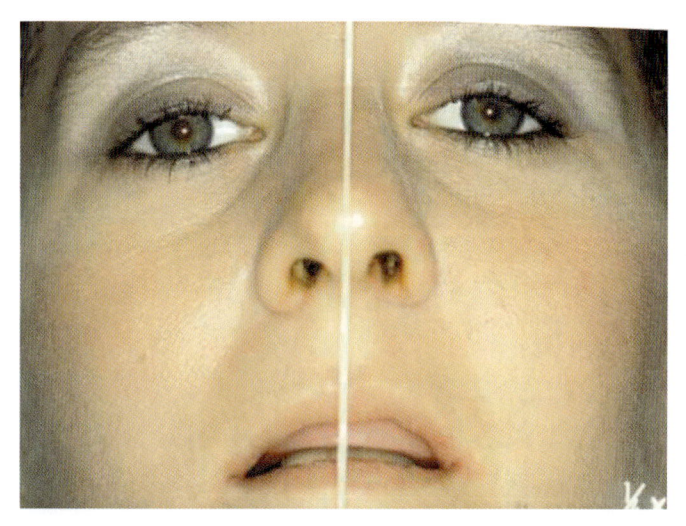

Figure 19.14 **(D)** The midline is marked.

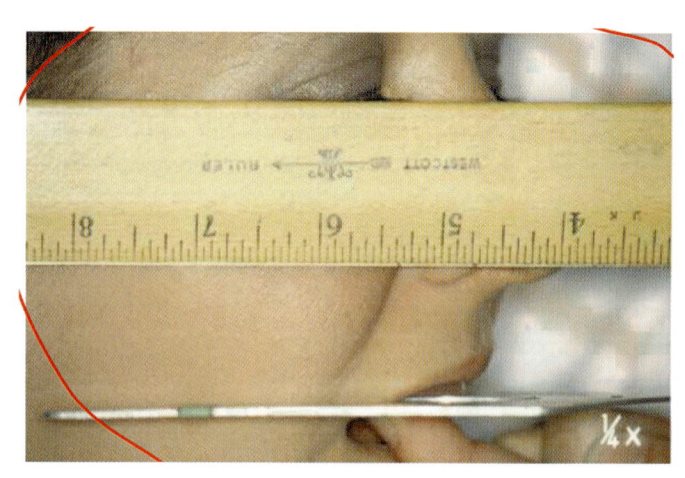

Figure 19.14 **(E)** The maxillary bite rim is built parallel to Camper's line.

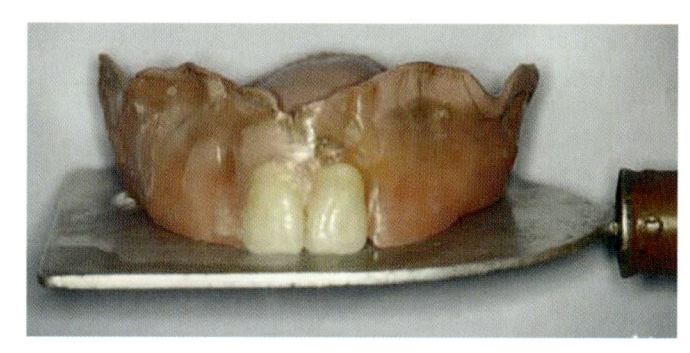

Figure 19.14 **(F)** The maxillary central incisors are set to the previously determined midline and the horizontal and vertical determinants. *Source:* Reproduced with permission from Turbyfill.[11]

arrangement. The cuspid begins to be tucked closer to the ridge as the corner is turned from the anterior ridge to the posterior area of the ridge. The result is a much improved esthetics of the finished denture. Figure 19.14 K shows the superior esthetics that has been achieved using this approach.

Once the maxillary teeth are set to anatomic harmony and the dentist is satisfied with this position, the mandibular anterior teeth are set so that they exhibit 0.5–1 mm of clearance as the sibilant sounds are being enunciated (Figure 19.14 L). The vertical dimension of occlusion is recorded by arcing the mandible in the arc of closure in centric relation and closing the vertical down until the anterior stop comes into contact (Figure 19.14 M).

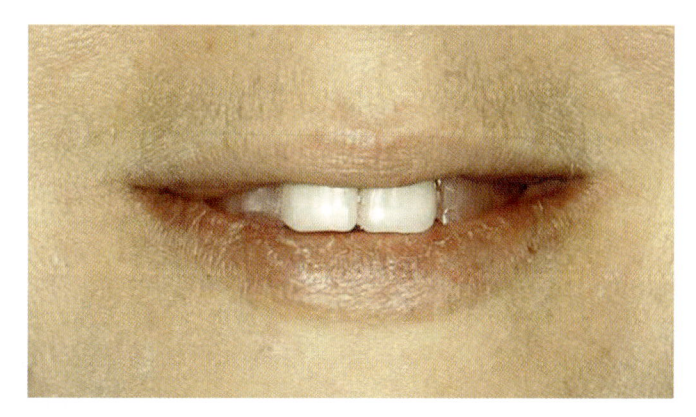

Figure 19.14 **(G)** The central incisor position is verified in the patient's mouth as to tooth display and midline.

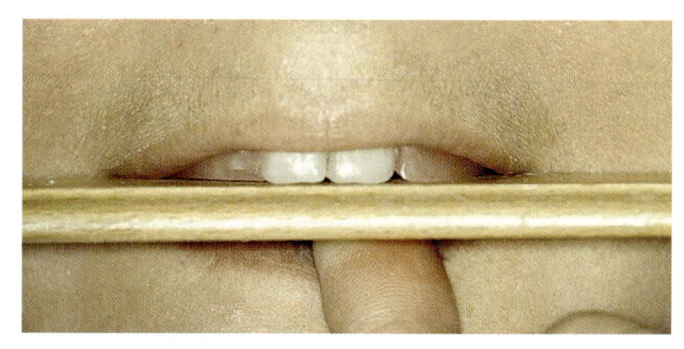

Figure 19.14 **(H)** The level of the central incisors is verified. *Source:* Reproduced with permission from Turbyfill.[11]

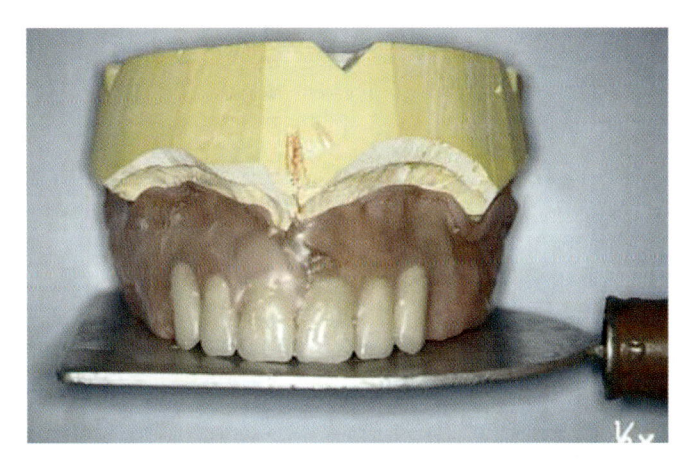

Figure 19.14 **(I)** The maxillary anterior tooth position is completed.

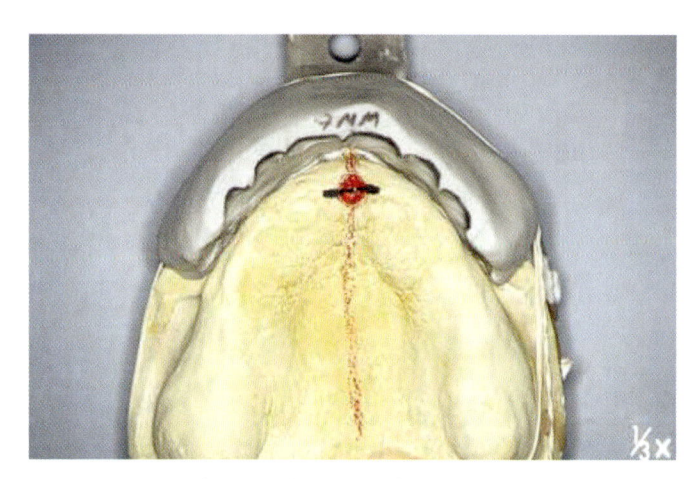

Figure 19.14 **(J)** The natural position of the maxillary teeth to the edentulous ridge.

A denture may appear to be reasonably esthetic at first glance, as is the maxillary denture shown in Figure 19.15A–C. The denture was remade because of poor function and comfort. The teeth are now set to a position more in keeping with anatomic harmony. This position is 20 mm down from the height of the maxillary vestibule and 10 mm out from the center of the incisive papilla. Figure 19.15D–F shows the subtle but exquisite improvement in esthetics and maxillary lip support.

Placement of the mandibular anterior teeth

The mandibular anterior teeth are set using phonetics. Dawson[30] noted that the vertical dimension of occlusion that has been lost can be regained by noting the closest speaking level and then establishing the vertical dimension of occlusion slightly more closed from that closest speaking position. Pound[31] referred to this as the vertical dimension of speech, and since the teeth are not to touch while a person is speaking, then the vertical dimension of occlusion should be slightly more closed than the "S" position. Further, the "S" position is the most forward, most closed position the mandible ever assumes during speech.

Two mandibular incisors are set to the "S" position. Pound defined the "S" position as the most intimate relationship of the teeth during speech.[31] There are intimate relationships that occur

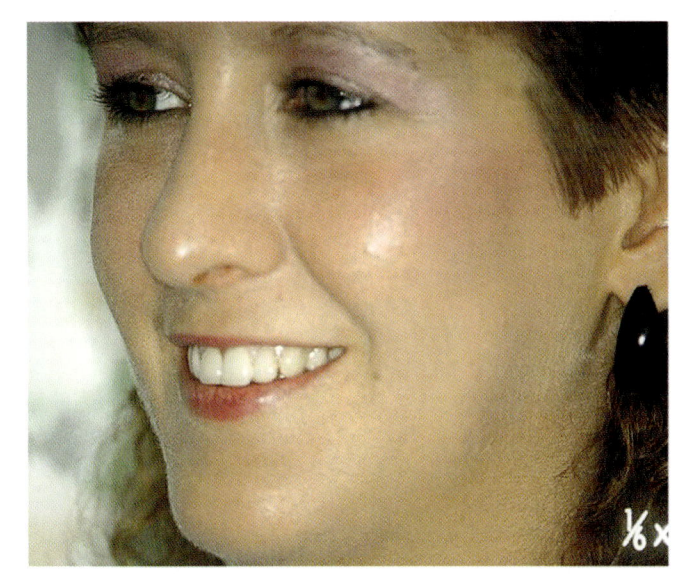

Figure 19.14 **(K)** The superior esthetic results achieved by placing the maxillary anterior teeth to anatomic harmony.

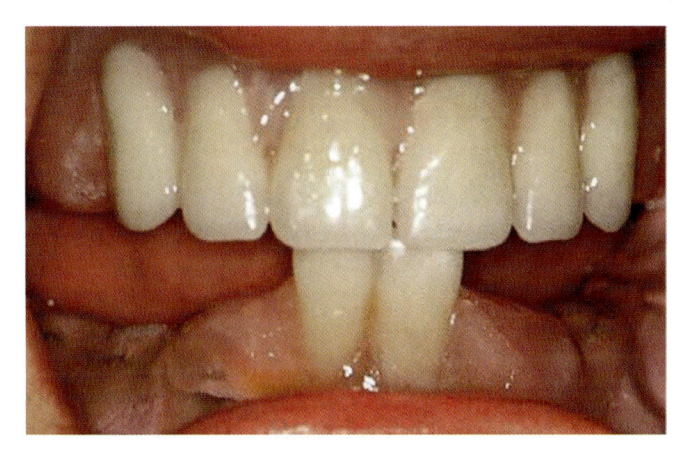

Figure 19.14 **(L)** The mandibular anterior teeth are positioned to exhibit a 0.5–1 mm clearance with the maxillary anterior teeth as the patient enunciates "S" sounds.

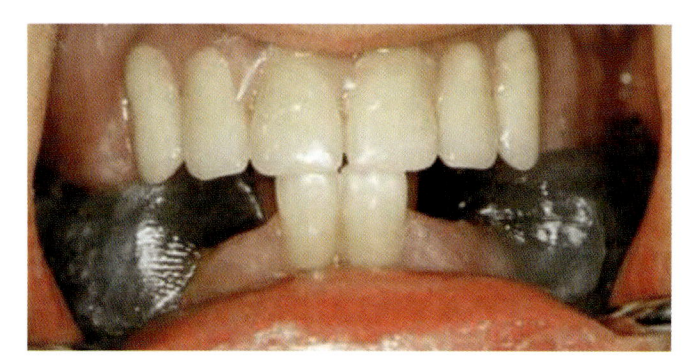

Figure 19.14 **(M)** The mandibular position of centric relation is determined by a simple wax recording. This is considered a treatment position, and final centric relation determination is achieved by using a central bearing point and Gothic arch tracing.

between the incisal edges of the mandibular teeth and the incisal edges and lingual surfaces of the maxillary anterior teeth. This allows the dentist to verify the accuracy of the maxillary tooth arrangement and place the mandibular incisors in an anatomically natural position that produces an articulate speech pattern. After this position is verified, the anterior stop has been reestablished (see Figure 19.14 L).

Anterior denture occlusion

No anterior teeth should be in contact when the posterior teeth are in maximum occlusion. This anterior pressure will cause destruction of the bone of the premaxilla. It also causes instability of the dentures. Once the anterior teeth are set to exhibit a phonetic clearance when the "S" sounds are enunciated, the centric relation registration is then taken with the anterior stop in contact. In Class I and II jaw relationships, the mandible leaves the centric relation posture position and moves forward to the phonetic "S" position. Therefore, the articulator pins are opened slightly on Class I and II occlusions so that the anterior teeth will not contact in the centric relation. Since the mandible always moves forward in phonetics, the condylar guidance will keep the posterior teeth from contacting in speech. In Class III occlusion, there is no forward movement of the mandible during speech. Slight anterior contact in the Class III jaw relationship is inevitable. The occlusal contact should be heavier in the posterior than in the anterior.

Vertical dimension

I use phonetics and the closest speaking position to develop the incisal edge position of the mandibular anterior teeth, and the vertical dimension of occlusion is determined from this. It must be understood that this method is not always accurate. Some patients exhibit an adapted position that is obviously overclosed. In cases like this, the vertical is opened on the trial bases until the facial profile looks more normal. In other words, the patient should not look older below the nose than above the nose. Since all patients are treated with a provisional treatment denture, this "arbitrary" vertical dimension is tested before denture finalization. Even though phonetics is not accurate in every case, it is still the preferred way because the different movements of the mandible for the different classes of occlusion help to position the incisal edges in a more natural position.

There are many ways to establish the vertical dimension of occlusion on dentures, such as phonetics, relaxation of the mandible to establish the resting level of the mandibular freeway space, having the patient wet the lips and breathe out, and measuring dots on the nose and chin and other facial dimensions. Volumes have been written about vertical dimension. The subject of vertical dimension is a very emotional one, and some heated arguments can erupt over it.

The most important thing that the dentist must remember about vertical dimension is that if the vertical is opened too far so as to cause the posterior teeth to hit as the patient speaks, a failure will always result. Another important observation is that the dentist should give each denture patient the greatest vertical dimension possible. The patient will look, chew, and feel better. Improper vertical dimension can have a profound effect on esthetics. In Figure 19.16A, the patient looks prognathic and old below the nose with a vertical dimension that is overclosed. Figure 19.16B shows excellent esthetics when the vertical dimension is properly restored. Figure 19.16C demonstrates the poor esthetics created by improper vertical and horizontal positioning of the maxillary anterior teeth and the denture look. Figure 19.16D shows the improved esthetics with proper maxillary anterior tooth positioning.

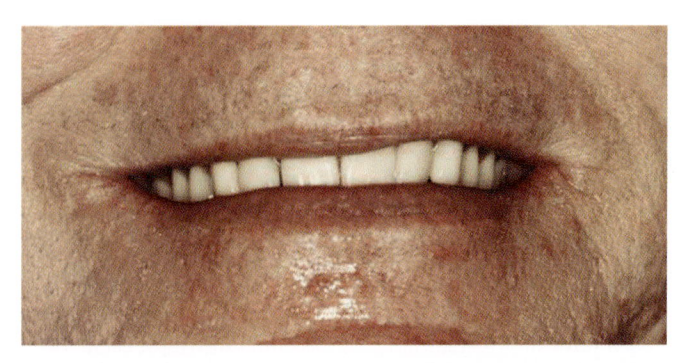

Figure 19.15 **(A)** A denture with a poor maxillary anterior tooth position.

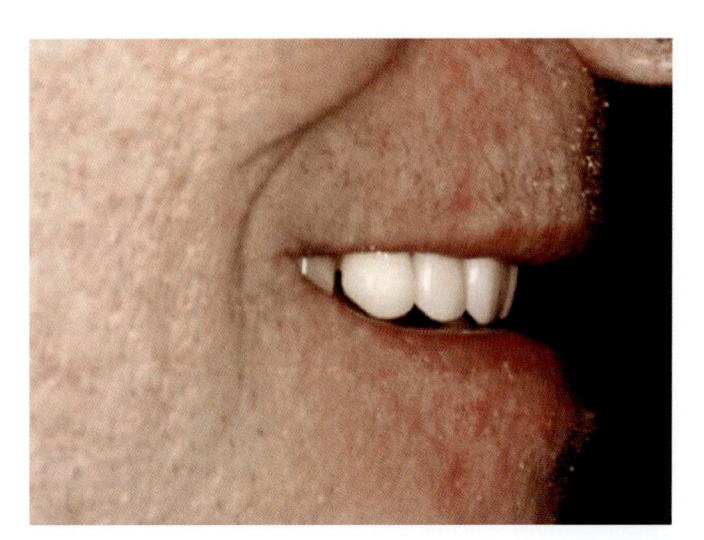

Figure 19.15 **(B)** Note the depressed position of the incisors.

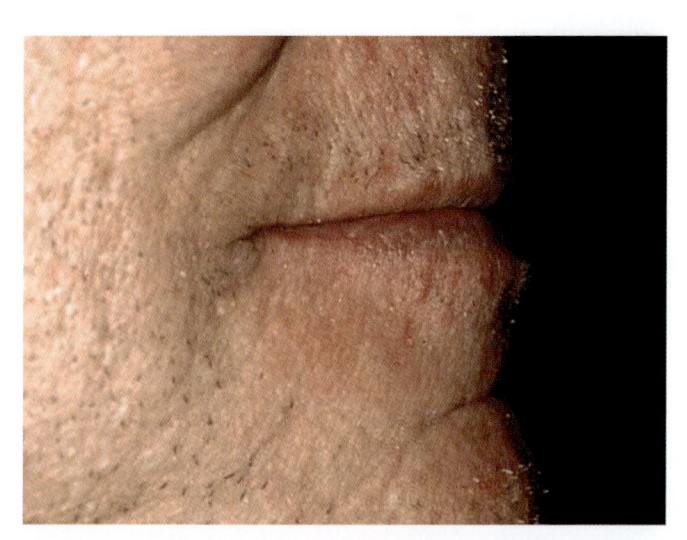

Figure 19.15 **(C)** Note the look of the maxillary lip support.

Consideration of the vertical dimension of the occlusion for the edentulous patient as it differs from the patient with natural teeth needs to be addressed. Patients with natural teeth are very adaptive to changes in the vertical dimension of the occlusion because of the exquisite proprioception of natural teeth. Many times, a slight opening of the vertical dimension is needed to facilitate restorative procedures. Edentulous patients do not adapt nearly as well. Generally, when the closest speaking position is determined, any opening from that position should be done while the patient is wearing the provisional training denture. An excessive vertical dimension of the occlusion in complete dentures results in a restriction of normal muscle activity, and the posterior and anterior teeth will hit during speech. When opened experimentally using the training denture, if the teeth continue to hit during speech for 1 week, then adaptation is not possible, and the teeth will hit during speech forever.

Posterior occlusion as it relates to denture esthetics

One area often overlooked or misunderstood is the effect of the posterior tooth position on esthetics. An extremely poor esthetic denture can result by establishing the posterior plane of

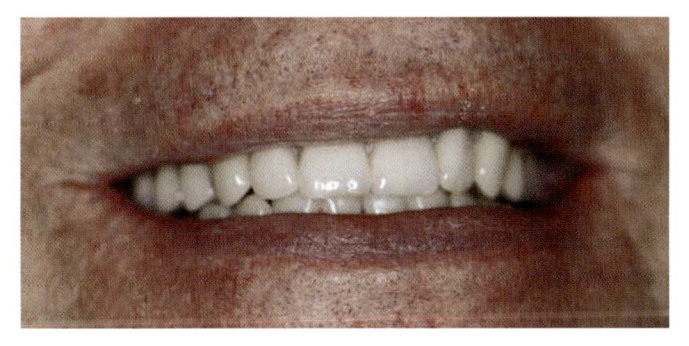

Figure 19.15 (D) An esthetic denture with the maxillary central incisors set to the 10 × 20 rule.

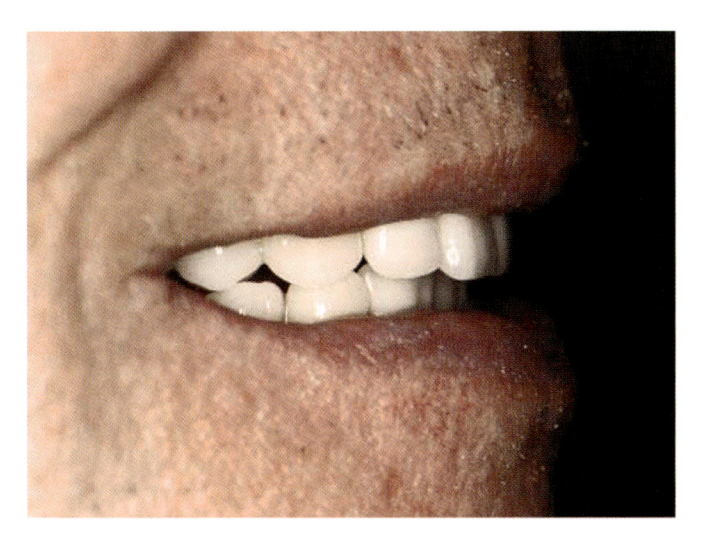

Figure 19.15 (E) Note the more natural tooth position.

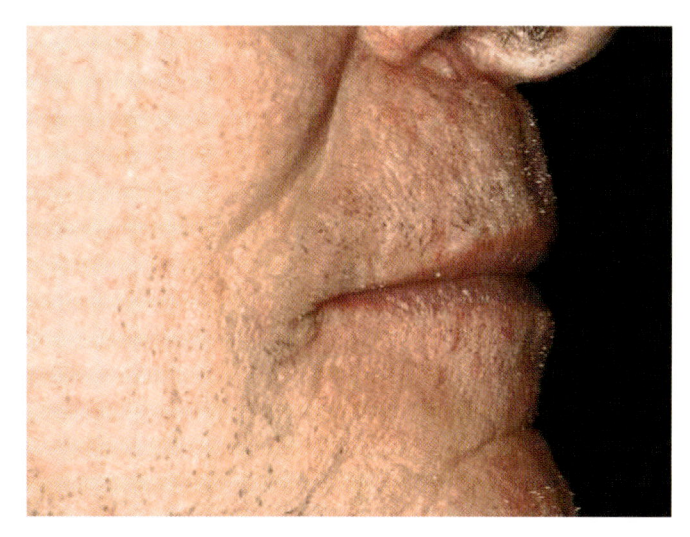

Figure 19.15 (F) Note the improved lip support.

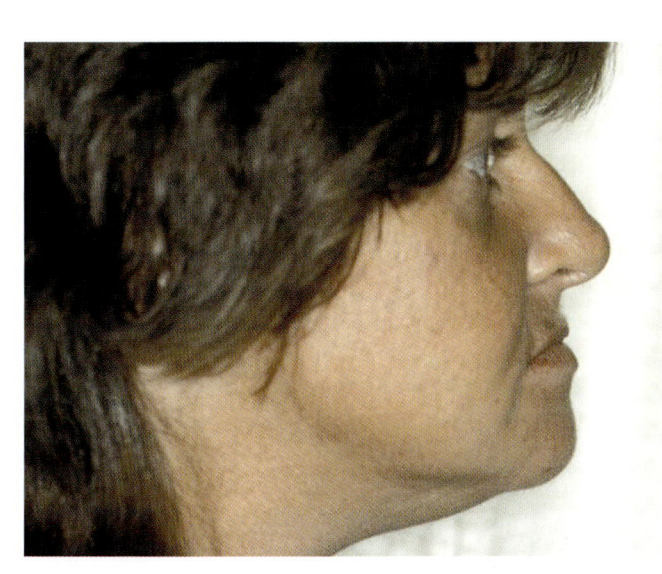

Figure 19.16 (A) Overclosure of the vertical dimension of the occlusion. Note the prognathic appearance and decreased lower facial length.

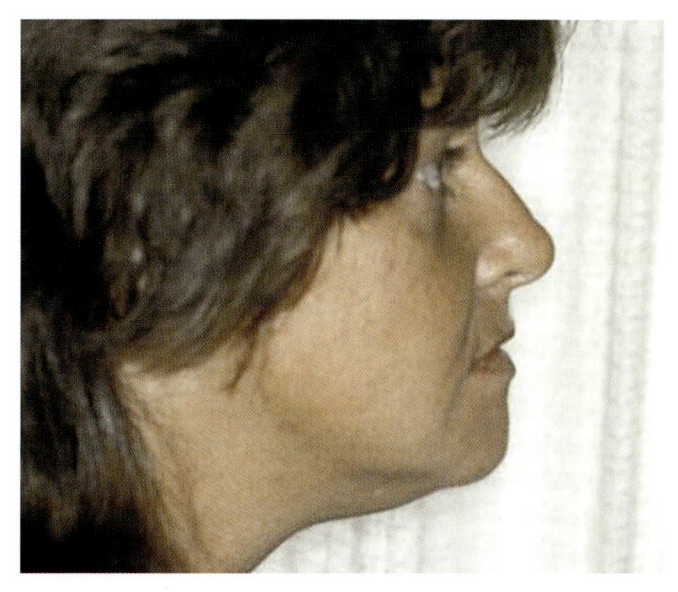

Figure 19.16 (B) Proper vertical dimension of occlusion. Note how much younger the patient appears.

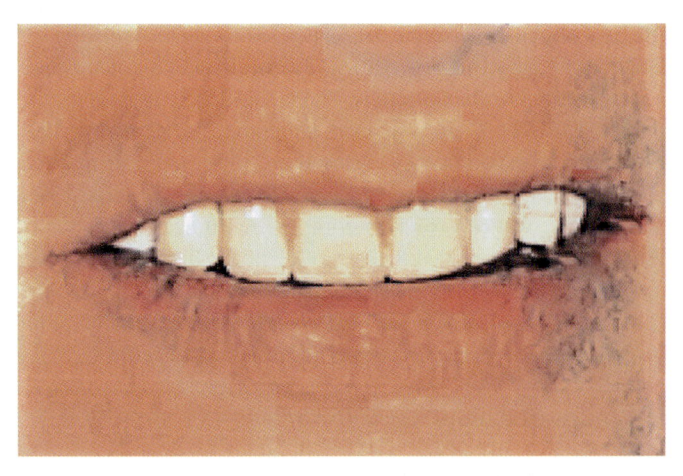

Figure 19.16 **(C)** Everything looks bad: the denture look.

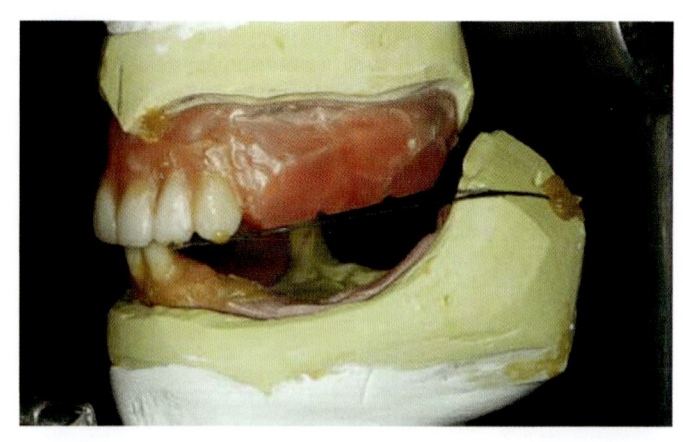

Figure 19.17 Posterior occlusal plane lines up from the maxillary incisal edges to a point halfway up the retromolar pad (Camper's line).

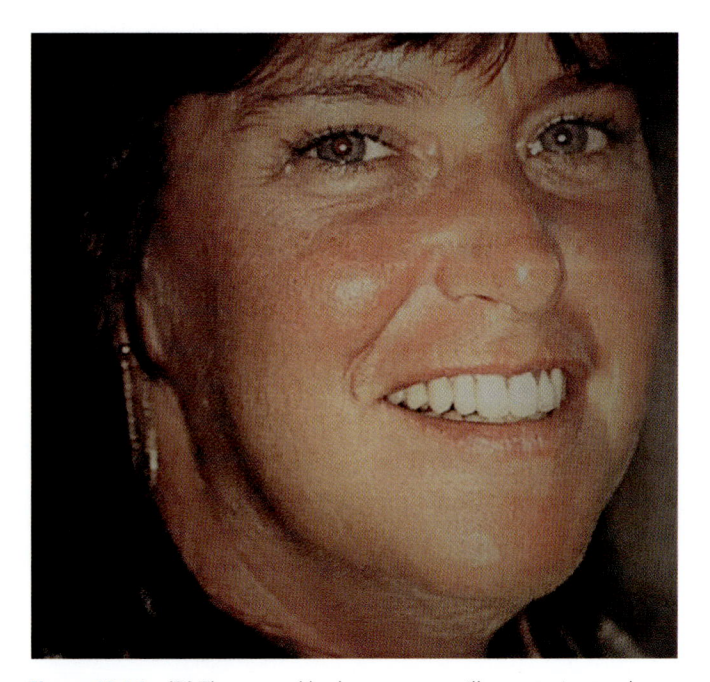

Figure 19.16 **(D)** The natural look: correct maxillary anterior tooth placement and correct vertical dimension of occlusion.

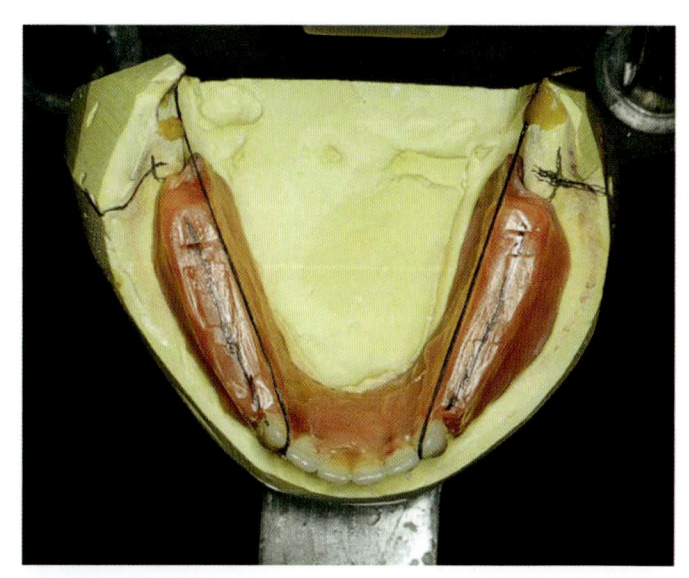

Figure 19.18 Buccolingual placement of the posterior occlusal plane. The lingual control line runs from the mesial contact of the cuspid to the lingual aspect of the retromolar pad.

occlusion too high or too low. This is demonstrated by the patient who smiles, and the maxillary posterior teeth can be seen hanging down below the plane of the maxillary incisors. Camper's line will position the posterior occlusal plane on a line beamed from the maxillary anterior incisal edge posterior to the middle of the retromolar pad (Figure 19.17).

The buccolingual placement of the posterior teeth can also affect esthetics. If the maxillary teeth are placed too far to the buccal aspect, then the buccal corridor between the maxillary posterior teeth and the corner of the mouth is lost. If the maxillary teeth are placed too far lingually or palatally, then they appear not to exist. Either extreme produces unacceptable esthetics. The guideline for the maxillary posterior tooth position is found in the mandibular arch. The lingual central line is from the mesial contact of the cuspid to the lingual aspect of the retromolar pad. The lingual surface of the mandibular posterior teeth should fall on this line. The mandibular posterior teeth are positioned closer to the tongue than this line (Figure 19.18).

Tips for tooth arrangement

1. The position of the maxillary central incisors is the key to denture esthetics. Once they are placed and accepted, all other tooth positions are a product of these two teeth.
2. Placement of the anterior teeth must be done at chairside in the presence of the patient. The author never lets the patient see the results of this initial placement because the setting is a very straight-line prosaic setup and represents basic tooth position. Detailed esthetics is done at the laboratory bench.
3. The appointment for this initial setting is from 1 to 1.5 h. The rapport that is built with the patient at this time is unbelievable. The patient will always say, "I've never had a dentist spend so much time with me."

4. The "S" position is the most intimate relationship of any teeth during speech.[32,33] As the "S" sounds are formed, the anterior teeth will exhibit a space of 1–1.5 mm. The "S" sounds are produced by forcing air between the incisal edges of the maxillary incisors and the mandibular incisors. The "S" sounds can also be produced by forcing air between the incisal edges of the mandibular incisors and the lingual surfaces of the maxillary incisors, as will be found in many Class II occlusal relationships. It should be remembered that the teeth do not touch when the "S" sounds are being enunciated.

5. The vertical dimension of occlusion is very easy to determine since it is always less than the vertical dimension of speech.[34–36] Therefore, when the anterior teeth are set to the "S" position, the mandible is retruded and closed down 2 mm to tooth contact or, if no teeth touch, merely closes in a centric relation 2 mm less than the vertical dimension of speech.

6. The "F" and "V" sounds are produced when the incisal edges of all six maxillary anterior teeth make a fleeting seal at the vermilion border or the wet–dry line of the lower lip. If the maxillary teeth are placed in anatomic harmony, the "F" and "V" position will always be correct. This is an extremely valuable check on the accuracy of the maxillary anterior tooth placement.

7. The anterior teeth, both maxillary and mandibular, should appear as if they are coming from the bone at a slightly different angle. Sharry[37] wrote, "There is one prominent guide for providing an excellent arrangement of anterior teeth; they must be separate." Bilateral symmetry is not found in nature. The laterals can be mesially lapped or winged out distally. Laterals can be set to be shorter than the centrals or cuspids; however, the older the patient is, the more even the incisal edges should be. If photographs are available and show diastemas, they can be placed subject to patient approval. It should be remembered that the younger the patient is, the more open the incisal embrasures.

8. Always keep the incisal plane level and slightly curved to follow the smile line of the lower lip. There is nothing more unesthetic than a slanted occlusal or incisal plane.

9. In a few patients, flaring of the cuspid can be esthetic, but in most cases it is best to set the cuspid so that only the mesial surface can be seen.

10. It should be remembered that the first introduction of dental esthetics to dental students and dental technology students was a Columbia Dentiform.

11. Pictures of "pretty" people should be used to show how beautiful smiles are made in nature. Dentists should point out the asymmetry and how prominent the teeth appear in a full smile.

12. Some interesting studies have been done concerning the arrangement of teeth for the edentulous patient by the use of cephalometric radiographs.[38] Orthodontists use the method of fixed bony landmarks to determine the ideal placement of natural teeth. It seems that this would be a valuable aid for tooth placement in complete denture prosthetics, particularly in the advanced resorbed dental arch.

13. I use "heart and imagination" in selecting and arranging teeth. In the laboratory, there should be a large selection of teeth, and as the dentist looks at the basic tooth position set at chairside, they must picture the patient in their mind's eye and set and select teeth to what they feel will be pleasing.

Denture base

The denture base is important in esthetics.[39,40] Its normal contour aids in support of the soft tissues of the lips and face. If the patient has a short upper lip and would normally show gingival tissues in a broad smile, an unesthetic denture base can destroy an otherwise esthetically successful denture. An anatomically accurate denture base is important to function, since "form and function are one." The food tables that we find facially at the tooth neck in normal healthy tissue help the buccinator muscles keep food out of the vestibule and up onto the occlusal surfaces. The form of the lingual surfaces is important, in that it imparts a feeling of naturalness to the tongue. It is also paramount that the neutral zone of the tongue not be violated by an overcontoured mandibular lingual flange. The denture base that copies nature is also self-cleaning. The interdental papilla is full and rounded, and there are no "festoons." They only create food traps and prevent a sweeping of the tongue from its cleaning action. Tinting of the denture base is important in several respects (Figure 19.19). A natural-looking base is desirable on the facial aspect and on the palatal as well. Nothing gives away a denture faster than an individual laughing with head held back as the slick mono color of the palate is viewed by others (Figure 19.20).

Tips on creating a natural-looking denture base

1. Casts of human tissue should be studied, noting stippling, gingival collars, and the interdental papilla. There should be no slick, flat, and shiny surfaces in human gingival tissues.

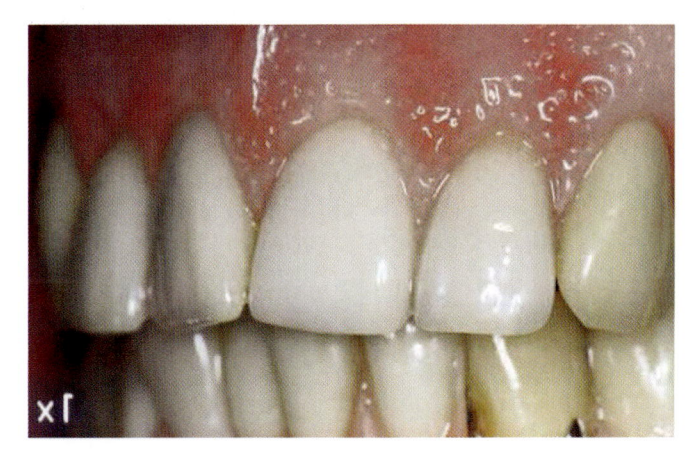

Figure 19.19 Denture base carved and tinted to appear natural.
Source: Reproduced with permission from Turbyfill.[10]

2. Whatever is wanted in the finished base should be carved in wax. No carving with rotary acrylic finishers can be done after it is processed (Figures 19.21, 19.22, and 19.23).
3. The denture should be invested with the same degree of care as was used in investing an inlay (Figure 19.24).
4. A denture base tinting acrylic (Kay-See Dental Manufacturing, Kansas City, MO) should be used (Figure 19.25).
5. Tints should be placed in eye dropper bottles with the glass droppers turned upside down to control the placement of the tints.

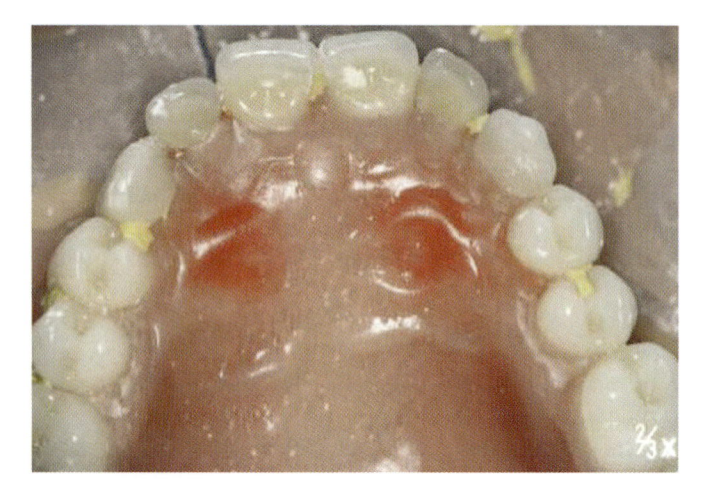

Figure 19.20 Correct anatomy of the palate with singulum carved on anterior teeth and lingual surfaces carved on the posterior teeth. The palate is also tinted.

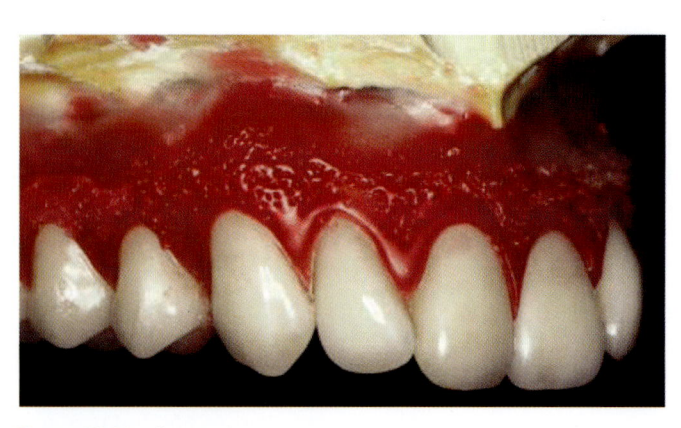

Figure 19.21 Anatomic wax-up.

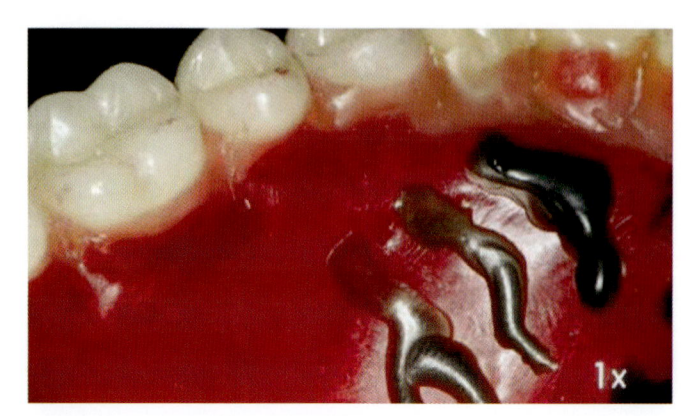

Figure 19.22 Anatomic wax-up.

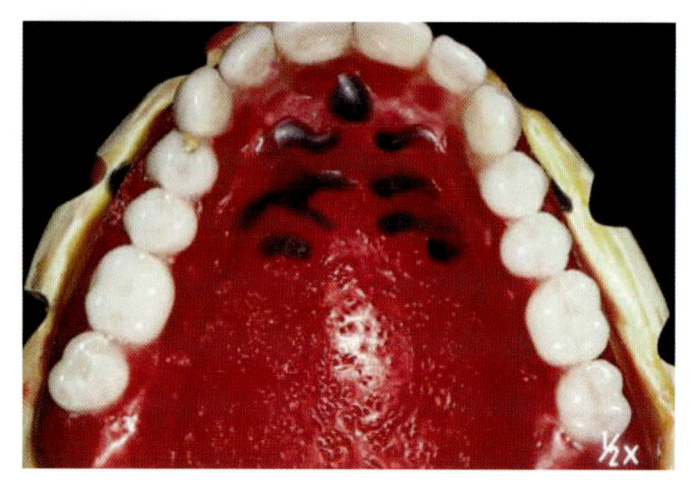

Figure 19.23 Anatomic wax-up. Note that the palate is lightly stippled so as not to appear shiny.

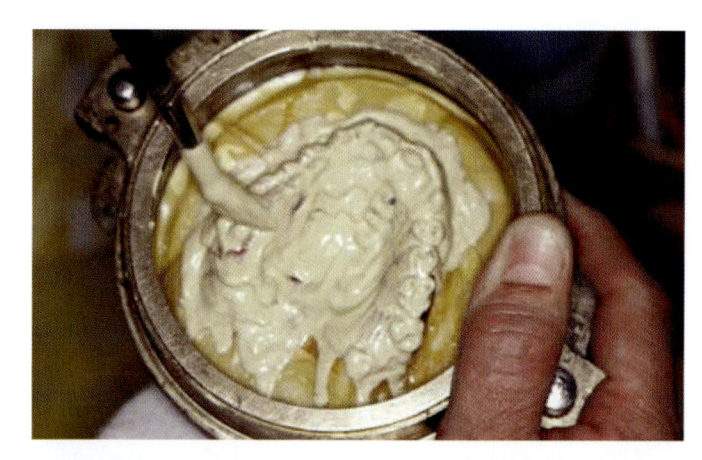

Figure 19.24 Investment is poured using a sable brush to capture the full anatomic wax-up.

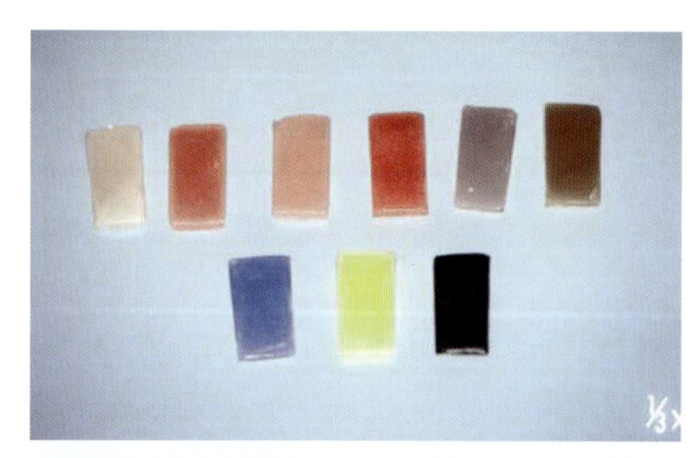

Figure 19.25 Shades of tints available for the wax-up. There is no carving of the base with rotary instruments.

6. The tints are sifted into the boiled out flasks and then are wet with monomer as the technician goes around the arch three or four teeth at a time (Figures 19.26, 19.27, and 19.28).
7. Cases are tinted in four basic shades: (1) light-complexion blue-eyed blonds, (2) medium-complexion brunettes, (3) dark-complexion brunettes, and (4) nonwhites.

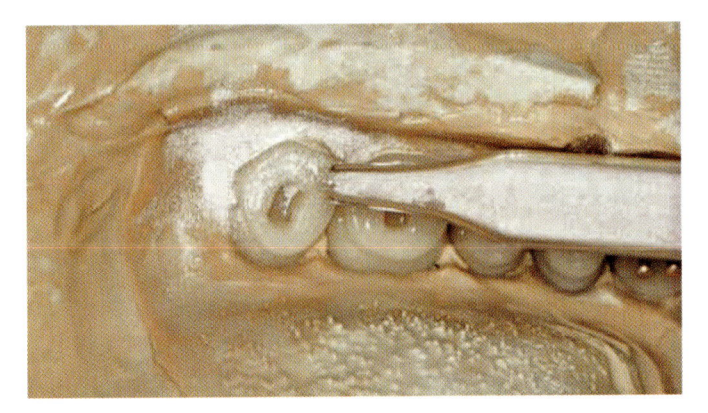

Figure 19.26 Tints are sifted around teeth.

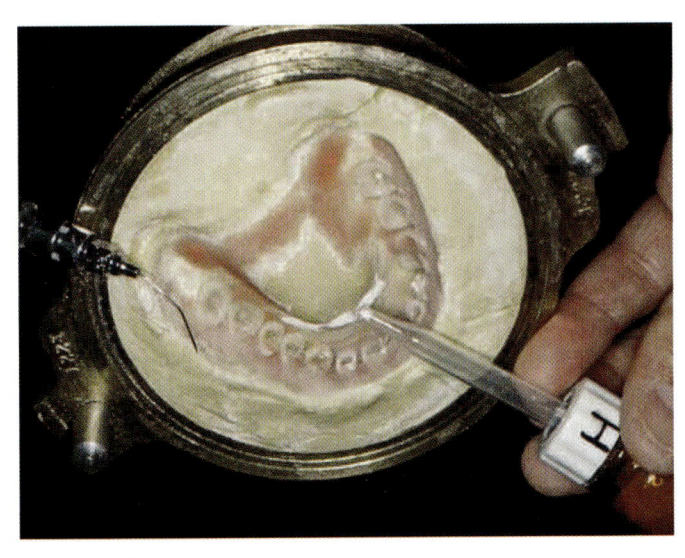

Figure 19.27 The palate is tinted.

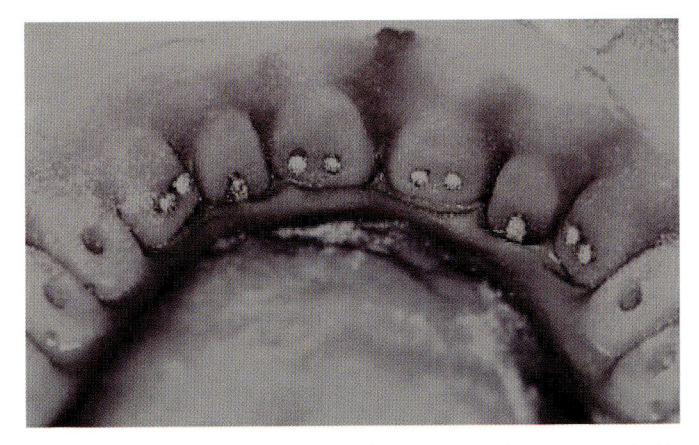

Figure 19.28 The maxillary case tinted. Dentures are then processed with acrylic of a color to complement the overall complexion of the patient.

Clinical examples of esthetic dentures

Figure 19.29A–F presents examples of esthetic dentures.

Bone quantity and quality dictate every procedure

Dentistry is the art and science of keeping people dentally healthy. This involves keeping patients comfortable, esthetic, and functional. This is a daunting task. In earlier times, when life expectancy was maybe 65–70 years of age, most patients could be somewhat comfortable and functional without too much trouble. We are now seeing patients who live often 90 years and older. Keeping patients comfortable, functional, and esthetic may not be possible. Patients who have good dental genes and who are resistant to dental disease are very fortunate. The increasing age of patients makes the art and science of removable prosthodontics more important than ever before. As I have observed over the years, there is less and less time and effort spent with dental students on this subject. Teaching partial and full denture prosthodontics for over 40 years has led me to the conclusion that the skills in removable prosthodontics are totally lost.

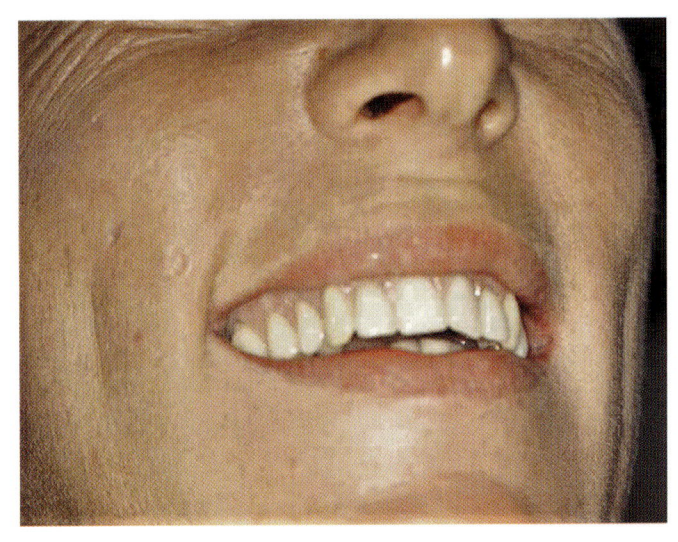

Figure 19.29 **(A)** Full-smile view of esthetic dentures.

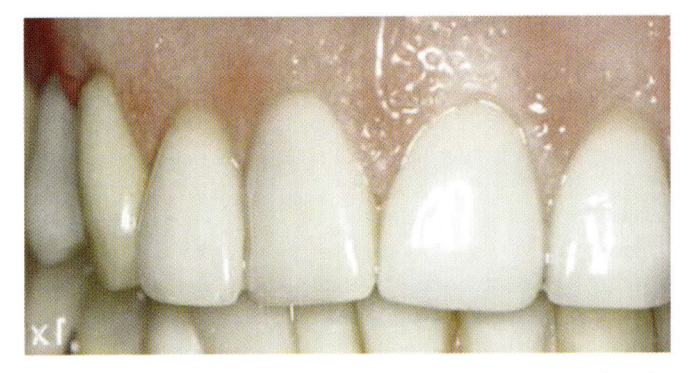

Figure 19.29 **(B)** Close-up of esthetic dentures. *Source:* Reproduced with permission from Turbyfill.[41]

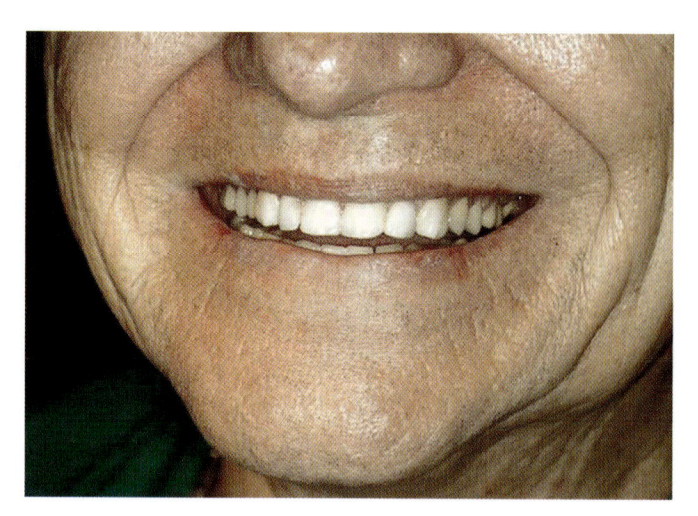

Figure 19.29 (C) Full-smile view of esthetic dentures.

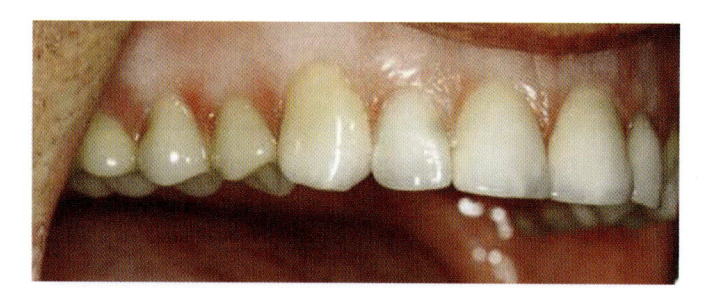

Figure 19.29 (D) Close-up of esthetic dentures.

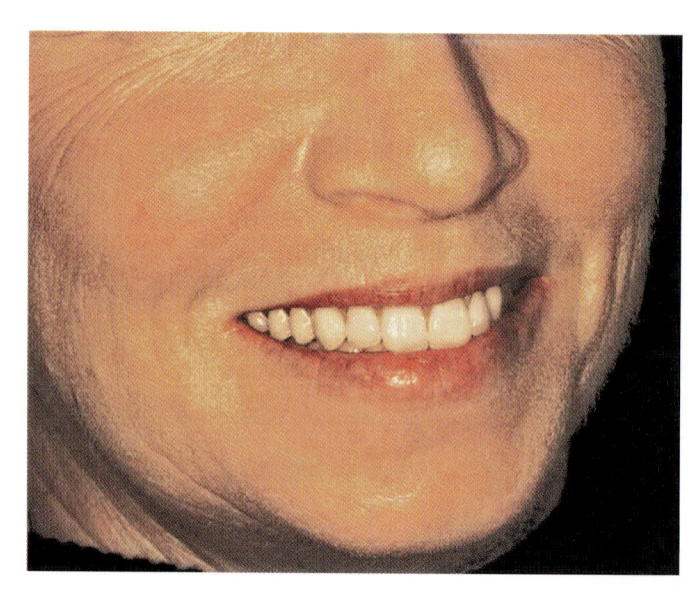

Figure 19.29 (E) Full-smile view of esthetic dentures.

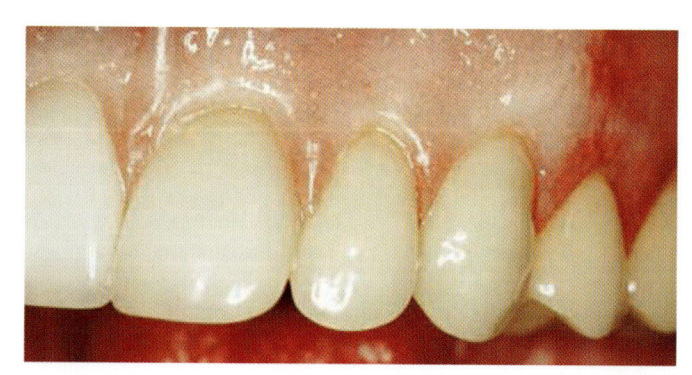

Figure 19.29 (F) Close-up of esthetic dentures.

Everything in dentistry depends on bone. Bone quantity and quality dictates everything that a dentist does. When there is no bone, then the only option is removable prosthodontics. With no bone, the endodontist, periodontist, orthodontist, fixed restorative dentist, and implant surgeon are out of work. No bone makes the treatment provided by the removable prosthodontist far less than satisfactory. There are now predictable methods to grow bone through grafting procedures, but so many patients have systemic health problems and financial limitations that the long process makes this option available to very few.

Porcelain versus plastic

The way removable prosthetics are constructed has an effect on preservation of bone. If you believe or have been taught that porcelain denture teeth destroy the bone, that is incorrect and there are no peer-reviewed studies to support that. American tooth manufactories have all but stopped making porcelain denture teeth. Technicians dislike using porcelain teeth because it is difficult, and broken sets of porcelain teeth are not returnable for credit. The widespread use of plastic teeth in my opinion is one of the shames of modern prosthodontics.

For example, this is a typical clinical scenario that proves my point. A patient loses all of the maxillary teeth and requires a maxillary complete denture. Now that patient may be a candidate for implants, but any thinking dentist will provide a conventional denture for that patient to establish acceptable esthetics, vertical dimension, and make sure that the patient has no serious problems accepting a prosthesis. Anytime there is a maxillary complete denture, the occlusion is a denture occlusion. It makes no difference what is in the mandible; if the maxillary is a complete denture, it must be a denture occlusion, which is as follows. To review, the definition of denture occlusion is *no anterior contact of the maxillary anterior teeth in centric closure, chewing, or speaking.*

The dentist makes a maxillary denture with all plastic teeth against a full complement of mandibular natural teeth. If the denture is properly made with good occlusal contact, the patient can chew very well. So with function, the posterior teeth will wear four times faster than the anterior teeth, and with the possibility of continuous eruption of the mandibular anterior teeth, it will not take long before the anterior teeth are bumping like crazy. Now the Kelly triad does its nasty work and the maxillary and premaxillary bones are destroyed, leaving only the nasal spine. The maxillary anterior teeth disappear under the upper lip, and because of a fibrous down growth of the posterior tuberosity, the posterior teeth seem to drop down.

Properly used porcelain denture teeth will preserve the bone. I have been using porcelain denture teeth for 40 years, and my experience is that the bone is preserved. The widespread use of plastic denture teeth in my opinion is one of the downfalls of removable prosthodontics as it is taught and handed down in dentistry over the years. The companies that make denture teeth are halting their manufacturing and sales of porcelain denture teeth. They claim that porcelain denture teeth can be "special ordered," but I am still awaiting delivery of my last "special order." The denture in the patient in Figure 19.30A–D has been in function for 28 years with no relines. Notice that the ridges look healthy, with no apparent bone destruction.

For a denture to function for this many years with no bone destruction, the envelope of anterior function should be in total freedom. This means that the anterior teeth do not hit during chewing, closing into maximum intercuspation, and there is no contact during speech. The only time that the anterior teeth will function is in straight protrusion, and then if a patient learns to control the back of the dentures with the tongue as they incise on the front teeth.

Another interesting observation is that the only border movement of concern is straight protrusion. Lateral check bites and so-called group working and group balance are not only impossible but also a waste of time (Figure 19.31A).

What destroys the bone is the unstable occlusal stops. The plastic teeth are not stable stops. If these two patients had worn their dentures for the years that they have, the plastic posterior teeth would have worn faster than the anterior teeth, and the anterior teeth on both of these patients would have been pounding on the anterior bone for many years, making them dental cripples.

Closing on cotton rolls takes out of the equation the possibility of a deflective interference being felt as a pressure area (Figure 19.31B). The second photo was taken 32 years later. The patient is still wearing the same denture with no relines or adjustment (Figure 19.31C). The centric stops of the sharp maxillary lingual cusps into the mandibular central fossa are a bit larger. There has been some wear of the porcelain teeth (Figure 19.31D). The porcelain teeth have done their job and kept the anterior envelope of function totally free (Figure 19.31E). The patient admits that her love for red wine and cigarettes is responsible for the staining (Figure 19.31D and E). The ridges are as healthy as can be—if there has been bone destruction, it is minimal (Figure 19.31 F and G).

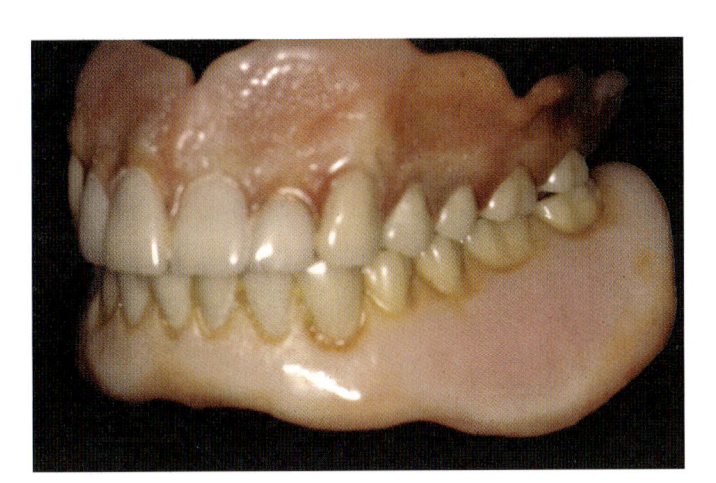

Figure 19.30 (A) Denture has served patient for 28 years.

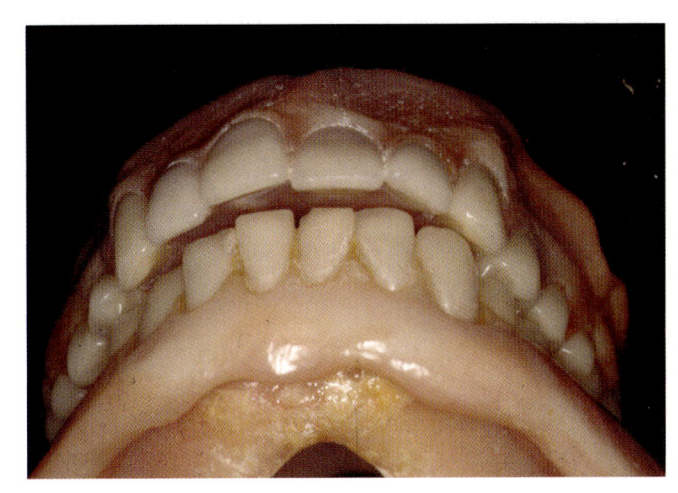

Figure 19.30 (C) Anterior occlusal relation maintained by porcelain teeth.

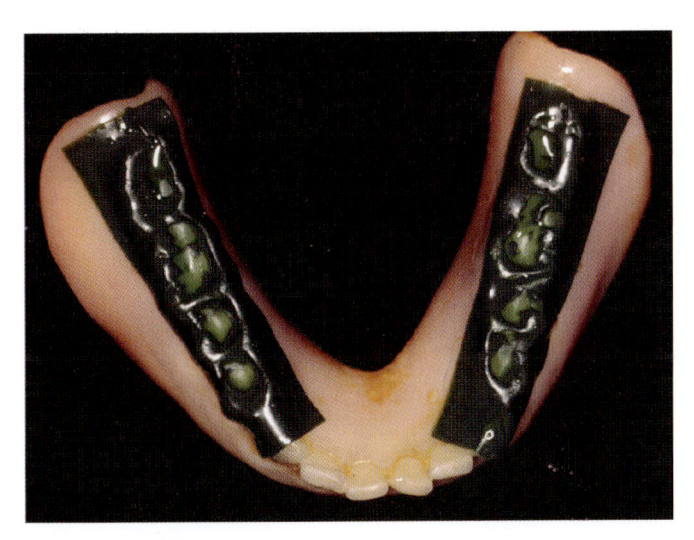

Figure 19.30 (B) Stable occlusal contacts.

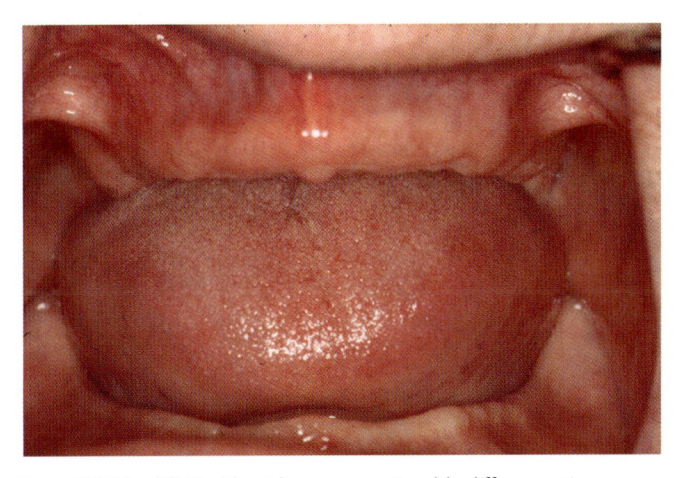

Figure 19.30 (D) Healthy ridges—no noticeable differences in 28 years.

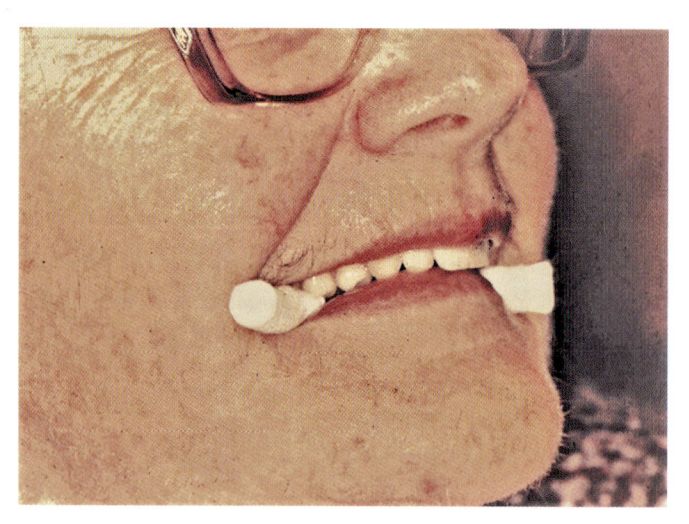

Figure 19.31 (A) New denture delivered—biting on cotton rolls to determine comfort.

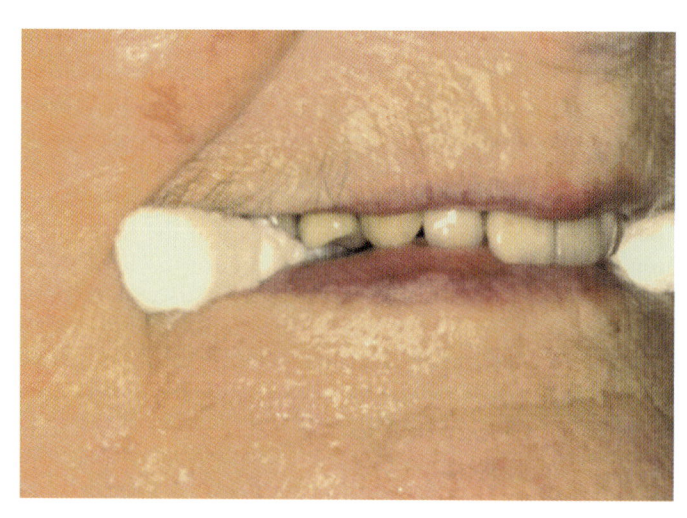

Figure 19.31 (B) Same denture 32 years later.

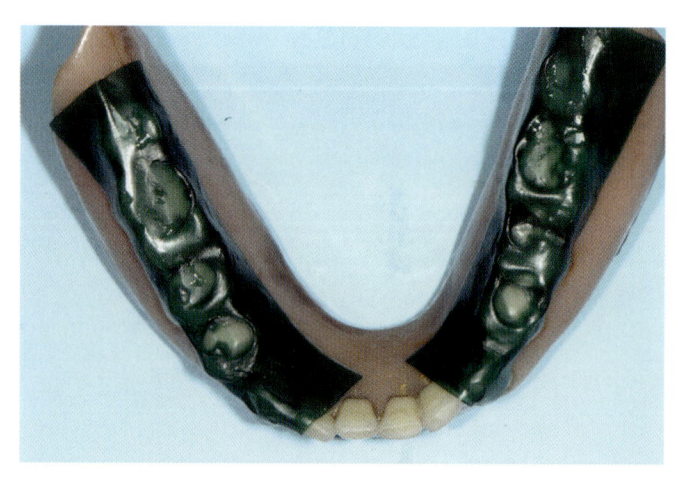

Figure 19.31 (C) Stable occlusion.

Dentures that oppose natural teeth

One of my patients told me, "I was told by my dentist that if I continue to wear an upper denture that if later on I decide to upgrade my dentistry with dental implants that there would be no bone." I looked at his denture and told him if he keeps wearing that denture then what he was told would be absolutely true (Figure 19.32A–F). This patient was treated 40 years ago and has been wearing an upper complete denture and a lower distal extension partial. The denture has all porcelain teeth. The lower partial could have had porcelain teeth but there was not enough room, so custom metal occlusals were placed on the lower partial. The defect on the left maxilla was due to a traumatic accident that evulsed the left cuspid and bone. This is the second denture and partial done in those 40 years. The case shows a distal extension

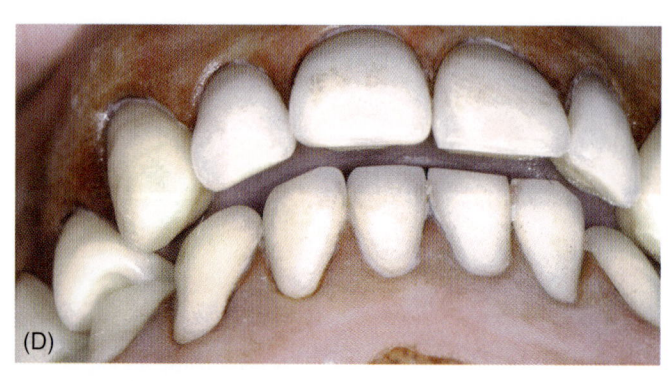

Figure 19.31 (D, E) Red wine and cigarette staining.

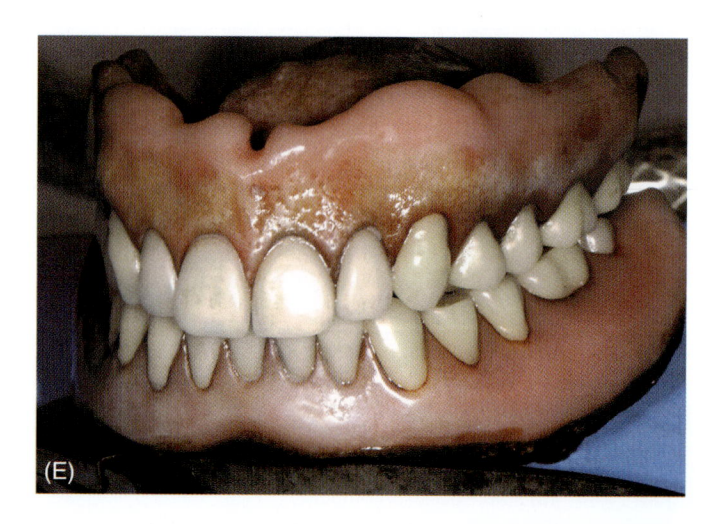

Chapter 19 The Complete Denture

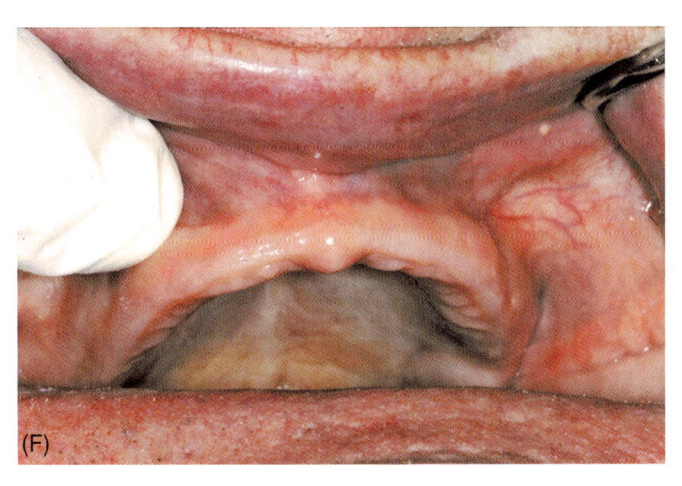

Figure 19.31 **(F, G)** The ridges are healthy.

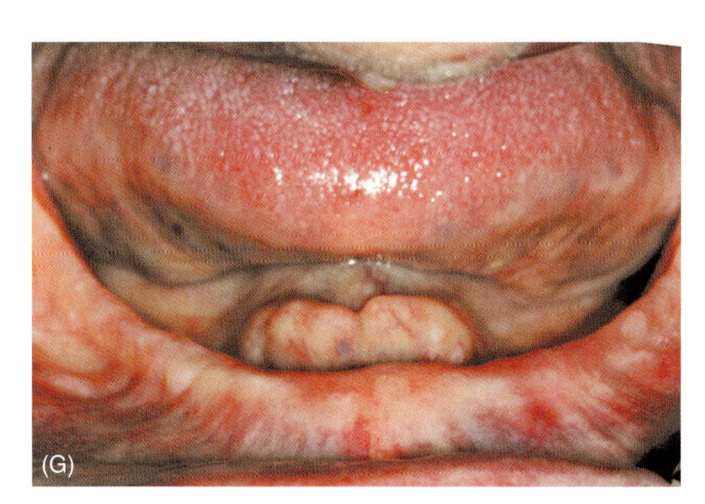

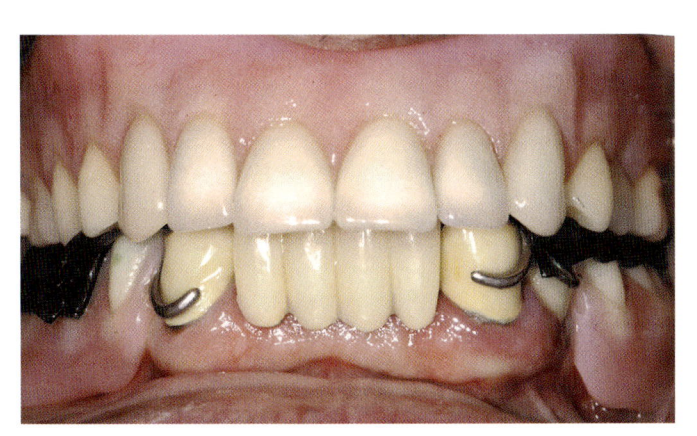

Figure 19.32 **(A)** Maxillary denture—mandibular anterior natural teeth and a free-end partial denture.

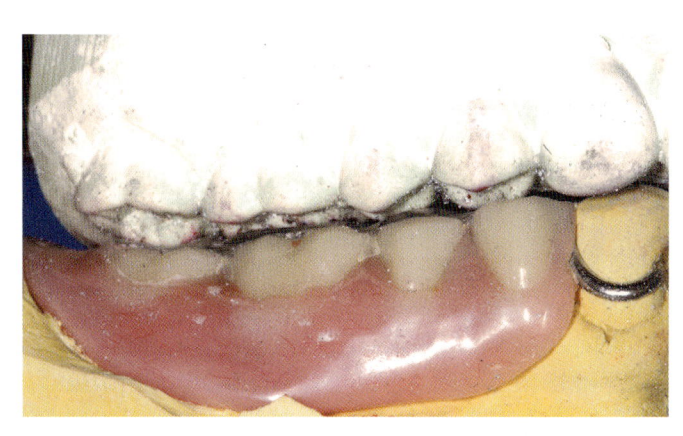

Figure 19.32 **(C)** Lingualized occlusion in posterior segment. Note: mandibular plastic teeth had to be used because of little space.

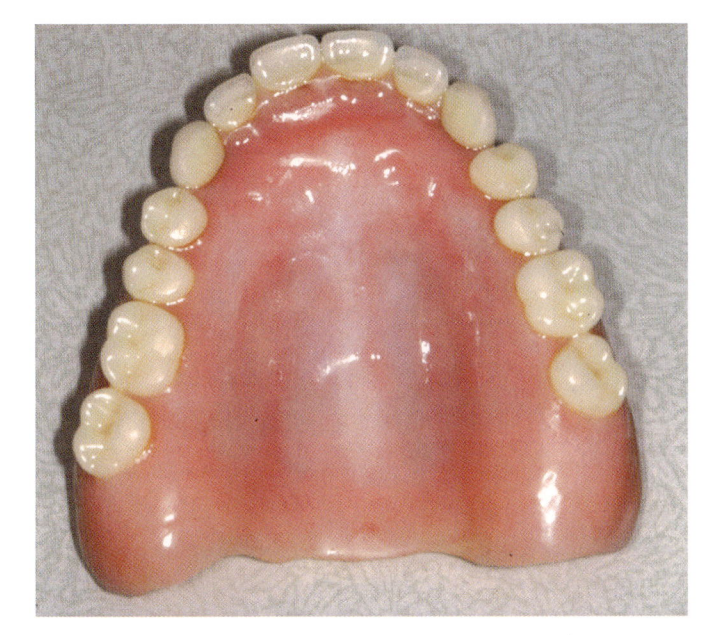

Figure 19.32 **(B)** Maxillary denture with all porcelain teeth.

mandibular partial that occludes with a maxillary complete denture.

The photos in Figure 19.33A–E are from patients who have a full complement of mandibular teeth that occlude with a maxillary full denture. To preserve the bone of the maxilla, it is necessary to provide an occlusal design to maintain the denture occlusion. This will prevent the combination syndrome from destroying the maxillary bone.

Implants and complete dentures

All patients who present for full denture prosthesis should be given the opportunity to know the possibility of dental implants. After the patient has been successfully treated with the diagnostic or provisional denture, they must be given the choice of conventional dentures or implants. At this point, we know the patient. Placing implants prolongs the treatment process. If the patient has been difficult and unreasonable in accepting any treatment, the dentist can advise away from implants or inform of the limitations. The patient in Figure 19.34A–D had no problems and was entirely satisfied with the treatment denture that

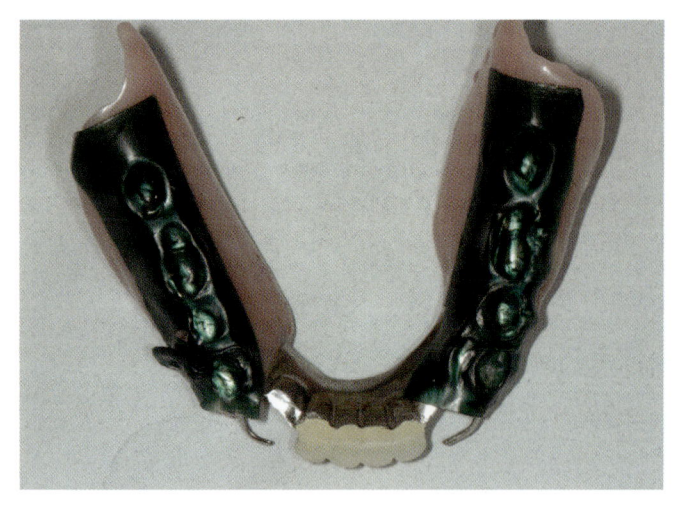

Figure 19.32 **(D)** Stable posterior contacts in centric.

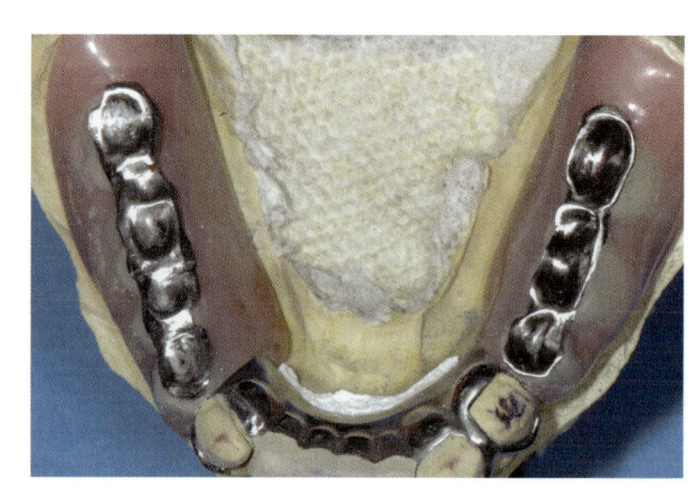

Figure 19.32 **(E)** With no space for porcelain teeth on partial, custom metal stops are used.

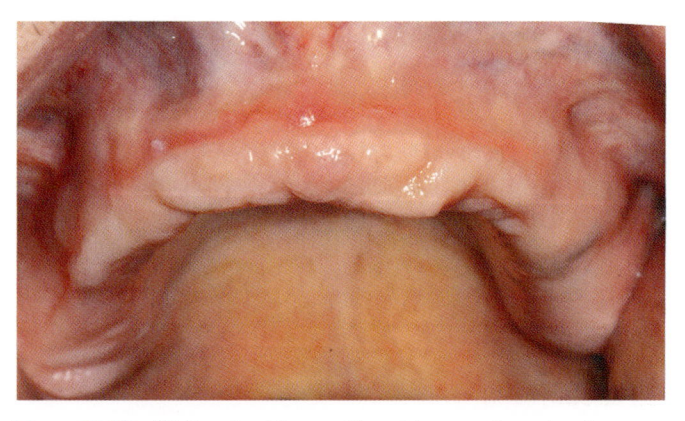

Figure 19.32 **(F)** Note healthy maxillary ridge—no bone loss in 40 years of maxillary denture.

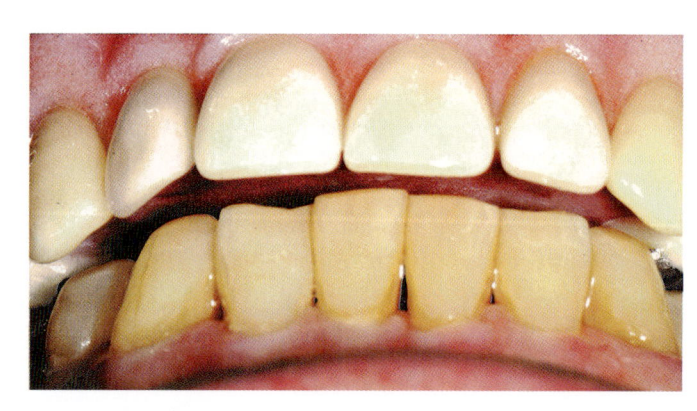

Figure 19.33 **(B)** Anterior denture occlusion.

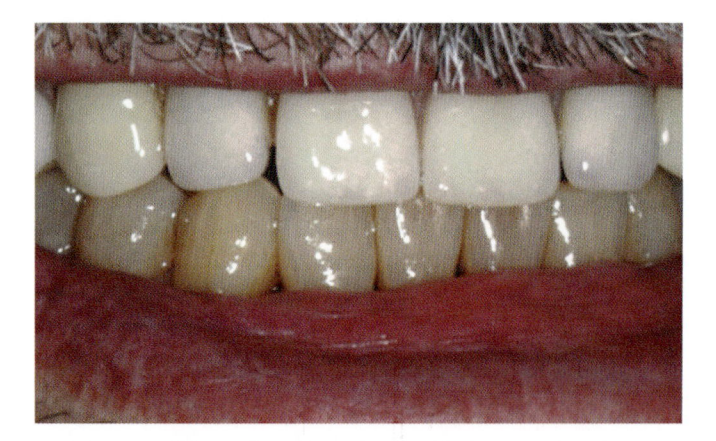

Figure 19.33 **(A)** Maxillary denture—mandibular natural teeth.

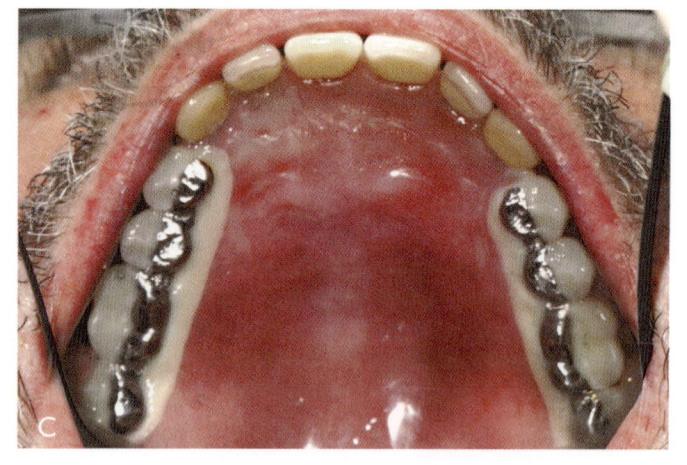

Figure 19.33 **(C)** Porcelain denture teeth cannot be used against natural teeth—custom metal occlusion.

she almost decided against the implants. Clear duplicates are made of the treatment dentures and can be used as surgical guides. We have found that the functional impression material that lines the dentures shows up on a computed tomography scan the same as hard acrylic. There is no need to make clear duplicates (Figure 19.34E–H). The implants have been placed using the clear duplicates of the patient-approved treatment dentures (Figure 19.34I–N).

Chapter 19   The Complete Denture

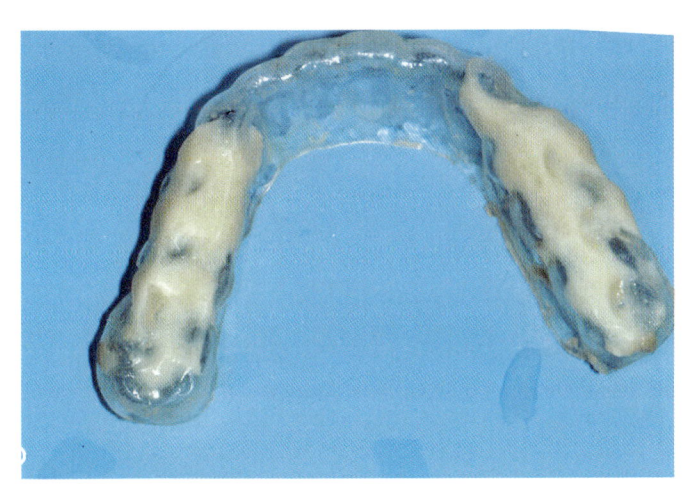

Figure 19.33 **(D)** Nightguard splint to prevent mandibular natural teeth from super eruption.

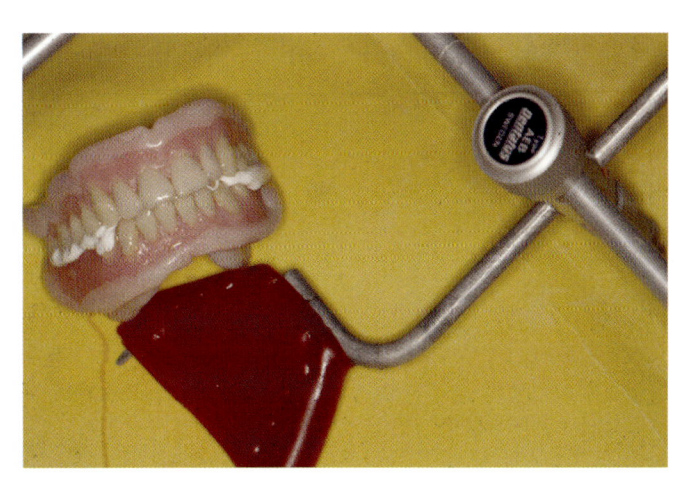

Figure 19.34 **(B)** Patient has worn the trial dentures for several months to gain approval. Clear duplicates will be constructed to use as surgical guides.

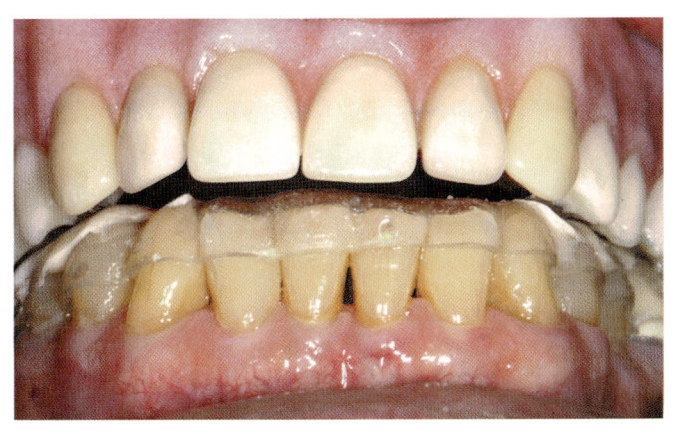

Figure 19.33 **(E)** Nightguard in patient's mouth—also in denture occlusion.

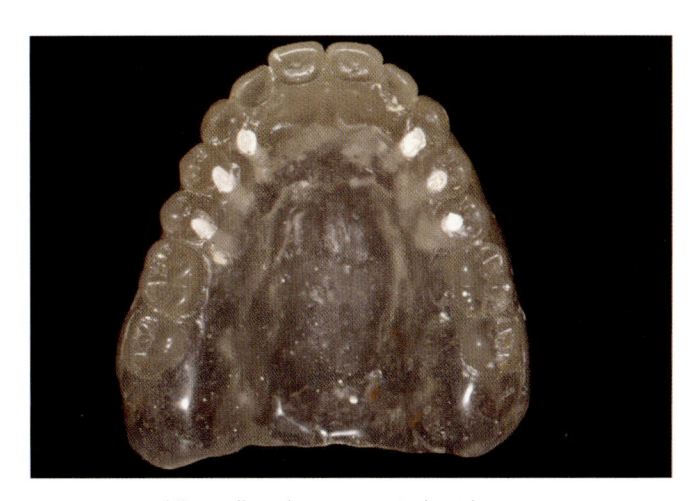

Figure 19.34 **(C)** Maxillary denture surgical guide.

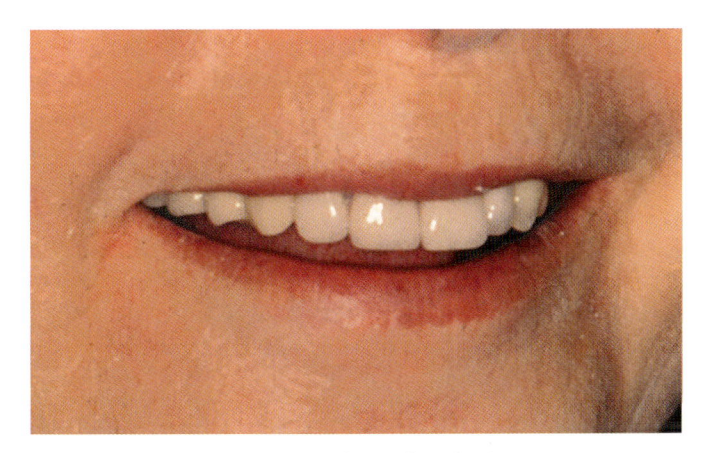

Figure 19.34 **(A)** Implant-assisted complete denture.

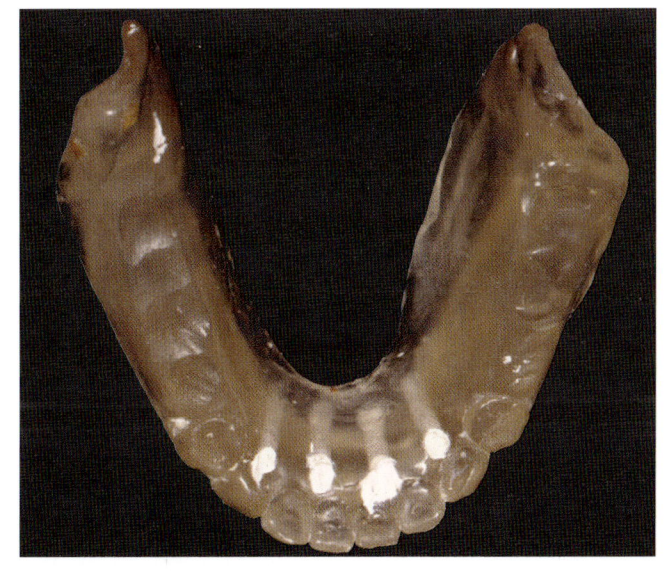

Figure 19.34 **(D)** Mandibular denture surgical guide. Gutta percha markers placed to show ideal implant position.

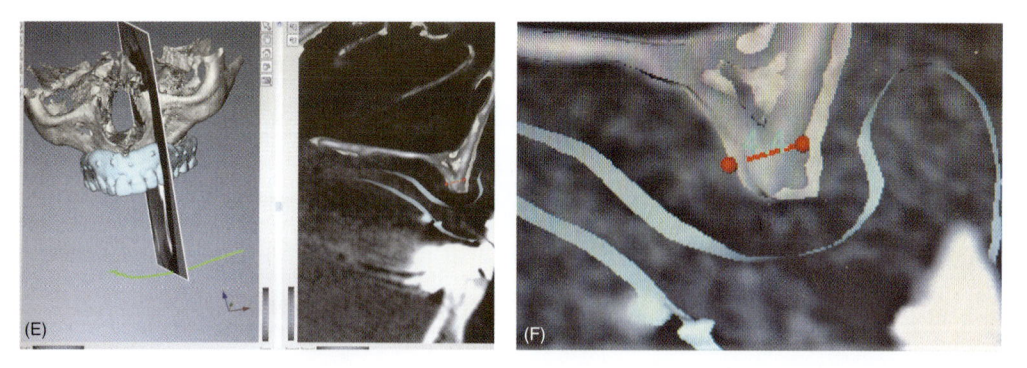

Figure 19.34 **(E, F)** The trial denture that has been approved by the patient can be used to scan. The functional impression material shows on the scan like hard acrylic.

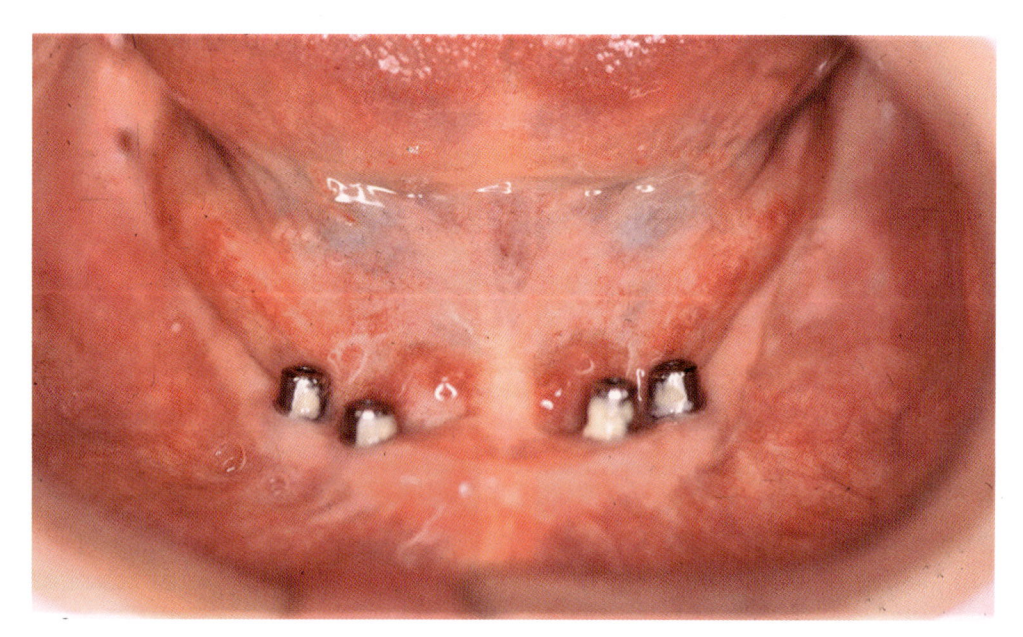

Figure 19.34 **(G)** Mandibular healing cap.

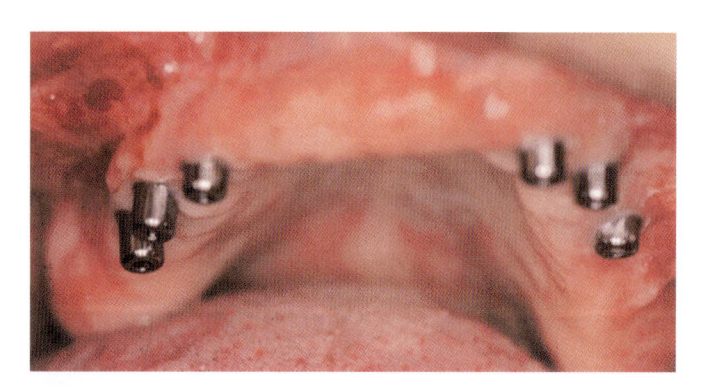

Figure 19.34 **(H)** Maxillary healing cap.

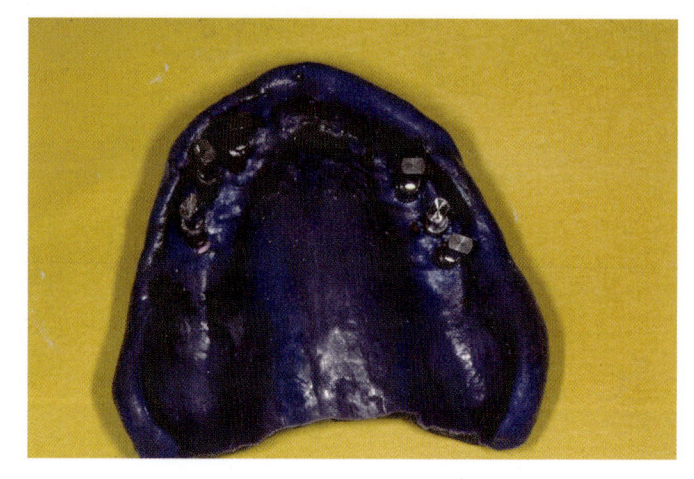

Figure 19.34 **(I)** The clear duplicates that were used as surgical guides are now used like custom impression trays.

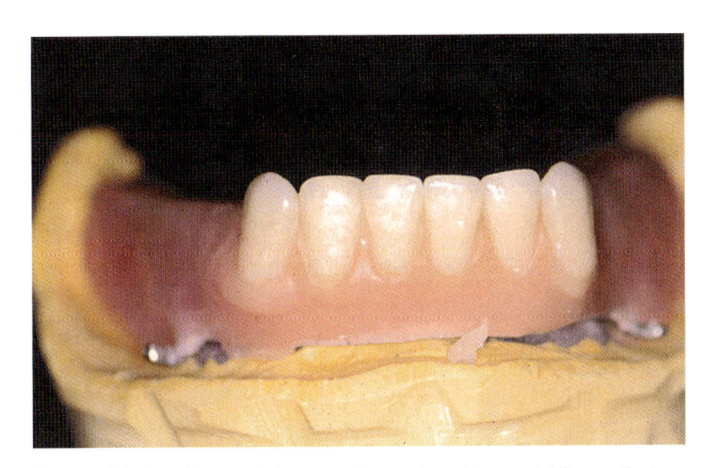

Figure 19.34 (J) Mandibular anterior teeth set to partial frame that fits implant bar.

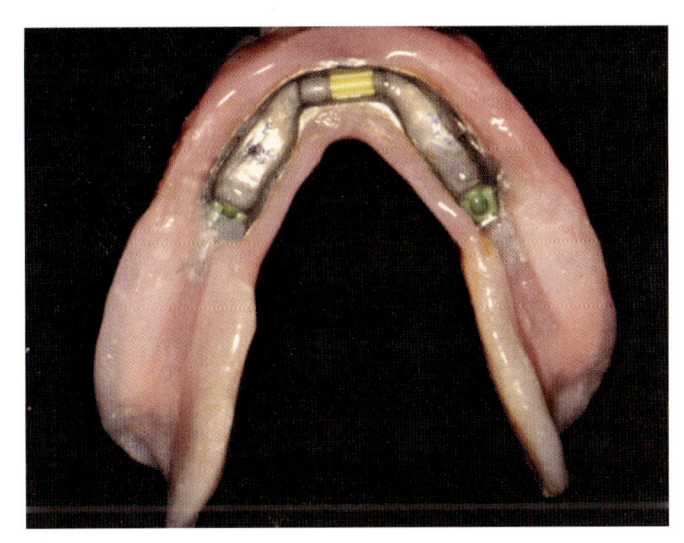

Figure 19.34 (M) Mandibular implant-assisted overdenture. Note the separate fit of the free-end saddle.

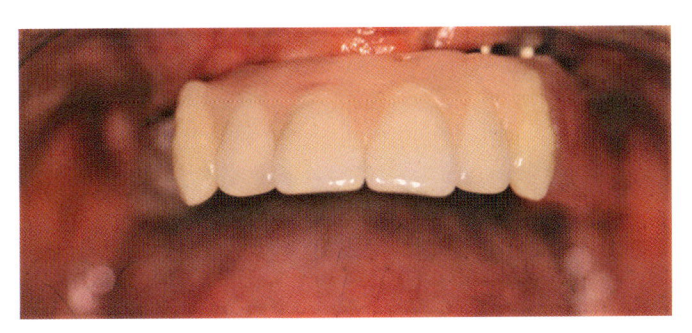

Figure 19.34 (K) Maxillary anterior teeth set to partial frame that fits implant bar.

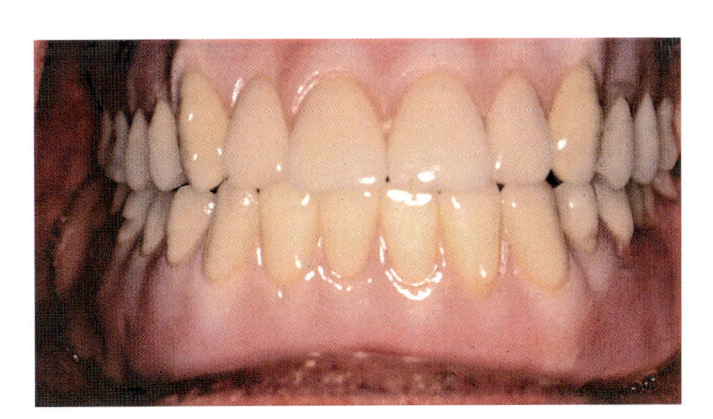

Figure 19.34 (N) Completed case.

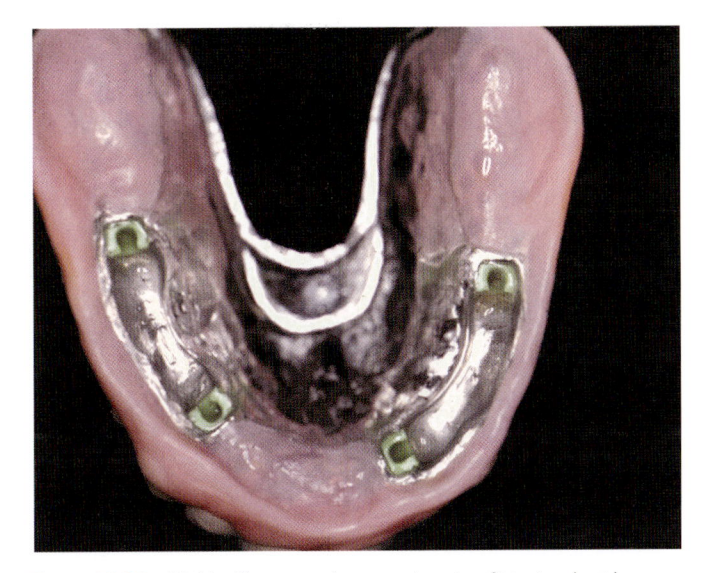

Figure 19.34 (L) Maxillary overdenture showing fit to implant bar.

References

1. Berg E, Johnson TB, Ingebretsen R. Patient motives and fulfillment of motives in renewal of complete dentures. *Acta Odontol Scand* 1984;42:235–240.
2. Fisher RD. Personalized restorations vs. plates. *J Prosthet Dent* 1973;30:513–514.
3. Goldstein RE. Study of need for esthetics in dentistry. *J Prosthet Dentist* 1969;6:589–598.
4. Boucher CO. Complete denture prosthodontics—the state of the art. *J Prosthet Dent* 1975;34:372–383.
5. Appelbaum MB. The practical dynamics of the interim denture concept: a comparison with the conventional immediate denture technique. *J Am Dent Assoc* 1983;106:826–830.
6. Hansen CA. Diagnostically restoring a reduced occlusal vertical dimension without permanently altering the existing dentures. *J Prosthet Dent* 1985;54:671–673.
7. Pound E. Preparatory dentures: a protective philosophy. *J Prosthet Dent* 1965;15:5–18.

8. Pound E, Murrell GA. An introduction to denture simplification. *J Prosthet Dent* 1971;26:570–580.
9. Pound E, Murrell GA. An introduction to denture simplification. Phase II. *J Prosthet Dent* 1973;29:598–607.
10. Turbyfill WF. Regaining pleasure and success with complete denture services. *Int J Prosthet* 1989;2:472–482.
11. Turbyfill WE. Denture aesthetics: the union of natural contour, color, and shape. *Signature* 1995;(Fall):14–17.
12. Lieb ND, Silverman SI, Garfinkel L. An analysis of soft tissue contours of the lips in relation to the maxillary cuspids. *J Prosthet Dent* 1967;18:292–303.
13. Marunick MT, Chamberlain BB, Robinson CA. Denture aesthetics: an evaluation of laymen's preferences. *J Oral Rehabil* 1983;10:399–406.
14. Mavroskoufis F, Ritchie GM. The face-form as a guide for the selection of maxillary central incisors. *J Prosthet Dent* 1980;43:501–505.
15. Smith BJ. The value of the nose width as an esthetic guide in prosthodontics. *J Prosthet Dent* 1975;34:562–573.
16. Turner LC. The profile tracer: method for obtaining accurate pre-extraction records. *J San Antonio Dent Soc* 1970;25:13.
17. Ivy RS. Dental and facial types. In: Litch WF, ed. *American System of Dentistry*, vol. 2. Philadelphia, PA: Leaman Brothers; 1887.
18. Williams JL. The temperamental selection of artificial teeth, a fallacy. Dent Dig. 1914;20:63.
19. House MM, Loop JL. *Form and Color Harmony in the Dental Art*. Whittier, CA: MM House (privately printed); 1939.
20. LaVere AM, Marcroft KR, Smith RC, Sarka RJ. Denture tooth selection: an analysis of the natural maxillary central incisor compared to the length and width of the face. Part 1. *J Prosthet Dent* 1992;67:661–663.
21. Frush JP, Fisher RD. Introduction to dentogenic restorations. *J Prosthet Dent* 1955;5:586–595.
22. Abrams L. *Male or Female—Can You Tell by the Teeth? Report of Sexual Dimorphism Study*. San Francisco, CA: American Academy of Esthetic Dentistry; 1981.
23. Ruffino AR. Personality projection in complete dentures: traits transmissible to the viewer through variations in maxillary anterior tooth arrangement. *J Prosthet Dent* 1984;50:661–662, 664.
24. Clough HE, Knodle JM, Leeper SH, et al. A comparison of lingualized occlusion and monoplane occlusion in complete dentures. *J Prosthet Dent* 1983;50:176–179.
25. Hirsch B, Levin B, Tiber N. Effects of patient involvement and esthetics preference on denture acceptance. *J Prosthet Dent* 1972;28:127–132.
26. Tau S, Lowenthal U. Some personality determinants of denture preference. *J Prosthet Dent* 1980;44:10–12.
27. Krajicek D. Guides for natural facial appearance as related to complete denture construction. *J Prosthet Dent* 1969;21:654–662.
28. Pound E. Apply harmony in selecting and arranging teeth. *Dent Clin North Am* 1962:241–258.
29. Pound E. Fine arts in the fallacy of the ridge. *J Prosthet Dent* 1954:4(1).
30. Dawson P. *Evaluation, Diagnosis, and Treatment of Occlusal Problems*. St. Louis, MO: CV Mosby; 1989.
31. Pound E. Mandibular movements of speech and their seven related values. *J Prosthet Dent* 1966;16:835–843.
32. Pound E. Controlling anomalies of vertical dimension and speech. *J Prosthet Dent* 1976;36:124–135.
33. Pound E. Utilizing speech to simplify personalized denture service. *J Prosthet Dent* 1970;24:586–600.
34. Murray CG. Re-establishing natural tooth position in the edentulous environment. *Aust Dent J* 1978;23:415–421.
35. Murrell GA. Phonetics, function, and anterior occlusion. *J Prosthet Dent* 1974;32:23–31.
36. Sherman H. Phonetic capability as a function of vertical dimension in complete denture wearers—a preliminary report. *J Prosthet Dent* 1970;23:621–632.
37. Sharry J. Essential concepts in denture esthetics. In: Goldstein RE, ed. *Esthetics in Dentistry*. Philadelphia, PA: JB Lippincott; 1976:326–329.
38. Rayson JH, Rahn AO, Wesley RC, et al. Placement of teeth in a complete denture: a cephalometric study. *J Am Dent Assoc* 1970;81:420–424.
39. Starcke EN Jr. The contours of polished surfaces of complete dentures: a review of the literature. *J Am Dent Assoc* 1970;81:155–160.
40. Zimmerman DE, Cotmore JM. Denture esthetics (I). Denture base contour. *Quintessence Int Dent Dig* 1982;13:543–549.
41. Turbyfill WFJ. The provisional denture: key to denture success. *Aurum Ceramic Classic News* 1995;8(2):1–4.

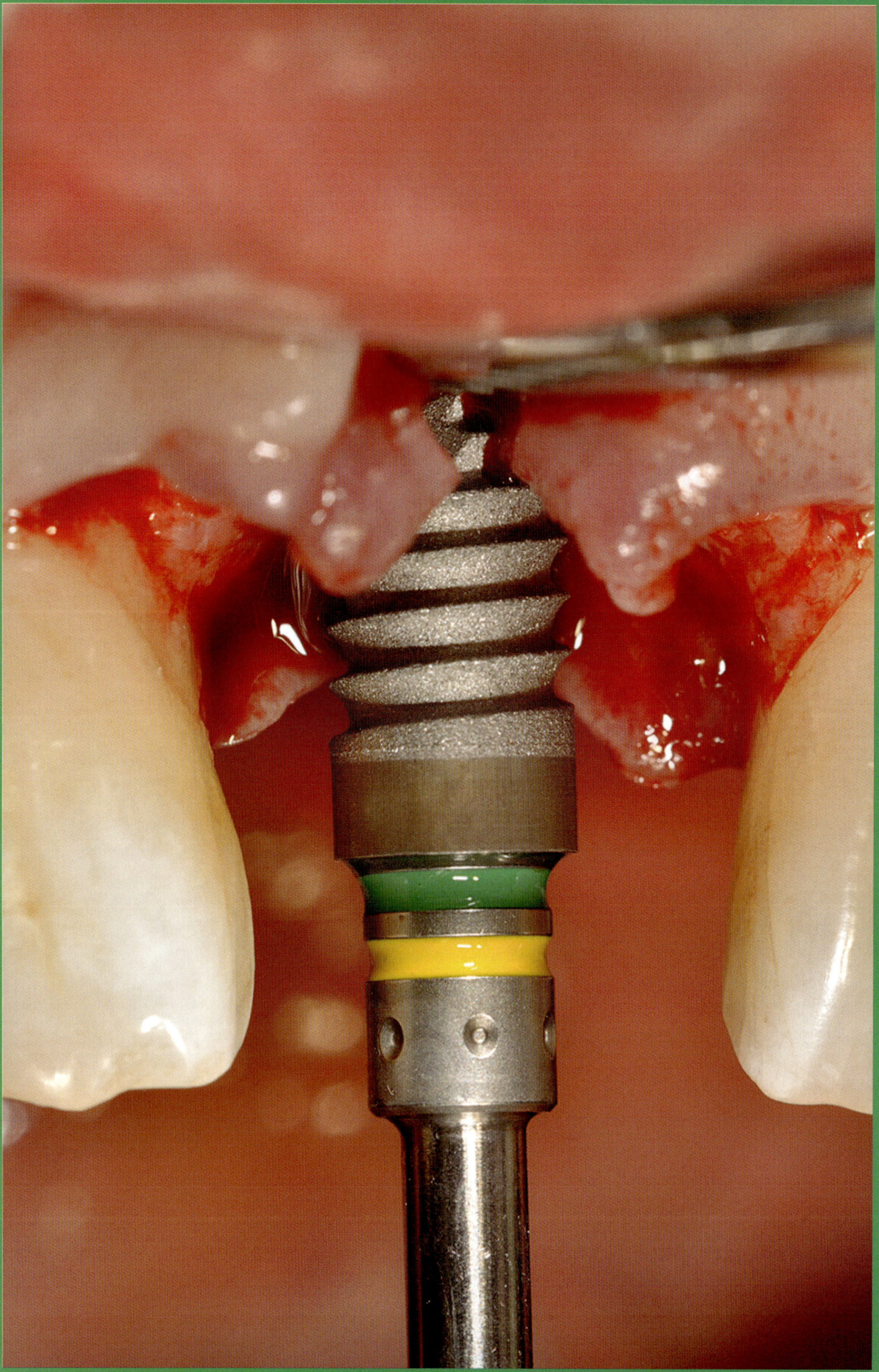

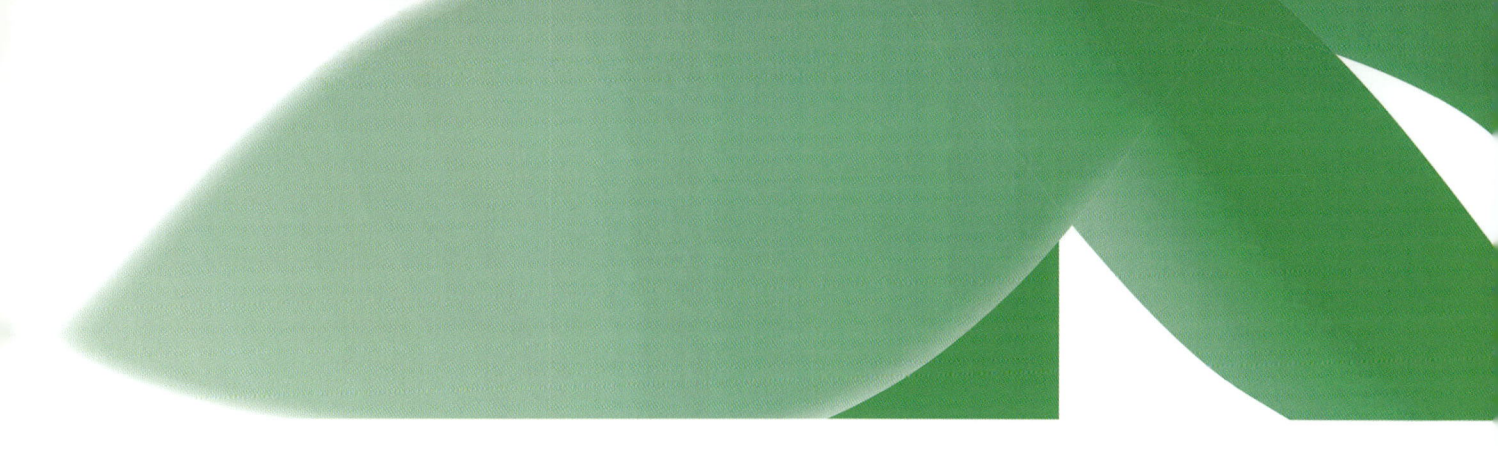

Chapter 20
Implant Esthetics: Concepts, Surgical Procedures, and Materials

Sonia Leziy, DDS and Brahm Miller, DDS, MSc

Chapter Outline

Smile line and lip dynamics	638	Buccolingual position	647
Ridge form and how ridge architecture impacts implant placement	638	Mesiodistal position	647
		Apicocoronal position (depth of implant placement)	653
Implant placement and restoration protocols: deciding the best strategy	643	Implant designs	653
Delayed or late implant placement (12 weeks or more following extraction)	643	Gingival biotype: assessment methods and enhancement procedures	654
Early implant placement (4–8 weeks following extraction)	643	Provisionalization: refinement of the gingival tissue architecture	656
Immediate implant placement (at the time of extraction)	643	Today's final "surgical step"	656
		Material choices: final abutments and restorations	657
Immediate implant restoration: functional (loaded) or nonfunctional (unloaded)	644	Abutments	657
		Implant restorations: ceramics	658
Implant position: a pivotal point in the treatment blueprint	646	Design and cementation	660

Implant-based therapy has dramatically impacted the way we can treat our patients, with a broad range of applications including the use of implants to restore single and small edentulous spans, as well as the fully edentulous patient. Implant treatment outcomes are commonly viewed in terms of implant survival and success rates.[1–6] This chapter will focus on the many criteria that must be considered for successful treatment outcomes in the esthetic zone.

Many tissue-related outcomes must be considered, including gingival tissue color/contour/texture, tissue level, and symmetry with adjacent and contralateral teeth, completeness of papilla fill, along with restoration form, color, and material characteristics as they relate to the natural dentition. Creating a harmonious transition between teeth and implant-supported restorations can be difficult and at times impossible to achieve. The measureable elements of the implant treatment process are emphasized and reported in the literature today, and yet, despite this, esthetically pleasing outcomes can still elude the clinician, sometimes due to treatment planning errors, at times the result of clinical errors, but often linked to biologic constraints that are not predictably correctable.

The experienced clinician or implant team will often develop a treatment plan based on experience and education, drawing on various materials and technology to achieve the desired outcome. For the less experienced clinician, the many factors that should be considered in an implant treatment plan in an esthetically sensitive area can be daunting due to a lack of awareness of the biologic variables related to ridge and soft-tissue form and quality, and implant and restorative material selection.

This chapter will highlight concepts and procedures important to achieving a desirable outcome, complications that can occur, prevention and management of these complications, and references for further study.

Smile line and lip dynamics

The lip can be considered friend or foe in any oral rehabilitation program, and it is generally accepted that the clinician must assess and document the lips at rest, and the lips in the posed or "forced" smile.[6] This is especially important in implant dentistry, where treatment planning and treatment errors can significantly impact soft-tissue level and form.[7]

It is obvious that a low lip line with little tooth and no gingival display can be very forgiving, as subtle or gross tissue-level problems are masked or not apparent during normal activities or expressions (Figure 20.1A–D). However, even the low lip line produces a challenge when a patient evaluates the treatment outcome with a mirror placed close to the face while lifting the lip with a finger to appraise the result of the treatment.

Ridge form and how ridge architecture impacts implant placement

Peri-implant bone volume and anatomy act as the foundation for the overlying soft-tissue form. With this in mind, it is important to understand that it is common for ridge resorption to develop following tooth extraction, which manifests as soft-tissue changes.[8] There is a high probability for horizontal bone loss after extraction, with the majority of this change occurring in the first 3 months, followed by gradual reduction in ridge volume thereafter. Figure 20.2A–C shows typical horizontal bone change as a result of tooth loss.[9–11]

Recent systematic reviews provide clear statements as to the ridge changes that occur in the 6 months after tooth extraction, as well as indications and contraindications for ridge preservation, and these are summarized in Table 20.1.[8,12,13]

Contributing factors to changes in ridge form and volume include bone loss or damage due to extraction complications or

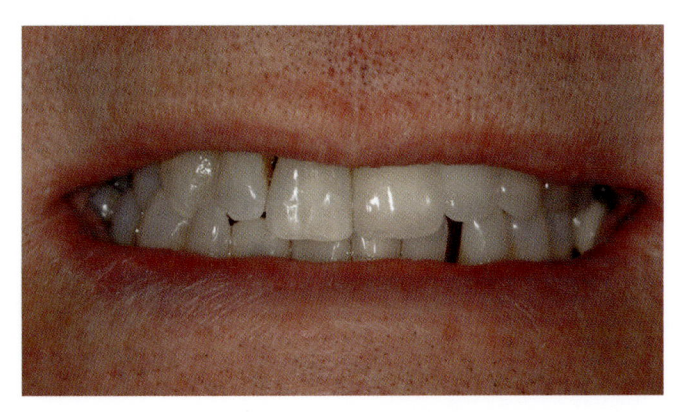

Figure 20.1 (A) Low lip line: no gingival display.

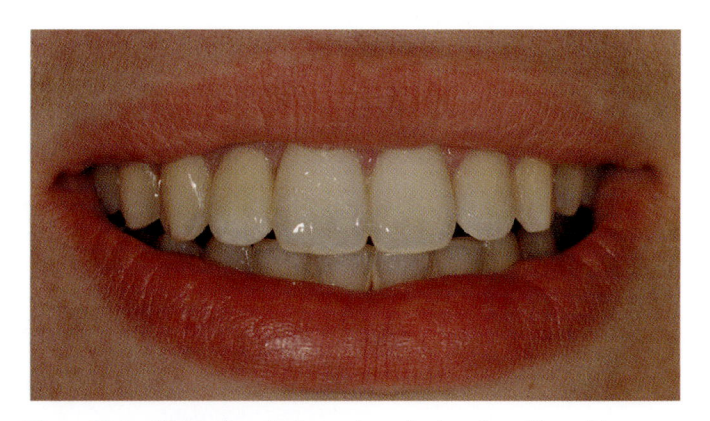

Figure 20.1 (B) Medium lip line: minor display of papilla and free gingival margins.

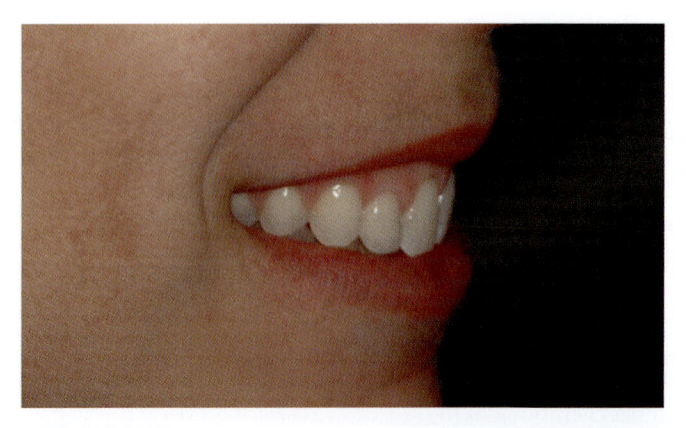

Figure 20.1 (C) High lip line: significant gingival display.

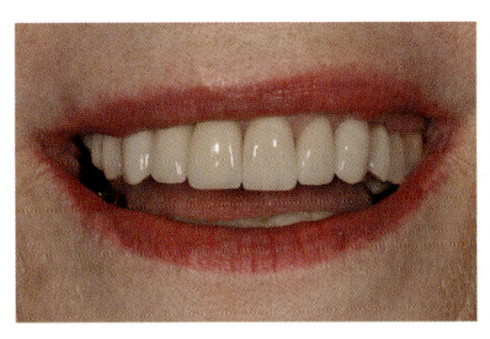

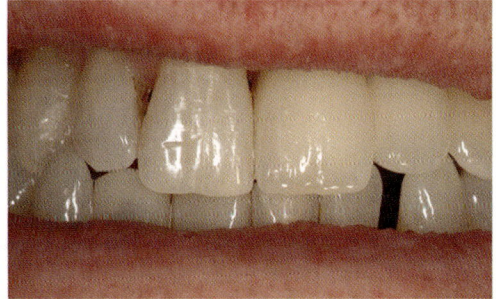

Figure 20.1 (D) Asymmetric lip with varying levels of gingival display.

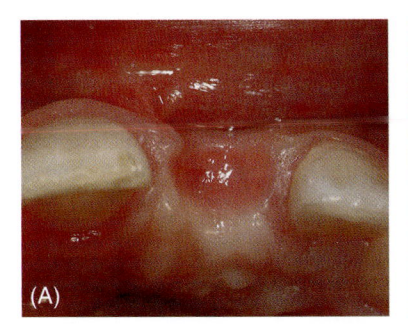

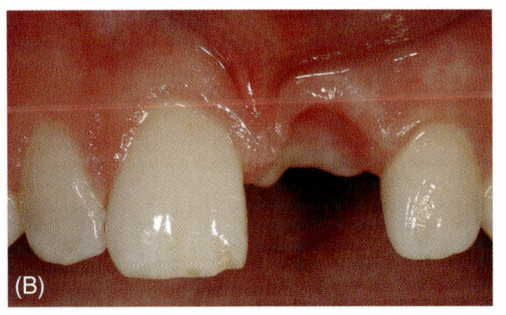

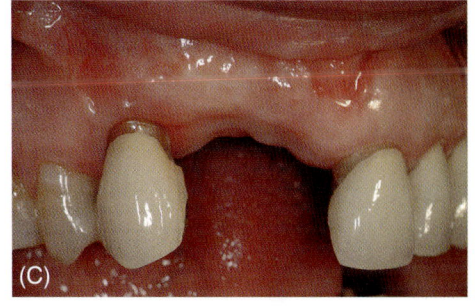

Figure 20.2 (A) Moderate facial ridge resorption (>3 mm) due to tooth extraction without ridge preservation. (B) Mild papilla blunting due to tooth loss and no ridge preservation. (C) Significant papilla blunting due to adjacent tooth loss and associated ridge remodeling.

Table 20.1 Ridge Changes and Indications and Contraindications for Ridge Preservation after Tooth Extraction[8,12,13]

Mean ridge resorption
Mean horizontal reduction in ridge width: 3.8 mm
Mean vertical reduction in ridge height: 1.24 mm

Rationale for ridge preservation procedures
Maintain existing soft-/hard-tissue envelope
Maintain stable ridge volume for optimized function and esthetic outcomes
Simplify treatment procedures subsequent to ridge preservation

Contraindications for ridge preservation procedures
General contraindications for oral surgery interventions
Patients taking bisphosphonates (controversial)
Local infections that cannot be eliminated or adequately treated
Radiation treatment history in the area of treatment

poor technique, poor vascularization of facial cortical bone due to thin buccal bone (commonly <1 mm in the anterior maxilla) (Figure 20.3A and B), as well as due to the impact of loss of the periodontal ligament and its blood supply, and loss of the periosteal blood supply in the case of flap elevation.[14,15]

In efforts to reduce ridge remodeling associated with extraction procedures, a number of conservative extraction approaches can be considered. Among these are new extraction tools, including vertical root extraction devices that eliminate luxation motion, periotomes, or piezotomes to effectively separate the root from the socket wall. Although there are controversial reports in the dental literature, minimizing flap elevation is often considered important to minimize disruption of the blood supply between periosteum and underlying bone. Coupled with this, it has become routine to consider ridge preservation procedures where bone or bone substitutes are placed in the extraction socket, coupled with membranes to confine a graft material in the case of dehisced, fenestrated, or damaged socket walls.[16,17] At this time, there is no clear consensus as to the most desirable product or product combination for the purpose of ridge preservation. For most clinicians, the decision on the type of product that is used is often based on experience, exposure to techniques and materials from lectures or media, and colleagues or opinion leaders. Figure 20.4A–H shows a typical procedure using a mineralized bone allograft and a resorbable membrane to correct a facial fenestration of the bone. It is important to remember that although ridge preservation procedures can reduce postextraction dimensional changes, they rarely completely prevent resorption.

Edentulous sites that have undergone remodeling often require buccal ridge augmentation to support long-term crestal bone stability and to satisfy esthetic treatment demands. The importance of adequate bone thickness to support facial and, to some degree, interproximal soft tissue was discussed by Grunder et al.;[18] a minimum of 2 mm bone thickness in all dimensions is recommended, but greater facial volumes are perhaps beneficial. To achieve this volume of bone mandates optimal implant position from a facial–lingual perspective; careful planning as to an appropriate implant diameter (bigger is not always better); and bone grafting, ridge splitting, or expansion procedures to enhance ridge volume. In Figure 20.5A, facial bone volume is ideal as viewed at the time of implant placement. This contrasts to commonly observed thin facial bone that may present with a dehiscence or fenestration, as shown in Figure 20.5B. Many materials and techniques have been described to increase the

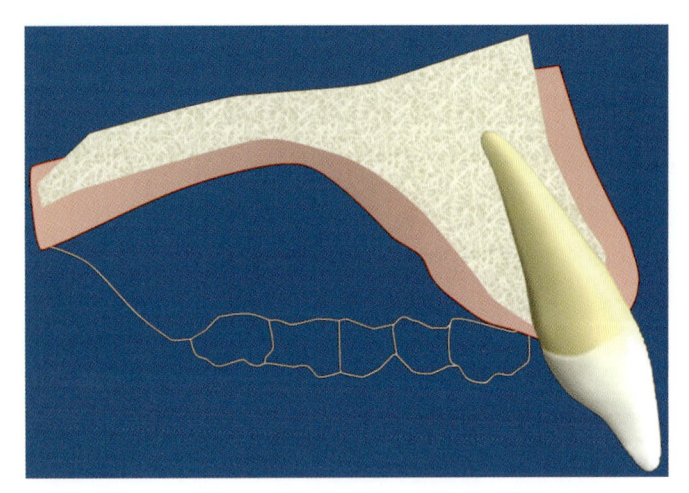

Figure 20.3 (A) In the premaxilla, the facial bone plate is generally thin (0.9 ± 0.4 mm). Thin bone is generally poorly vascularized due to its cortical nature. This translates into risk for postextraction resorptive changes.

buccolingual ridge volume. In contrast to vertical ridge augmentation, horizontal bone grafting is a relatively predictable event.[19–21] Perhaps more controversial is the subject of what type of material to use for this purpose. When ridge augmentation is carried out at the time of implant placement, it is the authors' opinion that structurally stable products with low substitution rates such as the xenograft Bio-Oss®, may offer a long-term

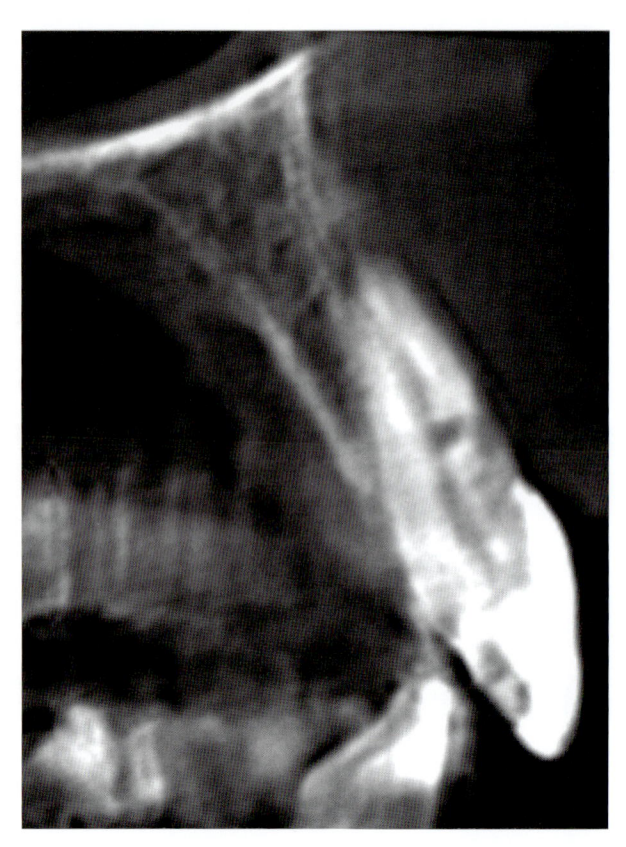

Figure 20.3 (B) Facial root inclination and position relative to the ridge midline is a common observation, resulting in thin facial bone.

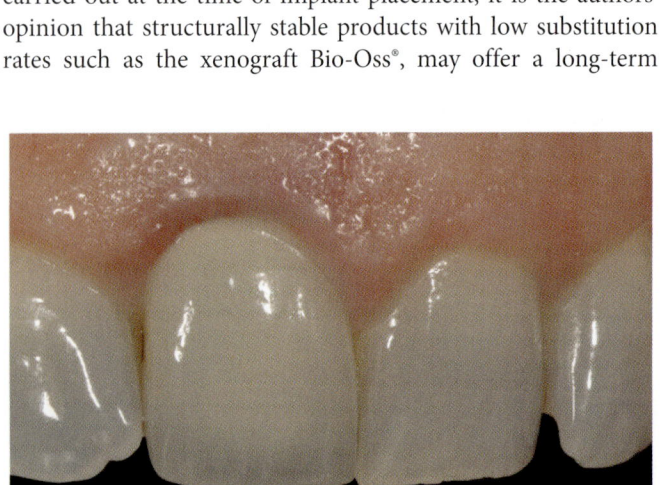

Figure 20.4 (A) Preoperative clinical photo.

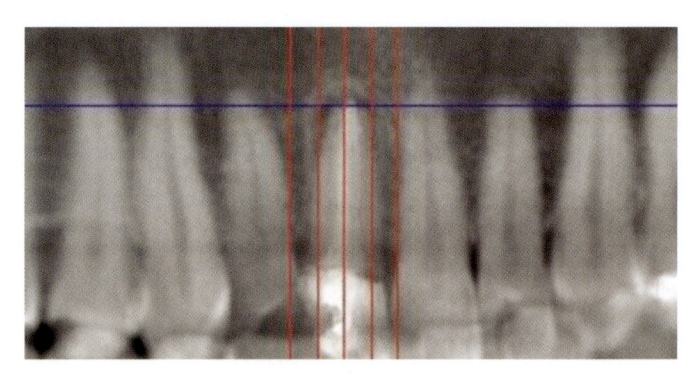

Figure 20.4 (B) Preoperative cone beam computed tomography (CBCT) scout view (panoramic) of tooth 8.

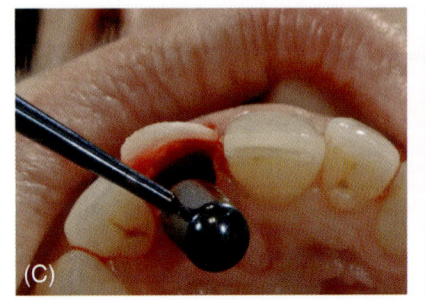

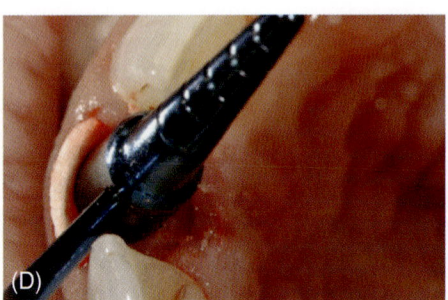

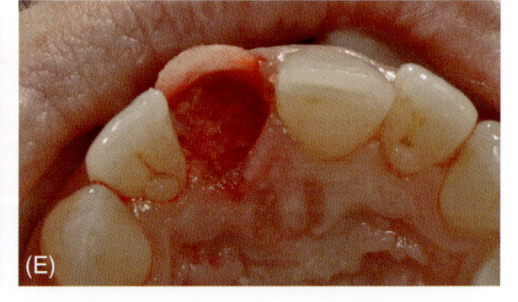

Figure 20.4 (C) A resorbable collagen membrane (Zimmer socket repair membrane) has been adapted palatal to the facial bone plate to seal a facial fenestration. A mineralized bone allograft (BioHorizons–Mineross cancellous allograft) is being condensed into the socket. **(D)** Same as Figure 20.4C, but lateral view. **(E)** Condensed bone graft, as viewed before crestal closure with the membrane.

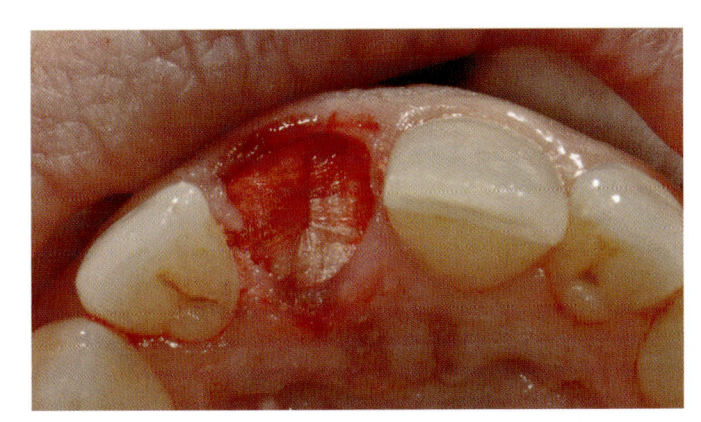

Figure 20.4 **(F)** Collagen membrane adaptation over the condensed mineralized allograft.

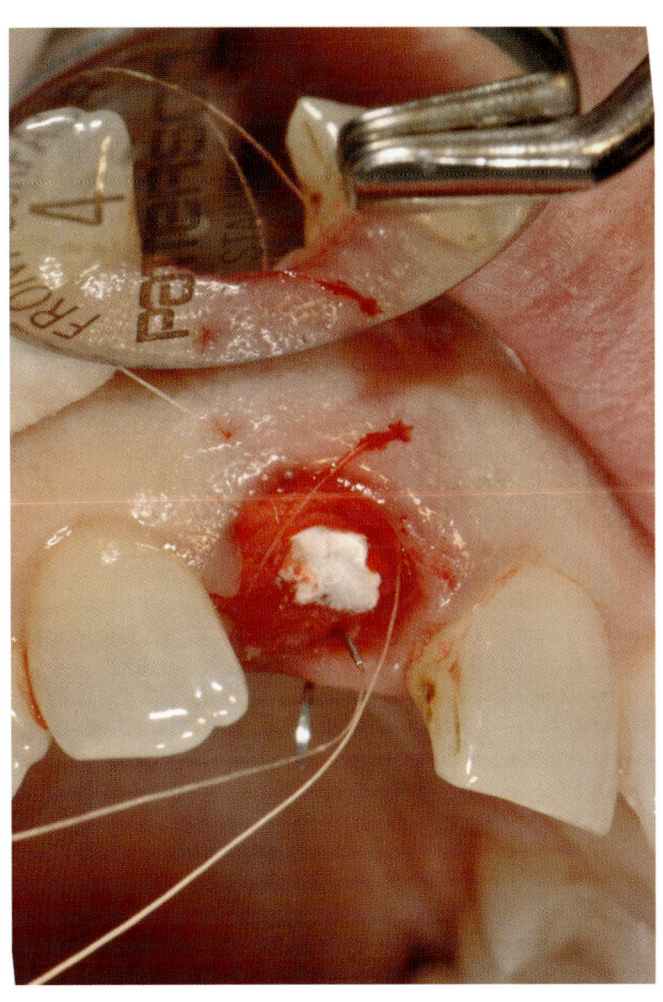

Figure 20.4 **(G)** Suturing with a resorbable figure-of-eight style suture (6-0 polyglycolic acid).

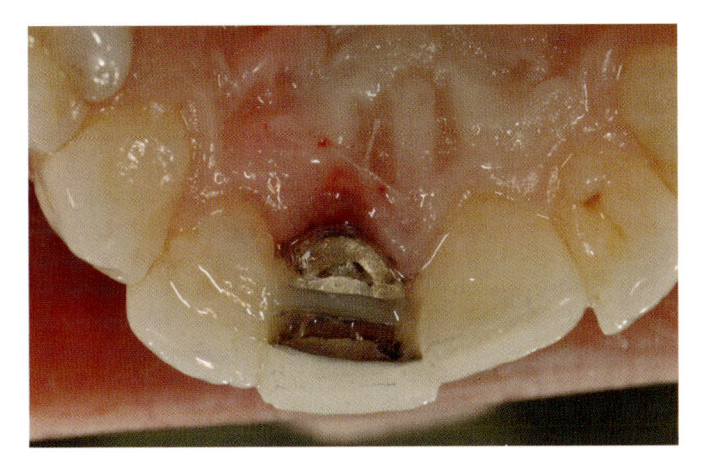

Figure 20.4 **(H)** Transitional provisionalization with a fiber-reinforced splinted crown (mirrored view).

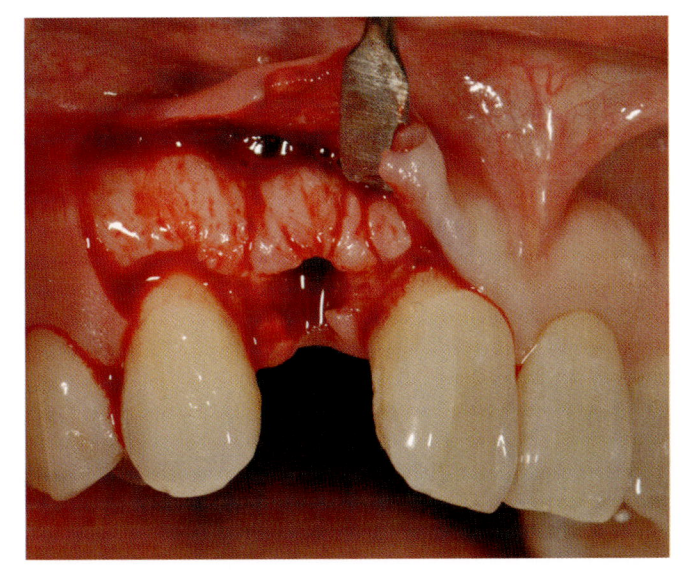

Figure 20.5 **(A)** Thick facial bone volume (>2 mm) at the time of tooth extraction. This ridge volume is unusual in the premaxilla.

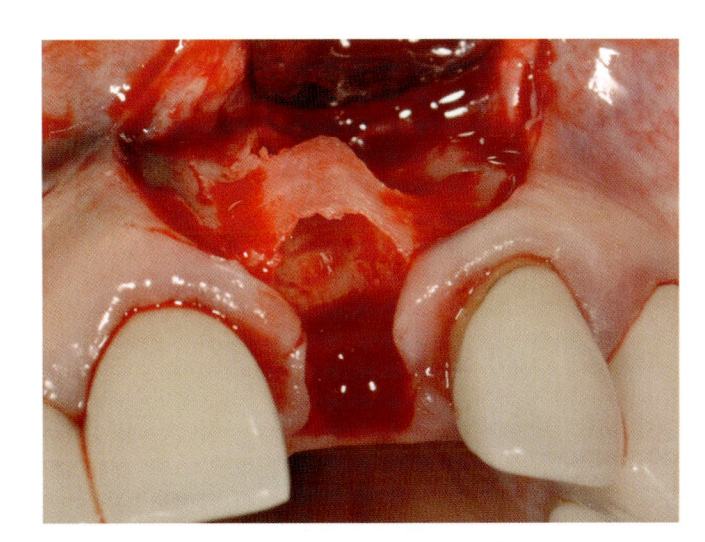

Figure 20.5 **(B)** Thin facial bone (<1 mm) coupled with a facial fenestration increases the treatment planning and treatment challenges. This type of clinical presentation increases the risk for adverse hard- and soft-tissue changes regardless of implant placement protocol selected (to be reviewed under implant placement protocols).

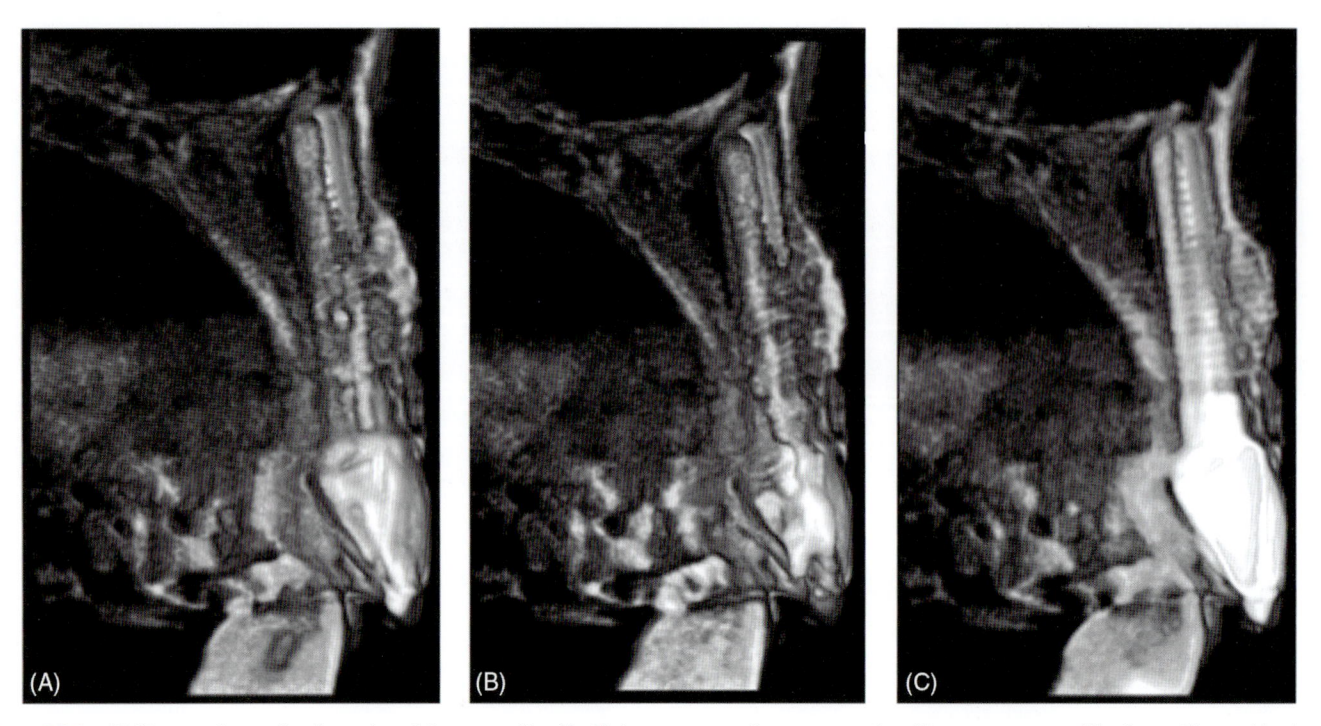

Figure 20.6 CBCT capturing an implant placed 8 years earlier: **(A–C)** three consecutive cross-sectional images separated by 1 mm. The residual horizontal defect had been grafted at the time of implant placement with a structurally stable xenograft product (Bio-Oss, Geistlich). This has predictably maintained the facial ridge contour.

advantage over other products that undergo faster replacement. CBCT cross-sectional images show the presence of a facial bone graft material and good bone volume 8 years after implant placement (Figure 20.6).

The challenge in bone grafting today continues to be the correction of vertical bone defects.[22] Despite many new materials and procedures to address ridge height deficiencies, vertical augmentation is not predictable for many clinicians. It is important to understand the limitation of vertical augmentation and to inform the patient of the likelihood that residual soft-tissue deficits will require prosthetic correction, including the use of longer contact areas or "pink" porcelain to replace the missing gingival tissue.

Bone substitutes in combination with a variety of membranes or meshes are increasingly used in efforts to reduce the treatment morbidity associated with autogenous graft procurement, and to thereby improve treatment acceptance. Figure 20.7A–C shows the use of bone allograft in block form to augment a horizontally and vertically deficient ridge.[23–26] An area of interest to the clinician struggling with vertical bone augmentation is the potential use of autogenous growth factors to enhance ridge augmentation results, with early reports on the use of recombinant growth

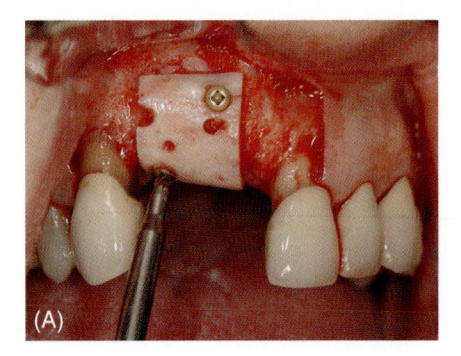

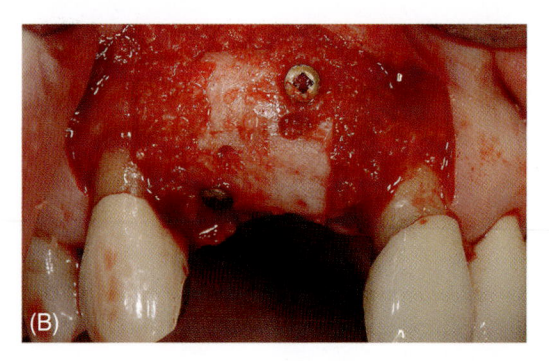

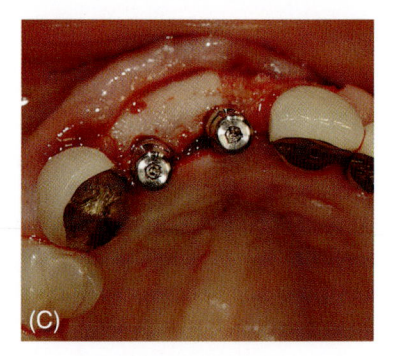

Figure 20.7 **(A)** A block allograft (Puros corticocancellous block, Zimmer) is shaped to intimately adapt to the underlying deficient ridge to regenerate both the buccal deficiency and height deficiency. Underlying cortical perforations improve blood supply to the graft. **(B)** Particulate mineralized graft material (Puros mineralized cancellous allograft, Zimmer) is adapted to fill proximal voids around the block graft. This is then confined and protected with a rapidly resorbed membrane, in this case, Bio-Gide (Geistlich). Other materials, including platelet-rich fibrin/autologous membranes or other resorbable membranes can be used. **(C)** Four-month reentry for implant placement illustrates ideal facial ridge volume. Implants have excellent primary stability (>45 N cm). Fixture level impressions were taken to fabricate lab-processed screw-retained provisional restorations.

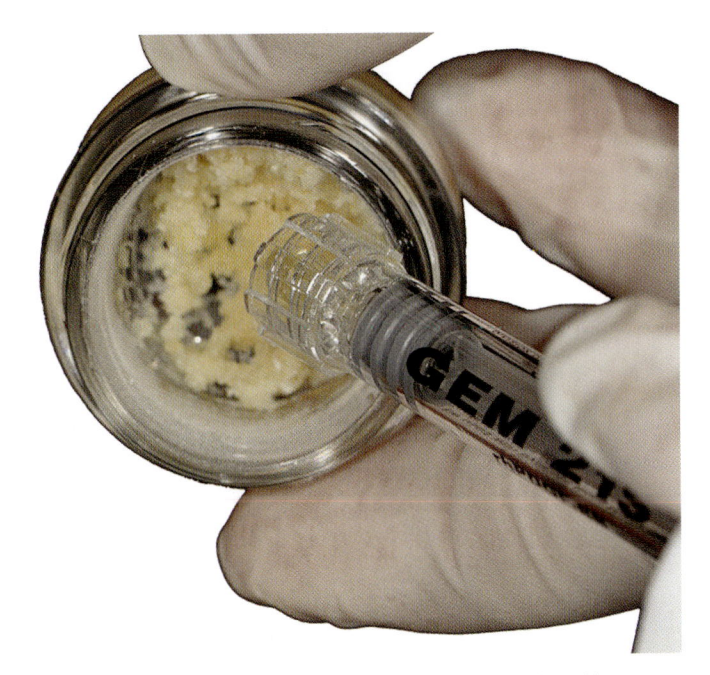

Figure 20.8 Autologous growth factors or factors produced by recombinant technology are increasingly incorporated into bone grafting procedures. In this illustration, a mineralized allograft is being reconstituted with platelet-derived growth factor-BB (off-label use of GEM-21S).

factors like platelet-derived growth factor-BB (shown in Figure 20.8), and BMP2 showing promise in select applications.[27,28] Most of the literature describing the use of these products has been in "space-making" defects that are generally considered predictable to treat with conventional treatment approaches.

Because of the potential difficulties and lack of predictability of grafting procedures, great care needs to be given to planning extraction procedures, in terms of timing, techniques, and instrumentation that will favor ridge preservation. In this respect, immediate implant placement and provisionalization may be beneficial to minimize bone and soft-tissue changes.

Implant placement and restoration protocols: deciding the best strategy

Many surgical and restorative treatment protocols are used in the management of single sites, small edentulous spans, and the fully edentulous arch. With respect to timing relative to tooth extraction, these range from late and delayed implant placement (4 months or more after extraction), early placement (8 weeks after extraction), to immediate placement at the time of extraction. In addition, restoration options include immediate or delayed provisionalization (postintegration). These restoration options can be combined in a variety of permutations with the surgical methodologies mentioned earlier.

Multiple factors influence these treatment-planning and procedural decisions. These approaches may not significantly affect the esthetic outcome of treatment if properly executed, although "stacked" or multiple procedures combined into one event increase the treatment complexity and the potential risk for adverse outcomes. From an esthetic perspective, adverse events often translate into unfavorable tissue changes. At this time, there is insufficient evidence to support one approach over another, as many of the reports are underpowered or of low quality. It is our opinion, however, that immediate and early implant placement do not result in a higher risk for failures or complications, as reported in some publications.[29]

Delayed or late implant placement (12 weeks or more following extraction)

In delayed implant placement (12–16 weeks after extraction) there is clinical and radiographic evidence of socket bone fill, and in late placement (more than 16 weeks) socket fill is complete. Varying degrees of resorption of the buccal plate and ridge height may be present, requiring augmentation procedures before or at the time of implant placement. These treatment approaches have commonly been used with long-term follow-up.[30] These protocols are generally implemented in cases where teeth have already been lost, or when in situations where immediate and early placement are contraindicated. In addition, it is frequently used by the inexperienced clinician. Figure 20.9A–C shows a typical case of implant placement into a healed ridge, including bone and soft-tissue management.

Early implant placement (4–8 weeks following extraction)

This treatment approach has been suggested as potentially advantageous, because it may benefit from the healing potential of the extraction socket, before the completion of ridge remodeling and resorption while providing soft-tissue closure. This treatment approach also creates a more favorable environment by allowing for resolution of infection prior to implant placement. Typically, additional bone augmentation and soft-tissue grafting procedures may be required to correct dimensional limitations and to enhance the quality and the volume of the soft tissue.[31–35]

Immediate implant placement (at the time of extraction)

Immediate implant placement is increasingly considered in esthetic sites. This decision may be driven in part by patient demands to minimize the number of interventions and decrease treatment time. It also provides an opportunity for immediate provisionalization, thus facilitating patient management during the osseointegration phase. Additional benefits include the potential for reduced treatment costs, more conservative surgical procedures, and, importantly, maximum bone volume compared with late or delayed treatment, where resorptive changes may develop. In our opinion, predictable outcomes are expected as long as adequate primary implant stability can be

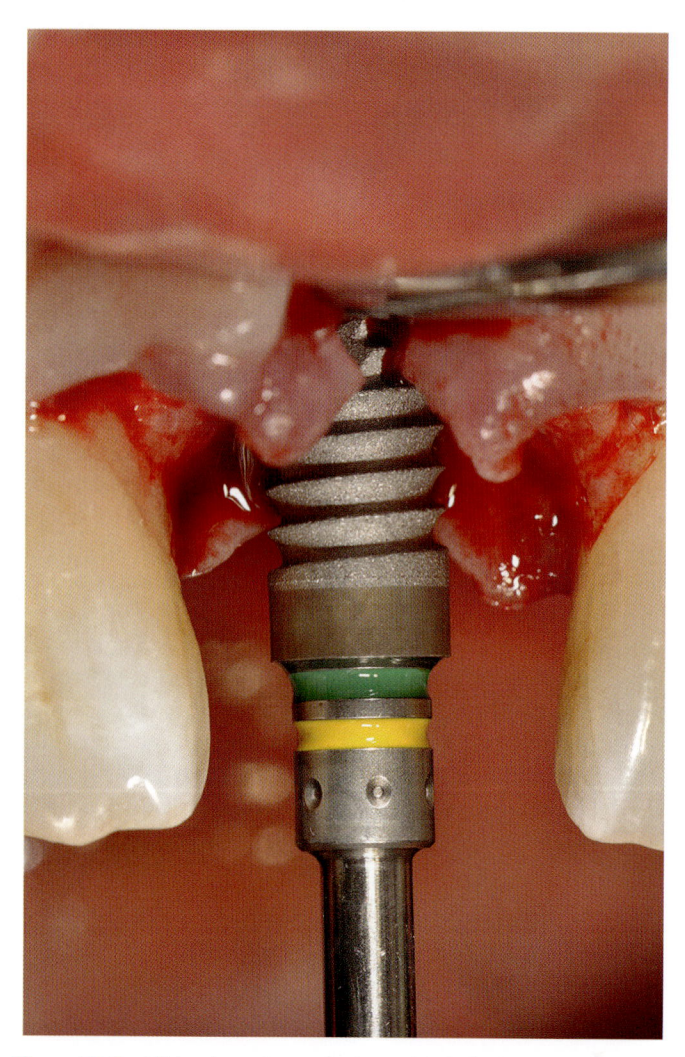

Figure 20.9 **(A)** Implant placement into a healed ridge, 4 months following ridge preservation. An implant design and thread form that offers high primary stability and the potential for enhanced long-term crestal bone stability with a unique laser-etched pattern (BioHorizons tapered internal implant) has been selected.

achieved, and bone and soft-tissue grafting procedures are incorporated to manage ridge defects and to enhance the soft-tissue biotype when necessary. Figure 20.10A–J shows immediate implant placement at the time of extraction, coupled with immediate provisionalization. Table 20.2 summarizes the findings and conclusions of two recent systematic reviews on the outcomes of implant placement at the time of extraction.[3,36]

Immediate implant restoration: functional (loaded) or nonfunctional (unloaded)

The use of provisional restorations is potentially beneficial in achieving esthetic implant treatment outcomes. One of the benefits is the ability to prosthetically guide the remodeling of the peri-implant soft-tissue contours. Figure 20.11A–C shows tissue form changes that can be developed though provisionalization.

Immediate provisional restorations (placed at the time of implant surgery) are being more frequently used in both healed ridges and extraction sites in single, small edentulous, or large edentulous spans. Immediate provisionalization of splinted and unsplinted restorations in the esthetic zone has not been shown to adversely impact osseointegration and implant survival rates as long as primary implant stability is adequate and the occlusion can be controlled.[36,37] In addition, patient education is important to prevent overload following surgery and before osseointegration.[38,39]

Significant differences in crestal bone levels have not been identified in most clinical studies that compare immediate provisionalization and conventional restoration methods. In addition to the advantage of avoiding a removable partial temporary denture, the positive impact on gingival integration

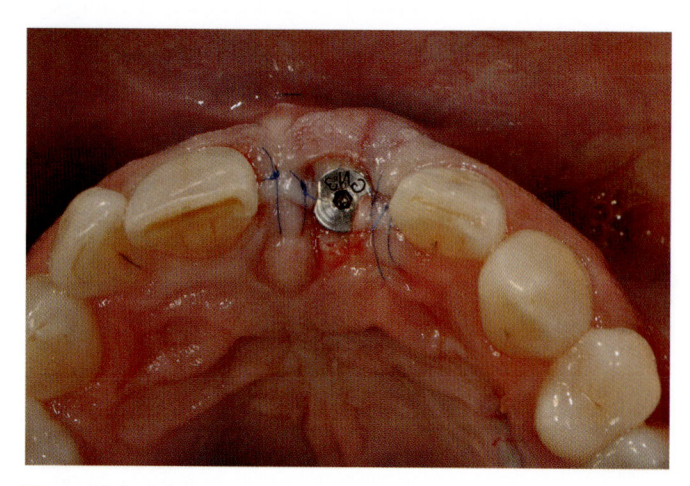

Figure 20.9 **(B)** A connective tissue graft adapted on the facial and extending around the healing abutment is used to augment the ridge volume and to enhance the gingival biotype. A lab-processed screw-retained provisional restoration will be inserted within 1 week of the surgical procedure.

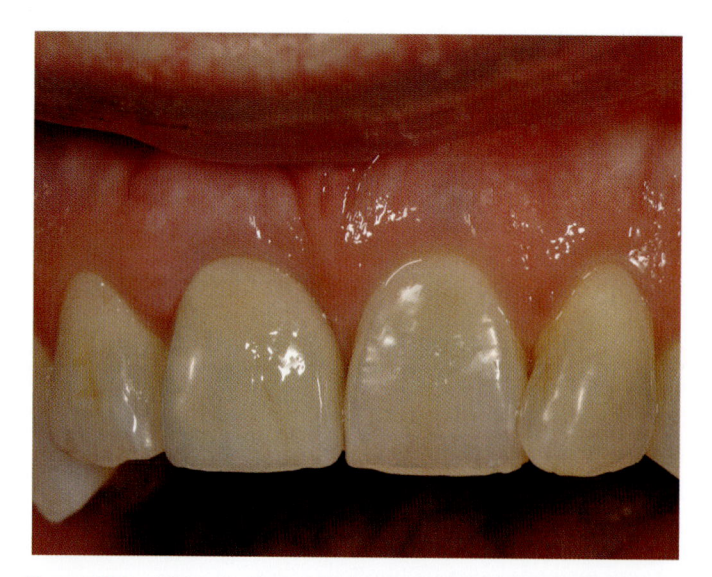

Figure 20.9 **(C)** Ideal soft-tissue outcome 6 months after delivery of the definitive restoration. Numerous factors contribute to the outcome, including tissue grafting and the tissue sculpting as defined by the provisional restoration.

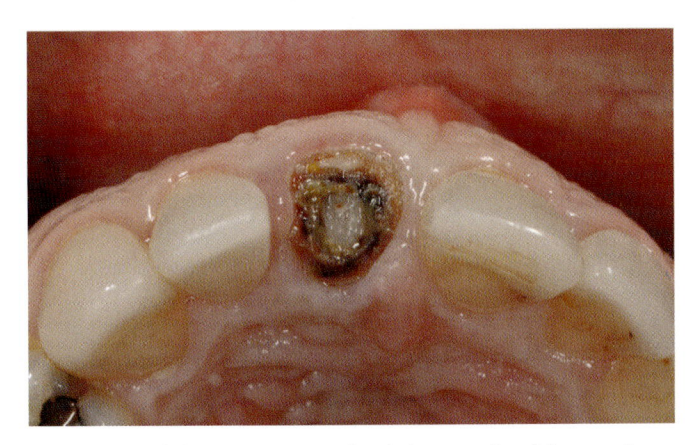

Figure 20.10 **(A)** Preoperative occlusal view: number 8 fractured to tissue level.

must also be considered.[40] Soft-tissue responses have been assessed and quantified both in terms of papilla development and facial gingival architecture in numerous studies. Papilla form tends to be maintained and/or developed more rapidly in immediate restoration cases compared with delayed restoration. In studies that have reported conflicting results in terms of the risk for mid-facial recession, excessive buccal position of the implant has been identified as the most deleterious risk factor.[41] In several studies, immediate implant placement and simultaneous restoration of single implants in the esthetic zone produced predictable treatment results in terms of papillary fill and mid-facial tissue levels.[42-44] Implant placement into a healed ridge and coordinated provisionalization are shown in Figure 20.12A–K.

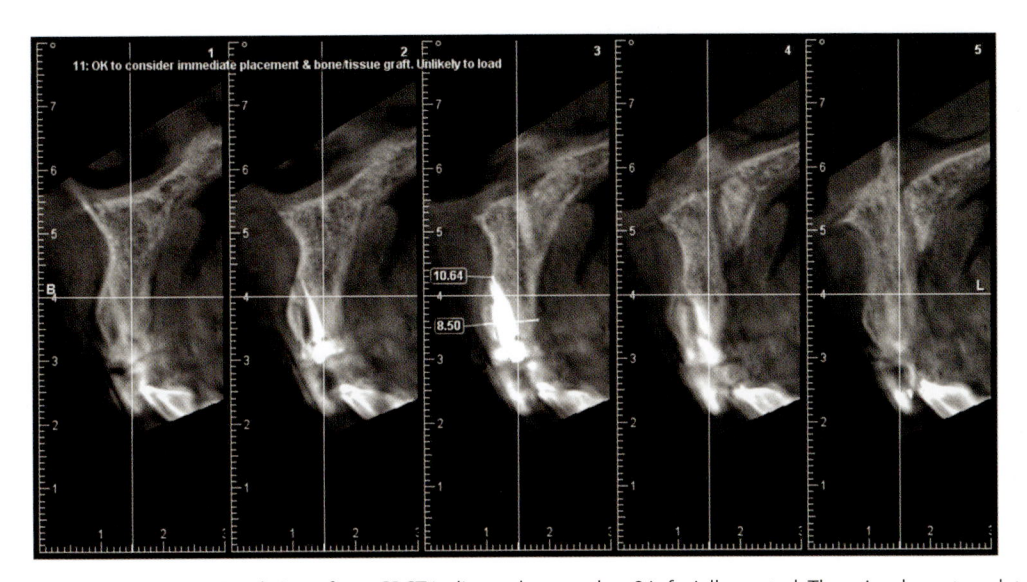

Figure 20.10 **(B)** Preoperative cross-sectional views from CBCT indicate that number 8 is facially canted. There is adequate palatal and apical bone for preparation of the osteotomy at the time of extraction.

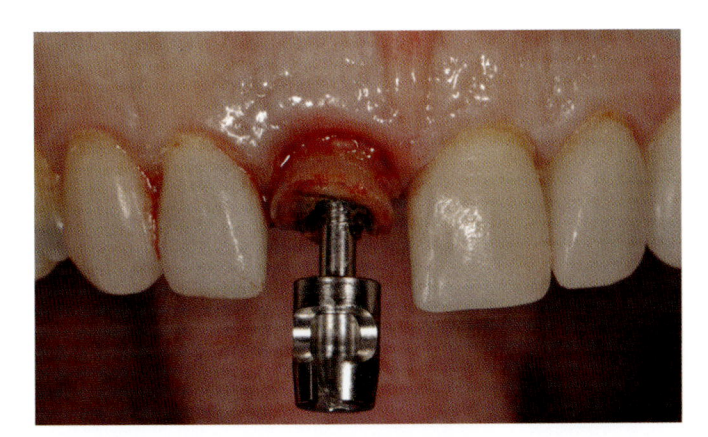

Figure 20.10 **(C)** Extraction of number 8 with a vertical extraction system (BENEX, Meisenger, Germany). This extraction device permits extraction without luxation, thereby preserving the thin facial bone.

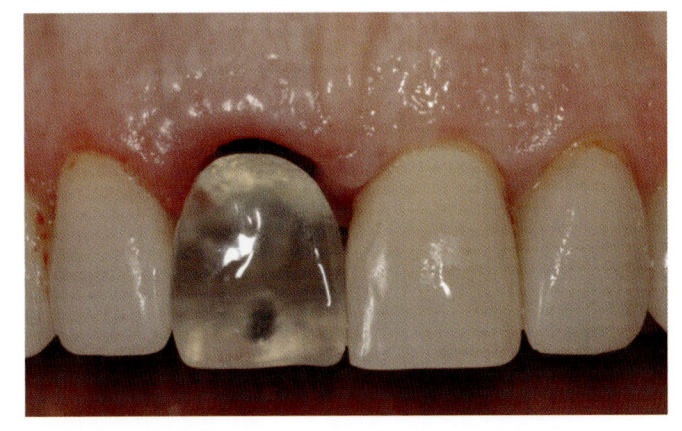

Figure 20.10 **(D)** Surgical guide: defines the preparation of the osteotomy in three dimensions.

Implant position: a pivotal point in the treatment blueprint

Implant placement is often discussed as a restoratively driven protocol; this underscores the importance of evaluation of the existing ridge anatomy, coupled with planning implant position based on the desired restoration and tissue outcome, and not just on the availability of bone.

The height of the papilla adjacent to a single implant is dictated for the most part by bone levels on adjacent teeth, whereas between implants it is dictated by interimplant bone height.[45] The potential impact of different implant–abutment connections, the spacing between implants, and the impact of prosthetic manipulation of the peri-implant tissues on bone height and long-term crestal bone stability will be discussed in this chapter.

It cannot be overemphasized how important it is to place the implant in the ideal location to achieve restorative success.[46] Given the broad literature relating to this aspect of treatment, it is not acceptable to make three-dimensional placement errors today. In Figure 20.13A–E, a distally and lingually canted implant cannot be restored and must be removed. Replacement and correction of implant position allows the use of a more appropriate implant diameter for the available restorative space. Poorly positioned implants not only jeopardize implant restorability and success but can also cause esthetic problems due to gingival recession and, significantly, can cause negative changes in the periodontium of adjacent teeth or implants.

Many surgical tools are available to help the clinician accurately plan and execute treatment, including CBCT to assess ridge anatomy, software planning systems using computer-aided design (CAD) that permit virtual implant placement and restoration, and surgical guides of varying degrees of precision.

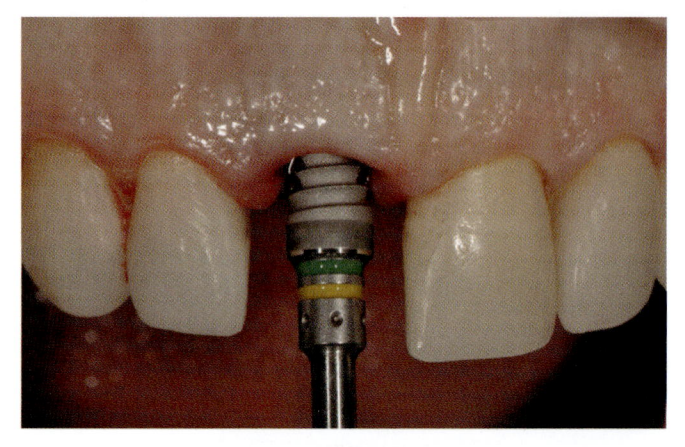

Figure 20.10 (E) Implant placement: a 4.6 mm diameter, 15 mm long BioHorizons tapered internal implant (BioHorizons, Birmingham, AL) engages the palatal and apical bone. This implant design—buttress threads and Laser-Lok surface technology—contributes to short-term high stability and long-term favorable crestal bone stability.

Figure 20.10 (F) Ideal implant placement. Note that there is a large buccal residual horizontal defect between the facial bone plate and the implant. This area must be grafted to ensure regeneration and to reduce the risk for facial bone remodeling.

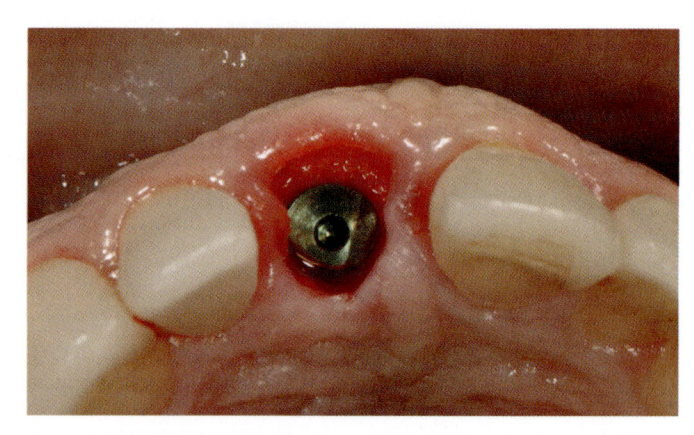

Figure 20.10 (G) Grafting of the residual horizontal defect with a structurally stable bone graft material. In this case, Bio-Oss (Osteohealth, Shirley, NY) was placed into the defect.

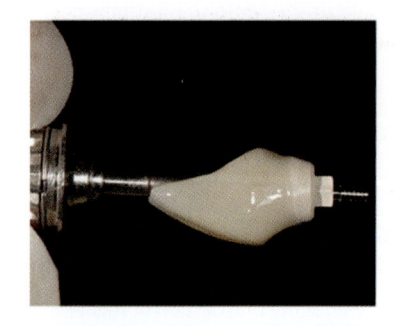

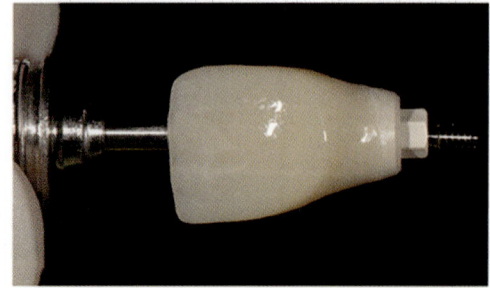

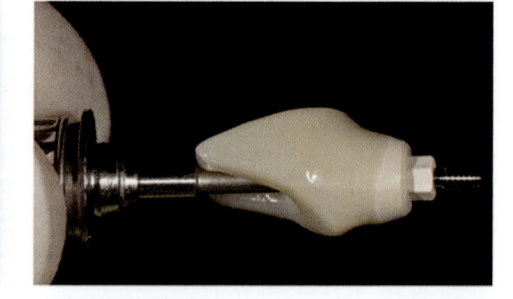

Figure 20.10 (H) Views of an ideally contoured screw-retained provisional restoration fabricated based on a fixture level impression taken at the time of surgery. Note the undercontouring of the crown in the subgingival area to avoid excess pressure that could induce recession.

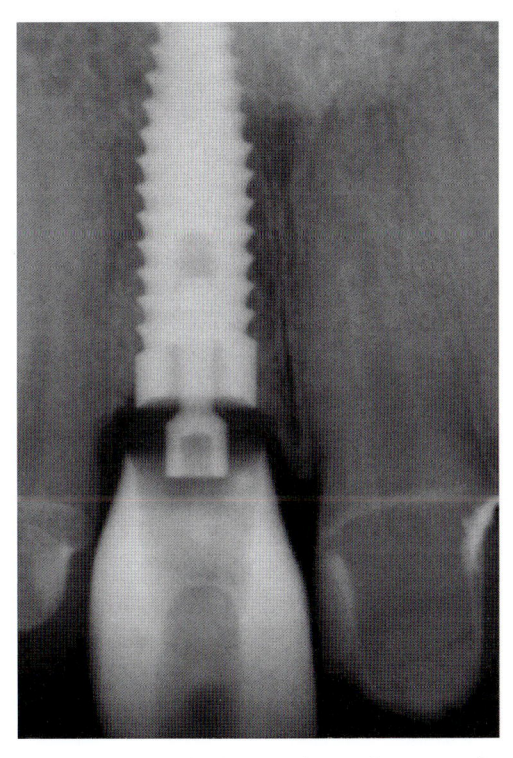

Figure 20.10 (I) Radiograph of the implant and provisional restoration after 4 months of healing. Note the radiopaque area correlates with the polyether ether ketone polymer abutment (BioHorizons, Birmingham, AL).

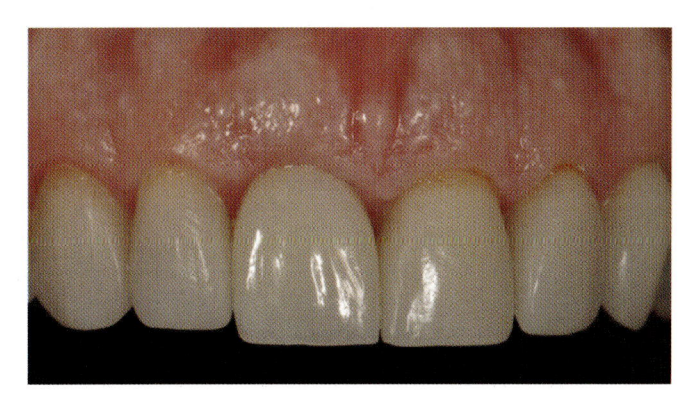

Figure 20.10 (J) Provisional restoration as viewed 4 months after surgery. Note that the gingival tissue has been developed and supported by the provisional restoration.

Table 20.2 Literature Findings and Risk Factors for Immediate Implant Placement Procedure[3,36]

Results of immediate implant placement procedure
High implant survival rates
High risk for mucosal recession (wide range reported in the literature)
Soft- and hard-tissue augmentation procedures are frequently necessary
This procedure should be used restrictively and by experienced clinicians
Recession risk factors
Smoking
Thin buccal bone (<1 mm thick), dehiscence/fenestration/damaged
Thin gingival biotype
Facial malposition of the implant

A conventional guide fabricated in the laboratory can drive the preparation of the osteotomy both buccolingually and mesiodistally, but as importantly can define the reference point for depth of implant placement if properly designed, as shown in Figure 20.14A and B. Stereolithographic surgical guides are more accurate and allow the greatest intraoperative precision Figure 20.15A–D) CAD/computer-aided manufacturing (CAM)-based surgical implant and restorative treatment is gradually penetrating clinical practice. This technology can improve surgical precision, reduce surgical time, minimize surgical invasiveness, and can be coupled with preplanned provisional or definitive restorations; however, subtle deviations in linear and angular implant position between planned and actual implant position are reported, albeit less than with conventional procedures.[47–50]

Currently, recommended surgical guidelines on three-dimensional implant placement include the following.

Buccolingual position

Implants should be positioned in a restoratively driven manner with the secondary goal of creating at least 2 mm of facial/buccal bone at the ridge crest and/or implant collar level.[18] Adequate facial bone volume enhances the long-term ridge crest stability, translating into stable gingival tissue levels.[51] Coupled with this, it is important to select implants of adequate diameter without reducing the buccal bone volume. Where large diameter implants may be used because of available bone, the impact on facial/buccal bone thickness must be considered because recession may be an unintended consequence. Figure 20.16A and B shows the impact of facially dominant implant position due to the use of a large implant diameter compared to an adjacent more appropriately sized implant.

Mesiodistal position

See Figure 20.17 for a graphic rendering.

- *Implants adjacent to teeth*: spacing of 1.5 mm from adjacent roots is recommended, based on efforts to minimize bone changes on adjacent roots due to the remodeling that occurs around the implant collar.[52] The redefinition of minimum spacing requirements may be forced by the introduction of new implant designs (platform-switching, one-piece, soft-tissue level implants), unique microtextured surface treatments that enhance crestal bone and soft-tissue stability (Laser-Lok®), or concept changes such as the placement of final abutments at the time of surgery to reduce the effect of repetitive disruptive prosthetic procedures that can contribute to the apical migration of bone and gingival tissues. If crestal remodeling and establishment of an apicalized biologic width is no longer a common outcome of the

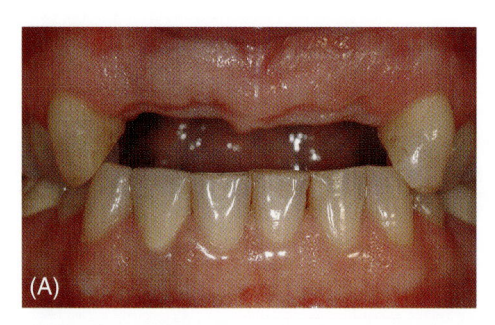

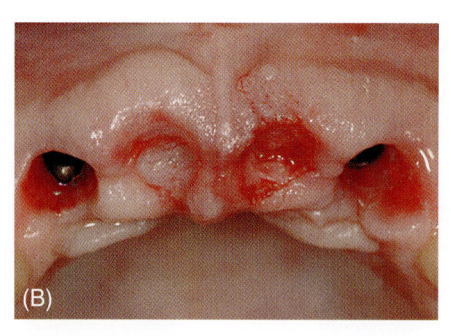

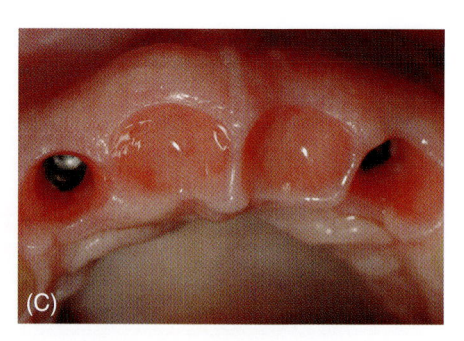

Figure 20.11 **(A)** Preoperative flat ridge anatomy due to longstanding partial edentulism. **(B)** Modification of the soft (and hard)-tissue anatomy at the time of implant placement, or after implant integration, can be accomplished using provisional restorations to guide the tissue form around implants and in pontic sites. Where necessary, tissue can be resected with burs, electrosurgery, or a laser and then guided with the provisional restoration. **(C)** Tissue form as viewed 3 months later on removal of the provisional restoration.

integration process, perhaps the minimum spacing requirements that were established with traditional implant designs need to be revisited. It will be interesting to assess whether reduced interproximal spacing (<1.5 mm separation from adjacent teeth) can be accepted in the future.

- *Adjacent implant placement and interimplant spacing:* separation between implants has historically been set at a 3 mm minimum, again to prevent coalescing of remodeling zones that occurred at the implant–abutment interface.[45]

With the introduction of platform switching, there is some evidence that reduced interimplant spacing may be acceptable since there is less crestal bone remodeling. It has been suggested that spacing of as little as 2 mm between implants does not result in an apical movement of the crestal bone. From this, one can extrapolate that the papilla should remain stable despite the closer proximity of implant placement. However, in our opinion, the effect of reduced space recommendations on soft-tissue volume or papillary form and size between implants and between implants and teeth needs to be considered.

Papilla height between an implant and tooth is defined by the bone height on the adjacent root and the location of the contact area, and not the proximal bone level next to the implant. It appears that the distance between the interproximal crest and the contact area is still the predominant factor determining the presence of the papilla. Between natural teeth, a distance of 5 mm or less will result in papilla fill. Between implants, however, this dimension decreases to 3.5 mm.[53,54]

Numerous techniques have been proposed to enhance the papillary architecture between implants, including bone and

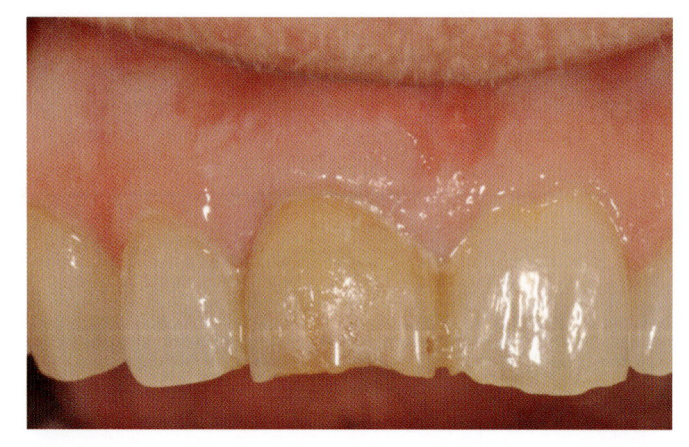

Figure 20.12 **(A)** Preoperative view: failing number 8 due to internal resorption.

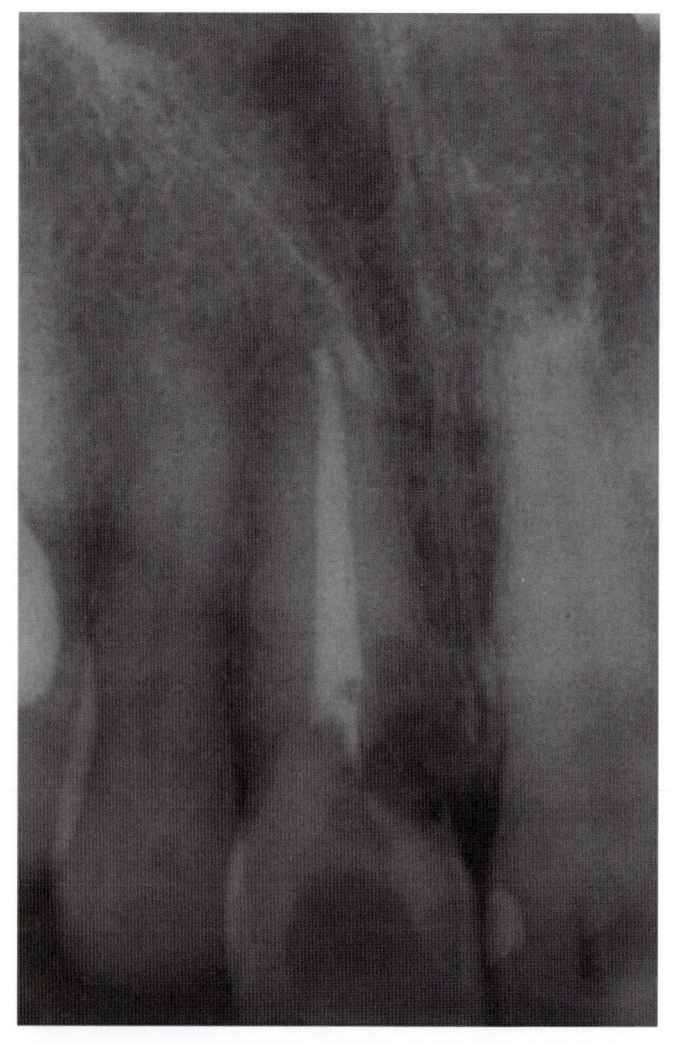

Figure 20.12 **(B)** Preoperative radiographic view. The large root size and length, along with the limited apical and palatal bone, do not permit immediate implant placement.

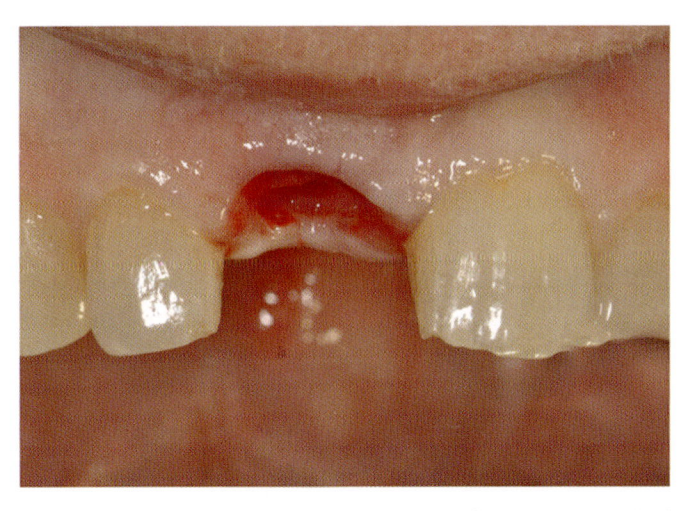

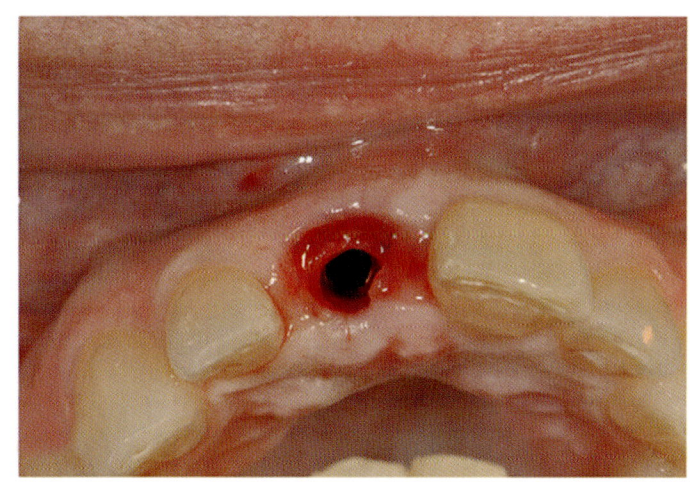

Figure 20.12 **(C)** Implant placement 4 months after extraction and ridge preservation.

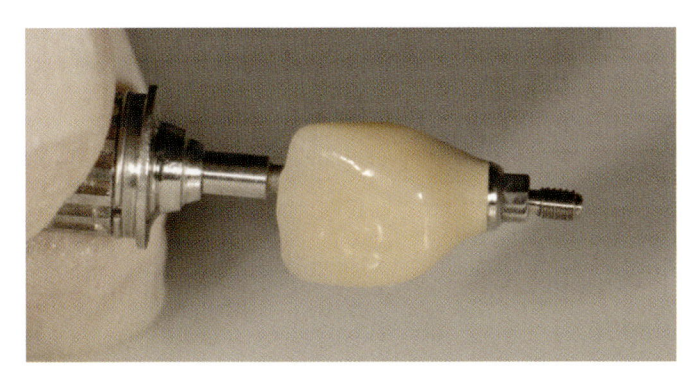

Figure 20.12 **(D)** A screw-retained provisional restoration is fabricated based on a fixture level impression taken at the time of surgery.

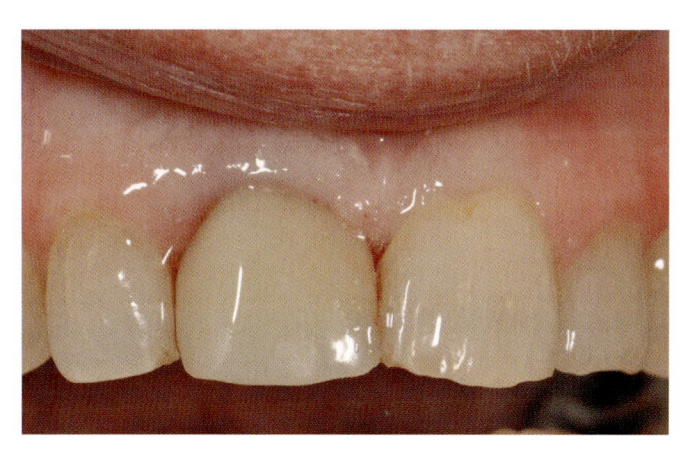

Figure 20.12 **(E)** The provisional restoration is delivered within 7 days of surgery. Its role is to coengineer the soft-tissue anatomy during the osseointegration period.

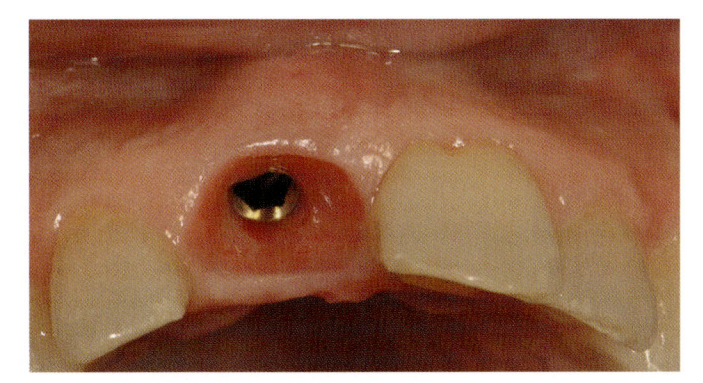

Figure 20.12 **(F)** Incisal view of the developed gingival anatomy after 12 weeks of healing.

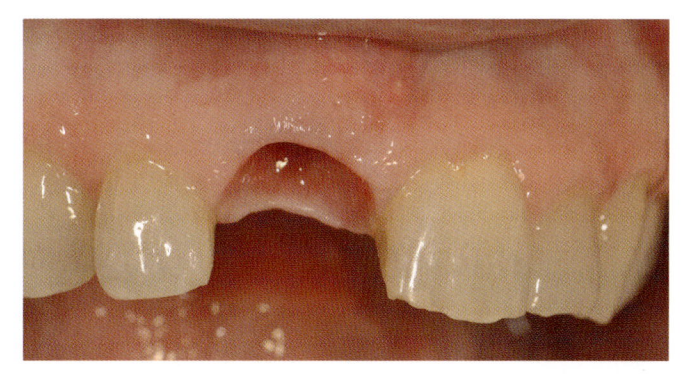

Figure 20.12 **(G)** Facial view of the developed gingival anatomy after 12 weeks of healing.

tissue grafting, correct three-dimensional implant position, implant and abutment design, and placement strategies. It has also been suggested that sequencing or staged implant placement may result in improved papilla form in contrast to simultaneous placement of side-by-side implants.[55] A comparative assessment of this and other commonly used surgical approaches, such as side-by-side implants placed in healed ridges, early implant placement (8 weeks of healing after extraction), and sequenced implant placement, did not identify significant esthetic benefits of one approach over another.[56]

The predictable achievement of adequate interimplant papillae still remains a significant clinical challenge.

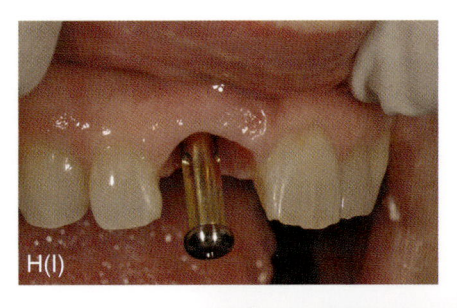

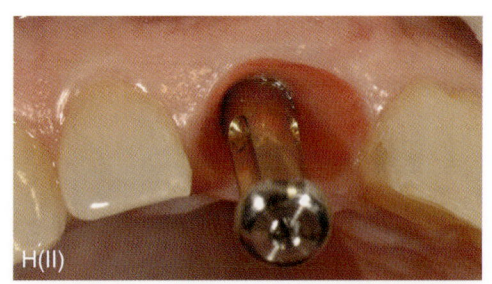

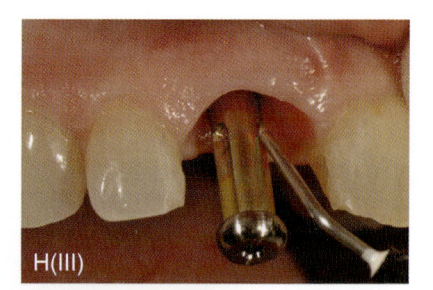

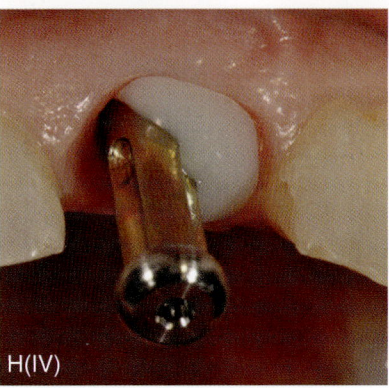

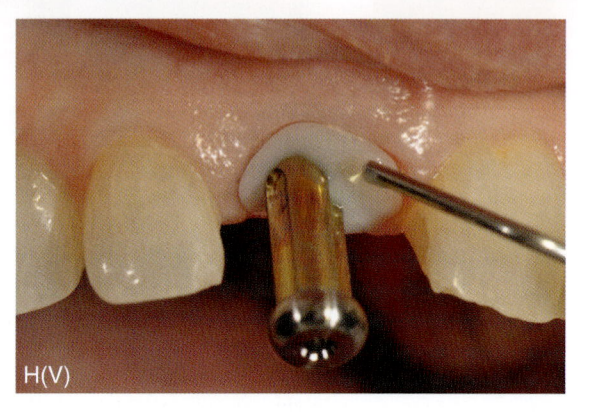

Figure 20.12 **(H)** Intraoral customizing of an impression coping used to record the implant position and the developed gingival anatomy. This technique works well when the gingival tissues are fibrous and stable. Thinner or more volatile tissues will collapse once a provisional restoration is removed, rendering the information less accurate for the technician. Extraoral indexing of the provisional restoration should be considered in this situation.

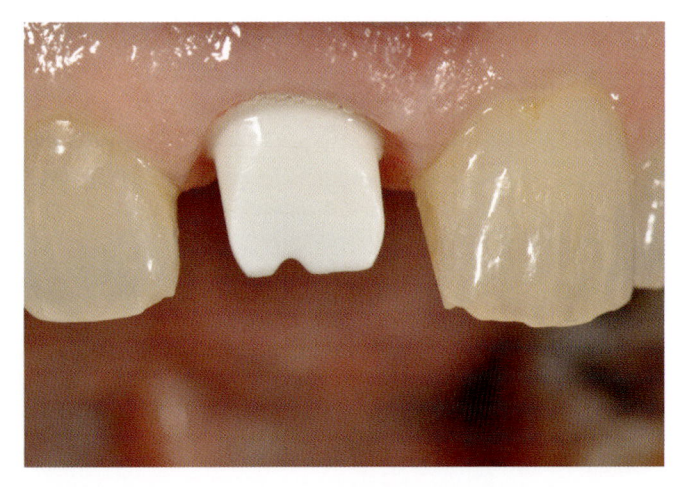

Figure 20.12 **(I)** Delivery of an ideally designed zirconia abutment in terms of support for the definitive restoration and position of the cement line.

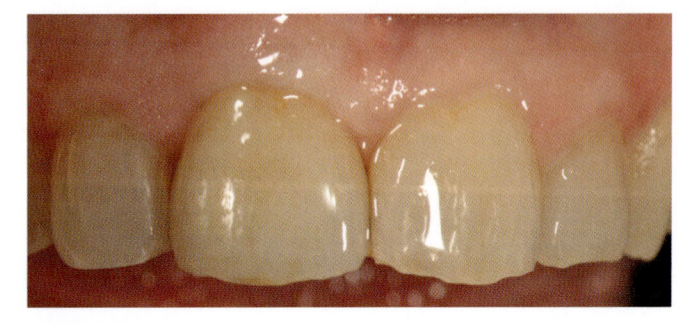

Figure 20.12 **(J)** Insertion of the definitive restoration (feldspathic porcelain-veneered zirconia crown).

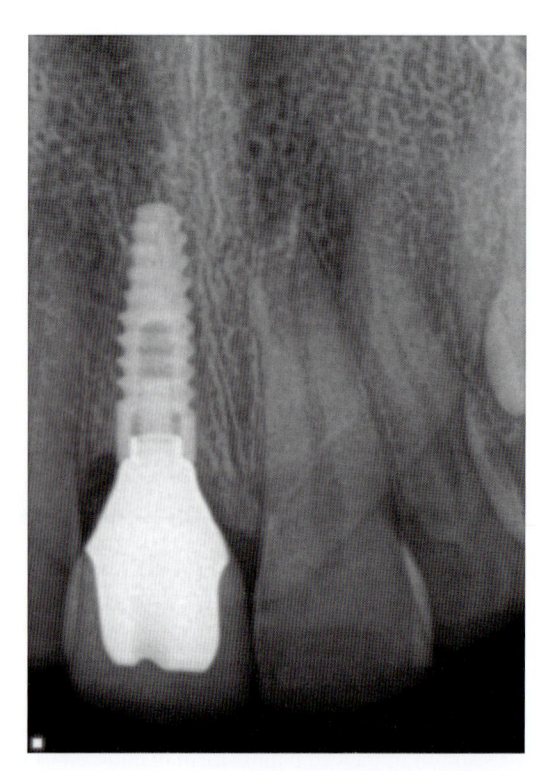

Figure 20.12 **(K)** Radiographic view of the definitive restoration following cementation.

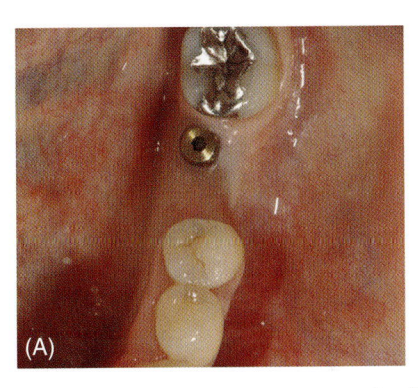

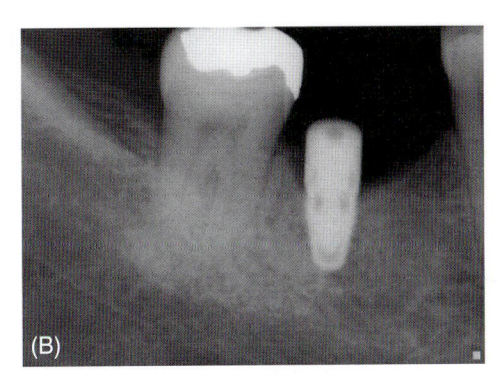

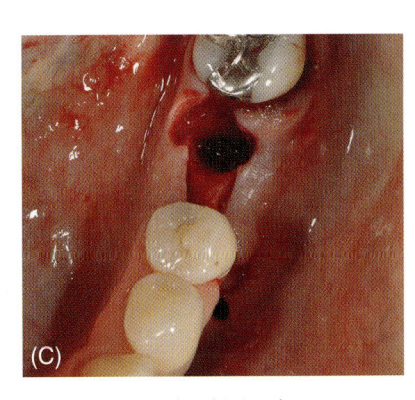

Figure 20.13 **(A)** Preoperative view: distally and lingually canted implant, and small diameter due to poor positioning render this implant unrestorable. **(B)** Preoperative radiographic view. **(C)** Removal of the implant can be accomplished with a variety of techniques, including reverse torque if not completely integrated, piezosurgery, or, in this case, removal with a hollow-core trephine.

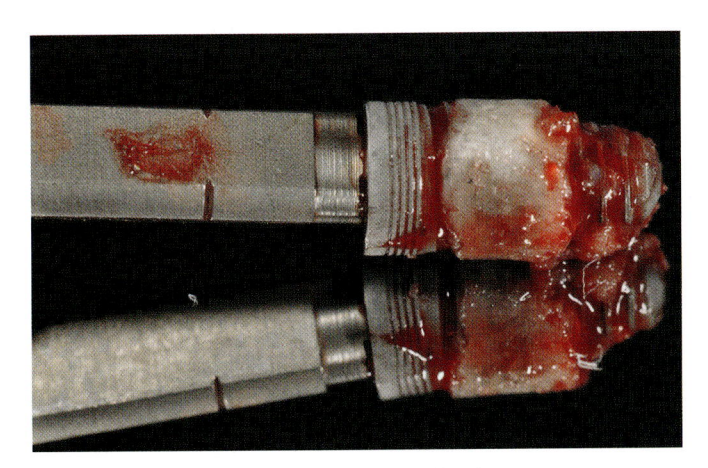

Figure 20.13 **(D)** This implant was removed with reverse torque following trephination of two-thirds of the implant length.

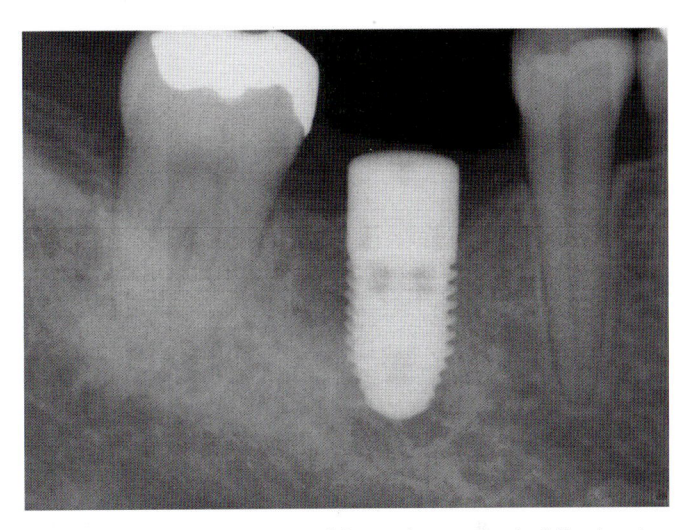

Figure 20.13 **(E)** Replacement of the implant 4 months following the implant removal and ridge augmentation. Radiographic view of the implant after a 3-month integration period. Note the improved position and larger diameter that could be placed due to the corrected position relative to the adjacent roots.

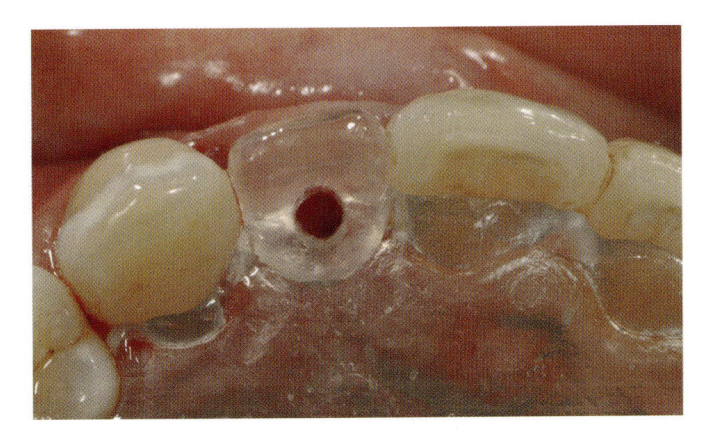

Figure 20.14 **(A)** A lab-processed surgical guide defines the mesiodistal and facial-palatal position for the future implant and restoration. Used at the time of surgery, this guides the preparation of the early drilling steps of the osteotomy preparation. With subsequent widening of the hole/access, larger drills can also be used to finalize the implant osteotomy.

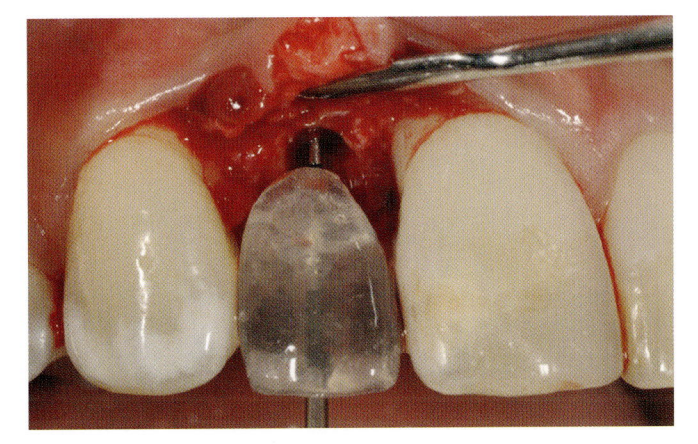

Figure 20.14 **(B)** An ideally designed surgical guide also defines the desired depth of implant placement. In this case, a probe placed through the guide to the head of the implant shows that the implant has been positioned 3 mm apical to the desired facial free gingival margin.

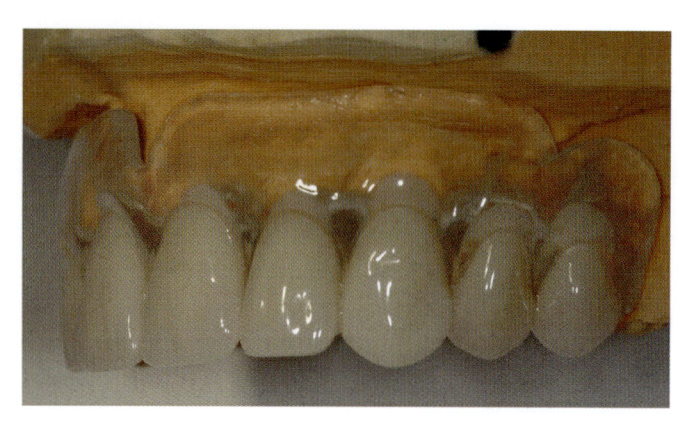

Figure 20.15 (A) Ideal tooth position as established in a provisional restoration is used to fabricate a radiographic template, before a CBCT.

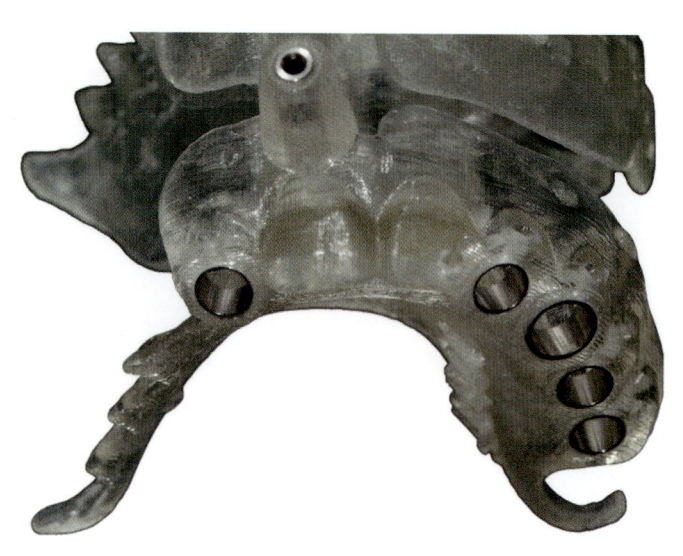

Figure 20.15 (B) A stereolithographic surgical guide is fabricated and will guide the implant site preparation and implant insertion.

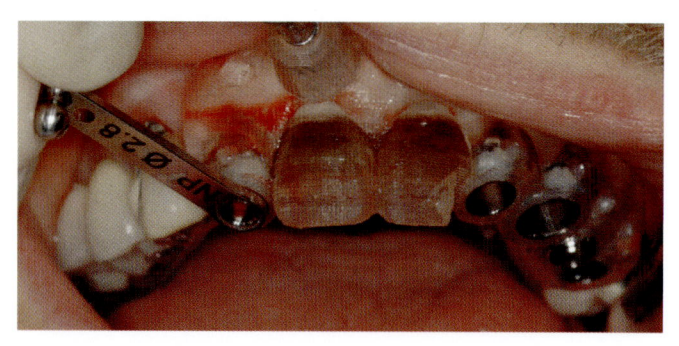

Figure 20.15 (C) Implant osteotomy preparation through a printed surgical guide improves the placement precision as planned virtually.

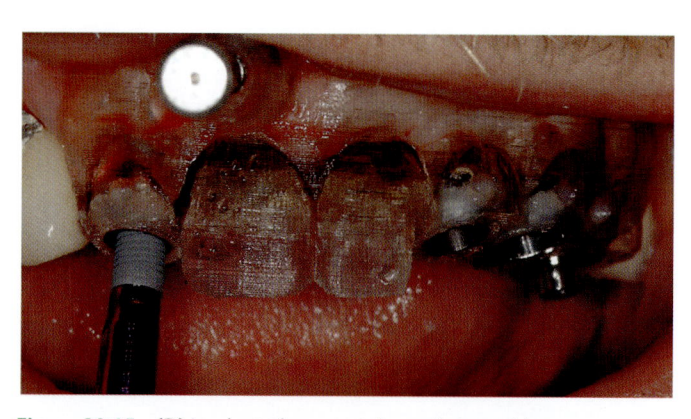

Figure 20.15 (D) Implant placement through the guide.

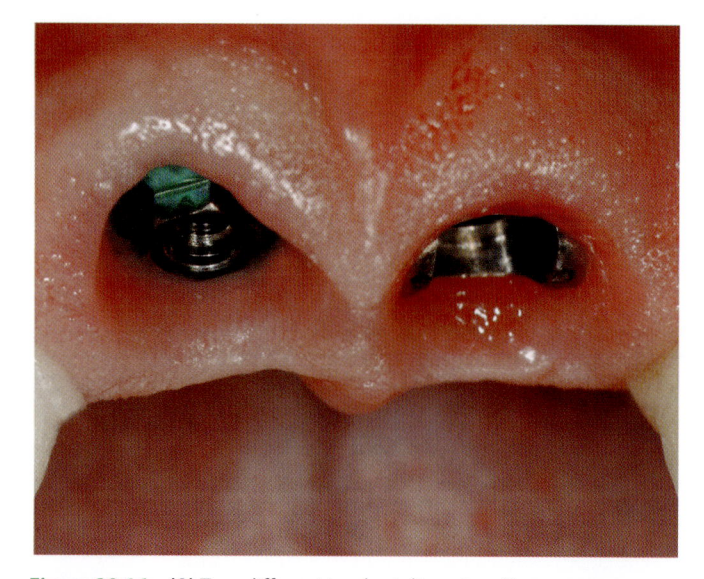

Figure 20.16 (A) Two different implant diameters (6 mm versus 4.3 mm) result in facial dominance of the larger implant, thinning of the buccal bone, and reduced restorative room for the abutment. This clearly translates into early negative soft-tissue level changes.

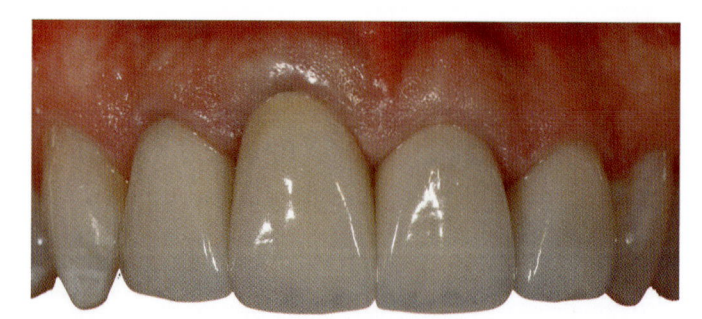

Figure 20.16 (B) The clear contrast in facial tissue level due to a treatment planning error on implant size, resulting in a long clinical crown, relative to the more normal and desirable tissue level in site number 9.

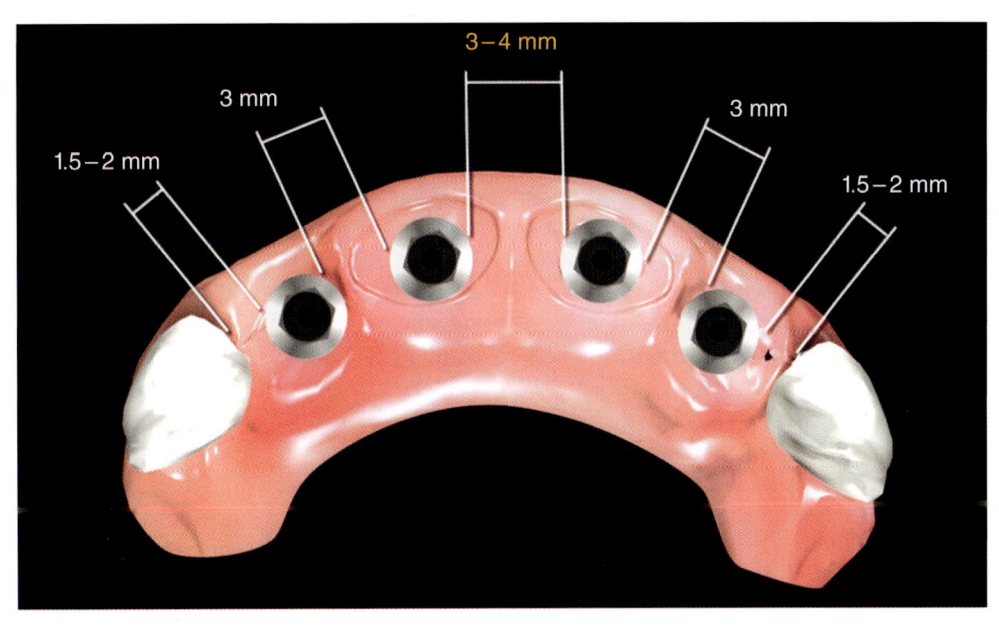

Figure 20.17 Graphic illustration showing ideal spacing between an implant and an adjacent root (1.5–2.0 mm) and between implants (3 mm).

Apicocoronal position (depth of implant placement)

In the esthetic zone, depth of implant placement is generally driven by the position of the desired future free gingival margin. Typically, the implant is positioned 3 mm apical to this position, allowing room for the transmucosal restorative components to develop both subgingival tissue contours and to support the desired marginal soft-tissue profile. As shown in Figure 20.14B, this is most predictably accomplished using surgical templates that define the gingival margin of the planned restoration. Some studies now also suggest that the use of implants with textured or grooved collars may benefit from slightly subcrestal placement, as it is suggested that this can lead to reduced crestal bone remodeling by placing the implant into a more protected or sheltered environment relative to bacterial challenge.[57–59]

Implant designs

The implant market offers a variety of designs, which are all basically evolutions of the original Brånemark root-form implant—a metal cylinder with screw threads. They are usually manufactured from commercially pure titanium or titanium alloy, although there have been recent attempts to use zirconia. Additional features have been incorporated into different implant designs, usually for the purposes of improved osseointegration, crestal bone preservation, and facilitating restoration.

A significant departure from the original Brånemark design is the incorporation of modified surfaces. Although early implants showed machined surfaces, most contemporary implants are treated to provide a roughened surface, for the purpose of improving bone-to-implant contact and enhancing the biologic response.[60] At this time, one surface technology has not been shown to be superior to another in terms of implant survival or success.

Another area where current implant designs differ from the Brånemark original is the abutment–implant interface. Root-form implants were initially manufactured with external connections. Over time, however, there has been a migration toward implant designs that feature internal connections. The reasons for this evolution range from attempts to decrease the bacterial load at the implant–abutment interface, to improving stress distribution at the bone–implant interface. Whether an implant has an external or an internal connection, however, does not seem to have an effect on implant success or survival rates.[61] Nevertheless, implants with internal connections show significant advantages from a restorative perspective. The most important may be the reduction in the incidence of screw loosening, mainly as a result of superior connection stability and axial support. In addition, they are more operator friendly, because it may be easier to properly seat abutments and other restorative components, particularly in areas of limited access.

Internal implant connections may be conical or parallel walled. There has been substantial disagreement as to whether or not conical connections provide a superior sealing ability from oral fluids, thereby decreasing bacterial contamination of the internal implant chamber, which may be beneficial in preventing crestal bone remodeling around implants. However, it appears that abutment micromotion may play a more important role with respect to the latter.[62]

Platform switching has been proposed as an alternative to improve crestal bone maintenance around implants. This concept incorporates the use of restorative components of a lesser diameter than that of the implant. In other words, the implant platform is "switched" to a narrower restorative platform. This results in a situation where the implant–abutment junction is located in a more medial location. Therefore, whether or not peri-implant bone remodeling is caused by bacterial leakage or abutment micromotion, platform switching places the potential etiologic factors further away from the implant–bone interface. The potential for platform switching to preserve crestal bone maintenance has been supported by extensive publications, including systematic reviews.[63–66]

In terms of macrogeometry (implant shape), "tapered implant designs" have recently gained in popularity. This may be due in part to their potential to achieve increased primary stability that offers significant advantages in terms of immediate placement and immediate restoration. For example, an implant design that routinely achieves outstanding primary stability may be used in more compromised situations, hence consolidating procedures and decreasing morbidity and treatment time. In addition, high primary stability facilitates immediate loading. Implant placement into fresh extraction sockets followed by immediate provisionalization has been increasingly used by clinicians because of the potential for predictable esthetic results by guiding tissues early in the treatment process.[42–44] Tapered implant designs are often advantageous when using this protocol.

Gingival biotype: assessment methods and enhancement procedures

The gingival biotype has long been recognized as an important parameter in treatment planning for the natural dentition, but it is just as essential a consideration for the health and esthetics of the peri-implant soft tissues.[50,67] Although success in terms of osseointegration is not impacted by gingival biotype, it has become clear that gingival margin stability, risk of recession, and maintenance of peri-implant soft-tissue health may be influenced by it.[68–71] Although there is a trend to focus on these issues in the esthetic zone or anterior maxillary dentition, it is important to assess tissue characteristics in nonesthetic areas as well.

The biotype can be described as thin (≤1.0 mm) or thick (>1 mm).[72–74] In the natural dentition, it is believed that a thin biotype is a contributing factor to recession and root exposure. A thick gingival tissue biotype has been suggested to protect underlying bone,[75,76] reduce the risk for postrestoration recession, improve esthetics, and mask the color of the underlying restorative. It is also important in facilitating oral hygiene procedures.[77]

A variety of techniques can be used to assess the thickness of the gingival tissue, including visual assessment, transmucosal probing under local anesthesia, sulcular probing and probe transparency, CBCT imaging, and experimental but not routinely used procedures such as ultrasound devices. In clinical practice, it is probably most common to use visual assessment to characterize the gingival biotype, but this is the least accurate method to assess tissue thickness.[78] Sulcular probing before tooth extraction, or around an implant, would be preferential as this allows the practitioner to estimate the tissue thickness based on the degree to which the probe can be visualized through the tissue, thus allowing an extrapolation to the potential impact of different restorative materials on gingival tissue color.[79] Similarly, transmucosal probing provides a numeric measurement, but can certainly be affected by probe or instrument size and tissue desiccation. Each of these procedures has pros and cons, as described in Table 20.3. Along with studies that emphasize the importance of the tissue thickness, other studies suggest that the width or height of the keratinized tissue band is also important to long-term facial tissue stability.[80]

Tissue thickness may also be influenced prosthetically. For example, undercontoured or concave emergence profiles, whether at the abutment or the restoration level, can be used to enhance the tissue thickness, offering potentially beneficial effects in terms of marginal tissue stability.[81,82] This concept will be reviewed in more detail in the "Provisionalization: refinement of the gingival tissue architecture" section.

Today, gingival and dermal grafting procedures are often incorporated into implant treatment plans to prevent mid-facial gingival recession, rather than using these procedures to remediate esthetic complications around implants (see Figure 20.18A–D). Connective tissue grafts,[83,84] and, to some degree, pediculated or rotated flaps[85,86] can be successfully used to enhance both tissue volume and quality before or at the time of implant placement. Although there is no supporting literature,

Table 20.3 Gingival Biotype: Strengths and Limitations of Assessment Techniques

Gingival Tissue Thickness Assessment Techniques	Pros	Cons
Visual assessment	Simple, inexpensive, noninvasive	Subjective (no numeric outcome)
Sulcular probing and probe transparency	Simple, inexpensive, noninvasive	Relatively subjective (no numeric outcome)
Transmucosal (gingival) probing	Simple, inexpensive, provides a numeric outcome or measurement	Requires local anesthesia, accuracy affected by probe size/form, tissue hydration
CBCT imaging (possibly coupled with radiopaque sulcular markers)	Simple, noninvasive	Expensive, accuracy influenced by type of CBCT device, marker size, restoration material scatter artifacts
Ultrasonic devices	Not available at present for routine clinical use	

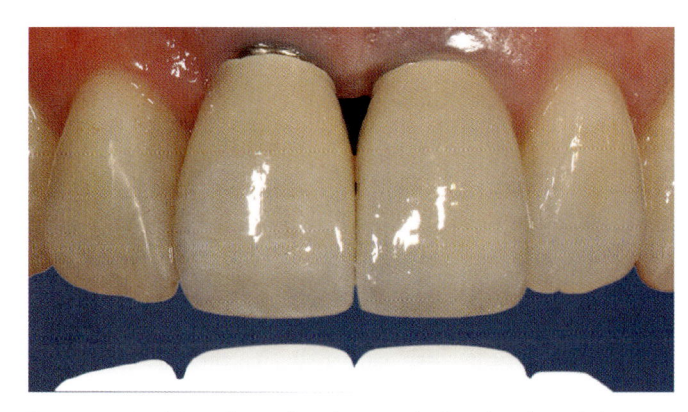

Figure 20.18 **(A)** Implants placed 8 years before this clinical photo were well positioned three-dimensionally. Embrasure between number 8 and number 9 shows deficient interimplant papilla typically associated with adjacent implants. The thin biotype was not addressed with a graft during the treatment, contributing to the recession, margin, and abutment exposure. Note the gray tissue color due to the underlying titanium abutment.

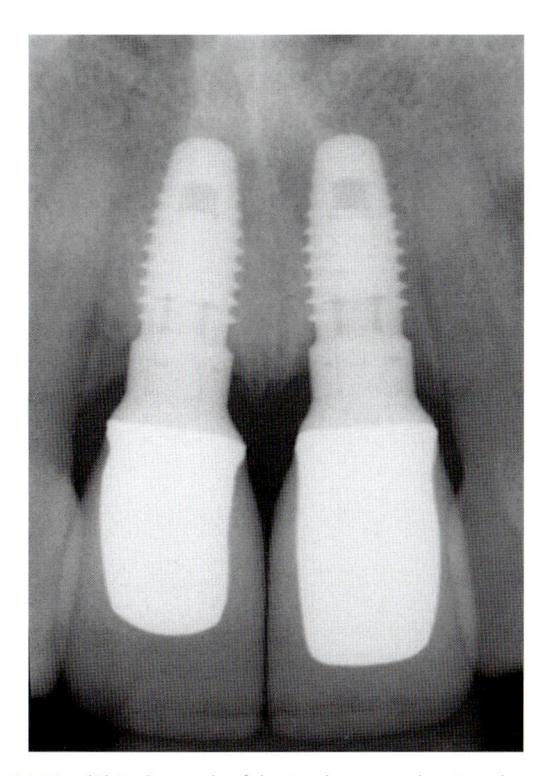

Figure 20.18 **(B)** Radiograph of the implants number 8 and number 9 after 8 years in function. Bone levels are normal with evidence of remodeling around this implant design to the first major thread (Nobel Replace Select, Nobel Biocare, Yorba Linda, CA).

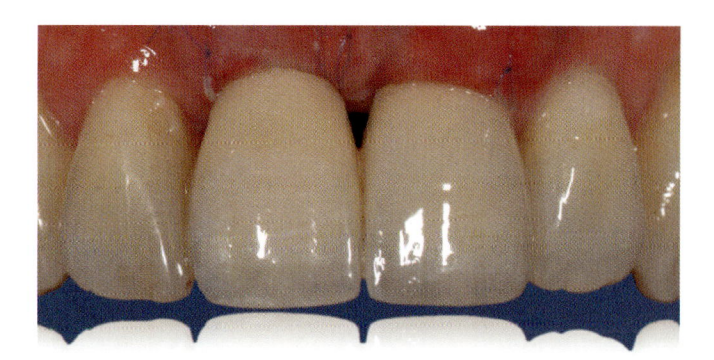

Figure 20.18 **(C)** Remedial connective tissue graft procedure using a microsurgical technique as viewed 10 days after surgery. The treatment goal is to enhance the tissue volume and quality before replacement of the restorations.

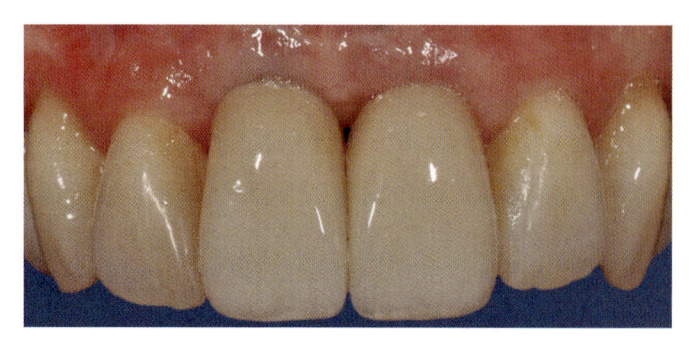

Figure 20.18 **(D)** Replacement of the restorations 4 months after the graft procedure. Note the long contact areas and long clinical crowns. Esthetic outcomes of treatment are rarely ideal when a corrective, rather than interceptive, approach is considered.

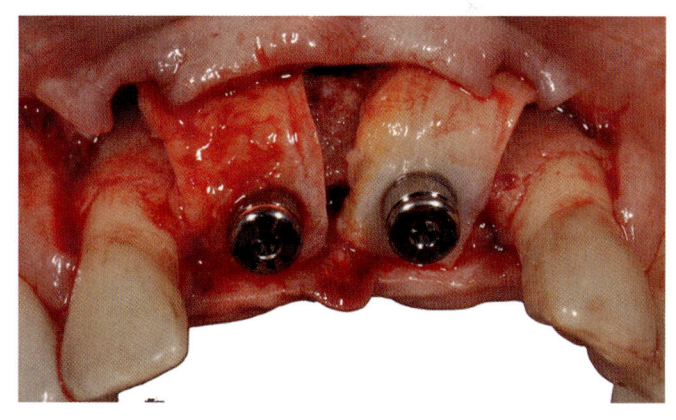

Figure 20.19 **(A)** Three-dimensional tissue augmentation to enhance the tissue biotype and the tissue volume. Palatal and proximal extension of the grafts improves the buccal tissue volume, the papillary form, and potentially protects the underlying ridge crest.

our clinical observations suggest that graft quality may play a role on the degree of tissue volume achieved, as well as its long-term stability. In this regard, gingival grafts with high fat content do not appear to perform as well as grafts composed of dense connective tissue. Figure 20.19A–C shows current graft techniques to three-dimensionally enhance tissue volume as well as the impact of variable graft quality on the maturation and potential impact on long-term tissue stability. It must be pointed out, however, that corrective soft-tissue procedures around implants may not offer predictable results or long-term peri-implant tissue stability.

In summary, although three-dimensional bone volume around implants is important to integration and crestal bone stability, the soft-tissue volume and quality are equally important in achieving optimal esthetics and peri-implant tissue health.

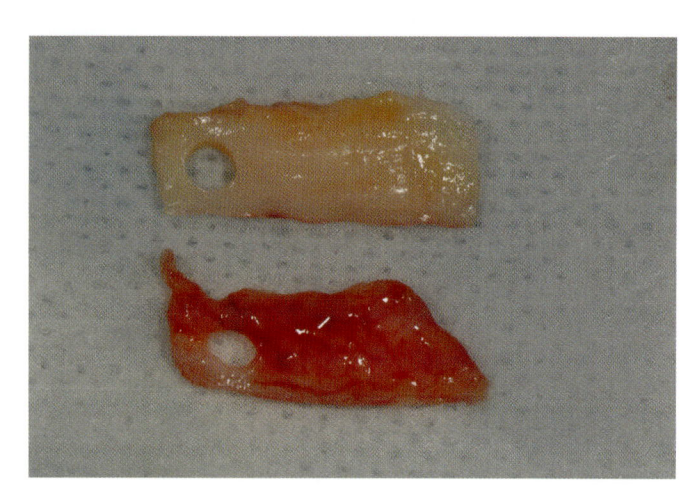

Figure 20.19 **(B)** Contrasting tissue quality, due to different graft harvesting techniques. One graft has a greater fatty component. We propose that grafts with lower fibrous composition heal in a different pattern and are not stable long term.

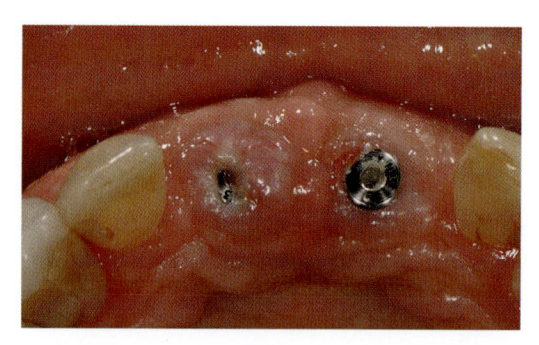

Figure 20.19 **(C)** Healing of the implants and grafts as viewed at 10 days postsurgery. Clear differences in healing patterns are noted between the fattier graft at site number 8 and the more fibrous graft at site number 9 early in the healing phase.

Provisionalization: refinement of the gingival tissue architecture

Today's final "surgical step"

Creating peri-implant tissues that are stable and look the same as those seen around healthy adjacent teeth requires (1) an understanding of how to preserve the existing hard and soft tissues and, if need be, regenerate them, (2) that the implant position be correct three-dimensionally, and (3) that the tissues be properly managed as they mature. Often overlooked is the importance of provisionalizing the implant and the distinct benefits of this step.

Provisionalization is generally thought of as the first step in the restorative phase of treatment, but it should perhaps be redefined as the final phase in surgery. Even if provisionalization is started after implant integration, its role is to define or finalize the tissue form in the transmucosal area and particularly at the gingival margin level.

As previously discussed, the temporary crown or fixed partial denture has the role of guiding and developing the transmucosal tissue form; this may be accomplished by using cemented provisional restorations on temporary or final abutments, or screw-retained provisional restorations.[87,88] Immediate provisionalization is advantageous for patients that object to the use of a removable temporary prosthesis. In addition, it may provide the benefit of preserving peri-implant tissue levels, particularly in the mid-facial aspect. Figure 20.20A–I shows the development of the tissue form with a provisional restoration that will subsequently serve as a template for the final restoration. Many studies report that immediate provisionalization outcomes are similar to those of conventional restoration protocols.[89] However, adverse soft-tissue changes presenting as advanced recession (>1 mm) have been reported as a risk in many studies. These undesirable sequelae are usually the result of labial implant position and/or inadequate restorative contours.[80,90,91]

Provisional restorations must be designed with appropriate supragingival contours for esthetics, but also in the subgingival area to develop the peri-implant tissue contours. As previously discussed, the contour of the provisional restoration must be optimized to support the desired gingival architecture. Overcontouring the implant restoration in the transmucosal area increases the risk for tissue recession, negatively impacting the esthetic outcome; in our opinion, this may be an important issue in studies that report gingival recession problems in immediate restoration scenarios. Conversely, undercontouring the implant restoration in the transmucosal area will result in coronal proliferation of the gingival margin.

In summary, implant provisionalization offers the following advantages for the patient and clinician:

1. Immediate gratification as the patient leaves with the tooth/teeth in place.
2. Time to assess the results of treatment; that is, evaluating the treatment plan.
3. If any additional treatment is required, such as soft-tissue revision, the provisional can be used to guide the healing process and to reevaluate the esthetic outcome.
4. The provisional can be modified to support the tissue or to change its form. Provisional materials that are typically used are acrylic resins such as polymethyl-methacrylates, bisacryl composite resins, and visible-light-cured urethane dimethacrylates. They are easily modified by using a shaping disc or bur or by adding adhesives and light-cured composites. In some cases, roughening and sand blasting before adhesive addition will help with the durability of the bond of the composite used to modify the provisional restoration.
5. The information as to the three-dimensional shape of the accepted emergence profile can be registered by either customizing a stock impression post directly in the mouth [shown in Figure 20.12H(i–v)] or indexing the provisional restoration itself (the latter requires a screw-retained provisional). If it is possible to pour the impression right away, an extended lab-screw can be substituted for the conventional temporary abutment screw and an open tray impression carried out. In this way the provisional acts as the impression post or coping, producing an exact replica of the subgingival tissue contours. The use of any of these techniques insures that the technician will have the required

information to design the ideal final abutment and crown contours. All too often, the technician is asked to guess at the final dimensions of the subgingival area, resulting in either under- or overcontoured definitive restoration.

Material choices: final abutments and restorations

Abutments

Final abutments for cemented restorations are generally available in either titanium or zirconium. The most widely used material is titanium, although each material offers distinct advantages. Titanium is a metal that can be alloyed to produce a strong, lightweight material for the production of both dental implants and abutments. It is corrosion resistant and has the highest strength-to-weight ratio of any metal available. It is less brittle than zirconia and has higher fracture toughness, and can be readily used in posterior regions of the mouth or where additional strength is required. The use of zirconia-based ceramics has emerged onto the scene in recent years for a wide range of clinical applications, including crowns, bridges, frameworks, and implant abutments. This has come under the banner of metal-free restorative materials, and the application of zirconia abutments has gained considerable interest because of its pleasing color, thus avoiding the "gunning" or "graying" appearance through the facial gingival tissues.

The physical and mechanical properties of zirconia oxide ceramics show a unique ability to resist crack propagation when properly handled and designed. Zirconia abutments in particular have been documented to resist fracture under normal occlusal loads.[92-94] The design of the abutments should allow for a minimal axial thickness of the crown of 1.2–1.5 mm and an occlusal or incisal thickness of 1.5–2.0 mm. The abutments should be created with rounded internal line angles. In other words, implant abutments should be designed with similar preparation guidelines to those of natural teeth. As a cautionary note, in situations where implant position demands that axial walls of the abutment be modified to the point where they become too

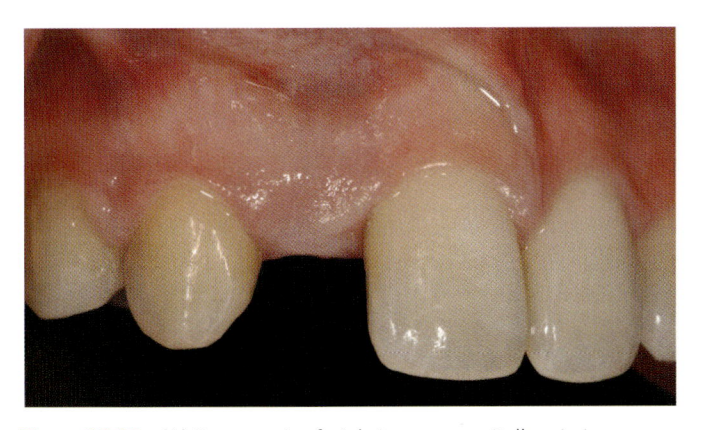

Figure 20.20 (A) Preoperative facial view: congenitally missing lateral incisor.

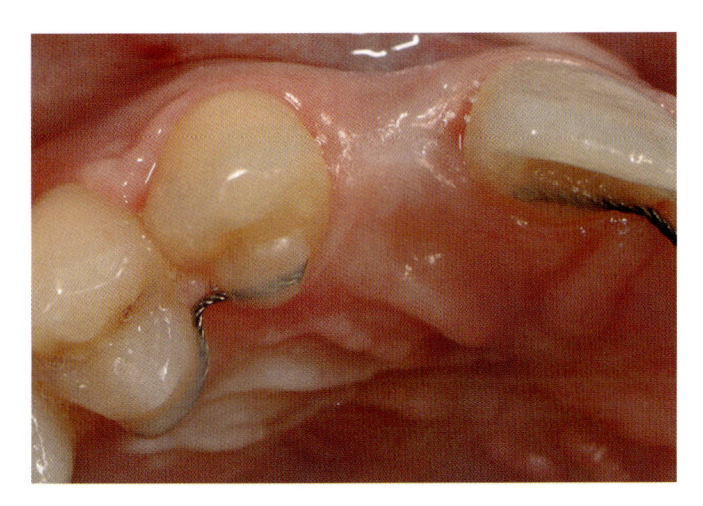

Figure 20.20 (B) Preoperative occlusal view.

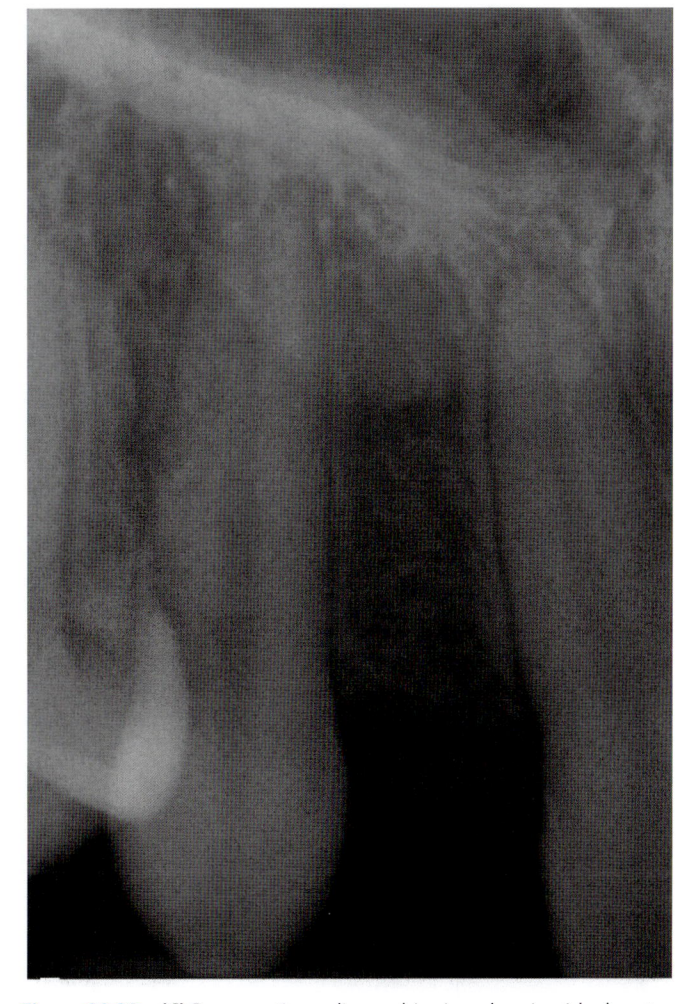

Figure 20.20 (C) Preoperative radiographic view showing ideal root alignment around the edentulous site. On the basis of clinical measurements and a CBCT, spacing of 6 mm permits 3 mm diameter implant placement, maintaining spacing of 1.5 mm on either side.

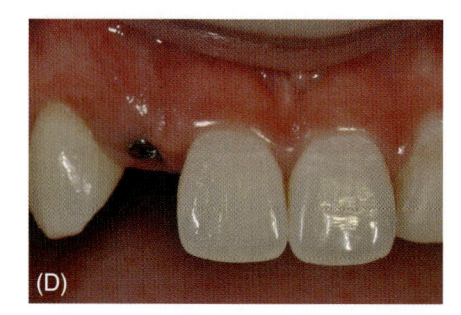

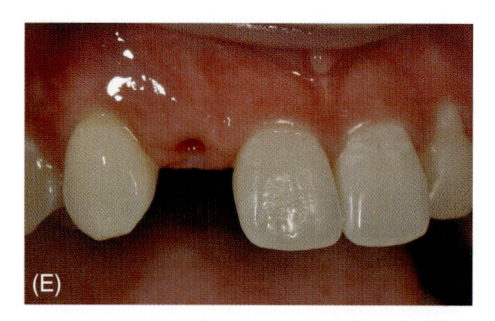

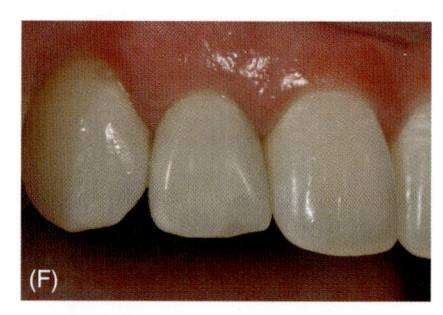

Figure 20.20 **(D)** Three months postsurgery: narrow healing abutment in place. **(E)** Three months postsurgery. Undeveloped tissue anatomy as defined by the healing abutment. A fixture level impression is taken to fabricate a screw-retained provisional restoration that will be used to define the marginal tissue anatomy. **(F)** Facial view after 3 months with the provisional restoration in place.

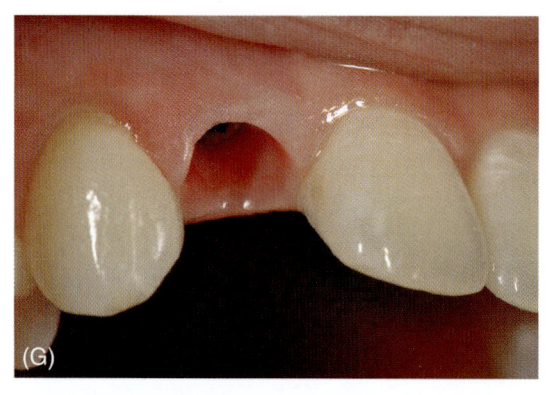

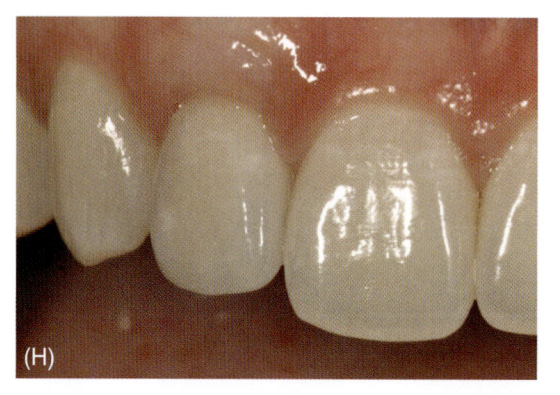

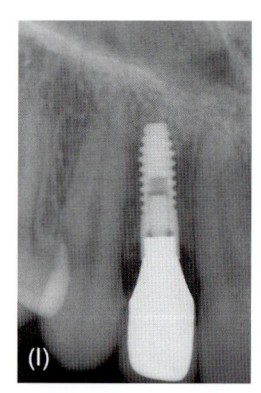

Figure 20.20 **(G)** Occlusal view of the subgingival prosthetic envelope and marginal tissue contours as developed by the provisional restoration. **(H)** Definitive restoration: postcementation clinical view. **(I)** Definitive restoration: postcementation radiographic view.

thin, particularly in the region of the head of the retaining screw, making it more prone to fracture, titanium is a better choice of material. Figure 20.21A indicates that adequate material volume around the head of the implant is necessary to avoid fracture of the abutment (as shown in Figure 20.21B) in the case of zirconia (one implant manufacturer suggests that a minimum thickness of 0.8 mm is necessary for the first 3 mm coronally from the head of the implant mating surface).

Both materials have been cited in the literature as showing adequate soft-tissue biocompatibility, with some evidence suggesting that zirconia is superior to titanium in this respect as suggested by lower bacterial colonization and reduced inflammation.[95–97] It is interesting to note, however, that zirconia biocompatibility may be affected by handling procedures, including polishing, veneering, or milling/preparation procedures.[98]

Zirconia abutments are increasingly used in the esthetic zone due to obvious color advantages compared with titanium or gold-hued abutments. The graying effect caused by titanium through the soft tissues can affect the esthetic outcome.[81,99] The use of zirconia also allows the clinician to locate the finish line just below the gingival margin to allow for easier isolation and control of cementation (Figure 20.22C). Zirconia abutments can also be colored to avoid the relatively opaque or white color if necessary. This may be an advantage in terms of creating color symmetry next to an adjacent tooth-supported restoration. Figure 20.22A and B compares the cement-line position on a titanium abutment to avoid the "graying" of the soft tissues, which invariably forces the final margin to be more deeply placed, compared with a more coronal position on a zirconia abutment.

This in turn places the veneering porcelain further into the tissue. This material has not been shown to be as biocompatible as zirconia. Furthermore, the deeper placement of the margin can result in the inability to thoroughly remove any residual cement, leading to possible peri-implantitis.[100,101] Figure 20.23A shows residual cement that can lead to inflammation in many cases, and to bone loss in some cases (as noted in Figure 20.23B).

Implant restorations: ceramics

Metal-based crowns and fixed partial dentures still constitute the majority of implant restorations today, especially where titanium abutments have been used. Again, in highly esthetically sensitive areas where zirconia abutments are used, it makes sense to couple this technology with metal-free restorations. Zirconia crowns are currently produced through CAD/CAM systems, which for the most part use partially sintered Y-TZP ceramics, where the crowns are dry milled and then undergo a final sintering process. The strength of zirconia is essentially higher than the functional forces that are generated in the mouth; however, the applied veneering porcelains, which have a high glass phase content to enhance translucency and esthetic properties, are significantly weaker than the zirconia coping and subject to crack growth and cumulative damage in a wet environment. The chipping of the

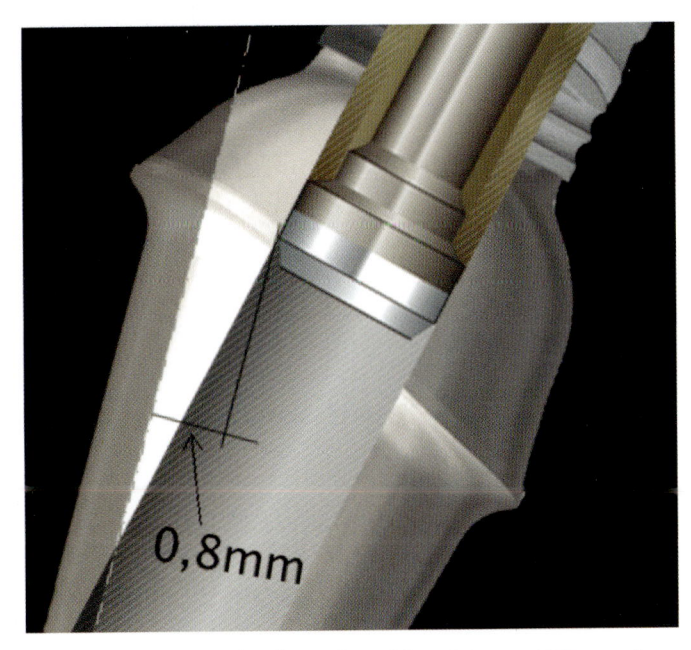

Figure 20.21 (A) Graphic illustration of the minimum thickness of zirconia required around the abutment screw head to avoid fracture under function.

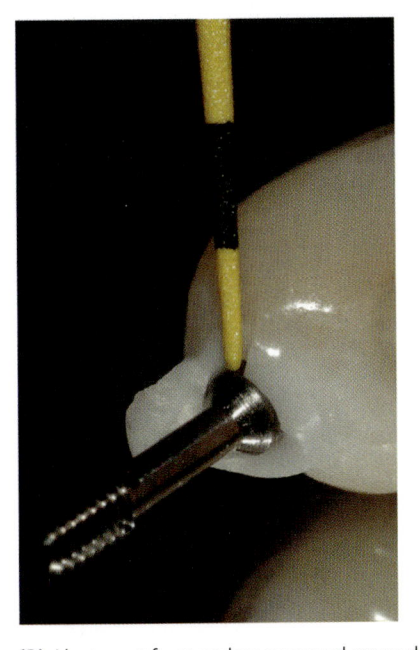

Figure 20.21 (B) Abutment fracture has occurred around the abutment screw due to thinning of the zirconia; this was deemed to be the result of the facial position of one of the implants supporting a fixed partial denture.

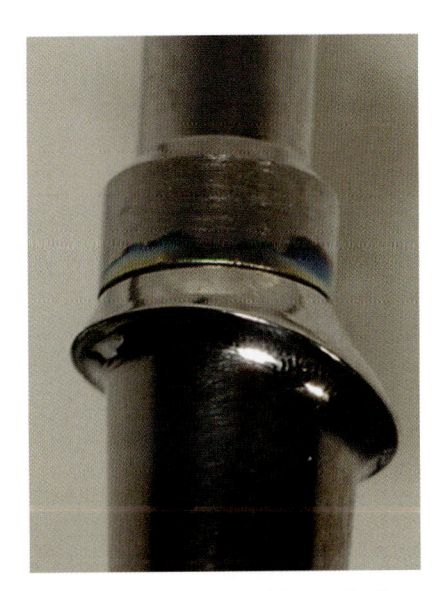

Figure 20.22 (A) Titanium abutment with an apically repositioned margin or cement line, in an effort to reduce the graying effect of titanium.

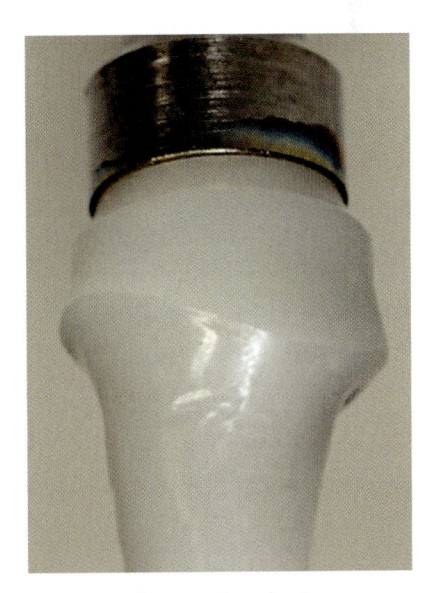

Figure 20.22 (B) In a similar case, zirconia allows a more coronal margin placement, because the white color of the zirconia will minimally impact the gingival tissue color.

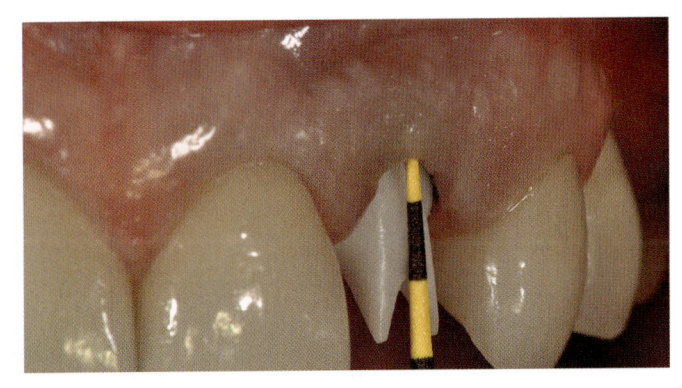

Figure 20.22 (C) An ideally designed abutment with a minimally submerged margin (0.5–1.0 mm) allows relatively easy access for cement removal.

feldspathic porcelain is commonly encountered in clinical practice and is attributable to several factors, including the bond between the veneering ceramic and zirconia substructure,[102–106] inadequate framework support design,[107,108] as well as residual stress buildup caused by the thermal mismatch between the veneering porcelain and the zirconia substructure. Tensile and compressive residual stresses can increase the occurrence of chipping.

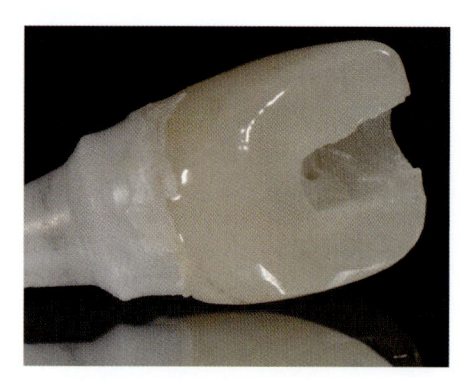

Figure 20.23 **(A)** Retrieved crown removed as a result of chronic marginal tissue discomfort. Note the retained cement circumferentially around the restoration margin.

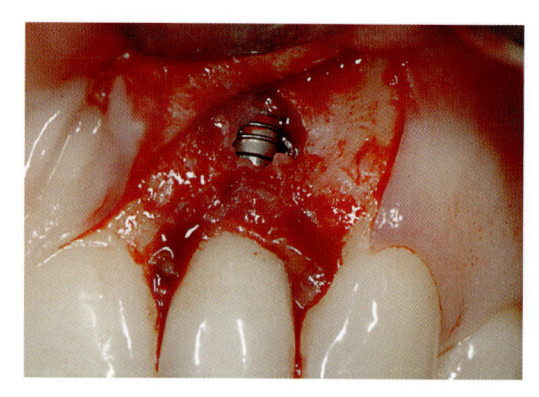

Figure 20.23 **(B)** Retained cement has resulted in extensive bone loss at the implant–abutment interface. Note crestal granulation tissue and thread exposure apical to this.

Design and cementation

The guidelines for zirconia crown dimensions are essentially the same for natural abutments and implants, effectively allowing room for adequate veneering porcelain application. The substructure copings of the crowns for zirconia crowns, if they are to be fully veneered, require anatomic designs and not just thimble-like shapes, which will result in unsupported veneering porcelain. Figure 20.24A–J shows ideal abutment design and cement-line position, which, coupled with careful placement of a retraction cord, minimizes the risk for subgingival cement trapping. Figure 20.25A–E shows a simple bench-top method to ensure adequate, but not excessive, cement before intraoral introduction to the abutment.[109]

Modified axial wall designs may allow better venting during cementation, thus allowing the crown to seat more fully. It can also minimize the cement thickness, which has been shown, at least in the case of zinc phosphate, to improve the retention of

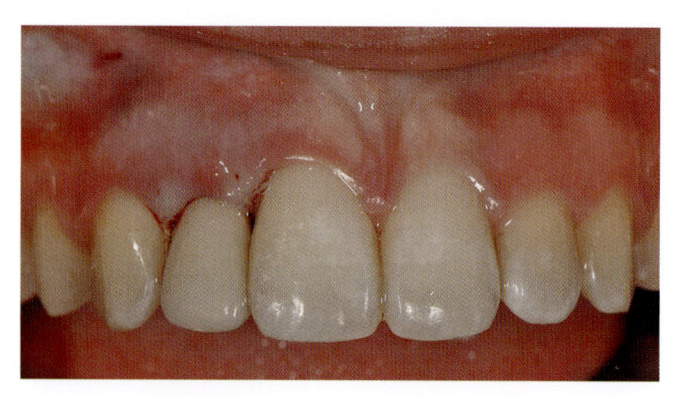

Figure 20.24 **(A)** Facial view: provisional restoration inserted at the time of implant placement.

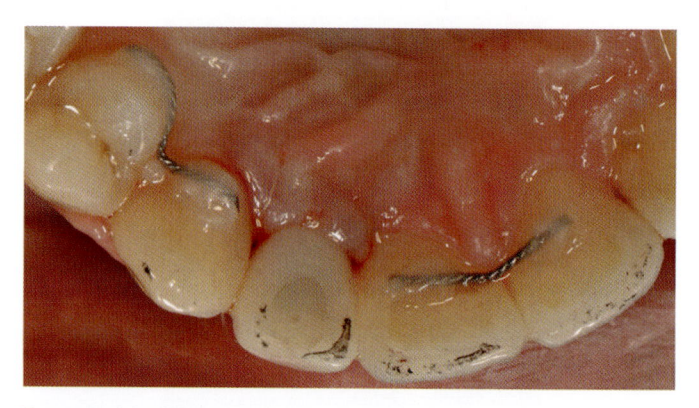

Figure 20.24 **(B)** Occlusal view: provisional restoration before elimination of eccentric contacts/guidance.

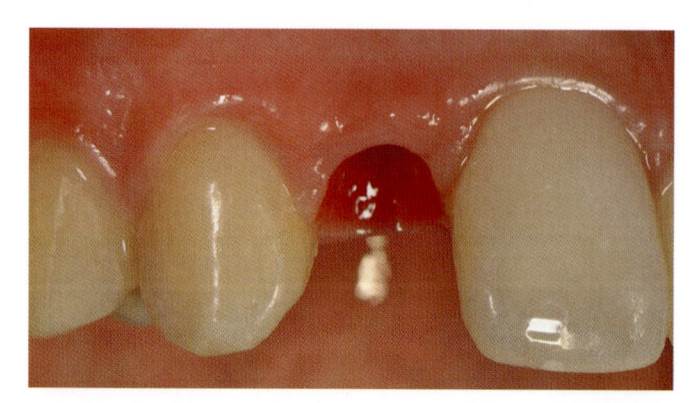

Figure 20.24 **(C)** Three months postsurgery: developed tissue as defined by the provisional restoration.

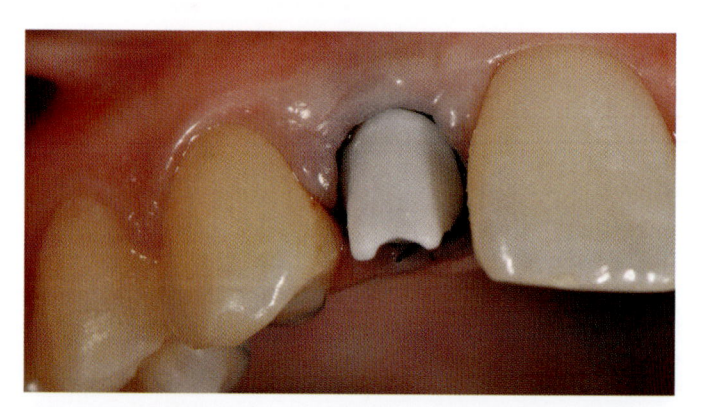

Figure 20.24 **(D)** Occlusal view 1: zirconia abutment delivered and torqued to 35 N cm. A retraction cord has been placed below the margin to deflect excess cement away from the sulcus.

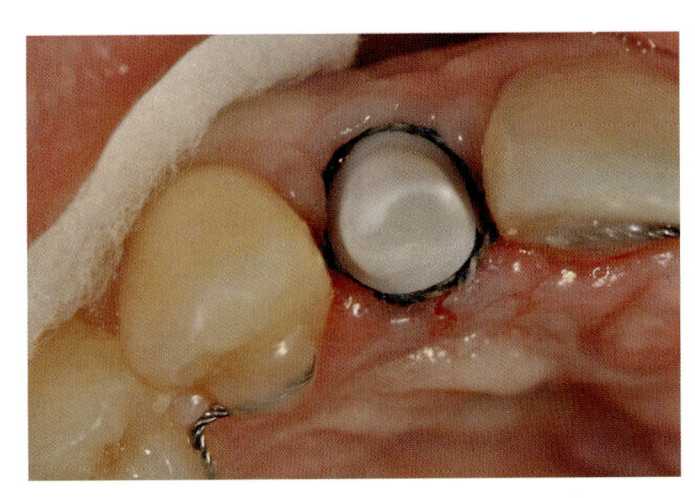

Chapter 20 Implant Esthetics: Concepts, Surgical Procedures, and Materials

Figure 20.24 (E) Occlusal view 2: complete visualization of the retraction cord.

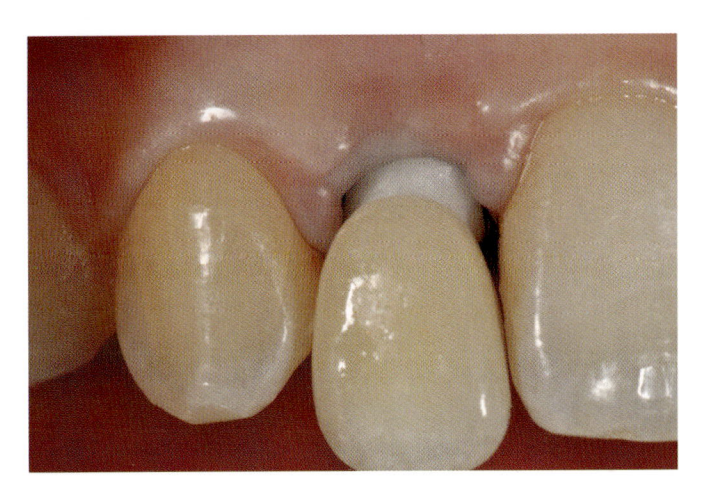

Figure 20.24 (F) Insertion of the definitive crown. Note that cement is not spilling out of the crown as adequate, but not excessive, cement has been placed in the crown.

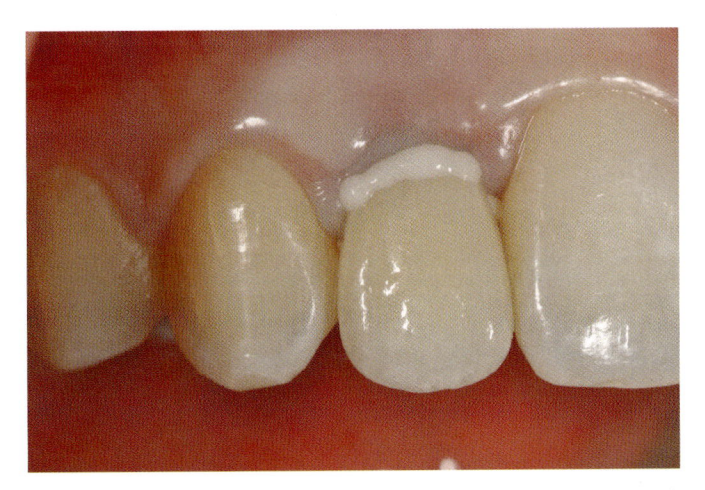

Figure 20.24 (G) Minor cement expulsion as the crown is fully seated.

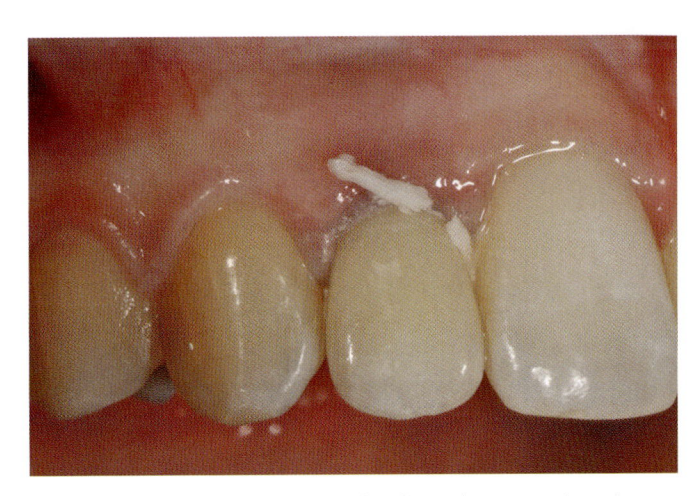

Figure 20.24 (H) Cement is trapped and introduction to the sulcus limited by the cord.

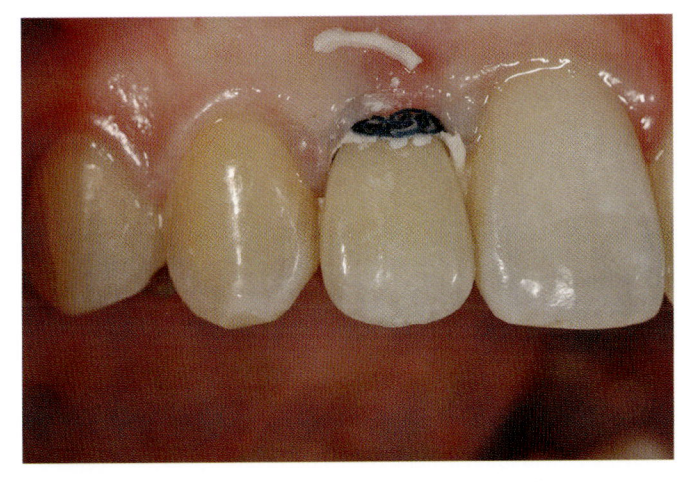

Figure 20.24 (I) Removal of the retraction cord with adherent cement.

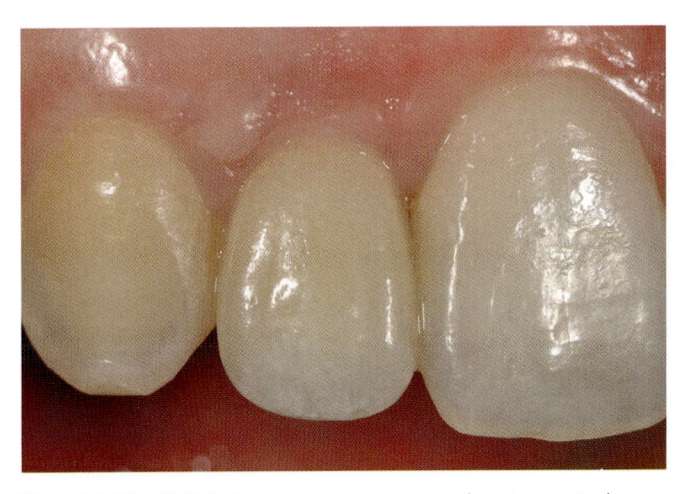

Figure 20.24 (J) Definitive restoration as viewed postoperatively.

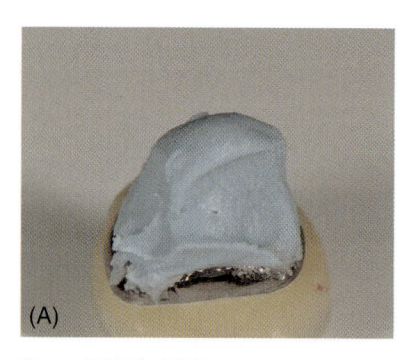

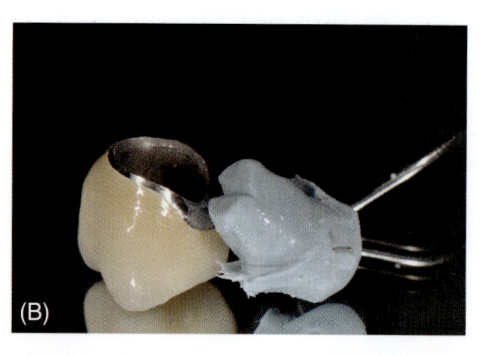

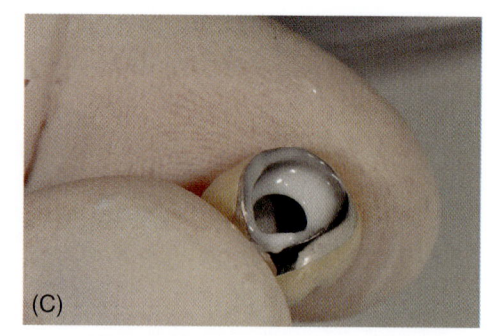

Figure 20.25 **(A)** Bite registration paste introduced into the restoration. **(B)** Retrieved impression of the intaglio surface of the definitive restoration. A notch is cut into the occlusal to create space for a cement to ensure sufficient, but not excess, volume. **(C)** Cement is introduced into the crown.

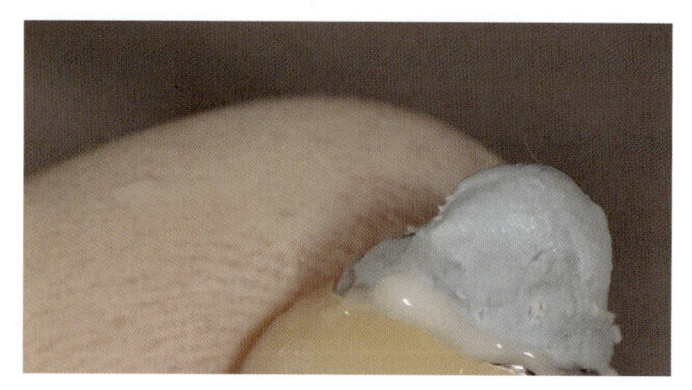

Figure 20.25 **(D)** Reintroduction of the bite registration index. Note that excess cement is expressed extraorally.

the crown. The cement layer must spread along the entire axial wall and margin of the abutment to achieve maximum retention.[110] In addition, resin cements show higher peak loads (better fracture resistance) than temporary cements or resin-modified glass ionomers, resulting in increased retention, better marginal adaptation, and less microleakage.[111] For effective bonding of zirconia to titanium or to zirconia itself, a cement containing methacryloyloxydecyl dihydrogen phosphate, adhesive, or silane or the use of tribochemical silica coating such as CoJet™ (3 M ESPE) or air particle abrasion with 30–50 μm aluminum oxide particles are recommended as these materials and techniques can improve the bond strength.

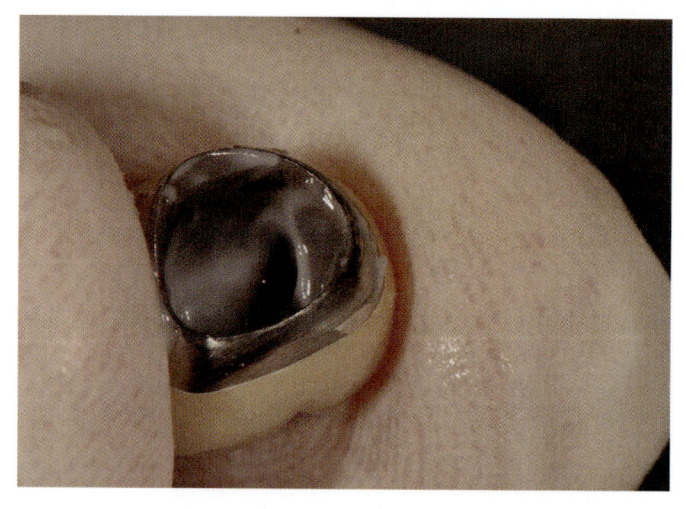

Figure 20.25 **(E)** Removal of the impression material reveals adequate and well-distributed cement. The crown is now ready for intraoral introduction to the abutment.

Lithium disilicate glass-based ceramics (e.max®, Ivoclar Vivadent, Liechtenstein), which allow surface modification through hydrofluoric acid etching, exhibit excellent clinical performance as a metal-free ceramic in restoration of the natural dentition and implants.[112,113] The etching of the glass results in additional adhesive strength, improving the fracture resistance of the crown, provided the zirconia abutment surface can be

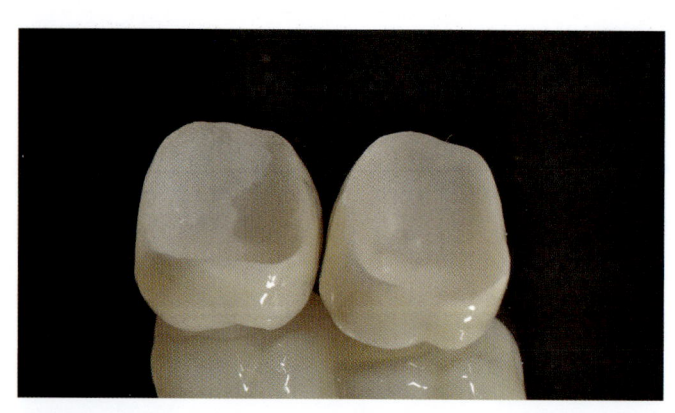

Figure 20.26 **(A)** Etchable lithium disilicate (EMAX, Ivoclar Vivadent, Lichtenstein) and a nonetchable full-contour (Wieland Zeno-Tec, Mannheim, Germany) zirconia crown.

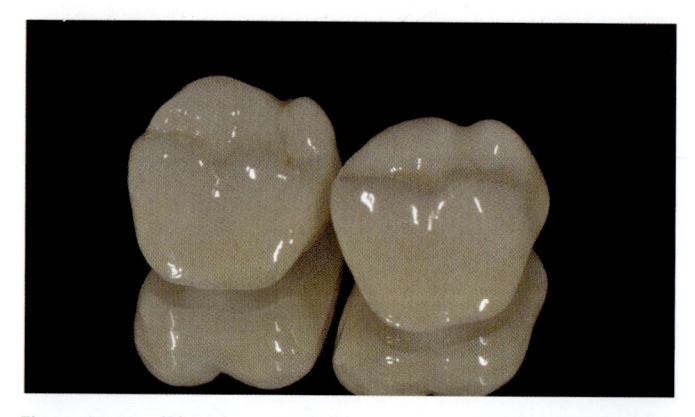

Figure 20.26 **(B)** Both restoration materials produce excellent esthetic results.

similarly modified. This material can be either stained in monolithic form or partially veneered in nonfunctional areas to improve esthetics.

More recently, manufacturers have improved the esthetic appearance of zirconia with increased translucency without having to add veneering feldspathic porcelain. Monolithic zirconia can be conventionally cemented and essentially can provide a fracture-free solution, particularly in the posterior regions of the mouth where isolation for resin bonding is more difficult. This has been described as the "full contour" or monolithic zirconia crown.[114,115] Figure 20.26A and B compares etchable lithium disilicate (e.max, Ivoclar) and a nonetchable zirconia crown (Wieland Zeno-Tec, Mannheim, Germany). Note that the esthetic results of the crowns are similar. Of importance, the full contour zirconia crown is virtually three times as strong as the lithium disilicate crown, making it a superior material for use in high-load areas such as molar regions or in individuals displaying parafunctional activities.

References

1. Chen ST, Buser D. Clinical and esthetic outcomes of implants placed in postextraction sites. *Int J Oral Maxillofac Implants* 2009;24(Suppl):186–217.
2. Grutter L, Belser UC. Implant loading protocols for the partially edentulous esthetic zone. *Int J Oral Maxillofac Implants* 2009;24(Suppl):169–179.
3. Lang NP, Pun L, Lau KY, et al. A systematic review on survival and success rates of implants placed immediately into fresh extraction sockets after at least 1 year. *Clin Oral Implants Res* 2012;23(Suppl 5):39–66.
4. Esposito M, Grusovin MG, Willings M, et al. The effectiveness of immediate, early, and conventional loading of dental implants: a Cochrane systematic review of randomized controlled clinical trials. *Int J Oral Maxillofac Implants* 2007;22(6):893–904.
5. Holm-Pedersen P, Lang NP, Muller F. What are the longevities of teeth and oral implants. *Clin Oral Implants Res* 2008;19(3):326–328.
6. Zachrisson BJ. Esthetic factors involved in anterior tooth display and the smile: vertical dimension. *J Clin Orthod* 1998;32(7):432–445.
7. Tjan, AHL, Miller GD. The JGP: some esthetic factors in a smile. *J Prosth Dent* 1984;51:24–28.
8. Tan WL, Wong TWL, Wong MCM, Lang NP. A systematic review of post-extractional alveolar bone dimensional changes in humans. *Clin Oral Implants Res* 2012;23(Suppl 5):1–21.
9. Schropp L, Wenzel A, Kostopoulos L, Karring T. Bone healing and soft tissue contour changes following single tooth extraction: a clinical and radiographic 12-month prospective study. *Int J Periodontics Restorative Dent* 2003;23:313–323.
10. Araujo MG, Lindhe J. Dimensional ridge alterations following tooth extraction. An experimental study in the dog. *J Clin Periodontol* 2005;32(2):212–218.
11. Nevins M, Camelo M, De Paoli S, et al. A study of the fate of the buccal wall of extraction sockets of teeth with prominent roots. *Int J Periodontics Restorative Dent* 2006;26:19–29.
12. Vignoletti F, Matesanz P, Rodrigo D, et al. Surgical protocols for ridge preservation after tooth extraction. A systematic review. *Clin Oral Implants Res* 2012;23(Suppl 5):22–38.
13. Hammerle CHF, Araujo MG, Simion M. Evidence-based knowledge on the biology and treatment of extraction sockets. *Clin Oral Implants Res* 2012;23(Suppl 5):80–82.
14. Lee SL, Kim HJ, Son MK, Chung CH. Anthropometric analysis of maxillary anterior buccal bone of Korean adults using cone-beam CT. *J Adv Prosthodont* 2010;2(3):92–96.
15. Fickl S, Zuhr O, Wachtel H, et al. Tissue alterations after tooth extraction with and without surgical trauma: a volumetric study in the beagle dog. *J Clin Periodontol* 2008;35(4):356–363.
16. Ten Heggeler JMAG, Slot DE, Van der Weijden GA. Effect of socket preservation therapies following tooth extraction in non-molar regions in humans: a systematic review. *Clin Oral Implants Res* 2011;22(8):779–788.
17. Morjaria KR, Wilson R, Palmer RM. Bone healing after tooth extraction with or without an intervention: a systematic review of randomized controlled trials. *Clin Implant Dent Relat Res* 2014;16(1):1–20.
18. Grunder U, Gracis S, Capelli M. Influence of the 3-D bone-to-implant relationship on esthetics. *Int J Periodontics Restorative Dent* 2005;25:113–119.
19. Buser D, Dula K, Hirt HP, Schenk RK. Lateral ridge augmentation using autografts and barrier membranes. a clinical study in 40 partially edentulous patients. *J Oral Maxillofac Surg* 1996;54:420–432.
20. Chiapasco M, Zaniboni M, Boisco M. Augmentation procedures for the rehabilitation of deficient edentulous ridges with oral implants. *Clin Oral Implants Res* 2006;17(Suppl 2):136–159.
21. Esposito M, Grusovin MG, Felice P, et al. The efficacy of horizontal and vertical bone augmentation procedures for dental implants: a Cochrane systematic review. *Eur J Oral Implantol* 2009;2(3):167–184.
22. Rocchietta I, Fontana F, Simion M. Clinical outcomes of vertical bone augmentation to enable dental implant placement: a systematic review. *J Clin Periodontol* 2008;35(Suppl 8):203–215.
23. Wallace S, Gellin R. Clinical evaluation of a cancellous block allograft for ridge augmentation and implant placement: a case report. *Implant Dent* 2008;17(2):151–158.
24. Nissan J, Mardinger O, Calderon S, et al. Cancellous bone block allografts for augmentation of the anterior atrophic maxilla. *Clin Implant Dent Relat Res* 2011;13(2):104–111.
25. Waasdorp J, Reynolds MA. Allogenic bone onlay grafts for alveolar ridge augmentation: a systematic review. *Int J Oral Maxillofac Implants* 2010;25:525–531.
26. Nissan J, Marilena V, Gross O, et al. Histomorphometric analysis following augmentation of the anterior atrophic maxilla with cancellous bone block allograft. *Int J Oral Maxillofac Implants* 2012;27:84–89.
27. Nevins ML, Reynolds MA. Tissue engineering with recombinant human platelet-derived growth factor BB for implant site development. *Compend Contin Educ Dent* 2011;32(2):18, 20–27.
28. Chang P-C, Seol Y, Cirelli J, et al. PDGF-B gene therapy accelerates bone engineering and oral implant osseointegration. *Gene Ther* 2010;17(1):95–104.
29. Esposito M, Grusovin MG, Polyzos IP, et al. Timing of implant placement after tooth extraction: immediate, immediate-delayed or delayed implants? A Cochrane systematic review. *Eur J Oral Implantol* 2010;3(3):189–205.
30. Adell R, Lekholm U, Rockler B, Branemark PI. A 15-year study of osseointegrated implants in the treatment of the edentulous jaw. *Int J Oral Surg* 1981;10:387–416.
31. Chen ST, Wilson TG Jr, Hammerle CH. Immediate or early placement of implants following tooth extraction: review of biologic basis, clinical procedures, and outcomes. *Int J Oral Maxillofac Implants* 2004;19:12–25.

32. Buser D, Bornstein MM, Weber HP, et al. Early implant placement with simultaneous guided bone regeneration following single-tooth extraction in the esthetic zone: a cross-sectional, retrospective study in 45 subjects with a 2- to 4-year follow-up. *J Periodontol* 2008;79:1773–1781.
33. Buser D, Chen ST, Weber HP, Belser UC. Early implant placement following single-tooth extraction in the esthetic zone: biologic rationale and surgical procedures. *Int J Periodontics Restorative Dent* 2008;28:441–451.
34. Buser D, Wittneben J, Bornstein MM, et al. Stability of contour augmentation and esthetic outcomes of implant-supported single crowns in the esthetic zone: 3-year results of a prospective study with early implant placement postextraction. *J Periodontol* 2011;82:342–349.
35. Sanz I, Garcia-Gargalio M, Herrara D, et al. Surgical protocols for early implant placement in post-extraction sockets. A systematic review. *Clin Oral Implants Res* 2012;23(Suppl 5):67–79.
36. Wang HL, Ormianer Z, Palti A, et al. Consensus conference on immediate loading: the single tooth and partial edentulous areas. *Implant Dent* 2006;15(4):324–333.
37. Atieh AMA, Atieh AH, Payne AG, Duncan WJ. Immediate loading with single implant crowns: a systematic review and meta-analysis. *Int J Prosthodont* 2009;22(4):378–387.
38. Cooper LF, Raes F, Reside GJ, et al. Comparison of radiographic and clinical outcomes following immediate provisionalization of single-tooth dental implants placed in healed alveolar ridges and extraction sockets. *Int J Oral Maxillofac Implants* 2010;25:1222–1232.
39. Den Hartog L, Slater JJ, Vissink A, et al. Treatment outcome of immediate, early and conventional single-tooth implants in the aesthetic zone: a systematic review of survival, bone level, soft-tissue, aesthetics and patient satisfaction. *Clin Periodontol* 2008;35:1073–1086.
40. Crespi R, Cappare P, Gherlone E, Romanos GE. Immediate versus delayed loading of dental implants placed in fresh extraction sockets in the maxillary esthetic zone: a clinical comparative study. *Int J Oral Maxillofac Implants* 2008;23:753–758.
41. Evans, CD, Chen ST. Esthetic outcomes of immediate implant placement. *Clin Oral Implants Res* 2008;19:73–80.
42. Block MS, Mercante DE, Lirette D, et al. Prospective evaluation of immediate and delayed provisional single tooth restorations. *J Oral Maxillofac Surg* 2009;67:89–107.
43. De Rouck T, Collys K, Wyn I, Cosyn J. Instant provisionalization of immediate single-tooth implants is essential to optimize esthetic treatment outcomes. *Clin Oral Implants Res* 2009;20(6):566–570.
44. Cosyn J, Eghbali A, De Bruyn H, et al. Immediate single-tooth implants in the anterior maxilla: 3-year results of a case series on hard and soft tissue response and aesthetics. *J Clin Periodontol* 2011;38(8):746–753.
45. Tarnow DP, Cho SC, Wallace SS. The effect of inter-implant distance on the height of inter-implant bone crest. *J Periodontol* 2000;71:546–549.
46. Bashutski JD, Wang HL. Common implant esthetic complications. *Implant Dent* 2007;16:340–348.
47. Van Steenberghe D, Naert I, Andersson M, et al. A custom template and definitive prosthesis allowing immediate loading in the maxilla: a clinical report. *Int J Oral Maxillofac Implants* 2002;17:663–670.
48. Ersoy AE, Turkyilmaz I, Oguz O, McGlumphy EA. Reliability of implant placement with stereolithographic surgical guides generated from computed tomography: clinical data from 94 implants. *J Periodontol* 2008;79:1339–1345.
49. Valente F, Schiroli G, Sbrenna A. Accuracy of computer-aided oral implant surgery: a clinical and radiographic study. *Int J Oral Maxillofac Implants* 2009;24:234–242.
50. Mandelaris GA, Rosenfeld AL, King SD, Nevins ML. Computer-guided implant dentistry for precise implant placement: combining specialized stereolithographically generated drilling guides and surgical implant instrumentation. *Int J Periodontics Restorative Dent* 2010;30:275–281.
51. Spray RJ, Black CG, Morris HR, Ochi S. The influence of bone thickness on facial marginal bone response: stage 1 placement through stage 2 uncovering. *Ann Periodontol* 2000;5:119–128.
52. Kan JY, Rungcharassaeng K, Umezu K, Kois JC. Dimensions of peri-implant mucosa: an evaluation of maxillary anterior single implants in humans. *J Periodontol* 2003;4:557–562.
53. Tarnow D, Elian N, Fletcher P, et al. Vertical distance from the crest of bone to the height of the interproximal papilla between adjacent implants. *J Periodontol* 2003;74(12):1785–1788.
54. Gastaldo GF, Cury PR, Sendyk WR. Effect of the vertical and horizontal distances between adjacent implants and between a tooth and an implant on the incidence of interproximal papilla. *J. Periodontol* 2004;75(9):1242–1246.
55. Kan JY, Rungcharassaeng K. Interimplant papilla preservation in the esthetic zone: a report of six consecutive cases. *Int J Periodontics Restorative Dent* 2003;23(3):249–259.
56. Leziy S, Miller B. The papilla between adjacent implants: treatment planning to optimize aesthetic outcomes. In: Cohen M, ed. *Interdisciplinary Treatment Planning*, vol. 2. Quintessence Publishing; 2011.
57. Barros RR, Novaes AB Jr, Muglia VA, et al. Influence of interimplant distances and placement depth on peri-implant remodeling of adjacent and immediately loaded Morse cone connection implants: a histomorphometric study in dogs. *Clin Oral Implants Res* 2010;21(4):371–378.
58. Tomasi C, Sanz M, Cecchinato D, et al. Bone dimensional variations at implants placed in fresh extraction sockets: a multilevel multivariate analysis. *Clin Oral Implants Res* 2010;21(1):30–36.
59. Caneva M, Salata LA, de Souza SS, et al. Influence of implant positioning in extraction sockets on osseointegration: histomorphometric analyses in dogs. *Clin Oral Implants Res* 2010;21(1):43–49.
60. Wennerberg A, Albrektsson T. On implant surfaces: a review of current knowledge and opinions. *Int J Oral Maxillofac Implants* 2009;24:63–74.
61. Gracis S, Michalakis K, Vigolo P et al. Internal vs. external connections for abutments or reconstructions: a systematic review. *Clin Oral Implants Res* 2012;23(Suppl 6):202–216.
62. Hermann JS, Schoolfield JD, Schenk RK et al. Influence of the size of the microgap on crestal bone changes around titanium implants. A histometric evaluation of unloaded non-submerged implants in the canine mandible. *J Periodontol* 2001;72(10):1372–1383.
63. Lazzara RJ, Porter SS. Platform switching: a new concept in implant dentistry for controlling postrestorative crestal bone levels. *Int J Periodontics Rest Dent* 2006;26(1):9–17.
64. Atieh MA, Ibrahim HM, Atieh AH. Platform switching for marginal bone preservation around dental implants: a systematic review and meta-analysis. *J Periodontol* 2010;81(10):1350–1366.
65. Annibali S, Bignozzi I, Cristalli MP, et al. Peri-implant marginal bone level: a systematic review and meta-analysis of studies comparing platform switching versus conventionally restored implants. *J Clin Periodontol* 2012;39(11):1097–1113.
66. Stafford GL. Evidence supporting platform-switching to preserve marginal bone levels not definitive. *Evid Based Dent* 2012;13(2):56–57.

67. Kois JC. Predictable single tooth peri-implant esthetics: five diagnostic keys. *Compend Contin Educ Dent* 2001;22:199–206.
68. Esposito M, Hirsch JM, Lekholm U, Thomsen P. Biological factors contributing to failures of osseointegrated oral implants: (1) Success criteria and epidemiology. *Eur J Oral Sci* 1998;106:527–551.
69. Lee A, Fu JH, Wang HL. Soft tissue biotype affects implant success *Implant Dent* 2011;20(3):e38–e47.
70. Fu HJ, Lee A, Wang HL. Influence of tissue biotype on implant esthetics. *Int J Oral Maxillofac Implants* 2011;26(3):499–508.
71. Zigdon H, Machtei EE. The dimensions of keratinized mucosa around implant affect clinical and immunological parameters. *Clin Oral Implants Res* 2008;19:387–392.
72. Olsson M, Lindhe J, Marinello CP. On the relationship between crown form and clinical features of the gingiva in adolescents. *J Clin Periodontol* 1993;20:570–577.
73. Müller HP, Heinecke A, Schaller N, Eger T. Masticatory mucosa in subjects with different periodontal phenotypes. *J Clin Periodontol* 2000;27:621–626.
74. Kan JY, Morimoto T, Rungcharassaeng K, et al. Gingival biotype assessment in the esthetic zone: visual versus direct measurement. *Int J Periodontics Restorative Dent* 2010;30:237–243.
75. Bouri A Jr, Bissada N, Al-Zahrani MS, et al. Width of keratinized gingiva and the health status of supporting tissues around dental implants. *Int J Oral Maxillofac Implants* 2008;23:323–326.
76. Linkevicius T, Apse P, Grybauskas S, Puisys A. The influence of soft tissue thickness on crestal bone changes around implants: a 1-year prospective controlled clinical trial. *Int J Oral Maxillofac Implants* 2009;24(4):712–719.
77. Chung DM, Oh TJ, Shotwell JL, et al. Significance of keratinized mucosa in maintenance of dental implants with different surfaces. *J Periodontol* 2006;77:1410–1420.
78. Eghbali A, De Rouck T, de Bruyn H, Cosyn J. The gingival biotype assessed by experienced and inexperienced clinicians. *J Clin Periodontol* 2009;36:958–963.
79. Jung RE, Sailer I, Hämmerle CH, et al. In vitro color changes of soft tissues caused by restorative materials. *Int J Periodontics Restorative Dent* 2007;27(3):251–257.
80. Kan JYK, Rungcharassaeng K, Lozada JL, Zimmerman G. Facial gingival tissue stability following immediate placement and provisionalization of maxillary anterior single implants: a 2- to 8-year follow-up. *Int J Oral Maxillofac Implants* 2011;26:179–187.
81. Rompen E, Touati B, Van Dooren E. Factors influencing marginal tissue remodeling around implants. *Pract Proced Aesthet Dent* 2003;15(10):754–757.
82. Redemagni M, Cremonesi S, Garlini G, Maiorana C. Soft tissue stability with immediate implants and concave abutments. *Eur J Esthet Dent* 2009;4(4):328–337.
83. Wiesner G, Esposito M, Worthington H, Schlee M. Connective tissue grafts for thickening peri-implant tissues at implant placement. One-year results from an explanatory split-mouth randomized controlled clinical trial. *Eur J Oral Implantol* 2010;3(1):27–35.
84. Lozada JL, Zimmerman G. Tissue and bone grafting in conjunction with immediate single-tooth replacement in the esthetic zone: a case series. *Int J Oral Maxillofac Implants* 2011;26:427–436.
85. Mathews DP. The pediculated connective tissue graft: a technique for improving unaesthetic implant restorations. *Pract Proced Aesthet Dent* 2002;14(9):719–724.
86. Yan JJ, Tsai AY, Wong MY, Hou LT. Comparison of acellular dermal graft and palatal autograft in the reconstruction of keratinized gingiva around dental implants: a case report. *Int J Periodontics Restorative Dent* 2006;26:287–292.
87. Leziy SS, Miller BA. Developing ideal implant tissue architecture and pontic site form. *Quintessence Dent Technol* 2007;30:143–154.
88. Priest G. A restorative protocol for implants replacing adjacent maxillary central incisors in a compromised site. *J Implant Reconstr Dent* 2009;1(1):15–19.
89. Lang LA, Turkyilmaz I, Edgin WA, et al. Immediate restoration of single tapered implants with nonoccluding provisional crowns: a 5-year clinical prospective study. *Clin Implant Dent Relat Res* 2014;16(2):248–258.
90. De Rouck T, Collys K, Cosyn J. Immediate single tooth implants in the anterior maxilla: a 1-year case cohort study on hard and soft tissue response. *J Clin Periodontol* 2008;35:649–657.
91. Raes F, Cosyn J, Crommelinck E, et al. Immediate and conventional single implant treatment in the anterior maxilla: 1-year results of a case series on hard and soft tissue response and aesthetics. *J Clin Periodontol* 2011;28(4):385–394.
92. Glauser R, Sailer I, Wohlwend A, et al. Experimental zirconia abutments for implant-supported single-tooth restorations in esthetically demanding regions: 4-year results of a prospective clinical study. *Int J Prosthodont* 2004;17:285–290.
93. Butz F, Heydecke G, Okutan M, Strub JR. Survival rate, fracture strength and failure mode of ceramic implant abutments after chewing simulation. *J Oral Rehabil* 2005;32:838–843.
94. Gehrke P, Dhom G, Brunner J, et al. Zirconium implant abutments: fracture strength and influence of cyclic loading on retaining-screw loosening. *Quintessence Int* 2006;27:19–26.
95. Rimondini L, Cerroni L, Carrassi A, Torricelli P. Bacterial colonization of zirconia ceramic surfaces: an in vitro and in vivo study. *Int J Oral Maxillofac Implants* 2002;17(6):793–798.
96. Scarano A, Piattelli M, Caputi S, et al. Bacterial adhesion on commercially pure titanium and zirconium oxide disks: an in vivo human study. *J Periodontol* 2004;75:292–296.
97. Nakamura K, Kanno T, Milleding P, Ortengren U. Zirconia as a dental implant abutment material: a systematic review. *Int J Prosthodont* 2010;23(4):299–309.
98. Mustafa K, Wennerberg A, Arvidson K, et al. Influence of modifying and veneering the surface of ceramic abutments on cellular attachment and proliferation. *Clin Oral Implants Res* 2008;19(11):1178–1187.
99. Watkin A, Kerstein RB. Improving darkened anterior peri-implant tissue color with zirconia custom implant abutments. *Compend Contin Educ Dent* 2008;29:238–240.
100. Thomas GW. The positive relationship between excess cement and peri-implant disease: a prospective clinical endoscopic study. *J Periodontol* 2009;80(9):1388–1392.
101. Tarica DY, Alvarado VM, Truong ST. Survey of United States dental schools on cementation protocols for implant crown restorations. *J Prosthet Dent* 2010;103:68–79.
102. White SN, Miklus VG, McLaren EA, et al. Flexural strength of a layered zirconia and porcelain dental allceramic system. *J Prosthet Dent* 2005;94:125–131.
103. Scherrer SS, Quinn JB, Quinn GD, Kelly JR. Failure analysis of ceramic clinical cases using qualitative fractography. *Int J Prosthodont* 2006;19:185–192.
104. Aboushelib MN, de Jager N, Kleverlaan CJ, Feilzer AJ. Microtensile bond strength of different components of core veneered all-ceramic restorations. *Dent Mater* 2005;21(10):984–991.
105. Aboushelib MN, Kleverlaan CJ, Feilzer AJ. Microtensile bond strength of different components of core veneered all-ceramic restorations. Part II: zirconia veneering ceramics. *Dent Mater* 2006;22(9):857–863.

106. Jung RE, Pjetursson BE, Glauser R, et al. A systematic review of the 5-year survival and complication rates of implant-supported single crowns. *Clin Oral Implants Res* 2008;19:119–130.
107. Strub JR, Stiffler S, Scharer P. Causes of failure following oral rehabilitation: biological versus technical factors. *Quintessence Int* 1988;19(3):215–222.
108. Choi Y-S, Kim S-H, Lee J-B, et al. In vitro evaluation of fracture strength of zirconia restoration veneered with various ceramic materials. *J Adv Prosthodont* 2012;4(3):162–169.
109. Wadhwani C, Pineyro A, Hess T, et al. Effect of implant abutment modification on the extrusion of excess cement at the crown–abutment margin for cement-retained implant restorations. *Int J Oral Maxillofac Implants* 2011;26(6):1241–1246.
110. Tan KM, Masri R, Driscoll CF, et al. Effect of axial wall modification on the retention of cement-retained, implant-supported crowns. *J Prosthet Dent* 2012;107(2):80–85.
111. Carnaggio TV, Conrad R, Engelmeier RL, et al. Retention of CAD/CAM all-ceramic crowns on prefabricated implant abutments: an in vitro comparative study of luting agents and abutment surface area. *J Prosthodont* 2012;21(7):523–528.
112. Silva NR, Thompson VP, Valverde GB, et al. Comparative reliability analyses of zirconium oxide and lithium disilicate restorations in vitro and in vivo. *J Am Dent Assoc* 2011;142(Suppl 2):4S–9S.
113. Albrecht T, Kirsten A, Kappert HR, Fischer H. Fracture load of different crown systems on zirconia implant abutments. *Dent Mater* 2011;27(3):298–303.
114. Preis V, Behr M, Hahnel S, et al. In vitro failure and fracture resistance of veneered and full-contour zirconia restorations. *J Dent* 2012;40(11):921–928.
115. Beuer F, Stimmelmayr M, Gueth JF, et al. In vitro performance of full-contour zirconia single crowns. *Dent Mater* 2012;28(4):449–456.

Appendix A Esthetic Evaluation Form Summary

The esthetic evaluation form is a tool for the clinician to identify the esthetic problem, visualize a solution, and then choose the appropriate technique. To *Identify the problems* and visualize the solution through a three-step analysis of the macro- and micro-esthetics and function, we use the Esthetic Evaluation Form as an esthetic checklist, digital pictures, and mounted study casts. We *Visualize the solution* through a diagnostic wax-up of the mounted study casts, and via intraoral mock-up. Once the solution is visualized, we *Choose the appropriate technique*, which means the most conservative option that will achieve your esthetic goals. The key objective of the Esthetic Evaluation Form is to establish the incisal edge position and the gingival margin of the maxillary central incisor, two critical landmarks while focusing on three views, facial, dentofacial and dental.

Aesthetic Evaluation Form©

Patient _____ Examiner _____ Date _____

1. Effective Questions

:A: If there was anything you could change about your smile, what would it be?
_____
_____

:B: Do you like the visual image of "Straight, White, Perfect", "Clean, Healthy, Natural", or "White and Natural" looking teeth?
_____
_____

:C: History of Aesthetic Change
_____
_____

:D: Previous Records – Do you have any photos of your smile, or any smile you like, to aid in aesthetic treatment planning?
○ Yes   ○ No

2 Facial Analysis

:A: Full Smile

1. **Interpupillary Line to Occlusal Plane**
   ○ Parallel
   ○ Canted right
   ○ Canted left

2. **Midline Relationship of Teeth** (Maxillary) **to Face** (Philtrum)
   ○ Coincident
   ○ Right of center
   ○ Left of center

3. **Relationship of Lips to Face** (Lip Symmetry)
   ○ Symmetrical
   ○ Left side higher
   ○ Right side higher

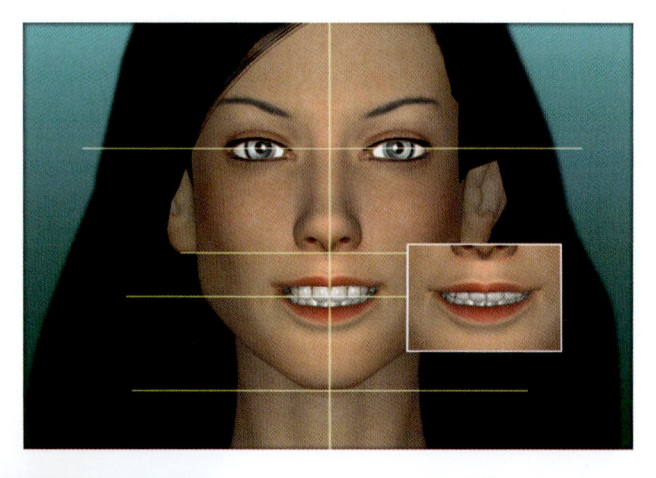

:B: Lips at Rest

1. **Upper Lip**
   ○ Full
   ○ Average
   ○ Thin

2. **Lower Lip**
   ○ Full
   ○ Average
   ○ Thin

3. **Lips**
   ○ Prominent
   ○ Retruded

4. **Tooth Exposure at Rest:**
   Maxillary _____ mm
   Mandibular _____ mm

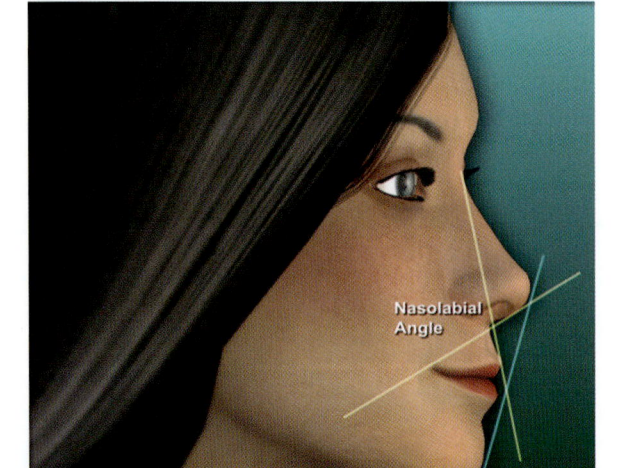

:C: Profile View: Facially – Directed Treatment Planning

1. **Nasolabial Angle**
   ○ Normal (approx. 90°)
   ○ Prominent Maxilla (<90°)
   ○ Retruded Maxilla (>90°)

2. **Ricketts E-Plane** (Drawn from tip of nose to chin)
   Upper Lip to E-Plane _____ mm (ideally 4 mm)
   Lower Lip to E-Plane _____ mm (ideally 2 mm)

3. **Profile Shape**
   ○ WNL   ○ Convex   ○ Concave

If maxilla is prominent, nasolabial angle is < 90°, or profile is convex, consider smaller, less dominant maxillary anterior restorations.

If maxilla is retruded, nasolabial angle is > 90°, or profile is concave, consider more dominant maxillary anterior restorations.

Aesthetic Evaluation Form created by Jonathan B. Levine, DMD

3. Dentofacial Analysis – Vertical and Horizontal Components

:A: Upper Smile Line
- ○ Average 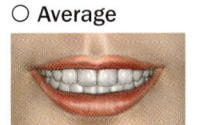
- ○ High 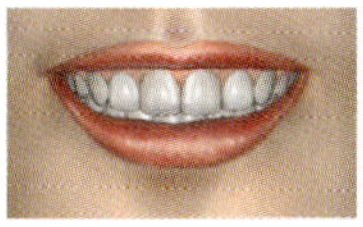
- ○ Low

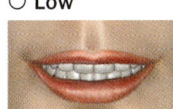

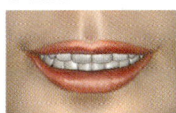

:B: Incisal Edges to Lower Lip
- ○ Convex Curve 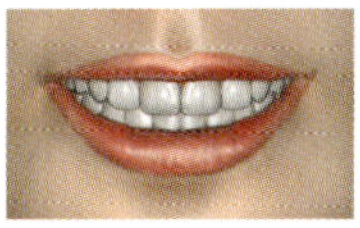
- ○ Straight 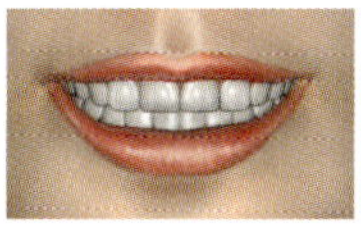
- ○ Reverse

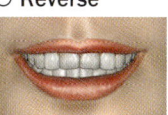

:C: Tooth – Lower Lip Position
- ○ Touching 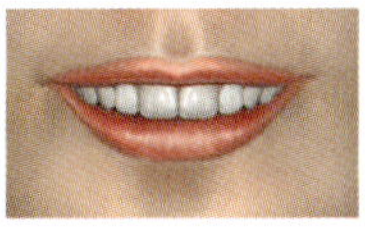
- ○ Not Touching 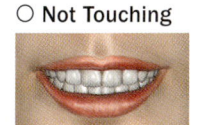
- ○ Slightly Covered

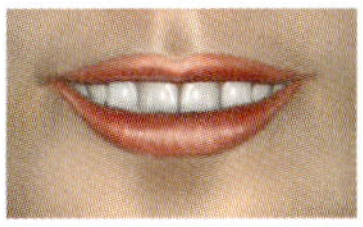

:D: Full Smile – Number of Teeth Displayed
- ○ 6
- ○ 8
- ○ 10
- ○ 12

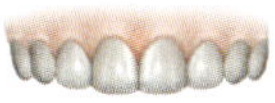

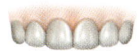

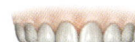

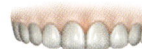

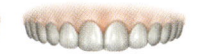

:E: Midline Location – Central Incisors to Philtrum
- ○ Center 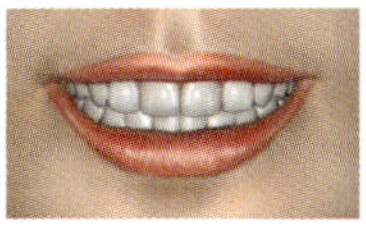
- ○ Right of Center 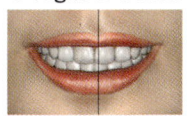
- ○ Left of Center

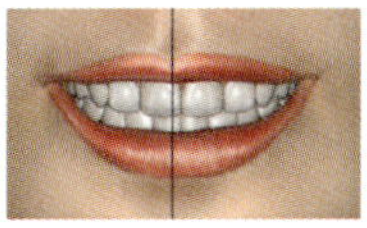

:F: Midline – Skewing to Left or Right
- ○ Right 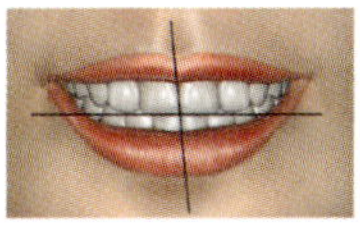
- ○ Left 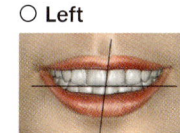
- ○ Straight

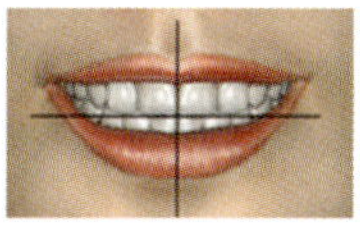

:G: Bilateral Negative Space
- ○ Normal 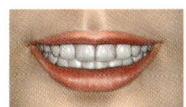
- ○ Increased

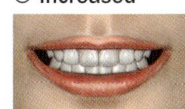

:H: Phonetics
1. **F** Sounds - Incisal edge of maxillary centrals on wet/dry line of lower lip?
   - ○ Yes ○ No
2. **S** Sounds - Closest speaking space – clear sound?
   - ○ Yes ○ No

4. Dental Analysis

:A: Starting shade
- Maxillary _____
- Mandibular _____

:B: Central Incisor Width/Height Ratio 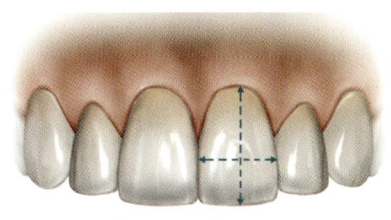
- ○ > 80% ○ < 80%

:C: Proportion of Central/Lateral/Canine

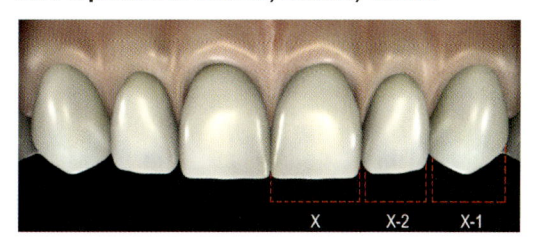

X   X-2   X-1

Central Width: _____ mm
Lateral Width: _____ mm
Cuspid Width: _____ mm

:D: Occlusal Analysis

1. Complete Occlusion 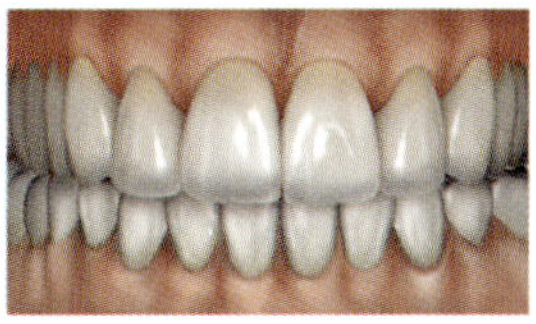
   - Interferences: _____

2. Incisive Position 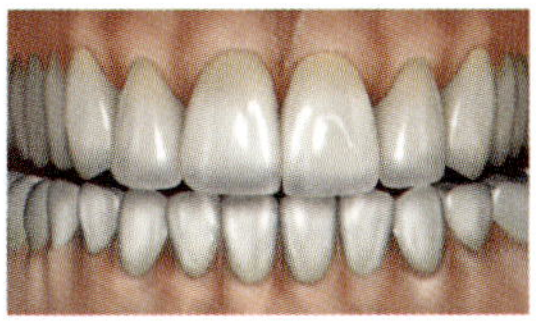
   - Interferences: _____

3. Left Working 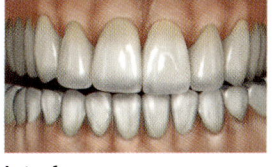
   - Interferences: _____
   - Guiding teeth: _____

4. Right Working 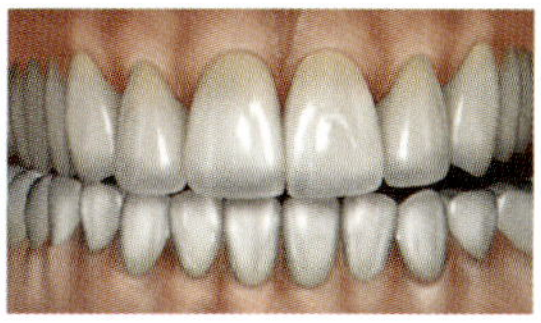
   - Interferences: _____
   - Guiding teeth: _____

Aesthetic Evaluation Form created by Jonathan B. Levine, DMD

:E: Micro-Aesthetic Elements: Acceptable or Not?

1. Incisal Edge Position   ○ Yes ○ No

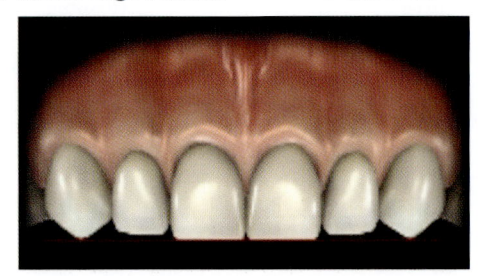

   Proposed changes: _____
   _____
   _____

2. Soft Tissue Symmetry   ○ Yes ○ No

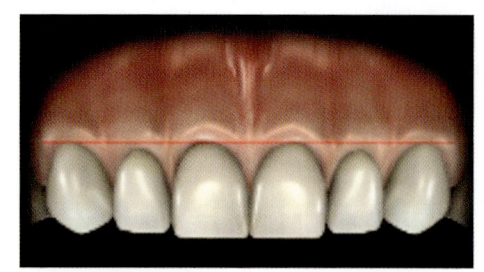

   Proposed changes: _____
   _____
   _____

3. Zenith Positions   ○ Yes ○ No

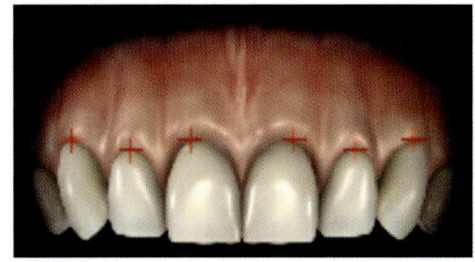

   Proposed changes: _____
   _____
   _____

4. Axial Inclination   ○ Yes ○ No

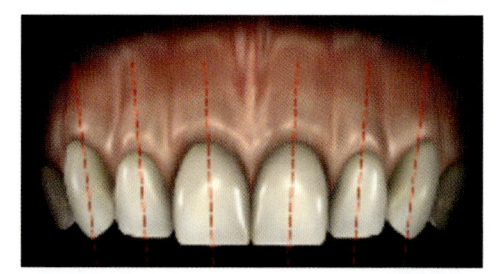

   Proposed changes: _____
   _____
   _____

5. Embrasures and Contacts   ○ Yes ○ No

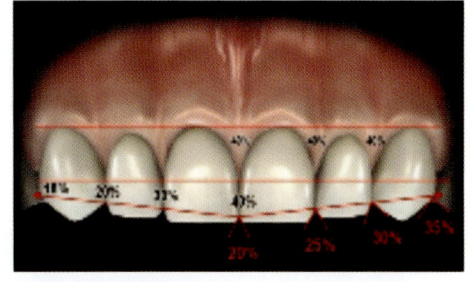

   Proposed changes: _____
   _____
   _____

6. Texture and Edge Contour   ○ Yes ○ No

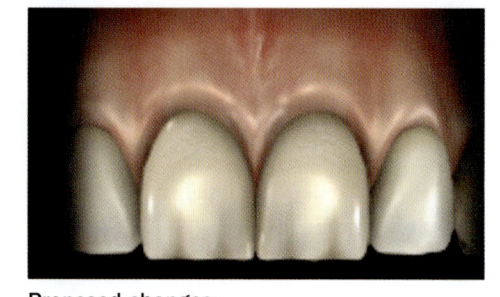

   Proposed changes: _____
   _____
   _____

:F: Diagnostic Wax-Up Information

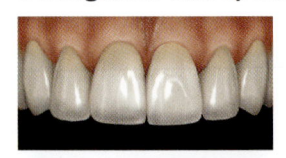

Proposed Max. Central Incisor Length:
_____ mm
Proposed Max. Central Gingival Position:
_____

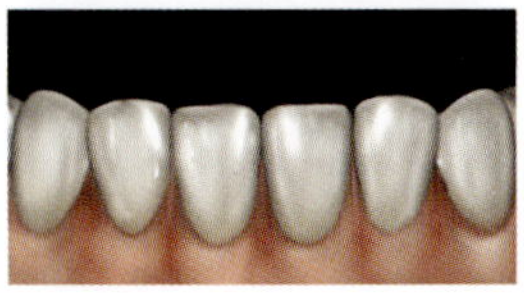

Proposed Mand. Central Incisor Length:
_____ mm
Proposed Mand. Central Gingival Position:
_____

Additional Notes to Guide Diagnostic Wax-Up:
_____
_____
_____
_____
_____
_____
_____

Aesthetic Evaluation Form created by Jonathan B. Levine, DMD

Appendix A

Esthetic Evaluation Form. Micro Esthetics

Incisal Edge Position

☐ a ☐ n/a

Soft Tissue Symmetry

☐ a ☐ n/a

Trigonal Shape and Zenith Points

☐ a ☐ n/a

Axial Inclinations

☐ a ☐ n/a

Tooth Proportion
75% to 85%

☐ a ☐ n/a

Tooth to Tooth Proportion
X   X-2   X-1

☐ a ☐ n/a

Aesthetic Evaluation Form created by Jonathan B. Levine, DMD and Anabella Oquendo, DDS

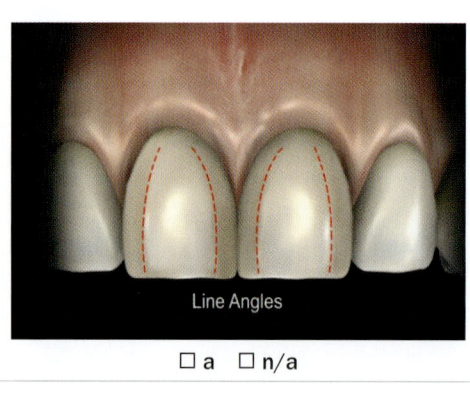

Line Angles

☐ a   ☐ n/a

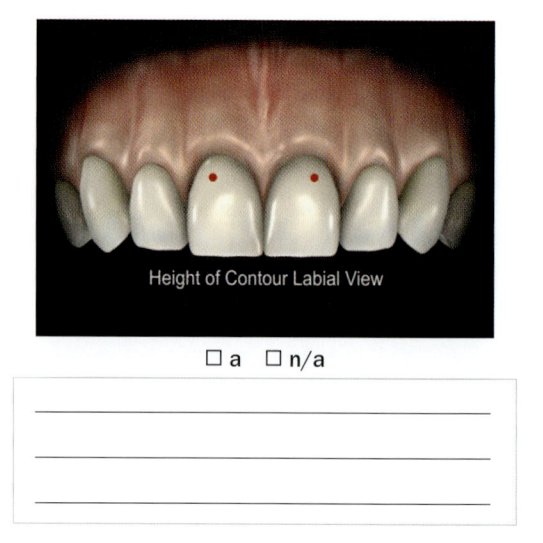

Height of Contour Labial View

☐ a   ☐ n/a

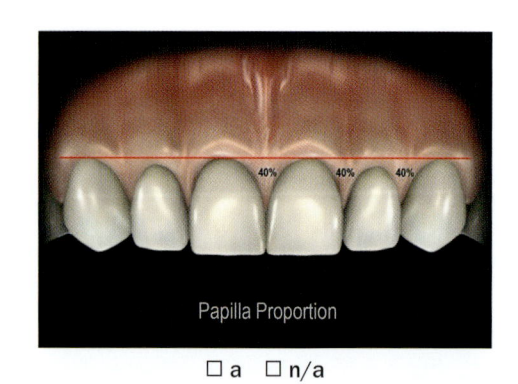

Papilla Proportion

☐ a   ☐ n/a

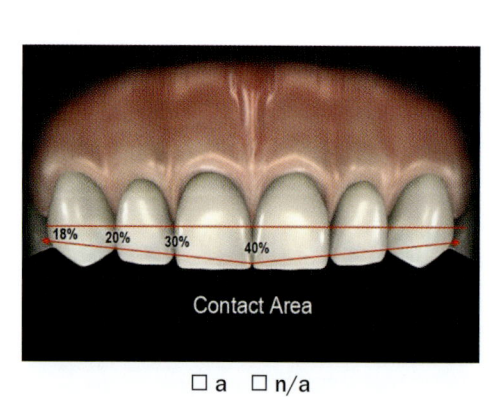

Contact Area

☐ a   ☐ n/a

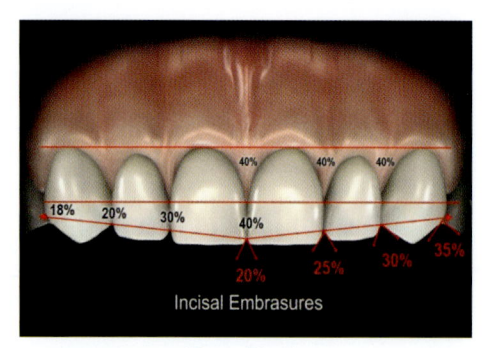

Incisal Embrasures

☐ a   ☐ n/a

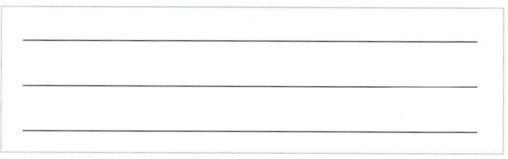

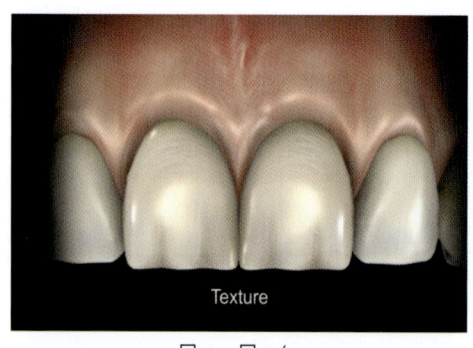

Texture

☐ a   ☐ n/a

Aesthetic Evaluation Form created by Jonathan B. Levine, DMD and Anabella Oquendo, DDS

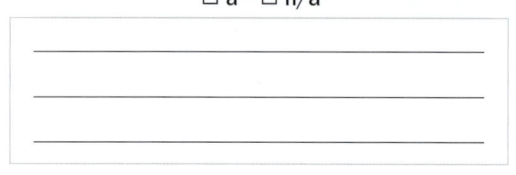

Appendix B: The Functional-Esthetic Analysis

FOR _____
DUE _____
DR. _____

UPPER ANTERIORS

INCISAL PLANE
- ☐ ALIGNED WITH BENCH-TOP
- ☐ SAME AS MOUNTED CAST OF TEMPS
- ☐ CENTRAL EMBRASURE VERTICAL

INCISAL EDGE POSITION
- ☐ FOLLOW E/O CAST
- ☐ COPY CAST of TEMPS
- ☐ COPY CAST of ORIGINAL
- ☐ NO CONTACT
- ☐ LABIALS ALIGNED IN PROTRUSIVE EDGE-TO-EDGE with AG TABLE

LABIAL EMBRASURES
- ☐ FORMED BY CONVEX PROXIMALS
- ☐ CUSPID MES-LAB LINE ANGLE FACES FORWARD
- ☐ INCISAL EDGES OUTLINED BY LINE ANGLES
- ☐ _____

EMERGENCE CONTOUR
- ☐ STRAIGHT or CONCAVE
- ☐ FOLLOW TISSUE MODEL
- ☐ NO BULGE AT MARGIN
- ☐ ALL SPACES CLOSED
- ☐ TRIGONAL SHAPE ON PONTICS
- ☐ GINGIVAL MARGIN SAME AS TEMPS
- ☐ CUSPID PROFILE

LABIAL CONTOUR
- ☐ ALIGNED WITH ALVEOLAR CONTOUR
- ☐ 2 PLANES FOR LABIAL CONTOUR
- ☐ COPY TEMPS
- ☐ DEFINITE STOP FOR LOWER ANTERIORS
- ☐ NO CONTACT

☐ SPECIAL INSTRUCTIONS
☐ SHADE INSTRUCTIONS

☐ CHECK CONTACTS ON SOLID MODEL

Esthetic Checklist ©1984 Peter E. Dawson, DDS

FOR _____
DUE _____
DR. _____

LOWER ANTERIORS

INCISAL PLANE
- ☐ COPY CAST of TEMPS
- ☐ INCISAL PLANE aligned with bench top
- ☐ LABIAL EMBRASURES aligned with VERTICAL
- ☐ _____

INCISAL EDGE POSITION
- ☐ FOLLOW E/O CAST
- ☐ COPY CAST of TEMPS
- ☐ COPY CAST of ORIGINAL
- ☐ INCISAL EDGES MEET DEFINITE STOP
- ☐ NO ANTERIOR CONTACT

INCISAL EDGES CONTOUR
- ☐ OUTLINED BY LINE ANGLES
- ☐ INCISAL EDGE HIGHER ON LINGUAL
- ☐ INCISAL EDGE WIDER AT LINGUAL
- ☐ DEFINITE LABIO-INCISAL LINE ANGLE
- ☐ LINGUAL STRAIGHT or SLIGHTLY CONCAVE

LABIAL EMBRASURES
- ☐ FORMED BY CONVEX PROXIMAL SURFACES
- ☐

LABIAL SILHOUETTE
- ☐ FORM SLIGHT OFFSET OF INCISAL EDGES
- ☐

INCISAL EDGES SILHOUETTE
- ☐ FORM SLIGHT ANGULATION OF FLAT EDGES
- ☐ PATIENT WANTS EVEN
- ☐

CUSPID
- ☐ MES-LAB LINE ANGLE POINTS FORWARD
- ☐ SHOW LINGUAL OF CUSPID FORM LABIAL VIEW

EMERGENCE CONTOUR
- ☐ RELATE TO SOFT TISSUE MODEL
- ☐ NO METAL EXPOSED
- ☐ PORCELAN MARGIN
- ☐ METAL EXPOSURE OK

LABIAL CONTOUR
- ☐ RELATE LABIAL CONTOUR TO E/O
- ☐ TO CAST OF ORIGINAL
- ☐ TO CAST OF TEMPS
- ☐ NO BULGE AT MARGIN

- ☐ SPECIAL INSTRUCTIONS
- ☐ SHADE INSTRUCTIONS
- ☐ CHECK CONTACTS ON SOLID MODEL

Esthetic Checklist ©1984 Peter E. Dawson, DDS

UPPER POSTERIORS

FOR _____
DUE _____
DR. _____

PLANE OF OCCLUSION
- [ ] ALIGN with BENCH
- [ ] COPY CAST of TEMPS
- [ ] COPY CAST of ORIGINALS
- [ ] _____

EMERGENCE CONTOUR
- [ ] USE TISSUE MODEL
- [ ] NEARLY VERTICAL
- [ ] STRAIGHT or SLIGHTLY CONVEX

BUCCAL CONTOUR
- [ ] OVERJET for CHEEK BITING PROTECTION
- [ ] TAPER BUCCAL CONTOUR IN
- [ ] CUSP TIP CONTACT (NO SURFACE to SURFACE)

LINGUAL CONTOUR
- [ ] TAPER LINGUAL INTO OCCLUSAL
- [ ] PROTECTION for TONGUE BITING

OCCLUSAL CONTOUR
- [ ] CONTOURS TAPER IN TO OCCLUSAL TABLE
- [ ] DEFINITE GROOVES
- [ ] MARGINAL RIDGES ALL EVEN
- [ ] BUCCAL SURFACES ALL ALIGNED
- [ ] FOSSAE OPENED FOR CUSP TIP

- [ ] SPECIAL INSTRUCTIONS

CONTACTS
- [ ] CHECK on SOLID CAST
- [ ] EACH CONTACT PROTECTS INTERDENTAL PAPILLA

- [ ] SPECIAL INSTRUCTIONS
- [ ] SHADE INSTRUCTIONS

- [ ] INDIVIDUALIZED CUSPS
- [ ] SHOW NO METAL in INTERPROXIMAL
- [ ] SHOW NO METAL at MARGIN
- [ ] METAL DISPLAY AT MARGIN OK
- [ ] CLOSE SPACES

Esthetic Checklist ©1984 Peter E. Dawson, DDS

LOWER POSTERIORS

FOR _____
DUE _____
DR. _____

PLANE of OCCLUSION
- ☐ COPY CAST of TEMPS
- ☐ ALIGN WITH BENCH
- ☐ DON'T ALTER
- ☐ USE FLAG
- ☐ _____

CUSP TIP POSITION
- ☐ AS MARKED ON UPPER CAST
- ☐ ALGIN with CENTRAL GROOVE OF UPPER
- ☐ _____

FOSSAE CONTOUR
- ☐ CR CONTACT ONLY
- ☐ USE FOSSA GUIDE
- ☐ _____

BUCCAL CONTOUR
- ☐ TAPER IN FOR CHEEK BITING PROTECTION
- ☐ HEIGHT OF CONTOUR AT JUNCTION of LOWER THIRD
- ☐ STRAIGHT or SLIGHTLY CONCAVE EMERGENCE CONTOUR
- ☐ VERTICAL EMERGENCE

LINGUAL CONTOUR
- ☐ TONGUE BITING PROTECTION
- ☐ TAPERED IN/ON LINGUAL
- ☐ CORRECT LINGUAL HEIGHT of CONTOUR

OCCLUSAL CONTOUR
- ☐ CONTOURS TAPER IN TO OCCLUSAL TABLE
- ☐ DEFINITE GROOVES
- ☐ MARGINAL RIDGES ALL EVEN
- ☐ FOSSAE OPENED FOR CUSP TIP CONTACT ONLY
- ☐ BUCCAL SURFACES ALIGNED and PARALLEL
- ☐ MESIAL 1/3 ALIGNED FACING FORWARD

FIRST PREMOLAR
- ☐ LINGUAL CUSP of FIRST PREMOLAR KEPT LOW

CONTACTS
- ☐ EACH CONTACT PROTECTS INTERDENTAL PAPILLA
- ☐ CHECK on SOLID CAST

☐ SPECIAL INSTRUCTIONS

☐ SHADE INSTRUCTIONS

- ☐ INDIVIDUALIZED CUSPS
- ☐ SHOW NO METAL IN INTERPROXIMAL
- ☐ SHOW NO METAL AT MARGIN
- ☐ METAL DISPLAY AT MARGIN OK
- ☐ CLOSE SPACES

Esthetic Checklist ©1984 Peter E. Dawson, DDS

THE FUNCTIONAL-ESTHETIC ANALYSIS

Are the TM Joints stable and healthy? Can they comfortably accept maximal load testing?	If '**Yes**' proceed with checklist.
	If '**No**' treat joint first.

5 Requirements for Occlusal Stability	Yes/No	Treatment Options
When in centric relation are there stable stops on **all teeth** or a substitute?		
Is the anterior guidance in harmony with the envelope of function? (CR contact to incisal edges)		
Is there immediate disclusion of the posterior teeth in protrusion?		
Do all the posterior teeth on the balancing side disclude during excursion toward the midline?		
Do all teeth on the working side disclude with the anterior guidance? ☐ *Group function may be indicated in cases of a compromised working side cuspid or implant in the cuspid site.*		

6 Elements of Global Esthetics	Yes/No	Treatment Options
Does the patient have an acceptable maxillo-mandibular relationship in centric relation (Face, Airway, Bite)?		
Is the embrasure between the centrals parallel with the midline and perpendicular to the occlusal plane?		
Is the lower posterior occlusal plane in harmony with the lower incisal plane?		
Are the vertical and horizontal edge positions of the maxillary central incisors related to the **inner** vermillion border (wet/dry line) of the lower lip?		
Is the buccal corridor (transverse relationship) within normal limits?		
Is the display of gingiva acceptable when smiling?		

6 Macro Esthetic Goals	Yes/No	Treatment Options
Is the gingival architecture appropriate and balanced?		
Are teeth 6-11 in proper proportion and contra-lateral balance?		
Is the width-to-length ratio of the central incisors 75-85%?		
Is the papillary position acceptable (without black triangles)?		
Are the axial inclinations of the anterior teeth acceptable esthetically?		
Is the depth of the incisal embrasures appropriate and do they graduate from anterior to posterior?		

Treatment options: Reshape, Reposition, Restore, Reposition a boney segment

©2013 The Dawson Academy • All Rights Reserved • www.TheDawsonAcademy.com

Appendix C Laboratory Checklist

LABORATORY CHECKLIST

M. FRADEANI   G. BARDUCCI

Patient _____ Age _____ Date ___/___/___ ☐ Male ☐ Female

ESTHETIC INFORMATION

PATIENT'S PHOTOGRAPH   PATIENT'S PHOTOGRAPH   PATIENT'S PHOTOGRAPH

■ **PHOTOGRAPHS** ☐ Old ☐ New   ■ **SMILE LINE** ☐ Average ☐ Low ☐ High

■ **ALIGNMENT** ☐ Yes ☐ No   ■ **APPEARANCE** ☐ Youth ☐ Adult ☐ Mature

■ **TOOTH TYPE** ☐ Ovoid   ☐ Triangular   ☐ Square

■ **TEXTURE** Macro ☐ None ☐ Slight ☐ Pronounced   Micro ☐ None ☐ Slight ☐ Pronounced

OCCLUSAL PLANE vs COMMISSURAL LINE – HORIZON

☐ Parallel   ☐ Slanted right   ☐ Slanted left
                    Maintain ☐   Maintain ☐
                    Modify   ☐   Modify   ☐

Indicate modifications: Mark with + to lengthen and – to shorten

(mm) 16 ___	15 ___	14 ___	13 ___	12 ___	11 ___	21 ___	22 ___	23 ___	24 ___	25 ___	26 ___ (mm)
(mm) 46 ___	45 ___	44 ___	43 ___	42 ___	41 ___	31 ___	32 ___	33 ___	34 ___	35 ___	36 ___ (mm)

Notes _____

COLOR

Shade Guide
☐ Vita   ☐ 3D Master
☐ Ivoclar ☐ Other

Spectrophotometer
☐ Yes   ☐ No

Value
High ☐ ☐ ☐ ☐ Low

Notes _____

This Laboratory Checklist is courtesy of Mauro Fradeani, MD, DDS; and Giancarlo Barducci, MDT
From: "Esthetic Rehabilitation in Fixed Prosthodontics" Vol 2, Quintessence Pub. 2008.

Appendix C

| SHAPE | Modifications | POSITION |

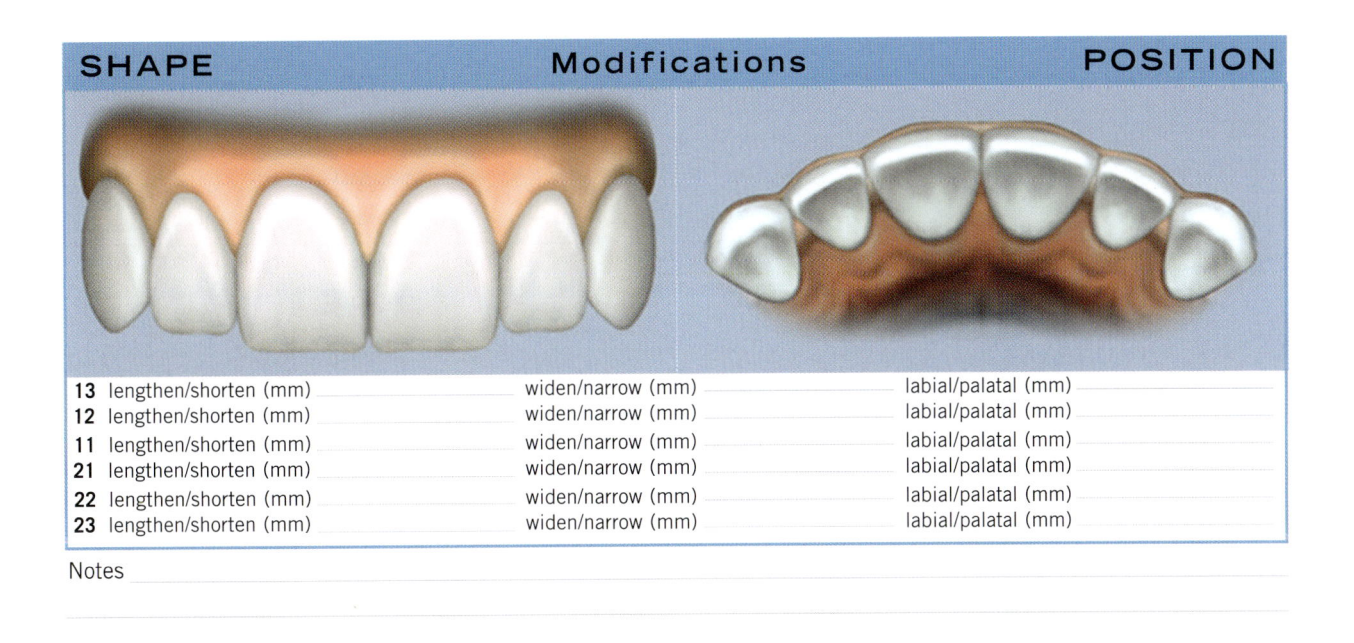

13 lengthen/shorten (mm)   widen/narrow (mm)   labial/palatal (mm)
12 lengthen/shorten (mm)   widen/narrow (mm)   labial/palatal (mm)
11 lengthen/shorten (mm)   widen/narrow (mm)   labial/palatal (mm)
21 lengthen/shorten (mm)   widen/narrow (mm)   labial/palatal (mm)
22 lengthen/shorten (mm)   widen/narrow (mm)   labial/palatal (mm)
23 lengthen/shorten (mm)   widen/narrow (mm)   labial/palatal (mm)

Notes

| SHAPE | Modifications | POSITION |

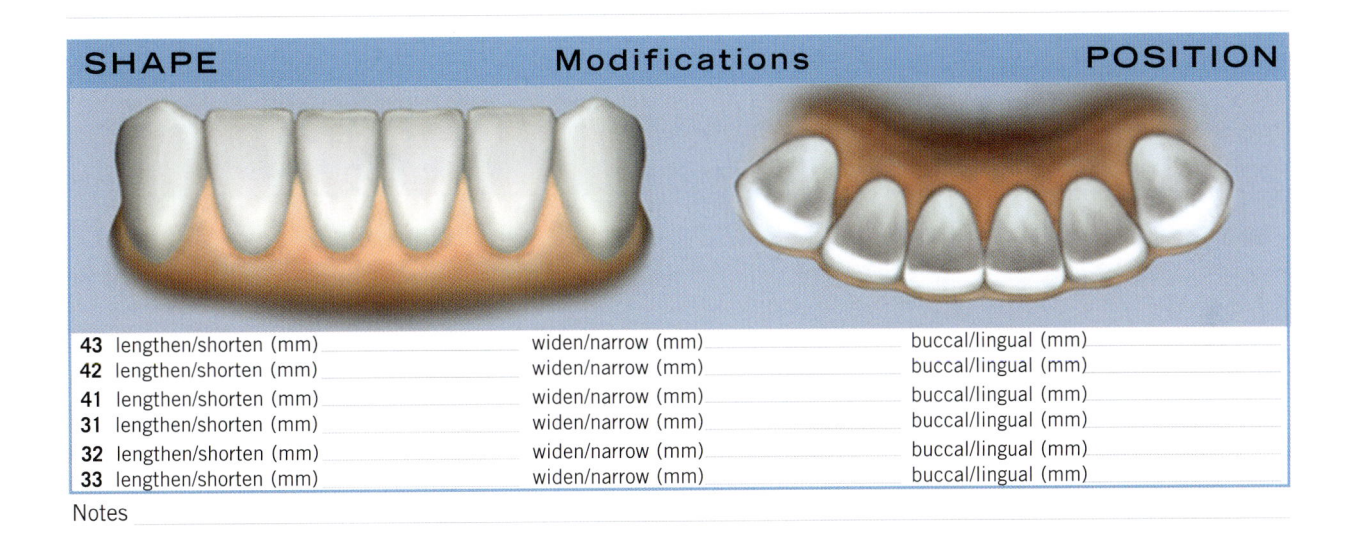

43 lengthen/shorten (mm)   widen/narrow (mm)   buccal/lingual (mm)
42 lengthen/shorten (mm)   widen/narrow (mm)   buccal/lingual (mm)
41 lengthen/shorten (mm)   widen/narrow (mm)   buccal/lingual (mm)
31 lengthen/shorten (mm)   widen/narrow (mm)   buccal/lingual (mm)
32 lengthen/shorten (mm)   widen/narrow (mm)   buccal/lingual (mm)
33 lengthen/shorten (mm)   widen/narrow (mm)   buccal/lingual (mm)

Notes

| OVERJET | Modifications | OVERBITE |

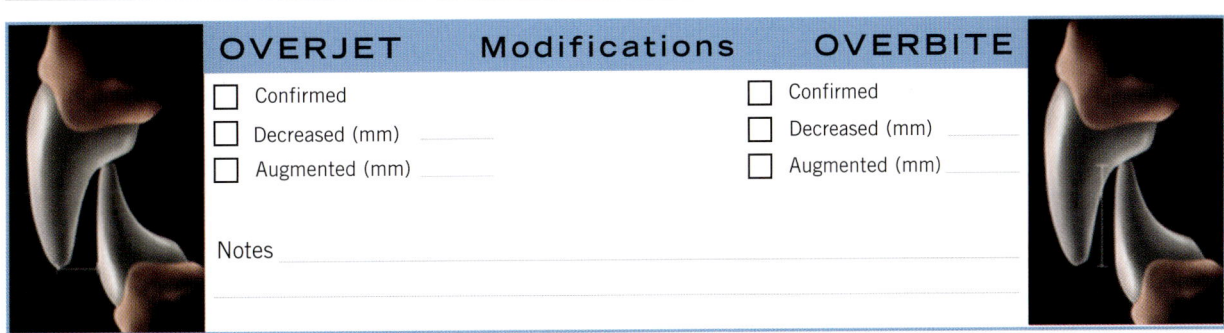

☐ Confirmed   ☐ Confirmed
☐ Decreased (mm)   ☐ Decreased (mm)
☐ Augmented (mm)   ☐ Augmented (mm)

Notes

Copyright © 2008 by Quintessence Publishing Co. Inc

FUNCTIONAL INFORMATION

■ STONE CASTS

- ☐ **Previous**
  - ☐ Maxillary ☐ Mandibular
- ☐ **Diagnostic**
  - ☐ Maxillary ☐ Mandibular
- ☐ **Provisional**
  - ☐ Maxillary ☐ Mandibular

■ OCCLUSAL RECORDS

☐ MI ☐ CR ☐ Protrusive interocclusal record ☐ Lateral interocclusal records

■ VERTICAL DIMENSION

☐ Unchanged ☐ Increase (mm) _____
- ☐ Maxillary (mm)
- ☐ Mandibular (mm)

☐ Decrease (mm) _____
- ☐ Maxillary (mm)
- ☐ Mandibular (mm)

■ FACEBOW   ■ Reference lines

☐ Arbitrary ☐ Kinematic ☐ Horizon ☐ Interpupillary ☐ Commissural ☐ Other _____

■ ARTICULATOR SET-UP

☐ **Semi-adjustable**
- ☐ Condylar inclination (degrees) _____ OR ☐ Protrusive interocclusal record
- ☐ Progressive mandibular lateral translation (degrees) _____ OR ☐ Lateral interocclusal records
- ☐ Immediate mandibular lateral translation (mm) _____

☐ **Fully adjustable**
- ☐ Mechanical pantograph
- ☐ Electronic pantograph

■ DISOCCLUSION

☐ Incisal guidance ☐ Canine guidance ☐ Group function ☐ Balanced occlusion

IMPRESSION

Recorded on ___/___/___   Time ___:___   Disinfected with _____

■ Impression materials

- ☐ **ALGINATE**
  - ☐ Maxillary ☐ Mandibular
- ☐ **POLYETHER**
  - ☐ Maxillary ☐ Mandibular
- ☐ **ADDITION SILICONE**
  - ☐ Maxillary ☐ Mandibular
- ☐ **POLYSULFUR**
  - ☐ Maxillary ☐ Mandibular
- ☐ **CONDENSATION SILICONE**
  - ☐ Maxillary ☐ Mandibular
- ☐ **OTHER** _____
  - ☐ Maxillary ☐ Mandibular

DOCUMENTATION

■ CASE HISTORY

- ☐ Contagious diseases
- ☐ Confirmed allergies
- ☐ Other medical device present
- ☐ Psychomotor handicap
- ☐ Bruxism
- ☐ Other _____

Notes _____

■ ATTACHMENTS

☐ Slides/Photographs ☐ Esthetic Checklist ☐ Other _____

LABORATORY WORK ORDER

Dr name _____	Dental lab name _____
Address _____	Address _____
City _____ State _____	City _____ State _____
Telephone _____	Telephone _____

Date ____/____/____   Work order no. _____

Patient/Code _____   Age _____ ☐ Male ☐ Female

■ **TYPE OF WORK**
☐ Diagnostic waxing   ☐ Indirect mock-up   ☐ Provisional   ☐ Fixed prosthesis   ☐ Removable prosthesis

■ **Description**
_____
_____
_____
_____

■ **SCHEMA**   o = Natural abutment   ☐ = Implant   X = Missing tooth

❶ 18 17 16 15 14 13 12 11 | 21 22 23 24 25 26 27 28 ❷
❹ 48 47 46 45 44 43 42 41 | 31 32 33 34 35 36 37 38 ❸

PFM: Porcelain-fused-to-metal	**PS1:** Presoldering	**PS2:** Postsoldering	**MM:** Metal margins
MCM: Metal-ceramic margin	**CS:** Ceramic shoulder	**PC:** Post and core	**ABU:** Abutment
AC: All-ceramic	**RB:** Resin-bonded	**V:** Veneer **IN:** Inlay	**ON:** Onlay

Alloy: _____
Ceramic: _____

COLOR

Shade Guide
☐ Vitapan
☐ 3D Master
☐ Ivoclar
☐ Other _____

Value
High ☐ ☐ ☐ ☐ Low

TRY-INS

Try-in _____	Date ___/___/___	Notes: _____	☐ Attachment No.
Try-in _____	Date ___/___/___	Notes: _____	☐ Attachment No.
Try-in _____	Date ___/___/___	Notes: _____	☐ Attachment No.
Delivery _____	Date ___/___/___	Notes: _____	☐ Attachment No.

Dentist's signature _____

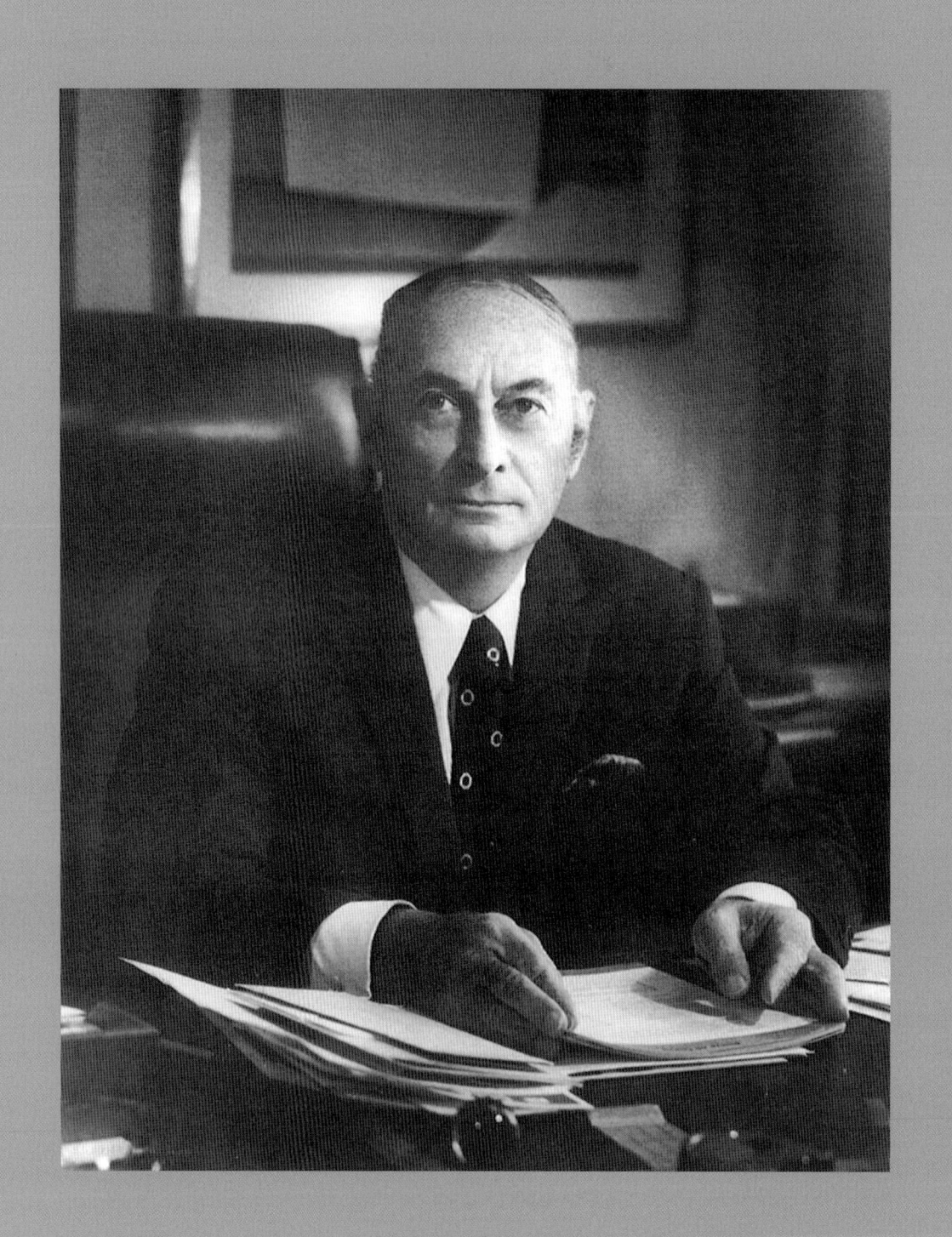

Appendix D Pincus Principles

Dedication

Dr Charles L. Pincus and I met for the first time in 1959 at the International Symposium in Knokke-Sur-Mer, Belgium, where we were the only Americans lecturing. From the beginning, a rapport was established and a friendship began that was to grow and endure until the day of Charlie's death on September 4, 1986.

As mentor as well as friend, Charlie nurtured my interest in esthetic dentistry in the early years of our friendship. In fact, had it not been for my strong family ties in Atlanta, I might have accepted his early invitation to enter practice with him in Beverly Hills. I did manage, however, to attend every course he taught and received much personal instruction.

Some 10 years later, I suggested to Charlie the need for a multidisciplinary organization comprising people who shared an interest in esthetic dentistry and who envisioned the important role it would play in the future of the profession. Together, we identified a group of approximately 50 leading dental educators and founded the American Academy of Esthetic Dentistry. That academy became the inspiration and stimulus for a worldwide expansion in esthetic dentistry, including the establishment of numerous other academies focusing on the same discipline, as well as the International Federation of Esthetic Dentistry.

In view of the pioneering contributions of this leader in the field, it is appropriate that we include some of the important principles that Charles Pincus taught the profession over the years. At the end of this chapter, Dr Pincus's autobiographical history, "The Development of Dental Esthetics in the Motion Picture Industry," appears. Thus, it is with a great deal of pride, nostalgia, and fond memories that I present this chapter.

Early contributions

Although his first published article appeared in a 1938 issue of the *Journal of the California Dental Association*,[1] Dr Charles Pincus actually began pioneering esthetic dentistry techniques some 10 years earlier when he was asked to solve a threefold problem presented to him by the heads of the makeup departments at Twentieth Century Fox and Warner Brothers Motion Picture Studios (see end of this appendix).

The problem stemmed from the emerging technology of talking movies, a technology that focused the camera and thus, the audience's attention, on the actors' mouths to a much greater extent than in silent movies. The makeup executives needed procedures for: (1) improving the photographic appearance of the actor's mouth; (2) developing appliances that would change the visual appearance of the performer, such as when playing Count Dracula or Frankenstein; and (3) creating esthetic restorations that would not degrade the quality of speech or be a hindrance to the actor. Although some work had been done in the area, it was altogether useless in the new "talkies."

Thus, Charles Pincus began the work that would consume much of his career and launch the field of esthetic dentistry. One of Dr Pincus's major contributions was to recognize the important principles of how teeth play a role in mouth personality. He also realized the vital role played by light reflection, surface texture, and tooth contour. He taught the basics of these theories throughout his career, constantly reminding us of how important they are in preventing esthetic failure. The remainder of this chapter is a distillation of the legacy he bequeathed to us.

Creation of mouth personality

Typically, dentists emphasize patient treatment outcomes related to function, articulation, and the like, with significantly lesser regard for the esthetic outcomes that affect the patient's visual personality. Said another way, many in our profession perceive the role of dentistry as functioning in three dimensions to achieve rehabilitation of the mouth. Factors associated with the dimensions of physiologic, biologic, and mechanical functions are the traditional concerns. The fourth dimension of effective mouth rehabilitation includes those psychologic factors that can be critically important to the self-concept of the patient.

Although their devotion to technical perfection is commendable, most dentists need to develop a greater sensitivity to the value of an attractive smile and the benefits it may hold for the patient. The opposite of the positive personality resulting from a smile that shows an even row of natural, white teeth is the inferiority felt by those with crooked, unattractive teeth. They tend to cover their mouths during speech or move their lips unnaturally to cover their teeth. This lack of confidence frequently accounts for the difference between success and failure in the lives of many people.

The importance of mouth personality is exemplified by the movie industry. Stars are provided with state-of-the-art makeup and costumes to maximize their attractive faces and figures. Writers and directors develop scripts for them that enable them to achieve precisely the desired dramatic effect. Yet, the entire illusion can be lost when those perfect lines proceed from a mouth full of crooked, protruding, or ill-spaced teeth. In realizing this, motion picture executives require that every prospective star have his or her mouth personality brought up to a level comparable to the actor's dramatic ability. Thus, while the need for attractive dental features among movie stars is obvious, the less obvious fact is that the same benefits are appreciated by the public. The effective dentist is the one who combines sensitive understanding of patient needs with knowledge of the principles of esthetic technique.

The importance of light

Basic to the practice of successful esthetic dentistry is a working knowledge of the properties of light. Unfortunately, there seems to be too little consideration given to this critically important factor. We must consider three characteristics of light if we expect to achieve superlative results with porcelain:

1. Direction of light
2. Movement of light
3. Color of light.

The direction and movement of light cast shadows and are the basic factors in the creation of cosmetic illusions. By varying the contour and facets on tooth surfaces we alter and affect the direction of light reflection. Shadows are created that are the basis of tooth illusion, as they affect porcelain restorations. As an example of the character of direction in light reflection, the shadows created are varied by the silhouette form of the teeth and the concavities and convexities of the enamel surface. Variation in the silhouette form can alter the color of the background by variation in the angle of lighting. The concavities and convexities of the enamel surface determine, partly, the surface texture, which influences the intensity and character of the reflected light by the way the surface absorbs or reflects the light. Shadows are used to dramatize a lighted area. The general lighting in one area may be deliberately played down by a darker shade of tooth or by darkening the interproximal areas as they curve into the contact areas. As an illustration, for an anterior fixed partial denture restoration, where insufficient depth can be attained interproximally to create the desired depth of shadow, the porcelain shade should be darkened interproximally to simulate the shadow, and thus create an illusion of depth.

Surface texture

Porcelain crowns and bridges should be fabricated so that the surface texture, including the convexities and concavities, matches the enamel surfaces of the adjacent natural teeth. This reproduces the characteristics of light reflection inherent in the patient's natural dentition (Figure D.1A and B). One of the very important things accomplished is lowering the value of the shade to the correct value for those teeth.

The character of color in light reflections

Tissue color—the color of the lips, cheeks, tongue, palate, and gingiva—reflects against and affects the color of the teeth. This causes variations in the appearance of the color and shade of the teeth. A high palatal vault will increase the translucency of a tooth with a thin incisal edge. With anterior porcelain restorations we grind away the linguoincisal and replace it with a translucent porcelain to simulate this very natural appearance when appropriate. When taking the shade, the hue, value (brilliance or amount of gray), and chroma (saturation) should be differentiated and matched. Concentrate on the tooth for only 5 s intervals, so as not to allow the phenomenon of adaptation of the retina of the eye to induce fatigue wherein all the shades tend to gray into one another. A florid (reddish) complexion will induce your judgment toward a green cast, while the patient with a sallow (yellowish-green) complexion will influence you toward a red cast. Also remember that the gingival color will influence your selection as well. With a dark gingiva you are apt to pick a shade that is too light. A light gingiva will usually result in a darker shade by contrast. The gingival tooth shade must be adapted to the influence of the gingival color. Pure north light or color-corrected fluorescent lighting is believed to reproduce shades and colors more accurately (Figure D.2). The final shade in the mouth should be checked with the patient in dynamic action. This is because a speaking patient affects the light reflections from the tooth surfaces differently (see Chapter 10).

The character of movement in light reflection

The movements of the lips, cheek, and tongue strongly influence light reflection. It varies with the differences in the width of the arch form of the teeth and the width of the vestibule. The narrower the arch form, as a rule, the wider the vestibule of

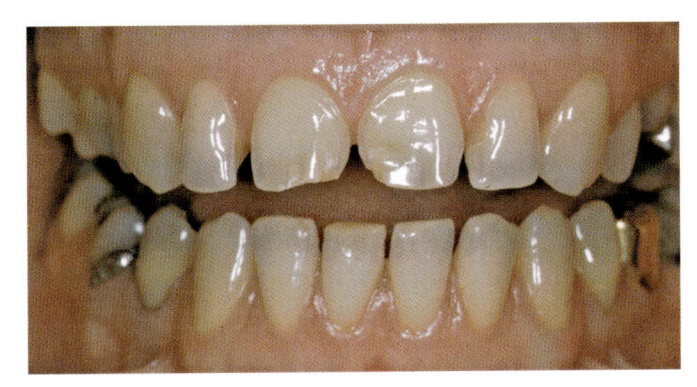

Figure D.1 (A) This patient with occlusal problems and broken teeth needed a metal framework to reinforce the porcelain.

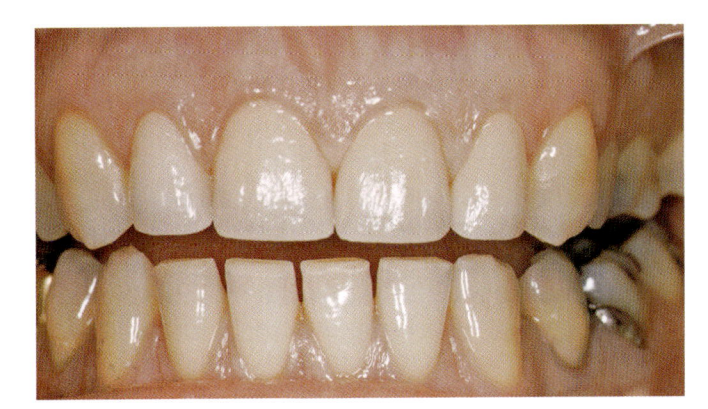

Figure D.1 (B) Four ceramometal crowns were constructed by Dr Pincus for this patient. Note how the delicate texture breaks up the light reflection for a more natural light.

MATCHING COLORS

CONCENTRATE ON THE TOOTH FOR SHORT FIVE SECOND PERIODS. IF YOU SPEND MORE TIME, COLORS TEND TO BLEND TOGETHER VISUALLY.

A FLORID (REDDISH) COMPLEXION WILL AFFECT YOUR JUDGEMENT TOWARD A GREEN CAST, WHILE THE PATIENT WITH A SALLOW (YELLOWISH-GREEN) COMPLEXION WILL INFLUENCE YOU TOWARD A RED CAST.

REMEMBER THAT THE GINGIVAL COLOR WILL INFLUENCE YOUR SELECTION. WITH DARK GINGIVAE YOU ARE MORE APT TO PICK TOO LIGHT A SHADE. WITH LIGHT GINGIVAE THE OPPOSITE IS TRUE. WE MUST ADAPT OUR GINGIVAL TOOTH SHADE TO THE INFLUENCE OF GINGIVAL COLOR.

THE COLOR OF THE LIGHT SOURCE WILL ALSO BE A FACTOR. PURE NORTH LIGHT OR COOL WHITE DELUXE FLUORESCENT LIGHTING WILL TEND TO REPRODUCE SHADES AND COLORS MORE CORRECTLY.

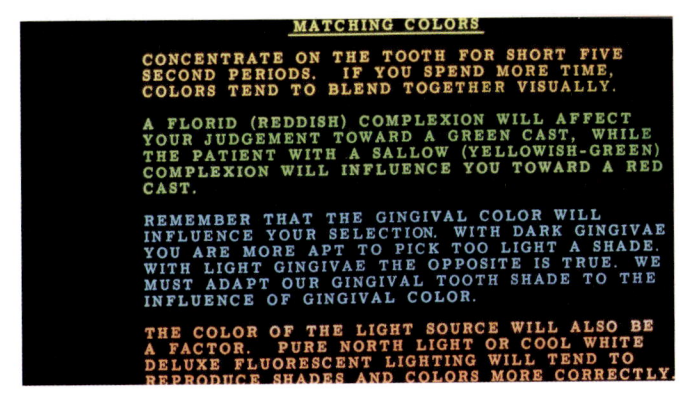

Figure D.2 Dr Pincus used bright colors in his teaching slides to illustrate his principles. Here, four tips were offered about matching colors.

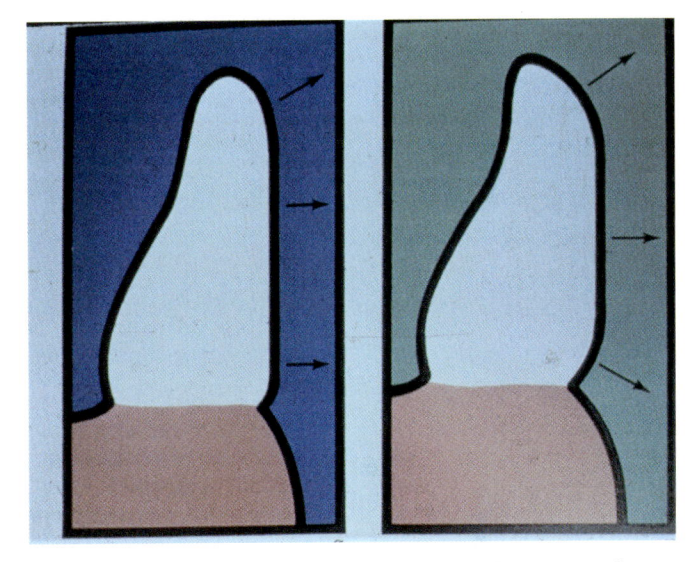

Figure D.3 This illustration shows how changing the contour of the labial surface alters the light reflection to make the tooth appear longer.

the cheek; and the light reflections will create more shadows posteriorly, so that the shade of the posterior porcelain teeth should be lightened. The wider the arch form, the narrower is the vestibule, so that very little or no shadows are produced by the light reflections on the teeth. As an example, a decalcified, whitish area added to a bicuspid crown in a narrow arch with a wide vestibule should be boldly placed, as otherwise it will not be visible in the mouth. The same addition in a mouth with a wide arch and a narrow vestibule requires a delicate placement to preclude it standing out role like a headlight. This explains why so often the insert, which looked so good on the model, defeats its purpose in the mouth. All of these factors must be communicated to the knowledgeable technician to ensure a superlative porcelain result.

Influence of contours on esthetic results

The contours affecting appearance

We create illusions to obtain the appearance of larger, smaller, longer, or shorter teeth in the same place. This is achieved in part by varying the outline or silhouette form, thus changing the character of light as the result of the direction and movement of light. To illustrate what is meant by the outline or silhouette form, consider that the mesial and distal highlights or marginal ridges of a maxillary central incisor tooth curve lingually from the ridges to the contact areas, reflecting light mesially or distally to the sides. The cervical one-fifth of the tooth curves lingually into the gingival sulcus, reflecting light upward. The incisal one-fourth curves lingually, reflecting and shadowing the light downward. When we speak of the outline or silhouette form of a tooth we describe that portion of a central incisor that reflects light forward or anteriorly. By reducing the portion of the tooth reflecting light forward, the silhouette form, we create the illusion of a smaller or shorter tooth in the same space. By enlarging the portion of the tooth reflecting light forward, the silhouette form, the illusion of a larger or longer tooth results (Figure D.3).

Incisal edge contour should conform to the dynamic action of the lips. This is checked in the mouth with the wax try-in. If one side of the lip raises more in speaking and smiling, the incisal line should also be raised on that side to make certain the teeth do not appear longer. Also check the median line. At the initial appointment, well before the restoration is started, it should be observed and noted whether the patient has a low, medium, or high lip line to determine how much gingiva is revealed.

Covering the exposed roots of the teeth can transform a simple case to one so difficult as to tax to the utmost the ability of the most skilled cosmetic dentist to obtain a superlative result.

The surface texture of the enamel

The convexities and concavities of the porcelain break up the surface and vary the reflection of light to a brilliance (value) that can be compared to the facets on a diamond. An actress with protrusive teeth, for example, photographed normally on screen because in dynamic action the lower anterior teeth did not allow the lower lip to fall under the upper teeth during speaking and smiling. Another actress with the same amount of protrusion photographed on screen with teeth extremely protrusive due to the lower anterior teeth being retrusive; this allowed the lower lip to hook under the upper teeth, thus exaggerating the defect. Contours have much effect on not only esthetic results but also on biologic and physiologic results, making it important not to overlook this area.

Basic cosmetic principles to achieve ultimate beauty in porcelain

a. Do not build on quicksand. Treat and resolve all inflammatory reactions and unstable periodontal conditions and allow healing before preparations are started. Sometimes it may require only a prophylaxis, other times several periodontal treatments.

b. Create models. In the parlance of the theatre, full-mouth casts should act as a "dress rehearsal" for the exact mouth preparations. Prepare the teeth on plaster or stone models as though you are working on a vital tooth, keeping in mind the relationship of the pulp to the preparation so as to retain vitality. After preparing, wax-up the correction on the study model. Very often it will be found that too much tooth structure was eliminated where it was not necessary, and not enough where it was important for the correction. In this way, we will know in advance each step in the preparation in the mouth to conservatively achieve the ideal porcelain correction.

c. Avoid tissue insults. In other words, do not injure the gingival tissues or periodontal fibers in preparation, impression taking, or treatment with chemicals before cementing. Otherwise, you may start a pattern of tissue recession that, once started, is difficult to stop. There are, of course, times when the preparation will include removing the epithelial lining of a periodontal pocket as part of the treatment plan. In most cases there should be "bloodless cutting"; no hemorrhaging during preparation.

d. Adapt the movement, color, and direction of light reflections to achieve the necessary illusions through varying the outline or silhouette form. Achieve the correct surface texture of the enamel for value in color. Adapt the placement and intensity of characteristic inserts to the presence of a wide or narrow vestibule of the cheeks.

e. Use a cast of soft resilient plastic to enable you to reproduce the gingival tissue and thus achieve the correct contour that will be biologically compatible with the soft tissues.

f. Have a wax try-in in the mouth to verify the fit of the pontics, the contact points, the length of the teeth, and arch form in relation to the dynamic action of the lips and illusions created.

g. The margins of the restoration should fit perfectly with appropriate contours to adequately deflect food and to provide support, not pressure, to the sulcular tissues (pressure would initiate a pathologic reaction). All of the margins and contours should be biologically compatible with the surrounding tissues.

h. The articulation should be free of prematurities, with the correct centric relation, and should not produce trauma to either the hard or soft tissues. To avoid additional stress on the investing tissues of the teeth by ceramometal restorations, create narrow occlusal tables with occlusal markings parabolic in form for minimal surface contact.

i. Proper maintenance, including a balanced diet (low in refined carbohydrates, high in protein), proper brushing, plaque control, vitamin and mineral supplements, and regular check-ups are vital to long-term success. The objective is good resistance and reparative ability, which is the greatest preventive factor of all.

j. The proximal surfaces should be properly contoured to allow a sufficient gingival papilla to regenerate or to be maintained (Figure D.4A). As much as possible, the crown contours should simulate the ideal physiologic pattern that existed, hopefully, before tooth preparation (Figure D.4B).

Three faults that can commonly occur during tooth preparation are illustrated in Figure D.4C:

1. Insufficient reduction of finish line.
2. Insufficient reduction on gingival half.
3. Insufficient rounding of buccal surface and linguo-occlusal line angle.

Interdisciplinary communication

Dentistry in general, and esthetic dentistry in particular, can greatly benefit from assuming an interdisciplinary perspective. There are many benefits that could result from a knowledgeable dialogue between the various disciplines. Some examples are:

1. Where a short lip would expose the entire gingival area in speech and smile, a knowledgeable dentist can try to prevent a future gingivectomy by recommending a conservative subgingival curettage or a conservative flap operation first.

2. When you have a short upper lip and maxillary anterior protrusion, correct the protrusion rather than extract the teeth. This will avoid the loss of the maxillary anterior ridge and prevent the creation of another dental cripple. Many of us have sweated blood and tears trying to arrive at an esthetic result on a similar case that had been irreparably ruined.

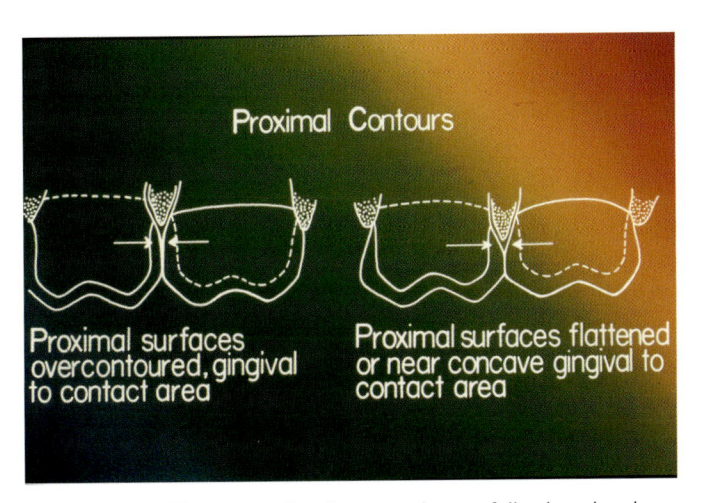

Figure D.4 **(A)** The proximal surface must be carefully planed and contoured to avoid impinging upon the gingival papilla.

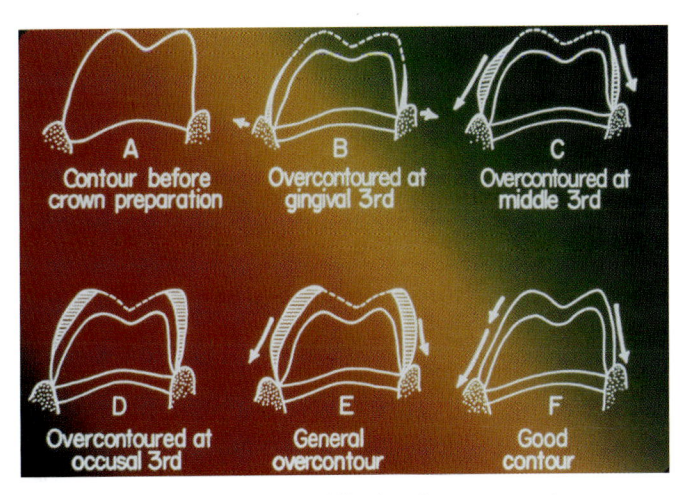

Figure D.4 **(B)** One of the most difficult tasks is to properly contour a full-crown replacement. This illustration shows proper contouring and the four common types of overcontouring.

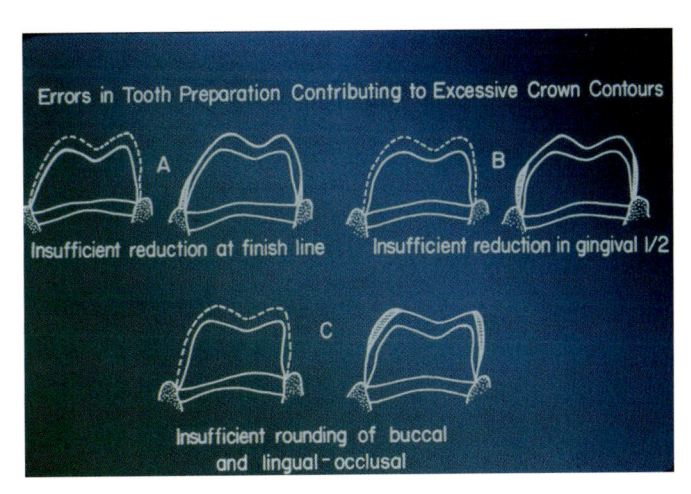

Figure D.4 **(C)** Errors in tooth preparation are a major factor in excessive crown contours.

We must stress cooperation and discussion among the various disciplines in advance of work being done! Intelligent discussion between experts from various disciplines could result in several additional choices for the cases described above; for example:

1. If the patient has sufficient time, adult orthodontics would be a good choice.
2. If the patient does not have the time for adult orthodontics and there is enough pulp recession to sufficiently shorten the teeth so that proper preparation can restore a cosmetic arch form, then crowning the teeth would be the restoration of choice.
3. In extreme cases, it would be good dentistry to treat the teeth endodontically, building the dowels lingually, so that the crowns may be placed in an esthetically pleasing arch form.

In these ways, a cosmetic result is achieved while retaining all the alveolar bone to keep normal lip support and actions.

Porcelain or plastic?

The use of porcelain crowns has been criticized by some dentists because of the frailty of the material. The reason for such frailty is that most dentists resort to porcelain only when the tooth has been badly broken down. By failing to build up the tooth with a casting in order to achieve a normal preparation to support the porcelain against stress, these dentists encounter breakage. Porcelain is only as strong as its underlying support. In contrast, acrylic crowns are much stronger and more resistant to breakage. When used on broken teeth, the preparation should be built up with a platinized gold casting.

Attention to detail

The single most important consideration when building mouth personality is attention to detail. The superior dentist, whose work stands apart from that of his average peers, is one who pays particular attention to every small detail, and it is this that explains why two dentists using exactly the same procedure will produce outcomes that are perfect in one case and marginal or unacceptable in the other. Although in the latter case we may believe we are following the procedure exactly, we may actually miss several tiny items, the sum of which results in a product that is less than we could have achieved had we painstakingly addressed each one.

Procedures for building mouth personality

Building mouth personality includes using one or more of the following five procedures:

1. **Porcelain or acrylic veneers.** Porcelain or acrylic veneers are thin facings that improve the appearance of incorrectly spaced, short, rotated, protruded, or retruded teeth. They were used exclusively in motion picture work, as they have very little strength to withstand the stresses induced by eating and other functions of daily living. In addition to improving the appearance of the actor's teeth, veneers are also used to build up teeth for the purpose of filling out narrow, sunken cheeks.

2. **Fixed porcelain or acrylic crown and bridge restorations (full-mouth reconstruction).** Although dentists may use the word "permanent" to describe porcelain or acrylic crown and bridge restorations, its use is misleading. Experienced clinicians understand that there are simply too many uncontrolled variables that can break down these esthetic restorations, such as a sudden and sustained craving for sweets that results in widespread caries in a patient who had been heretofore relatively free of caries, or psychosomatically induced breakdowns in healthy mouths brought on by anxiety and stress. Although these variables and others like them are the patient's responsibility, it is only ethical for the dentist to inform the patient when such a situation exists that might tend to break down esthetic restorations. They may prefer choosing a stronger, albeit less esthetic, material.

3. **Improving arch appearance.** Improving arch appearance is achieved through a combination of restorative procedures and cosmetic reshaping of the natural teeth (rounding cusp angles, shortening tooth lengths, etc.).

4. **Orthodontia.** Orthodontia may be easily accomplished with good results in children and adolescents in whom alveolar bone tissue is quick to regenerate. In general, adults do not respond as well, due in part to faulty bone regeneration that creates a predisposition to periodontosis. It is imperative for dentists, therefore, to identify the need for orthodontia during childhood. Patients who experienced previous root resorption secondary to orthodontia, hypothyroidism, or unknown causes usually can be esthetically corrected with porcelain crowns.

5. **Full or partial denture restorations.** Full and partial denture restorations constitute the final category of esthetic procedures that can be employed to build mouth personality. The emphasis in this appendix is on crown and bridge restorations and improving arch appearance, so if you want to study the various techniques included in this category, they are described in detail elsewhere in the dental literature.

The use of study models in treatment planning

The recommended starting point for patients needing esthetic treatment is to make a thorough diagnosis and treatment plan. The next step is taking an impression from which casts of both upper and lower jaws are poured and mounted for study. As mentioned earlier, the involved teeth are prepared and then correctly built up in wax in order to study the results that might be achieved and to ascertain the need for additional preparation. In this way, you can avoid excessive and unnecessary destruction of tooth structure. Full-mouth X-rays are always obtained at the start of the process; and in more extreme cases, additional radiographs are obtained at intervals in order to note the ever-closer proximity to the pulp as tooth structure is removed.

Frequently, 2–3 mm or more of tooth structure may be removed, especially in cases of excessive overbite with a short lip and recessive pulp. In contrast, patients with abnormally high and wide pulps may require shallow preparation in order to prevent death of the pulp. In these cases, the temporary crowns may be worn for as long as 2 years, during which time the pulp has time to safely recede, before making the final preparations.

A common mistake when treating widely spaced teeth with porcelain or acrylic crowns is to fill the entire space with only one crown, which typically results in a more unsightly outcome than the original problem. To create the best mouth personality, we must strive for a perfect, natural appearance that defies detection (Figure D.5A–C). Thus, just as abnormal spaces should be corrected by working with the teeth on either side of the space, protrusion should be corrected by bringing the protruded tooth in lingually and the adjacent retruded tooth (or teeth) out labially. Multiple tooth correction requires careful advance planning. One tooth may require more reduction on the distal surface to make room for a normal-sized tooth adjacent to it. Often the central incisor on one side is normally positioned with respect to the median line, and the other is responsible for most of the space. Again, with advanced planning and common sense, these situations can easily be corrected.

Conclusion

In addition to the benefits that accrue to the patient through the use of esthetic procedures, the benefit of an enhanced practice accrues to the dentist. Even simple procedures, such as rounding off long, sharp cusps to create a "softer" effect, will generate much enthusiasm in the patient. Such enthusiasm cannot help but result in loyalty and referrals. Thus, the clinician can enjoy expanded financial rewards and derive the personal satisfaction that comes from knowing that a patient's deep concern for his or her appearance has been met.

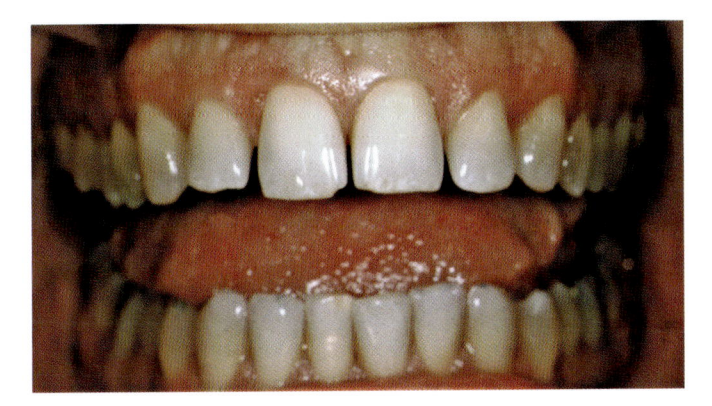

Figure D.5 **(A)** Dr Pincus taught that spaced teeth need to each be proportionally restored rather than create teeth that are too wide by treating only one or two of the teeth. Here, a patient with multiple spaces is shown.

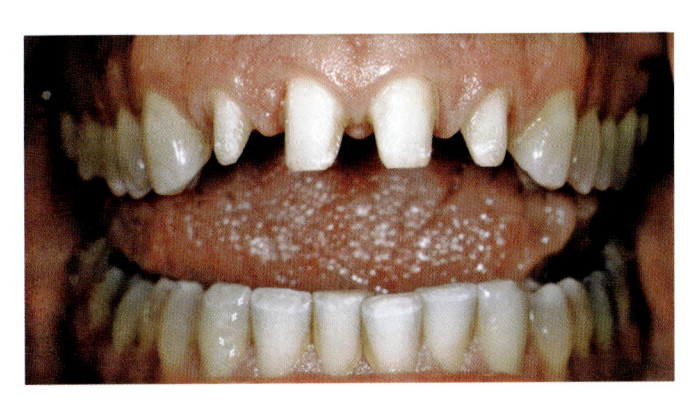

Figure D.5 **(B)** Four teeth were ideally prepared for full crowns. This patient was treated years before more conservative restorations (such as bonding with composite resin or porcelain/laminates) were available.

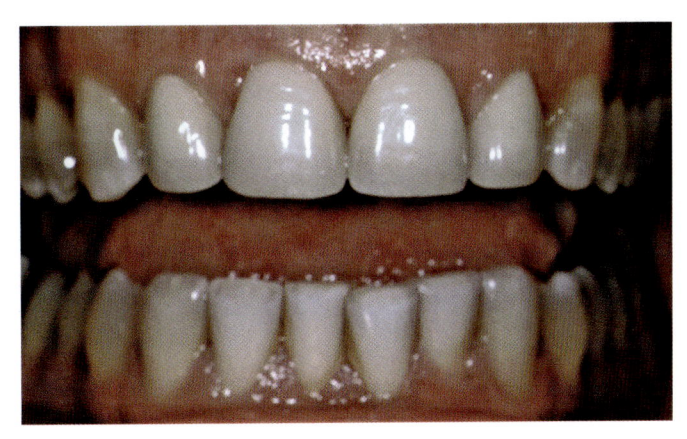

Figure D.5 **(C)** The final result shows four symmetrically placed, full porcelain crowns. Note how good the tissue response was to well-performed esthetic dentistry.

The development of dental esthetics in the motion picture industry[1]

Charles L. Pincus, DDS

Esthetic or cosmetic dentistry is actually the fourth dimension in addition to the biologic, physiologic, and mechanical factors—all of which must be achieved for the successful result. As one of the individuals responsible for the initial concepts and growth of esthetics, it might not be amiss for me to detail how it came about. Cosmetic dentistry was first brought to my attention around 1928 by Ern and Perc Westmore, who were then the executive heads of the makeup departments of Twentieth Century Fox and Warner Brothers Motion Picture Studios, respectively. They were referred to me with their problems by the top executives of the Max Factor makeup company who were patients of mine. Talking pictures were being born. Great dramatic stars were being imported from the legitimate stage and later from Europe. Quality in every phase of motion picture production was being stressed. Their requests were threefold:

1. They needed to know how to improve the photographic appearance of the mouth.
2. They wanted some form of appliance to change the visual appearance of the performer where a characterization (Dracula or Frankenstein) or dual role was required.
3. Most important was the fact that restorations could not interfere with speech or make the performer conscious of something foreign in the mouth, thereby affecting his dramatic ability.

Some crude work had been done in the past. However, this was completely unacceptable with the advent of sound and the emergence, as from a chrysalis, of motion pictures as a true art form. To solve their dilemma I pioneered and refined the "false front" we called veneers, now known as "Hollywood facings." These were very thin porcelain facings that were baked in a contour to cover the spaced, turned, or twisted teeth, so as to give the appearance of well-rounded arch form with normally positioned teeth, thus preventing the teeth from photographing black on screen. They were placed upon the teeth before the

---

[1] Originally written as an appendix for *Esthetics in Dentistry*, first edition, this section is reprinted here for its historical value.

actor appeared on camera, for interviews, or for personal appearances and were removed afterward. Ern and Perc Westmore were joined in their problems with me by a number of executive makeup heads (Jack Pierce of Universal Pictures, Jack Dawn of Metro-Goldwyn-Mayer, Clay Campbell of Columbia Pictures, and Mel Burns of RKO Studios). These men were the creative giants among the pioneers whose basic techniques formed the cornerstones that are responsible for so many of the makeup advances to date. We were called upon to look at screen tests at the studios and to recommend and produce the necessary changes. These improvements allowed the audience to focus on the beautiful performance presented by the actor or actress instead of being distracted by the defects in the mouth. Knowledge and techniques advanced with each challenge. For example, we learned that it was a simple matter to correct the arch form by placing facings on the two maxillary central incisors where they were in extreme lingual retrusion. Unfortunately, in covering the teeth to the incisal edge they would appear unduly long because the entire surface reflected light forward instead of only the gingival half, as before. Hence, it became necessary to bevel the incisal portion of the veneer from about 4 mm gingivally to the incisal edge of the natural central, so that a portion of the light would be reflected downward, thus creating the needed shorter appearance. This was the basis for all our subsequent work on illusions, varying tooth contours to change the light reflections and silhouette form, thereby making teeth appear longer, shorter, wider, or narrower in the same approximate space. It was also found that it was possible to cover short protrusive maxillary teeth from the lingual, lengthening the teeth without additional protrusion, and sometimes the correction of sibilation when it was present. Techniques were also evolved for shortening, evening, and recontouring teeth through judicious grinding with carborundum stones and Joe Dandy discs followed by polishing with fine sandpaper and crocus discs. In many instances this allowed mandibular buckled teeth to photograph normally on screen. Because of the time factor for performers, and the fact that "adult orthodontics" was not a technique of orthodontists in those days, a need arose for replacing long-term orthodontic therapy with simple and rapid techniques of illusion; hence, techniques for contouring turned or twisted anterior teeth or correcting diastemas were developed. The sum of all these experiences led to improved jacket crown restorative contours.

In Warner Brothers' *Man of Two Faces*, Edward G. Robinson played a dual role. In order to maintain suspense, a Frenchman had to be unrecognizable until the final scene. This posed quite a problem because of the short, square jaw, and thick lips that showed no teeth during speech or smile that were so unmistakably Robinson. Maxillary and mandibular removable castings were fabricated, opening the vertical dimension to create an elliptical face and longer teeth. Porcelain facings were placed so that teeth would show when he spoke and smiled. The makeup artist took over from there. Metro-Goldwyn-Mayer was in much the same difficulty with Lionel Barrymore in *Devil Doll*. He was to be disguised as a woman in a portion of the picture. The difficulty lay in the fact that the Barrymore characteristics were so strong that, in the screen test in his female disguise, he looked exactly like his sister, Ethel Barrymore. (As a matter of fact, as he was walking from the makeup department to the sound stage in female costume a mutual acquaintance who had just arrived from New York, rushed across the street calling him Ethel!) Impressions had to be taken on the set at the studio, as the picture was in production. A denture was constructed that modified the appearance of the lower third of his face. Much of the knowledge of what to avoid during contouring for natural-looking teeth was gleaned from these radical departures.

We were under contract to Twentieth Century Fox to ensure that Shirley Temple's mouth personality photographed the same in every film while she was a child star, regardless of the stage of primary tooth loss or eruption of the permanent teeth. It was vital that no picture production time be lost, as this would cost many thousands of dollars. The replacements varied from temporary dentures or very thin gold castings for retention with porcelain facings replacing missing teeth, to porcelain facings completely covering the partially erupted dentition. The latter were changed to labial facings as the teeth finally erupted.

Some motion pictures required character restorations to lend authority. A Twentieth-Century-Fox production *This Is My Affair* was about Theodore Roosevelt and his era. To create Roosevelt's protrusive and toothy appearance, and so create character authenticity, an appliance was constructed to overlay Sydney Blackmer's perfect arch of teeth. Thus, the teeth were lengthened and the arch widened without making him look too grotesque or stagey on camera and without interfering with his speech. Another character was built for Henry Hull in Universal Studios' *Great Expectations*, from the Charles Dickens classic. In this instance it was vital that there be a protrusive, bulldog effect of the lower jaw. For Paramount Studios' *The Years Are So Long*, starring Beulah Bondi and Victor Moore, we created a typical mouthbreather type of tooth protrusion for a brother and sister who were supposed to possess the same family characteristics. We were called upon to make the teeth for Frankenstein, Dracula, and the Wolf Man, and from the grotesque learned what not to do for the beautiful. Out of this motion picture proving ground emerged so many of the principles that contribute to the many beautiful results achieved today by the competent esthetic dentist.

Reference

1. Pincus CL. Building mouth personality. *J Calif Dent Assoc* 1938;14:125–129.

Additional resources

Blancheri RL. Optical illusions. *J Calif Dent Assoc* 1950;17:29.

Clark EB. An analysis of tooth color. *J Am Dent Assoc* 1931;18:2093.

Gill JR. Color selection—its distribution and interpretation. *J Am Dent Assoc* 1950;40:539.

Pincus CL. Cosmetics—the psychological fourth dimension in full mouth rehabilitation. *Dent Clin North Am* 1967;(March):71–88.

Pincus CL. New concepts in model techniques and high tempetature processing of acrylic resins for maximum esthetics. *J South Calif Dent Assoc* 1956;24:26–31.

Pincus CL. The role of jacket crown and fixed bridge restorations in the prevention and treatment of periodontal lesions. *J South Calif Dent Assoc* 1956;2:19–25.

Index

Page numbers in *italics* indicate figures; those in **bold** tables. Page numbers preceded by A, B, C or D refer to the appendices at the end of Volume 1.

abandonment, patient 145, 152
abfractions *704,* 704–708
    clinical cases 707–708, *707–708*
    differential diagnosis 711–712
    gingival recession and 1184
    mechanisms 704–707, *705–706*
    restorations 707
    scratch test 712
aboriginal populations 695–696
abrasion 708–709, *710*
    abfraction lesions 705, *706,* 707
    bleaching and 335
    differential diagnosis 711–712
    masticatory 708
    porcelain veneers 439
    restoration 708, *709*
    simulating tooth 219
abrasive strips, interproximal finishing 409
Absolute adhesive system 366
abutments
    fixed partial dentures 547, *548*
        cantilever bridges 555
        functional considerations 546–547
        partial-coverage retainers 549
        radiographic evaluation 544–545
        splinting 555
        telescoping crowns 555–562
    implant 657–658, *659*
        platform interface 1370, *1370–1371*

        restoration interface 1372–1374, *1373–1374*
        soft tissue interface 1370–1372, *1371–1372*
    removable partial dentures
        attachment 592, 594–595, 605
        clasp placement 584, *584*
        endodontic access 780
        radiographic evaluation 582
        selection 583–584
accelerated osteogenic orthodontics (AOO) 957–959
acceptability threshold 274
acetone-based primers, dentin bonding 359
acid demineralization, for root coverage 1183, 1185–1186
acid etching
    ceramic restorations *see* hydrofluoric acid etching
    dentin 359, *359*
        after laser ablation 972
        ceramic veneers 468, *471*
        composite resin bonding 403
    enamel 356, *356–357*
        after laser ablation 972
        ceramic restorations 468, *471, 1362, 1364*
        composite resin bonding 401, 403
    history of development 358
    pulpal irritation 134, 363, 401

    pulp capping with 769
    selective 358, 361, 403
    self-etch adhesives **357,** 357–358
    total (etch-and-rinse) 359, *359,* 403
acidic beverages/foods 710, 822–825
    dental erosion 33, 822–824, *824*
    erosion of veneers 477
    pH values **711**
Acromycin staining 755
acrylic (resin)
    A-splints 1320–1323
    camouflaging RPD clasps 590
    cosmetic stent, for actors 1155, *1156*
    crowns 502, *505*
    denture base 624, *624*
    denture teeth 616, 626–627, *627–629*
    implant provisionals 656
    occlusal registration 1305, *1306*
    overlays, for actors 1156–1160, *1158–1164*
    tissue inserts 1161, *1164,* 1323
    veneers 461, D7
actors *see* performers/actors
Adair, Peter 506
addition silicone (polyvinyl siloxane; PVS) impressions 1291, *1292,* 1388
    ceramic veneers 460, *460*
    disinfection 1302
    material properties **1293,** 1293–1294
    mixing 1292, *1293*

Ronald E. Goldstein's Esthetics in Dentistry, Third Edition. Edited by Ronald E. Goldstein, Stephen J. Chu, Ernesto A. Lee, and Christian F.J. Stappert.
© 2018 John Wiley & Sons, Inc. Published 2018 by John Wiley & Sons, Inc.

AdheSE adhesive 366, 368
adhesion 355–367
    aging of adhesive interface 363–365, *364*
    classification of adhesive systems 360–362, **362**
    definitions 356
    dentin *358*, 358–360, *361*
        after laser ablation 972–973
        ceramic veneers 452, 468, 471
        composite resins 403
        primers/priming adhesives 359–360
        priming of collagen network 360
        self-etch adhesives 360, *360*
        stabilization 360
        technique sensitivity 365–366, *366*
        tooth sensitivity after 366–367, 403
    enamel 356–358, 360, *361*
        after laser ablation 972–973
        ceramic restorations 1373
        ceramic veneers 439, 468, 471
        composite resin 401, 403
        conditioning/etching 356, 356–357
        historical development 358
        mechanisms 356–358, *357*
        self-etch adhesives **357**, 357–358
    failure prevention 367–368
    marginal gaps 355, *356*
    postoperative hypersensitivities 366–367
    prerequisites 356
adhesives 356
    air-thinning 404
    all-in-one *see under* self-etch adhesives
    biocompatibility 363
    ceramic veneers 471
    classification 360–362, **362**
    clinical recommendations 367–368
    dark-curing 361–362
    dentin bonding 359–360
    dual-curing 361–362, **362**
    etch-and-rinse *see* etch-and-rinse adhesive systems
    evaluation 363, *363*
    filled 362, *363*
    impression tray 1294
    self-etch *see* self-etch adhesives
    universal 361, **362**
    see also cement(s)
adjustment disorders 27, 41–42
adolescents
    tooth wear 696, *696*
    see also pediatric dentistry
advertising 124, 125–128, *126*
    word-of-mouth 115
agar hydrocolloid impressions 1302, 1388
agenesis of teeth (congenitally missing teeth) 982–983
    diastemas 843
    ectodermal dysplasia 982–983, *982–983*
    orthodontics 996, *996–997*
age-related changes
    crown restorations and 527, *527*
    facial thirds 245, *246*, 1101–1102, *1106–1107*
    incisal embrasures 247
    incorporating 219, *221–222*
    lower face 1137, *1138*
    midface 1133–1134, *1136*
    reducing 219–221, *223*
    smile design 248, *248*
    tooth appearance and **225**, *225*
    tooth exposure at rest 1119–1120, *1121*
    tooth size–arch length discrepancies 919–921
    see also older adults
aging, population 1015–1016, **1016**
air-abrasive technology 417–421
    caries management 417–419, *418*
    dulling metal restorations 1169
    prior to cementation 1356
    prior to composite resin bonding 396
    repair of existing restorations 419–421, 1227–1230, *1228*
    stained teeth 341, 670
air polishing 1417
air-thinning, bonding agents 404
alcohol abuse 825, *825*
Align Technology 1396–1397
all-ceramic crowns 506–514
    bilayer 1375
        glass ceramics 506, 1376
        oxide ceramics 507–510, *508–509*, 1377–1378, *1378*
        see also under porcelain veneers
    cementation 1361, *1362–1364*
    color matching 534, *535*
    crowded teeth **882**, 887–890, *888–889*, 1283
    endodontic access 778
    factors influencing choice 523, 525–526
    fixed partial denture retainers 550, *551–552*
    implants 658–663, *662*, 662–663
    longevity **513**, 1236, 1249–1250
    margins 553
    materials 506–514, 1264
    monolithic 506, 507–510, 1375, *1376*
    rubber dam placement 772–773, *773*
    technical failure 1255
    telescoping, as abutments 559
    tooth preparation 1263–1271
        esthetic depth determination 1268–1270, *1271–1276*
        positioning gingival margin *1267*, 1267–1268
        soft-tissue health 1264–1266, *1265–1267*
        thickness of marginal gingiva 1264
        tooth reduction 1268–1271, *1269–1276*
        types of margins 1277–1280
    troubleshooting **507**
    try-in 1341, *1341–1342*
    see also ceramic restorations; crowns
all-ceramic resin-bonded bridges 549–550, *550*
all-ceramic/zirconia fixed partial dentures 564
all-metal crowns
    as fixed partial denture retainers 550
    longevity 1244
    see also gold crowns
allogenic tissues, root coverage surgery 1184
alloplastic implant augmentation 959, *962*
Allport, Gordon 10, 11
alternative treatments
    cost issues 80
    obligations to disclose 48, 132–133
    patient decision making 48
    presentation to patients 63, *65*, 67
aluminum chloride 1236
aluminum oxide (alumina)
    densely sintered high-purity 1377
    endodontic access 777, *778*
    –feldspathic bilayer crowns 507–510, *508–509*, 1264
    glass-infiltrated 1377
    veneers 441
alveolar ridge *see* ridge
amalgam
    cosmetic replacement
        ceramic partial coverage restorations 480, *482–484*
        informed consent *136*, 137
    islands, bulimia nervosa 33, *33*
    prophylactic removal 136–137
    tissue discoloration (tattoo) 805, *807*
    tooth discoloration 379, *675*, 675–676, *677*
amelodentinal dysplasia 975, *975*
amelogenesis imperfecta
    tooth discoloration 330, 679, *680*
    tooth wear 697
American Academy of Esthetic Dentistry 303, 614, D2
American Association of Orthodontists (AAO) 899
American Board of Orthodontics (ABO), criteria for ideal occlusion 915
American Board of Plastic Surgery (ABPS) 1140
American Dental Association (ADA)
    classification of casting alloys 514
    color change units (ccu) 277
    Principles of Ethics and Code of Professional Conduct 138
    radiographic guidelines **1413–1414**
American Medical Association Code of Medical Ethics 138
American Society for Aesthetic Plastic Surgery (ASAPS) 14–16
American Society of Plastic Surgeons (ASPS) 14, 16
ammonium bifluoride etchant 506
anabolic steroids 825
Andrews, Lawrence F. 915

Index

anesthetic test, painful tooth 763–764
Angle classification, inadequacy 1076, *1077*
angle of correction, cosmetic contouring 305–306, *307*
angry patients 38, *39*
ankylosis 793–794
anorexia nervosa (AN) 26, 34–36, 822
    diagnostic criteria **32**
    signs 822, *823–824*
    worksheet for diagnosed **35–36**
anterior facial plane 1063, *1070*
anterior teeth
    cantilever fixed partial dentures 555, *556*
    complete dentures
        placement 616–620, *622*, 622–623
        size and form 614–615
    composite restorations 382–385, *384–389*
    fractured endodontically-treated 739–743
        options for restoring 732–733, *733–734*
        post and core options 739, **739**
        post-and-core restoration 739–743, *740–742*
    single missing 555, *555–557*
    too narrow 210–211, *212–213*
    too wide 208–209, *208–209*
    see also central incisors; mandibular anterior teeth; maxillary anterior teeth
antidepressant medications 28
antimicrobial rinses, implant patients 1421
anxiety mood disorders 26, 38
anxious patients 37–38
apexification 1219–1220
apical tooth forms, smile design 248, *250*
apnea–hypopnea index (AHI) 962
apologies 138
arch, dental
    age-related changes 919–921
    alignment, evaluation 56
    checking crown position 1345
    circumference, curve of Spee depth and 921–922
    irregularity
        correction 1094, *1097–1098*
        cosmetic contouring 319, *320–322*
        crowns 526, *526*
        special effects 218, *219–221*
    length 920–921
        pediatric patients 995–996
    orthodontic distalization 921
    perimeter 920–921, *921*
    space
        Berliner's formula 878, *879*
        deficiencies, crowded teeth 878, *878*
        maintenance in children 995–996
        measurement 921, *921*
archwires, esthetic 909
Arens, Donald E 750
A.R.T. Bond adhesive 366
arthritis 1022, 1024
artificial teeth *see* denture teeth
artistic skill, dentist's 80

A-splint, temporary immobilization 1320–1323, *1321–1323*
assisted-living residents 1036–1037
attachment removable partial dentures 590–606
    adjunctive procedures 593
    biomechanics and support 594–595
    classification 596, **596**
    cost 594, 597
    deciding to use 591–594
        contraindications 592–593, 594
        indications 592
        patient factors 592–593, 594
    definition 591
    extracoronal 596, 599–605
        advantages 599
        disadvantages 599–600
        types 600–605, *601–606*
    intracoronal 595–596, *596*, 597–599
        advantages 597
        disadvantages 597
        types 597–599, *598–599*
    nonprecision 591
    path of insertion 595
    placed in pontics 593, *594*
    precision 591
    retention 595, 596
    selection of type 595–597
    semiprecision 591
    special-use 605–606, *606–607*
    tooth preparation 595
    treatment planning 590–591
attitude, patient's 53
attractiveness *see* physical attractiveness phenomenon
attrition 696–702, *698–699*
    clinical cases *700–704*, 702–703
    differential diagnosis 711–712
    evaluation of tooth wear 697–698
    mechanisms 696–697
    treatment 699–702
aureomycin 682, *755*
avulsions, tooth 793–794, 1223–1224
    inflammatory root resorption after 794, *799–801*
    replantation 1223–1224, *1226*

baby boomers 1016–1017
background, tooth color matching 275–276
bacterial monitoring, implant health 1419, *1420*, 1427
Bali 298, *298*
base, complete dentures 623–625, *623–625*
base metal alloys 514, 571
Beaudreau's proportionate ratio 254
beauty
    commercial aspects 13–14
    concepts 3, 899–900
    esthetic dentistry and 1085–1086
    facial proportions *see* facial proportions
    facial symmetry and 1089–1090, *1089–1090*, 1094–1095

    rewards of 5–6
    trends 1005
    visual perception 1086, *1086*
    see also facial esthetics; physical attractiveness phenomenon
beauty pageant contestants 298, *1089*, 1154
Begg, P.R. 696, 920
Belushi, Jim *1157*
Bergen, S.F. 273
beryllium casting alloys 514
betel nut chewing 677, 816, *816*
beveled margin
    anterior veneers 442, *444*
    composite resin bonding 384, *389*, 398
    overlay technique 388, 398–400, *402*
    stained restorations 1252, *1256*
beveled shoulder margin, metal–ceramic restorations 516–517, *517*, 522, *522*
beverages
    acidic *see* acidic beverages/foods
    composite restoration longevity and 409–412
    in-office provision 118
    tooth discoloration 328, 675, *679*
billboard advertising 128
Biloc and Plasta attachments *596*, 597–599, *599*
Biodentine 769
biologic width invasion
    crown lengthening and 1205–1206
    legal considerations 149–150, *151*
    subgingival margins 1267, *1267*
bipolar disorder (BD) 26, 29–30
bipolar electrosurgery, gingival retraction 1291
bisphenol A-glycidyl methacrylate (bis-GMA) resin 360, 394
bite registration 1303–1307
    full-arch final 1306–1307, *1306–1307*
    occlusal registration 1303–1305, *1305–1306*
bite test 761–762, *761–762*, 799, 802
Black, G.V. 134
black lighting, effects of 1178
black line stain 674–675
black stains **671**, 677–678, 751
black triangles
    fixed partial dentures 548–549, 565–566, 570
    orthodontic aspects 902, 913–914, *914*
    patient preferences 138
    see also interdental spaces
bleaching 325–350, 687
    baseline color measurement 336, *337*
    calcified pulp chamber 788–789, *790–793*
    complications and risks 350
    endodontically-treated teeth *see under* endodontically-treated teeth
    home (without dental supervision) 345

bleaching (cont'd)
  in-office vital 331–341
    contraindications 331–332
    with matrix bleaching 341–343, *343–345*
    meeting expectations 332, *332*
    procedures 336–341, *338–340*
    results 341, *341*
    sequence of treatment 333–335, *333–335*
  localized brown stains 682–683, *685*
  matrix 341–345
  nonvital teeth 346–350, *347*
    color relapse 350
    complications and risks 350, 783–784, *785*
    continued treatment 349
    contraindications 346
    finishing 349
    inside-outside tray technique 348
    malpractice case 148, *150*
    nonnegligent risks 144
    out-of-office technique *348*, 348–349
    pediatric patients 988–989, *988–989*, 993
    precautions 144
    preparatory procedures 347–348
    results 349, *349*
    techniques 346–349
  older adults 331, 333–336, 1025, 1026, *1026*
  performers/actors 1167
  power/matrix combined 341–343, *343–345*
  prerestorative 844
  problem patients 78
  shade guides for monitoring 277–279, *279*, 336, *337*
  single dark tooth 682, *683–685*
  as stepping-stone to veneers 687
  tetracycline-stained teeth 328–329, *329–330*, 683–686, *686*, 687
  tooth color effects 274, 277–278
  vital teeth 326, 331–346
    children 335, *336*
    history 326, *327*
    in-office 331–341
    maintaining results 346
    nightguard 341–343
    older adults 335–336, 1025
    over-the-counter systems 345
    sequence of treatment 333–335, *333–335*
    tooth sensitivity during 345–346
  walking technique *348*, 348–349, 784–786, *786–787*
  white spots 332, 683, *685*
blepharoplasty 1132–1133, *1133–1135*
blood
  extravasation into pulp chamber 682, 751, *752*
  loss, orthognathic surgery 939
  pigments, dental staining 330–331, 681–682

Bluephase Meter 405, *406*
blue stains **671**
blushers, facial cosmetic 1150
bobby pins 825–826, *827*
body dysmorphic disorder (BDD) 26, 41, 42–44, *43*
body image 6, *8*, 10–11
body type, facial form and 930
Bolton's tooth-size relationships 923, **924**
bonding *see* adhesion
bonding agents *see* adhesives
bone
  condensation 582
  excessive alveolar 1205, *1205*
  grafts
    immediate implant placement 646
    ridge augmentation 642, *642–643*
    ridge preservation 639, *640–641*
  quantity and quality 1417
    complete dentures 625–629
    peri-implant changes 653–654, 1417, *1418*
    postextraction changes 638–639, **639**, *639–640*, 1200
    premaxilla 639, *640*, *641*
    removable partial dentures 582–583
  resection, crown lengthening 1205–1206, 1207–1208, *1207–1208*
bone morphogenetic protein 2 (BMP2) 643
botulinum toxin type A (Botox) 151, 898, 905
Bowen, R.L. 375, 394, 434
brachycephalic facial form 1058, *1061*, 1098, *1100*
brand, creating a 114
Brando, Marlon 1159, 1160
Brånemark root-form implant 653
bridges *see* fixed partial dentures
browlift 1132, *1132–1133*
brown stains **671**, 682–683, *685*
brushes
  interdental 1410, *1411–1412*, 1427
  tooth 1414, 1427
brushing *see* tooth brushing
bruxism 696–702, *698*, 814, 814–815
  clinical cases *700–704*, 702–703
  cosmetic contouring 300, 301, *301*, 814, *814*
  evaluation of tooth wear 697–698
  fractured restorations 1252, *1256–1257*
  intraoral appliances 413–415, *415*, 814, 815
  older adults 1034, *1034*
  sleep 697
  with temporomandibular joint pain 815, *815–816*
  treatment options 699–702
BruxZir materials 537
buccal corridors 1125
  patient esthetic standards 138
  preferences 899–900, *902*
budget-conscious patients 78, 80

bulimia nervosa (BN) 26, 31–34, 822
  case example 31
  dental erosion 33, *33–34*, 712–714, *713*, 822, *822–823*
  diagnostic criteria **32**
  parotid gland hypertrophy 32, *32*, 822, *824*
  signs 32–33, *32–33*
  worksheet for diagnosed **35–36**
bullying 11
Buonocore, Michael 356, 434, 1373
bupropion (Wellbutrin) 28
burs
  endodontic access cavity preparation 775–776
  see also carbide burs; diamond burs
Burstone line 1117, *1117*
butt joints
  metal–ceramic 516, *516*
  porcelain *see* porcelain butt-joint margins
  veneer preparation (Class 5) 442, *445*, 447–448
buyer's remorse 19

CAD/CAM *see* computer-aided design/ manufacturing
calcific degeneration/metamorphosis 767
  walking bleach technique 788–789, *790–793*
calcium hydroxide
  apexification therapy 1219–1220
  cavity base dressing 767
  endodontic treatment 780
  pulp capping 727, 769
  traumatically exposed dentin 1218
calculus 52
camcorders 181–182
cameras 155–156
  extraoral 59–60, *61*
  film vs digital 155–156
  intraoral *see* intraoral cameras
  point-and-shoot 158–159, *159*
  selection 158–163
  single-lens reflex *see* single-lens reflex cameras
  uploading images from 179, *180*
  wand-like 156, *156*
Camper's line 617, *618*, 622, *622*
canine protected occlusion (CPO) 915, 916
canines (cuspids)
  adjusting embrasures 1347
  age-related wear 221–222
  cosmetic contouring 314, *314–315*
  SPA factors 248, *249*
canine width (CW) 261
  ICW/CIW quotient for calculating 263, 265, **265**, *266–267*
  RED proportion for calculating 262, **262**
  in relation to other teeth 847
  too narrow 210, *212*
  too wide 208, *208*
carbamide peroxide 342, 343, 345, 348, 687

carbide burs
  endodontic access cavity 778
  finishing ceramic veneers 470, 473
  finishing composite restorations 406–407, 407–409
carbon dioxide (CO_2) laser 985
carbon fiber prefabricated posts **736**
Carestream system 490–492, 492–494
caries
  anorexia nervosa 34
  bleaching and 335
  bulimia nervosa 33
  detection
    air-abrasive technology 417–419, 418
    discolored deep grooves 670
    hand-held devices 55, 55
    intraoral camera 57, 59, 60
    pits and fissures 417, 417
  early childhood (ECC) 979
  pit and fissure see pit and fissure caries
  posterior ceramic partial coverage restorations 480
  prevention advice 1414–1415
  recurrent 1224, 1227, 1245–1248, 1247
    marginal leakage and 1250–1251
  risk assessment 536
  root
    older adults 1035, 1036
    soft tissue graft coverage 1194–1195, 1195
  susceptibility
    cosmetic contouring and 302
    follow-up care for crowns and 536
  tooth discoloration 330, 670, 674
  treatment
    air-abrasive technology 417–419, 418
    diamond burs 419
    hard tissue lasers 419, 419
    ozone therapy 971
    pediatric dentistry 973, 974, 974, 976, 976
Cariescan 55
caries management by risk assessment (CAMBRA) 1024
Carter, G.A. 920–921
case presentation 74–76, 74–77
  dentofacial deformity 935–937
  Digital Smile Design 87, 104–106
  marketing your services 120–121, 122
  role of photographs 159
cast glass-ceramic crowns 506, 507
  endodontic access 778
casting alloys 514
cast metal posts (custom made)
  anterior teeth 733, 734
    indications 739, **739**
    techniques 739, 742, 743
  crown preparation 744, 745
  design 734–735, 735
  premolars 743
casts, study see study models
cavitation, laser-induced 972

cavity preparation
  endodontic access see endodontic access cavity
  posterior ceramic partial coverage restorations 481–482
  pulpal response 764, 765, 766
  pulpal risk and depth 767, 769, 768
cavity test, pulp sensibility 758–759, 758, 759
CBCT see cone beam computed tomography
Celsus One salivary diagnostics 1423, 1424–1426
cement(s) 1355–1356
  Dicor restorations 506
  fluoride-containing 1247–1248
  In-Ceram crowns 506
  metal–ceramic crowns 521, 1355–1356
  pediatric dentistry 970
  removing excess 1358–1359, 1361
    ceramic veneers 469–470, 472, 473
    posterior ceramic partial coverage restorations 482–483
  residual
    checking for 1365, 1365, 1410, 1410
    implant–abutment interface 658, 660
  resin luting agents 1356, 1357–1358, 1361
  root canal 780
  self-adhesive 1361, 1362
  temporary restorations 1313, 1340, 1364
  see also adhesives
cementation 1355–1365
  all-ceramic crowns 1361, 1362–1364
  ceramic restorations 1361–1364, 1373
  ceramic veneers 468, 471–472, 1357–1358, 1361–1364
  CEREC restorations 487, 491
  implant crowns 660–662, 660–662
  metal–ceramic restorations 1358–1359, 1359–1361
  posterior ceramic partial coverage restorations 482–483
  posts 743
  preparation of surfaces for 1356, 1358
  radiographs after 1365, 1365, 1410, 1410
  tooth sensitivity after 1356
  try-in appointment 1352
central incisor length (CIL)
  complete dentures 615
  crowns 527, 527
  diastema closure and 846
  fixed restorations 1347, 1348
  ICW/CIW quotient chart method 263, 265, **265**, 266–267
  performers/actors 1174, 1176
  RED proportion to calculate 262, **262**
  width calculations and 261, 261–262, **262**
central incisors (maxillary)
  1/16th rules 249, 250, 614–615
  adjusting embrasures 1346, 1347
  black triangle between 137
  complete dentures 614–615, 616–617, 617–619
  crowning one 523–524, 524

  length see central incisor length
  overlapping, cosmetic contouring 315–316, 315–317
  post-and-core restorations 741–742
  reducing large 318, 318
  size in relation to face size 249–251, 250–251
  SPA factors 248, 248–249
  width see central incisor width
  see also incisors
central incisor width (CIW)
  1/16th rule 249, 250, 614–615
  complete dentures 614–615
  diastema closure and 846
  ICW/CIW quotient to calculate **263**, 263–265, 264–267, **265**
  RED proportion to calculate 261–262, 261–262, **262**
  in relation to other teeth 254–265
  see also intercanine width/central incisor width (ICW/CIW) quotient
central incisor width/length ratio 253, 256
  dentists' preferences 253, 256
  diastema closure and 846–847
  orthodontic esthetics and 902–903
  RED proportions and 257, 259
cephalometric analysis 253, 256
  dentofacial deformity 934, 935
  normal values 903–904, **904**
  orthodontics 901, 903–904, 904
  pediatric patients 1005–1006
cephalometric prediction tracings 934, 935–938
cephalometric radiographs 901, 903–904
  dentofacial deformity 934
ceramic(s)
  CEREC system 484–485, 1390
  endodontic access cavity preparation 776–778, 777–778
  failure rates of different 1253
  glass-infiltrated 1377
  high opacity 453
  prefabricated posts **736**
  veneers 434–435, 453
  see also glass-ceramics; oxide ceramics; porcelain; zirconia
ceramic orthodontic brackets 909
ceramic partial coverage restorations 433–492
  CAD/CAM technologies 483–492
  longevity 479
  posterior 478–483
    contraindications 481
    finishing 482–483
    impressions 482
    indications 480–481
    insertion 482
    patient instructions 483
    tooth preparation 481–482
    veneer onlay 482
  veneers see ceramic veneers
  see also porcelain veneers

ceramic restorations
  abutment–implant platform interface 1370, *1370–1371*
  abutment–soft tissue interface 1370–1372, *1371–1372*
  CAD/CAM systems *see* computer-aided design/manufacturing systems
  cementation 1361–1364, 1373
  digital laboratory workflow 1401–1402, *1401–1402*
  endodontic access 776–778, *777*, *778*
  occlusal interface 1374–1381
  partial coverage *see* ceramic partial coverage restorations
  principles of construction 1369–1382
  rebonding 1373, *1375*
  tooth or implant abutment interface 1372–1374, *1373–1374*
  see also all-ceramic crowns; ceramic veneers; metal–ceramic restorations
ceramic veneer onlays, posterior 482, *482–484*
ceramic veneers 433–492
  CAD/CAM fabricated 453
  fracture rates 473–474
  history 434–435
  impressions 459–460
  indications 440–441, 474, *474–481*
  longevity 439, *440*, 473–474
  placement 465–473
    cementation *468*, *471–472*, *1357–1358*, 1361–1364
    errors 472, *473*
    final insertion 464–465, *467–472*, *469–473*
    try-in *463*, 465–469, *466–467*
  post-treatment care 473–477
  pressable
    laboratory procedures 462–465
    longevity 474
    tooth preparation 453, *453–456*
  subgingival margins *see* subgingival margins
  temporary restorations 460–461, *461–463*
  tetracycline-stained teeth 440, 452, 453, 461–462, 687–688, *687–688*
  tooth preparation 442–459
    classic classes 442–446, *446–448*
    classic technique 456, *457–460*
    classification for anterior teeth 442–445, *442–448*
    mandibular anteriors 448–449, *449–451*
    novel classes 447–448
    novel extended technique *454*, 456–459, *475–476*
    tooth reduction 449–453, *457–459*
  traditional porcelain *see* porcelain veneers
ceramometal restorations *see* metal–ceramic restorations
Cercon all-ceramic crowns 507
CEREC system 483–490, 1389–1391

Bluecam 1389, 1390, *1390*
chairside fabrication 1390, *1391*
data acquisition 487, *487*, 1390, *1390*
design and milling 487, *487–490*, 1390, *1391*
hardware 1389, *1389*
material selection 484–485, 1390
Omnicam 484, *486*, 487, 1389, 1390, *1390*
placement of restorations 487, *491*
Planmeca PlanScan vs **1393**
research 487–490, *491*
shade selection 485, *485*
support and education 1390–1391
tooth preparation 485, *486*
cervical lesions, noncarious *see* abfractions
cervical root resorption *see* external root resorption
cervicomental angle 1067–1068, *1074–1075*
  correction of obtuse *1075*
chamfer margins
  all-ceramic crowns 1268
  metal–ceramic restorations 517, *517*, 522
  porcelain veneers 456
chamfer-shoulder preparation method 398, *399*, *400*
Chandler, T.H. 812
Change Your Smile (Goldstein) 49, *49*, *50*, 51, 54, 151
characterization *see* surface texture/characterization
check lines
  creating illusion of height 215, *215*
  simulation 196, *198–199*, **202**
cheek
  biting, habitual 819–821, *819–821*
  profile, pediatric patients 1008, *1008*
  projection, evaluation 1062
chemical bonding 356
chewing habits 816, *816*
children *see* pediatric dentistry
chin
  analysis of symmetry 1107
  asymmetry 1062, *1066*
  minimizing a double 1149–1150
  projection 1065–1068, 1115
  reshaping 959, *961–962*, 1137
chin–neck anatomy, evaluation 1063, *1068–1069*
chin–neck angle (cervicomental angle) 1067–1068, *1074–1075*
chin–neck length 1067–1068, *1074–1075*
chips *see* crown fractures
chlorhexidine
  mouthwashes, staining of teeth 673–674, *677–678*
  stabilization of bonding 364–365, 367
chroma 272–273, *273*
  effects of bleaching 277–278, **284**
chromium casting alloys 514
chronic illness, older adults 1020–1022, **1022**, 1024–1025
Chu esthetic guage 256

CIE (Commission Internationale de l'Éclairage) color notation system 273
circumferential fiberotomy of supracrestal gingival fibers (CSF) 915
citric acid demineralization, for root coverage 1183, 1185–1186
CK Diamond Endodontic Access Kit 775
Clark, E. Bruce 272, 276, *276*
clasps, removable partial dentures 584–588
  camouflage 590
  circumferential 584
  combination 588, *588*
  embrasure 588, *588*
  I-, Y-, T- or modified T-bar 584–585, *585*
  mesial groove reciprocation (MGR) 585, *587*, *588*
  placement 584, *584*
  rest–proximal plate–I-bar (RPI) 585, *587*
  ring 585–587
  unesthetic design 1238–1239, *1239*
Class 0 (no preparation) veneer 442, *442*
Class I restorations 379, *380–382*
  pediatric dentistry 974, *974*
  primary teeth 970
Class 1 (window) veneer preparation 442, *443*
Class II malocclusions *917*, 933
  comprehensive esthetic approach 1052–1053, *1053*
  diagnostic records 934
  profile angle 1113
  surgical–orthodontic correction 944–948, *946*
  vertical maxillary excess 950
Class II restorations 382, *383*
  durability 1251
  glass ionomer liners 403
  polymerization techniques 403, *405*
  primary teeth 970
Class 2 (feather) veneer preparation 442, *443*
Class III malocclusions 933
  alternative approach 1076, *1077*
  diagnostic records 934, *936–938*
  porcelain veneers 441
  profile angle 1113
  surgical–orthodontic treatment *939–941*, *940–942*, *943–944*
Class III restorations 382–384, *384–387*
Class 3 (bevel/small butt joint) veneer preparation 442, *444*
Class IV restorations 384–385, *387–389*
  excessively translucent 1251–1252, *1255*
Class 4 (incisal overlap) veneer preparation 442–446, *444*, *446–448*, *456–459*
Class V restorations 385, *389–390*, 408
  esthetic repair 690
  follow-up care 416
Class 5 (butt joint) veneer preparation 442, *445*, *447–448*

Class 6 (full) veneer preparation 442, *445, 447–448, 456–459*
cleaning
  ceramic veneers *467, 469*
  prior to composite resin bonding 396
clear aligner therapy 909
Clearfil SE Bond adhesive 362, *363,* 366, 368
Clearfil Tri-S-Bond adhesive system 366
cleft lip and palate 951, *952*
clinical examination 55–67
  components 55–56
  computer imaging 61–66
  esthetic evaluation chart 56, *58*
  extraoral camera 59–60, *61*
  intraoral camera 57–59, *59, 60*
  occlusal analysis 60
  periodontal charting 60–61
  pulpal health 751–762
  transillumination 56–57, *58*
  X-rays 60, *61, 62*
close-up repose image 174–175, *175*
close-up smile image 173, *174*
cocaine abuse 825
coca leaf chewing 816
coffee drinking 675, *679*
cognitive behavior therapy 43
cold sensitivity, bleached teeth 341
cold testing 754–756, *756–757*
collagen membrane, resorbable (Zimmer socket repair membrane) 640–641
collagen network, dentin
  durability after etching 364–365
  phosphoric acid etching 359, *359*
  priming 360
  technique sensitivity 365
color 271–292
  basics 272–273
  case study 289–292, *289–292*
  communicating 285–286
  in dentistry 273–274
  denture base 623–625, *623–625*
  dimensions 272–273, *273*
  education and training **287,** 287–288, *288–289*
  gingival 274
  hair 1147
  lipstick 1147, 1150–1151
  makeup 1149
  notation systems 273
  perception 272
  photographic management 157
  post-bleaching relapse 350
  skin 274
  tooth *see* tooth color
  triplet 272
  see also shade
color change units (ccu) 277
color difference (ΔE)
  CIELAB formula (ΔE*) 273, *273,* 274
  peri-implant tissues 1370, *1371*
color discrimination competency (CDC) 274

color matching *see* shade selection/color matching
color modification 286–287
  all-ceramic crowns 506, 510, 511
  ceramic veneers 467–469
  porcelain 286, 438
color rendering index (CRI) 275
color standards, dental *see* shade guides
color temperature, correlated (CCT) 275
color thresholds 274
combination clasp 588, *588*
commerce 12–16
Commission Internationale de l'Éclairage (CIE) color notation system 273
commissural line 1101, *1101*
  as plane of reference 1108, *1109,* 1111
communication
  Digital Smile Design tool 86
  function of teeth 11
  laboratory *see* laboratory, communication
  patients with poor 77
  practice website 122
  treatment planning phase 79
  try-in stage 1337
community relations 127, 128
complete dentures 611–630
  bone quantity and quality 625–629
  emergency repairs 1231–1232
  esthetics 611, *612,* 614–625
    clinical examples 625–626
    denture base 623–625, *623–625*
    tooth arrangement 616–623, *617–622*
    tooth color 616
    tooth size and form 614–616
  implants and 629–630
  occlusion 613, *613–614,* 620–622
    anterior 620
    posterior 621–622, *622*
    vertical dimension 620–621, *621–622*
  opposing natural teeth 628–629, *629–631*
  performers/actors 1156–1160, *1158–1164*
  porcelain vs plastic teeth 626–627, *627–629*
  provisional 612–613, *612–613*
complications of treatment
  disclosure of 132, 143–144
  "I'm sorry" legal protection 138
compomers 970–971, 1356
composite resin(s)
  camouflaging RPD clasps 590
  dual cure 403
  flowable 362, 403, *1227*
  hybrid 395, 862, 1416
  light curing 403, 404–405, *406*
  luting agents 1356
  materials for direct bonding 393–396
  microfilled *see* microfilled composites
  modification of RPD teeth 589
  nanofilled 396, 862
  pediatric dentistry 970
  polymerization *see* polymerization
  self cure 403
  small-particle macrofilled 395

composite resin bonding 375–421
  advantages and disadvantages **538**
  alternatives to 298–300, 376
  as alternatives to veneers 434, *434–438*
  basic categories 377, *379*
  broken tooth fragments 722–723, 726–727, 1220, *1220*
  case presentation 74
  chipped teeth *see under* crown fractures
  clinical use 375, *376,* 377–393
  cosmetic contouring with 319, *319*
    crowded teeth 883–884, *884–885*
  crowded teeth **882,** 883–884, *884–885*
  curing 403–406, *405*
    following final finish 404
    incremental layering 403, *405*
    shrinkage 405
    three-sited light-curing technique 403
  diastema closure 849–864
    large diastemata 856–862
    multiple diastemata 851, 853, *853, 857–858, 857–859*
    performers/actors 1173, 1175, *1175*
    posterior diastema 863–864, *863–865*
    prior orthodontics 853, 856, *856–857*
    simple diastemas 849–853, *850–852, 854–855, 854–856*
  finishing 406–409
    adding surface texture 407–408
    final polishing 407, *410–411*
    instrumentation 406–407, *407–411*
    interproximal 409
    problems 408–409, *412–415*
  fractured teeth *see under* crown fractures
  history of use 376
  informed consent 133, *134*
  inlays 393, *394*
  interdental tissue loss 226–228, *227*
  labial veneers 385–392, *393*
  materials 393–396
  older adults 1025–1028, *1027–1029,* 1030–1031, *1030–1031*
  pediatric dentistry 973
    amelodentinal dysplasia 975, *975*
    enamel hypoplasia 978, *978*
    extensive cavities 976, *976–977*
    preventive restoration 974, *974*
  pit and fissure caries 379, 417, *418–420*
  protective night appliances 413–415, *415*
  pulp capping with 769
  repair of existing restorations 392, 1224, 1226–1230, *1228–1230*
  shade selection 396–398, *397*
  techniques 396–409
    dentin bonding 403, *404*
    enamel bonding and acid etch 401, 403
    finishing 406–409, *407–412*
    incremental layering 403, *405,* 405–406
    laser-ablated tooth structure 972–973
    legal considerations 134
    overlay technique 398–400, *399–400,* 690

composite resin bonding (cont'd)
    polymerization 403–406
    sandwich technique 403, 404
    shade selection 396–398, 397
    tooth cleaning 396
  temporary 392
    performers/actors 1155, 1160–1163
    splinting 1317–1320, 1319–1320
    veneers 1316–1317, 1316–1317
  tooth preparation 398–399, 399–401
    air-abrasive technology 417, 418
    chamfer-shoulder method 398, 399, 400
    overlay method 398–399, 399–400
  transitional 377
composite resin cores **736**
  anterior teeth 740–742, 742
  posterior teeth 734, 735, 736, 739
  small premolars 743
composite resin restorations
  air bubbles/pockets 1252
  causes of failure 1250–1252
  Class I 379, 380–382
  Class II 382, 383
  Class III 382–384, 384–387
  Class IV 384–385, 387–389
  Class V 385, 389–390
  crowns 502, 505
  discoloration 689, 689, 690, 1167, 1252
  excessively translucent 1251–1252, 1255
  fractures 1252, 1256
  indirect posterior 382
  longevity 416, 1242–1243
    durability of adhesion 363–365, 364
    legal considerations 138
    posterior teeth 376, 377
  maintenance 409–421
    homecare 415, 416
    protective night appliances 413–415, 415
    recall visits 415–416
    scaling and polishing 415, 1416
  marginal staining 379, 380, 1252, 1256
    management 671, 674, 675–676, 689
    tooth preparation methods and 400, 400
  microleakage 379, 380, 401, 1250–1251, 1254
  performers/actors 1167–1169, 1169–1170
  preparation see composite resin bonding
  repairs to existing 690
    air-abrasive technology 419–421
    laser-assisted 987–988, 987–988
    marginal staining 671, 674, 675, 689
  veneers see direct composite veneers; indirect composite/acrylic veneers
composite resin stent/splint 1155, 1157
compound/copper band impressions 1302
computed tomography see cone beam computed tomography
computer-aided design/manufacturing (CAD/CAM) systems 483–492, 1387–1407

all-ceramic crowns 507, 512–514
Carestream system 490–492, 492–494
CEREC system see CEREC system
clinical cases 1403–1406, 1404–1406
comparison table **1393**
currently available 1389–1392
dedicated impression scanners vs 1389
digital impressions 459, 1303, 1389
fixed partial dentures 562–564
implant positioning 647
laboratory 1400–1402, 1401–1402
open vs closed architecture 1400
orthodontic appliances 909
Planmeca PlanScan 1391–1392, 1391–1393
temporary restorations 1315
computer imaging
  cosmetic contouring 304, 304–305
  dentofacial analysis 1056–1057, 1059
  disclaimers 61
  fixed partial dentures 546
  laboratory communication via 197
  older adults 1025
  orthodontics 909, 910–911
  proportional smile design 265–268, 267–268
  treatment planning 61–67, 65–66, 75
  trial smile 66–67
  see also images
computer imaging therapist 61
concealers, facial cosmetic 1150, 1151
concussion, tooth 1223
condensation impression materials 1292
condylar hyperplasia 951–955, 953–955
cone beam computed tomography (CBCT) 55
  endodontics 762, 764
  fixed partial dentures 564
  orthodontics 909, 910
  treatment planning 75–77
confidentiality 145
connective tissue (gingival) grafts
  fixed partial dentures 567
  implant patients 654–655, 655–656, 1195, 1196
  papilla reconstruction 1199, 1199
  ridge augmentation 1200–1201, 1202–1203, 1203–1204
  root coverage 1183–1195
    allogenic vs autogenous 1184
    harvesting 1189–1190, 1190–1191
    old restorations and root caries 1194–1195, 1195
    placement 1190–1191, 1192–1193
    postoperative care 1194, 1194
    potential for attachment 1185–1186, 1186
    quality and quantity of donor tissue 1195
    surgical technique 1186–1194
    sutures and dressing 1191–1194
    unesthetic 1183, 1183

connector area 247, 248
consent 27
  explicit and implicit 132
  informed see informed consent
consent forms 133, 134–137, 139
  video 139, 141
contact areas, try-in stage 1345, 1345
contaminants, causing restoration failure 1255
continuous positive airways pressure (CPAP) 959, 961
contouring, cosmetic 297–321
  bruxism 300, 301, 301, 814, 814
  chipped teeth 722, 723, 1217
  composite resin bonding with 319, 319
  crowded teeth 883–884, 884–885
  contraindications 301–303, 301–303
  crowded teeth 303, **882,** 883, 883
  early techniques 297–298, 298
  failure to perform 1239, 1241, 1241–1242
  indications 298–300, 299–300
  older adults 1025–1028, 1026
  performers/models 1166, 1167
  porcelain veneers 439
  principles 303–304
  techniques 305–319
    altering tooth form 313–314, 314–315
    angle of correction 305–306, 307
    arch irregularity 319, 320–322
    creating illusions 189–190, 305, 306–307
    reduction 306–313, 308–313
  too-wide teeth 207–209, 207–209
  treatment planning 304, 304–306
  try-in appointment 1347–1350, 1349–1351
contours, Pincus principles D4, D4–D5
coronal fractures see crown fractures
correlated color temperature (CCT) 275
corticotomy-assisted orthodontics 956–959
cosmetic adjuncts 1143–1151
cosmetic contouring see contouring, cosmetic
Cosmetic Contouring Kit, Shofu 310–311, 313
cosmetic dentistry 897–898, 898
cosmetics see makeup
cosmetics industry 13–14
cosmetic surgery 13, 14–16, 18
  see also plastic surgery
costs, financial see financial considerations
coverage error (CE) 280–281
cracked tooth syndrome (CTS) **722,** 794–804
  class I (incomplete vertical fracture) 798–799, 801–802
  class II (pulpal involvement) 799–801, 803–804
  class III (attachment involvement) 801–802
  class IV (complete separation of tooth fragments) 802–803
  class V (retrograde root fracture) 803

Index

diagnosis 794–798
discoloration 673
prevalence trends 797
see also crown fractures; microcracks, enamel; root fractures
Creation Porcelain 516
cross-bite 1061
crowded teeth 877–893
  clinical evaluation 877–881
    arch space 878, *878*
    Berliner's formula 878, *879*
    gingival architecture 878–879, *880*
    posttreatment oral hygiene 881
    root proximity 881
    smile line 881
  older adults 920
  pediatric patients 997, *997–1000*
  tooth preparation 1280–1283, *1282*
  treatment failure 1236, *1237*
  treatment options **882**, 883–890, 893
    composite resin bonding 883–884, *884–885*
    cosmetic contouring 303, 883, *883*
    crowning 887–890, *888–889*
    disking 883
    porcelain veneers 884–886, *886–887*
  treatment strategy 881–883
  unusual or rare presentations 890–893
crown fractures (and chips) 721–745, 1216–1221
  complicated (pulp involvement) 727–730, 1219–1221, *1220–1221*
  endodontics 790, *793*–794
  interdisciplinary approach 728–730, *729–731*
  pediatric patients 990, *990–993*
  treatment options **722**, 1219
  composite resin bonding 1218–1219, *1219*
    choosing 722, *723*, 725–726, **727**
    life expectancy 730–731, *731–732*
    long-term results 724–726, *728*
    posterior teeth 731–732
    techniques 384–385, *387–389*
  cosmetic contouring 722, *723*, 1217
  crowning **727**, 729, *730*
  diagnosis 56–57, 751, 755–756, 761–762
  enamel infractions 1216, *1217*
  endodontically-treated teeth 732–745
    anterior **739**, 739–743, *740–742*
    core materials **736**
    crown preparation 743–745, *744*
    post design 734–735, **736**
    posterior 736–739, *736–739*
    premolars 743, *743*
    principles 732–734, *733–734*
  incomplete 798–803
  pediatric 984–985
    intrusive luxation with complicated 990, *990–993*
    uncomplicated 986, *986–987*
    unsatisfactory treatment 987–988, *987–988*

porcelain veneers 722, 723–724, *723–724*, 726, **727**
posterior teeth 731–732
tooth fragment bonding 722–723, 726–727, 1219, 1220, *1220*
treatment 721–724
  conservative options 722, *723–724*
  factors influencing choice 722–724, *723–726*, **727**
  uncomplicated 1216–1219
    conservative bonding techniques 724–727, *728*
    enamel and dentin 1217–1219, *1219*
    enamel only 1216–1217, *1217–1218*
    endodontics 790, *793*, 1219
    pediatric patients 986, *986–987*
    treatment options **722**
see also cracked tooth syndrome
crown-lengthening procedures
  attachment RPDs 593
  biologic width and 1205–1206
  bruxism *701, 702*
  diastema closure and 846
  excessive gingival display 1204–1208, *1205*
  poorly contoured restorations 1245
  surgical procedure 1206–1208, *1206–1209*
crown–root fractures 740, 1221, *1222*
crown:root ratio, abutment teeth 582
crowns (prosthetic) 499–538
  advantages and disadvantages **538**
  all-ceramic *see* all-ceramic crowns
  all-metal *see* all-metal crowns
  alternatives to
    ceramic veneers 474, *474–481*
    cosmetic contouring 298–300
    importance of offering 143
  bleaching of adjacent natural teeth 687
  bruxism patients *701, 702*
  cementation 1352, 1358–1361
  crowded teeth **882**, 887–890, *888–889*
  diagnosis 500, *500–501*
  diastema closure 869–870, *872*
  emergency repairs 1224, *1230–1232, 1231–1232*
  failures
    dentinal staining 1236
    improper contours 1236–1238, *1238–1239*
    margin exposure 1236, *1237*
    material 1248–1250
    periodontal disease 1245, *1245*
    technical 1253–1255, *1257–1260*
  fractured teeth 731
    endodontically-treated 733, *733–734*
    pros and cons **727**
    with pulp involvement 729, *730*
  gold 502, *502–504*
  indications 499–500
  interdental tissue loss 227–228, *228–229*
  legal considerations

informed consent 133, *137*
  overcontoured crowns 147, *148–149*
  unnecessary placement 143, *143*
longevity 138, 500, *500*, 1244
  promoting 536
metal–ceramic *see* metal–ceramic restorations
metal inlay, fixed partial denture retainers 549
metal onlay, fixed partial denture retainers 549
older adults 1034–1035
patient maintenance 536
performers/actors 1173–1174
photographic records 500, *500*
porcelain-fused-to-metal *see* porcelain-fused-to-metal crowns
porcelain veneers for 441
posts and cores *see* post-and-core restorations
principles of esthetic 525–536
  arch irregularity 526, *526*
  final try-in 529
  inclination of teeth 526–527
  lip line 525–526, *526*
  natural appearance *527–528*, 527–529
  occlusal registration 531
  shade matching *532–535*, 532–536
  texture and characterization 532
  tooth arrangement 531–532
  tooth color 532
  tooth contour and shape 529, *530*
  tooth size *530*, 530–531
resin (acrylic and composite) 502, *505*
retention after endodontic therapy 779–780, *780*
selection 523–525, *524*, 525–526, *526*
technical considerations 501–514
telescoping 555–562
temporary 1313–1314
three-quarter, fixed partial denture retainers 549
tooth preparation 1263–1283
  pulp injury 767–769, *768–769*
try-in 1339–1352
  adding texture 1350, *1351*
  additional impressions 1343, *1344*
  contacts 1345, *1345*
  esthetic checks 1345–1347, *1346–1348*
  fitting to tooth 1341–1343, *1344*
  occlusal adjustment 1346
  shaping 1347–1350, *1349–1351*
  stuck on tooth 1341, *1342*
cultural aspects
  esthetics 3
  filing of teeth 298, *298*
curing *see* polymerization
curve of Spee 247, *247*, 921
  depth, ratio to arch circumference 921–922
  orthodontic leveling 944
Cushee rubber dam clamp cushions 773, *773*
cuspal fracture 797

cuspids *see* canines
customer service 117–119, *119–120*
Cvek pulpotomy 727, 1219
cystic fibrosis 328

Dalbo attachment system 600, *600–602*
DC-Zirkon 1253
decalcification spots *see* white spots
decision making, patient 48–49
    involving family/friends 1332
    older adults 1025
    role of temporaries 1312, *1313*
    see also case presentation; trial smile
dehydration, tooth
    post bleaching 340–341
    shade matching and 283, 396
demanding patients 38–40, *39*
dementia 1022, 1024, 1036
demographics, population 1015–1016, **1016**
Dentacolor 502
dental assistants
    computer imaging 61
    extraoral photographs 59
Dental Color Matcher (DCM) **287**, 287–288, *288–289*
dental education
    color **287**, 287–288, *288–289*
    Digital Smile Design 87
    role of photographs 158
    see also training
dental history 70
dental hygienists *see* hygienists
dental materials
    causing tooth discoloration 330
    color-related properties **286**, 286–287
dental midline
    canting 1101, *1102*, 1105–1106
    checking, at try-in 1345, *1346*
    deviations 1104–1106
        acceptability 137, 899–902, *902, 1094, 1095*
        correction 1094, *1096*
    diastema closure and 845
    Digital Smile Design 89, *89*
    facial midline and 1094, *1094*, 1104–1106
    to midsagittal plane 1061, *1065*
dental technicians
    communication with *see* laboratory, communication
    Digital Smile Design tool 86
dentifrices *see* toothpastes
dentin
    bonding *358*, 358–360, *361*
        after laser ablation 972–973
        ceramic veneers 452, 468, 471
        composite resins 403
        primers/priming adhesives 359–360
        priming of collagen network 360
        self-etch adhesives 360, *360*
        stabilization 360
        technique sensitivity 365–366, *366*
        tooth sensitivity after 366–367, 403

conditioning/acid etching *see* acid etching, dentin
    reparative 766–767, *767*
    secondary 767, *767*
    thickness, cavity preparations 767–768, *768*
    traumatic exposure 790, 1217–1219, *1219*
dentinoenamel junction (DEJ) scallop 705
dentinogenesis imperfecta
    tooth discoloration 330, 680–681, *681*
    tooth wear 697
dentist–patient relationship 51, 79, 145
    establishing rapport 750–751
    mistakes/errors and 138
dentists
    appearance 115–116, *119*
    correction of dentofacial deformity and 935
    identifying gender from tooth shape 614
    patient's right to choose 146–147, *146–147*
    preferences
        tooth-to-tooth width proportions 258–260, *260*
        tooth width/length ratio 253, 256
    responsibility for obtaining consent 144–145
    right to refuse treatment 145
    updating skills and practices 132
dentofacial analysis 1098, 1119–1125
    buccal corridors 1125
    facial landmarks 1053, *1054*
    incisal edges and lower lip 1120–1122
    orthodontic perspective 1057–1062, *1060–1067*
    papilla display during smiling 1124–1125
    smile line 1122–1124, *1122–1125*
    smile width 1125, *1125*
    tooth exposure at rest 1119–1120, *1119–1121*
    see also facial analysis; macroesthetic analysis; smile analysis
dentofacial deformity 929–965
    diagnostic records 934–935, *935–938*
    facial analysis 930–931, *931–932*
    first visit 933–935
    pediatric patients 933
    surgical–orthodontic correction 940–955
dentogenics 246
Dentsply Sirona 537
Dentsply tooth size facial guide *251*
dentures
    complete 611–630
    fixed partial 543–571
    performers/actors 1156–1160, *1158–1164*, 1176–1177, *1177*
    removable partial 581–606
denture teeth
    complete dentures 614–623
        arrangement 616–623
        color 616

        materials 616, 626–627, *627–628*
        size and form 614–616
    emergency repairs 1231
    removable partial dentures 589
Denzir all-ceramic restorations 1249–1250
depression 26, 27–29
    bipolar 30
    diagnosis 27, 28
dermabrasion 1140
dermal fillers 1137, *1140*
developing teeth, traumatic injuries to 986
developmental abnormalities
    cosmetic contouring 298, *299*
    porcelain veneers 440
    tooth discoloration 330
dexterity, patient 594
DiaComp Feather Lite composite polishers 407, *411*
Diagnodent 55, *55*, 971
diagnostic study models *see* study models
diagnostic wax-up *see* wax-up, diagnostic
diamond burs
    ceramic veneer finishing 470, *473*
    cosmetic contouring 308, *308*
    endodontic access cavity 776, *778*
    finishing composite restorations 406–407, *407*
    incisal embrasures 1346, *1347, 1347*
    pit and fissure caries 419
    tooth reduction
        all-ceramic crowns 1268–1271, *1269, 1271–1273*
        porcelain-fused-to-metal crowns *1278*, 1279
        veneers 456–457, *457–458*
    zirconia cutting 778
diamond impregnated polishing paste 473
diastemas 841–872
    diagnosis and treatment planning 843–844, *845*
    disguises used by patients 841, *842*
    etiology **842**, 842–843
    large 856–862, *860–861*
    multiple (diastemata)
        clinical case 857–858, *857–859*
        composite resin bonding 851, 853, *853*
        etiology **842**, 842–843
        porcelain veneers 867–869, *869–870, 871*, 871
        treatment 853, 857–858, *857–859*
    with narrow teeth 852–853, 856, *856–857*
    orthodontic therapy *see under* orthodontics
    periodontal surgery and 847, 915
    posterior 863–864, *863–865*
    removable veneers 841, *842*
    restorative treatment 844–870
        combination crowns/veneers 869–870, *872*
        composite resin bonding 849–864
        functional considerations 848–849

gingival esthetics 847
   illusions 847–848, *848–849*
   incisal edge position 846
   porcelain veneers 441, 864–869
   tooth proportion 846–847
simple
   clinical cases 854–856, *854–856*
   composite resin bonding 849–853, *850–852*
   orthodontics and direct bonding 856, *856–857*
   porcelain veneers 866–867, *868*
   temporary measures for performers 1155, 1173, 1175, *1175*
   tongue habits causing *816–817*, 817, 843, *843*
   see also interdental spaces
Dicor glass-ceramic crowns 506, *507*, **513**
dietary advice 712, 1414–1415
dietary factors
   dental erosion 710, **711**
   tooth discoloration 328, 675, *679*
dietary habits, poor 822–825
difficult patients *see* problem patients
Digital Facebow *87*, *88*
digital impressions 1302–1303, 1387–1407
   accuracy 1400
   bite registration 1307
   CAD/CAM systems 459, 1303, 1389
   ceramic veneers 459
   CEREC system 487, *487*, 1390
   clinical cases 1403–1406, *1404–1406*
   dedicated scanners 1389, 1393–1400
      3M True Definition 1394–1395, *1394–1396*
      3Shape TRIOS 1397–1400, *1398–1399*
      comparison table **1400**
      iTero Element scanner 1396–1397, *1396–1397*
      model fabrication 1394
   history 1388–1389
   open vs closed architecture 1400
digital mock-up, Digital Smile Design 94, *100*, *103–104*
digital models, orthodontics 909, *910*
digital photography *see* photography
digital radiographs *see* radiographs
Digital Smile Design (DSD) 85–94
   advantages 86–87
   clinical procedures *107–109*
   final results *109–110*
   presentation to patient *104–106*
   procedure 87–94, *87–104*
digital systems, integrated 67
digit sucking 811–813, *812*, 1004
Diller, Phyllis 1169, *1169–1170*
dimensional stability, impression materials **1293**, 1294
diode lasers
   gingival preparation for impressions 1291, *1292*
   pediatric dentistry 984–985

direct acrylic veneers 461
direct composite veneers
   combined with ceramic restorations 385–392, *393*
   diastema closure 862, *862–863*
   history 434
   provisional treatment 392
   temporary restorations 460–461, *461–463*
direct mail advertising 128
directories, telephone and online 125
discoloration
   soft tissue
      amalgam restorations 805, *807*
      around implants 655, 658, *659*, 1370
   tooth *see* stained/discolored teeth
discount shopping services, online group 128
disfigured face, makeup for 1151
disking, crowded teeth **882**, 883
displacement syndrome 16
disruptive technologies 1406
dissatisfied patients 19, 50, 147, 152
distal inclination, increasing 217–218
distal rotation of teeth 190, *191*, 209, *210–211*
distraction osteogenesis 933, 955–956
doctor *see* dentist
documentation 139–142
   chart 141–142
   role of photographs 157
   see also records, clinical
Dolder bar attachments 605, *607*
dolichocephalic facial form 1058, *1061*, 1098, *1100*
double tooth 1000, *1000–1003*
drinks *see* beverages
drug abuse 825
drug-induced problems *see* medication-induced problems

ears, prominent 1059, *1064*
eating disorders 26, 31–36, 822–825
   minors with 36
   worksheet for new patients **35–36**
eating habits, patients with ceramic veneers 474–477
ecstasy (methylenedioxymethamphetamine) 825
ectodermal dysplasia 982–983, *982–983*
edentulous areas
   Kennedy classification 582, *582*
   removable partial denture design 583
   ridge augmentation for implants 639–643, *641–642*
   tissue preparation for pontics 566–570, *569–570*
edentulous patients 611
education *see* dental education; patient education
Ehrmann, E.H. 727
elastic recovery, impression materials 1293, **1293**

elderly *see* older adults
electric pulp testing 756–757, *758*
   through test cavity *758*, 759
electromagnetic spectrum *272*
electronic health records (EHRs) 67, 142
electrosurgery, gingival 1290–1291, *1291–1292*
e-mail consultations 150
e.max *see* IPS e.max
embrasure clasp 588, *588*
embrasure spaces
   closure methods 1196
   see also papillae, interdental
emergencies 1215–1233
   avulsions 1223–1224
   crown fractures 1216–1221
   crown–root fractures 1221
   fractured restorations 1224–1230
   long-term preservation 1215–1216
   luxation injuries 1223
   patient evaluation 1216
   performers/actors 1176
   prosthesis fracture/failure 1231–1232
   root fractures 1221–1223
   see also traumatic injuries
empathy 38
employment 12, *13–14*
enamel
   acid etching *see* acid etching, enamel
   bonding 356–358, 360, *361*
      after laser ablation 972–973
      ceramic restorations 1373
      ceramic veneers 439, 468, 471
      composite resin 401, 403
      conditioning/etching 356, 356–357
      historical development 358
      mechanisms 356–358, *357*
      self-etch adhesives **357**, 357–358
   chips and fractures *see* crown fractures
   defects, stained 671, *673*
   fractures 1216–1217, *1217–1218*
   hypocalcification *see* hypocalcification, enamel
   hypoplasia
      restorative therapy 978, *978*
      tooth discoloration 330, *331*, 679, *679*
   infractions 1216, *1217*
   microcracks *see* microcracks, enamel
   mottled *see* fluorosis, dental
   reduction, ceramic veneers 452–453
   thickness
      cosmetic contouring and 302
      disking and 883
      radiographic measurement *879*, 883
Endo Access Kit 775
endodontic access cavity 774–780, *775*
   cavity shape and size 775, *775–776*
   coronal leakage 782, *783*, **783**, 785
   preparation and equipment 775–776
   restored teeth 776–780, *777–780*
   sealing 781–782, *781–782*

endodontically-treated teeth
  bleaching 347, 348, 682, 684–685, 783–789
    preventing resorption 786, 786–788, 788–789
    root resorption risks 350, 783–784, 785
    walking bleach technique 784–786, 786–787
  crowded tooth scenario 882
  discoloration 346, 682, 683, 786, 787
    prevention 780, 781
  posterior ceramic partial coverage restorations 480
  restoring fractured 732–745
    anterior teeth **739,** 739–743, 740–742
    crown preparation 743–745, 744
    post design 734–735, 735
    posterior teeth **736,** 736–739, 736–739
    post materials 735, **736**
    premolars 743, 743
    principles 732–734, 733–734
endodontics 749–807
  anesthetic test 763–764
  attachment RPDs 593
  clinical evaluation 750–764
  cracked tooth syndrome 794–804
  diagnosis 764
  indications for elective 767–771
  laser applications 973
  older adults 1030
  pediatric patients 996
  radiography 762–763, 763–765, 774
  restoration vs tooth removal 782–783, 784–785
  retreatment 805, 806
  tissue discoloration (tattoo) 805, 807
  trauma 728, 729–731, 790–794
  treatment planning 74, 750
  treatment protocols 771–783
    access cavity preparation 774–780
    coronal seal 781–782, 782
    instrumentation/debridement 780
    restored teeth 776–780
    rubber dam 771–774, 772–774
    sealing canal system 780–782, 781–782
endodontic surgery 804–805, 805–806
Endo-Ice 754–756, 757
Endo Safe access burs 776
Endo-Z bur 776
end-to-end bite, porcelain veneers and 441
enhancement of appearance 1051–1052
entertainers *see* performers/actors
environment, color matching 275–276
epinephrine 1288
E-plane, Ricketts 1117, 1117
erbium lasers 421, 971–973, 984
  see also lasers
erosion 709–711
  abfraction lesions 705, 706, 707
  alcohol and drug abuse 825
  bleaching and 335

bulimia nervosa 33, 33–34, 712–714, 713, 822, 822–823
ceramic veneers 477
clinical case 712–714, 713
definition 693, 709
differential diagnosis 711–712
etiology 709–710, **711,** 711
gastroesophageal reflux disease (GERD) 33, 712
habitual acid consumption 33, 822–824, 824
treatment 710–711
erythroblastosis fetalis 331, 682
esthetic analysis
  Digital Smile Design (DSD) tool 86
  see also macroesthetic analysis; microesthetics; miniesthetics
esthetic dentistry 3–20
  cosmetic dentistry vs 897–898, 898
  definition 3
  health science and service 6–8
  historical perspective 4–5, 4–5
  Pincus principles D2–D9
  social context 5–6, 6–7
  understanding patient's needs 8–9
esthetic depth determination
  all-ceramic crowns 1268–1270, 1271–1276
  porcelain-fused-to-metal crowns 1271–1272, 1277–1278
esthetic evaluation chart 56, 58
esthetic evaluation form A1–A6
esthetics
  defined 1085
  dental 3–20
  facial *see* facial esthetics
esthetic templates, fixed partial dentures 546, 547
Esthet-X shade guide 282
etch-and-dry systems 360
etch-and-rinse adhesive systems 361, **362**
  postoperative hypersensitivity 366
  recommendations for use 367–368, 367–368
  reliability and degradation 364, 364–365
  technique sensitivity 365
etch-and-rinse technique (total etching) 359, 359, 403
etching
  acid *see* acid etching
  laser 972
ethnic/racial differences
  facial form 930
  gingival display 1123
  interarch tooth size ratios 923
  lip position 1117
  nasolabial angle 1114
Etruscans 4, 4
eugenol cements 1313, 1364
expectations, high 78
"extension for prevention" philosophy 134–136
external root resorption

after bleaching 144, 350, 783–784, 785
  legal considerations 148, 150
  prevention 144, 786, 786–788, 788–789
avulsed/luxated teeth 794, 799–801, 1224
clinical evaluation 752
endodontic surgery 799–801, 804
orthodontic 144
extracoronal attachment removable partial dentures 596, 599–605
  advantages 599
  disadvantages 599–600
  types 600–605, 601–606
extractions
  after final impressions 1294, 1297–1298
  bone-conserving methods 639, 645
  crowded teeth 881
  early childhood caries 979
  endodontically-diseased teeth 782–783, 784–785
  implant placement at time of 643–644, 645–647, **647**
  microsurgical approach 1182, 1182
  performers/actors 1176
  pontic placement and 566
  ridge preservation 639, 640–641, 1200
  ridge resorption after 638–639, **639,** 639, 1182, 1182, 1200
extruded teeth, cosmetic contouring 300
extrusion, orthodontic
  cosmetic contouring after 298
  crown–root fractures 1221, 1222
  prior to implant placement 905, 907
  root segments 793, 798, 1223
eyebrow line 1099, 1101
eyebrows, makeup 1150
eyeglasses, harmful habits 831, 833
eye makeup 1150

facebow
  digital 87, 88
  transfer, casts 1303, 1303–1304
facelift (rhytidectomy) 1137, 1138
face size
  measurement 614–615, 614–615
  proportion of tooth size to 249–251, 250–252
facial analysis 56, 57, 1097–1119
  dentofacial deformity 930–931, 931–932
  diastemata restoration 844–845
  facial reference lines 1098–1101, 1101
  frontal view 1098–1113, 1100–1112
  importance 1086–1097
  oblique view 1113
  orthodontics 899–900
  profile view 1113–1119
  proportional 253–265
  records 1097–1098
  soft tissues 1005–1006
  see also dentofacial analysis; macroesthetic analysis
facial appearance, importance of 10–11, 10–11

facial asymmetry 951–955
　classification **953**
　clinical evaluation 1061–1062, 1065–1067
　esthetic *1090*, 1090–1091, *1092*, 1095
　location 1094, *1099*
　observation 1089–1090, *1089–1090*
　see also facial symmetry
facial components, ranking of importance 6, **8**
facial disfigurement, makeup for 1151
facial esthetics
　cosmetic adjuncts 1143–1151
　evaluation 930–931, *931–932*
　impact of orthodontics 898–905
　orthodontic perspective 1051–1083
　pediatric dentistry 1005–1010
　plastic surgery 1131–1140
　restorative dentistry 1085–1126
　three dimensions 1052, *1052*
facial expressions 1088–1089
facial fifths *see* fifths, facial
facial hair, male 1148, *1148*
facial image view evaluation (FIVE) 253, *255*
　calculating intercanine width 261, *262*
　tooth-to-tooth width proportions 257, *257*
facial index 1057–1058, *1060*
facial midline 1090–1094, *1091–1095*
　chin symmetry and 1107
　complete denture positioning 617, *618*
　dental midline and 1094, *1094*, 1104–1106
　diastema closure and 845
　digital smile design 87, 88, 94, *95–97*
　interpupillary line relationship 1099, *1101*
　nasal tip position and 1104
　perceived 1090, *1091*
facial photographs 1053–1056, 1098
　basic protocols 171–173
　dentofacial deformities 934
　frontal images 1053–1055
　　camera orientation 1053, *1055*
　　repose (at rest) 173, 1053, *1055*
　　smile (dynamic) 171–173, *173*, 1055, *1056*
　oblique images 1055–1056, *1057*
　profile images 173, 1056, *1058*
　submental image 1056, *1059*
facial profile
　convex 1113, *1114*
　denture tooth arrangement 620, *621*
　denture tooth selection 616
　diastema correction and 845
　facial analysis 1113–1119
　landmarks **1069**, *1069*, *1099*
　macroesthetic evaluation 1063–1068, *1069–1075*
　pediatric patients *1008–1009*, 1008–1010
　photographs 173, 1056, *1058*
　symmetry and proportion 931, *932*
facial profile angle 1113
facial proportions 245, 930–931
　aging effects 245, *246*, 1101–1102, *1106–1107*

golden proportion *see* golden proportion
　orthodontic esthetics 900–902
　pediatric patients *1007–1009*, 1007–1010
　rule of fifths *see* fifths, facial
　rule of sevenths 245, *245*
　rule of thirds *see* thirds, facial
　transverse 1058, *1059*, *1063–1064*
　vertical 1057–1058, 1101–1104
facial prostheses, shade guides 281
facial reference lines 1098–1101, *1101*
facial resurfacing 1140
facial shape (or form)
　classification 1058, *1060–1061*, 1098, *1100*
　denture tooth selection and 615, *616*
　female hairstyles and 1144–1147, *1144–1147*
　male 1147–1148, *1148*
　special effects influencing 218–219
facial symmetry 930–931, 1089–1097
　analysis using facial midline 1090–1094, *1091–1095*
　esthetic relevance 1094–1095
　pediatric patients *1006–1008*, 1007–1008
　see also facial asymmetry
facial taper 1058, *1062–1063*
facial thirds *see* thirds, facial
facial views *see* frontal view of face; oblique view of face; submental view of face
facilities, office, attractiveness 115, *116–118*
failures, esthetic 1235–1260
　compromised treatment plan 1240–1244
　eventual (restoration longevity) 1244–1260
　immediate 1236–1239
　prostheses 1231–1232
　reasons for 1235
family, patient's 1332
Faunce, F.R. 434
feather-edged veneer preparation 442, *443*
Federal Health Insurance Portability and Accountability Act 145
federal requirements 150
fees, dental 79–81
　factors determining 80–81
　patient education 49
　payment before completion 145
　payment planning 70
　raising, for problem patients 40, 77, 79
　refunds 147, *148*
　see also financial considerations
feldspathic porcelain
　all-ceramic crowns 502–505, 518, 1264
　bilayered ceramic restorations 507–510, *508–509*, 1264
　fused to metal 514
　milled restorations, tooth preparation 1264
　veneer onlay 482
　veneers 434, 502–505
　　diastema closure 867, *868*, 871, *871*
　　masking stained teeth 687, *687*
　　tooth preparation 446

feminine appearance
　cosmetic contouring 301, *301*, 303
　dentists' perceptions 614
　failure to incorporate 1237, *1238*
　ideal tooth widths 250–251, *252*
　incorporating 223, *225*
　size and shape of teeth 248, *249*, *250*
ferrule design, endodontically-treated teeth *744*, 745
fiber-polymer composite prefabricated posts **736**
fifths, facial 245, *246*
　orthodontics 902, *903*, 931, *931*, 1058–1059, *1063*
　prominent ears and 1059, *1064*
filing of teeth 5, *5*, 297–298, *298*
　see also contouring, cosmetic
film actors *see* performers/actors
financial considerations
　actors and entertainers 1154–1155, 1176
　attachment RPDs 594, 597
　choice of crown 523
　compromising esthetics 1242
　older patients 1025
　restorative choices 893
　restoring fractured teeth 724
　single-lens reflex cameras 159
　treatment planning 78, 79
　see also fees, dental
fingernail habits 825, *826*
finger sucking 811–813, *812*
first visit *see* initial visit
Fit Checker 1324, 1341, *1342*
FIVE *see* facial image view evaluation
fixed partial dentures (bridges; FPDs) 543–571
　after root fractures 793
　attachment RPDs placed on pontics 593, *594*
　attachments for conversion to RPDs 597–598, *599*
　cantilever 555, *556*
　ceramic connectors 1379, **1380**
　ceramic interdental inserts 228–230, *229*, 570, *572–573*
　diagnosis 543–547
　　clinical examination 544, *544*
　　diagnostic wax-up 545, *546*
　　esthetic considerations 545–546, *546–547*
　　functional considerations 546–547
　　interdisciplinary consultations 547
　　radiographic examination 544–545
　　study casts 545, *545*, *546*
　digital impressions 1403, *1404*
　endodontic access 779, *779*
　evolving technologies 562–563, *562–564*
　failure
　　emergency repair 1231–1232
　　framework 1250, *1250–1251*
　　technical 1254–1255, *1258–1260*
　　one missing anterior tooth 555, *555–557*

fixed partial dentures (bridges; FPDs) (cont'd)
    orthodontic-restorative treatment 909
    performers/actors 1173–1174
    pontics see pontics
    precision attachments 564, *564*
    prepless 549
    replacement of pre-existing 547, *548*
    resin-bonded 549
        diastema closure 863–864, *863–865*
        orthodontic-restorative therapy 909
    resin-bonded partial-veneer 549
    retainers 547–551
        complete coverage 550–551, *551–552*
        functional considerations 546–547
        margin location 551, *553*
        margin materials 552–553, *553–554*
        partial coverage 549–550, *549–550*
        porcelain–metal junction 553–554, *554*
        resin-bonded 549
    ridge augmentation 566–570, *569*, 1201–1204, *1201–1204*
    special impression technique 1294, *1295–1297*
    splinting and 555
    telescoping crowns as abutments 555–562
    temporary 1313–1314
    try-in 1341, *1343*, 1345
    zirconia frameworks *see under* zirconia
fixed prosthetic restorations
    performers/actors 1173–1174, *1173–1174*
    try-in principles 1339–1352
    see also crowns; fixed partial dentures; inlays/onlays; veneers
flash systems, camera
    selection 163, *164*, *165*
    settings 166–168, *169*, *170*
flexibility, impression materials 1293, **1293**
floss, dental 1410, 1414, *1415*
    composite restorations 409
    implant cleaning 1423–1427
    incorrect use 409, 827, 830–831, *831*, 1410, *1411*
    removing excess cement 1358–1359, *1361*
    rubber dam retention 772–773
fluoride
    acidic preparations 477
    -containing cement 1247–1248
    gel, vital bleaching 345
fluorosis, dental 679–680, *681*, 682
    bleaching 328, *328*, 682–683, *685*
    veneers 440, 441
follow-up care, patient's commitment 133
follow-up letters 139, *141*
food
    acidic *see* acidic beverages/foods
    stains 328, 675, *679*
Food and Drug Administration (FDA) 345
foreign objects, harmful habits 825–833
foundation, facial cosmetic 1150
FPDs *see* fixed partial dentures
fractures 721–745

crown *see* crown fractures
crown–root 740, 1221, *1222*
extracoronal **722**
intracoronal **722**
porcelain *see* porcelain fractures
restorations 1224–1230
root *see* root fractures
Frankfort plane 1113
frenectomy 915
frenum
    fibrous attachments 843
    prominent, gingival recession risk 1184
frontal view of face
    facial analysis 1098–1113, *1100–1112*
    facial asymmetry 1061–1062, *1065–1067*
    landmarks **1054**, *1054*, 1099
    macroesthetic evaluation 1057–1062, *1060–1067*
    pediatric patients *1006–1008*, 1007–1008
    photographs 1053–1055, *1054–1055*
        basic protocols 171–173, *173*
        camera orientation 1053, *1055*
    symmetry and proportion 930–931, *931*
f-stop 166–168, *169*, *170*
Fuji Bond LC adhesive 362
full veneer preparation design (Class 6) 442, 445, 447–448, 456–459
functional-esthetic analysis B1–B6
furcation involvement 1185, *1186*
fusion, tooth 1000, *1000–1003*

gastroesophageal reflux disease (GERD) 33, 712
G-Bond adhesive system 366
gender differences
    age-related arch changes 920, *921*
    color matching ability 274, **284**
    cosmetic contouring 301, *301*, 303
    facial index 1058
    interarch tooth size ratios 923
    nasolabial angle 1114
    tooth color 274
    tooth shape 303, 614
genetic testing 1423, *1424–1426*
genioplasty 959, *961–962*, 1137
geometric theory, tooth morphology 614
geresthetics 1015–1047
    see also older adults
Geristore resin ionomer 794, *800*
gingiva
    color 274
    effects on tooth appearance 186
    electrosurgery 1290–1291, *1291*
    implant patients *see* implants, gingival tissues
    porcelain biocompatibility 439
    prostheses *see* tissue inserts
    retraction prior to impressions 1288–1291, *1289–1292*
    shade guides 281
    see also soft tissues
gingival architecture

crowded teeth 878–879, *880*
implant provisionalization and 656–657
gingival augmentation
    indications 1185
    papilla reconstruction 1195–1199
    root coverage 1183–1195
    see also connective tissue grafts
gingival biotype
    assessment 654, **654**
    crown selection and 523
    esthetic crown-lengthening and 1205
    implant patients 654–655
    recession risk and *1185*
gingival display 1123
    crown selection and 523, 525–526, *526*
    diastema closure and 847
    excessive (gummy smile) 905, 1123–1124
        Botox therapy 905
        periodontal plastic surgery 1204–1208, *1205–1209*
        surgical–orthodontic correction *947*, 948
    orthodontic aspects 904–905, *905*
    patient/lay preferences 137–138, 899
    smile design 247, *247*
    see also smile line
gingival embrasures
    crowns 527–529, *528*
    diastema closure 849, *850*
    open *see* black triangles
    performers/actors 1174
    try-in appointment 1346, *1347*
gingival esthetics
    diastema correction 847
    orthodontics 909, 913–914
    patient preferences 137–138
gingival grafts *see* connective tissue grafts
gingival hypertrophy 1205, *1205*
    anabolic steroid abuse 825
    around restorations 1245, *1245*
gingival inflammation (gingivitis)
    excessive laser sculpting 149–150, *151*
    marginal fit of crown and 1267, *1268*
    prevention in older adults 1023
    recession risk 1184, *1185*
    try-in appointment 1339
gingival inserts *see* tissue inserts
gingival margins
    all-ceramic crowns 1267–1268
    ceramic veneers 456, *458*, 470, 473
    checking fit 1345
    composite restorations 408, 411–412
    fixed partial dentures 551–553, *553–554*
    free
        evaluating thickness 1264
        smile design 248, *250*
    metal–ceramic crowns 518–521, *520*, 1265–1266, *1267*
    orthodontics and 913
    poor fitting to 1236, *1237*
    porcelain-fused-to-metal crowns 1277–1280, *1280*
    see also subgingival margins

gingival recession
　around restorations 1245
　etiology 1184
　metal–ceramic crowns 519
　Miller classification 1184
　postimplant 655
　root coverage surgery 1183–1195
　tooth preparation for crowns and 1264–1266, 1267
gingival retraction cords 1288, 1288–1290
　ceramic veneers 469
　implant restoration 660–661
　metal–ceramic crowns 519
　one-cord technique 1289, 1289–1290
　placement 1288–1290
　problems 1290, 1290
　tooth staining caused by iron-impregnated 1236
　two-cord technique 1289, 1290
gingival sulcus
　choice of crowns and 523
　crown margin placement 1267, 1267–1268
　retraction cord placement 1288–1290, 1289–1290
gingivectomy
　attachment RPDs 593
　diastema correction and 847
gingivitis see gingival inflammation
glass-ceramics 1375–1377
　full coverage crowns 506, 507, 510–514
　posterior partial coverage restorations 481–482
　tooth preparation 1264
　veneers 434–435, 453, 462–465
　see also lithium-disilicate ceramic
glass-infiltrated ceramics 1377
glass ionomers
　adhesion to lased tooth structure 973
　cements 1356
　cores 736
　lining composite restorations 403
　pediatric dentistry 970
　polishing 1416
　see also resin-modified glass ionomers
glaze
　stain combined with 194–195, 197–198
　surface staining over 194
gloss, surface 284
glove materials 1292
Gluma Solid Bond adhesive 362
glycerin, ceramic veneer fitting 467, 472
gold
　collar, ceramometal crowns 1244
　factors influencing choice 523
　inlays, masking 1169
　pontics 571
　porcelain restorations opposing 479, 481
　powder, for spraying model casts 190, 190
　retainers for fixed partial dentures 549
gold crowns
　endodontic access 776
　partial or full coverage 502, 502–504

golden mean, Snow's 257, 257
golden proportion 243–245, 244, 1095–1097
　dentists' preferences 258–259, 260
　diastema closure and 846
　orthodontic esthetics and 902–903
　tooth to-tooth width ratios 254–257, 256
Goldstein, R.E.
　bleaching light 326, 327
　overlay method of tooth preparation 398–399, 399–400
　veneer onlays 482
Goldstein ColorVue Probe 61, 63
Goldstein veneer preparation kit 456, 457
gonial angle 1063, 1068–1069
gonion 1094, 1099
graying, peri-implant tissues 655, 658, 659, 1370
gray-stained teeth 671, 751, 753
　amalgam restorations 677, 679
　tetracycline staining 329, 329, 755
Grealy, Lucy 12
Greece, ancient 1095–1097
green stains 671, 672, 674, 678
grooves, discolored deep 670, 674
Grossman, David 506
group function occlusion 916
growth, craniofacial 1006
growth factors 642–643, 643
guarantees 79, 81, 137–138
guided tissue regeneration 1184
Gummy gingival indicator 281
gummy smile see gingival display, excessive
GUM Soft-Picks 1410, 1412
gutta-percha
　removal, for core retention 735, 737, 739–741
　root canal obturation 780, 781
Guy, Jasmine 1165

habits, oral 811–834
　adults 813–833
　ceramic veneers and 441, 474
　diagnosis 52, 833–834
　diastemas due to 816–817, 817, 843, 843
　effects on composite restorations 409–413
　fixed partial dentures and 554, 554
　pediatric patients 995
　porcelain veneers and 441
　questionnaire 828, 833–834
　signs 813
　tooth wear 697, 698, 708
　treatment 833–834
　see also bruxism; digit sucking
Hader vertical attachment 605
Hagger, Oskar 356
hair care services 14
hair color 1147
hairstyles 1144
　female 1144–1147, 1144–1147
　male 1147–1148, 1148
　minimizing a double chin 1150

Hannes anchor attachment 605
Hayashi shade guide 276
Hazard Communication Standard (HCS) 150
head-to-body height ratios 245, 245
heart disease 1023, 1024–1025
heart shaped face, hair styles 1144, 1146, 1148
heat testing 756
hematologic disorders 330–331, 682
hemifacial microsomia 955, 956–960
hemolytic disease of newborn (erythroblastosis fetalis) 331, 682
hemorrhage, pulp
　during canal instrumentation 780
　tooth color changes 682, 751, 752, 768
hepatic–biliary disorders 682
histogram, in photography 162, 165–166, 166–168, 168
history
　bleaching 326, 327
　contouring 297–298, 298
　esthetic dentistry 4–5, 4–5
　impression taking 1388–1389
Hollywood templates see esthetic templates
holographic group consultations 74
honesty 138
Hope, Bob 1155
horizontal 1/16th rule 249, 250
horizontal ridge augmentation 640–642, 642
House, M.M. 249, 614–615
hue 272, 273
　effects of bleaching 277–278, 284
Hulse, Tom 1160
Hybrid Bond adhesive system 366
hybrid composite resins 395, 862, 1416
hybrid ionomers 1356
hydrocolloid (agar) impressions 459, 1302, 1388
hydrofluoric acid etching
　ceramic fitting surfaces 1362, 1364
　ceramic veneers 467, 469
　fractured restorations 1228, 1230
　glass ceramics 1376
　intraoral repairs 1228, 1230
　porcelain butt margins 1356, 1358
hydrogen peroxide
　nonvital bleaching 346, 348
　vital bleaching 336, 340, 342, 343
hydroxyethyl methacrylate (HEMA) 360
hygienists 53–54, 54
　care of composite restorations 415
　care of crowns 536
　initial contact with 52
　maintenance appointments 1416, 1416–1417
　oral care advice 1412–1415
　polishing restorations 1416–1417
hypersensitive teeth see tooth sensitivity
hypertelorism 1058–1059
hypertension 1023, 1024

hypocalcification, enamel 679, *680–681*
    contouring 300, *300*, 302
    microabrasion *342*, 680–681
    see also white spots

I-bar clasp 584–585, *585*
iBond Self Etch adhesive system *363*, 366
ice chewing 831–833
ice pencil 754, *756*
IC plunger attachment 605, *606*
ICW *see* intercanine width
IL-1 gene mutation 1423
illuminance 275
illusions 188–192
    diastema correction and 847–848, *848–849*
    form and color creating 216, *217*, **218**
    principles 188–189, *188–189*
    resolving specific problems 206–229
    role of makeup 1149
    shaping and contouring creating 189–190, 305, *306–307*
    techniques for creating 189–192
    see also special effects
images
    editing 180, *180*
    file types 164–165
    importing to computer 179
    presentation 180
    resolution 160–161, *162, 163, 164*
    saving 179–180, *180*
    storage and presentation 179–181, *181*
    see also computer imaging; photographs
implant probes 1419, *1421*
implants 637–663
    abutments 657–658, *659*
        implant platform interface 1370, *1370–1371*
        restoration interface 1372–1374, *1373–1374*
        soft tissue interface 1370–1372, *1371–1372*
    clinical evaluation **1417**, 1417–1418, *1418*
    crestal bone loss 1417, *1418*
    crown–root fractures 1221, *1222*
    designs 653–654
    endodontically-diseased teeth 782–783, *784–785*
    fixed partial dentures as alternatives 555, *556–557*
    gingival tissues 654–655
        biotype assessment 654, **654**
        esthetics 1370–1372, *1371–1372*
        grafting 654–655, *655–656*, *1195, 1196*
        maintenance care 1419, 1423
        provisionalization and 644–645, 648–650, 656, 657–658
    informed consent 144
    intraoral examination 1419–1421
    mobility 1417
    older adults 1035–1036, *1037–1047*
    orthodontic extrusion prior to 905, *907*
    pain 1417
    position 646–653
        apicoronal (depth) 653
        buccolingual 647, *652*
        correcting errors 646, *651*
        mesiodistal 647–649, *653*
        surgical guides 646–647, *651–652*
    protocols 643–645
        delayed or late placement 643, *644*
        early placement 643
        immediate placement 643–644, *645–647*, **647**
        immediate restoration 644–645, *648–650*
    provisional restorations 656–657
        immediate 644–645, *646–650*, 656
        as impression posts 650, *656–657*
        Siltek method *1324, 1327–1328*
        soft tissue benefits 644–645, *648–650*, 656, *657–658*
    removal 651
    retained primary teeth 908
    smile line and lip dynamics 638
implant scalers 1422, *1422*
implant-supported dentures 629–630, *631–633*
    overpartial dentures 605
implant-supported restorations 658–663
    cement-retained 1372, *1373*
    design and cementation 660–662, *660–662*
    in-office hygiene care 1419–1423
    maintenance 1417–1428
    materials 658–659, *662*, 662–663
    patient self-care 1423–1428
    probing around 1418, *1418*
    retrievability 1379–1381
    screw-retained 1372–1373, *1374*, 1380–1381, *1381*
Impregum 1388
impressions 1287–1307
    analog vs digital 1400
    ceramic veneers 459–460
    concept 1388
    determining gingival form 1346
    digital *see* digital impressions
    Digital Smile Design 107
    disinfection 133–134, 1302
    gypsum die preparation 1302
    history 1388–1389
    interocclusal records 1303–1307
    materials 1291–1294, 1302
        history 1388
        manipulation 1294, **1294**
        properties **1293**, 1293–1294
    mounting casts 1303, *1303–1304*
    multiple backup 1302, *1303*
    posterior ceramic partial coverage restorations 482
    preimpression surface optimizer 1294, *1295*
    removal and trimming 1302
    soft-tissue preparation 1287–1291, *1288–1292*
    techniques 1294–1302
        dual viscosity 1298
        putty wash 1299, *1299–1302*
        single viscosity 1295
        special 1294, *1295–1298*
    try-in stage 1343, *1344*
impression tray adhesives 1294
impression trays 1294
"I'm sorry" legal protection 138
In-Ceram all-ceramic crowns 506, **513**
In-Ceram Zirconia restorations 1249–1250, 1253
incisal curve 1101
    lower lip relations 1121, *1122*
    reverse *1119*, 1122
incisal edges
    age-related wear 219, *221*
    close-up repose image 174–175, *175*
    determination of position 246–247, *246–247*
    diastema closure and 846
    esthetic shaping 314, *314*
    lengthening 1120, *1120*
    lower lip relationships 1120–1122, *1122*
incisal embrasures
    ceramic veneers 472, *473*
    cosmetic contouring 308, *310*, 316, *317*
    crowns 527, *528*
    performers/actors 1174, *1176*
    restorations 221, *224–225*
    smile design 247, *248*
    try-in appointment 1346–1347, *1347*
incisal exposure
    children 1008
    at rest 1119–1120, *1119–1121*
incisal overlap veneer preparation *see* overlapping incisal edge veneer preparation
incisal plane 246, *246*
    diastema closure and 846
    evaluation 1107–1110, *1110–1111*
incisors
    irregularity index 920
    proclination *922*, 923, 1076
    protrusion *see* protrusion, incisor
    shape and SPA factors 248, *248, 249*
    too narrow 210, *212*
    too wide *207*, 207–208
    width in relation to other teeth 254–265
    see also central incisors; lateral incisors
inclination, crown restorations 526–527
inclusion, dental 997, *997–1000*
inCoris TZI C 537
incremental layering technique, composite restorations 403, *405*, 405–406
indirect composite/acrylic veneers 434, 461, 502
infants 10
infection control, negligent practice 133–134
inferior alveolar nerve 942, 944–948

Index

informed consent 48, 132–137
    disclosure obligations 132–133, 143–144
    documentation 133, *134–137*, 139, *141*, 142
    less invasive procedures 145
    misinformed consent 144
    patient's commitment to follow-up 133
    responsibility for obtaining 144–145
    surgical–orthodontic correction of dentofacial deformity 933
infrabulge bar (I-bar) clasp 584–585, *585*
initial visit 51–67
    clinical examination 55–67
    important questions to ask 51–52
    patient observation 52–53
    prior to 48–51
    sequence of staff contacts 52, *52*
inlays/onlays 5, *5*
    ceramic
        cementation 1361–1364
        CEREC system 483–490, *486*
        endodontic access 778
        posterior 478–483, *482*
    ceramic veneer onlays 482, *482–484*
    composite resin 393, *394*
    jadeite 5, *5, 298, 298*
inside-outside tray bleaching technique 348
Insta-Dam Relaxed Fit 774
insurance, dental, for older adults 1017, 1025
integrated digital systems 67
intercanine width (ICW) 249–250, *251*
    determination 261, 262, *262*
    RED proportions and 257, *259*
    tooth width calculations from 260, *261*, 261–262, **262**
intercanine width/central incisor width (ICW/CIW) quotient 263–265
    chart **263**
    determination 263–264, *264, 266*
    example of clinical use 264–265, *265–267*
    method for using chart 263, **265**
interdental brushes 1410, *1411–1412, 1423*
interdental papillae *see* papillae, interdental
interdental spaces
    ceramic veneers 226–228, 452, *469*
    composite resin bonding 226–228, *227*
    crown restorations *227*–228, 228–229, 1280
    Pincus principles D7, *D8*
    see also black triangles; diastemas
interdental tissue inserts *see* tissue inserts
interdisciplinary approach
    facial esthetics 1089
    orthodontics 905–908, *905–909*
    papilla reconstruction 1196, *1197*
    Pincus principles D5–D6
interdisciplinary team
    communication 86
    consultations 73, *73*–74
inter-ear line 1099, *1101*
interincisal distance, crown restorations and 527, *527*

interior design 115, *116–118*
interlabial gap 1113
intermaxillary fixation (IMF) 937, 940
internal tooth resorption 682, *753*
    posttraumatic 980, *980*
interocclusal records 1303–1307
interpreters 144
interproximal areas
    ceramic veneer coverage 449, 452
    contacts with full crowns 519–521
    finishing
        ceramic veneers *471–472, 473*
        composite restorations 409
        posterior ceramic partial coverage restorations 483
    staining, to create tooth separation 218, *218*
interpupillary line 1099, *1101*
    assessing parallelism 1107–1110, *1109*
interzygomatic width (IZW) 249, *251*
intracoronal attachment removable partial dentures 595–596, *596*, 597–599
    advantages 597
    disadvantages 597
    types 597–599, *598–599*
intraoral cameras 55–56, *57–59, 59–60*
    alternatives to 158
    implant self-care 1427–1428
inverted "L" osteotomy 942
Invisalign 56, 890, 1169, 1396–1397
IPS e.max 512–514
    CAD
        CEREC inlays 484, *490–491*
        crowns 512–514
        crystalline structure 512–513, *513*
    Ceram 465
    implant restorations 662, *662*
    longevity **513**
    pressable (e.max Press)
        all-ceramic crowns *512*, 512–514
        crystalline structure 512, *513*
        posterior partial coverage restorations 481–482
        veneer onlays 482
        veneers *438–439*, 462
            as alternatives to full crowns 474–477
            laboratory procedures 463–465
            tooth preparation 453–456
IPS Empress
    all-ceramic crowns 510–513, *511*, **513**
    crystalline form 510, *510*
    veneers
        fabrication 462, *463*
        longevity 474
        tooth preparation *446*, 449–451
iron-impregnated gingival retraction cord 1236
irregularity index, incisor 920
irrigation, implant maintenance 1427, *1427*
ISO 164
Isosit-N crowns 502

iTero Element intraoral scanner 1396–1397, *1396–1397*, **1400**
Ivoclar Chromascop shade guide 279–280, *280*
Ivoclar Vivadent shade guides 281, *281*

jadeite inlays 5, *5, 298, 298*
Japan, *ohaguro* 4, *4*
jaundice, childhood 331, 682
jewelry, metal mouth 826, *829*
JPEG files 164–165
jury trials 151

Kahng Chairside Shade Guides 199–205, *204–207*
Katana all-ceramic crowns 507
Kennedy classification, edentulous areas 582, *582*
Keynote software 86, 87, *87*, 180
Kiel, Richard 1159, *1163–1164*
Kokich, Vincent 899, 902, 907–908, *909*, 1086–1087
Köle, H. 956–957
Kor whitening system 341–342
Kuwata, M. 500, 514

LAAXESS Diamond Bur 776
LAAXESS endodontic access kit 775
labial commissures 1111
labial rotation of teeth 213, *213–214*
labiomental angle 1065, *1072*, 1118–1119
labiomental sulcus 931, *932*, 1065
    excessively deep 1065, *1073–1074*
    pediatric patients 1009, *1009*
laboratory
    CAD/CAM systems 1400–1402
    checklist C1–C5
    communication
        color information 285–286
        crown color selection 535, *535*
        special effects and illusions 197–199
        try-in stage 1337, *1338*
        using photographs 157, *157*, 199
        verbal and written instructions 285
laboratory technician 53
lamina dura 582
laminates *see* veneers
Laminate Veneer System (LVS; Brasseler) 456, *457, 470, 473*
lanugo 822, *824*
laser-assisted new attachment procedure (LANAP) 1029, *1033*
laser conditioning 972
laser etching 972
lasers
    caries detection 55, *55*, 971
    classification **984**
    hard tissue ablation 971–972
        composite adhesion after 972–973
        discolored deep grooves 670
        pediatric dentistry 972
        pit and fissure caries 419, *419*

lasers (cont'd)
   pediatric dentistry 971–973
      amelodentinal dysplasia 975, *975*
      enamel hypoplasia 978, *978*
      extensive cavities 976, *976–977*
      preventive resin restoration 974, *974*
      trauma management 984–986
   soft-tissue applications
      gingival sculpting 148–149, *151*
      pediatric dentistry 973
      preparation for impressions 1291, *1292*
   tissue interaction 971
laser sintering, selective 1402
lateral incisors
   agenesis 441
      fixed partial dentures 549–550, *549–550*
      orthodontic–restorative treatment *905–906*
   peg-shaped, orthodontic–restorative treatment 905, *905–906, 907–908*
   post-and-core restorations 741
   SPA factors 248, *249*
   see also incisors
lateral incisor width (LIW) 261
   calculation using ICW/CIW quotient **263, 265**
   calculation using RED proportion 261, **262**, *262–263, 263*
   in relation to other teeth 254–265, 847
Lava 507
Lava Plus 537
Le Fort I osteotomy
   condylar hyperplasia 953
   macro- and miniesthetic approach 1080, *1080*
   maxillary deficiency 951, *951–952*
   vertical maxillary excess 948, *949–950*
left lateral arch image 176–178, *177*
legal considerations 131–152
   Botox use 151
   dentist's refusal to treat 145
   federal requirements and product warnings 150
   guarantee or warranty 137–138
   "I'm sorry" legal protection 138
   informed consent *see* informed consent
   jury trials 151
   malpractice examples 147–150, *148–151*
   nonnegligent risks and obligation to treat 144
   patient abandonment claims 145
   patient's choice of dentist 146–147
   records and documentation 139–142
   refunds 147, *148*
   standards of care 143–144
   telephone or e-mail consultation 150
   try-in appointment 138–139, *139*
   updating skills and practices 132
lemon consumption 33, 822–824, *824*
lenses, camera 160, *160, 161*
Leonardo da Vinci 243, *244*

leucite-reinforced ceramic 1264, 1376
   see also IPS Empress
lever forces 583
life event stress 27, 41–42
life expectancy 1016, **1016**
   active 1036
light 272, *272*
   color perception 272
   creating illusions 188, *188*
   effects on tooth appearance 185–187
   Pincus principles D3–D4, *D4*
   reflection, fixed restorations 1350
light curing 403, 404–405
   ceramic veneers 469, *472–473*
   equipment 405, *406*
   technique 404–405, *405*
light-emitting diodes (LED) 405
lighting conditions
   clinical photography 166–169
   color matching 275, *275*, 396, 397, *397, 532–533*
   esthetic try-in 1336
   performers and actors 1174, *1177*, 1178
   video recordings 182
light meters 405, *406*
lightness, effects of bleaching 277–278, **284**
light transmission *see* translucency
lines
   creating illusions 188–189, *188–189*
   tooth appearance and 189
lingually locked tooth 891–893
lip(s)
   appearance of teeth and 186–187
   augmentation 1137, *1140*
   biting, habitual 819–821, *819–821*
   closure, children 1008
   coloring *1150*, 1150–1151
   contours, changing with makeup *1150*, 1150–1151
   curvature, pediatric patients 1009, *1009*
   dynamics, implants and 638
   excess mucosal tissue 1112, *1112*
   incompetence, facial photographs 1053–1055
   oblique view 1063, 1113
   profile view 1064–1065, *1071*, 1115–1118
   reference lines 1101, *1101*
   symmetry 1111–1112, *1112*
   thickness 186–187, 1115
   wetting, habitual 819
lip length
   age-related increase 1120
   measurement 1112–1113
lip line
   asymmetric *1112*
   crown selection and 523, 525–526, *526*
   high 525, *526*, 638, *1123*
   low 526, *526*, 638, *1123*, 1124
   medium 525–526, *526*, 638, *1123*
   scar tissue affecting 1112, *1112*
   see also gingival display; smile line
lip position 1115–1118

   closed 1113
   complete dentures 619, *620–621*
   esthetic evaluation 1115–1117, *1116–1117*
   esthetic try-in 1336, *1336*
   repositioning methods 1115, 1117–1118
   rest 1113
   ridge replacement and 1118
   sagittal 1115–1117, *1117*
   tooth position and 1118
lip projection 1064–1065, *1071*
   esthetic evaluation 1115–1118
   reduction of excessive 1065, *1071–1072*
lipstick 1150–1151
   colors 1147, 1150–1151
   minimizing a double chin 1149–1150
   removal 283, 396, 533
lithium-disilicate ceramic 1264, 1376–1377
   bilayered 1376
   crowns
      endodontic access 778
      selection 523, 524, *525*
      technical considerations 512–514
   fixed partial dentures 550
   implant crowns *662*, 662–663
   monolithic *1376*, 1376–1377
   veneers
      indications 441
      laboratory procedures 463–465
      stained teeth 687–688, *687–688*
      tooth preparation 453, *453–456*
   see also IPS e.max
Lombardi, R.E. 1087
   guide to tooth arrangement 190–191, *191*
   repeated ratio 254
long-axis inclinations
   disguising 216–218, *218*
   prostheses for older patients 219, *222*
long face, hair styles 1147, *1147*, 1148
long teeth
   cosmetic contouring 306–313, *308–313*
   crowns 530, 1283
   illusions for 215–216, *215–216*
Loop, J.L. 249, 614–615
lost-wax method 462, 463, 506, 512
lower lip, incisal edge relationships 1120–1122, *1122*
low-level laser therapy (LLLT) 985–986
luting agents *see* cement(s)
lux (lx) 275
luxation injuries 1223
   clinical case 1225, *1225*
   endodontics 793–794
   extrusive 1223, *1224*
   intrusive 990, *990–993*, 1223
   laser-assisted management 993–994, *993–994*
   lateral 1223
LVS *see* Laminate Veneer System

macroesthetic analysis 1052–1076
   clinical case study 1076–1077, *1077–1079*
   facial asymmetry 1061–1062, *1065–1067*

Index

facial photographs 1053–1056, *1055–1059*
frontal view
  clinical examination 1057–1062, *1060–1067*
  landmarks 1053, **1054**, *1054*
  photographs 1053–1055, *1055–1056*
oblique view 1062–1063, *1068–1069*
  photographs 1055–1056, *1057*
pitch, roll and yaw 1072–1076, *1076*
profile view 1063–1068, *1069–1075*
  landmarks **1069**, *1069*
  photographs 1056, *1058*
smile dimensions and 1068–1072
submental view 1056, *1059*
technology and facial imaging 1056–1057, *1059*
see also facial analysis
macroesthetics 1052, *1052*
magnesium alumina, glass-infiltrated 1377
mail, direct 128
maintenance of restorations 1409–1428
makeup 1149–1151
  for facial disfigurement 1151
  for women 1149–1151
malocclusions
  diastemas 848–849
  digit sucking and 812–813
  pediatric patients 995
  porcelain veneers 441
  realistic orthodontic goals 916–919, *916–919*
  skeletal 930
    treatment in adults 916–917, *917*, 933
  tongue thrusting 816–817
  see also Class II malocclusions; Class III malocclusions; occlusion
malpositioned teeth 890–891
  porcelain veneers 441
malpractice claims 131–132
  example 147–150, *148–151*
  jury trials 151
  prophylactic measures 151–152
mamelons, nonfused 298, *299*
mandibular anterior teeth
  ceramic veneers 448–449, *449–451*
  complete dentures
    placement 618, *619*, 619–620, 623
    size and form 615
  cosmetic contouring 303–304, 305–306, *306–307*, 308, *308*
  crowding 890, 920
  fixed partial dentures 550, 551, 553–554
  incisal embrasures 1347
mandibular arch image 178–179
mandibular asymmetry 1061, *1067*
mandibular body osteotomy 942, *944–945*
mandibular deficiency (retrognathism) 942–948
  distraction osteogenesis 956
  orthodontics 944, *946*
  surgical correction 946–947

mandibular excess (prognathism) 940–942
  bimaxillary 940–941, *942*
  dentoalveolar 940
  maxillary deformities with 942, *945*
  orthodontics *939–941*, 940
  pseudo or false 941, 951
  surgical correction 941–942, *943–944*
mandibular plane 1078, *1078–1079*
mania 29, 30
manufacturer's instructions, failure to follow 1255–1260
marginal staining
  composite restorations *see under* composite resin restorations
  porcelain veneers 689–690
  restorations 330, 670–671, *674–676*
marketing 113–129
  creating a brand 114
  developing a plan 114
  Digital Smile Design tool 86
  external 122–129
  internal 115–122
marking, intraoral, cosmetic contouring 304, 308, *309*
masculine appearance
  cosmetic contouring 303
  dentists' perceptions 614
  ideal tooth widths 250–251, *252*
  incorporating 223, *226*
  size and shape of teeth 248, *249*, 250
matrix bleaching 341–345
matrix metalloproteinases (MMPs) 364–365
  inhibitors 364–365, 367
matrix strips
  fitting ceramic veneers 468, 471–472
  posterior ceramic partial coverage restorations 482–483
maxillary anterior teeth
  adjusting incisal embrasures 1346–1347, *1347*
  complete dentures 622
    placement 616–619, *617–621*, 622–623
    size and form 614–615
  cosmetic contouring 304
  size in relation to face size 249–251, *250–252*
  SPA factors 248, *248*
  width in relation to other teeth 254–265
  see also central incisors; incisors; lateral incisors
maxillary arch image 178, *178–179*
maxillary deficiency 948–951
  anteroposterior (horizontal) 951, *952*
  transverse 948
  vertical 951, *951*
maxillary excess 948
  see also vertical maxillary excess
maxillary osteotomy, Le Fort I *see* Le Fort I osteotomy
maxillomandibular asymmetry 1062, *1067*
Mayans 5, *5*, 298, *298*
McNamara, J.A. 920–921

medical history 67–68, *68–69*
  older adults 1022–1023
Medicare 1017, 1025
medication-induced problems
  older adults 1023
  tooth staining 328–330, *329–331*, **671**, 682, *682*, 751, *755*
  xerostomia 28, *29*, 30
men
  face shape and hairstyle 1147–1148, *1148*
  makeup for 1151
  see also gender differences; masculine appearance
mentocervical angle 931, *932*
mercury 136
mesial groove reciprocation (MGR) clasp 585, *587*, 588
mesial inclination, increasing 216–217, *218*
mesial rotation of teeth 190, *191*, 214, *214*
mesocephalic facial form 1058, *1060*, 1098, *1100*
metadata 142
metal–acrylic resin pontics 570–571
metal–ceramic butt-joint 516, *516*
metal–ceramic restorations 514–523
  adjunctive procedures 515–516
  advantages 515
  cementation 1358–1359, *1359–1361*
  choice of metals 514
  contraindications 514
  design
    metal substructure 516–518, *517–518*
    porcelain–metal junction 517–518, *520*
    porcelain thickness 518, *520*, *522*
  disadvantages 515, *515*
  discolored pulpless tooth 523–525
  esthetic considerations 516, *516*
  factors influencing choice 523, 525–526
  failures 518, *518–519*
    margin exposure 1244, *1245*
    metal thickness and 1253–1254, *1257*
  fixed partial denture retainers 551, 552
    margins 552–553, *553–554*
    porcelain–metal junction 553–554
  gingival health and 518–521, *520*
  history 514
  implants 658, *662*
  indications 514
  longevity 1236
  luting agents 521, 1355–1356
  margins *522*, 522–523
    see also metal collar margins; porcelain butt-joint margins
  repairs to existing *1231*
  rubber dam placement 772–773, *773*
  technical failure 1253–1254, *1257–1258*
  technical problems 514–515
  tooth preparation 518–522, *520*
    extent of occlusal reduction 510, *510*
  try-in 1341
  see also porcelain-fused-to-metal crowns
metal collarless crown 522

Page numbers 1–666 are in Volume 1; page numbers 667–1429 are in Volume 2.

metal collar margins 522
  FPD retainers 552, 553
  selection 525, 1265–1266, *1267*
metal mouth jewelry 826, *829*
metal–porcelain (covered metal)
    margins 552
metal restorations
  actors and entertainers 1169
  repairs to existing 1230, *1231*
  see also all-metal crowns; gold
metal stains 675, 1236
metamerism, color matching and 275
methylenedioxymethamphetamine
    (ecstasy) 825
microabrasion 341, *342*
  dental fluorosis 682
  hypocalcified areas *342*, 680–681
microcracks, enamel
  creating illusion of height 215, *215*
  ice chewing 831–833
  intraoral camera 57, *59*
  porcelain veneers 440
  simulation techniques 196, *198–199*, **202**
  staining 673
  transillumination 56–57, *58*
  see also cracked tooth syndrome
microdontia 843
microesthetics 1052, *1052*, 1077
microfilled composites 394, *395*
  diastema closure 862, *862–863*
  polishing 1416
microhybrid composites 394, 395, 862
microleakage
  access cavity repairs 782, *782–783*
  composite resin restorations 379, *380*, 401, 1250–1251, *1254*
micromechanical attachment 356–357, *357*
microsurgery 1182–1183
  instruments 1182–1183, *1183*
  papilla reconstruction 1196–1199, *1198–1199*
  ridge augmentation 1202, *1202–1203*
  root coverage 1188–1189, *1188–1189*
midface lift 1133–1134, *1136*
midline see dental midline; facial midline
midpupillary distance 1059
midsagittal plane
  maxillary dental midline to 1061, *1065*
  nasal tip to 1061, *1065*
Miller, P.D. 1183
Miller classification, gingival recession 1184
mineral trioxide aggregate (MTA)
  pulp capping 769, *769*
  pulpotomy 1219
  root resorption defects 794
miniesthetics 1052, *1052*
  clinical case study 1077, *1079*
  see also smile
minocycline staining 329–330, *331*, 683
minors
  eating disorders 36
  informed consent 144

mirrors
  clinical photography 169–170, *170–171*
  esthetic try-in 1332, *1335*, 1335–1336
  viewing results 80, *81*
misaligned teeth 890–891, 920
missing teeth
  congenitally see agenesis of teeth
  fixed partial dentures 543–571
  illusions, for actors 1158–1159
  orthodontic considerations 917
  pediatric dentistry
    advanced caries 979, *980*
    ectodermal dysplasia 982–983, *982–983*
    orthodontics 996, *996–997*
    pedodontic prostheses 979, *979–982*
    severe trauma 979, 980, *980–982*
  removable partial dentures 581–606
mixed dentition
  dental materials and techniques 970–971
  trauma management 983–986
mobility
  implants 1417
  root fractures 791, *795–796*, 1221
models
  diagnostic study see study models
  human professional see performers/actors
model spray 190, *190*
modification spaces 582
molars
  fractured endodontically-treated 736–739, *736–739*
  see also posterior teeth
monitor resolution 161, *163*, *164*
mood disorders 26, 27–31
morsicatio buccarum et labiorum 819
motion picture industry
  Pincus' work 434, 1153, 1155, D2, D8–D9
  see also performers/actors
motivations, patients' 16–19, 20, *20*
mouth breathing 821–822
mouthguards, protective see protective bite appliances
mouth rinses 1414
  staining of teeth 673–674, *677–678*
multidisciplinary approach see interdisciplinary approach
Munsell hue-value-chroma color notation system 273
myofascial pain 392

nail biting 825
nanofilled composites 396, 862
nanohybrid composites 395
nanoleakage 360, 364, *364*
narcissistic personality disorder (NPD) 26, 40–41
  case study 36–37
  diagnostic criteria **37**
narrow teeth
  diastema closure 853–854, 856, *856–857*
  illusions masking 209–214, *210–213*, 848
nasal projection 1064, *1071*

nasal tip
  analysis of position 1104
  elevation 1064, *1071*
  to midsagittal plane 1061, *1065*
nasofacial angle 931, *932*
nasofrontal angle 931, *932*
nasolabial angle 1063–1064, *1070*, 1114, *1115*
  orthodontic correction 1064, *1070*
  pediatric patients 1009
  restorative dentistry and 1114–1115, *1116*
nasomental angle 931, *932*
Natho classification of extrinsic dental stain 671
  type 1 (N1) 671, *676–677*
  type 2 (N2) 671, *677*
  type 3 (N3) 671, *678*
Nd:YAG lasers 984–985
needles, harmful habits 825–826, *827*
negative smile line see reverse smile line
negligent customary practice 133–137
neurotoxins 1137
neutral zone 616
nickel casting alloys 514
nifedipine 1023
nightguards see protective bite appliances
noble metals 514
nociceptive trigeminal inhibition tension suppression system (NTI-TSS) appliance 415
noncarious cervical lesions (NCCLs) see abfractions
nonvital teeth
  bleaching see under bleaching
  crowning 523–524
  discoloration 346
  temporary restorations 1315
  see also endodontically-treated teeth; pulp sensibility tests
no-preparation veneers 442, *442*
Nordland and Tarnow classification, papillary defects 1196, *1197–1198*
nose
  analysis of proportionality 1059
  plastic surgery see rhinoplasty
  prominence, pediatric patients 1009, *1009*
nose tip point (NTP)–gnathion (Gn)/ subnasal (Sn)–gnathion (Gn) ratio 1010
nursing bottle syndrome 979
nursing-home residents 1036–1037
nuts, cracking 833

object, color 272
oblique view of face
  clinical examination 1062–1063, *1068–1069*
  facial analysis 1113
  photographs 1055–1056, *1057*
observer, color 272
obsessive-compulsive disorder (OCD) 26, **30**, 30–31, *830*

Index

obstructive sleep apnea (OSA) 959–964, *962–964*
Obwegeser, Hugo 929–930
  sagittal splitting osteotomy 944–948, *946–947, 949–950*
Occlude-Pascal spray 1341, *1341–1342*
occlusal analysis
  cosmetic contouring 308, *308–309*
  crowns 531
  initial visit 60
  see also bite registration
occlusal plane
  assessment of pitch 1078, *1078–1079*
  evaluating inclination 1108–1110
  oblique view 1056
  surgical rotation 1079–1080, *1080*
occlusal registration 531, 1303–1305, *1305–1306*
occlusal registration strips *468, 472,* 1304, *1305*
occlusal splints, worn teeth 702
occlusion
  abfraction-inducing forces 705
  balanced 916
  bruxism and 697
  canine protected (CPO) 915, 916
  ceramic restorations and 1374–1381
  ceramic veneers and *470, 473*
  complete dentures 613, *613–614,* 620–622
    anterior teeth 620
    posterior 621–622, *622*
    vertical dimension 620–621, *621–622*
  cosmetic contouring and 302, 303–304, 313
  crown placement and 523, 531
    erroneous *1238, 1239*
  diastema closure and 848–849
  establishing a stable 1332
  group function 916
  ideal functional 915–916
  ideal static 915
  implant patients 1419–1421
  lingualized 613, *613–614*
  orthodontic goals 915–919, *916–919*
  removable partial dentures 583
  restoring fractured teeth and *724, 726*
  try-in appointment 1339, 1346
  vertical dimension *see* vertical dimension of occlusion
  see also malocclusions
Occupational Safety and Health Administration (OSHA) 133–134, 150
Octolink attachment system 600, *602–603*
office facilities, attractiveness 115, *116–118*
ohaguro 4, *4*
older adults 1015–1047
  attitudes to dental esthetics 1017–1020, 1024
  benefits of esthetic dentistry 1016, *1017–1020,* 1021, *1021–1022*
  bleaching 331, 333–336, 1025, 1026, *1026*

characteristics 1016–1017
chronic illness 1020–1022, **1022,** 1024–1025
demographic trends 1015–1016, **1016**
denture tooth selection 615
endodontics 1030
esthetic dental procedures 1025–1028
facial esthetics 904–905, 930
history and examination 1022–1023
implants 1035–1036, *1037–1047*
nursing-home or assisted-living residents 1036–1037
oral health maintenance 1023–1024
orthodontics 1029, 1031, *1031*
periodontal therapy 1029, 1032, *1032, 1033*
prevention and risk assessment 1023–1024
prosthodontics 1030–1035, *1032, 1034–1036*
tooth color 331, *332,* 616, 1025
tooth size–arch length discrepancies 919–921
tooth wear 696, 1025–1026, 1034–1035, *1034–1035*
treatment planning 1024–1025
see also age-related changes
oligodontia 982–983
Omega Ceramic 516
one-sixteenth (1/16th) rule
  combined with rule of thirds 249, *251*
  complete dentures 614–615, *615*
  horizontal 249, *250*
  vertical 249, *250*
onlays *see* inlays/onlays
online directories 125
online group discount shopping services 128
opalescent ceramic systems 516
opaquing
  crowns 524–525
  fractured restorations 1230, *1231*
  porcelain veneers 452, 461–462, 468–469
open bite
  abfraction 705
  caused by digit sucking 812–813
  mandibular excess with 940–941, 942, *942*
  pediatric patient 1004, *1004–1005*
OptiBond AIO adhesive 366
OptiBond FL adhesive 362, *363,* 367
OptiBond Solo Plus adhesive 362
OptiBond XTR adhesive 368
optical geometry, visual shade matching 283, *283*
Optradam Plus 774, *774*
oral cancer 1023
oral care products 1412–1415
oral habits *see* habits, oral
oral hygiene 1410–1415
  attachment RPDs 594
  bad habits 827, *830–831*
  bulimia nervosa 33
  ceramic veneers 477

composite restorations 409, 415, *416*
crowns 536
depressed patients 27, 28, *29*
implant self-care *1423,* 1423–1428, *1427–1428*
nursing-home residents 1036–1037
older adults 1023–1024
patient instruction 1412
pretreatment 1410
restoration of crowded teeth and 881
stained teeth due to poor *672,* 673, 674, 678
oral surgery 74
orange stains **671,** 674, *676*
Oraseal Putty 347, 773
orthodontic appliances
  bruxism 413–415, *415, 814,* 815
  digit sucking 813
  fingernail habits 825, *826*
  harmful oral habits 833
  lip or cheek biting *820,* 821, *821*
  pediatric trauma 980, *980–982*
  performers/actors 1169–1170, *1171–1172*
  postsurgical 939
  technological advances 909
  temporomandibular joint pain 815, *815–816*
orthodontics
  accelerated osteogenic (AOO) 957–959
  adult esthetic 897–923
  attachment RPDs 593
  bleaching combined with 334, *335*
  clinical records 899, *899–901*
  compromise 56, 72
  cosmetic contouring as alternative 300, 302, *302–303*
  cracked tooth syndrome 800–801, *803–804*
  crowded teeth **882,** 890, *892, 893*
  diastema closure 844, 849
    composite resin bonding after 853, 856, *856–857*
    periodontal surgery after 915
  esthetic vs cosmetic 897–898
  facial considerations 898–905, 1051–1083
    clinical case study 1076–1083
    dentofacial analysis 1057–1062
    evaluation in three dimensions *1052,* 1052–1054
    macroesthetic evaluation 1062–1068
    macroesthetics and smile dimensions 1068–1076
    photographs 1053–1056, *1055–1059*
    technology and facial imaging 1056–1057, *1059*
  fixed partial dentures and 545
  force requirements 911–912, *912–913*
  gingival recession due to 1184
  interdisciplinary approach *905–908,* 905–909
  malposed and misaligned teeth 890–891
  mandibular prognathism 939–941, 940

orthodontics (cont'd)
   mandibular retrognathism 944, *946*
   occlusal considerations 915–919, *916–919*
   older adults 1029, 1031, *1031*
   papillary defects 1196, *1197*
   pediatric 995–1004
      traumatic loss of teeth 980, *980–982*
   performers (actors) 1169–1170, *1171–1172*
   periodontal considerations 909–915, *911–914*
   periodontally accelerated osteogenic (PAOO) 912, *913*
   postsurgical 937–939
   presurgical 935–937, *939–940*
   referral for 70–72
   rejection by patient *1243*, 1243–1244
   root resorption risk 144
   skeletal malocclusions 933
   surgically assisted 956–959
   technological advances 909, *910*
   temporary restorations during 1312
   tongue thrusters 817
   tooth size–arch length discrepancies 919–923
   treatment planning 60
      three-dimensional approach *1052*, 1052–1056, *1054*
   vertical maxillary excess 948, *949*
   worn teeth 699–702
orthognathic surgery *see* surgical–orthodontic treatment
Osler, Sir William 751
otoplasty 1059, *1064*
oval face, hair styles 1144, *1144*, 1148
overextensions, potential 1339
overhead, financial 80–81
overlapping incisal edge veneer preparation (Class 4) 442–446, *444*, *446–448*, 456–459
overlapping teeth, cosmetic contouring 298, *299*, 315–316, *315–317*, 318, *318*
overlay dentures
   for actors 1156–1160, *1158–1164*
   comic 1176–1177, *1177*
overlay technique 398–400, *399–400*, 690
   removing stains *400*, 675
   repairing composite restorations 690
   tooth lengthening 399–400, *401*
overpartial dentures 605
overtreatment 1235
oxide ceramics 1377–1381
   veneers 434–435, 453
   see also aluminum oxide; zirconia
ozone therapy 971

pain
   anesthetic test 763–764
   clinical evaluation of dental 754–762
   implant-related 1417
palatal stent 1190, *1192*

palate, connective tissue harvesting 1189–1190, *1190–1191*
palpation, tooth 761, *761*
panoramic radiographs 762
   dentofacial deformity 934
   orthodontics *901*, 903
papillae, interdental
   crown lengthening and 1206–1207, *1207*
   display when smiling 1124–1125
   implant placement and 645, 648–649
   large diastemata 856–862
   loss of 1181–1182, *1182*
      concealing 225–229, *227–236*
      flossing-related 409, 827, *830–831*, 1410, *1411*
      gingival inserts *see* tissue inserts
   Nordland and Tarnow classification of defects 1196, *1197–1198*
   orthodontic aspects 913–914, *914*
   postextraction changes 639
   reconstruction 1195–1199
      multidisciplinary approach 1196, *1197*
      postoperative care 1199
      surgical technique 1196–1199, *1197–1199*
   reshaping, diastema closure 849–850
parafunctional habits *see* habits, oral
parents, consent by 144
parotid gland enlargement 31, 32, *32*, 822, *824*
passive fit 1378
patient education 898
   caries prevention 1414–1415
   implant self-care 1423–1428, *1428*
   marketing role 119–120, *121*
   oral hygiene 1412
   prior to treatment planning 49, *49–50*
   role of photographs 159
patients
   abandonment 145, 152
   commitment to follow-up 133
   decision making *see* decision making, patient
   esthetic perceptions 137–138
   motivations 16–18, 20, *20*
   personality types 48–49
   predicting response to treatment 19
   problem 36–41, 77–79
   psychological challenges 25–44
   response to abnormality 16
   right to choose a dentist 146–147, *146–147*
   smile design preferences 268
   types 16–19, 77–78
   understanding their needs 8–9
payment plans 70
pediatric dentistry 969–1010
   bleaching vital teeth 335, *336*
   dentofacial deformities 933
   facial harmony 1005–1010
   harmful habits 995
      digit sucking 811–813, *812*, 833
      mouth breathing 821–822

   laser-assisted minimally invasive 971–973
   materials and techniques 970–971
   operating procedures 973–983
      amelodentinal dysplasia 975, *975*
      early childhood caries 979
      ectodermal dysplasia 982–983, *982–983*
      enamel hypoplasia 978, *978*
      extensive cavities 976, *976–977*
      loss of teeth 979–982, *979–982*
      preventive resin restoration 974, *974*
   orthodontics 995–1004
   pedodontic prostheses *979*, 979–982
   tooth wear 696, *696*
   trauma management 983–986
      case studies 986–994, *986–995*
      hard tissues and pulp 984–985
      injuries to developing teeth 986
      laser applications 984
      loss of teeth 980, *980–982*
      periodontal tissues 985–986
      prevention 983–984
   see also minors
pedodontic prostheses *979*, 979–982
peg-shaped lateral incisors, orthodontic–restorative treatment 905, *905–906*, 907–908
pen/pencil chewing 827, *831–832*
perceptibility threshold 274
percussion, tooth 759–761, *760*
perfectionist patients 77, 332
performers/actors 1153–1178
   cosmetic procedures 1155–1165
      acrylic stent 1155, *1156*
      comic arrangement 1176–1177, *1177*
      composite resin bonding 1155, 1160–1163
      composite resin stent/splint 1155, *1157*
      creating characters 1156–1163
      overlay dentures 1156–1160, *1158–1164*
      removable dentures 1156
      removable porcelain veneers 1155, *1156*
   economic dental procedures 1154–1155
   emergency treatment 1176
   esthetic dentistry *1165–1166*, 1165–1178
      brighter/whiter teeth 1165–1169
      composite resin restorations 1167–1169, *1169–1170*
      cosmetic contouring *1166*, *1167*
      metal restorations 1169
      porcelain veneers 1167, *1168–1169*
   with imperfect teeth 1154, *1154*
   long-distance consultation 1176–1177
   orthodontics 1169–1170, *1171–1172*
   periodontal treatment 1171–1172, *1173*
   Pincus' work with 434, 1153, 1155, D2, D8–D9
   principles of treatment 1177–1178
   prosthetic treatment 1172–1174, *1173–1174*
   special issues for 1174–1176
periapical radiolucency 759, *759–760*

peri-implantitis 1418
   bacterial monitoring 1419, *1420*, 1427
   genetic susceptibility 1423
   locally applied chemotherapeutics 1421
peri-implant mucositis 1421, 1427
perimylolysis 33, *33*, 34
periodontal charting 60–61, *63*, *64*
   orthodontics 911, *912*
   voice activated 61, 67
periodontal disease
   bleaching and 335
   cosmetic contouring 300, 302
   diastemata due to 843–844
   endodontic lesions vs 759, *759–760*
   impact on tooth proportions 902
   metal–ceramic crowns 522
   mimicking, for actors 1161, *1164*
   older adults 1035, *1036*
   orthodontic patients 909–911, 919
   porcelain veneers 441
   restoration failure due to 1244–1245, *1245–1247*
   telescoping bridges 558–559, *558–559*, 560, *560–561*
   tooth preparation 1280, *1281*
periodontal evaluation 56
periodontal ligament
   avulsed/luxated teeth 793–794
   edentulous areas 583
periodontally accelerated osteogenic orthodontics (PAOO) 912, *913*
periodontal plastic surgery 1181–1208
   computer imaging 63, 65–66
   crown lengthening and sculpting 1204–1208
   microsurgical instruments 1182–1183, *1183*
   papilla reconstruction 1195–1199
   ridge augmentation *see* ridge augmentation
   root coverage 1183–1195
periodontal probing 61, *63*
   charting *see* periodontal charting
   endodontics 751–754
   gingival biotype assessment 654, **654**
   orthodontics 911, *912*
   peri-implant 1418, *1418*, 1419, *1421*
periodontal surgery
   concealing interdental tissue loss after 225–229, *227–236*
   diastema correction 847, 915
   fractured teeth 728, *729*
   older adults 1029, 1032, *1032*
   orthodontic patients 911, 912, *913*, 915
periodontal tissues
   traumatic injuries 985–986
   see also soft tissues
periodontics
   adult orthodontics and 909–915, *911–914*
   bleaching combined with 335
   cosmetic 847
   older adults 1029, 1032, *1032*, *1033*
   orthodontics 909–911

performers/actors 1171–1172, *1173*
   referral for 72–74
periodontist, consultation with 56
periradicular tests, pulp health 759–762
peroxyborate monohydrate 348
personality
   assessing patient's 48–49, *53*
   definition 37
   incorporating patient's 225, *227*, 1347
   mouth (Pincus) D3, D6–D7
   smile design and 248, *249*
personality disorders 26, 40–41
   see also narcissistic personality disorder
personality factors 26–27, 36–41
personal values 11–12
PFM crowns *see* porcelain-fused-to-metal crowns
Phillips, R.W. 375, 401, 403
phonetics
   denture tooth placement 619, *619–620*, 623
   temporary restorations and 1313
phosphoric acid etching *see* acid etching
photocuring *see* light curing
photographs, digital
   case documentation 157
   clinical applications 157–158
   color matching 157, 286, 533, *534*
   dental education 158
   editing 180, *180*
   extraoral
      close-up repose 174–175, *175*
      close-up smile 173, *174*
      Digital Smile Design 87–88, *87–89*
      full-face *see* facial photographs
      initial visit 59–60, *61*
      left and right lateral arches 176–178, *177*
      mandibular arch 178–179
      maxillary arch 178
      retracted closed 175, *175*
      retracted open 176, *176–177*
   facial *see* facial photographs
   functions 140–141, 156
   indications for 157
   intraoral
      dentofacial deformities 934
      Digital Smile Design 89–91, *89–94*
      initial visit 55–56, *57–59*, *59–60*
      new restorations 1410, *1412*
      post-and-core procedures 741
   laboratory communication 157, *157*, 199
   patient education 158
   privacy and confidentiality 145
   smile evaluation *see* smile analysis, photographic
   storage and presentation 179–180, *181*
   try-in appointment 1336, *1337*
   see also images
photography, clinical 155–182
   equipment 158–170
   image composition 171–179, *172*
   image storage and presentation 179–181
   see also cameras; photographs

physical attractiveness phenomenon 3–4, 8–10, **9**
   economics 12–16
   employment and 12, *13–14*
   functions of teeth 11
   personal values 11–12
   research methodology 9–10
   sexiness and 8–9, *9*
   see also beauty
piercings, oral 826, *829*
Pincus, Charles
   on cosmetic contouring 298
   gingival contour determination 1346
   principles of esthetic dentistry D2–D9
   work with film actors 434, 1153, 1155, D8–D9
pink spots 751, *752–753*
pins, harmful habits 825–826, *827*
pipe smokers 708, 831, *832*
pit and fissure caries 416–417
   detection 416–417, *417*
   treatment 417–419
      air-abrasive technology 417–419, *418*
      composite resin bonding 379, 417, *418–420*
      diamond burs 419
      hard tissue laser 419, *419*
      pediatric dentistry 974, *974*
pit and fissure stain 416–421
pitch 1072–1076, *1076*
pixels 160–161, *162*, *163*
Planmeca PlanScan 1391–1392, *1391–1393*, **1393**
plaque
   crown design and 529
   initial observation 52
   see also oral hygiene; scaling
plasma arc curing (PAC) lights 405
plastic *see* acrylic
plastic surgery 1131–1140
   broaching the subject 1089, 1143
   lower face 1137, *1138–1139*
   midface 1133–1134, *1136*
   nonsurgical 1137–1140, *1140*
   older adults 1020, 1025
   patient safety 1140
   upper face 1132–1133, *1132–1135*
   see also periodontal plastic surgery
platelet-derived growth factor-BB 643, *643*
platinum foil technique, porcelain veneer fabrication 461, *465–466*
plunger-type attachments 605, *606*
polishing
   ceramic restorations *470*, *473*, 1416
   composite restorations 407, *410–411*, 415, 1416
   glass ionomers 1416
   implants 1422
   pastes, grit size 1416
   prior to shade selection 396
   try-in appointment 1351

Polo, Mario 905
polyether impressions 1292
   ceramic veneers 459
   disinfection 1302
   history 1388
   material properties **1293,** *1293–1294*
polymerization
   ceramic veneer fixation *469,* 472–473
   composite restorations 403–406, *405*
      following final finish 404
      incremental layering 403, *405*
      three-sited light-curing technique 403
   shrinkage 405
   see also light curing
polysomnogram 962
polysulfide impressions 459, 1388
polyvinyl siloxane (PVS)
   impressions *see* addition silicone impressions
   interocclusal records 1304
pontics 565–571
   attachment RPDs 593, *594*
   conical or bullet-shaped 565
   design 565–566, *565–567*
   failure 1250, *1250–1251*
   hygienic (sanitary) 565
   incorrect height 1239, *1240–1241*
   materials 570–571, *571–573*
   modified ridge lap 565, 566, *566–567*
   ovate 565, 566, *567,* 1204
   ridge lap (saddle) 565, *566*
      conversion to ovate 1201, *1202*
   tissue preparation 566–570, *569–570*
   try-in 1345
   see also fixed partial dentures
population aging 1015–1016, **1016**
porcelain
   biocompatibility 439
   chipped or fractured *see* porcelain fractures
   color modification 286, 438
   denture teeth 616, 626–627, *627–629*
   feldspathic *see* feldspathic porcelain
   firings 196–197, 286
   metal–ceramic restorations *see* metal–ceramic restorations
   Pincus principles D5, D6, *D6*
   pitting by topical fluoride 440
   polishing 1416
   pontics 570, 571, *571–573*
   unglazed 1351
   see also ceramic(s)
porcelain butt-joint margins
   design 517, *517*
   esthetics 516, *516*
   facial margin *1280*
   FPD retainers 552–553
   preparation for cementation 1356, *1358*
   selection 522, *522,* 525–526, 1266
porcelain crowns (all-porcelain) 502–505, *505–506*
   contraindications 505
   crowded tooth situation 1283
   longevity 1248–1249
   troubleshooting **507**
   see also all-ceramic crowns
porcelain fractures 1248–1249, *1248–1249*
   composite resin bonding 392, 1226–1230, *1228–1230*
   esthetic emergencies 1224, 1226–1230
   legal considerations 138
   occlusal pressure detecting 1255, *1260*
   porcelain veneers to repair 440
   smoothing and polishing 1226
porcelain-fused-to-metal (PFM) crowns 514–523
   adjunctive procedures 515–516
   advantages 515
   choice of metals 514
   contraindications 514
   design
      metal substructure 516–518, *517–518*
      porcelain–metal junction 517–518, *520*
      porcelain thickness 518, *520, 522*
   disadvantages 515, *515*
   discolored pulpless tooth 523–525
   endodontic access via *758, 777, 778, 778*
   esthetic considerations 516, *516*
   factors influencing choice 523, 525–526
   failures 518, *518–519*
   history 514
   indications 514
   margins 522, *522–523*
   retention after endodontic therapy 779–780
   rubber dam clamps 772–773, *773*
   technical problems 514–515
   tooth preparation 1271–1280, *1277–1278*
      esthetic depth determination 1271–1272, *1277–1278*
      extent of occlusal reduction 510, *510*
      labial tooth reduction 1272–1277, *1279*
      types of margins 1277–1280, *1280*
   see also metal–ceramic restorations
porcelain partial coverage restorations *see* ceramic partial coverage restorations
porcelain pieces (sectional veneers) 867, *868*
porcelain veneers 438–442
   advantages 438–440, 505
   bilayer ceramic restorations 502–505, 1264
      alumina cores 507, *508–509*
      zirconia cores 507, 537, 1254–1255, *1259,* 1377
   contouring as alternative to 298–300
   contraindications 441
   coronal fractures 722, 723–724, *723–724,* **726, 727**
   crowded teeth **882,** 884–886, *886–887*
   diastema closure 441, 864–869
      crowning with 869–870, *872*
      minimal preparation 865–866, *865–866*
      multiple diastemata 867–869, *869–870, 871, 871*
      proximal finish line 866, *867*
      single midline diastema 866–867, *868*
   disadvantages 440
   evolution of use 376
   fracture-related failure 473–474, *1228–1230, 1248–1249*
   see also porcelain fractures
   history 434–435
   indications *438–439,* 440–441
   interdental space closure 226–228, 452, 469
   laboratory procedures 461–462
      platinum foil technique 461, *465–466*
      refractory die technique 461–462
      two-tier quattro technique 229, *232–236*
   legal considerations
      informed consent 133, *137*
      overbuilt 148, *150*
      subgingival margins 134–136
   longevity 439, *440,* 473–474, 1249
   marginal failures
      legal issues 135–136
      poor fit *1237*
      recurrent caries *1227*
      staining 472, *473,* 689–690
   older adults 1030–1034, *1032*
   performers/actors 1167, *1168–1169*
   Pincus principles D7
   placement 465–473
      errors 472, *473*
      final insertion *464–465,* 467–472, *469–473*
      try-in *463,* 465–469, *466–467*
   post-treatment care 473–477
   rebonding 1373, *1375*
   removable 1155, *1156*
   repairs to existing 440, *1252*
   resin luting cement *1357–1358*
   as retainers for fixed partial dentures 549
   shade selection 441–442
   temporaries 460–461, *461–463*
   tooth preparation 442–459
      classification for anterior teeth 442–448
      diastema closure 864–865, 867–869
      extent of reduction 449–453
      technique 456, *457–460*
   see also ceramic veneers
porphyria 331, 682
post-and-core restorations
   anterior teeth 739–743
      case example 728, *730*
      procedure 739–743, *740–742*
      treatment options 739, **739**
   core materials **736**
   crown preparation 743–745, *744*
   ferrule design *744,* 745
   posterior teeth 736–739, *738*
   premolars 743, *743*
   principles 733–734, *733–734*
   see also posts

posterior occlusal plane, complete dentures 621–622, *622*
posterior teeth
  adjusting embrasures 1347
  ceramic partial coverage restorations 478–483
  complete dentures *614*, 616, 621–622, *622*
  composite restorations 379–382, *380–383*
    direct and indirect inlays 393, *394*
    finishing 409, *413–415*
    indirect 382
    limitations 478–479
    longevity 376, *377*
  crowns 523
  diastema closure 863–864, *863–865*
  fractured endodontically-treated 736–739
    composite resin core 734, 735, *736*, 739
    options for restoring 733–734
    prefabricated posts 734, 736–739, *738*
  fractures 731–732
  metal–ceramic restorations *510*
  too narrow 210–211, *212–213*
  too wide 208–209, *208–209*
postoperative pain/edema 940
posts
  cast metal *see* cast metal posts
  design 734–735, *735*
  materials 735, **736**
  perforations, endodontic surgery 804, *805–806*
  prefabricated *see* prefabricated posts
  see also post-and-core restorations
potassium nitrate 345–346
Pound, E. 616
powder, facial cosmetic 1150
Powerpoint, Microsoft 86, 87, *87*, 180
practice, dental
  attractiveness 115, *116–118*
  marketing *see* marketing
  websites 122, 124, *124–125*, 125
precision attachments, for RPDs 591
precision milling, attachment RPDs 606
prefabricated posts
  anterior teeth 733, *734*
    indications 739, **739**
    procedure 739, *741*, *742*, *743*
  design 734–735, *735*
  materials **736**
  posterior teeth 734, 736–739, *738*
  premolars 743, *743*
prehistoric societies 696, 708, 920
premolars
  as abutment teeth 584
  fractured endodontically-treated 736–739, *736–739*, 743, *743*
pressable ceramic veneers *see* ceramic veneers, pressable
press releases 128
Preston proportion (naturally occurring) 257, *257*
  dentists' preferences 258–259, *260*
prevention

older adults 1023–1024
  patient education 1414–1415
primary dentition
  avulsions 1224
  complicated crown fractures 1220–1221
  dental materials and techniques 970–971
  luxation injuries 1223
  orthodontic management 995–996
  porcelain veneers 441
  retained teeth 908
  root fractures 1223
  tooth structure 976
  trauma management 983–986
primers
  ceramic veneers 471
  dentin bonding 359–360
  universal 361
privacy, patient 145
probing
  peri-implant sulcus 1418, *1418*, 1419, *1421*
  periodontal *see* periodontal probing
  pits and fissures 417, *417*
problem patients 36–41, 77–79
  managing 78–79
  raising your fees 40, 77, 79
  see also psychological disorders
Procera all-ceramic crowns 507, *508–509*
proclination, incisor *922*, 923, 1076
product warnings/liability 150
profile angle 1113
profile view of face *see* facial profile
prognostication, legal considerations 138
prominent teeth, gingival recession risk 1184
proportional dental/facial analysis 253–265
proportional smile design 243–268
proportionate ratio, Beaudreau's 254
ProRoot MTA, pulp capping 769, *769*
prostheses
  diastema closure 849
  emergency repairs 1231–1232, *1231–1232*
  older adults 1030–1035, *1032*, *1034–1036*
  performers/actors 1172–1174, *1173–1174*
  provisional 612–613, *612–613*
protective bite appliances (nightguards)
  ceramic veneers 441, 473
  composite restorations 413–415, *415*
  dentures opposing natural teeth 631
  fixed partial dentures 554, *554*
protrusion, incisor
  orthodontic *922*, 922–923
  restorative therapy 891, *891*
provisional prostheses 612–613, *612–613*
provisional restorations *see* temporary restorations
psychiatric team 27–28, 30–31, 34
psychological considerations
  cosmetic contouring 302
  facial appearance 10–11, *11*
  seeking treatment 16–19
  tooth reduction for veneers 452
  treatment planning 19

psychological disorders 25–44, **26**
  terms and concepts 26–27
public relations 124, *124*, 128–129
pulp
  calcific metamorphosis 767
  capping *769*, 769–770
    traumatic injuries 727, 1219
  clinical evaluation *751–756*, 751–762
  degeneration, percussion test 759–761
  exposure
    fractures **722**, 727–730, 790, *793*
    pulp capping 727, 769–770
    restorative dentistry 768–769, *769*
  healthy 765
  hemorrhage *see* hemorrhage, pulp
  injury
    acid etching 134, 363, 401
    dental procedures 134, 765–767, *766*, 768–769, *768–769*
    repair mechanisms 766–767, *767*
    root fractures 1221–1223
    tooth color changes 682, 751, *752–755*, 768
    uncomplicated crown fractures 1219
  necrosis
    complicated crown fractures 1219–1220
    cracked tooth syndrome 798, 800
    electronic pulp testing 759
    root fractures 1223
    visual tooth examination 751, *751*, *753*
  protection 767, 1313
  response to operative procedures 764–767, *766*
  stressed 770, *770–772*
pulp canals, large
  cosmetic contouring 301, *301*
  crown restoration and 529
  tooth reduction for veneers and 452
  vital bleaching 331
pulpitis
  anesthetic test 763–764
  bite test 762
  cold testing 754–755
  cracked tooth syndrome 798, 799–800
pulpotomy 727
  laser 985
  partial (Cvek) 727, 1219
pulp sensibility tests 754–759
  cavity test 758–759, *758–759*
  cold tests 754–756, *756–757*
  electric 756–757, *758*
  endodontic vs periodontal lesions 759, *759–760*
  heat tests 756
  pediatric dental trauma 984
Pythagoras 1097

quartz-tungsten-halogen (QTH) light sources 405

racial differences *see* ethnic/racial differences
radio advertising 128

radiographs (X-rays)
  cosmetic contouring 304
  enamel thickness 879, 883
  endodontics
    precementation 762–763, 765
    pretreatment 762, 763–764, 774
  fixed partial dentures 544–545
  implant evaluation 1417, 1418, 1419
  initial visit 60, 61, 62
  monitoring of restorations 1411–1412
  orthodontics 899, 901, 903–904
  porcelain restorations 440
  postcementation 1365, 1365, 1410, 1410
  recommendations for
      prescribing **1413–1414**
  removable partial dentures 582–583
  review prior to second visit 67
  traumatic injuries 1216
rapport, building 750–751
RAW files 164–165
RealSeal Sealer 780
reasonable patient standard 137, 143–144
reception area 51
  attractive decor 115, 116–117
  educational materials 49, 49
receptionist, dental 48
records, clinical 139–142
  adult orthodontics 899, 899–901
  dentofacial deformity 934–935, 935–938
  electronic 67, 142
  essential components 142
  facial analysis 1097–1098
  functions 139–141
  making corrections to 141–142
  role of photographs 157
  spoilation 142
recurring esthetic dental (RED)
      proportion 257, 258
  70% 257, 258
  computer simulation methods 265–267, 267–268
  dentists' preferences 258–260, 260
  diastema closure and 846–847
  intercanine width (ICW) and 257, 259
  tooth lengths and 260–261, 261
  tooth width calculations 260–265
    clinical use 261–263, **262**, 262–263
    simplified method **263**, 263–265, 264–267, **265**
red-colored teeth **671**, 751, 752
RED proportion see recurring esthetic dental
      proportion
referrals
  patient 121–122, 123
  problem patients 77–78
  psychological 31–32, 43–44
  source of patient's 52
  specialist 72–74
refractory die technique, porcelain veneer
      fabrication 461–462
refunds 147
refusal to treat, dentist's 145

release of all future claims form 148
removable complete dentures see complete
      dentures
removable partial dentures (RPD) 581–606
  abutments see abutments, removable
      partial dentures
  alternative treatments 589–590
  attachments see attachment removable
      partial dentures
  design principles 582–589
    biomechanics 583–584
    clasps see clasps, removable partial
      dentures
    flange 589
    other esthetic aspects 589
    problem situations 584
    replacement teeth 589
    rest seats 588–589, 589
    retention enhancement 588
    use of a surveyor 583
  digital impressions 1405–1406, 1405–1406
  distal extension 583–584
  emergency repairs 1231–1232
  esthetic failures 1238–1239, 1239–1241
  evaluating tissue support 582–583
  pedodontic prostheses 979, 979–982
  performers/actors 1156–1160, 1158–1164
  rest seats 588–589
  rotational path 590, 590–593
  tooth-supported 582
  tooth-tissue-supported 582
removable porcelain veneers 1155, 1156
repeated ratio, Lombardi's 254
reshaping, cosmetic tooth see contouring,
      cosmetic
Resilon 780
resin, composite see composite resin
resin-bonded fixed partial dentures 549
  diastema closure 863–864, 863–865
  orthodontic–restorative therapy 909
resin-bonded partial-veneer fixed partial
      dentures 549
resin luting agents 1356, 1357–1358, 1361
resin-modified glass ionomers (RMGI)
  caries prevention 1247–1248
  cements 970, 1356, 1358
  cores **736**
  traumatically exposed dentin 1218
resin tags 357, 357, 368
resolution, image 160–161, 162, 163, 164
resorption
  alveolar ridge see ridge resorption
  external root see external root resorption
  internal tooth 682, 753
restorations
  bleaching and 332, 342, 346, 687
  cementation 1355–1365
  color modification 286–287
  consent forms 135–137
  cosmetic contouring and 303
  Digital Smile Design 94, 108–109
  discoloration 689–690

  endodontic access via 776–780, 777–780
  endodontically-treated teeth 780–781
  factors influencing appearance 185–187
  failure 1244–1260
    contaminants 1255
    digital impression system 1403
    esthetic emergencies 1224–1230
    exposure of margins 1244, 1245
    to follow manufacturer's
        instructions 1255–1260
    legal considerations 138
    material 1248–1252, 1248–1257
    periodontal disease 1244–1245,
        1245–1247
    recurrent caries 1245–1248, 1247
    technical 1252–1255, 1257–1260
  fractured 1224–1230
  gingival graft coverage 1194–1195, 1195
  gingival recession due to 1184
  implant-supported see implant-supported
      restorations
  longevity 1244–1260
    informing patients 138, 1242–1243
  maintenance 1409–1428
  marginal staining 330, 670–671, 674–676
  margin exposure 1236
  orthodontic therapy and 917–919
  posttreatment visit 1410–1412
  pretreatment oral care 1410
  repairs to
    air-abrasive technology 419–421,
        1227–1230, 1228
    composite resin bonding 392, 1224,
        1226–1230, 1228–1230
    esthetic emergencies 1224–1230
restorative treatment
  bleaching combined with 333–334
  crowded teeth 877–893
  elective endodontics 767–770, 768–769
  facial considerations 1085–1126
  integrating orthodontics into 905–908,
      905–909
  papillary defect closure 1196, 1197
  pulp injury 764–766, 766
  vs removal of endodontically-diseased
      teeth 782–783, 784–785
rest–proximal plate–I-bar (RPI) clasp 585, 587
rest seats 588–589, 589
retainers, orthodontic 914, 914
  crowded teeth 881, 890
retention
  attachment RPDs 595, 596
  RPDs 584–588
retina, color perception 272
retracted closed image 175, 175
retracted open image 176, 176–177
retraction cords see gingival retraction cords
retractors
  clinical photography 171, 171
  left and right lateral images 176–177, 177
  mandibular arch image 178–179
  maxillary arch images 178, 179

retruded tooth 891
reverse (negative) smile line 186, *186*, 247, *247*, *902*, 1122, *1122*
Rhesus factor incompatibility 331
rhinoplasty 1081, *1081*, 1134, *1136*
rhytidectomy (facelift) 1137, *1138*
Ricketts E-plane 1117, *1117*
ridge augmentation *1200–1201*, 1200–1204
    facial considerations 1118
    fixed partial dentures 566–570, *569*, 1201–1204
    horizontal 640–642, *642*
    implants 639–643, *641–642*
    indications 1201
    surgical technique 1201–1204, *1201–1204*
    vertical 642–643
ridge deformities 1118, 1199–1200
ridge form and volume 1118
    fixed partial dentures 566–567
    implants 638–643, *639–642*
    see also bone, quantity and quality
ridge preservation 639, *640–641*, 1200
ridge resorption 1199–1200
    dentures opposing natural teeth 628–629
    facial considerations 1118, *1118*
    fixed porcelain interdental insert *228–230*, 229
    pontic design 567, *568–569*
    porcelain vs plastic denture teeth 626–627
    postextraction 638–639, **639**, *639–640*, *1182*, *1182*, 1200
    removable partial dentures 589
    Siebert classification 567
right lateral arch image 176–178
ring clasp 585–587
risks of treatment
    disclosure 132, 143–144
    misrepresentation 144
    nonnegligent 144
    see also informed consent
Rite-Lite 2 *1177*, 1178
roll 1072–1076, *1076*
root
    proximity, crowded teeth 881
    RPD abutment teeth 583–584
root canal therapy *see* endodontics
root caries
    connective tissue graft coverage 1194–1195, *1195*
    older adults *1036*
root coverage 1183–1195
    autogenous vs allogenic tissues 1184
    furcation involvement 1185, *1186*
    indications 1185
    old restorations and root caries 1194–1195, *1195*
    postoperative care 1194, *1194*
    potential for new attachment 1185–1186, *1186*
    quality and quantity of donor tissue 1195
    surgical technique 1186–1194
        graft positioning 1190–1191, *1192–1193*
        microincisions and gingival pouch 1188–1189, *1188–1189*
        root preparation 1186–1188, *1187–1188*
        sutures and dressing 1191–1194, *1193–1194*
        tissue harvesting 1189–1191, *1190–1191*
root fractures 790–793, *795–798*, 1221–1223
    apical third 791, *795*
    coronal third 793, *797–798*
    diagnosis 761–762
    endodontically-treated teeth *740*, 743–744
    mid root 791–793, *795–796*
    partial pulpotomy 727
    pediatric patients 985
    retrograde 803
    treatment options **722**
root preparation
    connective tissue graft coverage 1186–1188, *1187–1188*
    papilla reconstruction 1196
root resorption, external *see* external root resorption
root segments, extrusion 793, *798*
Rotadent
    bonded restorations 415, *416*
    implant cleaning 1421, *1421*, 1427
    interproximal cleaning *1423*, 1427
rotational path removable partial dentures 590, *590–593*
Roth #801 root canal cement 780
round face, hair styles 1144, *1145*
RPD *see* removable partial dentures
rubber cup polishing 473, 1416
rubber dam
    bleaching nonvital teeth 144, 347
    ceramic veneers 469
    endodontics 771–774
    isolation of multiple teeth 773, *774*
    pediatric dentistry 973
    protecting ceramic crowns 772–773, *773*
    selective vital bleaching 333, *333*
    smaller alternatives 774, *774*
Russell's sign 32, *33*

Sadoun, Michael 506
Safety Data Sheets (SDSs) 150
sagittal splitting osteotomy, Obwegeser's 944–948, *946–947*, *949–950*
salivary diagnostics
    genetic risks 1423, *1424–1426*
    peri-implantitis bacteria 1419, *1420*, 1427
salivary flow 671, 1023
sandwich technique 403, *404*
Sarver, David 899, 903
satisfaction, patient 18, 115, *123*
saturation, effects of bleaching 278, **284**
scaling
    ceramic veneers 473
    implant-supported restorations 1421–1422, *1422*

scars
    lip 1112, *1112*
    makeup for concealing 1151
Scharer, Peter 510
sclera exposure 1008
Scotchbond adhesives 363, 367
scratch test 712
sealants, surface
    composite resin restorations 689
    discoloration over time 670, *674*
second appointment
    preparation for 67–70
    treatment planning 70–77
segmental arch mechanics 911, *913*
selective serotonin reuptake inhibitors (SSRIs) 28
self-etch adhesives **357**, 357–358
    dentin bonding 360, *360*, 403
    development 358
    enamel bonding 357–358
    one-step (all-in-one) 360, 362, **362**, 365–366, *366*
    postoperative hypersensitivity 366–367
    recommendations for use 368
    reliability and degradation 365
    technique sensitivity 365–366, *366*
    two-step **362**, 366
self-image 6, *8*, 10–11, 1149
self-smile analysis 49–51, *51*, 70
semiprecision attachments, for RPDs 591
sensitivity, tooth *see* tooth sensitivity
separation of adjacent teeth, increasing 218, *218*
sertraline (Zoloft) 27, 28
setting time, impression materials 1293, **1293**
sevenths, facial 245, *245*
sewing needles/pins 825–826, *827*
sex, personality, age (SPA) factors 248, 614
sex characteristics
    apical tooth forms 248, *250*
    incorporating 223, *225–226*
    SPA factors 248, *249*
    see also feminine appearance; gender differences; masculine appearance
sexiness 8–9, *9*
shade
    staining techniques to alter **200–201**
    verification of final 1339, 1345
    see also color
shade charts 533, *533*
shade guides 199–205, *204–207*, 276–281
    checking completed prostheses 1339
    crowns 534–535, *535*
    custom-made 285–286
    facial prostheses 281
    modified 285
    monitoring bleaching 277–279, *279*, 336, *337*
    oral soft tissues 281
    porcelain veneers 442
    tooth 276–281

shade guides (cont'd)
   coverage error (CE) 280–281
   historical 276, *276*
   proprietary or classical-proprietary 279–280, *280–282*
   pros and cons 280–281, **282**
   VITA classical A1–D4 276–277, *277*
   VITA System 3D-Master 277–279, *277–279*
shade guide units (sgu) 277
Shademan, Nasser, two-tier quattro veneer construction 229, *232–236*
shade selection/color matching 271, 274–285
   bleaching 336, *337*
   case study 289–292, *289–292*
   composite resin bonding 379, 385, 396–398, *397*
     repairs 690
   crowns 532–536
     laboratory communication 535, *535*
     lighting 532–533
     records 533–534, *533–534*
     shade guides 534–535, *535*
     tips 535–536
   education and training **287, 287–288,** *288–289*
   to individual patient 678
   instrumental 284–285, *285*
   older patients 219–221, *223*
   performers/actors 1168–1169, *1169–1170*
   porcelain veneers 441–442
   role of photographs 157, 286
   unsatisfactory 1236, *1236*
   visual 274–284
     conditions 274–276
     individual variations 274
     method 282–284, *283*
     myths and facts 284, **284**
shadowing
   creating illusions 188, *188*
   lip thickness and 186–187
   tooth appearance and 189, 190
shaping, tooth
   illusional effects 189–190
   older patients 219
   too-long teeth 215–216, *215–216*
   too-narrow teeth 210–211, *212–213*
   too-short teeth *214*, 214–215
   too-wide teeth 207–209, *207–209*
   try-in appointment 1347–1350, *1349–1351*
   see also contouring, cosmetic
Shofu Cosmetic Contouring Kit 310–311, 313
short teeth
   crowns 530–531, 1283, *1283–1284*
   illusions for *214*, 214–215
   see also tooth length; tooth lengthening
shoulderless full porcelain crown 1268
shoulder margins
   all-ceramic crowns 1268, *1269, 1270–1271, 1273*
   metal–ceramic crowns 522–523, 525

porcelain-fused-to-metal crowns 1279–1280, *1280*
porcelain veneers 456
   try-in stage 1343, *1344*
shrinkage
   impression materials **1293,** 1294
   polymerization 405
Siebert classification of edentulous areas 567
silanation
   ceramic fitting surfaces *1362,* 1364
   ceramic veneers *467, 471*
   fractured restorations 1230
   porcelain butt margins 1356, *1358*
silicone impression materials 1291–1292, 1388
Siltek method
   implant temporaries 1324, *1327–1328*
   interim temporary restorations 1324, *1325–1327*
silver-containing materials
   endodontic therapy 780
   tooth discoloration 682, 751, *753*
single-lens reflex (SLR) cameras 158, *159,* 159–169
   cost 159
   flash systems 163, *164,* 165
   f-stop and flash settings 166–169, *169, 170*
   functions 161–162
   histogram 162, 165–166, *166–168,* 168
   image file types 164–165
   image resolution 160–161, *162, 163*
   intraoral images 158, *158*
   ISO 164
   lenses 160, *160, 161*
   lighting 166–169, *169–170*
   screen size 159–160
   selection 159–163
   setting up 163–166
   size-weight 162–163
   smile evaluation 252–253, *252–253*
   through the lens (TTL) vs aperture priority 165–166
   wand-like cameras vs 156, *156*
sinusitis, acute 759–761
skin care 1149
skin color 274
   shade guides 281
skin resurfacing, facial 1140
SLA models *see* stereolithography apparatus models
sleep bruxism 697
slip-cast aluminum oxide ceramic 506
SLR cameras *see* single-lens reflex cameras
smile
   asymmetric 1068–1071
   differing esthetic standards 138, 899–900, *902*
   historical perspective 4–5
   posed vs spontaneous 899, *901,* 1098
   width 1125, *1125*
smile analysis

crown selection 525–526, *526*
Digital Smile Design 88, *88*
facial context 1086–1088, *1087–1088*
horizontal planes of reference 1108
macroesthetic 1068–1072, 1077–1078, *1078–1079*
miniesthetic 1078, *1079*
orthodontics 899–900, *902*
photographic 251–253
   close-up image 173, *174*
   equipment 252–253, *252–253*
   facial image view evaluation (FIVE) 253, *255*
   full-face view 171–173, *173*
   standardized protocols 253, *254*
self-smile analysis 49–51, *51,* 70
smile arc 1071–1072, *1076*
   patient preferences 138
smile design
   computer simulation 88, *88,* 265–268, *267–268*
   digital *see* Digital Smile Design
   patient preferences and individuality 268
   performers/actors 1173–1174, *1176*
   principles 246–247
   proportional 243–268
smile line 931, 1122–1124
   crowded teeth 881
   diastema closure and 847
   high *905,* 1123, 1123–1124
   implant esthetics and 638
   low *905,* 1123, 1124, *1124–1125*
   medium *905,* 1123, *1123*
   orthodontic implications 904–905, *905*
   positive 186
   preferences 899–902, *902*
   reverse (negative) 186, *186,* 247, *247,* 902, 1122, *1122*
   see also gingival display; lip line
Smith and Knight's Tooth Wear Index **697**
smoking, tobacco 825
   older adults 1023
   pipe users 831, *832*
   stained teeth 675, *678*
   tooth color 274
   see also tobacco
Snap-On Smile 1332, *1333*
   disguising a diastema 842
   treatment planning 75, *76,* 844
Snow's golden mean 257, *257*
social context, esthetic dentistry 5–6, *6–7*
social media 128–129
Society for Color and Appearance in Dentistry (SCAD) **287**
socket repair membrane, Zimmer 640–641
sodium hypochlorite 780
sodium perborate 348
soft-tissue fillers 1137, *1140*
soft tissues (oral)
   discoloration
     amalgam tattoo 805, *807*
     peri-implant *655, 658, 659,* 1370

Index

edentulous areas 583
fixed partial dentures 551, *553*, 571
laser applications 973
peri-implant *see* implants, gingival tissues
preparation for impressions 1287–1291, *1288–1292*
preparation for pontics 566–579, *568–570*
prostheses *see* tissue inserts
retraction prior to impressions 1288–1291, *1289–1292*
sculpting
 excessive gingival display 1204–1208
 fixed partial dentures 570
 see also periodontal plastic surgery
shade guides 281
temporary restorations and 1313, *1313*
tooth preparation for crowns and 518–521, *520*, 1264–1266, *1265–1267*
traumatic injuries 985–986
see also gingiva; periodontal disease
space
 arch *see* arch, space
 attachment RPDs 596–597
 deficiencies, crowded teeth 878
 maintenance in children 995–996
 too narrow 209–214, *210–213*
 too wide 206–209, *207–209*
SPA (sex, personality, age) factors 248, 614
spark erosion technology 606
special effects 185–234
 illusions 188–192
 laboratory communication 197–199
 shade guides 199–205, *204–207*
 specific problems 206–229
  adding age features 219, *221–222*
  arch irregularity 218, *219–221*
  incisal embrasures 221, *224–225*
  incorporating personality 225, *227*
  influencing facial shape 218–219
  insufficiently differentiated teeth 218, *218*
  interdental tissue loss 225–229, *227–236*
  long-axis inclinations 216–218, *218*
  reducing age effects 219–221, *223*
  sexual differentiation 223, *225–226*
  too-long tooth 215–216, *215–216*
  too-narrow space 209–214, *210–213*
  too-short tooth 214–215, *214–215*
  too-wide space 206–209, *207–209*
  using form and color 216, *217*, **218**
 staining 193–197
 see also illusions
specialists, consultation with 70–74, *73*
spectacles, harmful habits 831, *833*
spectral power distribution (SPD) 275
Spectratone shade guide 276
spectrophotometers 284–285, *285*
SpectroShade Micro 284–285, *285*
Spee, F. Graf von 921

speech
 denture tooth placement 619–620, 621, 623
 vertical dimension of *619*, 619–620
splint bar attachments 605, *607*
splinting
 attachment RPDs 595, *604*, 605
 fixed partial dentures and 555
 luxation injuries 1223, 1225, *1225*
 orthodontically treated patients 914, *914*
 problem patients 78–79
 root-fractured teeth 791, *795–796*, 1221
 telescopic bridges 558–559, *558–559*
 temporary 1317–1323
splints
 composite resin 1155, *1157*
 fixed, try-in 1341, *1341–1342*, 1345
 occlusal, worn teeth 702
spoilation 142
square face, hair styles 1144, *1145*, 1148
"S" sounds, denture tooth placement *619*, 619–620, 623
stained/discolored teeth 669–690
 bleaching *see* bleaching
 ceramic veneers 440, 441, 687–688, *687–688*
  final color adjustments 468–469
  increasing opaqueness 452, 461–462
  tooth preparation 452, 453
 composite resin restorations 689, *689*, 690, 1252
 cosmetic contouring 300, *300*, 302
 crowns 523–524
 etiology 328–331, 346, 670, **671, 673**
 examination 326
 extrinsic staining 328, 670, 671–678
  causes 672–673, 673–674
  direct or nonmetallic 673
  indirect or metallic 673
  management 673, **673**, 678, 679
  Natho classification 671
  predisposing factors 671
  specific types 674–676
  whitening toothpastes 676–678
 gingival retraction fluid causing 1236
 indicating pulpal problems 751, *751–755*
 initial observation 52
 intrinsic staining 328, 670, 678–687
  causes 672, 678–686
  localized brown stains 682–683, *685*
  localized white spots 683, *685*
  management **673**, 687
  single tooth 682, *683–684*
  see also tetracycline-stained teeth
 mechanisms 326
 microabrasion 341, *342*
 older adults 331, *332*
 pediatric patients
  bleaching vital teeth 335, *336*
  previous subluxation injury 988–989, *988–989*
  previous trauma 994, *994–995*

pit and fissure stains 416–419, *418–420*
porcelain denture teeth 627, *628*
porcelain resistance 439
single dark tooth 682, *683–685*
tooth defects causing 670–671, *673*
 caries 670, *674*
 deep grooves 670, *674*
 leakage around restorations 670–671, *674–676*
treatment options *670*, **673**, 687–690
see also marginal staining
staining techniques 193–194, 193–205
 adding illusion of width 211, *212–213*
 communication with laboratory 197–199
 increasing apparent length 215, *215*
 in-office 193, 286
 masking extra width 209, *209*
 older patients 219, *221–222*
 reducing apparent length 216
 surface 194–197, *196–198*
  adding characterization **202–203**
  altering shade **200–201**
  IPS Empress crowns 510, 511
  tips 195–197, *198–199*
stainless steel prefabricated posts **736**
standards of care 131–132, 143–144
Steiner line 1117, *1117*
stents
 composite resin 1155, *1157*
 cosmetic acrylic 1155, *1156*
stereolithography apparatus (SLA) models 1390, 1394
 clinical cases 1403, *1404*, 1405, *1406*
Stern ERA attachment 600, *604–606*
Stern ERA-RV attachment 600, *606*
Stern G/A attachment 597, *598*
Stern G/L attachment 597, *598*
Stern McCollum attachment 597, *598–599*
Stern Type 7 attachment 597
Stim-u-dents, used as wedges 826, *829*
stress
 role in bruxism 814
 tensile, abfraction etiology 704–705, *705*
stressed pulp 770, *770–772*
stroke 1022, 1024
studio lighting 1178
study models 67
 cosmetic contouring 304, *306*
 dentofacial deformities 934–935
 digital
  laboratory systems 1401, *1401*
  orthodontics 909, *910*
 digitally-guided fabrication 1394
  3D printing 1394
  milling 1390, 1394, 1396
  TRIOS system 1399–1400
 digital scanning 1401
 Digital Smile Design 91–94, *101–102*
 fixed partial dentures 545, *545, 546*
 orthodontics *900*

study models (*cont'd*)
    Pincus principles D7
    preparation 1302
    SLA *see* stereolithography apparatus models
    surface characterization 190, *190*
subgingival margins
    all-ceramic crowns 1267, *1267–1268*
        try-in stage 1343, *1344*
    ceramic veneers 448–449, 452, 453, 456, *458*
        final placement 469
        legal considerations 134–136
    fixed partial dentures 551
    see also gingival margins
subluxation injury 1223
    tooth discoloration after 988–989, *988–989*
submental view of face, photographs 1056, *1059*
substructure materials 192, *192–193*, **193**
suicide 42
supernumerary teeth 1000, *1000–1003*
SureFil 403
surface roughness, role in adhesion 356
surface texture/characterization
    composite restorations 407–408
    crowns 532, *532*
    performers/actors 1174–1176
    Pincus principles D3, *D4*, *D5*
    planning 190, *190*
    staining techniques 194–197, *196–199*, **202–203**
    translucency/light transmission and 192, *192*
    try-in appointment 1350, *1351*
    visual matching 284
surgically assisted orthodontics 956–959
surgical–orthodontic treatment 929–965
    adjunctive procedures 959, *961–962*
    case presentation visit 935–937
    complications and risks 939–940
    dentofacial deformities 940–955
    distraction osteogenesis 955–956
    facial analysis 930–931, *931–932*
    first visit 933–935
    indications 933
    obstructive sleep apnea 959–964, *962–964*
    patient expectations 933
    pediatric patients 933
    postsurgical treatment 937–939
    presurgical orthodontics 935–937, 939–940
    presurgical visit 937
    three-dimensional approach 1079–1083, *1080–1082*
surround, tooth color matching 275, 276
surveyor, dental 583
suspensory sutures 1199, *1199*
SwissTac/Tach E-Z attachment 605
Syntac adhesive 363, 366, 367
systemic disorders, causing tooth discoloration 330–331

tattoo, amalgam 805, *807*
T-bar clasp 584–585, *586*
    modified 584–585, *586*
team, dental
    appearance 115–116, *119*
    customer service 117–119
tear energy, impression materials 1293, **1293**
technical skill, dentist's 80
teeth
    denture *see* denture teeth
    differentiation between adjacent 218, *218*
    examination 55–56, 751
    functions 11
Teflon tape 854, 855, *855*
telephone consultations 150
telephone directories 125
telescoping bridges 555–562
    advantages 555–558
    clinical examples 558–559, *558–559*, 560, *560–561*
    disadvantages 559–560
television 6, 10
    actors *see* performers/actors
    advertising 125–128
temperamental theory, tooth morphology 614
temporary anchorage devices (TADs) 933
temporary restorations 1311–1324
    acrylic crowns 502
    CAD/CAM construction 1315
    cements 1313, 1340, 1364
    composite resin bonding 392
    consent form 135
    crowded teeth 881–882
    decision-making role 1312, *1313*
    esthetic uses 1311–1314
    implant 656–657
        immediate placement 644–645, *646–650*, 656
        Siltek method 1324, *1327–1328*
        soft tissue benefits 644–645, *648–650*, 656, *657–658*
        used as impression posts 650, *656–657*
    orthodontic therapy and 1312
    phonetic concerns 1313
    previewing illusions 189–190, *191–192*
    protective function 1313, *1313*
    removal 1339
    requirements 1313–1314
    temporary (interim) 1323–1324, *1324–1325*
        secondary function 1324
        Siltek matrix 1324, *1325–1327*
    trial smile role 1312, *1313*
    vacuform technique 1315, *1315–1316*
    veneers 460–461, *461–463*, 1316–1317, *1316–1319*
temporary splinting 1317–1323
    A-splint 1320–1323, *1321–1323*
    composite resin 1317–1320, *1319–1320*
temporization, esthetic 1311–1324
    functions 1311–1314
    specific types 1315–1324

temporomandibular joint pain 815, *815–816*
tensile bond strength, porcelain veneers 439
tensile stress model, abfraction 704–705, *705*
Terramycin staining 755
tert-butanol 359
tetracycline paste, root surface demineralization 1188, *1188*
tetracycline-stained teeth 672, 683–686, *686*, 751, *755*
    bleaching 328–329, *329–330*, 683–686, *686*, 687
    ceramic veneers 440, 452, 453, 461–462, 687–688, *687–688*
1,1,1,2-tetrafluoroethane (Endo-Ice) 754–756, *757*
texture, surface *see* surface texture
theater actors *see* performers/actors
thermal pulp testing 754–756
Thermaseal Plus 780
thirds, facial 245, *246*, 1097, *1100*
    age-related changes 245, *246*, 1101–1102, *1106–1107*
    combined with 1/16th rule 249, *251*
    facial analysis 1101–1102, *1104–1105*
    orthodontic correction of dentofacial deformity 930–931, *931*
    orthodontics 900–902, *902*, 1057, *1060*
    pediatric patients 1007, *1007*
    profile view 1063
thread biting, habitual 826, *828*
three-dimensional (3D) technology
    CEREC system 484
    fixed partial dentures 564
    treatment planning 75–77
    see also computer-aided design/manufacturing systems; digital impressions
3M True Definition Scanner system 1394–1395, *1394–1396*, **1400**
3M zirconia 537
3Shape TRIOS system 1397–1400, *1398–1399*, **1400**
thumb sucking 811–813, *812*, 1004
TIFF files 164–165
tissue inserts
    acrylic 1161, *1164*, 1323
    cantilevered porcelain 229
    crown restorations 530
    fixed composite resin 229, *230–232*
    fixed partial dentures 228–230, 229, 570, *572–573*
    shade guides 281
tissues, oral soft *see* soft tissues (oral)
titanium
    implant abutments 655, 657–658, *659*
        ceramic interface 1370, *1370–1371*
        soft tissue interface 1370–1371
    implants 653
    prefabricated posts **736**
tobacco
    chewing 816
    oral cancer risk 1023

Index

stains 328, 675, *677, 678,* 687
  see also smoking, tobacco
tongue thrusting 816–817, *816–818,* 843, *843*
tooth appearance
  factors influencing 185–187
  lighting considerations for actors *1177, 1178*
  lip thickness and 186–187
  shaping and contouring and 189–190
  substructure materials and 192, *192–193,* **193**
  surface texture and 192, *192*
  tooth arrangement and 190–192, *191*
tooth arrangement
  complete dentures 616–623
  crowns 531–532
  illusional effects 190–192, *191*
  Lombardi's guide 190–191, *191*
  masking too-wide teeth 209, *210–211*
  narrow spaces 212–214, *213–214*
  too-short teeth 215
tooth brushes 1414, 1427
tooth brushing
  after bulimic vomiting 822
  ceramic veneers 477
  composite restorations 415, *416*
  gingival recession due to 1184
  implant care 1427, *1428*
  improper technique 1412, *1414*
  tooth abrasion 705, *706,* 708, *709,* 710, 827, *830*
tooth color 274
  complete dentures 616
  crowns 532
  evaluating pulpal health 751, *751–755*
  factors influencing perception 185–187, 678
  hair color and 1147
  matching *see* shade selection/color matching
  older adults 331, *332,* 616, 1025
  perceived aging and **225,** *225*
  performers/actors 1174
  shade guides *see* shade guides, tooth
Tooth Color Indicator (Clark) 276, *276*
tooth contour
  crowns 529, *530*
  see also contouring, cosmetic
tooth exposure, at rest 1119–1120, *1119–1121*
tooth form
  complete dentures 614, 615
  reshaping 313–314, *314–315*
  see also tooth shape
tooth fragments
  bonding original 722–723, 726–727, 1219, 1220, *1220*
  complete separation 802–803
tooth length
  1/16th rule 249, *250*
  contouring to reduce 306–313, *308–313*
  crown preparation and 530–531

fixed restorations 1347, *1348*
illusions for increasing 214–215, *214–215*
illusions for reducing 215–216, *215–216*
temporary restorations 1312
tooth width calculations and
  ICW/CIL quotient **263,** 263–265, *264–267,* **265**
  RED proportion 260, *261,* 261–262, **262**
  see also central incisor length
tooth lengthening
  composite resin bonding 400, *401–402*
  porcelain veneers 439, 441
tooth migration, pathologic 843
tooth molds 615
tooth morphology *see* tooth shape
toothpastes 1414
  relative dentin abrasivity **1415**
  whitening 676–678
toothpicks, harmful habits 826, *829*
tooth preparation 1263–1283
  all-ceramic crowns 1263–1271
  attachment RPDs 595
  ceramic veneers *see under* ceramic veneers
  CEREC system 485, *486*
  checklists 1283
  composite resin bonding 398–399, *399–401*
  crowded tooth situation 1280–1283, *1282*
  Digital Smile Design 94, *107*
  extremely short teeth 1283, *1283–1284*
  long crown/root ratio 1283
  metal–ceramic restorations 518–522, *520*
  periodontal disease 1280, *1281*
  porcelain-fused-to-metal crowns 1271–1280, *1277–1278*
  posterior ceramic partial coverage restorations 481–482
tooth proportion
  complete dentures 614–615, *615*
  cosmetic contouring and 303
  crowns *530,* 530–531
  diastema closure and 846–847
  Digital Smile Design 89–90, *90*
  orthodontics and 902–903, *903*
  periodontal disease impact 902
  in relation to face size 249–251, *250–252*
  restoring crowded teeth and 887–890
  see also tooth length; tooth-to-tooth width proportions; tooth width
tooth reduction
  all-ceramic crowns 1268–1271, *1269–1270*
  ceramic veneers 449–453, *457–459,* 885
  cosmetic contouring 306–313, *308–313,* 318, *318*
  metal–ceramic restorations 521
  porcelain-fused-to-metal crowns 1271–1277, *1277–1279*
  pulp injury 764–765
tooth sensitivity
  after dentin etching/bonding 366–367, 403
  cosmetic contouring 301

postcementation 1356
vital bleaching 331, 341, 342, 345–346
see also pulp sensibility tests
tooth shape
  apical forms 248, *250*
  complete dentures 614–616
  crowns 529, *530*
  diastema closure and 852–853, 856, *856–857*
  factors influencing perception 185–186
  gender differences 303, 614
  SPA factors 248, *248, 249*
  see also tooth form
tooth size
  1/16th rule 249, *250*
  Bolton's analysis 923, **924**
  complete dentures 614–616, *615*
  crowns *530,* 530–531
  interarch discrepancies in adults 923, *923*
  proportion to face size 249–251, *250–252*
  SPA factors 248, *248, 249*
  see also tooth length; tooth width
Tooth Slooth 761–762, *761–762*
tooth-to-tooth width proportions 254–265
  calculating ideal 260–265
  dentists' preferences 258–260, *260*
  diastema closure and 846–847
  orthodontics and 902–903, *903*
  RED proportion *see* recurring esthetic dental proportion
  theories 254–257, *256–257*
tooth wear *see* wear, tooth
Tooth Wear Index, Smith and Knight's **697**
tooth width
  1/16th rule 249, *250,* 614–615, *615*
  Bolton's analysis 923, **924**
  calculating ideal 260–265
    ICW/CIW quotient **263,** 263–265, *264–267,* **265**
    RED proportion 260–263, *261–263,* **262**
  diastema closure and 846–847, 850–851, *852*
  in relation to face size 249–251, *250–252*
  in relation to other teeth *see* tooth-to-tooth width proportions
  see also central incisor width; narrow teeth; wide teeth
tooth width/length ratio *see* central incisor width/length ratio
torque, removable partial dentures 582
torquing, ceramic veneers 472, *473*
tragion 1094
training
  CAD/CAM systems 1390–1391, *1392*
  color **287,** 287–288, *288–289*
  cost implications 80
  see also dental education
transformation toughening 550, 1377
transillumination 56–57
  enamel microcracks 56–57, *58*
  evaluation of pulpal health 751, *751*
  fractured teeth 751, *755–756*

Page numbers 1–666 are in Volume 1; page numbers 667–1429 are in Volume 2.

translucency
  esthetic failures 1251–1252, *1255*
  IPS Empress 510, 511
  surface texture and 192, *192*
  visual matching 284
  zirconia materials 537
transmetal burs 776, 778
transplantation, tooth 997, *997–1000*
transverse cant of maxilla 1062, *1067, 1068–1071*
traumatic injuries
  emergencies 1215–1224
  endodontic therapy 790–794
  patient evaluation 1216
  pediatric patients 983–986
    case studies 986–994, *986–995*
    hard tissues and pulp 984–985
    injuries to developing teeth 986
    laser applications 984
    loss of teeth 980, *980–982*
    periodontal tissues 985–986
    prevention 983–984
  surgical dental injuries 939
  tooth discoloration after 346, 683
  vital bleaching 333, *333*
  see also emergencies; fractures
tray adhesives, impression 1294
trays, impression 1294
treatment coordinator 70, *72*, 79, 80
  Digital Smile Design tool 86
treatment planning 47–81
  clinical examination 55–67
  compromised 1242–1244
  continuous communication 79
  costs of treatment 79–81
  decision making 48
  documentation 70, *71*, 139, *140*
  final case presentation see case presentation
  hygienist's role 53–54
  initial visit 51–53
  before initial visit 48–51
  preliminary 70
  preparation for second visit 67–70
  problem patients 78
  psychology and 19
  second appointment 70–77
  technology/integrated digital systems 67
  three-dimensional approach *1052, 1052–1056, 1054*
  treatment coordinator's role 70, *72*
  trial smile 66–67
trial smile 66–67, 75, 1332
  performers/actors 1177–1178
  removable appliance 75, *76*, 1332, *1333*
  temporary restorations as 1312, *1313*
trichion (Tr)–menton (Me)/zygion angle (ZA) (ZA ratio) 1008, *1008*
triethylene glycol dimethacrylate (TEGDMA) 357, 360
Trubyte Bioform shade guide 280, *280*

Trubyte Lucitone 199 shade guide (Dentsply) 281
truthfulness 138
try-in, esthetic 1331–1352
  additional appointments 1336–1337
  cementation 1352
  checklist 1339
  communication aspects 1337
  direct viewing by patient 1332–1336, *1334–1336*
  indirect viewing techniques 1336
  initial visualization 1332
  involving family/friends 1332
  legal considerations 138–139, *139*
  polishing 1351
  principles 1339–1352
    adding texture 1350, *1351*
    contact 1345, *1345*
    esthetic checks 1345–1347, *1346–1348*
    final shaping 1347–1350, *1349–1351*
    fitting to tooth 1341–1343, *1341–1344*
    occlusal adjustment 1346
    prior to insertion 1339
    prior to patient arrival 1339
    reevaluation 1350
  trial smile see trial smile
  unglazed restorations 1351
  written statement of approval 1337–1338, *1340*
Turner classification, tooth wear 697

ultrasonic scalers 1417, 1422
uncooperative patients 78
U/P Root Canal Sealer 780
urea peroxide 342, 343
urethane dimethacrylate (UEDMA) 360

vacuform matrix
  construction of temporaries 1315, *1315–1316*
  laboratory communication 198
  temporary temporaries 1323–1324, *1324–1325*
Valdez v. Worth, D.D.S. 142
validation, of patient's concerns 38
value, color 272, *273*
vampire teeth 1157, *1161–1162*
Variolink Esthetic LC System 472
veneer onlays, ceramic 482, *482–484*
veneers
  advantages and disadvantages **538**
  ceramic see ceramic veneers
  direct composite see direct composite veneers
  history of development 434–435
  indirect composite/acrylic 434, 461
  informed consent 133
  porcelain see porcelain veneers
  removable 841, *842*, 844
  temporary 460–461, *461–463*, 1316–1317, *1316–1319*
Venus shade guide 282

vertical 1/16th rule 249, *250*
vertical dimension of occlusion (OVD; VDO)
  age-related decrease 1021, *1021*, 1026
  analysis 1102, *1108–1109*
  complete dentures 618, 619, 620–621, *621–622*, 623
  concave profile 1113
  effects of bruxism 697–698, *698*, 702
  final bite registration 1306
  orthodontic patients 919, *919*
  tooth lengthening to restore 215, *215*
vertical dimension of speech 619, *619–620*
vertical maxillary deficiency 951, *951*
vertical maxillary excess (VME) 948
  gummy smile *947*, 948, 1204
  mandibular prognathism with 941
  surgical–orthodontic correction 948, *949–950*
vertical ramus osteotomy (VRO) 941–942, *943*
vertical ridge augmentation 642–643
vertical subcondylar osteotomy (VSO) *940*, 941–942, *943*
video camera recorders (camcorders) 181–182
video recordings 180–182
  Digital Smile Design 87
  informed consent 139, *141*
  initial visit 59–60, 67
  try-in appointment 1336, *1338*
Vintage Halo NCC shade guide 282
Vintage Opal Porcelain 516
vinyl polysiloxane 1324
Visio-Gem crowns 502
visual angle of subtense 275, 283
visual examination
  facial perspective 1087–1088, *1087–1088*
  teeth 55, 751
visual perception *1086*, 1086–1087
VITABLOCS Mark II 1264
VITA classical A1–D4 shade guides 276–277, *277*
  clinical use 280, **284**
  monitoring bleaching 336
  value scale 277, *277*
VITA Easyshade V 285, *285*
Vitality Scanner 756–757, *758*
vitality tests see pulp sensibility tests
VITA System 3D-Master Shade Guides 277–279
  Bleachedguide 277–279, *279*
  clinical use 280–281
  Linearguide 277, *278–279*
  Toothguide 277, *277*, 336
Vit-I-ecsence shade guide 282
voice-activated periodontal charting 61, 67
vomiting, self-induced 32–33, *33*, 822

walking bleach technique 348, 348–349, 784–786, *786–787*
Ward, Fred *1156*
warranty, treatment 79, 81, 137–138

water irrigation, implant maintenance 1427, *1427*
Wawira people, tooth filing 298
wax
    mortician's, diastema closure 1173, 1175
    tooth-colored 74, *74*, 197–198
wax printing 1401–1402, *1402*
wax-up, diagnostic 67
    complete dentures 624, *624*
    crowded teeth 881–882
    diastemas 844, *845*
    Digital Smile Design (DSD) 94, *102*
    digital systems 1401–1402, *1402*
    fixed partial dentures 545, *546*
    laboratory communication via 197
    orthodontic–restorative treatment 906, *908*
    presentation to patient 74–75, *75*
wear
    composite resins 376, 393, 502
    porcelain veneers 439
    tooth 693–714
        complete dentures 615
        differential diagnosis 711–712
        etiological factors 697
        evaluation 697, **697**
        low smile line 1124, *1125*
        older adults 696, 1025–1026, 1034–1035, *1034–1035*
        orthodontic esthetics and 902, *903*
        porcelain veneers for 441
        presentation 693, *694–695*
        reduced incisal exposure *1119*, 1120
        simulating 219, *221–222*
        Turner classification 697
        zirconia restorations 1378
    see also abfractions; abrasion; attrition; erosion
website, practice 122, 124, *124–125*, 125
Wedjets 772, *772–773*

wet bonding problem 359–360
wettability, impression materials 1293, **1293**
whitening, tooth *see* bleaching
whitening toothpastes 676–678
white spots **671**, *680–681*, 683
    bleaching 332, 683, *685*
    creating illusion of height 215
    dental fluorosis 328, 680
    see also hypocalcification, enamel
wide teeth, illusions masking 206–209, *207–209*, 847, *848–849*
Williams, J.L. 614
window veneer preparation 442, *443*
wine drinking 710
Wohlwend, Arnold 510
women
    facial shape and hairstyles 1144–1147, *1144–1147*
    makeup 1149–1151
    see also feminine appearance; gender differences
word-of-mouth advertising 115
working time, impression materials 1293, **1293**
wrinkle patients 78

Xeno III adhesive system 366
xerostomia
    antidepressant medications and 28, *29*, 30
    bulimia nervosa 33
    older adults 1022
XP Bond 359, *363*
X-rays *see* radiographs

yaw 1072–1076, *1076*
Y-bar clasp 584–585
yellow tooth discoloration **671**, *754*
yttrium-stabilized zirconia (Y-TZP) 550, 1253, 1377
    see also zirconia

zinc oxide–eugenol (ZOE) 1364
zinc phosphate cement 1355–1356
zirconia (zirconium oxide) 536–537, 1377–1379
    bilayered restorations 1377, *1378*
        crowns 507, 536–537
        failure rates 1254
        implants 658–659
        tooth preparation 1254
        wear of opposing teeth 1378
    cutting for endodontic access 778
    failure rates 1253, 1254
    fixed partial denture frameworks 550, *551–552*, 564
        coping design 550, *552*
        occlusal interface 1379, *1380*
        resin-bonded retainers 549–550, *549–550*
        telescoping crowns as abutments 559
    glass-infiltrated alumina with 1377
    implant abutments 657–658, *659*, 660–661
        platform interface 1370, *1370–1371*
        soft tissue interface 1370–1372, *1371–1372*
    implant restorations 658–662, *662*
        passive fit 1378
        retrievability 1379–1380, *1381*
    monolithic (all-zirconia) 507–510, 1377–1378
        crowns 537, *537*
        implant crowns *662*, 663
        screw-retained restorations 1379, *1379*
        tooth preparation 1265
        wear of opposing teeth 1378
    prefabricated posts **736**
    veneers 441, 453
    yttrium-stabilized (Y-TZP) 550, 1253, 1377
zygion 1094, *1099*